TUFTS UNIVERSITY LIBRARIES
W9-CPE-861

Sherris

# Medical Microbiology

## An Introduction to Infectious Diseases

Third Edition

*Editor*

**Kenneth J. Ryan, MD**
Professor and Associate Head
Department of Pathology
Professor of Microbiology and Immunology
College of Medicine
University of Arizona
Tucson, Arizona

**James J. Champoux, PhD**
Professor of Microbiology
School of Medicine
University of Washington
Seattle, Washington

**Stanley Falkow, PhD**
Professor of Microbiology and Immunology
Professor of Medicine
School of Medicine
Stanford University
Stanford, California

**James J. Plorde, MD**
Professor of Laboratory Medicine
Professor of Medicine
School of Medicine
University of Washington
Veterans Administration Medical Center
Seattle, Washington

**W. Lawrence Drew, MD, PhD**
Professor of Laboratory Medicine
Professor of Medicine
School of Medicine
University of California, San Francisco
Mount. Zion Medical Center
San Francisco, California

**Frederick C. Neidhardt, PhD**
Frederick G. Novy Distinguished University Professor of Microbiology and Immunology
Associate Vice President for Research
University of Michigan
Medical School
Ann Arbor, Michigan

**C. George Ray, MD**
Professor and Chairman
Department of Pediatrics
School of Medicine
St. Louis University
St. Louis, Missouri

*Consulting Editor*

**John C. Sherris, MD, FRCPath**
Professor Emeritus
Department of Microbiology
School of Medicine
University of Washington
Seattle, Washington

*Chapter 8, A Survey of Immunological Principles, contributed by*
**John J. Marchalonis, PhD**
Professor and Head
Departments of Microbiology and Immunology
College of Medicine
University of Arizona
Tucson, Arizona

*Chapter 62, Dental and Periodontal Infections contributed by*
**Murray R. Robinovitch, DDS, PhD**
Professor and Chairman
Department of Oral Biology
School of Dentistry
University of Washington
Seattle, Washington

*Sherris*

# Medical Microbiology

## An Introduction to Infectious Diseases

**Third Edition**

**Kenneth J. Ryan, Editor**

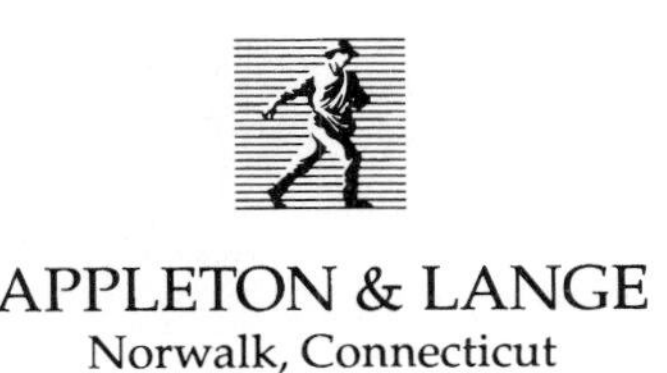

APPLETON & LANGE
Norwalk, Connecticut

Notice: The authors and the publisher of this volume have taken care to make certain that the doses of drugs and schedules of treatment are correct and compatible with the standards generally accepted at the time of publication. Nevertheless, as new information becomes available, changes in treatment and in the use of drugs become necessary. The reader is advised to carefully consult the instruction and information material included in the package insert of each drug or therapeutic agent before administration. This advice is especially important when using new or infrequently used drugs. The publisher disclaims any liability, loss, injury, or damage incurred as a consequence, directly or indirectly, of the use and application of any of the contents of this volume.

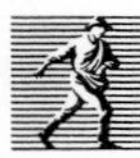



94 95 96 97 98 / 10 9 8 7 6 5 4 3 2 1

Prentice Hall International (UK) Limited, *London*
Prentice Hall of Australia Pty. Limited, *Sydney*
Prentice Hall Canada, Inc., *Toronto*
Prentice Hall Hispanoamericana, S.A., *Mexico*
Prentice Hall of India Private Limited, *New Delhi*
Prentice Hall of Japan, Inc., *Tokyo*
Simon & Schuster Asia Pte. Ltd., *Singapore*
Editora Prentice Hall do Brasil Ltda., *Rio de Janeiro*
Prentice Hall, *Englewood Cliffs, New Jersey*

**Library of Congress Cataloging-in-Publication Data**

Sherris medical microbiology / edited by Kenneth J. Ryan. —3rd ed.
p. cm.
Rev. ed. of: Medical microbiology / editor, John C. Sherris. 2nd ed. c1990.
Includes bibliographical references and index.
ISBN 0-8385-8541-8
1. Medical microbiology. 2. Communicable diseases. I. Ryan, Kenneth J. (Kenneth James), 1940– . II. Sherris, John C. III. Title: Medical microbiology.
[DNLM: 1. Communicable Diseases. 2. Microbiology. WC 100 S553 1994]
QR46.M473 1994
616.01—dc20
DNLM/DLC 94-14526
for Library of Congress CIP

Acquisitions Editor: Martin J. Wonsiewicz
Production Editor: Elizabeth C. Ryan
Designer: Michael J. Kelly

PRINTED IN THE UNITED STATES OF AMERICA

ISBN 0-8385-8541-8
90000
9 780838 585412

***Dedication***

*To the memory of*
*James Dillon Ryan*
*and the future of*
*James Dillon Truscott*

# Contents

# Preface

With this third edition, *Medical Microbiology* becomes *Sherris Medical Microbiology,* the name by which it has become known in the ten years since publication of the first edition. John Sherris has retired as editor and author and Lawrence Corey, another founder, as author. The continuing impact of Dr. Sherris' and Dr. Corey's writing on this volume is gratefully acknowledged by the current editor and by the authors who took over their chapters. At the same time we welcome Dr. W. Lawrence Drew of the University of California, San Francisco and Dr. Stanley Falkow of Stanford University as new authors. Dr. Sherris continues as consulting editor, acting as an advisor to all of us.

The goal of *Sherris Medical Microbiology* remains unchanged. This book is intended to be the primary text for students of medicine and medical science who are encountering microbiology and infectious diseases for the first time. The organization is the same as the second edition with basic topics followed by chapters on the major bacterial, viral, fungal, and parasitic pathogens. We have tried to improve the consistency of our presentation of pathogens to the student by placing the most important features of the organism (structure, metabolism, genetics), the disease (epidemiology, pathogenesis, immunity), and the clinical aspects (manifestations, diagnosis, treatment, prevention) in distinct sections and in the same order. Fourteen brief chapters at the end summarize the relevant clinical, diagnostic, and therapeutic information into the most common clinical infectious syndromes without the addition of new material. It is hoped that these chapters will be of particular value when the student prepares for case discussions or sees patients.

Marginal notations throughout the text have been revised and extended to capsulize major points as an aid for the student during review. The detail in tables and figures is for example or explanation and not intended to be learned unless included in the narative of the text. Reference material that may be useful at another time has been placed in appendices, including one at the end of the book that gives features of organisms and diseases too rare for the main text. An overview chapter on the immune response is included for continuity, but it is assumed this subject will be covered by one of the many excellent immunology texts available. The chapter on dental microbiology has been updated to serve the needs of dental students. Study questions, case studies, and problems have not been included as their fundamentally interactive nature is beyond the scope of this textbook and other excellent publications of this nature are available including multimedia electronic products.[1,2]

*Sherris Medical Microbiology* is designed to be read comprehensively, not as a reference work. In this regard all the pathogenic microorganisms we feel are important are included at a level of detail relevant for medical students. Much new material has been included, but in order to keep the student from being overwhelmed, older or less important information has been deleted to keep the size of this book approximately the same as the previous edition. As a rule of thumb, material on classic microbial structures, toxins, and the like not clearly linked to disease has been trimmed to make way for the newer molecular and genetic understanding of infectious diseases. At the same time, we have tried not to eliminate detail to the point of becoming synoptic and uninteresting. For example, adequate explanation of the pathogenesis of an infectious disease may require discussion of the roles played by multiple proteins, genes, and regulators. Where these features form a coherent picture we have tried to tell the complete story, particularly if it is instructive as a general principle.

A saving grace is that our topic is important, dynamic, and fascinating. Who could have predicted that AIDS, which occupied less than a page in the first edition (published in 1984), would become by the end of 1993 the leading cause of death of American men between the ages of 25 and 44 years? On a more positive note, gastritis and ulcers attributed to stress in the past are now being cured by antimicrobial therapy directed against *Helicobacter pylori,* an organism recognized for decades but not understood until recently. These and many other infectious agents and diseases old and new are described and explained in these pages. The student is invited to use them to begin a lifetime of learning in microbiology, infectious diseases, and medicine.

**Kenneth J. Ryan**
*Editor*

1. Gilligan PH, Shapiro DS, Smiley ML. Cases in Medical Microbiology and Infectious Diseases. Washington, DC: American Society for Microbiology; 1992.
2. Microbiology TextStack, Microbiology VideoIndex, Microbiology QuizBank. Blue Bell, PA: Keyboard Publishing.

# Acknowledgments

The authors wish to thank Drs. James Moulder, Richard Friedman, Rodney Adam, and Michael Schumacher for selected chapter review and helpful suggestions. Administrative support was provided by Sara Fisher and Alexa Suslow and was expertly coordinated by Cathy Crane. We also wish to acknowledge the professionalism of the Appleton & Lange staff, who took on this complicated new project and completed it with remarkable speed and flexibility.

New illustrations for this edition were prepared by Cindy Tinnes, whose skill and ability to creatively respond to the diverse needs of this text are gratefully acknowledged. Illustrations prepared for the first edition mycology and parasitology sections by Sam Eng have been carried over to this edition, as have many illustrations prepared for the second edition by Marilyn Pollack-Senura, with and without modifications done by Ms. Tinnes.

Finally, we wish to acknowledge our students, past and present, who provide the stimulation for continuation of this work, and our families who provide the encouragement and support that make it possible.

# Acknowledgments

[illegible]

Chapter 1

# Overview

*John C. Sherris and Kenneth J. Ryan*

> Humanity has but three great enemies: fever, famine and war; of these by far the greatest, by far the most terrible, is fever.
>
> Sir William Osler, 1896*

## DISCOVERY AND MEDICAL MICROBIOLOGY

Historical background

The science of microbiology as it applies to medicine dates back to the pioneering studies of Pasteur and Koch and is, thus, only a little over a century old. The period between 1875 and 1910 was the first golden age of medical microbiology. Many bacterial diseases and the organisms responsible for them were defined. Methods were developed for growing bacteria and studying their phenotypic characteristics. The existence of antibodies and complement as mediators of immune responses to infection were recognized, and the first steps were taken to extend the principles of vaccination for smallpox described by Jenner in 1796 to other infectious diseases. Other diseases were shown to be caused by filterable agents (viruses) that could not yet be grown but that caused disease in experimental animals and elicited immune responses. As a result of these developments, the aura of mysticism and helplessness that surrounded infectious diseases was dispelled, the epidemiology of infectious diseases was clarified, and avenues for control were opened. In the period from 1910 to 1944 many new pathogenic organisms were described, and there were great advances in public health and the epidemiologic control of infectious diseases, the discoveries of penicillin by Fleming in 1929 and of sulfonamides by Domagk in 1935 opened the way to the great developments in chemotherapy that were to come.

During the next four decades or so, there was a quantum leap in understanding of the structure, physiology, and genetics of microbes, the processes by which pathogens cause disease, and the elegant complexities of the defense mechanisms of the host. Electron microscopy clarified the ultrastructure of bacteria, fungi, and protozoa and demonstrated the shape and structure of viral particles. The science of molecular biology has led to an understanding of microbial genetics and of the processes by which bacteria control protein synthesis, maintain their identity, and adapt to different environments. In recent years these advances have been applied to the study of infectious diseases in ways that elucidate details of the precise molecules and mechanisms by which microorganisms cause disease. Numerous antimicrobial agents, some tailored to particular needs and targets, have been developed and provide the clinician with powerful weapons to control infections.

A major effect of the knowledge and understanding gained during this second golden age of microbiology is that phenomena that were learned simply as facts in the past can now be explained. The end result of these advances has been control of many of the infectious

* Osler W. *JAMA.* 1896;26:999.

scourges that have afflicted our species and a level of understanding that opens the way to controlling those that remain. Some of the most significant applied and basic research discoveries of the past century are listed in the Historical Appendix at the end of the book.

## DIVERSITY OF MICROORGANISMS

Entry into microbial world

At birth, the normal infant, previously protected from the environment by the mother's placenta and immune system, enters an enormously complex microbial world that has evolved over the past 3.5 billion years. Most of these microorganisms are free-living but a few have ecologic niches in the external, mucosal, and other surfaces of humans (and other creatures) often to their mutual benefit. A tiny minority become unwelcome guests through the expression of highly specialized features that give them the capacity to injure their host and thus cause disease. Understanding of the latter events and how they relate to the practice of medicine is the major goal of this book.

Roles of microorganisms in nature

Microorganisms, which are by definition invisible to the unaided eye, are responsible for much of the breakdown and natural recycling of organic material in the environment. Some can fix atmospheric nitrogen and synthesize nitrogen-containing inorganic and organic compounds that contribute to the nutrition of living things that lack this ability. Some can use atmospheric carbon dioxide as a source of carbon for organic compounds; others (the oceanic algae) produce oxygen through their use of atmospheric carbon dioxide for photosynthesis. Thus, microorganisms play central roles in the nitrogen and carbon cycles and contribute to maintaining the atmospheric oxygen level.

Microbial adaptation to diverse environments

Very few areas on the surface of the planet do not support microbial life, because microorganisms have an astounding range of metabolic and energy-yielding abilities, and many can exist under conditions that are lethal to other life forms. For example, some bacteria can oxidize inorganic compounds such as sulfur and ammonium ions to generate energy, and some can survive and multiply in hot springs at temperatures above 75°C. Many microorganisms can metabolize only fermentatively, using substances other than oxygen as terminal electron acceptors, and can thus multiply under highly reduced conditions. Some of these are cellulolytic and can multiply rapidly in masses of decaying vegetation in the absence of oxygen. To many, oxygen is rapidly lethal.

Microorganisms that plants interact with

Some microbial species have adapted to a symbiotic relationship with higher forms of life. For example, bacteria that can fix atmospheric nitrogen colonize root systems of legumes and of a few trees such as alders and provide the plant with its nitrogen requirements. When the plant dies or is plowed under, the fertility of the soil is enhanced by nitrogenous compounds originally derived from the metabolism of the bacteria. Ruminants can use grasses as their prime source of nutrition, because the abundant flora of anaerobic bacteria in the rumen break down cellulose and other plant compounds to usable carbohydrates and amino acids and synthesize essential nutrients including some amino acids and vitamins. These few examples illustrate the protean nature of microbial life and their essential place in our ecosystem.

Use of microbial diversity by humans

The metabolic heterogeneity and diverse synthetic abilities of microorganisms have led to their application to human purposes. These uses include alcoholic fermentation in the production of wines and beers, the area of Pasteur's initial studies, and production of complex molecules such as vitamin $B_{12}$ and various antibiotics. Through the use of recombinant DNA techniques, genes encoding the synthesis of substances such as human growth hormone and some immunologic mediators have been added to the genome of bacteria or yeasts, which then synthesize the desired product in culture. Because of this relatively simple and manipulable genetic structure, molecular biological studies on bacteria continue to help illuminate the complexities of cellular regulation and differentiation in higher life forms.

## MICROORGANISMS AND DISEASE: THE OFFENSE

It is because microorganisms are essential to the existence of life on our planet that the study of general microbiology and of their role in nature is of such great interest and importance.

This book, however, has a narrower anthropocentric focus and is concerned with those microorganisms directly involved in the maintenance of health or causation of disease in humans. Within this context, we consider the four broad classes of microorganisms that interact with humans: bacteria, fungi, viruses, and protozoa. We have extended the definition of microbiology to include some disease-producing multicellular parasites, the helminths and flukes, that are macroscopic at some stages of their life cycles; indeed, intestinal tapeworms can measure many feet in length and become discomfortingly obvious.

Focus on the classes of microorganisms that interact with humans

Among the microorganisms that infect or coexist with humans, the **fungi** and **protozoa** have many of the cellular characteristics of mammalian or plant cells: nuclear membranes, several chromosomes, mitotic apparatus, mitochondria, sterol-containing cell membranes, and, in many cases, the ability to reproduce sexually. These microorganisms are termed **eukaryotes** because of their "true" nuclear structure. Their size is quite variable; although width or diameter rarely exceeds 10 μm (0.01 mm), length may be much greater. Most fungi and some protozoa can be grown in culture on artificial media.

Fungi and protozoa are eukaryotic

The **bacteria** are generally smaller, simpler, and probably more primitive than the fungi and protozoa. Their nuclear material comprises a single, double-stranded, but very large DNA molecule without a structural nuclear membrane. They are thus described as **prokaryotic** and are haploid with no true sexual mode of reproduction. Many possess autonomous self-replicating smaller circular DNA molecules, termed **plasmids**, which are transmissible between bacteria and often encode properties that facilitate their survival under adverse conditions. Bacteria have no mitochondria, their cytoplasmic membranes generally contain no sterols, and they have a unique and usually very rigid cell wall structure. Most divide by binary fission and can be grown in artificial culture, often with extraordinary rapidity. For example, many bacteria have a doubling time under ideal conditions of about 20 minutes; thus, under optimal growth conditions, a single organism can yield a population of more than $10^9$ after only 8 hours. The major differences between prokaryotic and eukaryotic cells are listed in Table 1–1.

Bacteria are prokaryotic

The **viruses**, a totally distinct group of infecting agents, are strict intracellular parasites of other living cells, not only of mammalian and plant cells but also of simple unicellular organisms, including bacteria (the bacteriophages). The viruses are simple forms of replicating, biologically active particles that carry genetic information in either DNA or RNA molecules, but never both. Most mature viruses have a protein coat over their nucleic acid and sometimes a lipid surface membrane derived from the cell that they infect. They lack the protein-synthesizing enzymes and structural apparatus necessary for their own replication; they bear essentially no resemblance to a true eukaryotic or prokaryotic cell.

Viruses are strict intracellular parasites

Viruses replicate by using their genetically active nucleic acids to subvert the metabolic activities of the cell that they infect to bring about the synthesis and reassembly of their component parts. A cell infected with a single viral particle may thus yield many thousands of viral particles, which can be assembled almost simultaneously under the direction of the viral nucleic acid. With many viruses, cell death and infection of other cells by the newly formed viruses result. Sometimes, viral reproduction and cell reproduction proceed

Viral nucleic acid directs host cell synthetic activity

**TABLE 1–1. DISTINCTIVE FEATURES OF PROKARYOTIC AND EUKARYOTIC CELLS**

| Cell Component | Prokaryotes | Eukaryotes |
|---|---|---|
| Nucleus | No membrane, single circular chromosome | Membrane bounded, a number of individual chromosomes |
| Extrachromosomal DNA | Often present in form of plasmid(s) | In organelles |
| Organelles in cytoplasm | None | Mitochondria (and chloroplasts in photosynthetic organisms) |
| Cytoplasmic membrane | Contains enzymes of respiration; active secretion of enzymes; site of phospholipid and DNA synthesis | Semipermeable layer not possessing functions of prokaryotic membrane |
| Cell wall | Rigid layer of peptidoglycan (absent in *Mycoplasma*) | No peptidoglycan (in some cases cellulose present) |
| Sterols | Absent (except in *Mycoplasma*) | Usually present |
| Ribosomes | 70 S in cytoplasm | 80 S in cytoplasmic reticulum |

simultaneously without cell death, although cell physiology may be affected. The close association of the virus with the cell sometimes results in the integration of viral nucleic acid into the functional nucleic acid of the cell, producing a latent infection that can be transmitted intact to the progeny of the cell.

Integration may be an inherent property of the virus or may be facilitated by mutational changes in the host or viral nucleic acid. The integrated viral genome can be silent, producing no metabolic effect; can alter the expression of the genome of the host cell; or may encode the production of a biologically active protein. For example, diphtheria toxin is encoded by a bacteriophage integrated into the chromosome of the bacterium that causes diphtheria.

Viruses may lyse the host cell, modify its functions, or integrate into its genome

Carriage of viral nucleic acid may be passed not only to the progeny of cells within the host, but also longitudinally through each successive generation of inbred animals. Some latent viral infections are associated with a high incidence of specific tumors in animals, and some human tumors are associated with certain viral infections. The integrated viral nucleic genome can sometimes be activated by mutational or other stimuli, leading to production of complete viral particles and death of the host cell. Other types of viral latency occur. For example, latency between clinical attacks of herpes simplex infection may not be consequent to viral integration but probably to a balance between the ability of the virus to replicate and some immunologic response of the host: when host immunity declines, relapse occurs.

Latent state may be terminated by multiple factors

Although a few viruses can coexist with humans without causing disease, most of the known normal microbial inhabitants of humans are bacteria and fungi. The skin and the alimentary, upper respiratory, and vaginal tracts all play host to numerous bacteria that are amazingly well adapted to survive under the physiologic and nutritional conditions found in these sites. These organisms often maintain themselves by adhering specifically to epithelial cells and multiplying on their surfaces without damaging them. In some cases, organisms of the normal flora are directly beneficial to the host: they prime the immune system or synthesize nutritionally useful products, such as vitamin K. The normal flora also benefit the host indirectly by providing formidable competition to colonization and infection by pathogenic bacteria. Elimination of this competition by removal of normal floral organisms with antibiotic treatment increases susceptibility to many bacterial and fungal infections.

The human normal flora comprises primarily bacteria and yeasts

Many members of the normal flora have pathogenic potential and are included among organisms referred to as opportunistic pathogens; if sufficient numbers reach normally sterile areas of the body (eg, tissues, peritoneal cavity, bladder, or lower respiratory tract), they may cause severe or even fatal infections. These infections can begin with mechanical causes, such as a ruptured intestine, or from a congenital or acquired failure of some critical component of the immune system that normally helps to prevent organisms from transgressing body surfaces or removes them when the day-to-day minor accidents of life deposit them in the tissues. This process is largely affected by the phagocytic cell system and enhanced by the early inflammatory response. Likewise some environmental organisms have opportunistic potential. Changes in the way we live, even the advances of medical practice, may create new niches for opportunistic pathogens.

Endogenous infections can be produced by members of the normal flora

The initial stages of infection by extraneous organisms (those not part of the body's indigenous flora) may be secondary to structural or functional damage to surface structures that normally exclude them (eg, a third-degree burn of the skin, the bite of an insect vector, or damage to the bronchial ciliated epithelium from smoking). Other organisms can infect healthy individuals with intact epithelia, and these are particularly associated with epidemic spread. A major attribute of these pathogens is the ability to adhere to target epithelial cells and establish a primary site of colonization. Some organisms invade the target cell and replicate there, others pass through or between cells, and yet others produce cytotoxins that destroy cells. In some diseases toxins alter the physiology of the target cells without injury, for example, cholera toxin, which stimulates a massive outpouring of water and electrolytes into the intestine from the affected mucosal cells.

Exogenous infection requires multiple steps

Organisms that invade and multiply in the tissue of individuals with intact immune mechanisms have virulence determinants that allow them to avoid eradication by phagocytic cells. Some organisms produce surface molecules that confer resistance to opsonophagocytosis and others change their antigenic coat to confuse recognition, others produce substances that kill phagocytes or inhibit their migration, and still others confound

Virulence factors relate to the frequency, nature, and severity of disease the phagocyte's mechanisms of destruction once inside. Intracellular existence and multiplication protect viruses and some bacteria, fungi, and protozoa from immune mechanisms as long as they remain within the cell. Some bacteria produce enzymes that destroy surface-secreted antibody. In most cases, the ability to circumvent the body's defenses is relative, and organisms must be numerous to initiate an infection that may then progress with simultaneous destruction and multiplication of the infecting agent.

The mere presence of microorganisms multiplying in the tissues does not necessarily produce disease. Many produce toxic substances. Some of these toxins are highly potent and pharmacologically specific and facilitate spread of infection or damage local and remote organs. Viral diseases often result from direct or immunologic destruction of infected cells or from alterations in cellular function. Damage also results from the body's response to infection through inflammation, through immediate or delayed hypersensitivity to microbial antigens, or through local or remote tissue responses to immune complexes. Some organisms can cause disease without penetrating mucous membranes through the effects of their highly potent toxins. Such toxins are often produced in the intestinal tract or, in some cases, in food before ingestion.

Injury is produced by toxins, direct cell damage, or immunological mechanisms

## RESPONSE TO INFECTION: THE DEFENSE

During the course of an infection, the body's adaptive immune mechanisms, both specific and nonspecific, come into play. The local inflammatory reaction mobilizes phagocytes and serum antimicrobial factors. Polymorphonuclear leukocytosis often develops in bacterial infections and increases the number of available phagocytic cells. Antigen, often processed by macrophages, primes and leads to multiplication of specific immunologically active lymphoid cells of both the T and B series. Antibody with specific attachment sites for the infecting agent and for phagocytic cells increases the efficiency of phagocytosis or abrogates the effectiveness of antiphagocytic surface components of some bacteria, a process in which the normal serum complement system collaborates. In some cases, direct killing of the pathogen results from the action of complement on antibody-coated cells; in others, antibody blocks attachment sites on the surface of strict intracellular parasites such as viruses, thus halting the cycle of spread from cell to cell. Cytokine-activated cell-mediated immune mechanisms serve to increase the ability of macrophages to control the growth of intracellular pathogens. Interferon production, which plays a major role in blocking the intracellular replication of viruses, also appears to interact with natural killer cells to increase their efficiency in destroying virus-infected cells. These processes are but a few of the diverse and often interacting defense mechanisms that the body mounts against infecting agents.

A full range of immune responses are stimulated by infection

The outcome of an infection is determined by the size of the infecting dose, the site of infection, the virulence of the organism, and the speed and effectiveness of the immune response. Most infections transmitted between humans are ultimately controlled by the body's defenses, even without therapeutic intervention, because selective pressures over the course of human history have been toward a balanced state of parasitism that ensures survival of both host and parasite. This does not apply to infections with pathogens that have a primary reservoir in nonhuman hosts (eg, rabies) or to organisms that have not been previously or recently experienced by our species. These are frequently of unusual virulence. Examples are the 1918–1919 influenza pandemic that took more lives than World War I and the present pandemic of acquired immunodeficiency syndrome (AIDS). The origin of such "new" highly virulent organisms is uncertain, but may have arisen by mutation in pathogens of other species or by recombinational events within or between human and animal pathogens.

Outcome of infection is determined by complex host–parasite interactions

## SPREAD AND CONTROL OF INFECTIONS

Many infections may spread in epidemics ranging from those in small, closed communities or hospitals to massive, worldwide pandemics. To produce a transmissible epidemic, an organism must have a sufficient degree of infectivity and virulence, and conditions must exist that permit spread. These conditions may include direct contact (impetigo), aerial transmission (influenza), blood and body fluid transmission (AIDS), contaminated food or

Epidemic spread relates to virulence of organism and immunity of population

water (typhoid), and the presence of essential insect vectors (malaria). The degree of innate and acquired immunity in the population must be sufficiently low for the rate of infection to be amplified as the disease spreads.

Epidemic spread and disease are facilitated by malnutrition, poor socioeconomic conditions, natural disasters, and hygienic inadequacy. In previous centuries, epidemics, sometimes caused by the introduction of new organisms of unusual virulence, often resulted in high morbidity and mortality. The possibility of recurrence of old pandemic infections remains, and we are currently witnessing a new and extended pandemic infection in the case of AIDS. Understanding of the etiology, epidemiology, and immunology of individual diseases points the way to their control. As the focus of medicine moves increasingly toward prevention, it becomes even more important for all health care workers to understand the principles and control of epidemic spread.

## DIAGNOSIS OF INFECTIOUS DISEASES

Diagnosis remains primarily by isolation and identification of the infectious agent

Detection and identification of microorganisms or their products in clinical material are undertaken in clinical or public health microbiology laboratories. Most bacteria and fungi can be grown in artificial culture, studied for a variety of key taxonomic characteristics, and speciated within a day or two. Once grown, they can be tested for their susceptibility to antimicrobial agents and the results used in the rational selection of therapy. Most viruses can be grown in cultures of eukaryotic cells derived from human or mammalian tissues, then speciated by appropriate techniques, such as reactivity with specific antibodies. These processes take several days, and much more rapid diagnostic procedures are now being used increasingly. In some cases, antigenic components or metabolic products of infecting organisms can be detected in clinical specimens using chemical or immunologic techniques. In other cases, nucleic acid probes have been developed by gene cloning that can detect microbial genes in infected cells or clinical exudates. The sensitivity of these procedures has been vastly improved by amplification techniques such as the polymerase chain reaction (PCR) which can be primed from the genomic remains of even a single infectious particle.

Sometimes, diagnosis of an infection is practicable only by detecting antibodies produced by the patient in response to the infecting organism (serodiagnosis). Procedures for accomplishing this have been in use for some diseases since the turn of the century but have now increased greatly in sensitivity and specificity. This approach is still the primary diagnostic means for infections such as syphilis and AIDS in which the causative organism either cannot be recovered or can only be isolated with great difficulty and expense. Serodiagnosis has limited value in the diagnosis of acute life-threatening infections because of the inherent delay in mounting an immune response. It is, however, of great value epidemiologically in detecting and tracing the occurrence of epidemic diseases, especially those caused by viruses.

Serodiagnosis uses the immune response for diagnosis

The isolation or detection of a potentially pathogenic organism, particularly in material from a site with a normal flora, often does not provide sufficient evidence of etiology. Knowledge of potential sources of contamination, the constituents of the normal flora, and the probability of a particular pathogen's association with the clinical manifestation must all be considered in arriving at a probable or confirmed diagnosis. Likewise, interpretation of the significance of antibodies to an organism in a patient's serum involves recognition that they could result from a previous infection or sometimes from cross-reaction with another organism. Informed judgment thus plays a critical role in presumptive laboratory diagnosis of many specific infectious diseases and in the interpretation of all laboratory results. It is essential that the student grasp the principles, methods, and pitfalls of these approaches if the potentialities of the laboratory are to be applied correctly and errors and misinterpretations avoided.

Correlation of laboratory results with other factors is important

## TREATMENT AND PREVENTION

Over the past 50 years, therapeutic tools of remarkable potency and specificity have become available for the treatment of bacterial infections. These include all the antibiotics and an array of synthetic chemicals that kill or inhibit the infecting organism, but have minimal or acceptable toxicity for the host. These antibacterials exploit the structural and metabolic differences between bacterial and eukaryotic cells to provide the selectivity necessary for good antimicrobial therapy. Penicillin, for example, interferes with the synthesis of the bacterial cell wall, a structure that has no analog in human cells. After Fleming's discovery of penicillin, the earlier effective antibiotics were discovered by screening many fungi and bacteria for their possible production of antimicrobial agents. This approach yielded a rich harvest that included, among many others, such agents as streptomycin, chloramphenicol, the tetracyclines, and erythromycin. More recently, research and development have focused on molecular modification of naturally occurring agents to improve their ranges of activity, to enhance their pharmacologic characteristics, or to make them insusceptible to the resistance mechanisms that some bacteria have developed to their earlier congeners. There are fewer antifungal and antiprotozoal agents, because of closer metabolic and structural similarities between the eukaryotic cells of the host and those of the parasite. Nevertheless, there are a series of significant differences, and effective therapeutic agents have been discovered or developed to exploit them.

Chemotherapy can be specifically directed at the infective agent

Specific therapeutic attack on viral disease has posed more complex problems, because of the intimate involvement of viral replication with the metabolic and replicative activities of the cell. Thus, most substances that inhibit viral replication have unacceptable toxicity to host cells. In recent years, however, advances in molecular virology have identified specific viral targets that can be attacked. Some successful antiviral agents have resulted, including agents that interfere with the liberation of viral nucleic acid from its protective protein coat or with the processes of viral nucleic acid synthesis and replication. Some experimental antiviral agents act indirectly by stimulating production of interferons, a group of antiviral proteins usually produced by virally infected host cells.

The response of bacteria, and to a lesser extent of protozoa and fungi, to the widespread use of specific antimicrobial agents in therapy and prophylaxis reflects their extraordinary genetic plasticity. Resistant strains have appeared among many species that were previously fully susceptible to a particular agent. This resistance has resulted from mutation in the microbial genome and, in the case of bacteria, from the acquisition of genetic determinants of resistance on extrachromosomal, self-replicating portions of DNA (plasmids). Some individual genetic sequences can move from plasmid to plasmid or from plasmid to chromosome or vice versa (transposons). Some plasmids carry multiple resistance determinants against several antibiotics and can be transferred within or between bacterial species. Thus, the selective pressure of a single antimicrobial agent can lead to the predominance of multiple resistance in a previously fully susceptible strain. These developments have had major implications for successful prevention and treatment of many bacterial infections, and the selective factors that have contributed to the spread of resistance must be understood and acted on if some of the benefits of the antibiotic revolution are not to be lost through excessive or inappropriate use. Mutational resistance to antivirals is also encountered and poses problems in the treatment of AIDS because of the remarkable mutability of the HIV virus.

Microbial resistance has complicated chemotherapy

As indicated previously, new developments and understanding in medicine are increasing the emphasis on prevention of disease, and nowhere is this more important than in infectious diseases. Specific immunization by parenteral injection of nonliving purified or complex antigens has long been shown effective in preventing diphtheria, tetanus, pertussis, poliomyelitis, and influenza infections. More recently, vaccines incorporating purified capsular polysaccharides have been highly effective in preventing major causes of acute bacterial meningitis and pneumonia.

Immunization is the mainstay of epidemic disease prevention

Live vaccines, using organisms of reduced virulence (attenuated) that undergo limited multiplication in the body, have also been used for many decades in the prevention of smallpox, rabies, poliomyelitis, and tuberculosis. This approach has been extended more recently to measles, rubella, and mumps and has effected dramatic changes in the overall occurrence of childhood infections with their toll of poor health, school absences, serious complications, and even death. Live vaccines provide prolonged immunologic stimuli and thus reduce the need for boosters.

Many infectious diseases have not yet been controlled by vaccines, either because effective immunizing antigens have not been discovered or because the parenteral routes of immunization are ineffective. Particular attention is being paid to the development of vaccines that stimulate local (sIgA) antibody at the initial site of infection. Some are mutants that have lost certain determinants of virulence but continue to produce the immunizing antigen and thus resemble the oral poliomyelitis vaccine. Another promising avenue is the production of hybrid organisms by genetic engineering in which genes encoding immunizing antigens of the pathogen are introduced into nonpathogenic organisms capable of colonizing the susceptible area of the body. These approaches are being applied particularly to intestinal diseases such as cholera and dysentery.

Chemoprophylaxis is a means of prevention in certain circumstances

Other methods of prevention are being exploited. Chemoprophylaxis with specific antibiotics for brief periods has extended the range of surgical procedures that can be performed safely; for example, patients with implanted heart valves or artificial hips can be protected from infection by organisms that gain access during surgery and may then lead to loss of the prosthesis. Knowledge of the chemical nature of receptor–ligand relationships of bacterial toxins or viruses may allow their action to be blocked prophylactically or therapeutically. Perhaps most importantly, there is increasing emphasis on stimulation of the body's nonspecific phagocytic and cytotoxic immune system and on the physiologic and nutritional factors that influence resistance to infection. For example, it has been shown that a key factor in preventing the severely burned patient from succumbing to infection is the maintenance of general nutritional balance by parenteral feeding with essential nutrients. Those who have read George Bernard Shaw's *The Doctor's Dilemma* will deduce that we are coming full circle and that "stimulation of the phagocytes," a major focus of research in the 1920s, is highly relevant today.

It is hoped that this overview will help the reader to understand how the different topics in this book relate to one another and the reasons why the authors believe that a student who will practice in any branch of medicine should understand the material presented. There is much specific information in the book, some of which illustrates principles that must be understood and some of which presents important microorganism/disease features to be learned. We offer no apologies for the fact that some memorization is essential. For example, one cannot deduce the major characteristics of a staphylococcus and how they relate to the manifestation of a staphylococcal infection from principles alone. They must be learned, and memory continually reinforced and extended. Memorization without understanding, however, is no basis for the application of a discipline to the care of patients and to the diagnosis and treatment of disease. It is essential that the underlying principles be firmly grasped.

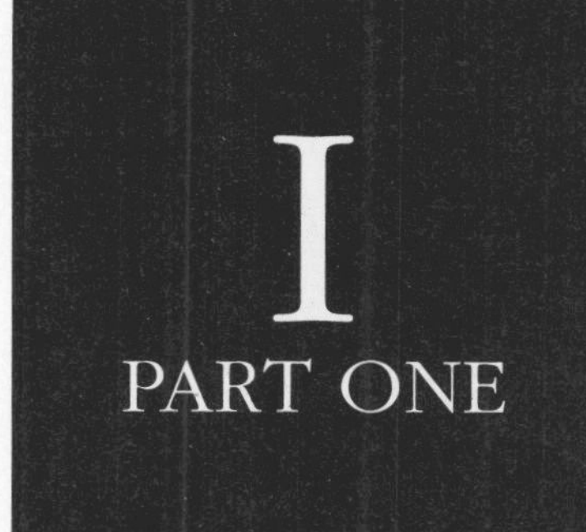


# The Bacterial Cell

Chapter 2

# Bacterial Structures

*Frederick C. Neidhardt*

## GENERAL MORPHOLOGY, BODY PLAN, AND COMPOSITION

The bacterial cell that is seen today is closer in form to the primordial cells of our planet than is any animal or plant cell. Despite this similarity, bacteria are the product of close to 3 billion years of natural selection and have emerged as immensely diverse and successful organisms colonizing almost all parts of the world and its inhabitants. Because they have remained microscopic, it can be concluded that very small size per se is not a disadvantage in nature and may very well provide unique opportunities for survival and reproduction. Thus, the first major principle to help us understand bacteria is their small size.

Bacteria are by far the smallest living cells, and some are considered to have the minimum possible size for an independently reproducing organism. Individuals of different bacterial species that colonize or infect humans range from 0.1 to 10 μm (1 μm = $10^{-6}$ m) in their largest dimension. Most spherical bacteria have diameters of from 0.5 to 2 μm, and rod-shaped cells are generally from 0.2 to 2 μm wide and 1 to 10 μm long. At the lower end of the scale, some bacteria (rickettsias, chlamydia, and mycoplasmas) overlap with the largest viruses (the poxviruses), and at the upper end there are some rod-shaped bacteria with a length equal to the diameter of some eukaryotic cells (Fig 2–1). As a shorthand approximation, bacteria are sole possessors of the 1-μm size.

Most bacteria are in the range of 1–8 μm

A wealth of structural detail cannot be discerned in bacteria even with the best of light microscopes because of their small size and because they are nearly colorless and transparent and have a refractive index similar to that of the surrounding liquid. Shape, however, can easily be discerned with appropriate microscopic techniques, and distinctive shapes are characteristic of broad groupings of bacteria (Fig 2–2). The major forms that can be recognized are spheres, rods, bent or curved rods, and spirals. Spherical or oval bacteria are called **cocci** (singular: **coccus**). Rods are called **bacilli** (singular: **bacillus**). Very short rods that can sometimes almost be mistaken for cocci are called **coccobacilli**. Some rod-shaped bacteria have tapered ends and are therefore termed **fusiform**, whereas others are characteristically club-shaped at one end. Short rods that are curved or bent are sometimes referred to as **vibrios**. Spiral-shaped bacteria are called **spirilla** if the cells are rigid and **spirochetes** if they are more flexible and undulating.

In addition to shape, distinctive arrangements of groups of cells can readily be observed for some bacterial genera (Fig 2–3). The reason one can speak of arrangements of unicellular organisms is that there is a tendency, varying with different genera, for newly divided cells to stick together. The nature of the aggregates formed depends on the degree of stickiness (which can vary with growth conditions) and on the plane of successive cell divisions. Among the cocci, pairs (**diplococci**), chains (**streptococci**), cubical arrays (**sarcinae**), and irregular clusters (**staphylococci**) are found. A few genera of bacteria were named for their distinctive shape or cell arrangement. There are many thousands of species of bac-

Variety of shape and cell arrangements

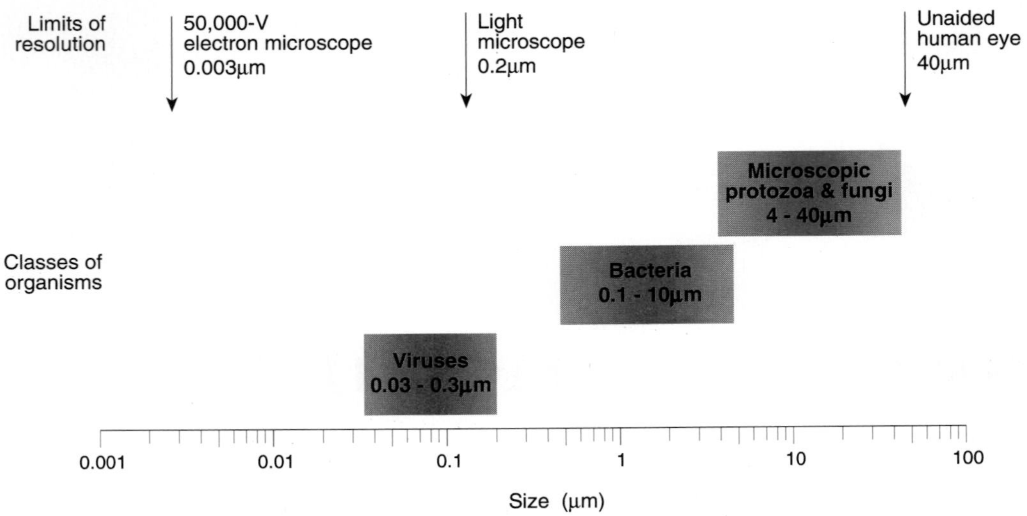


**Figure 2–1.** Relative sizes of microorganisms.

Some antimicrobics affect cell morphology

teria, however, so it should be clear that the shape and arrangement of cells cannot be taken far in identifying the particular organism in a given sample or culture. A further caution for medical microbiologists is the tendency of some bacteria to take on altered shapes and arrangements when in contact with various antimicrobics.

Whatever the overall shape of the cell, the 1-µm size could not accommodate the familiar eukaryotic cell plan. There is insufficient room for mitochondria, nucleus, Golgi apparatus, lysosomes, endoplasmic reticulum, and the like in a cell that is itself only as large as an average mitochondrion. The design of the bacterial cell must thus differ fundamentally from that of other cells. This is precisely the case, and the unique design is designated **prokaryotic**.

Prokaryotic cell design is unique

Chemical similarities to eukaryotic cells

A generalized bacterial cell is shown in Figure 2–4. The major structures of the cell belong either to the multilayered **envelope** and its **appendages** or to the interior core consisting of the nucleoid (or nuclear body) and the **cytosol.** In contrast to the alien nature of this body plan, the general chemical nature of the bacterial cell is more familiar to a eukaryotic cell biologist. Greater than 90% of its dry mass consists of five macromolecular-like substances similar to those found in eukaryotes: proteins (about 55% of the dry mass); RNA, consisting of the familiar messenger (mRNA), transfer (tRNA), and ribosomal (rRNA) RNAs (about 20%); DNA (about 3%); carbohydrate (about 5%); and phospholipid (about 6%). In addition there are a few macromolecules unique to prokaryotes: a peptidoglycan called **murein** is found in all walled bacteria, and a few other unique molecules (lipopolysaccharide and teichoic acids) are found in specific groups of bacteria.

Small size and simple design facilitates rapid growth

As we shall see, it is small size and extraordinarily simple design that help explain the success of bacteria in nature. Small size facilitates rapid exchange of nutrients and metabolic byproducts with the environment, whereas simplicity of design facilitates the assembly of cell structures and the formation of new cells by division. Both features contribute to a distinctive functional property of bacteria, their ability to grow at least an order of magnitude faster than eukaryotic cells. At the molecular level, however, bacteria are far from simple, and it is necessary to learn something of their complexity at this level to understand the ability of some of them to colonize humans or to cause disease.

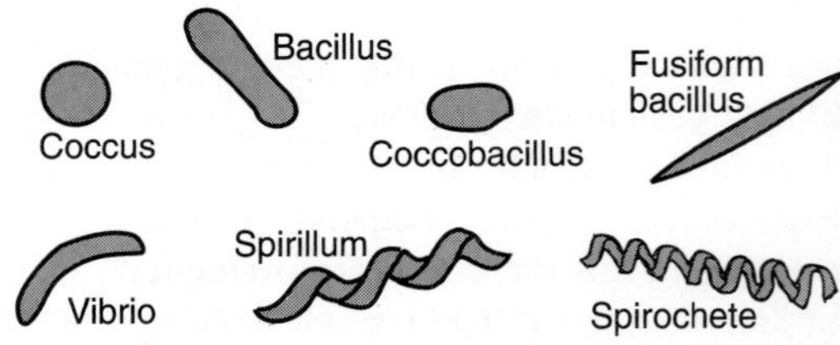


**Figure 2–2.** Shapes of some different bacteria.

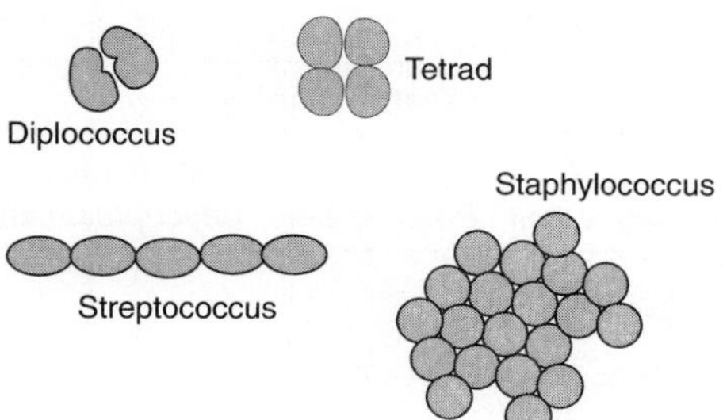


**Figure 2–3.** Arrangement of spherical bacterial cells.

## ENVELOPE AND APPENDAGES

As a first approximation, bacteria can be said to have a plain interior and a fancy exterior. The cell core, consisting solely of nucleoid and cytosol, is incredibly simple and almost structureless compared with the interior of a eukaryotic cell. It fits our notion that simplicity facilitates rapid growth. The envelope, on the other hand, is an exceedingly baroque part of the cell, consisting of structures of great complexity that vary in detail among the different major groups of bacteria. This can be readily understood by appreciating three important principles of bacterial functional anatomy: (1) the envelope is responsible for many cellular processes that are the province of the internal organelles of eukaryotic cells; (2) the envelope is the primary site of functions that protect the bacterial cell against chemical and biological threats in its environment; (3) the envelope and certain appendages make possible the colonization of surfaces by bacteria.

Complexity of prokaryote structure and function of cell envelope

Differences in envelope structure and composition (Table 2–1) are the basis of the assignment, described next, of all eubacterial species to one of three major groups: Gram-negative bacteria, Gram-positive bacteria, and the mollicutes (mycoplasma). Figure 2–5 shows schematically these major differences.

### Capsule

Many bacterial cells surround themselves with one or another kind of hydrophilic gel. This layer is often quite thick; commonly it is thicker than the diameter of the cell. Because it is

Capsule is a hydrophilic gel; not readily stained

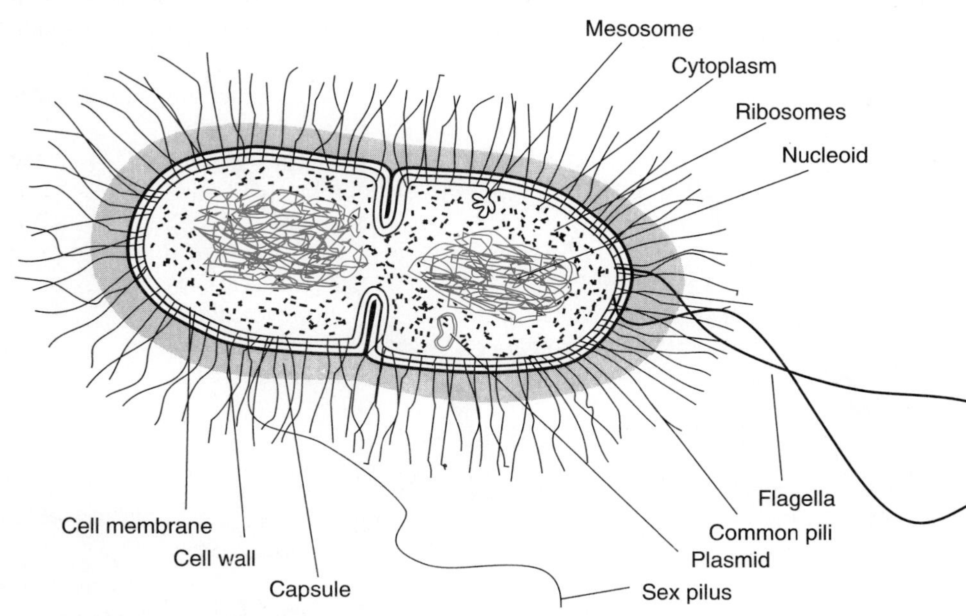


**Figure 2–4.** Schematic of structures of a dividing bacterium.

**TABLE 2–1. COMPONENTS OF BACTERIAL CELLS**

| Structure | Composition | Distribution[a] | | |
|---|---|---|---|---|
| | | ***Gram-Negative Cell*** | ***Gram-Positive Cell*** | ***Mollicutes (Mycoplasmas)*** |
| **Envelope** | | | | |
| Capsule (slime layer) | Polysaccharide or polypeptide | + or – | + or – | – |
| Wall | | + | + | – |
| Outer membrane | Proteins, phospholipids, and lipopolysaccharide | + | – | – |
| Peptidoglycan layer | Murein (+ teichoate in Gram-positive cells) | + | + | – |
| Periplasm | Proteins and oligosaccharides in solution | + | – | – |
| Cell membrane | Proteins, phospholipids | + | + | + |
| Appendages | | | | |
| Pili (fimbriae) | Protein (pilin) | + or – | + or – | – |
| Flagella | Proteins (flagellin plus others) | + or – | + or – | – |
| **Core** | | | | |
| Cytosol | Polyribosomes, proteins, carbohydrates (glycogen) | + | + | + |
| Nucleoid | DNA with associated RNA and proteins | + | + | + |
| Plasmids | DNA | + or – | + or – | + or – |
| **Endospore** | | | | |
| All cell components plus dipicolinate and special envelope components | | – | + or – | – |

[a] "+" indicates the structure is invariably present; "–" indicates it is invariably absent; "+ or –" indicates that the structure is present in some species or strains and absent in others.

Most capsules are polysaccharide; a few are polypeptide or protein

transparent and not readily stained, this layer is usually not appreciated unless made visible by its ability to exclude particulate material, such as India ink. If the material forms a reasonably discrete layer, it is called a **capsule**; if it is amorphous in appearance, it is referred to as a **slime layer**. Almost all bacterial species can make such material to some degree. Most capsules or slime layers are polysaccharides made of single or multiple types of sugar residues; some are simple (though unusual) polypeptides, such as the polymer of D-glutamic acid, which forms the capsule of *Bacillus anthracis*, the causative agent of an-

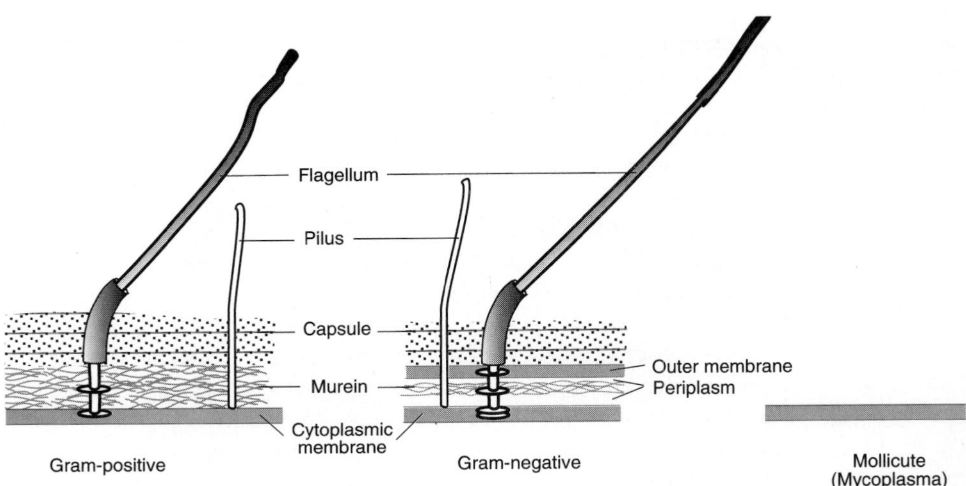


**Figure 2–5.** Schematic representation comparing the envelopes of Gram-positive bacteria, Gram-negative bacteria, and mollicutes.

thrax (see Chapter 17); a few are proteins. When cultured on solid media (see Chapter 14) encapsulated bacteria give rise to smooth, often mucuslike colonies, but unencapsulated variants are common, particularly with long-term laboratory cultivation. Their colonies are nonmucoid and described as "rough."

Capsules can protect bacteria. Within animal and human hosts capsules impede ingestion by leukocytes. *Streptococcus pneumoniae*, the causative agent of pneumococcal pneumonia, in large measure owes its virulence to the ability of its copious polysaccharide capsule to interfere with opsonophagocytosis (see Chapter 16). The pneumococcal polysaccharide, as is the case with most capsular material, is antigenic (see Chapter 8), and when specific antibody attaches to it, phagocytosis can occur. A mouse–pneumococcus experimental model is instructive. Unencapsulated pneumococci are tolerated by mice; however, a single encapsulated cell injected intraperitoneally will kill a mouse unless the mouse has been immunized with capsular material of the specific antigenic type of the infecting pneumococcus, in which case it is protected. More than 80 capsular serotypes of this organism are known, reflecting a diverse genetic capacity of the species to produce capsular polysaccharides of differing chemical structure.

Antiphagocytic effect of some capsules is major virulence determinant

Protection against phagocytosis is only part of the much broader function of bacterial capsules in nature, which is to aid colonization, primarily by assisting the cell to attach to surfaces. For example, the ability of *Streptococcus mutans* and *Streptococcus salivarius* cells to adhere to the surface of teeth is in large measure a function of the polysaccharide capsules of these oral bacteria (see Chapter 62).

Role of some capsules in adherence and colonization

Capsules do not contribute to growth and multiplication and are not essential for cell survival in artificial culture. Capsule synthesis is greatly dependent on growth conditions. For example, the capsule made by the caries-producing *S. mutans* consists of a dextran–carbohydrate polymer made only in the presence of sucrose.

Capsule synthesis depends on growth conditions

## Cell Wall

Internal to the capsule (if one exists), but still outside the cell proper, a rigid **cell wall** surrounds all eubacterial cells except mollicutes (mycoplasmas). The structure and function of the bacterial wall is so distinctive as to constitute a hallmark of the prokaryotes; nothing like it is to be found elsewhere. Unlike the capsule, which is dispensable for survival outside the body of the host, the wall has vital functions. It protects the cell from mechanical disruption and from being burst by the turgor pressure resulting from the hypertonicity of the cell interior relative to the environment. The wall also provides a barrier against certain toxic chemical and biological agents. Being rigid, its form is responsible for the shape of the cell.

Rigid structure unique to prokaryotes

Prevents osmotic lysis, determines shape, and protects against toxins

Bacterial evolution has led to two major solutions to the challenge of constructing a wall that can protect a minute, fragile cell from chemical and physical assault while still permitting the rapid exchange of nutrients and metabolic byproducts required by rapid growth. Long before these solutions were understood in ultrastructural terms, it was recognized that bacteria could be divided into two groups depending on their reaction to a particular staining procedure devised a century ago by the Danish microbiologist Hans Christian Gram. This procedure, the Gram stain, is described in detail in Chapter 14. It depends on the differential ability of ethanol or ethanol–acetone mixtures to extract iodine–crystal violet complexes from bacterial cells. These complexes are readily extracted from one group of bacteria, termed **Gram-negative**, which can be subsequently stained red with an appropriate counterstain. They are retained by the other, termed **Gram-positive**, which are thus stained violet by the retained crystal violet. The positive or negative Gram stain response of a cell reflects which of the two types of wall it possesses.

Significance of Gram stain reactions

Virtually all of the eubacteria with walls can be assigned a Gram response. The few exceptions, however, include some medically important organisms. For example, the mycobacteria (such as *Mycobacterium tuberculosis*, the causative agent of tuberculosis) are Gram positive on the basis of their wall structure, but fail to stain because of interference by special lipids present in their walls. The spirochetes, including *Treponema pallidum* (the causative agent of syphilis), although Gram negative by structure, are too thin to be resolved in the light microscope when stained by simple stains.

Bacteria without walls, whether natural forms (the mollicutes or mycoplasmas) or artificial products of procedures that remove the wall, exhibit a Gram-negative staining response. Furthermore, some bacteria that are Gram positive on the basis of wall structure and staining response may lose this property and appear Gram negative if they have been held under nongrowing conditions. These examples emphasize that being Gram positive is a distinct property that can be temporarily lost because it depends on the integrity of the cell wall; a Gram-negative bacterial cell, on the other hand, does not have a staining property to lose.

## Gram-Positive Cell Wall

Gram-positive walls contain peptidoglycan and teichoic acid

The Gram-positive cell wall contains two major components, peptidoglycan and teichoic acids, plus additional carbohydrates and proteins depending on the species. A generalized scheme illustrating the arrangement of these components is shown in Figure 2–6.

Murein comprises linear glycan chains of alternating NAG and NAM cross-linked in three dimensions by peptide chains

The chief component is **murein,** a peptidoglycan, which is found nowhere except in prokaryotes. Murein consists of a linear glycan chain of two alternating sugars, *N*-acetylglucosamine (NAG) and *N*-acetylmuramic acid (NAM), in 1:4 linkages (Fig 2–7). Each muramic acid residue bears a tetrapeptide of alternating L- and D-amino acids. Adjacent glycan chains are crosslinked into sheets by peptide bonds between the third amino acid of one tetrapeptide and the terminal D-alanine of another. The same crosslinks between other tetrapeptides connect the sheets to form a three-dimensional, rigid matrix. The crosslinks involve perhaps a third of the tetrapeptides and may be direct or may include a peptide bridge, as, for example, a pentaglycine bridge in *Staphylococcus aureus.* The crosslinking extends around the cell, producing a scaffoldlike giant molecule, termed the **murein sac**, or **sacculus.** Murein is much the same in all bacteria, except that there is diversity in the nature and frequency of the crosslinking bridge and in the nature of the amino acids at positions 2 and 3 of the tetrapeptide.

Scaffold-like murein sac surrounds cell

The murein sac derives its great mechanical strength from the fact that it is a single, covalently bonded structure; other features contributing strength are the ß-1,4 bonds of the polysaccharide backbone, the alternation of D- and L-amino acids in the tetrapeptide, and extensive internal hydrogen bonding. Biological stability is contributed by components of murein that are not widely distributed in the biological world or in fact are unique to murein. These include muramic acid, D-amino acids, and diaminopimelic acid (an amino acid found in the tetrapeptide of some species). Most enzymes found in mammalian hosts and other biological systems do not degrade peptidoglycan; one important exception is lysozyme, the hydrolase present in tears and other secretions, which cleaves the ß-1,4 glycosidic bond between muramic acid and glucosamine residues (see Figure 2–7). On the other hand, bacteria themselves are rich in hydrolases that degrade peptidoglycan, because the murein sac must be constantly expanded by insertion of new chains as the cell grows and forms a crosswall preparatory to cell division. As we shall learn, disruption of the fine control that bacteria exert over the activity of these potentially lethal enzymes is the means by which a large number of antibiotics and other chemotherapeutic compounds work (see Chapter 13).

Rare or unique components of murein provide resistance to most mammalian enzymes

Bacterial enzymes insert new murein chains during growth and provide targets for antimicrobics

The role of the murein component of the cell wall in conferring osmotic resistance and

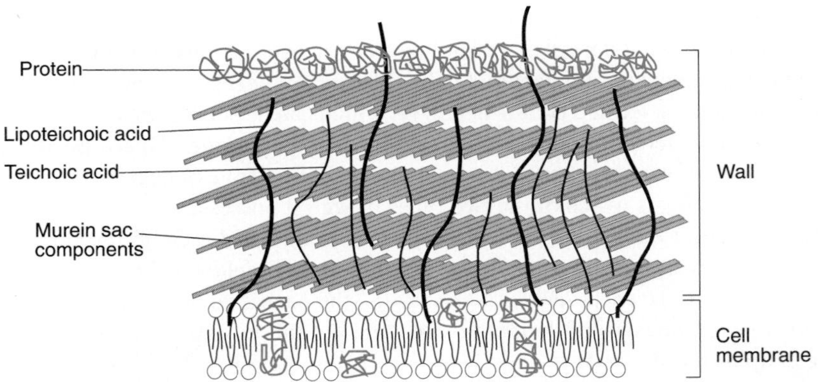


**Figure 2–6.** Schematic representation of the wall of Gram-positive bacteria.

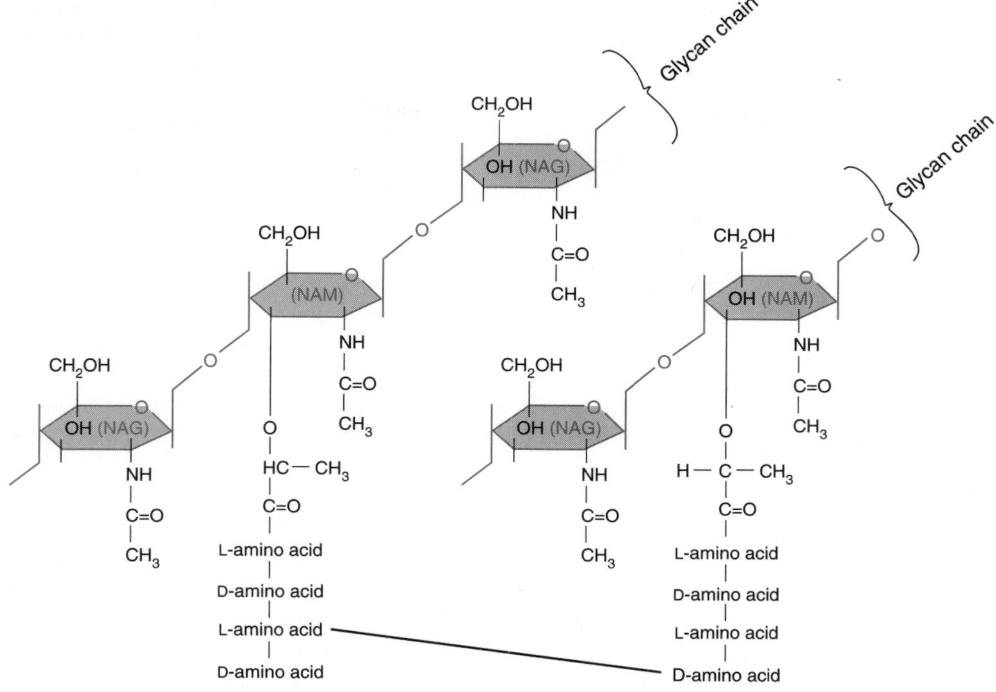


**Figure 2–7.** Schematic representation of the peptidoglycan murein. NAG, *N*-acetylglucosamine; NAM, *N*-acetylmuramic acid.

shape on the cell is easily demonstrated by removing or destroying it. Treatment of a Gram-positive cell with penicillin (which blocks formation of the tetrapeptide crosslinks and activates the cell's own murein hydrolases) or with lysozyme (which directly hydrolyzes the glycan chains) destroys the murein sac, and the wall is lost. Prompt lysis of the cell ensues. If the cell is protected from lysis by suspension in a medium approximately isotonic with the cell interior, such as 20% sucrose, the cell rounds up and forms a sphere called a **protoplast.** Some protoplasts can grow, and their formation from classic bacteria within patients treated with penicillin-type antibiotics (L-forms) has been postulated to account for some persistent infections. Superficially, protoplasts resemble the mollicutes (mycoplasmas) that are naturally wall-less bacteria.

Loss of cell wall leads to lysis in hypotonic media or protoplasts in isotonic media

A second component of the Gram-positive cell wall is a **teichoic** acid. These compounds are polymers of either glycerol phosphate or ribitol phosphate, with various sugars, amino sugars, and amino acids as substituents (Fig 2–8). The lengths of the chain and the

Teichoic and lipoteichoic acids are components of Gram-positive cell wall

```
            D-alanine
                |
   OH       H   O   H       OH
   |        |   ||  |       |
-O-P-O-C-C-C-O-P-O-
   ||       |   |   |       ||
   O        H   H   H       O
 |_________________________|
      Repeating subunit
A

            R   D-alanine
            |      |
   OH    H  O  OH  O   H     OH
   |     |  |  |   |   |     |
-O-P-O-C-C-C-C-C-O-P-O-
   ||    |  |  |   |   |     ||
   O     H  H  H   H   H     O
 |_______________________________|
        Repeating subunit
B
```

**Figure 2–8.** Schematic reproduction of teichoic acids. **A.** Glycerol teichoic acid. **B.** A ribitol teichoic acid in which R may be glucose or succinate in different species.

nature and location of the substituents vary from species to species and sometimes between strains within a species. Up to 50% of the wall may be teichoic acid, some of which is covalently linked to occasional NAM residues of the murein. Of the teichoic acids made of polyglycerol phosphate, much is linked not to the wall, but to a glycolipid in the underlying cell membrane. This type of teichoic acid is called **lipoteichoic acid** and seems to play a role in anchoring the wall to the cell membrane and as an epithelial cell adhesin. Teichoic acids are found only in Gram-positive cells and constitute major antigenic determinants of their cell surface individuality. For example, *S. aureus* polysaccharide A is a teichoic acid and *Enterococcus faecalis* group D carbohydrate is a lipoteichoic acid.

Different teichoic acids occur in different Gram-positive genera

Beside the major wall components—murein and teichoic acids—Gram-positive walls usually have lesser amounts of other molecules. Some are polysaccharides, such as the group-specific antigens of streptococci; others are proteins, such as the M protein of group A streptococci. The detailed arrangement of the various antigens in some of the more complex Gram-positive walls is still being worked out, but minor components are thought to protect the peptidoglycan layer from the action of such agents as lysozyme and, sometimes, to promote colonization by sticking the bacteria to the surfaces of host cells.

Other cell wall components may offer protection and promote colonization

### Gram-Negative Cell Wall

The second kind of cell wall found in bacteria, the Gram-negative cell wall, is depicted in Figure 2–9. Except for the presence of murein, there is little chemical resemblance to cell walls of Gram-positive bacteria, and the architecture is fundamentally different. In Gram-negative cells, the amount of murein has been greatly reduced, with some of it forming a single-layered sheet around the cell and the rest forming a gel-like substance, the **periplasmic gel**, with little crosslinking. External to this **periplasm** is an elaborate outer membrane.

Thin murein sac is imbedded in periplasmic murein gel

Historically the cell wall was regarded as the structure external to the cell membrane (excluding the capsule), and for Gram-positive bacteria this conception is certainly appropriate. Examination of Figures 2–5 and 2–9 shows the dilemma in applying the same term to the Gram-negative envelope. There is some reason to apply the same definition used for the Gram-positive situation, in which case the cell wall of Gram-negative bacteria consists of periplasm with its murein sac plus the outer membrane. This convention is used in Table 2–1 and in the text of this chapter. An alternative convention is to consider that the cell wall of Gram-negative bacteria is simply the structure chemically most like the Gram-positive wall, namely, the thin murein sac, with perhaps its attendant periplasmic gel. The student will quickly realize the underlying truth that **cell wall** is not a very satisfying term. Some microbiologists use cell envelope and envelope layers and avoid using the term cell wall altogether for Gram-negative bacteria.

Earlier electron micrographs had suggested that the small amount of murein in Gram-

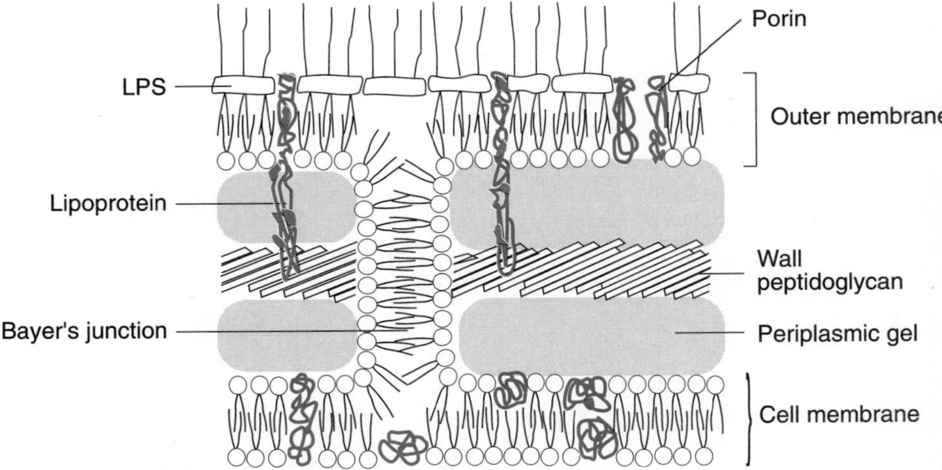


**Figure 2–9.** Schematic representation of wall of Gram-negative bacteria. LPS, lipopolysaccharide with endotoxic properties.

negative cells, such as *Escherichia coli*, formed a single sheet around the cell, and that this murein sac was floating in a space, the periplasmic space, containing a fairly concentrated solution of proteins and oligosaccharides. Recent evidence modifies this picture and indicates that the "space" is a gel formed by murein peptidoglycan chains with little or no crosslinking.

Whatever its precise nature, the periplasm contains a murein sac, with a unit peptidoglycan structure quite similar to that in Gram-positive cells. Despite its reduced extent in the Gram-negative wall, the murein sac still is responsible for the shape of the cell and is vital for its integrity. As in the case of Gram-positive cells, removing or damaging the peptidoglycan layer leads to cell lysis. If the cells are protected from osmotic lysis during lysozyme or penicillin treatment, they assume a spherical shape. Because such spheres cannot be totally stripped of wall material, they are called **spheroplasts,** in contrast to the protoplasts formed from Gram-positive cells. Spheroplasts of some species can multiply.

Structural significance of murein sac; removal results in spheroplasts

The proteins in solution in the periplasm consist of enzymes with hydrolytic functions (such as alkaline phosphatase), sometimes antibiotic-inactivating enzymes, and various binding proteins with roles in chemotaxis and in the active transport of solutes into the cell (see Chapter 3). Oligosaccharides secreted into the periplasm in response to external conditions serve to create an osmotic pressure buffer for the cell.

Periplasmic proteins have transport, chemotactic, and hydrolytic roles

The periplasm is an intermembrane structure, lying between the cell membrane (discussed later) and a special membrane unique to Gram-negative cells, the **outer membrane.** This has an overall structure similar to most biological membranes with two opposing phospholipid–protein leaflets. In composition, however, the outer membrane is unique in all biology. Its inner leaflet consists of ordinary phospholipids, but these are replaced in the outer leaflet by a special molecule called **lipopolysaccharide** (LPS). LPS is extremely toxic to humans and other animals and is called **endotoxin;** even in minute amounts, such as the amount released to the circulation during the course of a Gram-negative infection, this substance can produce a fever and shock syndrome called **Gram-negative shock**, or **endotoxic shock** (see Chapter 68).

Gram-negative outer membrane is phospholipoprotein bilayer

Outer layer is LPS endotoxin

LPS consists of a toxic **lipid A** (a phospholipid containing glucosamine rather than glycerol), a **core polysaccharide** (containing some unusual carbohydrate residues and fairly constant in structure among related species of bacteria), and **O antigen polysaccharide side chains** (Fig 2–10). The last component constitutes the major surface antigen of Gram-negative cells (which, it is recalled, lack teichoic acids).

Lipid A is toxic moiety of LPS; polysaccharides are antigenic determinants

The presence of LPS in the outer leaflet of the outer membrane results in the covering of Gram-negative cells by a wall that should block the passage of virtually every organic molecule into the cell. Hydrophobic molecules (such as some antibiotics) would be blocked by the hydrophilic layer of O antigen; hydrophilic solutes, including most nutrients, such as sugars and amino acids, would face the barrier created by the lipid portion of the outer membrane. Clearly this is a trade-off that cannot be made; the Gram-negative cell, for whatever benefit is afforded by possessing a wall with an outer membrane, must make provision for the rapid entry of nutrients. Active transport (described in Chapter 3) is part of the solution, and another part is contributed by a particular structural feature of the outer membrane. Special proteins, called **porins** or **matrix proteins**, form pores through the outer membrane that make it possible for hydrophilic solute molecules of molecular weight less than about 800 to diffuse through it and into the periplasm.

Impermeability of outer membrane is overcome by active transport and porins

The outer membrane does not contain the variety of proteins present in the cell membrane, but those that are present are quite abundant. In addition to the porins, there is a protein called **Braun's lipoprotein** or **murein lipoprotein**, which is probably the most abundant outer membrane protein in Gram-negative cells, such as *E. coli.* This protein is covalently attached at its amino end to a lipid embedded in the outer membrane. About one third of these lipoprotein molecules are covalently attached at their carboxyl end to the third amino acid in the murein tetrapeptide. It is believed that this forms the major attachment of the murein layer to the outer membrane of the wall in *E. coli* (Fig 2–9).

Murein lipoprotein is an abundant component

The innermost leaflet may well be contiguous, in places, with the outermost leaflet of the cell membrane (see Fig 2–9), because under the electron microscope preparations of the outer membrane and the cell membrane can be seen to adhere to each other at **zones of adhesion** (also called **Bayer's junctions**). Evidence has been found for other zones of

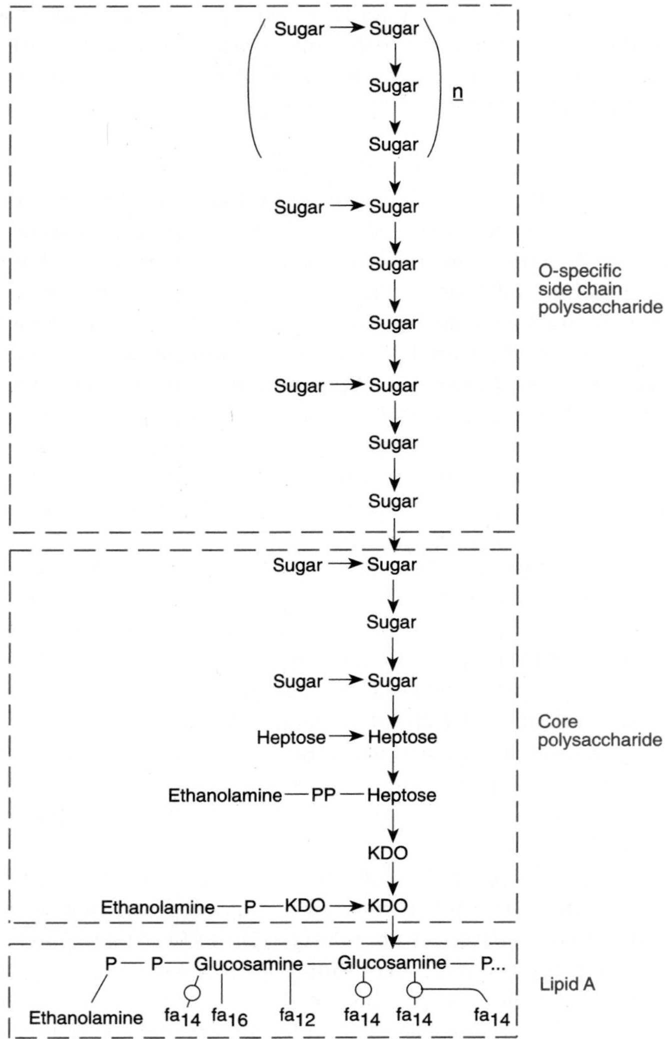


**Figure 2–10.** Schematic representation of lipopolysaccharide. The O-specific side chain is highly variable among species and subspecies and is a major determinant of antigenetic specificity.

adhesion girding the whole circumference of *E. coli* and related species. Because these annular rings tend to form about the cell division septum, they have been called **periseptal annuli.**

Outer membrane has many functions

In evolving a cell wall containing an outer membrane, Gram-negative bacteria have succeeded in (1) creating the periplasm, which holds digestive and protective enzymes and proteins important in transport and chemotaxis; (2) presenting an outer surface with strong negative charge, which is important in evading phagocytosis and the action of complement; and (3) providing a permeability barrier against such dangerous molecules as host lysozyme, ß-lysin, bile salts, digestive enzymes, and many antibiotics.

## Cell Membrane

Basic structure is phospholipid-protein bilayer membrane

Sterols are absent

Generally the cell membrane of bacteria is similar to the familiar bileaflet (trilaminar) membrane, containing phospholipids and proteins, that is found throughout the living world. There are, however, important differences. The bacterial cell membrane is exceptionally rich in proteins (up to 70% of its weight) and does not (except in the case of mycoplasmas) contain sterols. It may in some species possess convoluted infoldings called **mesosomes.** The biological significance of mesosomes has been questioned; they may be artifacts of fixation. The bacterial chromosome is attached to the cell membrane, which plays a role in segregation of daughter chromosomes at cell division, analogous to the role of the mitotic apparatus of eukaryotes. The membrane is the site of synthesis of DNA, cell wall polymers, and membrane lipids. It contains the entire electron transport system of the cell (and, hence, is functionally analogous to the mitochondria of eukaryotes). It contains receptor proteins that function in chemotaxis. Like cell membranes of eukaryotes, it is a permeability barrier and contains proteins involved in selective and active transport of solutes. It is also involved in secretion to the exterior of proteins (exoproteins), including exotoxins and hydrolytic enzymes involved in the pathogenesis of disease. The bacterial cell membrane is therefore the functional equivalent of most of the organelles of the eukaryotic cell and is vital to the growth and maintenance of the cell.

Role in synthetic, homeostatic, and electron transport processes and cell division

Cell membrane is functional equivalent of many eukaryotic organelles

The cell membranes of Gram-positive and Gram-negative cells are similar in composition, structure, and function except for the modification, already described, in Gram-negative cells that places the outer membrane of the wall and the cell membrane in intimate contact (Bayer's junctions).

## Flagella

Flagella are molecular organelles of motility found in many species of bacteria, both Gram positive and Gram negative. They may be distributed around the cell (an arrangement called peritrichous from the Greek **trichos** for "hair"), at one pole (**polar** or **monotrichous**), or at both ends of the cell (**lophotrichous**). In all cases, they are individually helical in shape and propel the cell by rotating at the point of insertion in the cell envelope. The presence or absence of flagella and their position are important taxonomic characteristics.

Flagella are rotating helical organs of locomotion

The flagellar apparatus is complex, but consists entirely of proteins, encoded in genes called *fla* (for flagella). They are attached to the cell by a **basal body** consisting of several proteins organized as rings on a central rod (see Fig 2–5). In Gram-negative cells, there are four rings: an outer pair that serve as bushings through the outer membrane and an inner pair located in the peptidoglycan gel and the cell membrane. In Gram-positive cells, only the inner pair is present. The **hook** consists of other proteins organized as a bent structure that may function as a universal joint. Finally, the long **filament** consists of polymerized molecules of a single protein species called **flagellin** (Fig 2–11).

Flagella have bushing rings in cell envelope

Flagellar filament is composed of flagellin protein

Motility and chemotaxis, both important properties contributing to colonization, are discussed in Chapter 3.

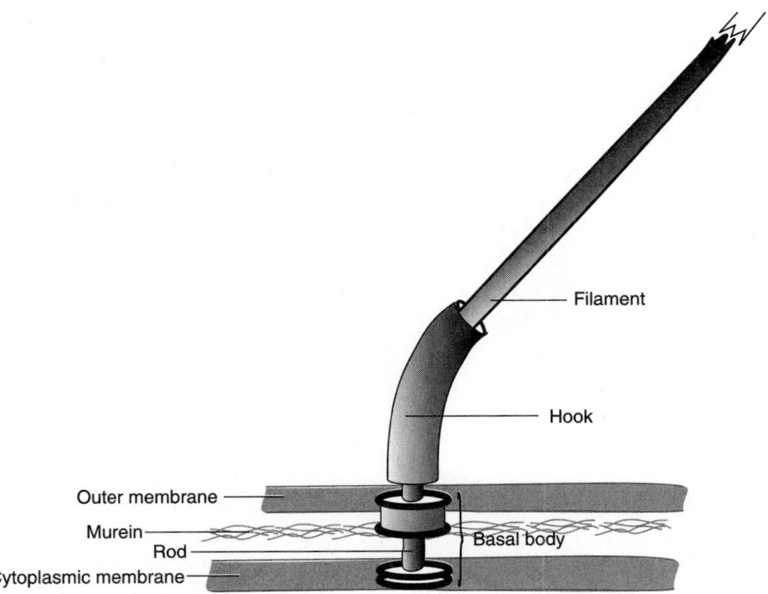


**Figure 2–11.** Schematic representation of the flagellar apparatus. (After DePamphilis ML, Adler J. Fine structure and isolation of hook-basal body complex of flagella from *Escherichia coli* and *Bacillus subtilis*. *J Bacteriol.* 1971; 105:384–359.)

## Pili

Pili are proteinaceous hairlike projections

Common pili have adherence roles

Male Gram-negative cells of some species have single tubular sex pili

Some pili are plasmid encoded

Pili are molecular hairlike projections found on the surface of cells of many Gram-positive and Gram-negative species. They are composed of molecules of a protein called **pilin** arranged to form a tube with a minute, hollow core. There are two general classes, common pili and sex pili (Fig 2–12). **Common pili** cover the surface of the cell. They are, in many cases, **adhesins,** which are responsible for the ability of bacteria to colonize surfaces and cells. To cite only one example, the pili of *Neisseria gonorrhoeae* are necessary for the attachment to the urethral epithelial cells prior to penetration; without pili, the bacterium cannot cause gonorrhea. Thus, common pili are often important virulence factors. Some bacteriologists use the name **fimbriae** to refer to common pili. The sex pilus is diagnostic of a male bacterium and is involved in exchange of genetic material between some Gram-negative bacteria. There is only one per cell. The function of the sex pilus is discussed in Chapter 4. Some pili are encoded not by chromosomal, but by plasmid genes (see Chapter 4). This fact means that both sex and virulence are properties conferred on many bacteria by a foreign genome.

## CORE

In contrast to the structural richness of the layers and appendages of the cell envelope, the interior seems relatively simple in transmission electron micrographs of thin sections of bacteria (Fig 2–13). There are two clearly visible regions, one granular (the cytosol) and one fibrous (the nucleoid). In addition, many bacteria possess plasmids that are circular, double-stranded DNA bodies in the cytosol separate from the larger nucleoid; plasmids are too small to be visible in thin sections of bacteria.

## Cytosol

The dense **cytosol** is bounded by the cell membrane. It appears granular because it is densely packed with ribosomes, which are much more abundant than in the cytoplasm of eukary-

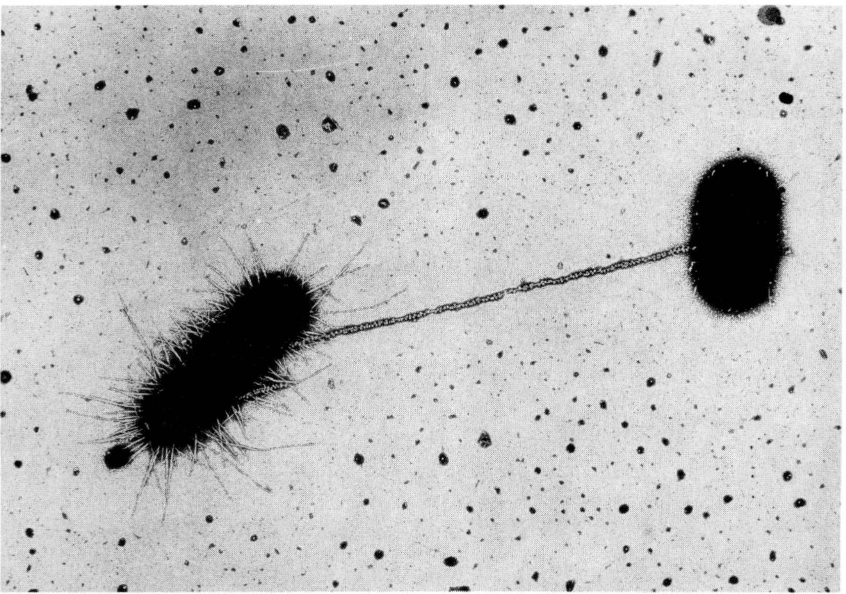

**Figure 2–12.** On the left-hand side is a "male" *Escherichia* coli cell exhibiting many common (somatic) pili and a sex pilus by which it has attached itself to a "female" cell that lacks the plasmid encoding the sex pilus. As discussed in Chapter 4, the sex pilus facilitates exchange of genetic material between the male and female *E. coli.* In this preparation, the sex pilus has been labeled with a bacterial virus that attaches to it specifically. (*Courtesy of Charles C. Brinton and Judith Carnahan.*)

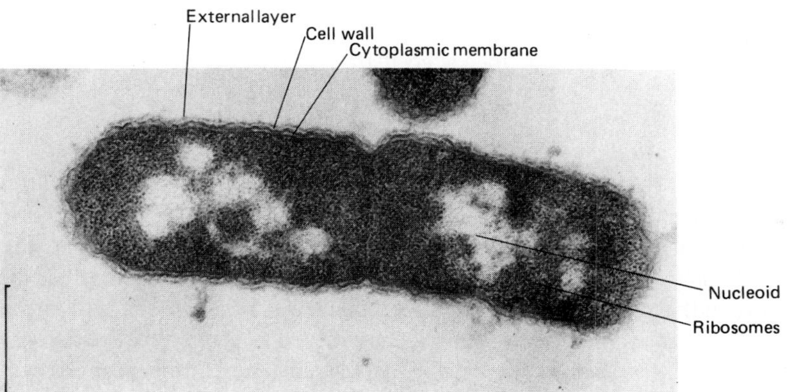


**Figure 2–13.** Electron micrograph of a Gram-negative bacterium. (*Courtesy of the late Dr. E. S. Boatman.*)

otic cells. This is a reflection of the higher growth rate of bacteria. Each ribosome is a ribonucleoprotein particle consisting of three species of rRNA (5 S, 16 S, and 23 S) and about 56 proteins. The overall subunit structure (one 50 S plus one 30 S particle) of the 70 S bacterial ribosome resembles that of eukaryotic ribosomes (which are 80 S, composed of one 60 S and one 40 S particle), but is smaller and differs sufficiently in function that a very large number of antimicrobics have the prokaryotic ribosome as their target. The number of ribosomes varies directly with the growth rate of the cell (see Chapter 3). At all but the slowest growth rates about 70% of the ribosomes at any one time exist as polysomes and are engaged in translating mRNA.

Abundant 70S ribosomes with 50S and 30S subunits that are targets for some antimicrobics

Except for the functions associated with the cell membrane, all of the metabolic reactions of the cell take place in the cytosol. Accordingly it is found to be the major location of a great fraction of the 2000 to 3000 different enzymes of the cell.

The cytosol of some bacterial species also contains nutritional storage granules called **reserve granules.** The most prevalent kinds consist of glycogen or polymetaphosphate. Their presence and abundance depend on the nutritional state of the cell.

## Nucleoid

The bacterial genome resides on a single chromosome and typically consists of about 4000 genes encoded in one, large, circular molecule of double-stranded DNA containing about 5 million nucleotide base pairs. This molecule is more than 1 mm long, and it therefore exceeds the length of the cell by some 1000 times. Needless to say, tight packing is necessary, and it is this packing that displaces all ribosomes and other cytosol components from the regions that appear clear or fibrous in electron micrographs of thin sections of bacterial cells (see Fig 2–13). Each region thus contains a chromosome, coated usually by polyamines and some specialized DNA-binding proteins, but not with the structural organization of a eukaryotic chromosome. Because it is not surrounded by a membrane, it is not correctly called a nucleus, but rather a **nucleoid** or **nuclear body**. The manner in which the DNA molecule is packed to form a nucleoid is not yet totally known. It is known that the DNA is attached to the cell membrane and that the double-helical DNA chain is twisted into supercoils. Evidence indicates that the entire chromosome is attached to some central structure, perhaps RNA, at a large number of points (12–80), creating folds of DNA, each of which is independently coiled into a tight bundle. Gentle methods of lysing cells permit nucleoids to be isolated as compact particles from which DNA loops can be sprung out.

Large circular chromosome of supercoiled double-stranded DNA

Bacteria have no nuclear membranes

Nucleoid is attached to cell membrane and central structures

Each nuclear body corresponds to a DNA molecule. The number of nuclear bodies varies as a function of growth rate; resting cells have only one, rapidly growing cells may have as many as four. As is described in Chapter 4, bacteria are genetically **haploid,** because all the chromosomes are identical and are segregated at random into daughter cells.

Cell may contain 2–4 nucleoids during growth

The absence of a nuclear membrane confers on the prokaryotic cell a great advantage for rapid growth in changing environments. As described in Chapter 3, ribosomes can be translating mRNA molecules even as the latter are being made; no transport of mRNA from where it is made to where it functions is needed.

## Plasmids

Plasmids are nonchromosomal, small, circular, double-stranded DNA molecules

Many encode protective enzymes, virulence determinants, and transmissibility

Many bacteria contain small, circular, covalently closed, double-stranded DNA molecules separate from the chromosome. More than one type of plasmid or several copies of a single plasmid may be present in the cell. Many plasmids carry genes coding for the production of enzymes that protect the cell from toxic substances. For example, antibiotic resistance is often plasmid determined. Many attributes of virulence, such as production of some pili and of some exotoxins, are also determined by plasmid genes. Some plasmids code for production of a sex pilus by which they promote cell conjugation and thereby accomplish their own intercellular transmission. They are thus "infectious," are nonhomologous to the bacterial chromosome, and provide a rapid method for acquisition of valuable genetic traits. This topic is considered in more detail in Chapter 4.

## SPORES

Endospores are resistant, quiescent forms of some Gram-positive bacteria

**Endospores** are small, dehydrated, metabolically quiescent forms that are produced by some bacteria in response to nutrient limitation or a related sign that tough times are coming. Very few species produce spores (the term is loosely used as equivalent to endospores), but they are particularly prevalent in the environment. Some sporing bacteria are of great importance in medicine, causing such diseases as anthrax, gas gangrene, tetanus, and botulism. All spore formers are Gram-positive rods. Some grow only in the absence of oxygen (eg, *Clostridium tetani*), some only in its presence (eg, *Bacillus subtilis*).

Spore allows survival of cell under adverse conditions

The bacterial endospore is not a reproductive structure. One cell forms one spore under adverse conditions (the process is called **sporulation**). The spore may persist for a long time (centuries) and then, on appropriate stimulation, give rise to a single bacterial cell (**germination**). Spores, therefore, are survival rather than reproductive devices.

Resistance due to dehydrated state, calcium dipicolinate, and specialized spore coats

Spores of some species can withstand extremes of pH and temperature, including boiling water, for surprising periods of time. The thermal resistance is brought about by the low water content and the presence of a large amount of a substance found only in spores, **calcium dipicolinate**. Resistance to chemicals and, to some extent, radiation is aided by extremely tough, special coats surrounding the spore. These include a **spore membrane** (equivalent to the former cell membrane); a thick **cortex** composed of a special form of peptidoglycan; a **coat** consisting of a cystein-rich, keratin-like, insoluble structural protein; and finally an external lipoprotein and carbohydrate layer called an **exosporium.**

Germination reproduces cell identical to that which sporulated

The metabolic signal for sporulation is not fully understood. A nucleoid and its surrounding cytosol become walled off initially by invagination of the cell membrane, and later the special spore layers are added. Germination begins with activation (by heat, acid, and reducing conditions). Initiation of germination leads eventually to outgrowth of a new vegetative cell of the same genotype as the cell that produced the spore.

## ADDITIONAL READING

Neidhardt FC, Ingraham JL, Schaechter M. *Physiology of the Bacterial Cell: A Molecular Approach.* Sunderland, MA: Sinauer Associates; 1990. A very readable description of the composition, organization, and structure of the bacterial cell is presented in Chapters 1 and 2. A good list of references for further reading is included.

Chapter 3

# Bacterial Processes

*Frederick C. Neidhardt*

In this chapter we examine how the structural and chemical components of bacteria function in the growth and survival of these cells and in their colonization of the human host.

## CELL GROWTH

Growth of single-celled organisms is accomplished by an orderly progress of metabolic processes followed by cell division by binary fission. The subject of growth has three areas for study: metabolism, which produces cell material from the nutrient substances present in the environment; regulation, which coordinates the progress of the hundreds of independent biochemical processes of metabolism to result in an orderly and efficient synthesis of cell components and structures in the right proportions; and cell division, which results in the formation of two independent living systems from one.

Bacterial growth requires metabolism, regulation, and division by binary fission

### Bacterial Metabolism

We do not review in depth the many aspects of (mostly mammalian) metabolism customarily learned in biochemistry courses. Many of the principles, and even some of the details of metabolism, are universal. Indeed, the principle known as the **unity of biochemistry** is underscored by the fact that much of what we know of metabolic pathways is derived from work with *Escherichia coli*. We focus, rather, on the unique aspects of bacterial metabolism that are important in medicine.

The broad differences between bacteria and human eukaryotic cells can be summarized as follows:

1. The metabolism of bacteria is geared to rapid growth and proceeds 10 to 100 times faster than in cells of our bodies.
2. Bacteria are much more versatile than human cells in their ability to use various compounds as energy sources and in their ability to use oxidants other than molecular oxygen in their metabolism of foodstuffs.
3. Bacteria are much more diverse than human cells in their nutritional requirements, because they are more diverse with respect to the completeness of their biosynthetic pathways.
4. The simpler prokaryotic body plan makes it possible for bacteria to synthesize macromolecules by far more streamlined means than our cells employ.
5. Some biosynthetic processes, such as those producing murein, lipopolysaccharide (LPS), and teichoic acid, are unique to bacteria.

Metabolism of prokaryotic cells is more active, versatile, and diverse than that of human cells

Each of these differences contributes to the special nature of the human/microbe encounter, and each provides a potential means for designing therapeutic agents to modify the outcome of this interaction.

Bacterial metabolism is highly complex. The bacterial cell synthesizes itself and generates energy for active transport, motility (in some species), and other activities by as many as 2000 chemical reactions. These reactions can be helpfully classified according to their function in the metabolic processes of **fueling, biosynthesis, polymerization,** and **assembly.**

## Fueling Reactions

Fueling reactions provide the cell with energy and with the 12 precursor metabolites used in biosynthetic reactions (Fig 3–1).

Nutrients enter despite envelope permeability barriers

The first step is the capture of nutrients from the environment. Both Gram-positive and Gram-negative cells have surrounded themselves with envelopes designed in part to exclude potentially harmful substances and, therefore, have had to evolve a number of ways to ensure rapid transport of selected solute molecules through the envelope. Methods used by Gram-negative cells are summarized in Figure 3–2.

Facilitated diffusion across cell membrane requires shuttling by carrier protein

Almost no important nutrients enter the cell by **simple diffusion**, because the cell membrane is too effective a barrier to most molecules (the exceptions are carbon dioxide, oxygen, and water). Some transport occurs by **facilitated diffusion** in which a protein carrier in the cell membrane, specific for a given compound, participates in the shuttling of molecules of that substance from one side of the membrane to the other. Glycerol enters *E. coli* cells in this manner, and in bacteria that grow in the absence of oxygen (anaerobic bacteria, see below) it is reasonably common for some nutrients to enter the cell and for fermentation byproducts to leave the cell by facilitated diffusion. Because no energy is involved, this process can work only with, never against, a concentration gradient of the given solute.

Active transport can move nutrients against concetration gradient

**Active transport**, like facilitated diffusion, involves specific protein molecules as carriers of particular solutes, but the process is energy linked and can therefore establish a concentration gradient (active transport can pump "uphill"). Active transport is the most common mechanism in aerobic bacteria. Gram-negative bacteria have two kinds of active transport systems. In one, called **shock-sensitive** because the components are released from the cell by osmotic shock treatments, solute molecules cross the outer membrane either by diffusion through the pores of the outer membrane (as in the case of galactose) or by a special protein carrier (as in the case of maltose). In the periplasm the solute molecules bind to

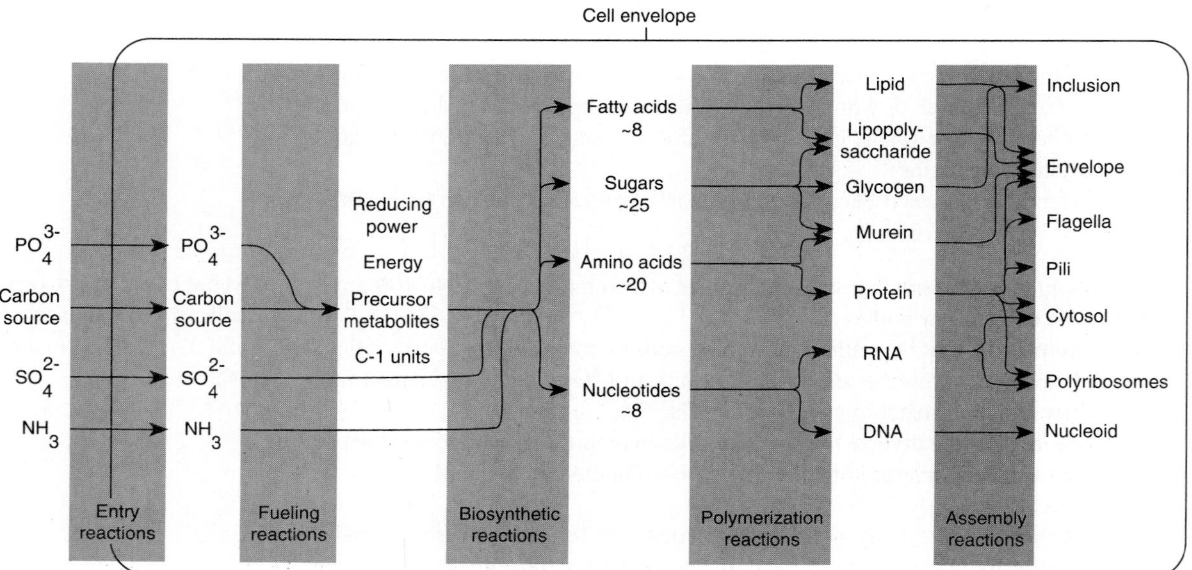


**Figure 3–1.** General pattern of metabolism leading to the synthesis of a bacterial cell from glucose.

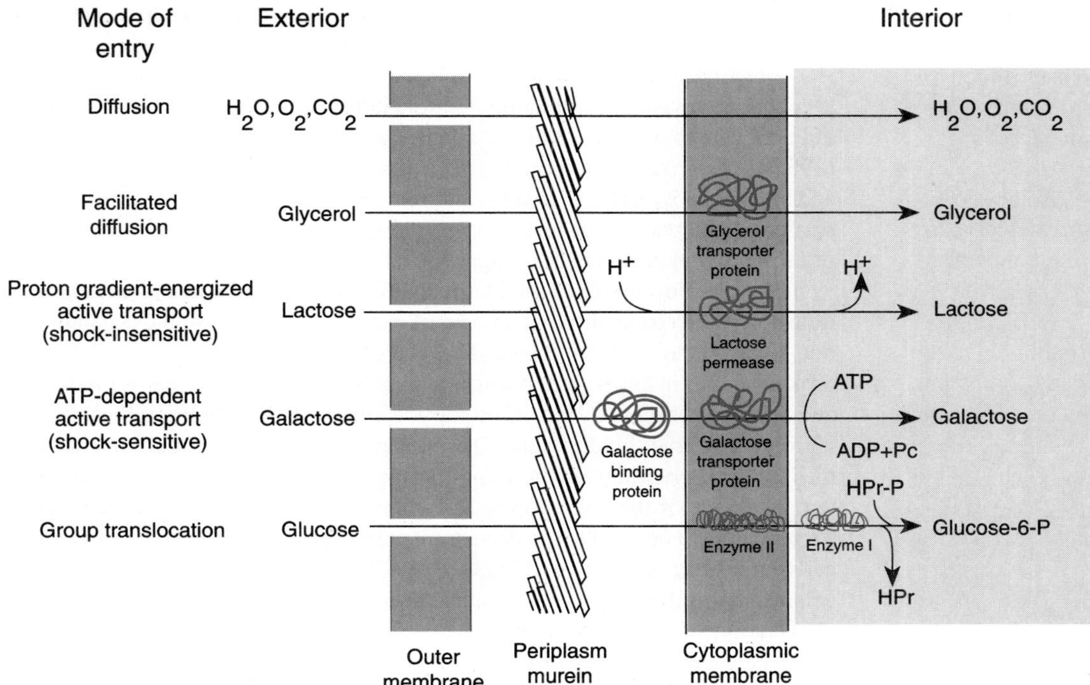


**Figure 3–2.** Schematic representation of the various modes of carbohydrate transport by *Escherichia coli.* Facilitated diffusion is demonstrated by glycerol transport; proton gradient-energized transport, by lactose uptake; shock-sensitive ATP-dependent transport, by galactose uptake; and group translocation, by glucose uptake.

specific **binding proteins**, which interact with carrier proteins in the cell membrane. Shock-sensitive systems couple the transport across the cell membrane with the hydrolysis of ATP.

Shock-sensitive transport involves periplasmic binding proteins and ATP-derived energy

The other type of active transport involves only cell membrane components (and, hence, is **shock insensitive**) and is distinctive in that solute transport is coupled to the simultaneous passage of protons ($H^+$) through the membrane. The energy for this type of active transport is therefore derived not from ATP hydrolysis, but from the proton gradient set up by electron transport within the energized cell membrane.

Shock-insensitive transport at cell membrane requires proton gradient energy

Finally, **group translocation** is an extremely common means of transport in the absence of oxygen. It involves the chemical conversion of the solute into another molecule as it is transported. The phosphotransferase system for sugar transport, which involves the phosphorylation of sugars such as glucose by specific enzymes, is a good example.

Group translocation involves chemical conversion of transported molecule

The transport of iron and other metal ions needed in small amounts for growth is special and of particular importance in virulence. There is little free $Fe^{3+}$ in human blood or other body fluids, because it is sequestered by iron-binding proteins (eg, **transferrin** in blood and **lactoferrin** in milk). Bacteria must have iron to grow, and their colonization of the human host requires capture of iron. Bacteria secrete **siderophores** (iron-specific chelators) to trap $Fe^{3+}$; the iron-containing chelator is then transported into the bacterium by specific active transport. One example of a siderophore is **aerobactin** (a citrate type of hydoxamate), another is **enterobactin** (a catechol). Some siderophores are produced as a result of enzymes encoded not in the bacterial genome, but in the genome of a plasmid, providing another example of the many ways in which plasmids are involved in virulence.

Iron is an essential nutrient, but is sequestered by host Fe-binding proteins

Bacterial siderophores chelate the iron and are actively transported into cell

Once inside the cell, sugar molecules or other sources of carbon and energy are metabolized by the Embden–Meyerhof glycolytic pathway, the pentose phosphate pathway, and the Krebs cycle to yield the carbon compounds needed for biosynthesis. Some bacteria have central fueling pathways (eg, the Entner–Doudoroff pathway) other than those familiar in mammalian metabolism.

Unidirectional central fueling pathways produce biosynthetic precursors

The central fueling pathways function unidirectionally to produce the 12 precursor metabolites, but connections to **fermentation** and **respiration** pathways allow the reoxidation of reduced coenzyme nicotinamide adenine dinucleotide (NADH) to $NAD^+$ and the generation of ATP. Bacteria make ATP by substrate phosphorylation in fermentation or by

Fermentation and respiration pathways regenerate ATP and NAD+

a combination of substrate phosphorylation and oxidative phosphorylation in respiration (photosynthetic bacteria are not important in medicine).

Fermentation uses direct electron and proton transfer to final organic receptor

**Fermentation** is the transfer of electrons and protons via $NAD^+$ directly to an organic acceptor. Pyruvate occupies a pivotal role in fermentation (Fig 3–3). Fermentation is an inefficient way to generate ATP, and consequently huge amounts of sugar must be fermented to satisfy the growth requirements of bacteria anaerobically. Large amounts of organic acids and alcohols are produced in fermentation. Which compounds are produced depends on the particular pathway of fermentation employed by a given species, and therefore the profile of fermentation products is a diagnostic aid in the clinical laboratory.

Fermentation produces organic acids and alcohols; low ATP-generating efficiency

Respiratory chain of electron carriers; oxygen usually the terminal acceptor

**Respiration** involves fueling pathways in which substrate oxidation is coupled to the transport of electrons through a chain of carriers to some ultimate acceptor, frequently, but not always, molecular oxygen. These are efficient generators of ATP. Respiration in prokaryotes as in eukaryotes occurs by membrane-bound enzymes (quinones, cytochromes, and terminal oxidases), but in prokaryotes the cell membrane rather than mitochondrial membranes serve this function. The passage of electrons through the carriers is accompanied by the secretion from the cell of protons, generating an $H^+$ differential between the external surface of the cell and the cell interior. This differential, called the **protonmotive force**, can then be used to (1) drive transport of solutes by the shock-insensitive systems of active transport (see above); (2) power the flagellar motors that rotate the filaments and result in cell motility in the case of motile species; and (3) generate ATP by coupling the phosphorylation of adenosine diphosphate (ADP) to the passage of protons inward through special channels in the cell membrane. The last pathway, facilitated by the enzyme anachronistically called **membrane ATPase**, can in fact function in either direction, coupling ADP phosphorylation to the inward passage of protons down the gradient or hydrolyzing ATP to accomplish the secretion of protons to establish a protonmotive force. The latter process explains how cells can generate a protonmotive force anaerobically (in the absence of electron transport).

Respiration is efficient energy producer

Varying responses to oxygen

In evolving to colonize every conceivable nook and cranny on this planet, bacteria have developed distinctive responses to oxygen. They are conveniently classified according to their fermentative and respiratory activities, but much more generally by their overall response to the presence of oxygen. The response depends on their genetic ability to ferment or respire, but also on their ability to protect themselves from the deleterious effects of oxygen.

Production of peroxide and toxic oxygen radicals; detoxifying enzymes

Oxygen, though itself only mildly toxic, gives rise to at least two extremely reactive and toxic substances, **hydrogen peroxide** ($H_2O_2$) and the **superoxide anion** ($O^{2-}$). Peroxide is produced by reactions (catalyzed by flavoprotein oxidases) in which electrons and protons are transferred to $O_2$ as final acceptor; the superoxide radical is produced as an in-

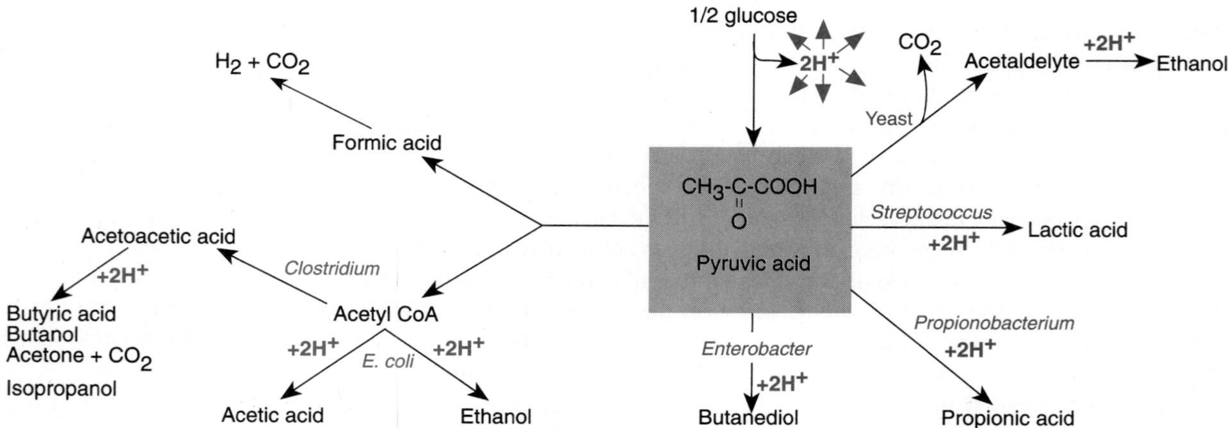


**Figure 3–3.** Some pathways of fermentation of sugars by various microorganisms. The protons ($H^+$) generated by the conversion of glucose to pyruvate by the Embden–Meyerhoff pathway are transferred to NAD. Oxidized NAD must be regenerated by reducing pyruvate and its derivatives.

termediate in most reactions that reduce molecular $O_2$. Superoxide is partially detoxified by an enzyme, **superoxide dismutase**, found in all organisms (prokaryotes and eukaryotes) that survive the presence of oxygen. Superoxide dismutase catalyzes the reaction

$$2O^{2-} (+)\ 2H^+ \rightarrow H_2O_2\ (+)\ O_2.$$

Hydrogen peroxide is degraded by peroxidases by the reaction

$$H_2O_2\ (+)\ H_2A \rightarrow 2H_2O\ (+)\ A$$

where A is any of a number of chemical groups (in the case in which $H_2A$ is another molecule of $H_2O_2$, the reaction yields $2H_2O + O_2$, and the peroxidase is called catalase). Bacteria that lack the ability to make superoxide dismutase and catalase are exquisitely sensitive to the presence of molecular oxygen and, in general, must grow anaerobically using fermentation. Bacteria that possess these protective enzymes can grow in the presence of oxygen, but whether they use the oxygen in metabolism or not depends on their ability to respire. Whether these oxygen-resistant bacteria can grow anaerobically depends on their ability to ferment.

Superoxide dismutase and peroxidase allow growth in air; absence requires strict anaerobiosis

Organisms growing in air may or may not have respiratory pathway

Various combinations of these two characteristics (oxidation resistance and the ability to use molecular oxygen as a final acceptor) are represented in different species of bacteria, resulting in the five general classes shown in Table 3–1. There are important pathogens within each class. Both the nature of the diseases they cause and the methods for cultivating and identifying these pathogens in the laboratory are dictated to a large extent by their response to oxygen.

Aerobes, anaerobes, facultatives, indifferents, and microaerophils

## Biosynthesis

Biosynthetic reactions form a network of pathways that lead from 12 precursor metabolites (provided by the fueling reactions) to the many amino acids, nucleotides, sugars, amino sugars, fatty acids, and other building blocks needed for macromolecules (see Fig 3–1). In addition to the carbon precursors, large quantities of reduced nicotinamide adenine dinucleotide phosphate (NADPH), ATP, amino nitrogen, and some source of sulfur are needed for biosynthesis of these building blocks. These pathways are similar in all species of living things, but bacterial species differ greatly as to which pathways they possess. Because all cells require the same building blocks, those that cannot be produced by a given cell must be obtained preformed from the environment. Nutritional requirements of bacteria, there-

Biosyntheses require 12 precursor metabolites, energy, amino nitrogen, and sulfur

Nutritional requirements differ

**TABLE 3–1. CLASSIFICATION OF BACTERIA BY RESPONSE TO OXYGEN**

| Type of Bacteria | Growth Response: Aerobic | Growth Response: Anaerobic | Possession of Catalase and Superoxide Dismutase | Comment | Example |
|---|---|---|---|---|---|
| Aerobe (strict aerobe) | + | – | + | Requires oxygen; cannot ferment | *Mycobacterium tuberculosis*<br>*Pseudomonas aeruginosa*<br>*Bacillus subtilis* |
| Anaerobe (strict anaerobe) | – | + | – | Killed by oxygen; ferments in absence of $O_2$ | *Clostridium botulinum*<br>*Bacteroides melaninogenicus* |
| Facultative | + | + | + | Respires with $O_2$; ferments in absence of $O_2$ | *Escherichia coli*<br>*Shigella dysenteriae*<br>*Staphylococcus aureus* |
| Indifferent (aerotolerant anaerobe) | + | + | + | Ferments in presence or absence of $O_2$ | *Streptococcus pneumoniae*<br>*Streptococcus pyogenes* |
| Microaerophilic | (+)[a] | + | (+)[a] | Grows best at low $O_2$ concentration; can grow without $O_2$ | *Campylobacter jejuni* |

[a] (+) indicates small amounts of growth or catalase and superoxide dismutase.

fore, differ from species to species and serve as an important practical basis for laboratory identification.

There are relatively few unique reactions in the domain of biosynthesis that form the basis for specific therapeutic attack on the microorganism rather than the host. The effectiveness of sulfonamides and trimethoprim is one of these exceptions; the requirement of many bacteria to synthesize folic acid rather than being able to use it preformed from their environment as human cells do renders bacteria susceptible to these agents, which interfere with the biosynthesis of folic acid.

## Polymerization Reactions

Bidirectional semiconservative DNA replication occurs at replication forks

**Polymerization** of DNA is called **replication.** In bacteria it involves 12 or more proteins acting at a small number of sites (replication forks) where DNA is synthesized from activated building blocks (dATP, dGTP, dCTP, and dTTP). Replication always begins at special sites on the chromosome called *oriC* (in *E. coli* for origin of replication) and then proceeds bidirectionally around the circular chromosome (Fig 3–4). Synthesis of DNA at each replication fork is termed **semiconservative** because each of the DNA chains serves as the template for the synthesis of its complement, and, therefore, one of the two chains of the new double-stranded molecule is conserved from the original chromosome. One of the two new strands must be synthesized in chemically the opposite direction of the other; this is accomplished by having each new strand made in short segments, 5′ to 3′, which are then ligated by one of the DNA-synthesizing enzymes (see Fig 3–4). Interestingly, an RNA primer is involved in getting each of these segments initiated. The two replication forks meet at the opposite side of the circle. The frequency of initiation of chromosome replication (and, therefore, the number of growing points) varies with cell growth rate; the chain elongation rate is rather constant.

DNA gyrase inhibitors

Some chemotherapeutic agents derive their selective toxicity for bacteria from the unique features of prokaryotic DNA replication. The antibiotic **novobiocin** and the synthetic quinolone compounds inhibit DNA gyrase, one of the many enzymes participating in DNA replication.

One RNA polymerase synthesizes all forms of bacterial RNA

**Transcription** is the synthesis of RNA. Transcription in bacteria differs from that in eukaryotic cells in several ways. One way is that all forms of bacterial RNA (mRNA, tRNA, and rRNA) are synthesized by the same enzyme, RNA polymerase. Like the several eukaryotic enzymes, the single bacterial RNA polymerase uses activated building blocks (ATP, GTP, CTP, and UTP) and synthesizes an RNA strand complementary to whichever strand of DNA is serving as template.

Bacterial mRNA needs no special means of transport to ribosomes

A second major difference is that bacterial mRNA need not be transported to the cytoplasm through a nuclear membrane, and hence no poly(A) cap is needed and no special means of transport exists. In fact, because each mRNA strand is directly accessible to ribosomes, binding of the latter to mRNA to form polysomes begins at an early stage in the synthesis of each mRNA molecule (Fig 3–5).

RNA polymerase σ subunit recognizes promoters

RNA polymerase is a large, complicated molecule with a subunit structure of $\alpha_2\beta\beta^1\sigma$. The σ subunit is the one that locates specific DNA sequences, called promoters, which precede all transcriptional units. Bacterial RNA polymerases generally possess more than one σ subunit, each designed to recognize a different set of related promoters, which provides a simple means to activate groups of related genes that cooperate in such cellular processes as sporulation, nitrogen acquisition, heat shock response, and adaptation to nongrowth conditions.

As in eukaryotic cells, all stable RNA molecules are made from giant precursor molecules that must be processed by nucleases and then extensively modified to produce the mature product (the tRNAs and rRNAs).

Rifampin inhibits RNA polymerase

Bacterial RNA polymerase is the target of the **rifamycin** series of antimicrobics (including the semisynthetic compound **rifampin**). They block initiation of transcription. Other substances of biological origin block extension of RNA chains or inhibit transcription by binding to DNA. They have been of great value in molecular biological studies, but are toxic also to human cells and thus are not used in human therapy.

**Translation** is the name given to protein synthesis. Bacteria activate the 20-amino-

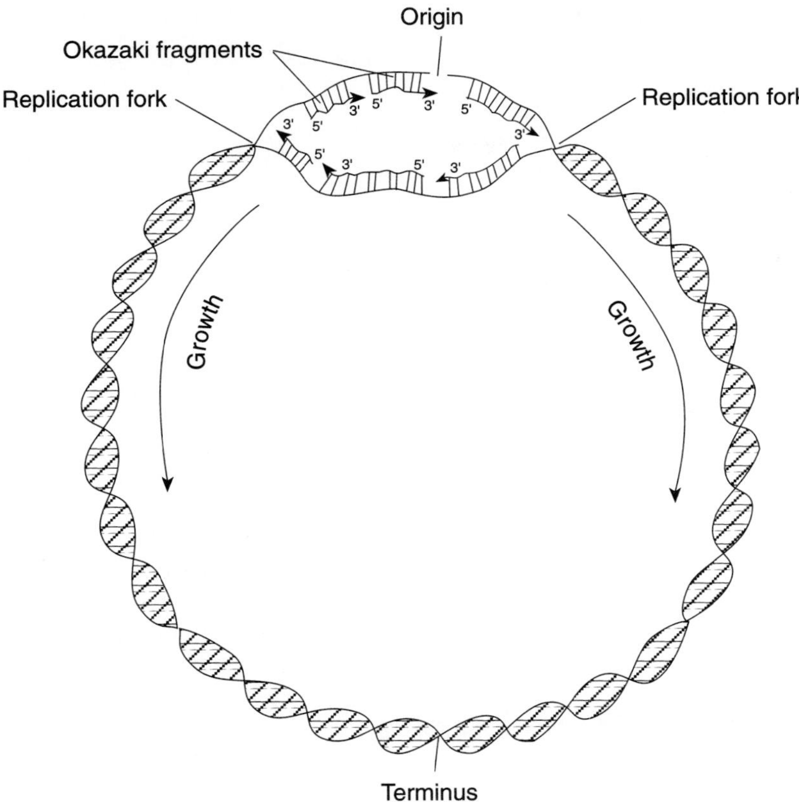


**Figure 3–4.** Schematic representation of DNA replication in bacteria. Shown is a portion of a replicating chromosome shortly after replication has begun at the origin. The newly polymerized strands of DNA are synthesized in the 5′ to 3′ direction (indicated by the arrows) using preexisting DNA strands as templates. The process creates two replication forks that travel in opposite directions until they meet on the opposite side of the chromosome.

acid building blocks of protein in the course of attaching them to specific transfer RNA molecules. The aminoacyl-tRNAs are brought to the ribosomes by soluble protein factors, and there the amino acids are polymerized into polypeptide chains according to the sequence of codons in the particular mRNA that is being translated. Having donated its amino acid, the tRNA is released from the ribosome to return for another aminoacylation cycle.

Proteins made by polymerizing amino acid residues from specific tRNAs

This description fits translation in eukaryotic as well as prokaryotic cells, but major differences do exist. The initiation of translation of a new polypeptide chain requires fewer proteins in bacteria. The ribosomes of bacteria are smaller and simpler in structure. Bacterial mRNA is largely polycistronic, that is, each mRNA molecule is the transcript of more than one gene (cistron) and, therefore, directs the synthesis of more than one polypeptide. No processing or transport of the mRNA is necessary. RNA polymerase makes mRNA at about 55 nucleotides per second (at 37°C), and ribosomes make polypeptide chains at about 18 amino acids per second. Therefore, not only does translation of each mRNA molecule occur simultaneously with transcription, but it occurs at the same linear rate (55 nucleotides per second/3 nucleotides per codon = 18 amino acids per second). This means that ribosomes are traveling along each mRNA molecule as fast as RNA polymerase makes it. This coupling plays a role in several aspects of regulation of gene expression unique to bacteria.

Bacterial mRNA is polycistronic; requires no processing or transport

mRNA translation and transcription occur simultaneously

These special features of translation in bacteria contribute to the streamlined efficiency of the process. The bacterial cytosol is packed with polyribosomes. Each ribosome functions near its maximal rate, and therefore, the faster the growth rate of the cell, the more ribosomes are needed for protein production. It can be estimated that during growth in rich media, more than half the mass of the *E. coli* cell consists of ribosomes and other parts of the translation machinery.

Many antimicrobics derive their selective toxicity for bacteria from the unique features of the prokaryotic translation apparatus. In fact, protein synthesis is the target of a greater

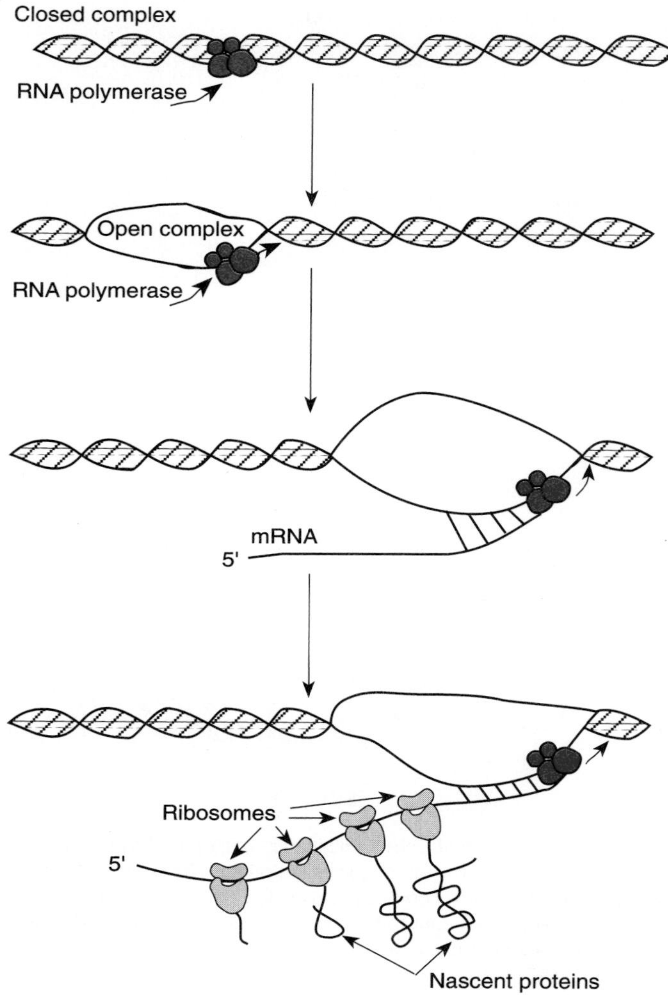


**Figure 3–5.** Schematic representation of the coupling of transcription and translation in bacteria.

Many antimicrobics act on translation mechanisms

variety of antimicrobics than is any other metabolic process (see Chapter 13). Some inhibit the ribosomal large subunit (eg, **chloramphenicol, lincomycin,** and **erythromycin**), some the small subunit (eg, **tetracyclines, streptomycin,** and **spectinomycin**), and some the soluble protein factors involved in initiation or elongation steps of peptide synthesis (eg, **fusidic acid**).

Other polymerization reactions involve synthesis of peptidoglycan, phospholipid, LPS, and capsular polysaccharide. All of these reactions involve activated building blocks that are polymerized or assembled within or on the exterior surface of the cytoplasmic membrane.

**Peptidoglycan (murein)** synthesis occurs in three compartments of the cell (Fig 3–6).

N-Acetyl muramic acid and attached peptide synthesized in cytosol; attached to carrier bactoprenol

1. In the cytosol a series of reactions leads to the synthesis, on a nucleotide carrier (UDP), of an *N*-acetylmuramic acid residue bearing a pentapeptide (the tetrapeptide found in mature murein plus an additional terminal D-alanine).

N-Acetyl glucosamine and bridge amino acids added in cell membrane

2. This precursor is then attached, with the release of UMP, to a special, lipidlike carrier in the cell membrane called **bactoprenol** (or **undecaprenol**). Within the cell membrane *N*-acetylglucosamine is added to the precursor, along with any amino acids that in this particular species will form the bridge between adjacent tetrapeptides.

Glycan polymer and peptide cross-links formed in periplasm or wall

3. Outside the cell membrane (in the periplasm of Gram-negative cells and the wall of Gram-positive cells), this disaccharide subunit is attached to the end of a growing glycan chain, and then crosslinks between chains are formed by a transpeptidization using the energy transduced by the release of the terminal D-alanine—the

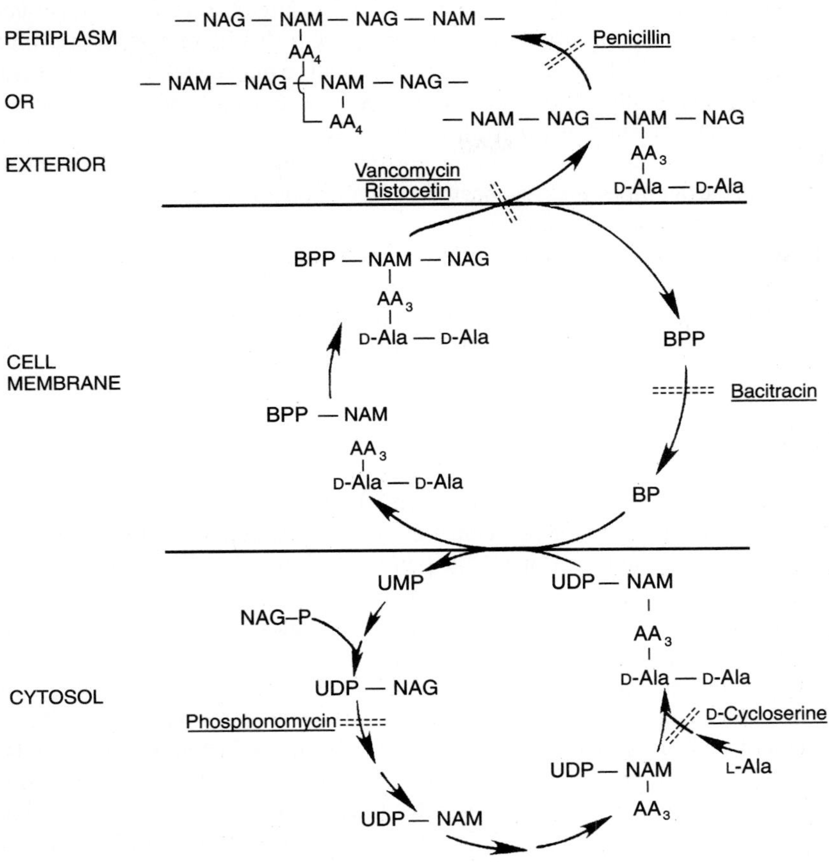


**Figure 3–6.** Schematic representation of murein synthesis with sites of action of some antibiotics. NAG, *N*-acetylglucosamine; NAM, *N*-acetylmuramic acid; BP and BPP, bactoprenol phosphate and bactoprenol pyrophosphate, respectively; $AA_3$, tripeptide residue that in *Escherichia coli* is L-alanyl-D-glutamyl-*m*-diaminopimelic acid; D-Ala and L-Ala, D-alanine and L-alanine, respectively; UMP and UDP, uridine mono- and diphosphate, respectively. Some of the arrows represent more than one chemical reaction. See the text for a description of this process.

extra amino acid on the tetrapeptide. Eventually, release from the carrier occurs. Many enzymes, called **penicillin-binding proteins** (PBPs) for their property of combining with this antibiotic, are involved in forging, breaking, and reforging the peptide crosslinks between glycan chains. This dynamic process is necessary to permit expansion of the murein sac during cellular growth, to shape the envelope, and to prepare for cell division. It is this process that goes awry in the presence of penicillin and related antimicrobics, the action of which can be broadly stated as preventing formation of stabilizing peptide crosslinks.

PBPs are involved in murein assembly, expansion, and shaping

The whole process of synthesizing peptidoglycan (murein), which is completely absent from eukaryotic cells, offers many vulnerable attack points for antibiotics and other chemotherapeutic agents. Some of these are shown in Figure 3–6; others are described more fully in Chapter 13.

Uniqueness of wall offers target for several antimicrobics

## Assembly Reactions

Assembly of cell structures occurs both by spontaneous aggregation (**self-assembly**) and by special, specific mechanisms (**guided assembly**). Some macromolecules are made at the sites of assembly (such as LPS in the outer membrane), and others must be transported to them (porin is made in the cytosol but ends up in the outer membrane). Self-assembly is illustrated by two cell structures that will spontaneously assemble in a test tube from their

Self-assembly (eg, of ribosomes) can occur in vitro

Guided assembly requires transport of components within cell

component macromolecules: flagella and ribosomes. Guided assembly is illustrated by the formation of the envelope. A problem is posed by the difficulty of getting macromolecules out of the cell and into their proper place in the wall, outer membrane, and capsule. This process is only beginning to become understood. Important parts of envelope assembly include special mechanisms for the secretion of proteins, the use of Bayer's zones of adhesion (see Chapter 2, Fig 2–9) to form the phospholipid/protein leaflets of the membranes, and the use of carrier molecules (eg, bactoprenol) to transport hydophilic compounds within the lipid portions of the membrane.

**Bacitracin** and **vancomycin** interfere with the function of bactoprenol as a carrier in polymerization and assembly reactions. The polymyxins partially disassemble the cell membrane, leading to an interference in envelope assembly but, probably more importantly, causing leakage of essential compounds from the cell.

## Cell Division

Many genes involved

Bacteria multiply by binary fission. More than 30 genes in *E. coli* are known to be involved in the process that involves the polar separation of the daughter chromosomes, the formation of the cross-wall and envelope at the point of cell division, and ultimately the separation of the two newly formed cells. In rich medium at 37°C the entire process in *E. coli* and many other pathogenic species is completed in 20 minutes. The most astounding aspect of this feat is that the replication of the chromosome in these cells takes approximately 40 minutes, largely independently of the nature of the medium. The trick of dividing faster than the chromosome can replicate is accomplished by a mechanism that triggers the start of a new round of replication before an earlier one has been completed. In other words, during rapid growth there are multiple pairs of replication forks at work on a given chromosome, and a newborn cell inherits chromosomes that have already been partially replicated. Bacteria maintain a constant cell mass:DNA ratio, and because rapidly growing cells have extra DNA (due to the multiple replication forks), cell size obviously is related to growth rate; the faster bacteria grow, the larger is their average size.

Multiple replication forks allows faster cell division than chromosome replication

Cell division must be precisely coordinated with the completion of a round of DNA replication, or nonviable offspring will be produced. This coordination does not just happen; it requires a special regulatory system. Mutants are known that are defective in this regulation. Under some growth conditions, such mutants fail to synchronize cell division with DNA replication, and one of the daughter cells, called a **minicell,** is born without a chromosome. Minicells are useful research tools to study metabolic processes in the absence of instruction from endogenous chromosomal DNA or to study the specific functions of plasmids (including recombinant plasmids) introduced into them.

Uncoordinated division and DNA replication yields anucleate minicells

The complexity of cell division would lead one to expect that it might be easily disrupted by chemotherapeutic agents. This is the case. Nonlethal concentrations of antimicrobics that act, even indirectly, on the polymerization or assembly reactions of the cell wall cause the formation of bizarre and distorted cells. Long filaments can result from incomplete cell division in the case of rod-shaped bacteria such as *E. coli.* Such forms are frequently encountered in direct examination of specimens from patients treated with antimicrobics.

Division and morphology distorted by some antimicrobics

## GROWTH OF BACTERIAL CULTURES

Definitions

Solutions of nutrients that support the growth of bacteria are called **media** (singular, **medium**), which can be solidified by the incorporation of agar. The introduction of live cells into liquid sterile media or onto the surface of solidified media is called **inoculation**. A population of bacterial cells is referred to as a **culture**. If the population is genetically homogeneous (ie, if all cells belong to the same strain of the same species), it is called a **pure culture**. Study of bacteria usually requires pure cultures which can be obtained in several ways. The most common is to spread a very dilute suspension of a mixed culture on the surface of medium solidified with agar. Growth of individual cells deposited across the surface of solidified medium leads to visible mounds of bacterial mass called **colonies.** The

Bacteria grow as colonies on solid media

cells in a colony are usually descended from a single original cell and, in this case, constitute a **clone**. There is little difference between a pure culture and a clone, except that a pure culture may have been produced by the original inoculation of several identical cells. Colonies of different species and strains show marked differences in size, form, and consistency resulting from differences in growth rates, surface properties of the organisms, and their response to the gradients of nutrients and metabolites that develop within the colony as it enlarges. This facilitates subculturing to pure cultures. The diagnostic application of these techniques is discussed in Chapter 14.

Difference in colonial morphologies and consistency

Growth of a liquid bacterial culture can be monitored by removing samples at timed intervals and placing suitable dilutions in or on solidified medium to obtain a count of the number of colonies that develop. The count can be directly extrapolated to the number of viable units in the original sample (which, because certain bacteria clump or form chains, may not represent the number of bacterial cells). Growth can also be measured by determining the number of **total cells** in each sample. Direct count with a microscope is simple but tedious; more sensitive and accurate counts can be made with the aid of an electronic particle counter. More often, the turbidity of the culture is measured, because bacterial cultures above approximately $10^6$ cells/mL are visibly turbid, and turbidity is proportional to the total mass of bacterial protoplasm present per milliliter. Turbidity is quickly and easily measured by means of a spectrophotometer.

Monitoring growth in liquid media by colony counts

Monitoring growth turbidimetrically

The growth rate of a bacterial culture depends on three factors: the species of bacterium, the chemical composition of the medium, and the temperature. The time needed for a culture to double its mass or cell number is in the neighborhood of 30 to 60 minutes for most pathogenic bacteria in rich media. Some species can double in 20 minutes (*E. coli* and related organisms), and some (eg, some mycobacteria) take almost as long as mammalian cells, 20 hours. In general, the greater the variety of nutrients provided in the medium, the faster growth occurs. This superficially simple fact actually depends on the operation of metabolic regulatory devices of considerable sophistication, which, as we shall see in the next section, ensure that building blocks provided in the environment not be wastefully synthesized by the cells. For each bacterial species, there is a characteristic optimum temperature for growth, and a range, sometimes as broad as 40°, within which growth is possible. Most pathogens of warm-blooded creatures have a temperature optimum for growth near normal body temperature, 37°C; growth often occurs at room temperature, but slowly; therefore, incubators set at 35 to 37°C are employed for culture of most clinical specimens. Exceptions to this rule include some organisms causing superficial infections for which 30°C is more suitable. As a group, bacteria have the widest span of possible growth temperatures, extending virtually over the entire range of liquid water, 0°C to 100°C. Bacteria that grow best at refrigerator temperatures are called **psychrophiles**, those that grow above 50°C are called **thermophiles**; in between are the **mesophiles,** including all pathogens.

Some species can divide every 20 minutes, others much more slowly

Growth rate dependent on nutrient availability, pH, and temperature

Wide ranges of growth temperatures

When first inoculated, liquid cultures of bacteria characteristically exhibit a **lag period** during which growth is not detectable. This is the first phase of what is called the **culture growth cycle** (Fig 3–7). During this lag, the cells are actually quite active in adjusting the levels of vital cellular constituents necessary for growth in the new medium. Eventually net growth can be detected, and after a brief period of **accelerating growth,** the culture enters a phase of constant, maximal growth rate, called the **exponential** or **logarithmic phase** of growth, during which the generation time is constant. During this phase, cell number, and total cell mass, and amount of any given component of the cells increase at the same exponential rate; such growth is called **balanced growth**, or **steady-state growth.** The full reproductive potential of bacteria is exhibited during this phase: one cell gives rise to 2 cells in 1 generation, to 8 cells after 3 generations, to 1024 cells after 10 generations, and to about 1 million cells in 20 generations. For a bacterial species with a generation time of 20 minutes, therefore, it takes less than 7 hours in the exponential phase of growth to produce a million cells from one.

Phases of growth; metabolic activity in lag phase

Consequences of exponential growth

By use of an equation for exponential growth it can be demonstrated that 2 days of growth at this rate would be sufficient to generate a mass of bacteria equal to 500 times the mass of the earth. Fortunately this never occurs, but not because the equation is faulty. Constant growth rate requires that there be no change in the supply of nutrients or the concentration of toxic byproducts of metabolism (such as organic acids). This constancy can exist for only a short time (hours) in an ordinary culture vessel. Then growth becomes progres-

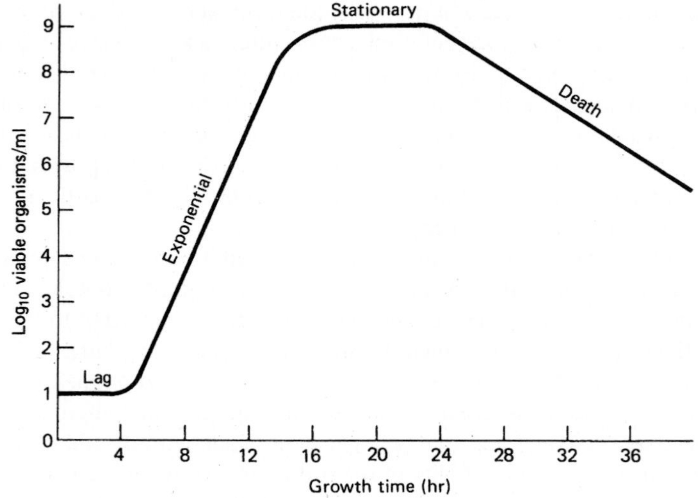


**Figure 3–7.** Phases of bacterial growth in liquid medium.

Nutrient depletion or metabolite accumulation terminate exponential phase

Cultures of most species die slowly after the stationary phase

Continuous exponential growth in chemostat

sively limited (**decelerating phase**) and eventually stops (**stationary phase**). Cells in the stationary phase are different from those in the exponential phase. They are smaller, they have a different complement of enzymes (to deal with survival during starvation), and they have fewer ribosomes per unit mass. When an inoculum of such cells is placed into fresh medium, exponential growth cannot resume immediately, and hence the lag period is observed. Note that there is no lag phase if the inoculum consists of exponential-phase cells. Prolonged incubation of a stationary-phase culture leads to cell death for many bacterial species (such as the pneumococcus), though many (such as *E. coli*) are hardy enough to remain viable for days. During the **death phase** or **decline** of a culture, cell viability is lost by exponential kinetics as described in Chapter 11. As already noted, for those Gram-positive species that can sporulate, entry into the stationary phase usually triggers this event.

One way to maintain a culture in exponential, steady-state (balanced) growth for long periods is to use a device in which fresh medium is continuously added but the total volume of culture is held constant by an overflow tube. One such constant-volume device is called a **chemostat**; it operates by infusing fresh medium containing a limiting nutrient at a constant rate, and the growth rate of the cells is set by the flow rate (Fig 3–8). A similar constant-volume device is the **turbidostat**; it operates by the infusion of fresh medium by

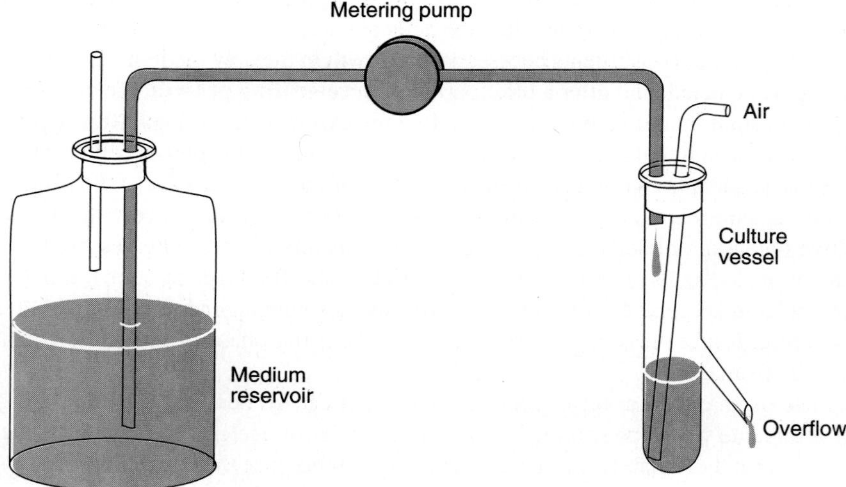


**Figure 3–8.** Schematic diagram of a chemostat. This continuous-culture device consists of a constant-volume growth chamber into which fresh sterile medium is fed at a constant rate by a pump.

a pump controlled indirectly by the turbidity of the culture. Although such devices may sound artificial, they mimic many situations of interest to medical microbiologists. Most of the places in which bacteria live on and within our bodies, in health and disease, provide conditions more closely resembling those of nutrient-limited continuous-culture devices than of enclosed flasks.

## REGULATION AND ADAPTATION

Metabolic reactions must proceed in a coordinated fashion. It would not do to have them governed solely by the laws of "mass action" by which the concentrations of reactants and products determine the rate of reactions. Furthermore, it would not do to have rates of individual reactions set at some fixed levels. Bacteria can do little to control their environment, and any change in environment (in temperature, pH, nutrient availability, osmolarity, etc) would disrupt the preset synchronization or render it inappropriate. Bacteria must, therefore, not just coordinate reactions, but must do so in a flexible, adjustable manner to make growth possible in a changing environment.

Flexible coordination of metabolic reactions in response to environmental changes

Bacteria have evolved many regulatory mechanisms. Some operate to control **enzyme activity**, some to control **gene expression.**

### Control of Enzyme Activity

Although there are many examples of covalent modification of enzymes (eg, by phosphorylation, methylation, or acylation) to alter their activity, by far the most prevalent means by which bacterial cells modulate the flow of material through fueling and biosynthetic pathways is by changing the activity of **allosteric enzymes** through the reversible binding of low-molecular-weight metabolites (**ligands**). In fueling pathways it is common for AMP, ADP, and ATP to control the activity of enzymes by causing conformational changes of allosteric enzymes, usually located at critical branch points where pathways intersect. By this means, the flow of carbon from the major subtrates through the various pathways is adjusted to be appropriate to the demands of biosynthesis. For example, the **energy charge** of the cell, defined as (ATP + ½ ADP)/(ATP + ADP + AMP), is kept very close to 0.85 under all conditions of growth and nongrowth. In biosynthetic pathways, it is common for the end product of the pathway to control the activity of the first enzyme in the pathway. This pattern, called **feedback inhibition** or **end-product inhibition,** ensures that each building block is made at exactly the rate it is being used for polymerization. It also ensures that building blocks supplied in the medium are not wastefully duplicated by synthesis. Because many biosynthetic pathways are branched and have multiple end products, special arrangements must be made to produce effective regulation. These include the production of multiple isofunctional enzymes for the controlled step; the design of allosteric enzymes, that require the cumulative effect of all end products to be completely inhibited; and sequential inhibition of each subpathway by its last product (Fig 3–9).

Most metabolic processes controlled by allosteric enzymes

Fueling pathway enzymes controlled by AMP, ADP, and ATP concentrations to maintain energy charge

Feedback inhibition control of biosynthetic pathways allows economy and efficiency

### Control of Gene Expression

To a far greater extent than eukaryotic cells, bacteria regulate their metabolism by changing the amounts of different enzymes. This is accomplished chiefly by governing their rates of synthesis, that is, by controlling gene expression. This works rapidly for bacteria because of their speed of growth; shutting off the synthesis of a particular enzyme results in short order in the reduction of its cellular level due to dilution by the growth of the cell. Also, bacterial mRNA is degraded rapidly. With an average half-life of 2–3 min at 37°C, the mRNA complement of the cell can be totally changed in a small fraction of a generation time. The synthesis of a given enzyme can therefore be rapidly turned on and just as rapidly turned off simply by changes in the rate of transcription of its gene.

Changes in rate of transcription can rapidly change enzyme concentration

Most, although not all, of the regulation of gene expression occurs at or near the beginning of the process: the initiation of transcription. That is, gene expression is not regu-

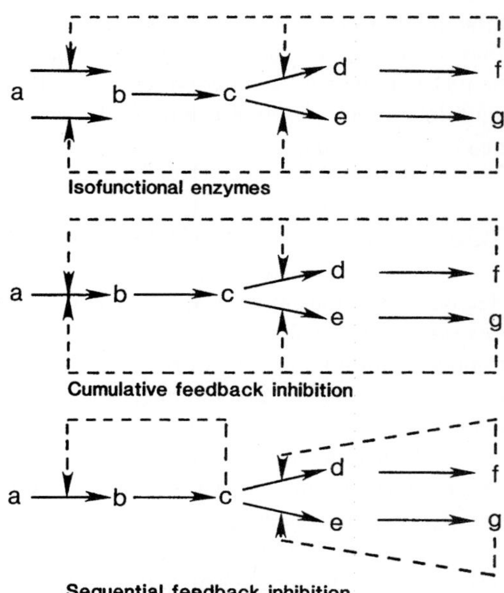


**Figure 3–9.** Patterns of end-product inhibition in branched biosynthesis pathways.

Regulation frequently operates at initiation of transcription

lated by changing the rate of mRNA chain elongation; once started, transcription proceeds at a more or less constant rate. Regulation occurs by a decision of whether to initiate or not, or what amounts to the same thing, by setting the frequency of initiation.

Transcription steps

A closer look at transcription is necessary to understand how it is controlled. Most of the genes we know about in bacteria are organized as **multicistronic operons.** A **cistron** is a segment of DNA encoding a polypeptide. An **operon** is the unit of transcription; the cistrons that it comprises are cotranscribed as a single mRNA. The structure of a typical operon (Fig 3–10) consists of a **promoter** region, an **operator** region, component cistrons, and a **terminator**. In the best-studied bacterium, *E. coli*, RNA polymerase, programmed by the major replaceable σ subunit σ-70, recognizes the –35 and –10 regions of the promoter and binds to the DNA. Initially the binding is a closed complex, but this can be converted into an open complex in which the two strands of DNA are partially separated. Strand separation exposes the nucleotide bases and permits initiation of synthesis of a mRNA strand complementary to the sense strand of the DNA. In a simple case, transcription continues through the cistrons of the operon until the termination signal is reached. In some cases recognition of the termination signal requires another removable subunit of RNA polymerase, ρ. This process is shown in Figure 3–10.

Mecanisms of repression and induction of gene transcription

Near the promoter in many operons is an operator to which a specific **regulator protein** can bind. In some cases the binding of this regulator blocks initiation; in such a case of negative control, the regulator is called a **repressor**. Repressors are allosteric proteins, and their binding to the operator depends on their conformation, which is determined by the binding of ligands that are called **corepressors** if their action permits binding of the repressor and **inducers** if their action prevents binding. In some cases, the regulator protein is required for initiation of transcription, and it is then called an **activator.** The functioning of both types of regulator proteins on transcription initiation is illustrated in Figure 3–11 using the regulation of the *lac* operon as an example. This operon encodes proteins necessary for the use of lactose as a carbon and energy source.

Some regulator proteins bend DNA on binding, and this can bring together what would otherwise be distant sites of the DNA. In this manner, proteins bound at sites called **enhancers** far upstream or downstream of a promoter can be brought into physical contact with RNA polymerase and influence its activity. One such DNA bender in **E. coli** is called the **integration host factor** (IHF).

Attenuation as a means of controlling biosynthetic operons

Once transcription is initiated it may continue uneventfully, but in some operons another site of control is quickly encountered. After transcription of a **leader region,** the RNA polymerase encounters a region known as an **attenuator**. Synthesis of mRNA is aborted at the attenuator; only a small percentage of the RNA polymerase molecules reaching the attenuator can successfully pass through it. The activity of the attenuator can, however, be

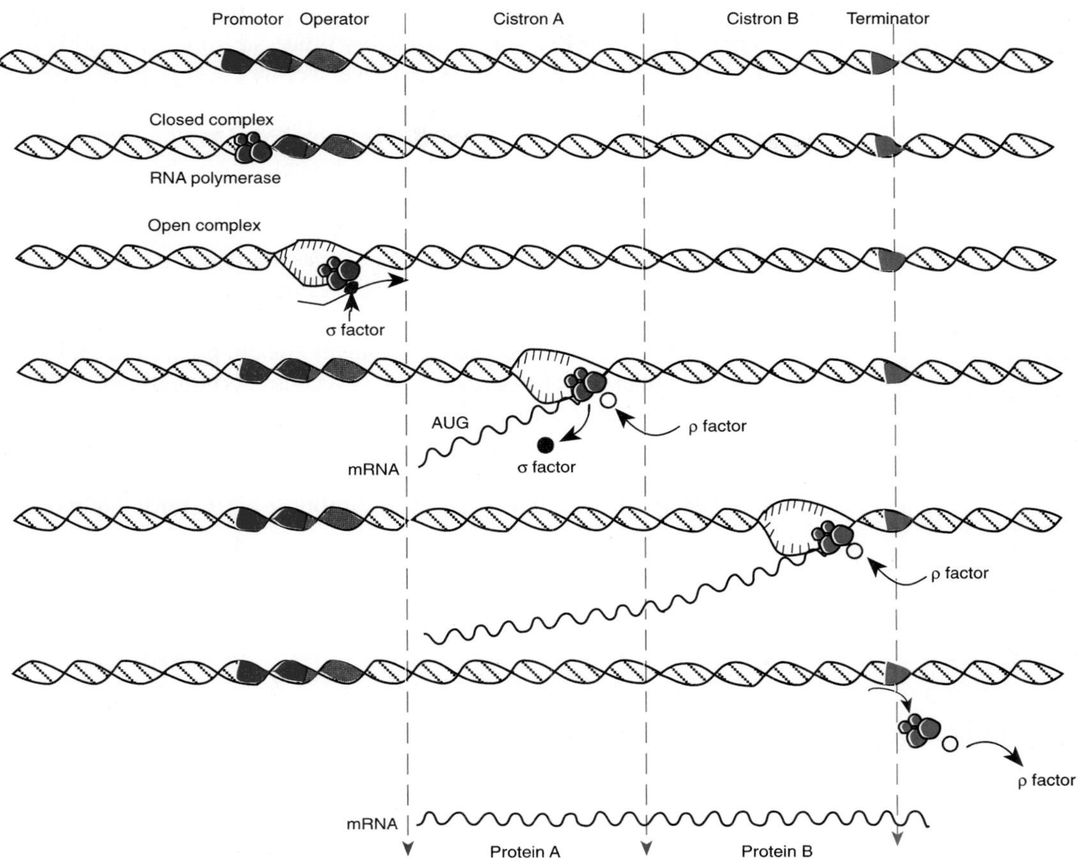


**Figure 3–10.** Control of transcription. Schematic representation of a bacterial operon and its transcription by RNA polymerase.

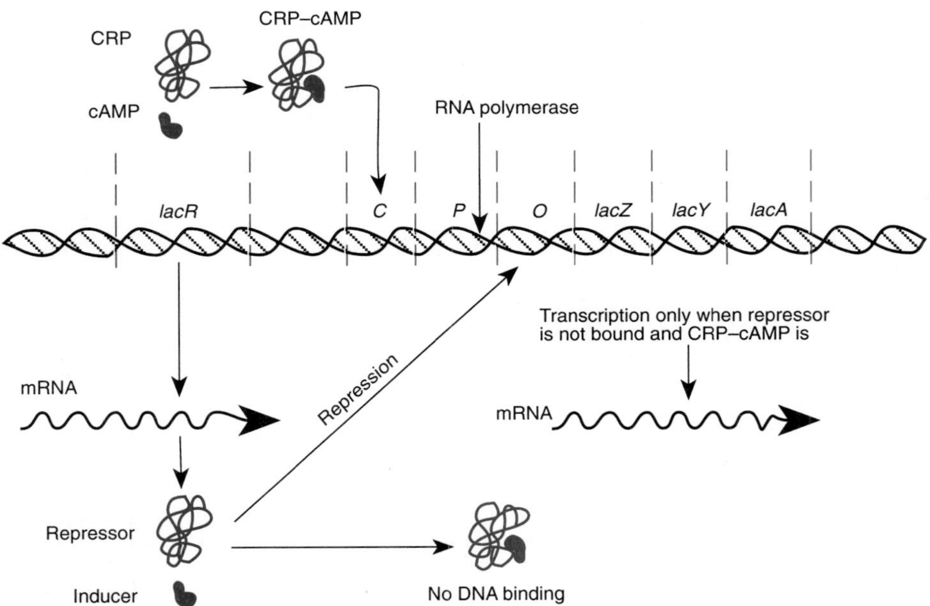


**Figure 3–11.** Schematic representation of the control of transcription initiation by repressor and activator proteins. The example chosen is the *lac* operon of *Escherichia coli. lacR* (or I), gene encoding the lac repressor protein; C, CAP region (binding site of cAMP receptor protein); P, promoter region (binding site of RNA polymerase); O, operator region (binding site of repressor); *lacZ*, gene encoding ß-galactosidase; *lacY*, gene encoding permease for ß-galactosides; *lacA*, gene encoding galactoside acetylase.

modified by a process that involves not a regulator protein, but rather changes in the secondary structure of the mRNA. This regulatory process is illustrated in Figure 3–12 using the *his* operon, which encodes the enzymes necessary for the biosynthesis of the amino acid L-histidine, as an example. In enteric bacteria, attenuation is a common means of controlling biosynthetic operons. Note that it differs from the repression mechanism in that it requires no special regulatory gene or regulatory proteins.

The catabolite repression regulon ensures optimal use of preferred substrates

There are many instances known in which groups of genes that are independently controlled as members of different operons must cooperate to accomplish some response to an environmental change. When such a group of genes is subject to the control of a common regulator, the group is called a **regulon**. One such regulon, or **global control system**, is catabolite repression. Its function is to prevent the cell from responding to the presence of alternative carbon sources when the environment already provides a more than adequate supply from the preferred substrate, glucose. This control is brought about as follows. Operons that encode catabolic enzymes (those responsible for initiating the use of carbon sources, such as lactose, maltose, arabinose, and other sugars and amino acids) have weak promoters that need help to promote high-level initiation of transcription by RNA polymerase. The help is supplied by a regulator protein called **catabolite activator protein** (CAP) or **cAMP**

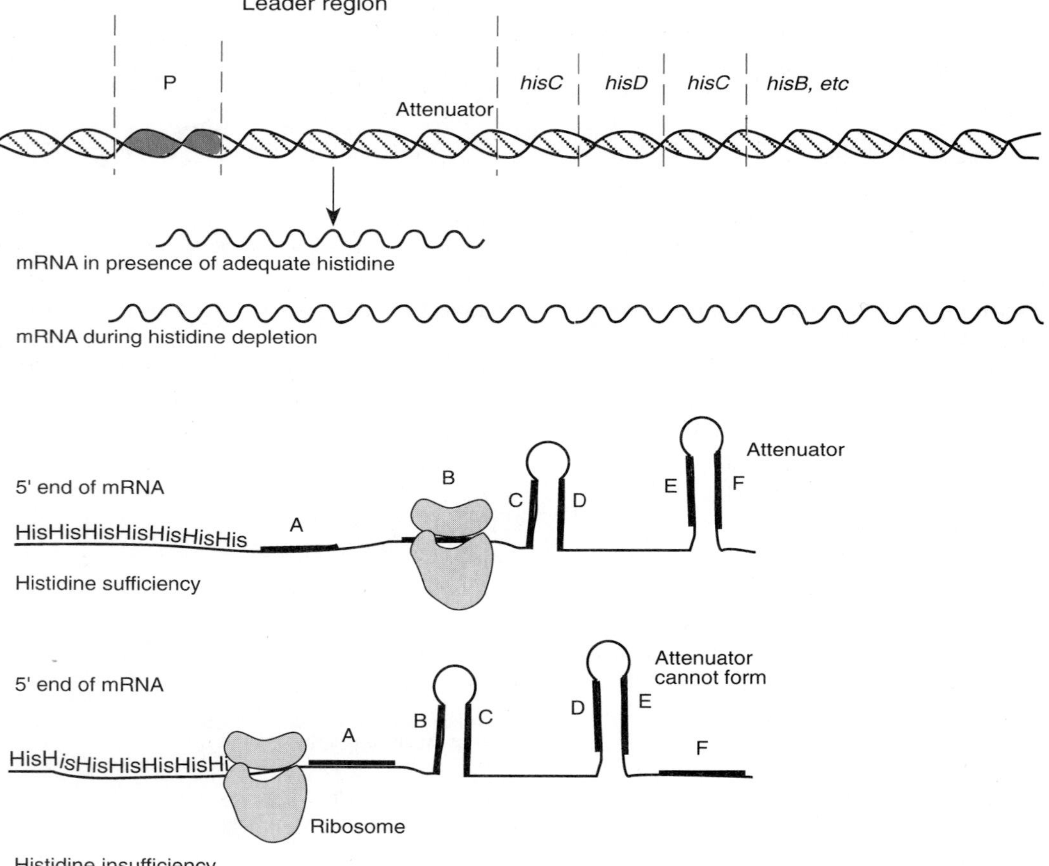


**Figure 3–12.** Schematic representation of the control of transcription by the process of attenuation. The example chosen is the *his* operon of *Escherichia coli.* How attenuation works is fascinating. The leader region is always transcribed and translated into a small oligopeptide. The peptide near the attenuator site has a string of seven *his* codons. Movement of the first ribosome coming behind the polymerase is drastically affected by the supply of charged *his* tRNA. If there is an adequate supply, the ribosome is not delayed, and an attenuator loop forms in the mRNA, causing transcription to terminate. With a shortage of histidine, the first ribosome gets hung up over the *his* codons, and the attenuator loop is not formed, because alternate loops form. As a result, transcription proceeds, the complete *his* mRNA is made, and the biosynthetic enzymes can be made in large quantities. The upper portion of the figure illustrates the difference in transcription of the *his* operon in histidine sufficiency and insufficiency; the lower two diagrams depict the molecular mechanism of attenuation.

**receptor protein** (CRP). This protein, if and only if cyclic AMP is bound to it, binds slightly upstream from the promoter and permits high-level expression if the operon is specifically induced (ie, and repressor has been removed by induction). Because cAMP levels are very low during growth on glucose or other favored substrates, there is insufficient cAMP–CRP complex to activate catabolic operons even if their inducers are present in the environment. As a result, the cells ignore the induction signal if they have an adequate supply of glucose.

## CELL SURVIVAL

### Cell Stress Regulons

The catabolite repression regulon is in essence a means by which the cell can optimize its synthesis of catabolic enzymes by making only those that contribute to growth. But this regulon can also be viewed as a survival device, helping the cell to respond to the nutritional stress of running out of glucose. If an alternative source of carbon is present in the environment, the cell can redirect its pattern of gene expression to make a suitable adjustment to the nutritional stress.

From studies with *E. coli*, it is becoming appreciated that cells have many regulons involved in survival responses during difficult circumstances. One is the **SOS system**, a set of 17 genes that are turned on when the cell suffers damage to its DNA. The products of these genes are involved in several processes that repair damaged DNA and prevent cell division during the repair.

SOS system repairs damaged DNA and prevents multiplication during repair

Another prominent bacterial cell stress regulon is responsible for the **heat-shock response.** It encompasses some 20 genes, which are transcriptionally activated on a shift up in temperature or on imposition of several kinds of chemical stress, including alcohol. In the case of *E. coli*, the heat-shock regulator protein is a special subunit of RNA polymerase, σ-32, which replaces the normal σ-70 subunit and locates the special promoters of the heat-shock genes. At least half of the heat-shock genes encode proteins that either are proteases or are **protein chaperones** that assist in the processing, maturation, or export of other proteins. It is thought that these chaperones and proteases are needed for normal protein processing at all temperatures, but are required in higher amounts to counteract the effects of high temperature on protein folding and protein–protein interactions. The bacterial chaperones are highly similar to their mammalian counterparts. For example, HtpG, DnaK, and GroEL of *E. coli* correspond to the mammalian hsp90, hsp70, and hsp60 families of chaperones, respectively. The precise involvement of the heat-shock response in infectious disease is still being explored, but it is a striking fact that antibodies directed against bacterial heat-shock proteins constitute a major component of the serologic response of humans to infection or vaccine administration. Fever in humans can elevate body temperature sufficiently to induce the heat-shock response, and it is suspected that this response may affect the outcome of various infections. Also, some viruses both of bacteria and of humans use the heat-shock proteins of their host cells to promote their own replication.

Heat-shock genes are expressed at high temperature and allow cell survival

Heat-shock response involves production of protein chaperones

Other regulons deal with cell survival in the face of such stresses as osmotic shock, high or low pH, oxidation damage, presence of toxic metal ions, and restrictions for fundamental nutrients (phosphate, nitrogen, sulfur, and carbon). A large number of these responses involve teams of proteins that sense the environment, generate a signal, transmit that signal by protein–protein interactions, and activate the appropriate response regulon. In a striking number of cases, a response system includes a **protein kinase** that becomes phosphorylated by ATP on a particular conserved histidine residue in response to an environmental stimulus. This kinase is teamed with a second protein called a **phosphorylated response regulator**. The phosphate residue from the kinase is transferred to an aspartic acid residue of the response regulator, usually converting this protein into an activator of transcription of the appropriate genes. Members of these two families of **signal transduction proteins** share highly conserved domains throughout distantly related bacteria.

Response to environmental change frequently involves phosphorylation of protein kinases

Two of the most elaborate bacterial survival responses involve the transition of growing cells into a form that can survive long periods without growth. In a few Gram-positive bacterial species, this involves **sporulation**, the production of an **endospore,** as we saw in

Sporulation involves sequential activation of interrelated regulons

Chapter 2. This process, extensively studied in a few species, involves cascades of σ subunits activating sequentially several interrelated regulons that cooperate to produce the elaborately encased spore, which though metabolically inert is capable of germinating into a growing (vegetative) cell. For all other bacteria, however, a process surprisingly analogous to sporulation occurs as they prepare for the transition from exponential-phase growth to the stationary phase. The product is certainly far different morphologically from an endospore, but a tough and metabolically quiescent cell is produced that looks distinct from its growing counterpart. And here again cascades of signals and responses involving the sequential activation of sets of genes appear to be involved.

A final bacterial survival response system to be described is **chemotaxis**, motility directed toward an **attractant** chemical or away from a **repellent.**

## Motility and Chemotaxis

Motility in most bacterial species is the property of swimming by means of flagellar propulsion. The complex structure of a flagellum—its filament, hook, and basal body—was presented in Chapter 2. The helical filament functions as a propeller, the hook possibly as a universal joint, and the basal body with its rod and rings as a motor anchored in the envelope. The flagellar motors turn the filaments using energy directly from the electrochemical gradient (protonmotive force) of the cell membrane rather than from ATP. The filament can be rotated either clockwise or counterclockwise. Whatever the number of flagella on a cell and whatever their arrangement on the surface (polar, peritrichous, or lophotrichous), all are synchronized to rotate simultaneously in the same direction. Only counterclockwise rotation results in productive vectorial motion, called a **run.** Clockwise rotation of the flagella causes the cell to **tumble** in place. The flagella alternate between periods of clockwise and counterclockwise rotation according to an endogenous schedule. As a result, motile bacteria move in brief runs interrupted by periods of tumbling.

Flagellar motor uses protonmotive force energy

Direction of flagellar rotation determines a run or a tumble

**Chemotaxis** is directed movement toward chemical attractants and away from chemical repellents. It is accomplished by a remarkable molecular sensory system that possesses many of the characteristics that would be expected of behavioral systems in higher animals, including memory and adaptation. Beside the genes of the flagellar proteins (called *fla*, for flagella) more than 30 genes (called *mot*, for motility, and *che*, for chemotaxis) encode the proteins that make this system work: receptors, signalers, transducers, tumble regulators, and motors.

Multiple genes required for chemotoctic ability

Whether a cell is moving toward an attractant or away from a repellent, chemotaxis is achieved by **biased random walks**. These result from alterations in the frequency of tumbling. When a cell is, by chance, progressing toward an attractant, tumbling is suppressed and the run is long; if it is swimming away, tumbling occurs sooner and the run is brief. It is sheer chance in what direction a cell is pointed at the end of a tumble, but by regulating the frequency of tumbles in this manner, directed progress is made.

Changes in duration of runs and tumbles determine chemotactic response

The mechanism of chemotaxis is fairly well understood from work with *E. coli*. Small molecules diffuse through the pores of the outer membrane and bind to protein **receptors** in the cell membrane, either directly or after binding to specific **binding proteins** in the periplasm. Dozens of such chemoreceptors are known. The stimulant–receptor complex interacts with one or another **methyl-accepting chemotaxis protein** (MCP). The MCPs are in fact members of the family of protein kinases described in the preceding section. On presentation of a stimulant–receptor complex to an MCP, autophosphorylation occurs, followed by a cascade of signal transduction through five proteins that appear to be signal transducers passing along the information that an attractant has been sensed. At the end of the line, the phosphorylated form of a **tumble response regulator protein** (called CheY in *E. coli*) is released from a tumble complex, binds to a flagellar motor protein, and causes the productive (counterclockwise) rotation of the flagella. Even in the continued presence of the stimulant, however, the response regulator soon returns to its inactive state. This occurs because the phosphorylation signal ceases when the MCP becomes methylated and thus less active as a kinase. This so-called accommodation results in the release of a different protein from the tumble complex, one that combines with another flagellar motor protein to cause clockwise rotation and, hence, tumbling. But, if by now the cell is in a higher

Molecular memory recognizes change in attractant concentration and ensures progress toward it

concentration of stimulant (as by having moved up a gradient), a new positive signal is generated faster than the endogenous schedule would have produced.

All this can be summarized as follows: Binding of an attractant alters the endogenous routine schedule of runs and tumbles by initiating a **phosphorylation cascade** that prolongs the runs. Accommodation by methylation restores the endogenous schedule and resets the cell's sensitivity to the attractant to require a higher concentration to prolong the run. This constitutes a **molecular memory.** The bacterial cell senses a concentration gradient not by measuring a difference between the concentration at each end of the cell, but by a molecular memory that enables it to compare the concentration now with what it was a short time ago. Escape from a repellent occurs in an analogous fashion.

Chemotaxis is both a survival device (for avoiding toxic substances) and a growth-promoting device (for finding food). It can also be a virulence factor in facilitating colonization of the human host by bacteria.

Chemotaxis serves survival, growth-promoting, and, sometimes, pathogenetic roles

## SPECIAL ATTRIBUTES OF THE COLONIZERS OF HUMANS

The abilities to grow and to survive harsh conditions are possessed by most bacteria. Yet of the thousands of bacterial species, only a small percentage are associated with humans as part of the natural flora or as causative agents of disease. This fact generates the question that has been central to medical microbiology from the very start: What makes a bacterium pathogenic? The answer is not simple, because it turns out that many properties are necessary for a bacterial cell to gain entrance to a human, evade its defense systems, and establish an infection. Virulence is a multigene property.

Many bacterial structures and activities contribute to virulence

The structures and activities described in Chapter 2 and this chapter bear directly on virulence attributes of bacteria. They include the ability to colonize and penetrate epithelial surfaces, evade phagocytic and immunologic attack, secrete toxic proteins, and survive adverse conditions both within and outside the body. These aspects are considered further in Chapter 10.

## ADDITIONAL READING

Neidhardt FC, Ingraham JL, Schaechter M. *Physiology of the Bacterial Cell: A Molecular Approach.* Sunderland, MA: Sinauer Associates; 1990. Chapters 3 to 8 present bacterial metabolism and physiology in a manner similar to what was done here, but in more detail.

Chapter 4

# Bacterial Genetic Determinants

*Frederick C. Neidhardt*

## BACTERIAL VARIATION AND INHERITANCE

It was rather difficult to establish that many of the same rules of heredity apply to bacteria as well as to plants and animals. This may seem strange, because the most spectacular advances in molecular genetics have been achieved almost exclusively through work on *Escherichia coli* and its viruses. During the 1940s and early 1950s, however, serious experimental efforts were still being directed toward determining whether mutations in bacteria were random or specifically directed by the environment.

The difficulty of establishing the basis of heredity in bacteria grew out of their inherent properties and their manner of growth. First, because bacteria are **haploid,** the consequences of a mutation, even a recessive one, are immediately evident in the mutant cell. Because the generation time of bacteria is short, it does not take many hours for a mutant cell that has arisen by chance to become a significant component of a culture under appropriate selective conditions. This can lead to the false conclusion that the environment has directed a genetic change. Second, as was noted in Chapter 3, bacteria, to a far greater extent than animals and plants, respond to change in their chemical and physical environment by altering their pattern of gene function, thereby taking on previously unexpressed properties. For example, *E. coli* cells make the enzymes for lactose metabolism only when grown with this sugar as carbon source. Superficially this might suggest that lactose changes the cell's **genotype** (its complement of genes), when instead it is only the **phenotype** (the characteristics actually displayed by the cell) that has been changed by the environment. Finally, even when rather exceptional technical measures are taken to ensure a pure culture, contamination can occasionally occur. With cultures containing more than one bacterial species, different conditions of growth can cause one or another species to predominate (by, for example, a million to one ratio), suggesting to the unwary observer that the characteristics of "the bacterium" under study are very unstable and dependent on the environment.

Mutations are rapidly expressed; mutants quickly predominate under selective conditions

Environment can influence phenotype expression of genotype

Progress in bacterial genetics was rapid once it was recognized that mutation and selection can quickly change the makeup of a growing population and that bacterial cells inherit genes that may or may not be expressed depending on the environment. Even so, it was not until the discovery in the 1980s of transposable genetic elements and insertion sequences (to be discussed later in this chapter) that certain examples of high-frequency variation, the so-called **phase transition,** could be satisfactorily explained within the framework of classic genetic principles.

Several experiments were particularly important in establishing that mutations occur in nature as random events and are not guided by the environment. The most convincing

Proof of random occurrence of bacterial mutations

introduced the technique of replica plating and was used to show how a population of cells totally resistant to an antimicrobic could be isolated from an initially sensitive population without ever exposing them to the toxic agent (Fig 4–1). This clarified the mechanism of an important clinical problem.

## MUTATION AND REPAIR

The spontaneous development of mutations is a major factor in the evolution of bacteria. Mutations occur in nature at a low frequency, on the order of one mutation in every million cells for any one gene.

### Kinds of Mutations

**Mutations** are heritable changes in the structure of genes. The normal, usually active, form of a gene is called the **wild-type allele;** the mutated, usually inactive, form is called the **mutant allele.** There are several kinds of mutations, based on the nature of the change in nucleotide sequence of the affected gene(s). **Replacements** involve the substitution of one base for another. **Microdeletions** and **microinsertions** involve the removal and addition, respectively, of a single nucleotide (and its complement in the opposite strand). **Insertions** involve the addition of many base pairs of nucleotides at a single site. **Deletions** remove a contiguous segment of many base pairs. **Inversions** change the direction of a segment of DNA by splicing each strand of the segment into the complementary strand. **Duplications** produce a redundant segment of DNA, usually adjacent (tandem) to the original segment.

Change in nucleotide sequence

By recalling the nature of genes and how their nucleotide sequence directs the synthesis of proteins, one can understand the immediate consequence of each of these biochemical changes. If a replacement mutation in a codon changes the mRNA transcript to a different amino acid, it is called a **missense mutation** (eg, an AAG [lysine] to a GAG [glutamate]). The resulting protein may be enzymatically inactive or very sensitive to environ-

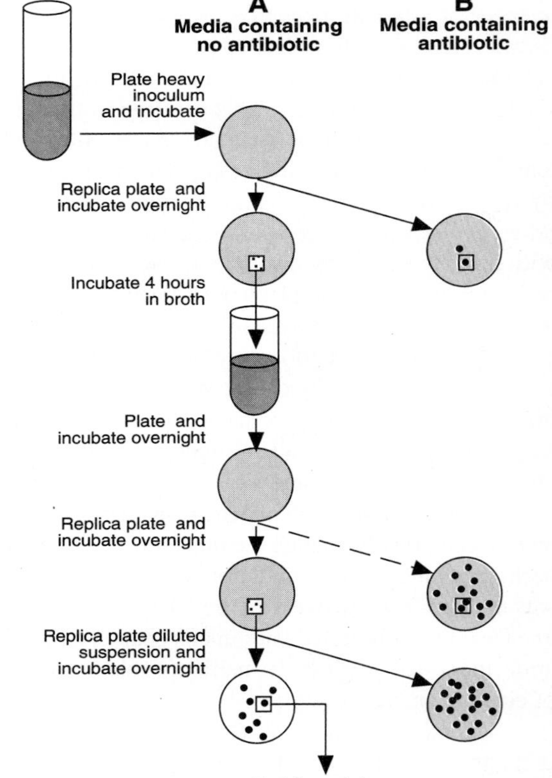


**Figure 4–1.** Lederberg technique for indirect selection of antimicrobic resistant mutants. Growth on plates in the left-hand column **(A)** is replicated to antimicrobic-containing plates in the right-hand column **(B)**. If resistant mutants arise in the absence of antimicrobic **(A)**, the position of colonies on antimicrobic-containing plates would indicate their position on the plates that do not contain antimicrobic. By selecting growth from this position and repeating the process with appropriate inoculum dilutions, resistant mutants that have never been exposed to the antimicrobic can be directly selected **(A)**.

mental conditions, such as temperature. If the replacement changes a codon specifying an amino acid to one specifying none, it is called a **nonsense mutation** (eg, a UAC [tyrosine] to UAA [STOP]), and the truncated product of the mutated gene is called a **nonsense fragment.** Microdeletions and microinsertions cause **frame shift mutations,** changes in the reading frame by which the ribosomes translate the mRNA from the mutated gene. Frame shifts usually result in polymerization of a stretch of incorrect amino acids until a nonsense codon is encountered, so the product is usually a truncated polypeptide fragment with an incorrect amino acid sequence at its N terminus. Deletion or insertion of a segment of base pairs from a gene shortens or lengthens the protein product if the number of base pairs deleted or inserted is divisible evenly by 3; otherwise it also brings about the consequence of a frame shift. Inversions of a small segment within a gene inactivate it; inverting larger segments may affect chiefly the genes at the points of inversion. Duplications, probably the most common of all mutations, serve an important role in the evolution of genes with new functions. These mutations are summarized in Table 4–1.

Frame shift mutations usually result in truncated polypeptide

One unexpected biochemical consequence of gene mutation is that many mutations, particularly if they occur near the end of a gene, prevent the expression of all genes downstream (away from the promoter) of the mutated gene. Such **polar mutations** are thought to exert their effect on neighboring genes by the termination of transcription of downstream genes when translation of the mRNA of the mutated gene is blocked by a nonsense codon.

Mutations may affect neighboring genes by termination of transcription

There is a certain natural frequency of mutations brought about by errors in replication, but various environmental and biological agents can increase the frequency greatly. Different types of mutations are increased selectively by different agents, as listed in Table 4–1.

Mutagenic agents

Mutations may also be classified according to their biological consequences. Some mutations change the susceptibility of a cell to an antimicrobic or other toxic agent; these **resistance mutations** might, for example, affect the structure of certain cell proteins in such a way that the agent cannot enter the cell or cannot inactivate its normal target. Some mutations, called **auxotrophic mutations**, affect the production of a biosynthetic enzyme and result in a nutritional requirement of the mutant cell for the amino acid, nucleotide, vitamin, or other biosynthetic product it can no longer make for itself. The wild type from which the mutant was derived is said to be **prototrophic** for that nutrient. Some mutations affect a gene whose product is essential for growth and cannot be bypassed nutritionally; these are called **lethal mutations.** If the product of a mutated gene is active in some circum-

Mutations may affect entry to the cell or biosynthetic mechanisms

Mutations in essential genes are lethal

**TABLE 4–1. MUTATIONS**

| Type | Causative Agent | Consequence |
|---|---|---|
| **Replacement** | | |
| Transition: pyrimidine replaced by a pyrimidine or a purine by a purine | Base analogs, ultraviolet radiation, deaminating and alkylating agents, spontaneous | Transitions and transversions: nonsense codon formed, truncated peptide; missense codon formed, altered protein |
| Transversion: purine replaced by a pyrimidine or vice versa | Spontaneous | |
| **Deletion** | | |
| Macrodeletion: large nucleotide segment deleted | $HNO_2$, radiation, bifunctional alkylating agents | Truncated peptide; other products possible, such as fusion peptides |
| Microdeletion: one or two nucleotides deleted | Same as macrodeletions | Frame shift, usually resulting in nonsense codon and truncated peptide |
| **Insertion** | | |
| Macroinsertion: large nucleotide segment inserted | Transposons or insertion sequence (IS) elements | Interrupted gene yielding truncated product |
| Microinsertion: one or two nucleotides inserted | Acridine | Frame shift, usually resulting in nonsense codon yielding a truncated product |
| **Inversion** | IS or IS-like elements | Many possible effects |

stances, but inactive under others (eg, high or low temperature), the mutation is called **conditional** (meaning **conditionally expressed**). The most common kind of conditional mutation is one in which the protein product of the mutated gene is inactive at a normally physiologic temperature, but active at a higher or lower temperature; these are called **temperature-sensitive mutations.**

## Reversion and Suppression of Mutations

Back mutations rare because highly specific corrections are needed

Suppressor mutations reestablish phenotype of mutated wild type

A **reversion**, or **back mutation**, is the conversion of a mutated gene back to its original wild-type allele. True back mutation can occur, but at a low frequency, because a very specific and improbable event is required. Much more commonly observed is the conversion of a mutant cell into one that is phenotypically identical to the original wild-type bacterium for the affected character, but still retains the original mutation. These **suppressor** mutations can arise in several ways. Within the mutated codon a second mutation can create a new codon specifying the original amino acid. Alternatively, secondary mutations in other codons of the mutated gene can lead to a change in amino acid sequence that results in an active product despite the continued presence of the original amino acid error. Suppressing mutations can occur even in genes other than the one that was originally mutated. For example, when two proteins interact to perform a function, the mutant form of one may be active when combined with a mutant form of the other. Another example involves tRNA molecules, the translators of the genetic code, which can themselves be altered by mutation; it is possible for a mutant tRNA to "mistake" a mutant codon and insert the original correct amino acid, a case of two wrongs making a right.

## Repair of DNA Damage

Multiple genes involved in DNA repair; damage recognized by mispairing of strands

Many mutagenic agents directly alter the structure of DNA, and some are ubiquitous components of our environment (heat, sunlight, acid, oxidants, and alkylating agents). It is therefore not surprising to learn that bacteria have evolved multiple biochemical mechanisms for repairing damaged DNA. In *E. coli*, for example, more than 30 genes are known to be involved in DNA repair; many of these are members of the SOS response discussed in Chapter 3. Collectively these repair systems can remove thymine dimers produced by ultraviolet (UV) irradiation, can remove methyl or ethyl groups placed on guanine residues, can excise bases damaged by deamination or ring breakage and replace them with authentic residues, and can recognize and repair DNA depurinated by acid or heat. In large measure these repair systems use the fact that DNA is double stranded. Damage is recognized by the mispairing it causes, and the information on one strand is used to direct the proper repair of the damaged strand. Also, a proofreading process operates during DNA replication to detect any mismatch between each newly polymerized base and its mate in the template strand. Mismatches are excised to permit repolymerization with the properly matched nucleotide. Failures of this proofreading process can be detected and handled by an excision and resynthesis system similar to those that recognize and repair chemically damaged DNA.

One system bypasses DNA damaged by UV irradiation when repair has failed. It directs replication to proceed across a region badly damaged by the formation of thymine dimers. This **error-prone replication** is responsible for the mutations induced by UV light.

# GENETIC EXCHANGE

Mutation and selection are important factors in bacterial evolution, but evolution proceeds far faster than it could by these processes alone. For instance, the probability that the process of random mutation alone can produce a cell that, let us say, requires five mutations for optimal growth in a new environment is terribly low. It is in fact the product of the individual mutation frequencies (eg, $10^{-6} \times 10^{-6} \times 10^{-6} \times 10^{-6} \times 10^{-6} = 10^{-30}$), and that essentially pre-

Bacterial evolution is speeded by exchange of genetic material

cludes a natural population from ever acquiring the new property in this manner. Such alterations occur, however, because organisms exchange genetic material, thereby permitting combinations of mutations to be collected in individual cells.

Processes of genetic transfer

Despite the fact that bacteria reproduce exclusively asexually, the sharing of genetic information within and between related species is now recognized to be quite common and to occur in at least three fundamentally different ways. All three processes involve a one-way transfer of DNA from a **donor cell** to a **recipient cell.** The molecule of DNA introduced into the recipient is called the **exogenote** to distinguish it from the cell's own original chromosome, called the **endogenote**.

Transformation, transduction, and conjugation

One process of DNA transfer, called **transformation**, involves the release of DNA into the environment by the lysis of some cells, followed by the direct uptake of that DNA by the recipient cells. By another means of transfer, called **transduction**, the DNA is introduced into the recipient cell by a nonlethal virus that has grown on the donor cell. The third process, called **conjugation**, involves actual contact between donor and recipient cell during which DNA is transferred as part of a plasmid (an autonomously replicating, extrachromosomal molecule of circular double-stranded DNA); in conjugation, donor and recipient cells are referred to as male and female respectively. The three means of gene transfer are summarized in Figure 4–2.

Transformation, transduction, and conjugation mediated by chromosomal, viral, and plasmid genes, respectively

Species of bacteria differ in their ability to transfer DNA, but all three mechanisms are distributed among both Gram-positive and Gram-negative species; however, only transformation is governed by bacterial chromosomal genes. Transduction is totally mediated by virus genes, and conjugation, by plasmid genes.

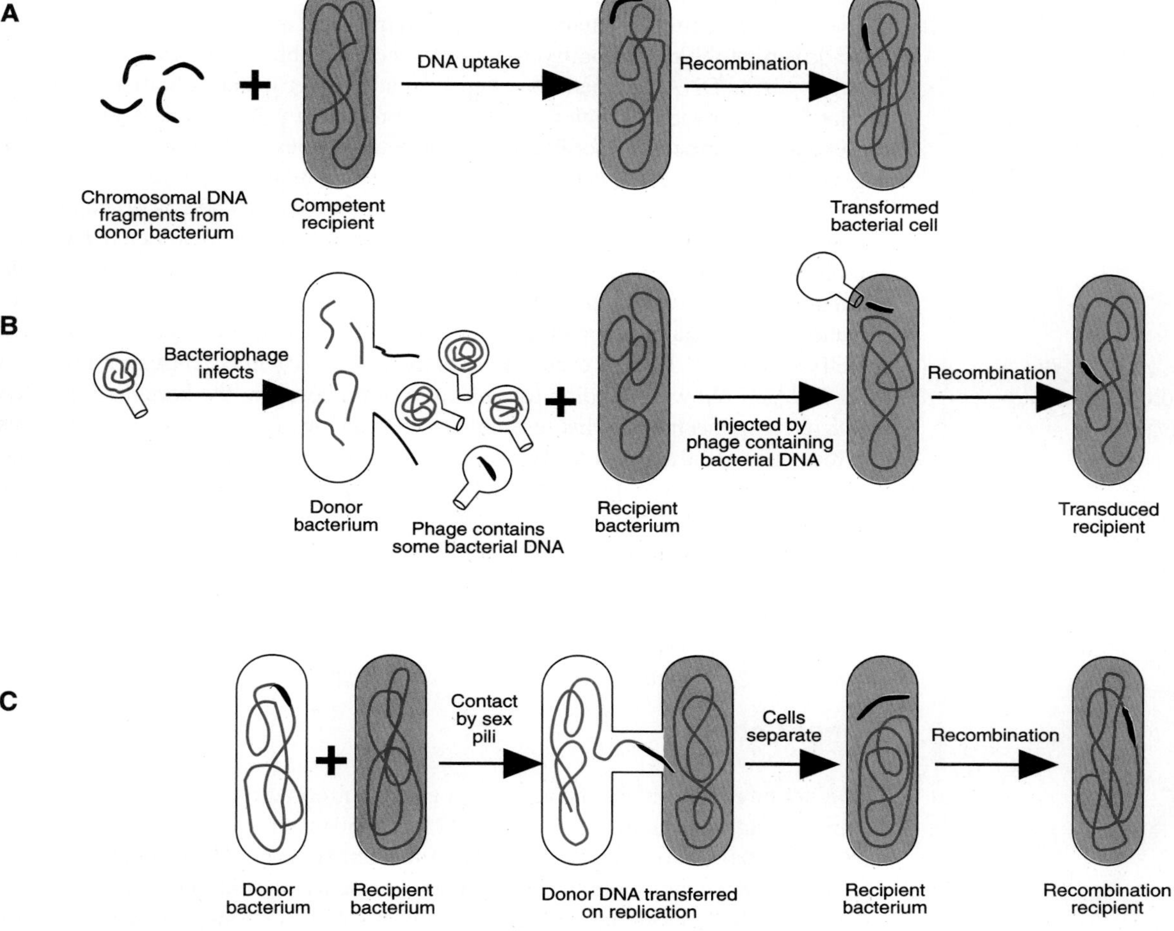


**Figure 4–2.** Chromosomal gene transfer mechanisms in bacteria. **A.** Transformation. **B.** Transduction. **C.** Conjugation.

## Transformation

Transformation was first demonstrated in 1928 by F. Griffith (a British public health officer) who showed that virulent, encapsulated *Streptococcus pneumoniae* (pneumococci) that had been killed by heat could confer on living, avirulent, nonencapsulated pneumococci the ability to make the polysaccharide capsule of the killed organisms and thus become virulent for mice. Subsequent work in 1944 by O. T. Avery, C. M. MacLeod, and M. McCarty at the Rockefeller Institute revealed that the "transforming factor" from the dead pneumococci was nothing other than DNA. This discovery had enormous impact on biology, because it was the first rigorous demonstration that DNA is the macromolecule in which genetic information is encoded. It opened the door to modern molecular genetics.

Early studies on pneumococcal transformation

The ability to take up DNA from the environment is called **competence**, and in many species of bacteria, it is encoded by chromosomal genes that become active under certain environmental conditions. In such species, transformation can occur readily and is said to be natural. Other species cannot enter the competent state, but can be made permeable to DNA by treatment with agents that damage the cell envelope making an **artificial transformation** possible.

Genes encoding competence activated by environmental conditions

Natural transformation must be important in nature, judged by the variety of mechanism that different bacteria have evolved to accomplish it. Two of the best-studied systems are those of the Gram-positive pneumococcus and a Gram-negative rod, *Haemophilus influenzae*. Pneumococcal cells secrete a protein **competence factor** that induces many of the cells of a culture to synthesize special proteins necessary for transformation, including an autolysin that exposes a cell membrane DNA-binding protein. Any DNA present in the medium is bound indiscriminately; even salmon sperm DNA can be bound and taken up as readily as DNA from another pneumococcal cell. The surface-bound double-stranded DNA is cleaved into fragments of about 6 to 8 kilobases (kb). One strand is degraded by a nuclease, while the complementary strand of each fragment is taken up by a process that seems to be driven by the protonmotive force of the cell membrane (see Chapter 3). The fate of the internalized DNA fragment then depends on whether it shares homology (the same or similar in base sequence) with a portion of the recipient cell's DNA. If so, recombination can occur by a process described later, but heterologous DNA (no similarity to the endogenote) is degraded and causes no heritable change in the recipient.

Pneumococcal competence exposes a protein that binds any DNA

Portion of DNA strand combines with any homologous chromosomal DNA

Transformation in *H. influenzae* is somewhat different. There is no competence factor, and cells become competent merely by growth in an environment rich in nutrients. Only homologous DNA (ie, DNA from the same or a closely related species of *Haemophilus*) is taken up, and it is taken up in double-stranded form. The selectivity is brought about by the presence of a special membrane protein that binds to an 11-base pair (bp) sequence (5′-AAGTGCGGTCA-3′) that occurs frequently in *Haemophilus* DNA and infrequently in other DNAs. Following binding to molecules of this protein, the homologous DNA is internalized by a mechanism that resembles membrane invagination, resulting in the temporary residence of the exogenote in cytoplasmic membrane vesicles. Although the DNA taken up is double stranded, only one of the two strands participates in the subsequent recombination with the endogenote.

*H. influenzae* endocytoses only homologous double-stranded DNA

The common use of *E. coli* as a host cell in which to clone genes on hybrid plasmids (see DNA Restriction and Genetic Engineering) depends on procedures involving treatment with salt and temperature shocks to bring about artificial transformation; this organism has no natural competence mechanism.

Artificial transformation of *E. coli* for gene cloning

## Transduction

Transduction is virus-mediated transfer of genetic information from donor to recipient cell. To understand transduction and its several mechanisms, it is necessary to preview the nature of bacterial viruses, a topic dealt with more extensively in Chapters 5, 6, and 7.

Viruses are capable of reproduction only inside living cells. Those that grow in bacteria are called **bacteriophages**, or simply **phages.** They are minimally composed of protein and nucleic acid, although some may have a very complex structure and composition. The individual virus particle or virion consists of a protein capsid enclosing genomic nucleic

Bacteriophage structure, infection, and replication

acid, which is either RNA or DNA, but never both. Virions infect sensitive cells by adsorbing to specific receptors on the cell surface and then, in the case of phages, injecting their DNA or RNA. Phages come in two functional varieties according to what happens after injection of the viral nucleic acid. **Virulent** (-lytic) **phages** cause lysis of the host bacterium as a culmination of the synthesis of many new virions within the infected cell. **Temperate phages** may initiate a lytic growth process of this sort or can enter a quiescent form (called a **prophage**) in which the infected host cell is permitted to proceed about its business of growth and division, but passes on to its descendents a prophage genome capable of being **induced** to produce phage in a process nearly identical to the growth of lytic phages. The bacterial cell that harbors a latent prophage is said to be a **lysogen** (capable of producing lytic phages), and its condition is referred to as **lysogeny**. Lysogens are immune to infection by virions of the type they harbor as prophage. Occasionally lysogens are spontaneously induced and lysed by the phage and release mature virions (as many as 75 to 150 or more per cell) into the environment. When triggered by UV irradiation or certain chemicals, an entire population of lysogens are induced simultaneously to initiate reproduction of their latent virus followed by lysis of the host cells. Infection of a sensitive cell with the temperate phage can lead to either lysis or lysogeny. How this choice comes about is described in Chapter 7.

Bacteria can be lysogenized with prophage from temperate phage

Prophage induction yields lytic phage

The prophage of different temperate phages exists in one of two different states. In one, the prophage DNA is physically integrated into a bacterial chromosome; in the second, it remains separate from the chromosome as an independently replicating, circularized, molecule of DNA. Prophages of this sort are in fact plasmids.

Some prophages integrate; others behave as plasmids

For the most part, transduction is mediated by temperate phage, and the two broad types of transduction result from the different physical forms of prophage and the different means by which the transducing virion is formed. These are termed **generalized transduction,** by which any bacterial gene stands an equal chance of being transduced to a recipient cell, and **specialized** or **restricted transduction,** by which only a few genes can be transduced.

Transduction mediated by temperate phage

### Generalized Transduction

Some phages package DNA into their capsids in a nonspecific way, the headful mechanism, in which any DNA can be stuffed into the capsid head until it is full. (The head is the principal structure of the virion to which, in some cases, a tail is attached. See Chapter 5.) An endonuclease then trims off any projecting excess. If fragments of host cell DNA are around during the assembly of mature virions, they can become packaged in place of virus DNA, resulting in **pseudovirions**. Pseudovirions are the transducing agents. They can adsorb to sensitive cells and inject the DNA they contain as though it were viral DNA. The result is the introduction of donor DNA into the recipient cell.

Occasional phages carry a random piece of host DNA to a recipient

Any given gene has an equal probability of being transduced by this process. With the temperate phage P1 of *E. coli*, this probability is approximately one transduction event per $10^5$ to $10^8$ virions, because nearly 1 out of every 1000 phage particles made in a P1 lytic infection are pseudovirions, and the bacterial DNA fragments packaged are 1 to 2% of the length of the chromosome. Cotransduction of two bacterial genes by a single pseudovirion occurs only if they are located close together within this small length of the chromosome, and this fact facilitates mapping the position of a newly discovered gene.

Any gene has equal but low probability of being transduced

Once injected into the host cell, the transduced DNA will be lost by degradation unless it can recombine with the chromosome of the recipient cell, usually by homologous recombination (see Genetic Recombination) in which both strands of the exogenote cross into and replace the homologous segment of the recipient's chromosome. Sometimes, however, the exogenote can persist without degradation by assuming a stable circular configuration. In this interesting situation, called **abortive transduction**, there is only linear transmission of the exogenote to one of the two daughter cells of the transduced recipient, one of the four granddaughters, one of the eight great-granddaughters, and so on.

Generalized transduction involves homologous recombination

### Specialized Transduction

It has been noted that the prophage of some phages is integrated into the lysogen's chromosome. This integration does not occur haphazardly, but is restricted to usually one site, called the *att* (attachment) site. When a lysogen carrying such a prophage is induced to pro-

Specialized transduction involves prophage integration at specific site

Induction occasionally leads to incorporation of adjacent bacterial genes in phage

duce virions, excision of the viral genome from the bacterial chromosome occasionally (eg, in 1 of $10^5$ to $10^6$ lysogens) occurs imprecisely, resulting in a pickup of genes of the bacterium adjacent to the *att* site. The resulting virion may be infectious (if no essential phage genes are missing) or defective (if one or more essential genes are missing). In either case, adsorption to a sensitive cell and injection of the DNA can occur, and integration of the aberrant phage genome into the chromosome of the new host cell results in the formation of a lysogen containing a few genes that have been transduced as hitchhikers with the phage genome. Integration of the phage genome automatically accomplishes the recombinational event needed to guarantee reproduction of the transduced genes. Only genes that border the *att* site stand a chance of being transduced by this process, which is why it is called specialized or restricted transduction.

Hitchhiker genes cointegrated in chromosome with phage genes

Because the original pickup event is rare, the first transducing process is termed **low-frequency transduction** (LFT); however, when a lysogenic transductant is, in turn, induced to produce phage, all of the new virions carry the originally transduced bacterial gene. The resulting mixture of lysed cells and virions now brings about **high-frequency transduction** (HFT) of the attached genes.

All phages produced by lysogenic transductants carry original transduced gene

Bacterial geneticists have learned to move genes of interest near the phage integration site and thereby construct specialized transducing phages containing these genes. Such transducing phages are valuable aids to cloning and sequencing genes and to studying their function and regulation. Obviously a temperate phage that could form a prophage by integrating randomly at any site in the bacterial chromosome would be of special use. The temperate phage Mu of *E. coli* has this property.

Value of specialized transduction in gene cloning and sequencing

Although both generalized transduction and specialized transduction can be regarded as the result of errors in phage production, transfer of genes between bacterial cells by phage is a reasonably common phenomenon. It occurs at significant frequency in nature; for example, genes conferring antimicrobic resistance in staphylococci are often transduced from strain to strain in this way. Transduction is also used extensively as a tool in molecular biology research.

Significance of transduction in nature

## Conjugation

Conjugation is plasmid encoded; requires cell contact

Conjugation leading to transfer of chromosomal genetic information from donor to recipient bacterial cell is plasmid mediated. Cell contact is required; hence, the process is frequently called mating, but all of the genes that govern it reside on plasmids resident within the donor (male) cells rather than on their chromosomes. Conjugation appears to differ between Gram-negative and Gram-positive species, as judged by its characteristics in two well-studied examples, *E. coli* and *Enterococcus faecalis.*

### Conjugation Among Gram-Negative Bacteria

Conjugation has been most studied in *E. coli*, in which it is most often brought about by a plasmid called F (for fertility). These studies have been of particular importance because of the light they have thrown on the biology of plasmids generally.

Like all plasmids, the F plasmid consists of circular double-stranded DNA that is capable of replicating in the bacterial cell and being passed on to the daughter cells at the time of division. The F plasmid is also one of a class of plasmids called **conjugative** because they have the genetic ability to bring about their own transfer from one cell to another by conjugation. A cell harboring the F plasmid is designated $F^+$; one lacking it, $F^-$. Genes on this plasmid encode proteins that change the surface properties of the cell by producing a **sex pilus.** This structure, which is longer and thicker than a common pilus, facilitates the capture of an $F^-$ cell and the formation of a conjugation bridge through which DNA passes from the $F^+$ cell (called male) to the $F^-$ cell (called female). This transfer of DNA is accomplished by a special replication of the F plasmid, called **transfer replication**. Transfer replication always begins at a point on the plasmid DNA called *oriT* (for origin of transfer). One strand directs synthesis of its complement within the donor ($F^+$, male) cell; the other strand is driven through the conjugation bridge into the recipient ($F^-$, female) cell. Synthesis of a strand complementary to the transferred strand occurs in the recipient cell while the transfer is in progress (Fig 4–3). The completed molecule circularizes, its genes are expressed, and it maintains itself by replication in the recipient cell, which is thus converted

*E. coli* F plasmid encodes sex pilus, which binds $F^+$ to $F^-$ cell

F plasmid DNA passes from $F^+$ to $F^-$ through conjugative bridge

Single DNA strand transferred; complementary strands resynthesized in recipient and donor

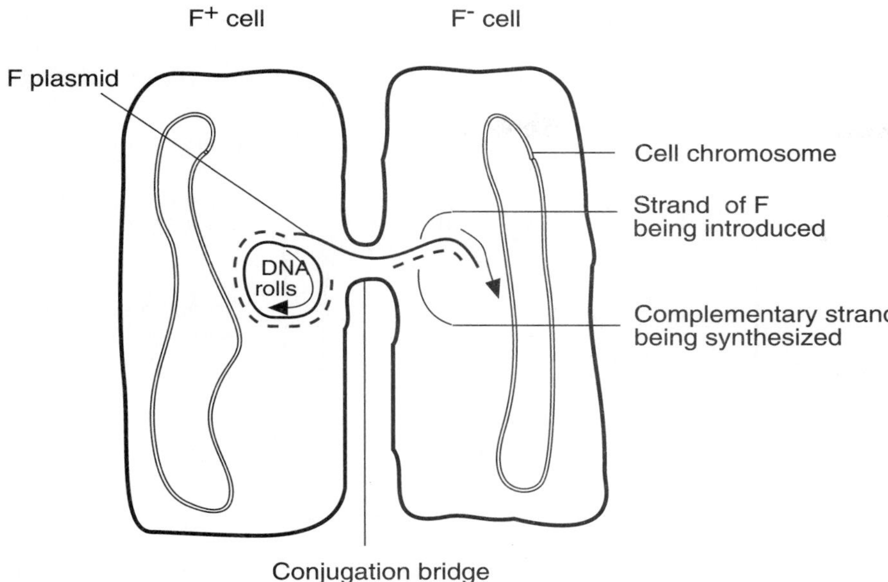


**Figure 4–3.** Bacterial conjugation resulting in the introduction of an F plasmid into an $F^-$ cell by replicative transfer from an $F^+$ cell.

from $F^-$ (female) to $F^+$ (male). The recipient cell and all of its descendents then have the ability to conjugate with any $F^-$ cells they encounter. The original donor $F^+$ cell remains $F^+$ because transfer replication has left an intact double-stranded F plasmid (see Fig 4–3).

$F^-$ recipient converted to $F^+$; donor remains $F^+$

It is only the absence of the sex pilus that determines the mating behavior of the recipient cells, because if the sex pilus is lost from $F^+$ cells by physical shearing or by incubation of the cells for several hours in stationary phase, these genetically $F^+$ cells behave as though they were $F^-$; that is, encounter with an $F^+$ cell leads to conjugation. Cells that contain the F plasmid but have lost their sex pilus are called $F^-$ **phenocopies** (because their phenotypic behavior in mating copies that of genetically $F^-$ cells).

Conjugation of an $F^+$ cell and an $F^-$ cell thus normally leads to transfer of plasmid DNA, but does not involve chromosomal DNA. How are bacterial chromosomal genes transferred?

Transfer of chromosomal genes by conjugation is the result of encounters between $F^-$ cells and rare cells in an $F^+$ culture termed **high-frequency recombination** (Hfr) **cells** that contain an F genome integrated into the chromosome. Integration occurs at a very low frequency at one of seven or eight chromosomal sites and results in linearization of the plasmid DNA as part of the giant circular chromosomal molecule. A cell with an integrated F factor resembles an $F^+$ male cell in many respects, including the synthesis of the sex pilus and the ability to form a conjugation bridge with an $F^-$ cell. Likewise, the usual transfer replication is initiated; however, this process cannot readily transfer the complete F plasmid genome, because the F plasmid and the bacterial chromosome became integrated by a recombinational event that occurred at a site other than *oriT*. Thus, breaking the integrated plasmid DNA at *oriT* results in the formation of a linear strand in which the entire bacterial chromosome lies between two portions of the F genome (Fig 4–4). Transfer replication drives the leading segment of the F genome into the $F^-$ cell, followed by bacterial genes one after the other. The conjugation bridge usually ruptures long before the entire bacterial chromosome with the trailing half of the F genome can be introduced into the $F^-$ cell. As a result, only one part of the F genome and a variable length of the bacterial chromosome extending from the original site of integration of the F plasmid are transferred. Thus, conjugation between an Hfr and an $F^-$ cell almost always leaves the recipient still $F^-$ and the donor still Hfr. The Hfr cell remains Hfr because it retains a copy of the chromosome with its integrated F genome.

F plasmid may integrate into chromosome to give Hfr cells

DNA transfer from Hfr to $F^-$ cells carries partial plasmid and chromosomal genes

Incomplete transfer of F genome leaves recipient $F^-$ in Hfr mating

In the absence of $F^-$ cells, Hfr cells grow and divide normally, and every offspring of an Hfr cell has the same chromosomal configuration, with the F genome integrated at the same site and in the same clockwise or counterclockwise orientation. It is possible to select a colony derived from a single Hfr cell and thereby establish a pure culture in which every

All Hfr offspring have F genome integrated at same site

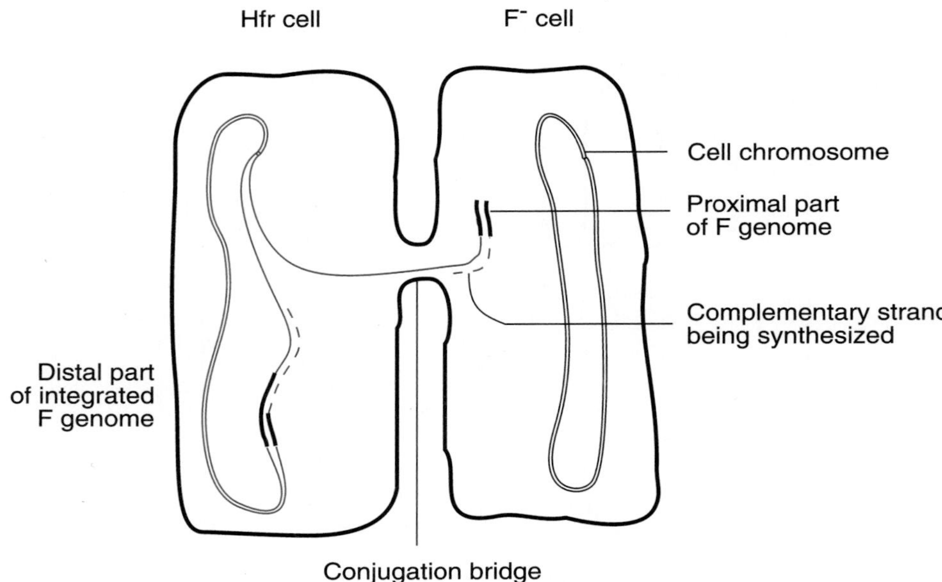


**Figure 4–4.** Bacterial conjugation resulting in the introduction of chromosomal genes and a portion of the F plasmid genome into an $F^-$ cell by replicative transfer from a high-frequency recombination (Hfr) cell.

Every cell in an Hfr culture can transfer genes

cell has an integrated F genome. In contrast to cultures of $F^+$ strains, every cell in an Hfr culture has the ability to transfer chromosomal genes during mating.

Excision of integrated F genome may include host genes in F′ plasmid

Sexduction involves transfer of F′ plasmid to $F^-$ cell

There is an additional wrinkle to chromosome transfer by conjugation in *E. coli.* It involves a process termed **sexduction** by which an F plasmid transfers from one cell to another a few bacterial chromosomal genes that it happens to contain. Here is how it comes about. The F genome in an Hfr cell can excise itself occasionally from the bacterial chromosome and recircularize into plasmid form. Sometimes this excision is imperfect, and as a result, one or a few of the neighboring bacterial genes are included in the plasmid (Fig 4–5). The resulting hybrid plasmid is called F′ to note its content of some bacterial DNA. The cell in which the F′ particle is formed is still haploid for all its genes, because the few incorporated into the F′ plasmid are missing from the chromosome. Transfer of the F′ plasmid into a normal $F^-$ cell is called sexduction. The new F′ cell is designated a **secondary F′** cell because it differs from the donor in being diploid for the genes introduced by the F′ plasmid. These cells are useful because they afford the opportunity to construct mutations in one copy of an essential gene while maintaining one functional copy for cell survival.

It is important to stress that one or all of these phenomena described for *E. coli* apply to other Gram-negative genera and species. They have simply been less well studied in detail. Furthermore, it must be understood that most transfers of genetic information by plasmids involve genes carried on the plasmid rather than on the chromosome. This is considered later in the chapter.

## Conjugation Among Gram-Positive Bacteria

*S. faecalis* coupling results from adhesin–receptor interactions

Plasmid encoded *S. faecalis* adhesin is produced in response to recipient pheromone

Conjugation in *E. faecalis* is mediated by plasmids, but there is also an involvement of chromosomal genes in the process. Donor and recipient cells do not couple by means of a sex pilus, but rather by the clumping of cells that contain a plasmid with those that do not. This clumping is the result of interaction between a proteinaceous **adhesin** on the surface of the donor (plasmid-containing) cell and a **receptor** on the surface of the recipient (plasmid-lacking) cell. Both types of cells make the receptor (possibly cell wall lipoteichoic acid), but only the plasmid-containing cell can make the adhesin, presumably because it is encoded by a plasmid gene. Interestingly, donor cells make the adhesin only when in the vicinity of recipient cells, because the recipients secrete small peptide **pheromones** that serve to notify the donor cells of the presence of recipients. Donor cells promptly make adhesin when they sense the pheromone, and, as a result, clumps are formed and plasmid DNA is trans-

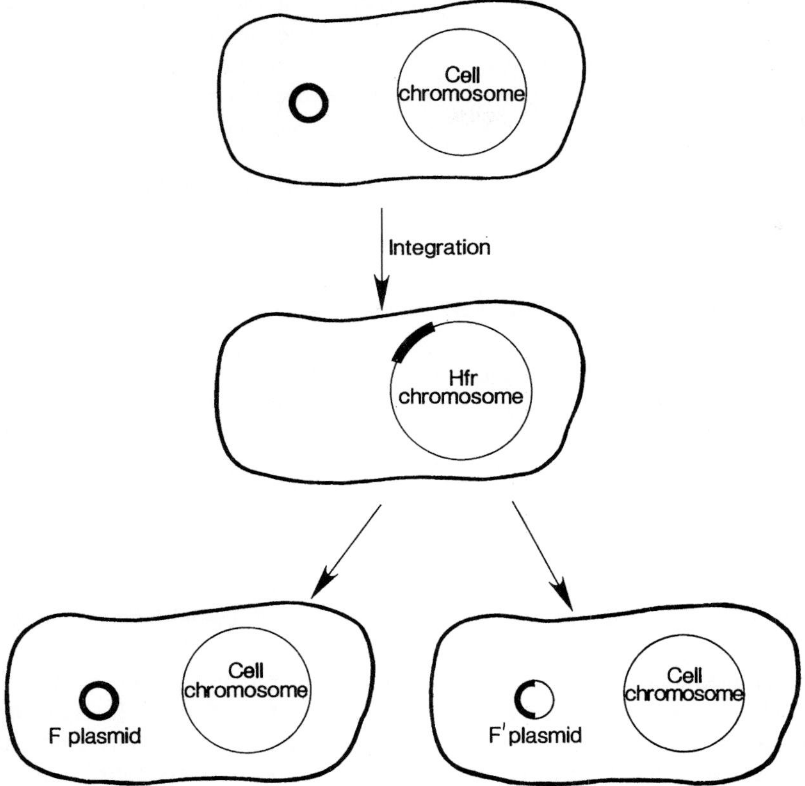


**Figure 4–5.** Integration of the F plasmid into a bacterial chromosome to form a high-frequency recombination (Hfr) chromosome, followed either by exact excision to re-form the F plasmid or by inexact excision to form an F′ plasmid containing some bacterial chromosome genes.

ferred across conjugation bridges into the recipient cells held in the clumps. Pheromones are widely distributed among insects and other animals as sexual and other attractants.

All *E. faecalis* cells are genetically capable of making several (five or more) pheromones, each encoded by a chromosomal gene, but each specific for a different plasmid. Acquisition of a particular plasmid represses the synthesis of the pheromone specific for that plasmid. As a result, the cell containing a given plasmid no longer informs its neighbor that it is a potential recipient for that plasmid, but continues to send out pheromone signals for other plasmids that it could still receive by conjugation with a suitable donor. As a further guarantee that it and its neighbors will not respond to the pheromone specific for the plasmid already present in these cells, a competitive inhibitor is synthesized under the direction of a plasmid gene.

In addition to streptococcal species, species of *Bacillus*, *Staphylococcus*, and *Clostridium* have been found to contain conjugative plasmids. Conjugative transfer of genes has also been observed in a number of Gram-positive species in the apparent absence of plasmid DNA. In several instances these transfers involve conjugative transposons (to be discussed later in this chapter), and it appears that a plasmid intermediate is formed, though only transiently.

Plasmid transfer of resistance and virulence genes

Plasmids carrying genes encoding antimicrobic resistance, common pili and other adhesins, and some exotoxins are readily transferred by conjugation among Gram-positive bacteria in the natural environment as well as in the laboratory.

## GENETIC RECOMBINATION

By whatever means an exogenote is conveyed into a recipient cell, its effect depends on what happens after transfer. There are basically three possible fates. The exogenote DNA may be degraded by a nuclease, in which case no heritable change is brought about. It may

Exogenote may be degraded, circularized, or integrated in recipient chromosome

be stabilized by circularization and remain separate from the endogenote. In this case, if it is unable to replicate, it will be unilinearly inherited (eg, abortive transduction), but if it is capable of self-replication, it will become established as an autonomous, inherited plasmid. The third possible fate is **recombination** between exogenote and endogenote, resulting in the formation of a partially hybrid chromosome with segments derived from each source. These possibilities are diagrammed in Figure 4–6.

In this section we examine some aspects of the third process, the formation of recombinant chromosomes following transformation, transduction, or conjugation.

## Homologous Recombination

Recombination of double-stranded DNA requires nucleotide similarity and crossover integration

One mechanism by which an exogenote can recombine with the bacterial chromosome is called **homologous recombination.** This term reflects one of the two requirements for this process: (1) The exogenote must possess reasonably large regions of nucleotide sequence identity or similarity to segments of the endogenote chromosome, because extensive base pairing must occur between strands of the two recombining molecules. (2) The recipient cell must possess the genetic ability to make a set of enzymes that can bring about the covalent substitution of a segment of the exogenote for the homologous region of the endogenote. Not all the details are known, but the latter process includes breaking one strand of each recombining molecule at a time and pairing it with the unbroken, complementary strand of the other molecule. The ends of the broken strands are partially digested, then repaired and joined so that the rejoined strands are now continuous between the chromosomes. A protein known as RecA (recombination) controls the entire process. The same **breakage** and **reunion** process then links the second strand of each recombining DNA molecule. This **crossover** event repeated further down the chromosome results in the substitution of the exogenote segment between the two crossovers for the homologous segment of the endogenote. This process is schematically presented in a very simplified form in Figure 4–7.

Homologous recombination is responsible for integration of DNA fragments trans-

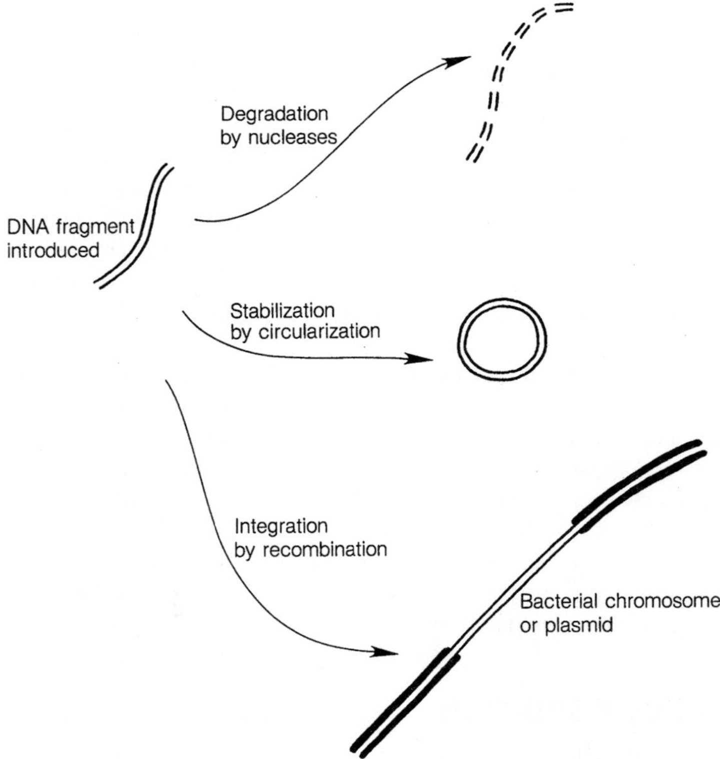


**Figure 4–6.** Possible fates of a DNA fragment after transfer into a bacterial cell.

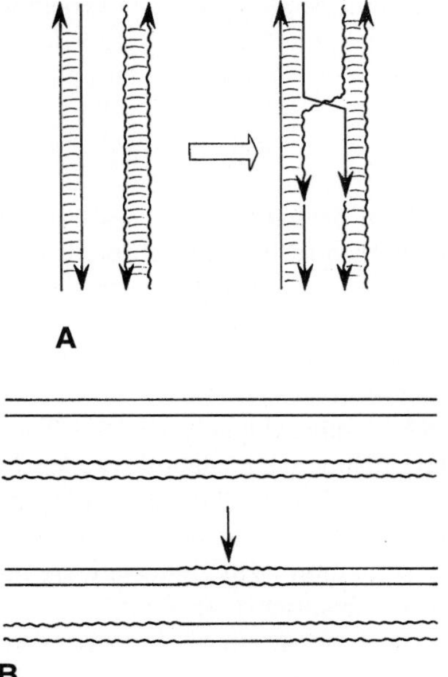


**Figure 4–7.** Homologous recombination. **A.** Central event in homologous recombination. Extensive base pairing between homologous regions of strands of two DNA molecules is illustrated. Events that accompany or follow this event include strand nicking, migration of the crossover point with partial digestion of the nicked strands, and resynthesis and ligation. Both strands of both recombining molecules must participate to effect a crossover event. **B.** Result of homologous recombination. Two crossover events are necessary to achieve the exchange of segments shown.

ferred by generalized transduction (eg, by phage P1) and by plasmid-mediated conjugation (eg, by Hfr-mediated conjugation). Recombination between the chromosome and DNA introduced by natural transformation likewise requires homologous pairing of DNA strands, but in this case it is only single-stranded exogenote DNA that pairs with the appropriate region of the complementary strand of the endogenote. The exogenote strand then displaces its nearly identical homolog, and breakage and reunion result in the formation of a partially **heterozygous** chromosome in which, at the region of recombination, one strand is original and the other is derived from the exogenote. At the next round of DNA replication, one of the daughter chromosomes will therefore be a **homozygous** recombinant.

Recombination of single-stranded DNA produces heterozygous chromosome

One daughter cell is homologous for transferred segment

## Site-Specific Recombination

RecA independent and occurs only at specific site

The second major type of recombination is actually a group of separate mechanisms that are RecA independent, that rely on only limited DNA sequence similarity at the sites of crossover, and that are mediated by different sets of specialized enzymes designed to catalyze recombination of only certain DNA molecules. Hence, one name for this group of mechanisms is **specialized recombination.** The more common name, **site-specific recombination,** reflects the fact that these recombinational events are restricted to specific sites on one or both of the recombining DNA molecules.

One good example of site-specific recombination has already been shown. The integration of some phage genomes into the chromosome occurs only at one site on the bacterial chromosome and one site on the phage chromosome. It was noted briefly that some phages, notably phage Mu, differ in being able to integrate almost anywhere in the bacterial chromosome. Because the site of recombination (the crossover site) in the Mu genome is the same in all cases, this, too, is a case of site-specific recombination.

Exogenote-encoded enzymes involved in site-specific integration

The RecA-related set of enzymes apparently are sufficient only when extensive base pairing can occur. The enzymes that bring about site-specific recombination work on a different principle: unique DNA sequences are recognized and acted on by specific recombination-generating enzymes. The unique DNA structures form the borders of the specific sites of integration or recombination; the specialized enzymes are usually encoded by genes on the exogenote.

Prophage and transposable element integration

In addition to the special kind of recombination represented by prophage integration, a particular form of site-specific recombination occurs in other situations of enormous consequence to medical microbiology. These involve special genetic units called **transposable elements**, which have proven to be so important in the life of bacteria, particularly in their roles in the pathogenesis of infectious disease, that a separate section must be devoted to their description.

## Transposable Elements

Genetic units that move within and between chromosomes and plasmids

Transposable elements are genetic units that are capable of mediating their own transfer from one chromosome to another, from one location to another on the same chromosome, or between chromosome and plasmid. This **transposition** relies on their ability to synthesize their own specific recombination enzyme.

The three major kinds of transposable elements are **insertion sequence** (IS) elements, **transposons** (or Tn elements), and certain phages, such as Mu.

IS elements encode only their own insertion

**Insertion sequence elements** are segments of DNA of approximately 1000 bp. They encode enzymes for site-specific recombination and have distinctive nucleotide sequences at their termini. Different IS elements have different termini, but, as illustrated in Figure 4–8, a given IS element has the same sequence of nucleotides at each end, but in an inverted order. Only genes involved in transposition and in the regulation of its frequency are included in IS elements, and they are therefore the simplest transposable elements.

Transposition is by copy of original IS element; occurs at low frequency

IS elements bounded by identical sequence derived from site of insertion

Transposition, which occurs infrequently (approximately once every $10^5$ to $10^7$ generations), involves recognition by the transposition enzymes of the ends of the IS element and the selection of a target area into which a new copy of the IS element will be inserted. The original copy remains at its original site. Because transposition involves duplication of the IS element, the process is sometimes called **replicative recombination.** The molecular mechanism of transposition results in a duplication also of the nucleotide sequence of the chromosome at the site of insertion. Each IS element is therefore bounded by a short identical sequence (4–12 bp) on each end, and this duplicated sequence is different at each site of insertion of a particular IS element.

Insertion of IS element into a gene causes mutation

Because IS elements contain only genes for transposition, their presence in a chromosome is not always easy to detect. If, however, an IS element transposes to a new site that is within a gene, this insertion is actually a mutation that alters or destroys the activity of the gene. Because most IS elements contain a transcription termination signal, the insertion also eliminates transcription of any genes downstream in the same operon. This property of IS elements led to their first recognition. Reversion of insertion mutations can occur by deletion, not transposition, because the latter does not delete the inserted element. The frequency of deletion is 100- to 1000-fold lower than that of insertion.

Base pairing between copies of IS elements can mediate homologous recombination

Numerous IS elements reside naturally at different locations in the *E. coli* chromosomes and in *E. coli* plasmids, for instance, and this has many consequences for the cell. Because their size is sufficient to permit strong base pairing between different copies of the same IS element, they can provide the basis for RecA-mediated homologous recombination. In this manner, the presence of particular IS elements in both the F plasmid and the bacterial chromosome provides a means for the formation of Hfr molecules by cointegration using IS sequence homology and the RecA system.

Transposons comprise genes usually flanked by IS elements

One of the major aspects of IS elements is that they are components of **transposons,** which are transposable segments of DNA containing genes beyond those needed for trans-

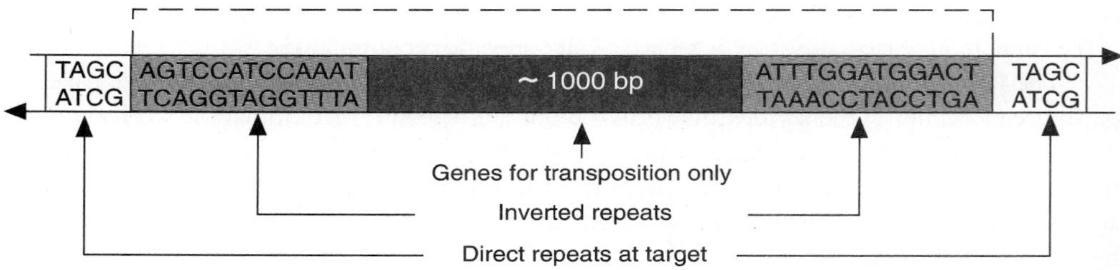


**Figure 4–8.** Structure of an insertion sequence (IS) element. The general features of bacterial IS elements are illustrated. As an example, IS2 has a total of 1327 bp, of which there are terminal inverted repeat sequences of 41 bp flanking the central region that encodes the one or two proteins required for transposition of IS2. A direct repeat of 5 bp was created at the site of insertion of the element. Approximately five IS2 elements are found in the chromosome of many strains of *Escherichia coli.*

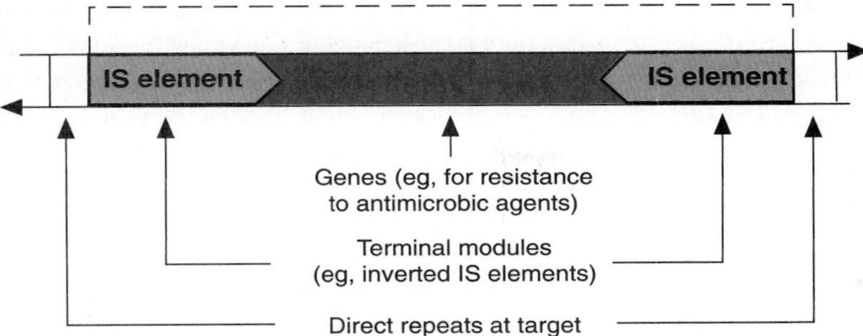


**Figure 4–9.** Structure of a transposon (Tn). The general features of bacterial transposons are illustrated. As an example, Tn9 has a total of 2500 bp. It consists of terminal direct-repeat IS1 elements flanking a central region that contains a gene for chloramphenicol resistance and genes needed for transposition.

position. Transposons are as much as 10-fold larger than IS elements, because they are composite structures consisting of a central area of genes bordered by IS elements. The genes may code for such properties as antimicrobic resistance, substrate metabolism, or other functions. Some transposons are known in which the flanking regions are not exactly the same as independent IS elements, but strongly resemble them. A generalized transposon structure is shown in Figure 4–9.

Transposons can encode antimicrobic resistance

The IS or IS-like elements of a transposon are responsible for its transposability by replicative recombination. Besides the primary insertion reaction that was described for IS elements, all transposable units promote other types of DNA rearrangements, including deletion of sequences adjacent to a transposon, inversion of DNA segments, fusion of separate plasmids within a cell, similar fusions that integrate plasmids with cell chromosome, and repeated duplications that result in **amplification** of genes within transposons. All of these events have great significance for understanding the formation and spread of antimicrobic resistance through natural populations of pathogenic organisms. These subjects are dealt with in the description of plasmids in the next section.

Transposable units can produce genetic rearrangements, duplications, and amplification

Some strains of streptococci harbor transposon-like elements that contain drug resistance genes and are located on the chromosome that can mediate their own transfer to other cells by conjugation. One such conjugative transposon is Tn916, found originally in a strain of *E. faecalis*. This element, approximately 16 kb in size, contains a gene for tetracycline resistance. It and similar elements resemble transposons in many respects, including size, multiple target sites, ability to transfer from a chromosome to a plasmid, and ability to be removed from a plasmid or a chromosome by precise excision. What is unusual, however, is their ability to mediate their own intercellular transfer. It now appears that Tn916, and presumably similar elements, can form a transient plasmidlike structure as part of the process of conjugational transfer.

Some transposons mediate their own intercellular transfer

The third type of transposable element is **transposable prophage,** such as that of bacteriophage Mu, which has the alternative of lytic growth or of lysogeny. During lysogeny the prophage of Mu can insert virtually anywhere in the *E. coli* chromosome and later can transpose itself from one location to another. It is, in fact, a transposon. When it integrates within a bacterial gene, it inactivates it in the same manner as any other transposable element. It was originally recognized as a virus that causes mutation, hence its name.

Transposable phage Mu integrates and causes mutations at many sites

This concludes the discussion of the two main types of bacterial genetic recombination, homologous recombination and site-specific recombination, but it would not be complete without mention of the fact that a third sort of recombinational process exists. It has been called **illegitimate recombination** (because it does not obey the legitimate laws governing homologous and site-specific recombination). Little is known other than it results in some types of gene duplications and deletions.

## Recombination Regulation of Gene Expression

A fascinating aspect of DNA rearrangements brought about by genetic recombination is that the expression of some chromosomal genes important in virulence are actually con-

Gonococcal pilus variation involves moving new pilin gene to promoter

trolled by recombinational events. All the known cases involve **phase variation** of surface antigens. In *Neisseria gonorrhoeae*, the bacteria causing gonorrhea, various genes encoding antigenically different pili are expressed depending on which one has been brought into a special expression site; the genes are otherwise silent because they lack effective promoters. Insertion of a pilin gene into the expression site and its replacement by another gene copy at a later time occur by a process somewhat related to site-specific recombination. The whole process resembles the insertion of cassette tapes into a tape player and, therefore, is referred to as the **cassette mode** of gene regulation.

Invertible element encodes H2 *Salmonella* flagellin and repressor for H1

Invertible element allows expression of H1 and inactivates H2 promoter

A different DNA rearrangement is responsible for the alternation of expression of antigenically distinct flagellins, H1 and H2, in *Salmonella* species. An **invertible element** of 995 bp lies between the two flagellin genes. The H2-encoding gene lies in an operon that also encodes a repressor for the H1-encoding gene. The latter gene is, therefore, active only if the former operon is inactive. Activity of the H2 operon, which lacks its own promoter, depends on a promoter within the invertible element. In one orientation, this promoter can initiate transcription of the H2-encoding gene; in the other orientation transcription, if it starts, proceeds in the opposite direction, and the H2-encoding gene is silent, allowing the H1-encoding gene to work. In this manner, excision of the invertible element and its reinsertion at the same site but in the opposite orientation lead to a shift from one flagellar form to the other (ie, to antigenic phase variation). The invertible element encodes its own site-specific **recombinase enzyme** that catalyzes the inversion in response to currently unknown signals.

Expression of structural gene for *E. coli* common pili controlled by inversion

The third example involves an invertible element too small to encode its own recombinase. It is a 314-bp segment located on the *E. coli* chromosome adjacent to the gene *fimA* encoding the structural protein for type 1 (common) pili. These pili function as an adhesin in mediating the binding of *E. coli* to eukaryotic cells, thereby aiding the early stages of colonization of various tissues by these bacteria. The *fimA* gene has no promoter other than one within the invertible element; therefore, the gene is turned off and on by inversion of the element.

Site-specific DNA rearrangements allow escape from immune response

It is believed that antigenic variation mediated by these site-specific DNA rearrangements provides a selective advantage to the bacteria in allowing invading populations to include individuals that can escape the developing immune response of the host and thus continue the infectious process. Similar strategies are employed by some eukaryotic parasites of humans, notably the trypanosomes (see Chapter 54).

## MORE ABOUT BACTERIAL PLASMIDS

One of the unanticipated features of microbial genetics has been the revelation that many virulence factors and much clinically significant resistance to antibiotics are the result of the activities not of bacterial chromosomal genes, but of the accessory genomes present in plasmids. In a certain sense, the health professional treating infectious disease is frequently coping with autonomous self-replicating DNA molecules. Many of the properties of plasmids have already been touched on, but the information is now consolidated and considered in more detail.

### Properties of Plasmids

Self-replicating plasmids found in most species

Conjugative plasmids can facilitate transfer of nonconjugatives

Some plasmids can integrate and replicate with chromosome

Plasmids are autonomous extrachromosomal elements composed of circular double-stranded DNA. They are found in most species of Gram-positive and Gram-negative bacteria and in most environments. A single organism can harbor several distinct plasmids. Like the chromosome, they have the property of governing their own replication by means of special sequences and regulatory proteins.

Many plasmids (the F plasmid of *E. coli* is an example) are able to bring about their own transfer by the products of a group of genes called *tra* (for transfer); such plasmids are called **conjugative plasmids.** Other plasmids, called **nonconjugative**, lack this ability. Conjugative plasmids may facilitate the transfer of certain nonconjugative plasmids or, in the case of the F plasmid, may mobilize the cell's chromosome. Some plasmids, again including the F factor, can replicate either autonomously or as a segment of DNA integrated into the chromosome. These are sometimes termed **episomes.** Certain prophages can exist as plasmids, but most plasmids are not viruses, because at no point of their life cycle do they exist as a free viral particle (**virion**). Most plasmids show little or no DNA homology with the chromosome and can, in this sense, be regarded as foreign to the cell.

Most plasmids are nonhomologous with the chromosome

Plasmids usually include a number of genes in addition to those required for their replication and transfer to other cells. Where their function has been established, these genes have been found to code for such properties as antimicrobic resistance and certain determinants of virulence that are not needed by the cell in all environments. In fact, they add a small metabolic burden to the cell, and in many cases, a slightly reduced growth rate results. Thus, under conditions of laboratory cultivation where the properties coded by the plasmid are not required, there is a tendency for **curing** of a strain to occur because the progeny cells that have not acquired a plasmid (or have lost it) have a selective advantage during prolonged growth and subculture. Conversely, where the property conferred by the plasmid is advantageous (eg, in the presence of the antimicrobic to which the plasmid determines resistance), selective pressure favors the plasmid-carrying strain.

Many plasmid genes facilitate survival under certain conditions

The origin of plasmids remains uncertain. They could possibly be descendents of bacterial viruses that evolved a sophisticated means of self-transfer by conjugation and then lost their unneeded protein capsid. Alternatively, they may have evolved as separated parts of a bacterial chromosome that could provide both the means for genetic exchange and a way to amplify certain genes of special value in a particular environment (eg, coding for an adhesin) or to dispense with them where they are superfluous.

Possible origins of plasmids

## Varieties of Plasmids

A great many bacterial plasmids are known. Some show similarity with each other in nucleotide sequence; thus, plasmids can be classified by their degree of apparent relatedness. Unrelated plasmids can coexist within a single cell, but closely related plasmids become segregated during cell division and eventually all but one are eliminated. For this reason, a group of closely related plasmids that exclude each other are referred to as an **incompatibility group.**

Only unrelated plasmids can coexist within the cell

Plasmids show a great variety in size, in the mode of control of their replication, and in the number and kinds of genes they carry. Naturally occurring plasmids span the range from below $5 \times 10^6$ daltons to more than $100 \times 10^6$ daltons, but even the largest are only a few percent of the size of the bacterial chromosome. The regulation of replication of a plasmid is said to be **stringent** if it is somehow closely tied to cell or chromosomal division so that few molecules of the plasmid exist per cell. Some plasmids are said to have **relaxed** regulation of replication, and many copies (even dozens) may be found in each cell, with a consequent increase in the products of the genes that they carry. In general, small plasmids have relaxed regulation, and large ones, stringent regulation. Each plasmid, by definition, must have genes sufficient to govern its own replication (including, eg, a genetic region called *ori*, or origin of replication). In addition, a conjugative plasmid must have genes that mobilize its DNA and mediate its transfer into a recipient cell. Finally, plasmids may have one or many genes unrelated to these functions, but important to the cell under certain environmental conditions.

Difference in plasmid sizes and control of replication

Small plasmids often have many copies

The variety of cellular properties associated with plasmids is very great and includes fertility (the capacity for gene transfer by conjugation), production of toxins, production of pili and other adhesins, resistance to some antimicrobics, resistance to other toxic chemicals, production of bacteriocins (toxic proteins that kill some other bacteria), production of siderophores for scavenging $Fe^{3+}$, and production of certain catabolic enzymes important in biodegradation of organic residues.

Wide range of properties encoded by plasmids

## R Plasmids

Plasmids that include genes conferring resistance to antimicrobics are of great significance to medicine. They are termed **R plasmids** or **R factors** (**resistance factors**). The genes re-

R plasmids usually encode antimicrobic-inactivating enzymes or reduced permeability

sponsible for resistance usually code for enzymes that inactivate antimicrobics or reduce the cell's permeability to them. In contrast, resistance conferred by chromosomal mutation usually involves modification of the target of the antimicrobics (eg, RNA polymerase or the ribosome).

Some R plasmids transmissible between species and genera; encode multiresistance

R plasmids occupy center stage in approaches to chemotherapy because of the constellation of properties they possess. Those of Gram-negative bacteria can be transmitted across species boundaries and, at lower frequency, even between genera. Many encode resistance to several antimicrobics and can thus spread multiple resistance through a diverse microbial population under selective pressure of only one of those to which they confer resistance. Nonpathogenic bacteria can serve as a natural reservoir of resistance determinants on plasmids that are available for spread to pathogens.

New R genes acquired by plasmid fusion or from transposons

R plasmids evolve rapidly and can easily acquire additional resistance-determining genes from fusion with other plasmids or acquisition of transposons. Many have the capability of amplifying the number of copies of their resistance genes either by gene duplications within each plasmid or by increasing the number of plasmids (copy number) per cell. By these means resistance can be achieved to very high concentrations of the antimicrobic. One process of gene amplification is based on the ability of some conjugative plasmids to dissociate their components into two plasmids, one (called the **resistance transfer factor** [RTF]) containing genes for replication and for transfer and another (called the **resistance** or **r determinant**) containing genes for replication and for resistance. Subsequent relaxed replication of the r determinant expands the cell's capacity to produce the resistance-conferring enzyme (Fig 4–10).

Gene amplification by increasing copy number

Over the past two decades many of the molecular feats of R plasmids have been explained on the basis of known genetic and evolutionary mechanisms. The discovery of transposable elements (insertion sequences and transposons) and their properties provides an explanation for many of these phenomena. Most plasmids, and all R factors, contain many IS elements and transposons. In fact, virtually all the resistance determinant genes on plasmids are present as transposons. As a result, these genes can be amplified by tandem duplications on the plasmid and can hop to other plasmids (or to the bacterial chromosome) in the same cell. Combined with the natural properties of many plasmids to transfer themselves by conjugation (even between dissimilar bacterial species), the rapid evolutionary development of multiple drug resistance plasmids and their spread through populations of pathogenic bacteria during the past three decades can be seen as a predictable result of natural selection resulting from the widespread and intensive use of antimicrobics in human and veterinary medicine (see Chapter 13).

Resistance spread facilitated by transposition of R genes

Selective pressure of antimicrobic use

The properties of transposons can explain the present-day ubiquity and mobility of resistance genes, but not their origin. Two facts help point to at least a direction in which

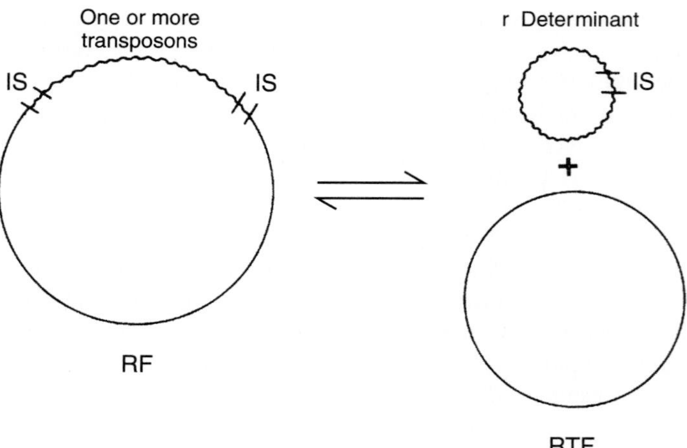


**Figure 4–10.** Structure and dissociation of an R-factor (RF) plasmid. The RF plasmid is shown with its two components: the r determinant, which contains one or more genes for antibiotic resistance (frequently present as transposons), and the resistance transfer factor (RTF), which contains the genes necessary for replication of the plasmid and its transfer to other cells.

to search for an answer. First, R plasmids carrying the genes encoding antimicrobic-inactivating enzymes have been found in bacterial cultures preserved by lyophilization (freeze-drying) since before the era of antimicrobic therapy; an accelerated evolutionary development need not be invoked. Second, the enzymes themselves are remarkably similar to those found in certain bacteria (*Streptomyces* spp) that produce many clinically useful antimicrobics. Perhaps a long time ago there was a cross-genus transfer of genetic information (by transformation?) that became stabilized on plasmids under the selection pressure of an antimicrobic released into the environment under natural conditions.

Resistance genes preexisted antimicrobic use

## Detection of Plasmids

A number of physical, morphologic, and functional tests can be used to reveal the presence of plasmids in a bacterial population. The rapid transfer of characteristics, such as resistance to antimicrobics, from strain to strain or, alternatively, the rapid loss of such traits is a hallmark of plasmid-encoded characteristics. When several genetically distinct characteristics are transferred simultaneously in the laboratory into cells known not to have possessed them previously, the evidence is very strong that a plasmid is responsible. Plasmids, including nonconjugative plasmids and those coding for no presently known trait, can be demonstrated directly by agarose gel electrophoresis. These methods and their diagnostic application are discussed in Chapter 14. Electron microscopy can also be used to visualize plasmids, to measure the length of their DNA, and to see the forms they take on hybridization to other nucleic acid molecules (Fig 4–11).

Rapid transfer of multiresistance indicates plasmid involvement

Plasmid DNAs separable electrophoretically

Bacterial plasmids, including R factors, have become valuable markers for comparing closely related strains of bacteria in epidemiologic studies. In outbreaks, spread of an epidemic strain can sometimes be followed more easily and more accurately by monitoring the profile of plasmids carried in strains isolated from different patients than by using traditional typing methods (Fig 4–12). This approach is particularly useful in studying outbreaks of nosocomial (hospital-acquired) infections. Likewise, the spread of an R plasmid between different species can be followed by showing that they carry an identical plasmid conferring the same pattern of antimicrobic resistance. The plasmid comparison can be carried

Methods for tracing plasmids epidemiologically

Plasmids compared by endonuclease digestion

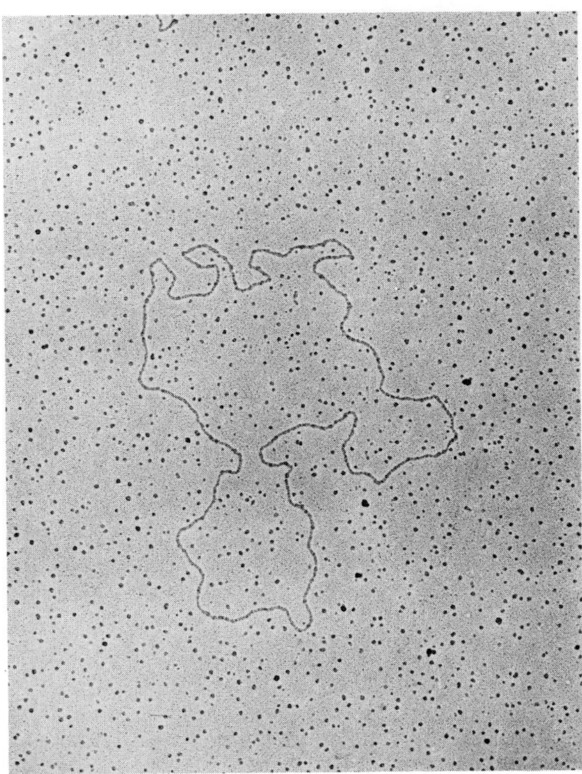

**Figure 4–11.** Electron micrograph of an R plasmid from *Escherichia coli*. The plasmid is 64 megadaltons and contains about 40 kilobase pairs. (*Courtesy of Dr. Jorge H. Crosa.*)

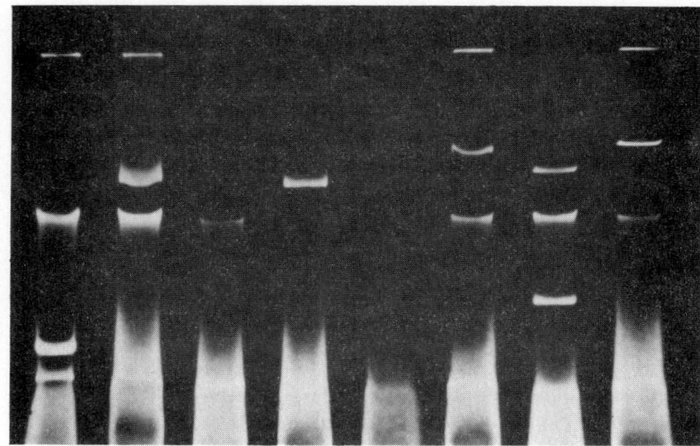

**Figure 4–12.** Agarose gel electrophoresis of various strains of staphylococci isolated from patients in a large metropolitan hospital. Each vertical lane displays the DNA of a separate isolate. The sharp bands visible in the upper half of most lanes are plasmids. The broad smear of DNA in the lower half is chromosomal DNA. The results illustrate the prevalence of multiple plasmids in freshly isolated bacterial strains. Most isolates contain more than one plasmid. (*Courtesy of Dr. D. R. Schaberg, University of Michigan.*)

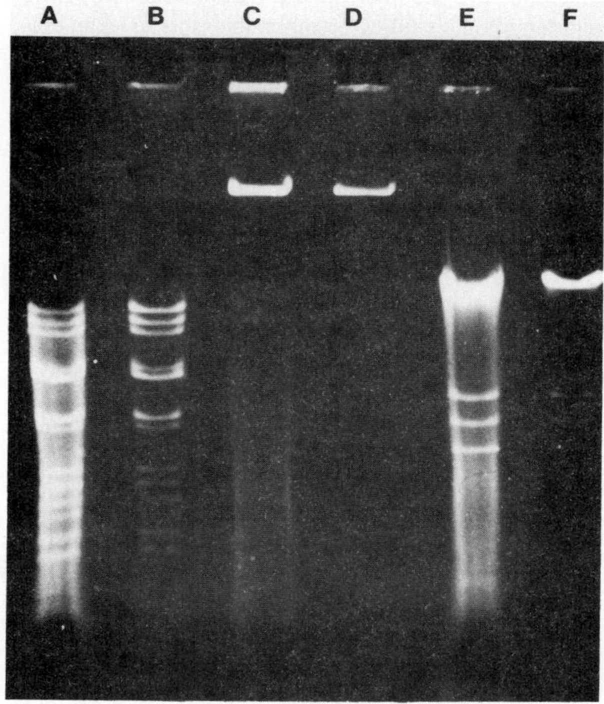


**Figure 4–13.** Use of agarose gel electrophoresis in molecular epidemiology. During an outbreak of bacteremia in infants in a neonatal intensive care unit, strains of *Klebsiella aerogenes* and *Enterobacter cloacae* were isolated that harbored R-factor plasmids of similar electrophoretic mobility and conferred resistance to some aminoglycosides, ampicillin, and chloramphenicol. To learn if an identical plasmid had established itself in both bacterial species, a restriction digest analysis was performed and the products were separated by electrophoresis. Lanes C and D display the intact plasmid DNA isolated form *K. aerogenes* and *E. cloacae*, respectively. Lanes A and B display the fragments produced by the action of the restriction enzyme *Bam*HI on the plasmids, and lanes E and F display the fragments produced by the restriction enzyme *Eco*RI. For each pair of treated samples, the plasmid DNA from *K. aerogenes* is on the left (ie, lanes A and E). The identical restriction patterns make it almost certain that the plasmids from the two bacterial species are identical, and raise the possibility that the epidemic itself was caused by the chance introduction and spread of this R plasmid. (*Kindly provided by Dr. D. R. Schaberg, University of Michigan.*)

one step further in specificity by cutting the plasmid DNA with specific restriction endonucleases (see next section) and examining the resulting fragments by agarose gel electrophoresis (Fig 4–13). Variations of this procedure enable even the spread of specific genes among a variety of plasmids to be detected.

## DNA RESTRICTION AND GENETIC ENGINEERING

The phenomena of DNA **modification** and **restriction** suggest that there is competition among the different replicons (prophages, plasmids, and chromosomes) for residence in a bacterial cell. Each of these genetic elements may possess genes for a restriction modification system, which serves to attach protective groups to its own DNA and to degrade other unprotected DNA.

**Restriction modification** systems are widespread in bacteria. Literally hundreds of bacterial **restriction enzymes** are now known. All are nucleotide-specific endonucleases that act on double-stranded DNA. They fall into three broad categories. **Type I** systems are large enzymes of great biochemical complexity. They recognize specific, unprotected nucleotide sequences, but cut the DNA molecule at variable distances from the recognized sequence. The enzymes have both endonuclease and methylating activity. They can modify DNA by methylating it at specific residues shortly after synthesis, thereby protecting it, but can cut mature DNA molecules that lack protection.

DNA restriction endonuclease enzymes common in bacteria

**Type II** systems are simpler enzymes. Each binds to and cuts at a specific nucleotide sequence. Some restriction enzymes of this type make a cut straight across the double-stranded DNA molecule, creating fragments with strands of equal length and therefore **blunt ended.** Others make a **staggered cut,** leaving single-stranded tails at the end of the fragment. These tails, being complementary to each other, can be reannealed under suitable conditions, making them exceptionally useful in **gene cloning** (Fig 4–14). Type II systems must always include a gene for an appropriate modifying methylase to protect the resident DNA.

Many enzymes make staggered cuts in double-stranded DNA

**Type III** systems resemble type I systems in that methylase and endonuclease activities reside in one enzyme, and the endonucleolytic cut is made at a site distant from the specific sequence recognized by the enzyme; they differ from type I systems by making the cut at a fixed rather than variable number of residues from the recognized sequence.

Restriction enzymes of the type II variety are extremely useful in gene cloning and other aspects of genetic engineering. The fundamental procedures in **recombinant DNA technology** are the **splitting** and **recombining** of different DNA molecules in vitro. Before the discovery of type II restriction enzymes, such splicing was possible only by a somewhat laborious process in which a tail of A residues was attached to one molecule and a tail of T residues to another to create sticky or **cohesive ends** by which the two could be held together by **annealing** (base pairing) before covalently linking them by DNA ligase. Type II restriction endonucleases provided a shortcut, because many of these enzymes, by making staggered cuts, create cohesive ends on the fragments of DNA that they restrict. As a result, DNA fragments from any source can be readily spliced together if they have been restricted by the same type II endonuclease.

Cohesive ends of different DNAs cut with the same enzymes can be spliced

The application of this procedure to splice a fragment of foreign DNA into the DNA of a bacterial plasmid is illustrated in Figure 4–14. To clone a gene from any biological source (ie, to prepare multiple exact copies of it separate from its usual neighboring genes), it is customary to prepare suitable DNA fragments with a restriction endonuclease for which there is a recognition site in a particular *E. coli* plasmid or phage molecule, called a **vector**. The cohesive ends created by the action of the endonuclease on the foreign DNA and the vector DNA facilitate their annealing, and the action of DNA ligase creates a hybrid vector (ie, one containing a fragment of the foreign DNA). The vector can then be introduced into a recipient *E. coli* cell by artificial transformation (see Transformation). If the vector is an R factor, cells successfully transformed can be selectively grown, and nontransformed cells eliminated, by plating the mixture on solid medium containing the antimicrobic against which the R factor has a resistance gene. Vectors with desirable restriction sites and genes for facilitating the recognition of desired recombinant molecules can be constructed by a multitude of powerful in vivo and in vitro techniques using transposons and various enzymes that cut, extend, and ligate DNA molecules.

Foreign genes can be spliced into plasmid or phage vector

Insertion of vector into bacteria by artificial transformation; selection and cloning

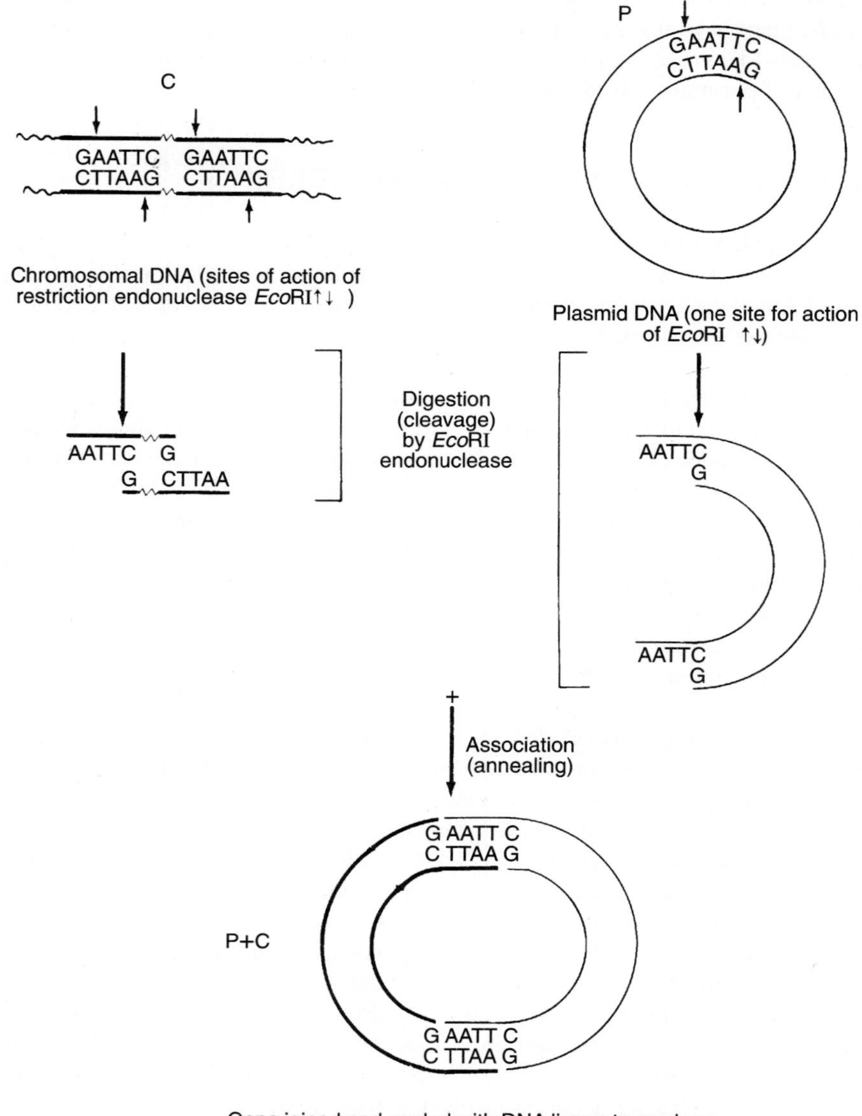


**Figure 4–14.** Construction of a recombinant DNA molecule. C, chromosomal fragments; P, plasmid.

Some foreign gene products may be produced in bacteria

When combined with information about the mechanism of transcription of genes in bacteria and the regulation of expression, recombinant DNA technology has made it possible to engineer *E. coli* cells to produce products from a variety of genetic sources. As a result medicine is now gaining the ability to produce efficiently large quantities of human enzymes and hormones, complex viral and bacterial products for vaccine production, and other useful biological products, many of which could only be obtained with great difficulty in the past and sometimes with significant risk to the recipient.

## BACTERIAL GENETICS AND CLASSIFICATION

Bacteria are classified into genera and species according to a binomial Linnean scheme similar to that used for higher organisms. For example, in the case of *Staphylococcus aureus*, *Staphylococcus* is the name of the **genus** and *aureus* is the **species** designation. Some genera with common characteristics are further grouped into **families**. Bacterial classification, however, has posed many problems. Morphologic descriptors are not as abundant as in higher plants and animals, there is little readily interpreted fossil record to help establish phylogeny, and there is no elaborate developmental process (ontogeny) to recapitulate the evolutionary path from ancestral forms (phylogeny). These problems are minor compared with others: bacteria mutate and evolve rapidly, they reproduce asexually, and they exchange genetic material over wide boundaries. The single most important test of species, the ability of individuals within a species to reproduce sexually by mating and exchanging genetic material, cannot be applied to bacteria. As a result, bacterial taxonomy developed pragmatically by determining multiple characteristics and weighting them according to which seemed most fundamental; for example, shape, spore formation, Gram reaction, aerobic or anaerobic growth, and temperature for growth were given special weighting in defining genera. Such properties as ability to ferment particular carbohydrates, production of specific enzymes and toxins, and antigenic composition of cell surface components were often used in defining species. As presented in Chapter 14, such properties and their weighting continue to be of central importance in identification of unknown isolates in the clinical laboratory, and the use of determinative keys is based on the concept of such weighted characteristics. These approaches are much less sound in establishing taxonomic relationships based on phylogenetic principles.

Weighted classification schemes valuable for identification but not for taxonomy

The recognition that sound taxonomy ought to be based on the genetic similarity of organisms and to reflect their phylogenetic **relatedness** has led in recent years to the use of new methods and new principles in taxonomy. The first approach was to apply **Adansonian** or **numeric taxonomy**, which gives equal weighting to a large number of independent characteristics and allocates bacteria to groups according to the proportion of shared characteristics as determined statistically. Theoretically, a significant correspondence of a large number of phenotypic characteristics could be considered to reflect genetic relatedness.

Sound taxonomy based on degrees of genetic similarity

A more direct approach available in recent years involves analysis of chromosomal DNA. Analysis can be somewhat crude, such as the overall ratio of A–T to G–C base pairs; differences of greater than 10% in G–C content are taken to indicate unrelatedness, but closely similar content does not imply relatedness. Closer relationships can be assessed by determining base sequence similarity, as by DNA–DNA hybridization, in which single strands of DNA from one organism are allowed to anneal with single strands of another. Some clinical laboratory tests have been devised based on the ability of DNA from a reference strain to undergo homologous recombination with DNA from an unknown isolate (see Chapter 14). Overwhelmingly, however, the molecular genetic technique that is introducing the greatest change in infectious disease diagnosis is the comparison of nucleotide sequences of genes highly conserved in evolution. Of these, in particular the sequences of the 16 S ribosomal RNA genes are proving the most valuable. So successful have been the deductions of phylogenetic relatedness based on these sequences that the absence of a fossil record is now regarded as insignificant. Part of the excitement in this field is that the use of polymerase chain reaction (PCR) to amplify the DNA of cells has made it possible to identify even infectious organisms that cannot be cultivated in the laboratory (see Chapter 14).

Phylogenetic relationships clarified by analyses of DNA base composition and base sequences

Ribosomal RNA analysis can reveal pylogenetic relationships

## POPULATION GENETICS OF PATHOGENS

One of the most striking discoveries to come from the application of molecular diagnostic tools to infectious diseases is the clonal nature of many infectious diseases. That is, over long periods and large geographic distances, the organisms of a given species isolated from clinical samples tend to be so similar in chromosomal genetic makeup and in their plasmid profiles that one is forced to envision that a clone of bacteria descended from a relatively recent common ancestor is responsible for all the disease incidence. This evidence comes partly from studies of **plasmid profiles**, but mostly it is a conclusion drawn by examining the specific alleles of various genes present in a population of cells using the technique of **multilocus enzyme electrophoresis**. By this technique differences in electrophoretic migration are used to detect subtle differences in amino acid sequence in a battery of two to three dozen different enzymes. The results have been striking. For example, isolates of *Bordetella pertussis* from the United States represent a single clone, whereas in Japan there is a slightly different clone. In another study it was determined that only 11 multilocus geno-

Clonality of bacteria revealed by enzyme profiles

types (clones) of *Neisseria meningitidis* have been responsible for the major epidemics of serogroup A organisms worldwide over the past 60 years. These discoveries provide an entirely new method for study of the epidemiology of infectious disease.

## ADDITIONAL READING

Selander RK, Musser JM, Caugent DA, Gilmour MN, Whittam TS. Population genetics of pathogenic bacteria. *Microb Pathog.* 1987;3:1–7. This article describes the technique of multilocus enzyme electrophoresis and summarizes some of the early findings using this technique.

Eisenstein BI. New molecular techniques for microbial epidemiology and the diagnosis of infectious diseases. *J Infect Dis.* 1990;161:595–602.

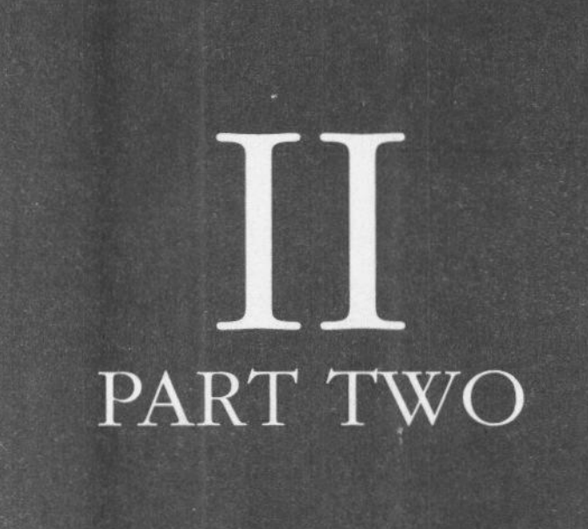


# Biology of Viruses

Chapter 5

# Virus Structure

James J. Champoux

A virus is a set of genes, either DNA or RNA, packaged in a protein-containing coat. The resulting particle is called a **virion.** Viruses that infect humans are considered as part of the general class of animal viruses; viruses that infect bacteria are referred to as bacteriophages, or phages for short. Virus reproduction requires that a virus particle infect a cell and program the cellular machinery to synthesize the macromolecular constituents required for the assembly of new virions. Thus, a virus is considered an intracellular parasite. The infected host cell may produce hundreds to hundreds of thousands of new virions and usually dies. Tissue damage as a result of cell death accounts for the pathology of many viral diseases in humans. In some cases, the infected cells survive, resulting in persistent virus production and a chronic infection that can remain asymptomatic, produce a chronic disease state, or lead to relapse of an infection.

A virus is an intracellular parasite composed of DNA or RNA and a protein coat

In some circumstances, a virus fails to reproduce itself and instead enters a latent state, often by integration into the host cell genome (called **lysogeny** in the case of bacteriophages), from which there is the potential for reactivation at a later time. A possible consequence of the presence of viral genes in a latent state is a new genotype for the cell. Some determinants of bacterial virulence and some malignancies of animal cells are examples of the genetic effects of latent viruses. Apparently vertebrates have had to coexist with viruses for a long time because they have evolved the special nonspecific interferon system, which operates in conjunction with the highly specific immune system to control virus infections.

Instead of reproducing, the virus may enter a latent state by integrating into the host genome

In the discussion to follow, the biologic and genetic bases for these phenomena are provided. Three themes are emphasized: (1) Different viruses can have very different structures, and this diversity is reflected in their replicative strategies. (2) Because of their small size viruses have achieved a very high degree of genetic economy. (3) Although viruses depend to a great extent on host cell functions and, therefore, are difficult to combat medically, they do exhibit unique steps in their replicative cycles, which are potential targets for antiviral therapy.

## VIRION SIZE AND DESIGN

Viruses are approximately 100- to 1000-fold smaller than the cells they infect. The smallest viruses (parvoviruses) are approximately 20 nm in diameter (1 nm = $10^{-9}$ m), whereas the largest animal viruses (poxviruses) overlap the size of the smallest bacterial cells (*Chlamydia* and *Mycoplasma*), having a diameter of approximately 300 nm. This means that viruses generally pass through filters designed to trap bacteria, and this property can, in principle, be used as evidence of a viral etiology.

Viral size ranges from 20 to 300 nm

Unenveloped viruses have a nucleic acid genome within a protein capsid

Enveloped viruses have a nucleocapsid of nucleic acid complexed to protein

Some viruses have surface protein or glycoprotein spikes

The basic design of all true viruses places the nucleic acid genome on the inside of a protein shell called a **capsid**. Some animal viruses are further packaged into a lipid membrane, or **envelope**, which is usually acquired from the cytoplasmic membrane of the infected cell during egress from the cell. Viruses that are not enveloped have a defined external capsid and are referred to as **naked capsid viruses.** Enveloped viruses contain a nucleic acid–protein complex called a **nucleocapsid** surrounded by a matrix protein that serves as a bridge between the nucleocapsid and the inside of the membrane envelope. Protein or glycoprotein structures called **spikes** often emanate from the surface of virus particles. These basic design features are illustrated schematically in Figure 5–1 and in the electron micrographs in Figure 5–2, and Figure 5–3.

Two shapes: cylindrical and spherical

The protein shell forming the capsid or the nucleocapsid assumes one of two basic shapes, cylindrical or spherical. Some of the more complex bacteriophages combine these two basic shapes. Examples of these three structural categories can be seen in the electron micrographs in Figure 5–2.

Outer shell is protective and aids in entry and packaging

The outer shell of viruses functions (1) to protect the nucleic acid genome from damage during the extracellular passage of the virus from one cell to another, (2) to aid in the process of entry into the cell, and (3) in some cases to package enzymes essential for the early steps of the infection process.

Genome of naked virus is condensed in core with basic proteins

Enveloped viral genome is condensed in nucleocapsid

In general, the length of the viral nucleic acid genome is hundreds of times the longest dimension of the complete virion. It therefore follows that the viral genome must be extensively condensed during the process of virion assembly. For naked capsid viruses this condensation is achieved by the association of the nucleic acid with basic proteins to form what is called the **core** of the virus (see Fig 5–1). The core proteins are usually encoded by the virus, but in the case of some DNA-containing animal viruses, the basic proteins are histones scavenged from the host cell. For enveloped viruses, the formation of the nucleocapsid serves to condense the nucleic acid genome.

Plant viroids are infectious RNA molecules

Prions are infectious proteins

Two classes of infectious agents exist that are structurally simpler than viruses. **Viroids** are infectious circular RNA molecules that lack protein shells; they are responsible for a variety of plant diseases. **Prions**, which apparently lack any genes and are composed only of protein, are agents that appear to be responsible for some chronic severe neurologic diseases such as scrapie in sheep and Creutzfeldt–Jakob syndrome in humans.

## GENOME STRUCTURE

DNA or RNA genomes may be single or double stranded

Structural diversity among the viruses is most obvious when the makeup of viral genomes is considered. Genomes can be made of RNA or DNA and be either double stranded or single stranded. For viruses with single-stranded genomes, the nucleic acid can be either of the same polarity (indicated by a +) or of a different polarity (–) from that of the viral mRNA produced during infection. In the case of adeno-associated viruses, the particles are a mixture: about half contain (+)DNA; the other half contain (–)DNA. The arenaviruses and bunyaviruses are unusual in apparently having an RNA genome, of which part has the same polarity as the mRNA and part is complementary to the corresponding mRNA.

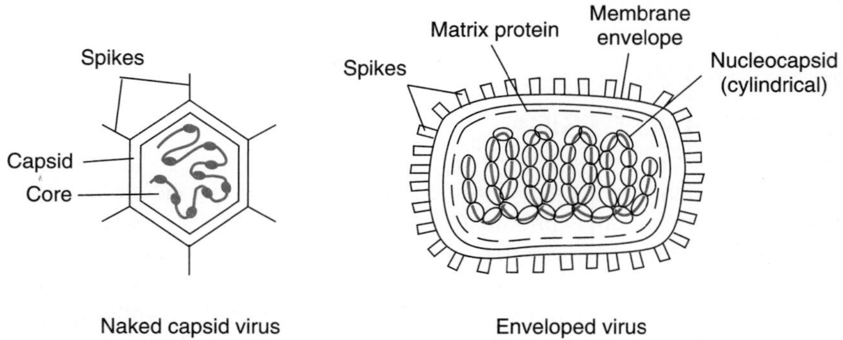


**Figure 5–1.** Schematic drawing of two basic types of virions.

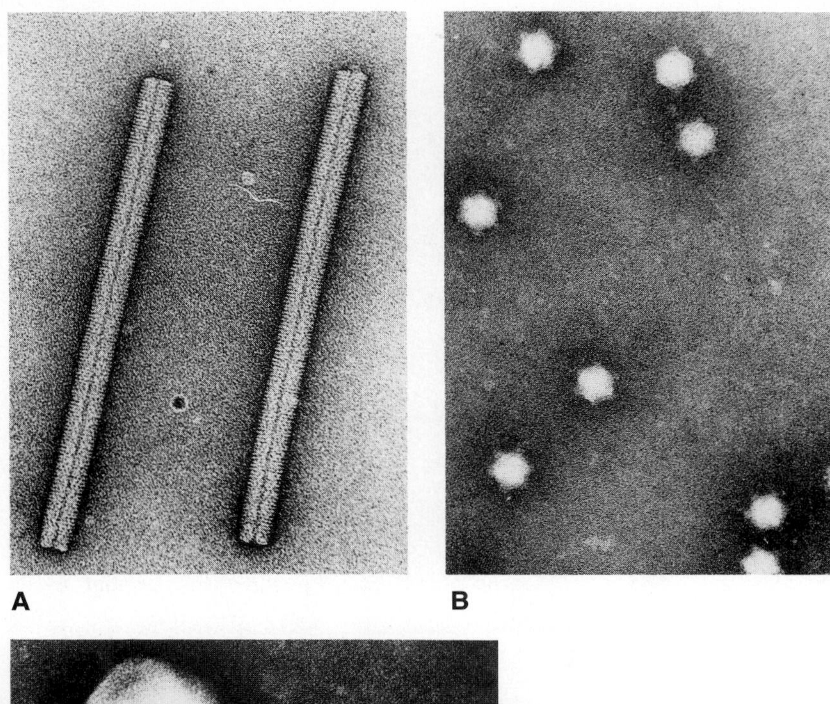


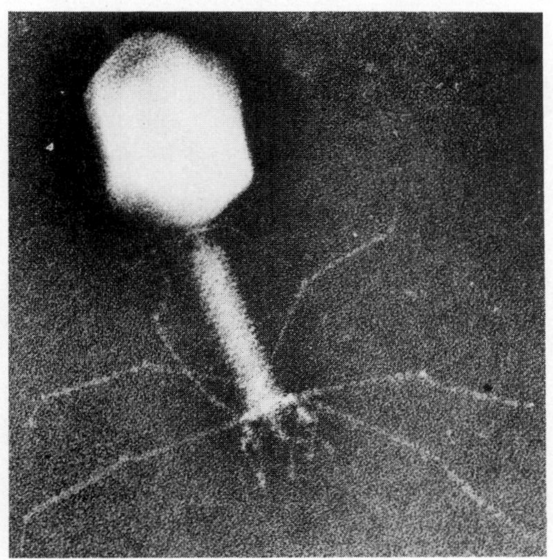


**Figure 5–2.** Three basic virus designs: **A.** Tobacco mosaic virus. **B.** bacteriophage øX174. **C.** Bacteriophage T4. (*Kindly provided by Dr. Robley C. Williams.*)

Both linear and circular genomes are known. Whereas most viruses have a single nucleic acid molecule for their genome, in some cases several pieces of nucleic acid constitute the complete genome. Such viruses are said to have segmented genomes. One virus class (retroviruses) carries two identical copies of its genome and is therefore diploid. A few viral genomes (picornaviruses, hepatitis B virus, and adenoviruses) contain covalently attached protein on the ends of the polynucleotide chains. As is discussed in Chapter 6, the terminal protein molecules as well as other special genome structures found in other viruses play key roles in the replication process.

Genomes may be linear or circular and single or segmented molecules

## CAPSID STRUCTURE

### Subunit Structure of Capsids

The capsids or nucleocapsids of all viruses are composed of many copies of one or at most several different kinds of protein subunits. This fact follows from two fundamental considerations. First, all viruses code for their own capsid proteins, and it turns out that even if the entire coding capacity of the genome were to be used to specify a single giant capsid protein, the protein would not be large enough to enclose the nucleic acid genome. Thus, multiple protein copies are needed, and, in fact, the simplest spherical virus contains 60

Capsids and nucleocapsids are composed of multiple copies of protein molecule(s) in crystalline array

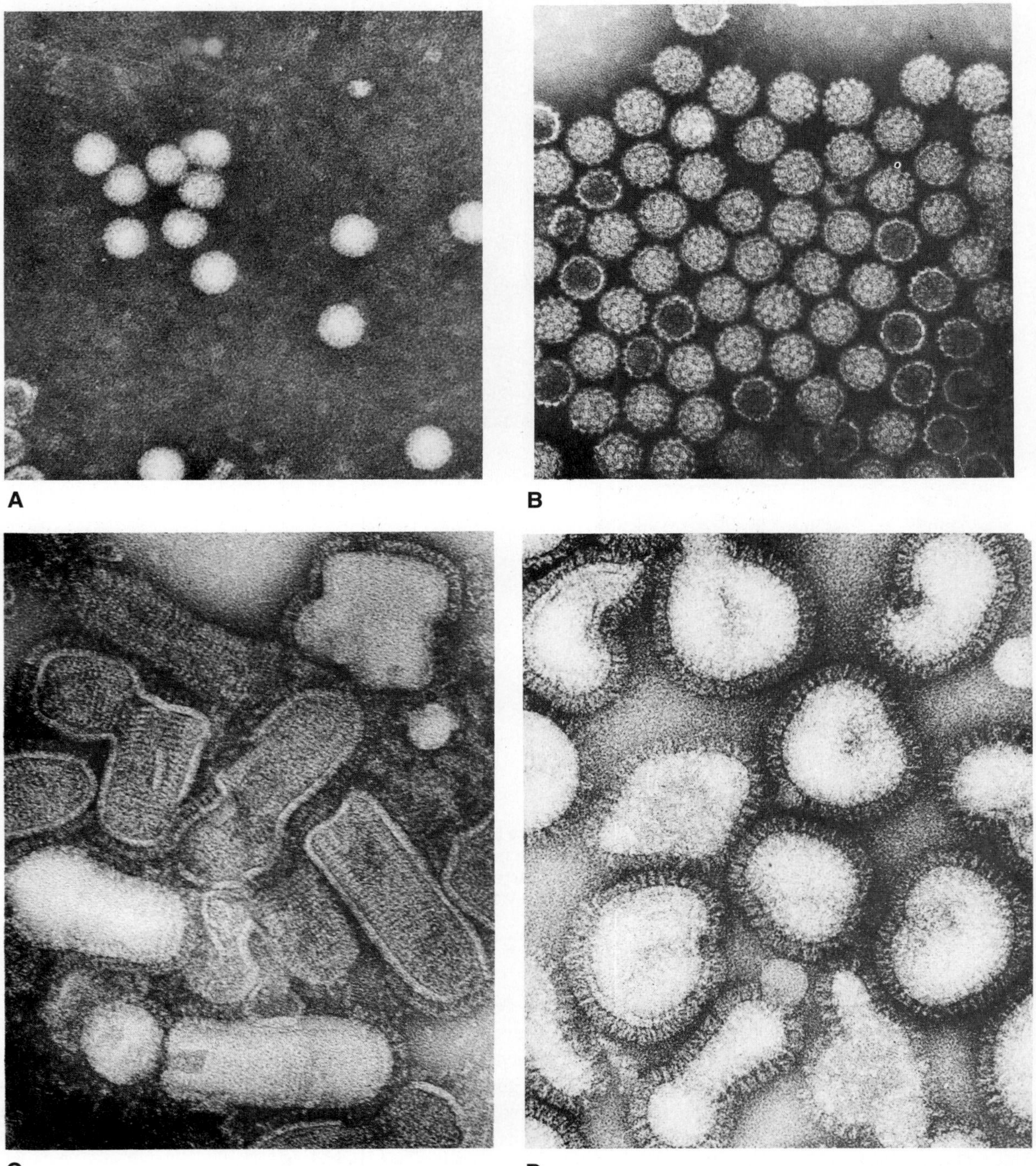

A

B

C

D

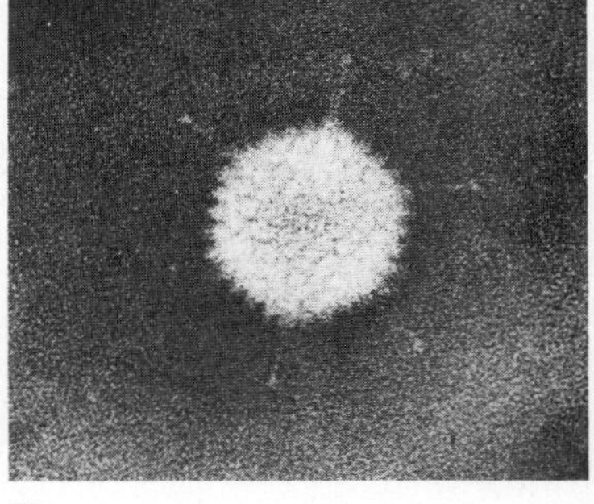

E

**Figure 5–3.** Representative animal viruses: **A.** Poliovirus. **B.** Simian virus 40. **C.** Vesicular stomatitis virus. **D.** Influenza virus. **E.** Adenovirus. (*Kindly provided by Dr. Robley C. Williams.*)

identical protein subunits. Second, viruses are such highly symmetric structures that it is not uncommon to visualize naked capsid viruses in the electron microscope as a crystalline array (eg, simian virus 40 in Fig 5–3B). A polypeptide chain that constitutes the basic subunit is, however, intrinsically irregular in shape. The only way to construct a regular symmetric structure out of irregular subunits is to follow the rules of crystallography and form an aggregate involving many identical copies of the irregular subunits, where each subunit bears the same relationship to its neighbors as every other subunit.

The presence of many identical protein subunits in viral capsids or the existence of many identical spikes in the membrane of enveloped viruses has important implications for adsorption, hemagglutination, and recognition of viruses by neutralizing antibodies (see Chapter 6).

## Cylindrical Architecture

A cylindrical shape is the simplest structure for a capsid or a nucleocapsid. The first virus to be crystallized and studied in structural detail was a plant pathogen, tobacco mosaic virus (TMV) (see Fig 5–2). The capsid of TMV is shaped like a rod or a cylinder, with the RNA genome wound in a helix inside it. The capsid is composed of many copies of a single kind of protein subunit arranged in a close-packed helix, which places every subunit in the same microenvironment. Because of the helical arrangement of the subunits, viruses that have this type of design are often said to have helical symmetry. Although less is known about the capsid structures of animal viruses with helical symmetry, it is likely their structures follow the same pattern as TMV. Thus, the nucleocapsids of influenza, measles, mumps, rabies, and poxviruses (Table 5–1) are probably constructed with a helical arrangement of protein subunits in close association with the nucleic acid genome.

Cylindrical viruses have a helical arrangement of genome and capsid protein molecules

## Spherical Architecture

The construction of a spherically shaped virus similarly involves the packing together of many identical subunits, but in this case the subunits are placed on the surface of a geometric solid called an **icosahedron**. An icosahedron has 12 vertices, 30 sides, and 20 triangular faces (Fig 5–4). Because the icosahedron belongs to the symmetry group that crystallographers refer to as cubic, spherically shaped viruses are said to have cubic symmetry. (Note that the term **cubic**, as used in this context, has nothing to do with the more familiar shape called the cube.)

Spherical viruses exhibit icosahedral symmetry

When viewed in the electron microscope, many naked capsid viruses and some nucleocapsids appear as spherical particles with a surface topology that makes it appear that they are constructed of identical ball-shaped subunits (see Fig 5–3C). These visible structures are referred to as **morphological subunits**, or **capsomeres**. A capsomere is composed of either five or six individual protein molecules, each one referred to as a **structural subunit**, or **protomer.** In the simplest case of a virus with cubic symmetry, five protomers are placed at each one of the 12 vertices of the icosahedron as shown in Figure 5–4 to form a capsomere called a **pentamer**. Thus, the capsid is composed of 12 pentamers, or a total of 60 protomers. It should be noted that as in the case of helical symmetry, this arrangement places every protomer in the same microenvironment as every other protomer.

Capsomeres are surface structures composed of five or six protein molecules

To accommodate the larger cavity required by viruses with large genomes, the capsids contain many more protomers. These viruses are based on a variation of the basic icosahedron in which the construction involves a mixture of pentamers and hexamers instead of only pentamers. A detailed description of this higher level of virus structure is beyond the scope of this text.

## Special Surface Structures

Many viruses have structures that protrude from the surface of the virion. In virtually every case these structures are important for the two earliest steps of infection, adsorption and penetration. The most dramatic example of such a structure is the tail of some bacterio-

Surface structures are important in adsorption and penetration

**TABLE 5–1. CLASSIFICATION OF RNA ANIMAL VIRUSES**

| Family | Virion Structure | Genome Structure and Molecular Weight | Representative Members |
|---|---|---|---|
| Hepatitis δ | Cubic, enveloped | ss circular (–) ($6 \times 10^5$) | Human hepatitis δ virus |
| Picornaviruses | Cubic, naked | ss linear (+) ($2–3 \times 10^6$); protein attached | Human enteroviruses: poliovirus, coxsackievirus, echovirus; rhinoviruses; bovine foot and mouth disease virus; hepatitis A |
| Arenaviruses | Helical, enveloped | 2 ss linear segments (+/–) ($3 \times 10^6$) | Lassa virus; lymphocytic choriomeningitis virus of mice |
| Caliciviruses | Cubic, naked | ss linear (+) ($2.6 \times 10^6$) | Vesicular exanthema virus, Norwalk-like viruses of humans |
| Rhabdoviruses | Helical, enveloped | ss linear (–) ($3–4 \times 10^6$) | Rabies virus; bovine vesicular stomatitis virus |
| Retroviruses | Cubic, enveloped | ss linear (+), diploid ($3–4 \times 10^6$) | RNA tumor viruses of mice, birds, and cats; visna virus of sheep; human immunodeficiency viruses (human T-cell leukemia and acquired immunodeficiency syndrome) |
| Togaviruses | Cubic, enveloped | ss linear (+) ($4 \times 10^6$) | Alphaviruses: Sindbis virus and Semliki Forest virus; flaviviruses: dengue virus and yellow fever virus; rubella virus; mucosal disease virus |
| Orthomyxoviruses | Helical, enveloped | 8 ss linear segments (–) ($5 \times 10^6$) | Type A, B, and C influenza viruses of humans, swine, and horses |
| Coronaviruses | Helical, enveloped | ss linear (+) ($5–6 \times 10^6$) | Respiratory viruses of humans; calf diarrhea virus; swine enteric virus; mouse hepatis virus |
| Filoviruses | Helical, enveloped | ss linear (–) ($5 \times 10^6$) | Marburg and Ebola viruses |
| Bunyaviruses | Helical, enveloped | 3 ss linear segments (+/–) ($6 \times 10^6$) | Rift Valley fever virus; bunyamwera virus; hantavirus |
| Paramyxoviruses | Helical, enveloped | ss linear (–) ($6–8 \times 10^6$) | Mumps; measles; Newcastle disease virus; canine distemper virus |
| Reoviruses | Cubic, naked | 10 ds linear segments ($15 \times 10^6$) | Human reoviruses; orbiviruses; Colorado tick fever virus; African horse sickness virus; human rotaviruses |

Abbreviations: ss, single stranded; ds, double stranded.

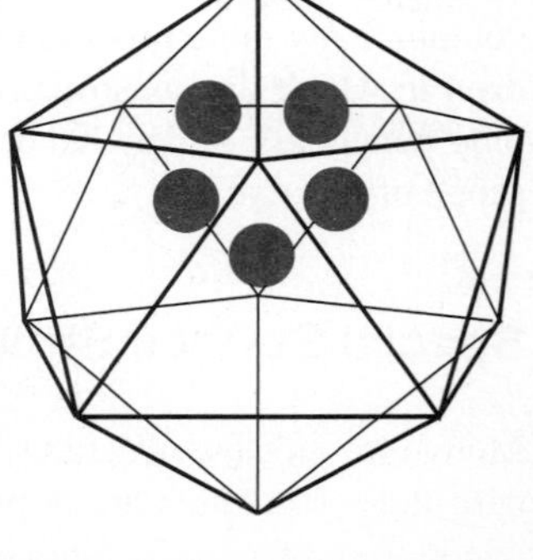

**Figure 5–4.** Diagram of an icosahedron showing 12 vertices, 20 faces, and 30 sides. The heavy dots indicate the position of protomers forming a pentamer on a spherical virus.

**TABLE 5–2. CLASSIFICATION OF DNA ANIMAL VIRUSES**

| Family | Virion Structure | Genome Structure and Molecular Weight | Representative Members |
|---|---|---|---|
| Parvoviruses | Cubic, naked | ss linear ($1–2 \times 10^6$) | Minute virus of mice; adeno-associated satellite viruses |
| Hepatitis B | Cubic, enveloped | ds circular ($2 \times 10^6$), gap in one strand; protein attached | Hepatitis B virus of humans; woodchuck hepatitis virus |
| Papovaviruses | Cubic, naked | ds circular ($3–5 \times 10^6$) | Papillomaviruses; polyomavirus (mouse); SV40 (monkey) |
| Adenoviruses | Cubic, naked | ds linear ($20–25 \times 10^6$); protein attached | Human and animal respiratory disease viruses |
| Herpesviruses | Cubic, enveloped | ds linear ($80–130 \times 10^6$) | Herpes simplex virus types 1 and 2; varicella–zoster virus; cytomegalovirus; Epstein–Barr virus; human herpesvirus type 6 |
| Poxviruses | Helical, enveloped | ds linear ($160–200 \times 10^6$) | Smallpox; vaccinia; molluscum contagiosum; fibroma and myxoma viruses of rabbits |

Abbreviations: ss, single stranded; ds, double stranded.

phages (see Fig 5–2), which, as described in Chapter 6, acts as a channel for the transfer of the genome into the cell. Other examples of surface structures include the spikes of adenovirus (see Fig 5–3E) and the glycoprotein spikes found in the membrane of enveloped viruses (see the influenza virus in Fig 5–3D). Even viruses without obvious surface extensions probably contain short projections, which, like the more obvious spikes, are involved in the specific binding of the virus to the cell surface (see Chapter 6).

## CLASSIFICATION OF VIRUSES

Tables 5–1 and 5–2 present a classification scheme for animal viruses that is based solely on their structure. The viruses are arranged in order of increasing genome size. It is important to bear in mind that phylogenetic relationships cannot be inferred from this taxonomic scheme. The tables should not be memorized, but instead used as a reference guide to virus structure. In general, viruses with similar structures exhibit similar replication strategies as is discussed in Chapter 6.

Representative and important bacteriophages are listed along with their properties in Table 5–3.

**TABLE 5–3. SOME IMPORTANT BACTERIOPHAGES**

| Bacteriophage | Host | Genome Structure and Molecular Weight | Comments |
|---|---|---|---|
| MS2 | *Escherichia coli* | ss linear RNA ($1.2 \times 10^6$) | Lytic |
| Filamentous (M13, fd) | *Escherichia coli* | ss circular DNA ($2.1 \times 10^6$) | No cell death |
| øX174 | *Escherichia coli* | ss circular DNA ($1.8 \times 10^6$) | Lytic |
| ß | *Corynebacterium diphtheriae* | ds linear DNA ($23 \times 10^6$) | Temperate, codes for diphtheria toxin |
| λ | *Escherichia coli* | ds linear DNA ($31 \times 10^6$) | Temperate |
| T4 | *Escherichia coli* | ds linear DNA ($108 \times 10^6$) | Lytic |

Abbreviations: ss, single stranded; ds, double stranded.

Chapter 6

# Virus Multiplication

## *James J. Champoux*

A typical virus multiplication cycle is divided into discrete phases of (1) adsorption to the host cell, (2) penetration or entry, (3) uncoating to release the genome, (4) virion component production, (5) assembly, and (6) release from the cell. This series of events, sometimes with slight variations, describes what is called the **productive** or **lytic response;** however, this is not the only possible outcome of a virus infection. Some viruses can also enter into a very different kind of relationship with the host cell in which no new virus is produced, the cell survives and divides, and the viral genetic material persists indefinitely in a latent state. This outcome of an infection is referred to as the **nonproductive response**. The nonproductive response is called lysogeny in the case of bacteriophages and may involve oncogenic transformation by animal viruses. (This use of the term **transformation** is to be distinguished from DNA transformation of bacteria discussed in Chapter 4.) In addition, there may exist examples of viruses that can transiently infect a cell, cause some permanent change, and then be lost. Such an encounter between a virus and a cell is called a **hit-and-run infection.**

Viral infection of cells may be productive or nonproductive

Animal viruses may cause oncogenic transformation

The outcome of an infection depends on the particular virus–host combination and on other factors such as the extracellular environment, multiplicity of infection, and physiology and developmental state of the cell. Those viruses that can enter only into a productive relationship are called **lytic** or **virulent viruses.** Viruses that can undergo both the productive and nonproductive responses are referred to as **temperate viruses.** Some temperate viruses can be reactivated or "induced" to leave the latent state and enter into the productive response. Whether induction occurs depends on the particular virus–host combination, the physiology of the cell, and the presence of extracellular stimuli.

Lytic viruses destroy cells

Temperate viruses may enter a latent state

The remainder of this chapter is concerned with the details of the steps of the lytic response. In Chapter 7 the topics of lysogeny and oncogenic transformation are considered.

## GROWTH AND ASSAY OF VIRUSES

Viruses are generally propagated in the laboratory by mixing the virus and susceptible cells together and incubating the infected cells until lysis occurs. After lysis, the cells and cell debris are removed by a brief centrifugation and the supernatant is called a **lysate.**

The growth of animal viruses requires that the host cells be cultivated in the laboratory. To prepare cells for growth in vitro, a tissue is removed from an animal and the cells are disaggregated using the proteolytic enzyme trypsin. The cell suspension is seeded into a plastic petri dish in a medium containing a complex mixture of amino acids, vitamins, minerals, and sugars. In addition to these nutritional factors, the growth of animal cells requires components present in animal serum. This method of growing cells is referred to as **tissue culture,** and the initial cell population is called a **primary culture.** The cells attach

Viruses are cultivated in cell cultures derived from mammalian tissues

to the bottom of the plastic dish and remain attached as they divide and eventually cover the surface of the dish. When the culture becomes crowded, the cells generally cease dividing and enter a resting state. Propagation can be continued by removing the cells from the primary culture plate using trypsin and reseeding a new plate.

Permanent cell lines are useful for growing viruses

Cells taken from a normal (as opposed to cancerous) tissue cannot usually be propagated in this manner indefinitely. Eventually most of the cells die; a few may survive, and these cells often develop into a permanent cell line. Such cell lines are very useful as host cells for isolating and assaying viruses in the laboratory, but they rarely bear much resemblance to the tissue from which they originated. When cells are taken from a tumor and cultivated in vitro, they display a very different set of growth properties reflecting their tumor phenotype (see Chapter 7).

Cytopathic effects are characteristic of viruses

When a virus is propagated in tissue culture cells, the cytologic changes induced by the virus, which usually culminate in cell death, are often characteristic of a particular virus and are referred to as the **cytopathic effect** of the virus (see Chapter 14).

Viruses are quantitated by plaque assay

Viruses are quantitated by a method called the plaque assay (see Plaque Assay under Quantitation of Viruses for a detailed description of the method). Briefly, viruses are mixed with cells on a petri plate such that each infectious particle gives rise to a zone of lysed cells called a **plaque.** From the number of plaques on the plate, the titer of infectious particles in the lysate is calculated. Virus titers are expressed as the number of plaque-forming units per milliliter.

## ONE-STEP GROWTH EXPERIMENT

High multiplicity of infection allows study of synchronous viral replication

To describe an infection in temporal and quantitative terms it is useful to perform a one-step growth experiment (Fig 6–1). The objective in such an experiment is to infect every cell in a culture so that the whole population proceeds through the infection process in a synchronous fashion. The ratio of infecting plaque-forming units to cells is called the multiplicity of infection. By infecting at a high multiplicity (eg, 10 as in Fig 6–1), one can be certain that every cell is infected.

Shortly after infection, a virus loses its identity (eclipse phase)

The time course and efficiency of adsorption can be followed by the loss of infectious virus from the medium after removal of the cells (solid line, in Fig 6–1). In the example shown, adsorption takes about a half-hour and all but 1% of the virus is adsorbed. If samples of the culture containing the infected cells are treated so as to break open the cells prior to assaying for virus (broken line in Fig 6–1), it can be observed that infectious virus initially disappears, because no particles are detectable above the background of unadsorbed virus. The period of infection in which no infectious viruses are found is called the **eclipse phase** and serves to emphasize that the original virions lose their infectivity soon after entry into the cells. Infectivity is lost because, as is shown later, the virus particles are dis-

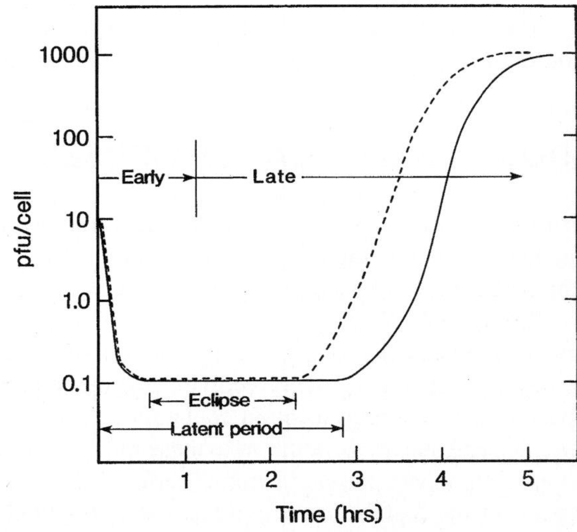


**Figure 6–1.** One-step growth experiment. pfu, plaque-forming unit.

mantled as a prelude to their reproduction. Later, infectious virus particles rapidly reappear in increasing numbers and are detected inside the cell prior to their release into the medium (see Fig 6–1). The length of time from the beginning of infection until progeny virions are found outside the cells is referred to as the **latent period.** Latent periods range from 15 minutes to hours for bacteriophages and from a few hours to many days for animal viruses.

Infectious virus reappears increasingly inside the cell

The time in the infection at which genome replication begins has often been used to divide the infection operationally into early and late phases. Early viral gene expression is restricted to producing those proteins required for genome replication; later, the proteins synthesized are primarily those necessary for construction of the new virus particles.

Proteins for replication are produced early, and those for construction, late

The average number of plaque-forming units released per infected cell is called the burst size for the infection. In the example shown, the burst size is about 1000. Burst sizes range from less than 10 for some relatively inefficient infections to millions for some highly virulent viruses.

## ADSORPTION

The first step in every viral infection is the attachment or adsorption of the infecting particle to the surface of the cell. A prerequisite for this interaction is a collision between the virion and the cell. Viruses do not have any capacity for locomotion and so the collision event is simply a random process determined by diffusion. Therefore, like any bimolecular reaction, the rate of adsorption is determined by the concentrations of both the virions and the cells.

Only a small fraction of the collisions between a virus and its host cell lead to a successful infection. This is because adsorption is a highly specific reaction that involves protein molecules on the surface of the virion called **virion attachment proteins** and certain molecules on the surface of the cell called **receptors.** Typically there are $10^4$ to $10^5$ receptors on the cell surface. Receptors for some bacteriophages are found on pili, although the majority adsorb to receptors found on the bacterial cell wall. The receptors for animal viruses are usually glycoproteins located in the plasma membrane (also called cytoplasmic membrane), which carry out normal cellular functions. In the case of bacteriophages with tails, virion attachment proteins are found at the very end of the tails or the tail fibers (see Fig 5–2). It appears that surface protrusions in general, such as the spikes found on adenoviruses and on virtually all of the enveloped animal viruses, contain the virion attachment proteins. Receptors for some animal viruses are also found on red blood cells of certain species and are responsible for the phenomena of hemagglutination and hemadsorption discussed later.

Adsorption involves virion attachment proteins and cell protein receptors

Viral spikes and phage tails carry attachment proteins

Some receptors are found on red blood cells

The repeating subunit structure of capsids and the multiplicity of spikes on enveloped viruses are probably important in determining the strength of the binding of the virus to the cell. The binding between a single virion attachment protein and a single receptor protein is relatively weak, but the combination of many such interactions leads to a strong association between the virion and the cell. The fluid nature of the animal cell membrane may facilitate the movement of receptor proteins to allow the clustering that is necessary for these multiple interactions.

Adsorption is enhanced by multiplicities of attachment and receptor proteins

A particular kind of virus is capable of infecting only a limited spectrum of cell types called its **host range.** Thus, although a few viruses can infect cells from different species, most viruses are limited to a single species. For example, dogs do not contract measles, and humans do not contract distemper. In many cases, animal viruses infect only a particular subset of the cells found in their host organism. Clearly this kind of tissue tropism is very important in determining the pathology of the infection. In most cases studied, the specific host range of a virus and its associated tissue tropism are determined at the level of the binding between the cell receptors and virion attachment proteins. Thus, these two protein components must possess complementary surfaces that fit together in much the same way as a substrate fits into the active site of an enzyme. It therefore follows that adsorption occurs only in that fraction of collisions that lead to a successful binding interaction between receptors and attachment proteins and that the inability of a virus to infect a cell type is usually due to the absence of the appropriate receptors on the cell. The exquisite specificity of these interactions is well illustrated by the case of a particular mouse reovirus, where it has been found that the tissue tropism and, therefore, the resultant pathology are altered by a

Differences in host range and tissue tropism are due to presence or absence of receptors

point mutation that changes a single amino acid in the virion attachment protein. A few cases are known in which the host range of a virus is determined at a step after adsorption and penetration, but these are the exceptions rather than the rule.

Neutralizing antibodies are usually specific for attachment proteins

Once a virus particle has penetrated to the inside of a cell, it is essentially hidden from the host immune system. Thus, if protection from a virus infection is to be accomplished at the level of antibody binding to the virions, it must occur before adsorption and prevent the virus from attaching to and penetrating the cell. It is therefore not surprising that most neutralizing antibodies, whether acquired as a result of natural infection or vaccination, are specific for virion attachment proteins.

## ENTRY AND UNCOATING

Viruses are dismantled before being replicated

The eclipse phase is a direct consequence of the fact that viruses are dismantled prior to being replicated. As is shown later, the uncoating step may be simultaneous with entry or may occur in a series of steps. Ultimately the nucleocapsid or core structure must be transported to the site or compartment in the cell where transcription and replication will occur.

### The Bacteriophage Strategy

Bacteriophage capsids are shed and only the viral genome enters the host cell

The processes of penetration and uncoating are simultaneous for all bacteriophages. Thus, the viral capsids are shed at the surface and only the nucleic acid genome enters the cell. In some cases, a small number of virion proteins may accompany the genome into the cell, but these are probably tightly associated with the nucleic acid or are essential enzymes needed to initiate the infection.

Tailed phages attach by tail fibers and DNA is injected through the tail

Bacteriophages with tails have evolved these special appendages to facilitate the entry of the genome into the cell. The process of penetration and uncoating for bacteriophage T4 is shown schematically in Figure 6–2. The tail fibers extending from the end of the tail are responsible for the attachment of the virion to the cell wall, and, in the next step, the end of the tail itself makes intimate contact with the cell surface. Finally the DNA of the virus is injected directly into the cell through the hollow tail structure. The process has been likened to the action of a syringe, but the energetics and the nature of the orifice in the cell surface through which the DNA travels are poorly understood.

### Enveloped Animal Viruses

There are two basic mechanisms for the entry of an enveloped animal virus into the cell. Both mechanisms involve fusion of the viral envelope with a cellular membrane, and the end result in both cases is the release of the free nucleocapsid into the cytoplasm. What distinguishes the two mechanisms is the nature of the cellular membrane that fuses with the viral envelope.

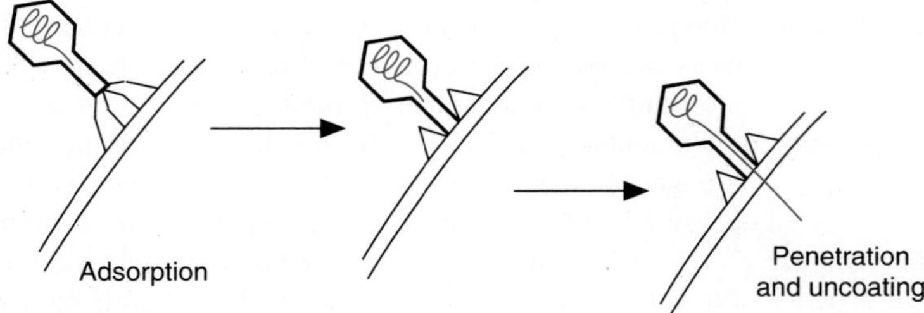


**Figure 6–2.** Bacteriophage entry.

Figure 6–3 depicts the entry mechanism for paramyxoviruses such as the measles virus. The envelopes of these viruses contain protein spikes that promote fusion of viral envelopes with the plasma membrane of the cell, releasing the nucleocapsid directly into the cytoplasm. Because the viral envelope becomes incorporated into the plasma membrane of the infected cell and still possesses its fusion proteins, infected cells have a tendency to fuse with other uninfected cells. Cell–cell fusion is a hallmark of infections by paramyxoviruses and can be important in the pathology of a disease such as measles.

Some enveloped viruses enter cells by membrane–envelope fusion

The mechanism for the entry of most of the remaining enveloped animal viruses, such as orthomyxoviruses (eg, influenza viruses), togaviruses (eg, rubella virus), rhabdoviruses (eg, rabies), and herpesviruses, is shown in Figure 6–4. Following adsorption, the virus particles are taken up by a cellular mechanism called **receptor-mediated endocytosis,** which is normally responsible for internalizing growth factors, hormones, and some nutrients. When it involves viruses, the process is referred to as **viropexis.**

Other enveloped and naked viruses are taken in by receptor-mediated endocytosis (viropexis)

In viropexis the adsorbed virions become surrounded by the plasma membrane in a reaction that is probably facilitated by the multiplicity of virion attachment proteins on the surface of the particle. Pinching off of the cellular membrane by fusion encloses the virion in a cytoplasmic vesicle termed the **endosomal vesicle.** The nucleocapsid is now surrounded by two membranes, the original viral envelope and the newly acquired plasma membrane. The surface receptors are subsequently recycled back to the plasma membrane, and the endosomal vesicle is acidified by an unknown mechanism. The low pH of the endosome leads to a conformational change in a viral spike protein, which results in the fusion of the two membranes and release of the nucleocapsid into the cytoplasm. In some cases, the contents

Acidified endosome releases nucleocapsid to cytoplasm

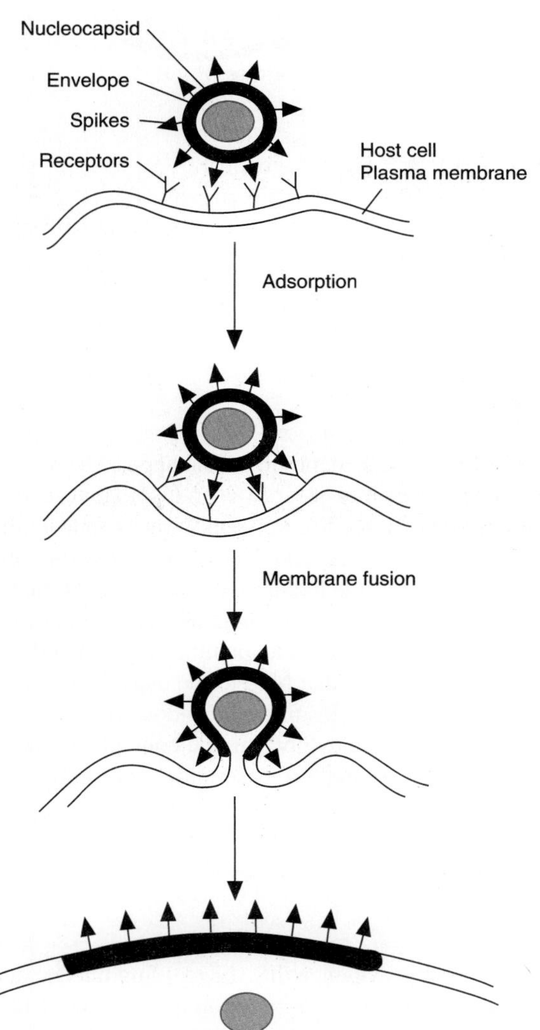


**Figure 6–3.** Paramyxovirus entry.

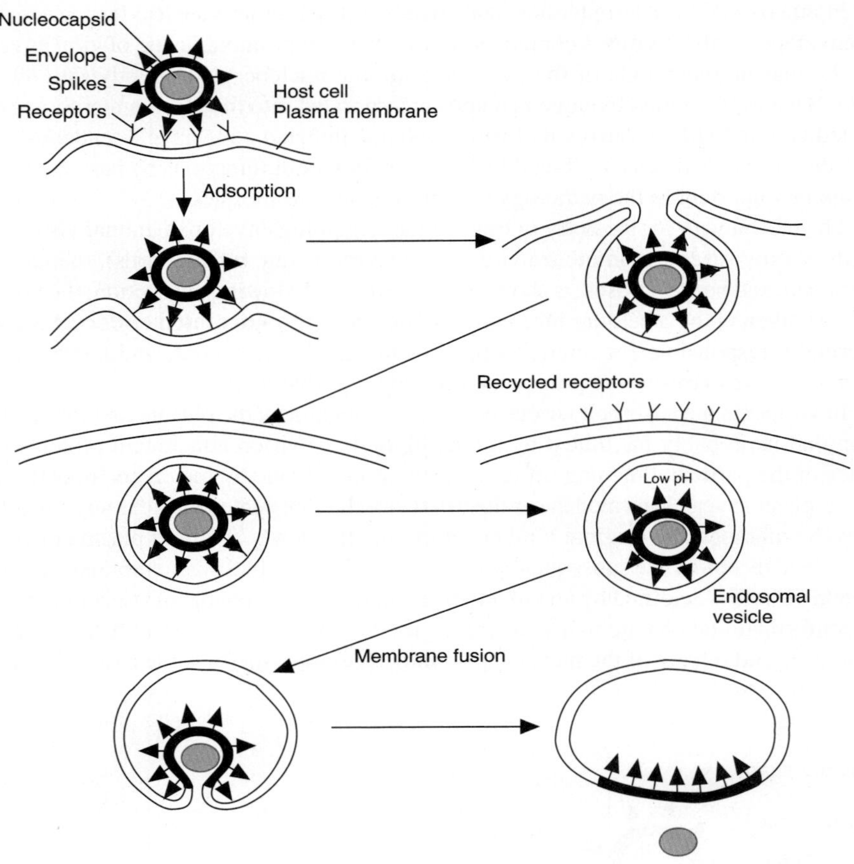


**Figure 6–4.** Viropexis.

of the endosomal vesicle may be transferred to a lysosome prior to the fusion step that releases the nucleocapsid.

## Naked Capsid Animal Viruses

Virions may escape endosome by dissolution

Naked capsid viruses, such as poliovirus, reovirus, and adenovirus, also appear to enter the cell by viropexis. In this case, however, the virus cannot escape the endosomal vesicle by membrane fusion as described earlier for enveloped viruses. For poliovirus it appears that the viral capsid proteins in the low-pH environment of the endosome expose hydrophobic domains, which results in the binding of the virions to the membrane and release of the nucleic acid genome into the cytoplasm. In other cases the virions may escape into the cytoplasm by promoting the dissolution of the vesicle. This step is a potential target of antiviral chemotherapy, and recently drugs have been developed that bind to the capsids of certain picornaviruses and prevent the release of the virus particles from the endosome.

Reovirus is unusual in that prior to release into the cytoplasm, the contents of the endosome are transferred to a lysosome where the lysosomal proteases strip away part of the capsid proteins and activate virion-associated enzymes required for transcription.

## Fate of Intracellular Particles

Nucleic acid must be directed to target sites

Even in the relatively simple bacterial cell, there is evidence that the entering nucleic acid must be directed to a particular cellular locus to initiate the infection process. **Pilot proteins** have been described that accompany the phage genome into the bacterial cell and serve the function of "piloting" the nucleic acid to a particular target, such as a membrane site where transcription and replication are to occur.

The ultimate fate of internalized animal virus particles depends on the particular virus and on the cellular compartment where replication occurs. Most RNA viruses with the exception of influenza viruses and the retroviruses replicate in the cytoplasm, the immediate site of entry. Retroviruses, influenza viruses, and all the DNA viruses except the poxviruses must move from the cytoplasm to the nucleus to replicate. The larger DNA viruses, such as herpesviruses and adenoviruses, must uncoat to the level of cores prior to entry into the nucleus. The smaller DNA viruses, such as the parvoviruses and the papovaviruses, enter the nucleus intact through the nuclear pores and subsequently uncoat inside. The largest of the animal viruses, the poxviruses, carry out their entire replicative cycle in the cytoplasm of the infected cell.

Most RNA viruses replicate in cytoplasm

Influenza viruses, retroviruses, and DNA viruses except poxviruses replicate in the nucleus

## THE PROBLEMS OF PRODUCING mRNA

### From Genome to mRNA

An essential step in every virus infection is the production of mRNAs by transcription. The virus-specified mRNAs program the cellular ribosomes to synthesize viral proteins. Besides the structural proteins of the virion, viruses must direct the synthesis of enzymes and other specialized proteins required for genome replication, gene expression, and virus assembly and release. The production of the first viral mRNAs at the beginning of the infection is a crucial step in the takeover of the cell by the virus.

Virus-specified mRNAs direct synthesis of viral proteins

For some viruses the presentation of mRNA to the cellular ribosomes poses no problems. Thus, the genomes of most DNA viruses are transcribed by the host DNA-dependent RNA polymerase to yield the initial mRNAs. The (+)-strand RNA viruses, such as the picornaviruses, the togaviruses, and the coronaviruses, possess genomes that can be used directly as mRNAs and are translated (at least partially, as is discussed later) immediately on entry into the cytoplasm of the cell.

Most DNA virus mRNA is synthesized by host polymerase

(+)-strand RNA virus genome serves as mRNA

For many viruses, however, the production of mRNA starting from the genome is not so straightforward. The fact that poxviruses replicate in the cytoplasm means that the cellular RNA polymerase is not available to transcribe the genome. Moreover, no cellular machinery exists that can use either single-stranded or double-stranded RNA as a template to synthesize mRNA. Therefore, viruses with these types of genomes must provide their own transcription enzymes to produce the initial mRNAs at the beginning of the infection process. This is accomplished by synthesizing the transcriptases in the later stages of viral development in the previous host cell and packaging the enzymes into the virions, where they remain associated with the genome as the virus enters the new cell and uncoats. In general, the presence of a transcriptase in virions is indicative that the host cell is unable to use the viral genome as mRNA or as a template to synthesize mRNA. At later times in the infection of the cell, any special enzymatic machinery required by the virus, and not initially present in the cell, can be supplied among the proteins translated from the first mRNA molecules.

Other RNA viruses synthesize and package transcription enzymes to produce initial mRNAs

The pathways for the synthesis of mRNA by the major virus groups are summarized in Figure 6–5 and related to the structure of viral genomes. The polarity of mRNA is designated as (+) and the polarity of polynucleotide chains complementary to mRNA as (–). The black arrows denote synthetic steps for which host cells provide the appropriate enzymes, whereas the red arrows indicate synthetic steps that must be carried out by virus-encoded enzymes. Several additional points need to be emphasized. The parvoviruses and some phages have single-stranded DNA genomes. Although the RNA polymerase of the cell requires double-stranded DNA as a template, these viruses need not carry special enzymes in their virions because host cell DNA polymerases can convert the genomes into double-stranded DNA. Note that the production of mRNA by the picornaviruses and similar (+)-strand viruses requires the synthesis of an intermediate (–)-strand template. The enzyme required for this process is produced by translation of the genome RNA early in infection.

There are a variety of pathways for synthesis of mRNA by different virus groups

Single-stranded viral DNA can be converted to double-stranded DNA by host cell polymerases

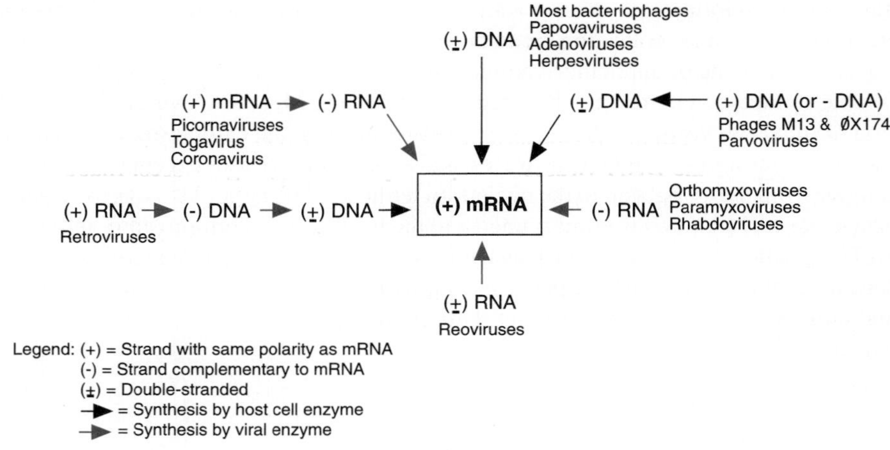


**Figure 6–5.** Pathways of mRNA synthesis for major virus groups.

Retroviral RNA is copied to DNA by virion reverse transcriptase; host RNA polymerase transcribes DNA into more RNA

The retroviruses are a special class of (+)-strand RNA viruses. Although their genomes are of the same polarity as mRNA and could in principle serve as mRNAs early after infection, their replication scheme apparently precludes this. Instead, the RNA genomes of these viruses are copied into (–)DNA strands by an enzyme carried within the virion called **reverse transcriptase**. The (–)DNA strands are subsequently converted by the same enzyme to double-stranded DNA in a reaction that requires the degradation of the original genomic RNA by the RNase H activity of the reverse transcriptase. The DNA product of reverse transcription is ultimately transcribed by the host RNA polymerase to complete the replication cycle as well as produce viral mRNA. The need to package reverse transcriptase in the virion apparently derives from the fact that translation of the genomic RNA to produce the enzyme early after infection would prevent the use of the RNA as a template for reverse transcription (see Chapter 41).

## The Monocistronic mRNA Rule in Animal Cells

Prokaryotic mRNA (and, thus, phage RNA) can be polycistronic

The ribosome requires input of information in the form of mRNA. For a viral mRNA to be recognized by the ribosome, its production must conform to the rules of structure that govern the synthesis of cellular mRNAs. Prokaryotic mRNA is relatively simple and can be polycistronic, which means it can contain the information for several proteins. Each cistron is translated independently beginning from its own ribosome binding site. In fact, the genome of the well-studied *Escherichia coli* RNA phage is just such a polycistronic mRNA.

Eukaryotic mRNAs are more complex, containing a special 5′-cap structure and a 3′-poly(A) attachment. In addition, their synthesis often involves removal of internal sequences by a process called **splicing**. Most importantly, virtually all eukaryotic mRNAs are monocistronic. Eukaryotic translation is initiated by the binding of the ribosome to the 5′-cap, followed by movement of the ribosome along the RNA until the first AUG initiation codon is encountered. The corollary to this first AUG rule is that the eukaryotic ribosome generally cannot initiate translation at internal sites on a mRNA. In special circumstances, it appears that this rule is broken, allowing one or more AUG sites to be skipped before initiation occurs. For the most part, however, animal viruses must program the synthesis of mRNAs that are translated to produce only a single polypeptide chain by initiation of translation near the 5′ end of the mRNA.

Animal virus mRNAs are monocistronic

Because most DNA animal viruses replicate in the nucleus, they adhere to the monocistronic mRNA rule either by having a promoter precede each gene or by programming the transcription of precursor RNAs that are processed by nuclear splicing enzymes into monocistronic mRNAs. The virion transcriptase of the cytoplasmic poxviruses apparently must synthesize monocistronic mRNAs by initiation of transcription in front of each gene.

Some RNA viruses have segmented genomes or splice precursor RNAs

RNA-containing animal viruses have evolved three different strategies to circumvent or conform to the monocistronic mRNA rule. The simplest strategy involves having a segmented genome. Each genome segment of the orthomyxoviruses and the reoviruses corresponds to a single gene; therefore, the mRNA transcribed from a given segment constitutes a monocistronic mRNA. The orthomyxovirus virus influenza A, unlike most RNA viruses, replicates in the nucleus and some of its monocistronic mRNAs are produced by splicing of precursor RNAs.

A second solution to the monocistronic mRNA rule is very similar to the strategy employed by cells and the DNA viruses. The paramyxoviruses, togaviruses, rhabdoviruses, and coronaviruses synthesize monocistronic mRNAs by initiating the synthesis of each mRNA at the beginning of a gene. In most cases, the transcriptase terminates mRNA synthesis at the end of the gene so that each message corresponds to a single gene. For the coronaviruses, RNA synthesis initiates at the beginning of each gene and continues to the end of the genome so that a set of mRNAs is produced. Each mRNA, however, is functionally monocistronic and is translated to produce only the protein encoded near its 5′ end.

Some viruses make monocistronic RNA by initiating synthesis at the start of each gene

The picornaviruses have evolved yet a third strategy to deal with the monocistronic mRNA requirement (Fig 6–6). The (+)-strand genome contains just a single ribosome binding site near the 5′ end and is translated into one long polypeptide chain called a **polyprotein.** The polyprotein is subsequently broken into the final set of protein products by a series of proteolytic cleavages. In fact, the required proteolytic activities reside within the polyprotein itself.

Picornaviruses make a polyprotein that is cleaved later

Several viruses employ more than one of these strategies to conform to the monocistronic mRNA rule. For example, the retroviruses and the togaviruses synthesize multiple mRNAs, each one coding for a polyprotein.

# GENOME REPLICATION

## DNA Viruses

Cells obviously contain the enzymes and accessory proteins required for the replication of DNA. In bacteria these proteins are present continuously, whereas in the eukaryotic cell they are present only during the S phase of the cell cycle, and they are restricted to the nucleus. The extent to which viruses depend on cell replication machinery depends on the size of their genome and, thus, on their protein-coding potential.

The smallest of the DNA viruses, the parvoviruses, are so completely dependent on host machinery that they require the infected cells to be dividing so that a normal S phase will occur and replicate their DNA along with the cellular DNA. At the other end of the spectrum are the largest of the viruses, which are relatively independent of cellular functions. The largest bacteriophages, such as T4, degrade the host cell chromosome early in infection and replace all of the host replication machinery with virus-specified proteins. The

The smallest DNA viruses depend exclusively on host DNA replication machinery

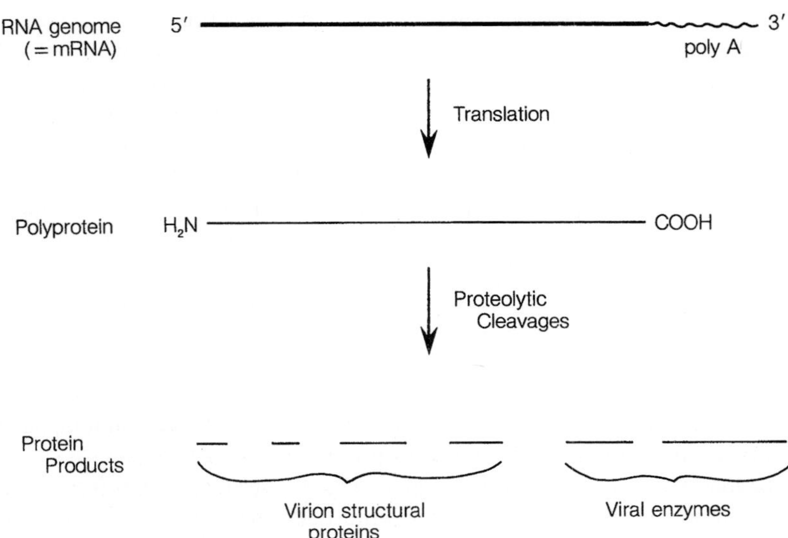


**Figure 6–6.** Poliovirus gene expression.

The largest DNA viruses code for enzymes important for DNA replication

largest animal viruses, the poxviruses, are similarly independent of the host. Because they replicate in the cytoplasm, they must code for virtually all of the enzymes and other proteins required for replicating their DNA.

The remainder of the DNA viruses are only partially dependent on host machinery. For example, bacteriophages øX174 and λ code for proteins that direct the initiation of DNA synthesis to the viral origin. The actual synthesis of DNA, however, occurs by the complex of cellular enzymes responsible for replication of the *Escherichia coli* DNA. Similarly the small DNA animal viruses, such as the papovaviruses, code for a protein that is involved in the initiation of synthesis at the origin, but the remainder of the replication process is carried out by host machinery. The slightly larger adenoviruses and herpesviruses, in addition to providing origin-specific proteins, also code for their own DNA polymerases and other accessory proteins required for DNA replication.

Herpesvirus-encoded DNA polymerase is a target of chemotherapy (eg, acyclovir)

The fact that the herpesviruses code for their own DNA polymerase has important implications for the treatment of infections by these viruses and illustrates a central principle of antiviral chemotherapy. Certain antiviral drugs (adenine arabinoside and 5′-iododeoxyuridine) have been found to be effective against herpesvirus infections (see Chapter 37), because they are sufficiently similar to natural substrates that the virally encoded DNA polymerase mistakenly incorporates them into viral DNA resulting in an inhibition of subsequent DNA synthesis. The host cell enzyme is more discriminatory and fails to use the analogs in the synthesis of cellular DNA; thus, the drugs do not kill uninfected cells. The antiviral drug acyclovir (acycloguanosine) preferentially kills herpesvirus-infected cells because the viral enzyme thymidine kinase, unlike the cellular counterpart, phosphorylates the thymidine analog, converting it to a form that when incorporated into DNA by DNA polymerases inhibits further DNA synthesis. In principle, any viral process that is distinct from a normal cellular process is a potential target for antiviral drugs. As more becomes known about the details of viral replication, more drugs will become available that are targeted to those processes unique to the virus.

All DNA viruses except parvoviruses can transform host cells

As noted earlier, with the exception of the poxviruses, all of the DNA animal viruses are at least partially dependent on host cell machinery for the replication of their genomes. Unlike the parvoviruses, however, the other DNA viruses do not need to infect dividing cells for a productive infection to ensue. Instead, all of these viruses code for a protein expressed early in infection that induces an unscheduled cycle of cellular DNA replication (S phase). In this way, these viruses ensure that the infected cell makes all of the machinery required for the replication of their DNA. It is noteworthy that all of the DNA viruses except the parvoviruses are capable, in some circumstances, of transforming a normal cell into a cancer cell (see Chapter 7). This correlation suggests that the unlimited proliferative capacity of the cancer cells may be due to the continual synthesis of the viral protein(s) responsible for inducing the unscheduled S phase in a normal infection. Therefore, the fact that these DNA viruses can induce oncogenic transformation of cell types that are nonpermissive for viral multiplication may simply be an accident related to the need to induce cellular enzymes required for DNA replication during lytic infection.

Replication on linear DNA has termination restraints

All DNA polymerases, including those encoded by viruses, synthesize DNA chains by the successive addition of nucleotides onto the 3′ end of the new DNA strand. Moreover, all DNA polymerases require a primer terminus containing a free 3′-hydroxyl to initiate the synthesis of a DNA chain. In cellular replication, a temporary primer is provided in the form of a short RNA molecule. The priming RNA is synthesized by an RNA polymerase, and after elongation by the DNA polymerase it is removed. With circular chromosomes, such as those found in bacteria and many viruses, the unidirectional chain growth and primer requirement of the DNA polymerase pose no structural problems for replication. As illustrated in Figure 6–7, however, when a replication fork encounters the end of a linear DNA molecule, one of the new chains (heavy lines in Fig 6–7) cannot be completed at its 5′ end, because there exists no means of starting the DNA portion of the chain exactly at the end of the template DNA. Thus, after the RNA primer is removed, the new chain is incomplete at its 5′ end. This constraint on the completion of DNA chains on a linear template is sometimes called the **end problem** in DNA replication.

It is beyond the scope of this text to detail all of the strategies viruses have evolved to deal with this problem, but it is worthwhile pointing out some of the structural features found in linear viral genomes whose presence is related to the solutions to this problem. Some of

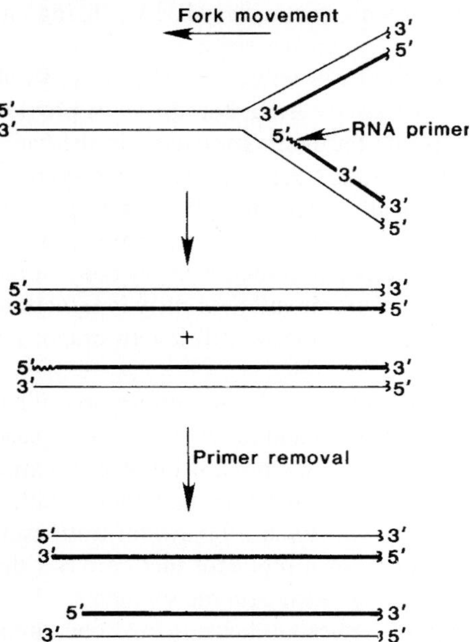


**Figure 6–7.** The end problem in DNA replication.

these structures are diagrammed schematically in Figure 6–8. The linear double-stranded genome of bacteriophage λ possesses 12-bp single-stranded extensions that are complementary in sequence to each other and thus called **cohesive ends.** Very early after entry into the cell, the two ends pair up to convert the linear genome into a circular molecule in preparation for replication. The linear double-stranded adenovirus genome contains a protein molecule covalently attached to the 5′ end of both strands. These proteins provide the primers required to initiate the synthesis of the DNA chains during replication, circumventing the need for RNA primers and thus solving the end problem in replication.

Protein is also found attached to the hepatitis B genome, presumably a vestige of chain initiation by this virus as well. The single-stranded parvovirus genome contains a self-complementary sequence at the 3′ end that causes the molecule to fold into a hairpin, making it self-priming for DNA replication. The poxviruses contain linear double-stranded genomes in which the ends are continuous. In the latter two cases, the solution to the end problem creates additional problems that must be solved to produce replication products that are identical to the starting genomes.

## RNA Viruses

RNA animal viruses generally replicate in the cytoplasm, as nuclear functions are primarily designed for DNA metabolism. Influenza and the other orthomyxoviruses are exceptions to this rule. They replicate in the nucleus using pieces of newly synthesized cellular mRNAs

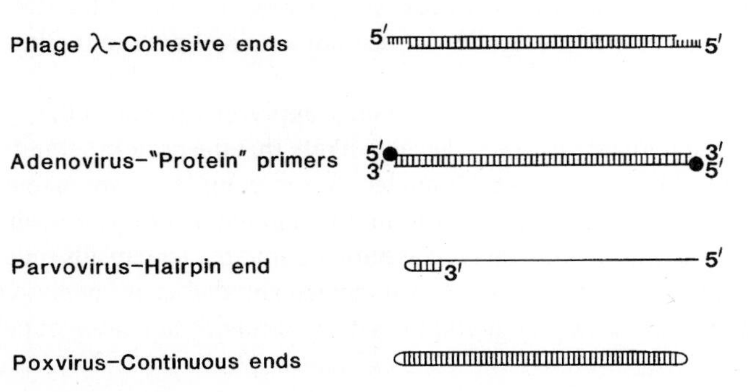


**Figure 6–8.** Some solutions to the end problem.

to prime their own mRNA synthesis. In addition, they use the nuclear RNA splicing enzymes in the synthesis of some of their mRNAs.

RNA viruses must encode their own transcriptases

Cells do not have RNA polymerases that can copy RNA templates. Therefore, RNA viruses not only need to code for transcriptases as discussed earlier, but also must provide the replicases required to duplicate the genomic RNA. Furthermore, except in the cases of the RNA phage and the picornaviruses, where transcription and replication are synonymous, the RNA viruses must temporally and functionally separate replication from transcription. This requirement is especially apparent for the rhabdoviruses, paramyxoviruses, togaviruses, and coronaviruses, where a complete genome, or complementary copy of the genome, is transcribed into a set of subgenomic monocistronic mRNAs early in infection. After replication begins, these same templates are used to synthesize full-length strands for replication.

Transcription and replication must be separated for most RNA viruses

Mechanisms for separating replication from transcription are varied

Two mechanisms exist to separate the process of replication from transcription. First, in many cases, transcription is restricted to subviral particles and involves a transcriptase transported into the cell within the virion. Second, the replication process involves a somewhat different set of enzymes that make full-length copies of the genome template rather than the shorter monocistronic mRNAs. In the case of reoviruses, the switch from transcription to replication appears to involve the synthesis of a replicase that converts the (+)mRNAs synthesized early in infection to the double-stranded genome segments.

Viral RNA polymerases synthesize chains in only one direction and generally without primers

Viral RNA polymerases, like DNA polymerases, synthesize chains in only one direction; however, RNA polymerases in general can initiate the synthesis of new chains without primers. Thus, there is no obvious end problem in RNA replication. There exists one exception to this general rule. The picornaviruses contain a protein covalently attached to the 5′ end of the genome called Vpg. It is clear that this protein is involved in priming the synthesis of new (−) strands as well as new (+)RNA viral genomes by a mechanism that appears to resemble the priming described earlier for adenoviruses.

## ASSEMBLY OF NAKED CAPSID VIRUSES AND NUCLEOCAPSIDS

Capsids and nucleocapsids self-assemble from preformed capsomeres

The formation of the capsid structure that surrounds the viral genome is called **encapsidation.** Four general principles govern the construction of capsids and nucleocapsids. First, the process generally involves self-assembly of the component parts. Second, assembly is stepwise and ordered. Third, individual protein structural subunits or protomers are preformed into capsomeres in preparation for the final assembly process. Fourth, assembly often initiates at a particular locus on the genome called a **packaging site.**

### Viruses With Helical Symmetry

Tobacco mosaic virus is a model for the construction of viral components

The assembly of the cylindrically shaped tobacco mosaic virus (TMV) has been extensively studied and provides a model for the construction of helical capsids and nucleocapsids. For TMV, donut-shaped disks containing many individual structural subunits are preformed and added stepwise to the growing structure. Elongation occurs in both directions from a specific packaging site on the single-stranded viral RNA (Fig 6–9). The addition of each disk involves an interaction between the protein subunits of the disk and the genome RNA. The nature of this interaction is such that the assembly process ceases when the end of the RNA is reached. The structural subunits as well as the RNA trace out a helical path in the final virus particle.

The basic design features worked out for TMV probably apply in general to the assembly of the nucleocapsids of enveloped viruses. Thus, it is likely that the protein subunits are intimately associated with the RNA and that the nucleoprotein complexes are assembled by the stepwise accretion of protein subunits. For influenza and the other viruses with segmented genomes, the various genome segments are assembled into nucleocapsids independently and then brought together during assembly by a mechanism that is as yet poorly understood. It is notable that virtually all of the animal RNA viruses with helical symmetry are enveloped.

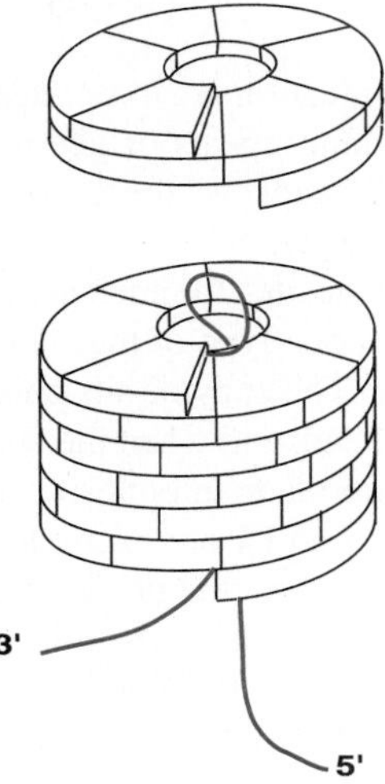


**Figure 6–9.** Tobacco mosaic virus assembly.

## Viruses With Cubic Symmetry

Icosahedral capsids are preassembled and the genomes are threaded in

For both phage and animal viruses, icosahedral capsids are preassembled and the nucleic acid genomes, usually complexed with condensing proteins, are threaded into the empty structures. Construction of the hollow capsids appears to occur by a self-assembly process, sometimes aided by other proteins. The stepwise assembly of components involves the initial aggregation of structural subunits into pentamers and hexamers, followed by the condensation of the capsomeres to form the empty capsid. In some cases, it appears that the structurally significant intermediates in assembly involve dimers or trimers of the structural subunits rather than pentamers and hexamers.

## Features Unique to Bacteriophages

Phage heads, tails, and tail fibers are synthesized separately and then assembled

The morphogenesis of a complex bacteriophage such as T4 involves the prefabrication of each of the major substructures by a separate pathway, followed by the ordered and sequential construction of the final particle from its component parts. Figure 6–10 diagrams the assembly process for T4 showing how the head, tail, and tail fibers are assembled and then brought together to form the completed phage (many steps are omitted).

An intermediate in the assembly of a bacteriophage head is an empty structure containing an internal protein network that is removed prior to insertion of the nucleic acid. The constituents of this network are often appropriately referred to as **scaffolding proteins.** The

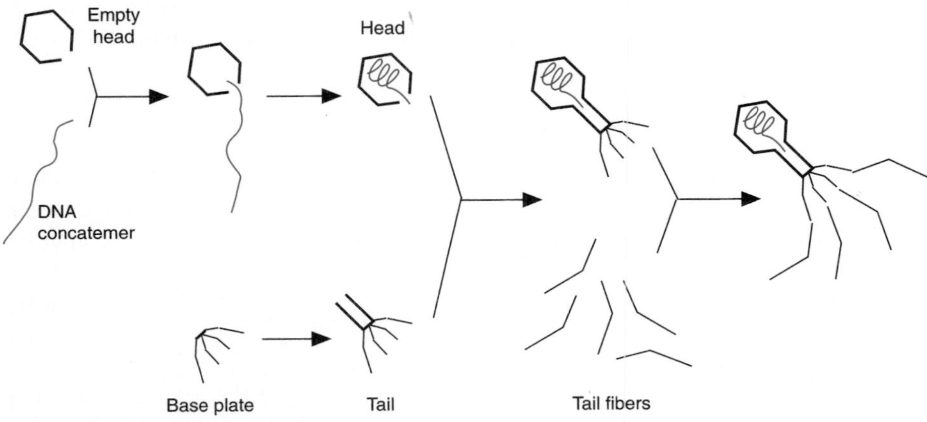


**Figure 6–10.** Assembly of bacteriophage T4.

scaffolding proteins apparently provide the lattice necessary to hold the capsomeres in position during the early stages of head assembly.

Some phage DNA is replicated to produce concatemers

For many DNA bacteriophages, the products of replication are long linear DNA molecules called **concatemers,** which are made up of tandem repeats of genome-size units. During the packaging of the DNA into the preformed capsids, these concatemers are processed by nuclease cleavages to generate genome-size pieces.

Mechanisms for cutting phage DNA during packaging involve site-specific nuclease or concatemer cuts

There are two mechanisms for determining the correct sites for nuclease cleavage during packaging of a concatemer. Bacteriophage λ typifies one type of mechanism in which the enzyme that makes the cuts is a site-specific nuclease. The enzyme sits poised at the orifice of the capsid as the DNA is being threaded into the head, and when the specific cut site is encountered, the DNA is cleaved. For λ, the breaks are made in opposite strands, 12 bp apart, to generate the cohesive ends. Bacteriophages T4 and P1 are examples of bacterial viruses that illustrate the second mechanism. For these phages, the nuclease does not recognize a particular DNA sequence, but instead cuts the concatemer when the capsid is full. Because the head of the bacteriophage can accommodate slightly more than one genome equivalent of DNA and packaging can begin anywhere on the DNA, the "headful" mechanism produces genomes that are terminally redundant (the same sequence is found at both ends) and circularly permuted. The fact that packaging is nonspecific with respect to DNA sequence explains why bacteriophage P1 is capable of incorporating host DNA into phage particles, thereby promoting generalized transduction (see Chapter 4). T4 does not carry out generalized transduction, because the bacterial DNA is completely degraded to nucleotides early in infection.

Host DNA may be incorporated by the headful mechanism, and generalized transduction results

## RELEASE

### Bacteriophages

Phages encode lysozyme or peptidases that lyse bacterial cell walls

Most bacteriophages escape from the infected cell by coding for an enzyme (or enzymes) synthesized late in the latent phase that causes the lysis of the cell. The enzymes are either lysozymes or peptidases, which weaken the cell wall by cleaving specific bonds in the peptidoglycan layer. The weakened cells burst as a result of the osmotic pressure.

### Animal Viruses

#### Cell Death

Naked capsid viruses lacking specific lysis mechanisms are released with cell death

Nearly all productively infected cells die (see below for exceptions), presumably because the viral genetic program is dominant and precludes the continuation of normal cell functions required for survival. The naked capsid animal viruses lack specific mechanisms for lysing the infected cell and apparently are released into the extracellular milieu simply as a consequence of cell death. Release may therefore be facilitated by the liberation of a variety of degradative lysosomal enzymes that aid in the dissolution of the dying cell.

#### Budding

Most enveloped viruses acquire an envelope during release by budding

With the exception of the poxviruses, all enveloped animal viruses acquire their membrane by budding either through the plasma membrane or, in the case of herpesviruses, through the nuclear membrane. Thus, for these viruses, release from the cell is coupled to the final stage of virion assembly. How the herpesviruses ultimately escape from the cell after budding through the nuclear membrane is unclear; they may travel through channels in the endoplasmic reticulum to get from the nucleus to the outside. The poxviruses appear to program the synthesis of their own outer membrane. How the poxvirus envelope is assembled on the nucleocapsid is not known.

Poxviruses synthesize their own envelopes

The membrane changes that accompany budding are just the reverse of the entry process described before for paramyxoviruses (compare Fig 6–3 and Fig 6–11). The region

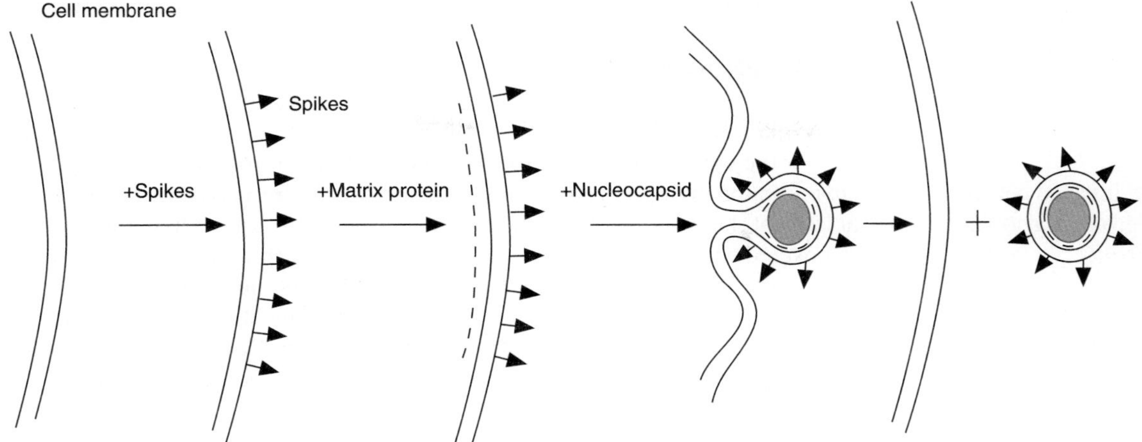


**Figure 6–11.** Viral release by budding.

of the cellular membrane where budding is to occur acquires a cluster of viral glycoprotein spikes. These proteins are synthesized by the pathway that normally delivers cellular membrane proteins to the surface of the cell by way of the Golgi apparatus. The presence of hydrophobic leader sequences on the amimo terminus tags the proteins for transport to the plasma membrane. At the site of the glycoprotein cluster, the inside of the membrane becomes coated with a virion structural protein called the **matrix** or **M protein.** The accumulation of the matrix protein at the proper location is probably facilitated by the presence of a binding site for the matrix protein on the cytoplasmic side of the transmembrane glycoprotein spike. The matrix protein attracts the completed nucleocapsid that triggers the membrane fusions that enclose the nucleocapsid in the envelope and at the same time release the completed particle to the outside (see Fig 6–11).

The membrane site for budding first acquires virus-specified spikes and matrix protein

For viruses that bud, it is important to note that the plasma membrane of the infected cell contains virus-specific glycoproteins that represent foreign antigens. This means that the infected cells become targets for the immune system. In fact, cytotoxic T lymphocytes that recognize these antigens can be a significant factor in combatting a virus infection.

The process of viral budding usually does not lead directly to cell death, because the plasma membrane can be repaired following budding. It is likely that cell death for most enveloped viruses, as for naked capsid viruses, is related to the loss of normal cellular functions required for survival. The causative agent of acquired immunodeficiency syndrome (AIDS) represents an exception to this generalization. The agent is a retrovirus (called human immunodeficiency virus type 1 [HIV-1]) that replicates in CD4+ T lymphocytes. It appears that the virus is latent in the host cell until triggered by external factors (see Chapter 41) to produce massive quantities of new virus. The cytotoxic nature of this virus, unlike most retroviruses, results from a combination of factors, including permanent membrane damage and the accumulation of unintegrated viral DNA in the cell.

The budding process rarely causes cell death

## Cell Survival

For retroviruses (except HIV-1) and the filamentous bacteriophages, virus reproduction and cell survival are compatible. Retroviruses convert their RNA genome into double-stranded DNA, which integrates into a host cell chromosome and is transcribed just like any other cellular gene (see Chapter 41). Thus, the impact on cellular metabolism is minimal. Moreover, the virus buds through the plasma membrane without any permanent damage to the cell (see above for HIV-1 exception).

Most retroviruses (except HIV) reproduce without cell death

Because the filamentous phages are nonenveloped viruses, cell survival is even more remarkable. In this case, the helical capsid is assembled onto the condensed single-stranded DNA genome as the structure is being extruded through both the membrane and the cell wall of the bacterium. How the cell escapes permanent damage in this case is unknown. As with the retroviruses, the infected cell continues to produce virus indefinitely.

Filamentous phages assemble during extrusion without damaging cells

## QUANTITATION OF VIRUSES

### Hemagglutination Assay

Virion and infected cell attachment proteins also bind red blood cells

For some animal viruses, red blood cells from one or more animal species contain receptors for the virion attachment proteins. Because both the receptors and attachment proteins are present in multiple copies on the cells and virions, respectively, an excess of virus particles coat the cells and cause them to aggregate. This aggregation phenomenon was first discovered with influenza virus and is called **hemagglutination.** The virion attachment protein on the influenza virion is appropriately called the **hemagglutinin.** Furthermore, the presence of the hemagglutinin in the plasma membrane of the infected cell means that the cells as well as the virions will bind the red blood cells. This reaction, called **hemadsorption**, is a useful indicator of infection by certain viruses (see Chapter 14).

The titer of hemagglutinin-containing virus can be measured by hemagglutination

Hemagglutination can be used to estimate the titer of virus particles in a virus-containing sample. Serially diluted samples of the virus preparation are mixed with a constant amount of red blood cells and the mixture is allowed to settle in a test tube. If there is insufficient virus to agglutinate the red blood cells, they will settle to the bottom of the tube and form a tight pellet; however, agglutinated red blood cells settle to the bottom to form a thin disperse layer of cells. The difference is easily scored visually and the endpoint of the agglutination is used as a relative measure of the virus concentration in the sample.

### Plaque Assay

Plaque assay: dilutions of virus are added to excess cells immobilized in agar

Replicated virus infects only neighboring cells, producing countable plaques

The plaque assay is a method for determining the titer of infectious virions in a virus preparation or lysate. The sample is diluted serially and an aliquot of each dilution is added to a vast excess of susceptible host cells. For an animal virus, the host cells are usually attached to the bottom of a plastic petri dish; bacterial cells are infected in suspension. In both cases the infected cells are immersed in a semisolid medium, such as agar, which localizes the infection to a particular site on the petri dish. Because of the agar, the virus released from the initial and subsequent infections can invade only the cells in the immediate vicinity of the initial infected cell. The end result is an easily visible clearing of dead cells at each of the sites on the plate where one of the original infected cells was localized. (Visualization in the case of animal cells usually requires staining the cells.) The clearing is called a **plaque** (Fig 6–12). By counting the number of plaques and correcting for the dilution fac-

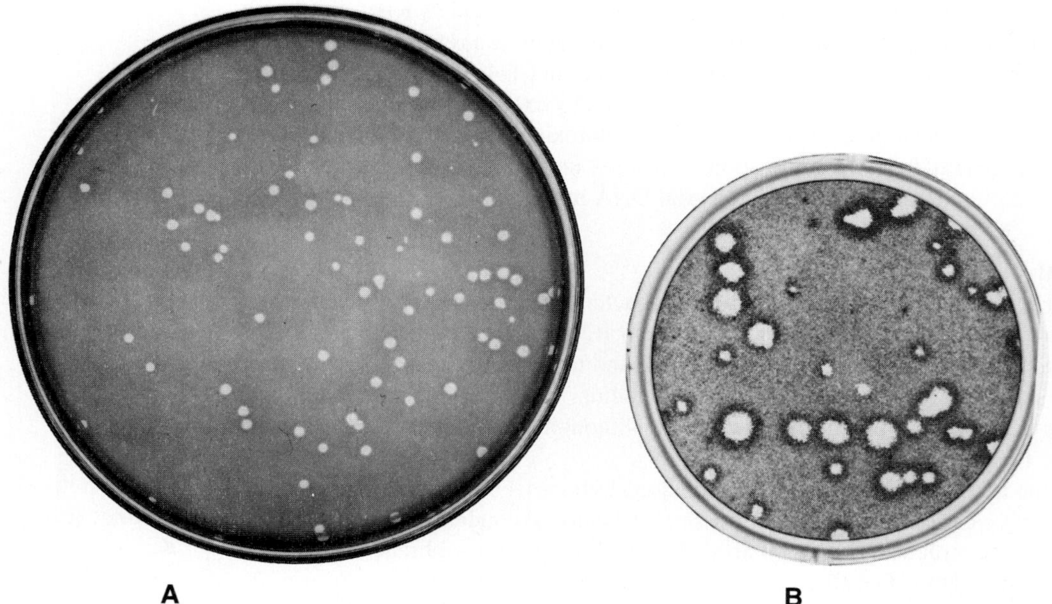


**Figure 6–12.** Plaque assays: **A.** Bacteriophage λ. **B.** Adenovirus.

tor, the virus titer in the original sample can be calculated. The titer is usually expressed as the number of plaque-forming units per milliliter (pfu/mL).

## INTERFERONS

Interferons are host-encoded proteins that provide the first line of defense against viral infections. Virus infection of all types of cells stimulates the production and secretion of an interferon that in turn acts on other infected cells to prevent virus production. Unlike immunity, interferon is not specific to a particular kind of virus; however, interferons usually act only on cells of the same species. Other agents stimulate the production of interferons by lymphoid cells. In this case interferon appears to play an important role in the immune system independent of any role as an antiviral protein (see Chapter 10).

Interferons are proteins from virally infected cells that inhibit viral production in other cells

Interferons are not virus specific

The signal that leads to the production of interferon by an infected cell appears to be double-stranded RNA. This conclusion is based on the fact that treatment of cells with purified double-stranded RNA or synthetic double-stranded ribopolymers results in the production of interferon. It is not obvious why double-stranded RNA should be present in an infected cell except in the case of reovirus. For the other RNA viruses, however, transcription and replication require complementary RNA molecules as templates. It is likely that complementary strands occasionally combine during the infection to produce sufficient quantities of double-stranded RNA to induce interferon. In the case of DNA viruses, double-stranded RNA may accumulate because transcription of a particular region of DNA occasionally occurs in both directions, producing complementary RNA strands. Alternatively, viral mRNAs may in general possess more secondary structure than the typical cellular mRNA.

Interferons are produced in response to accumulation of double-stranded RNA during viral synthesis

The viral inhibitory effects of interferon are not yet completely understood and what follows is at best an incomplete description of how interferon works. It appears that interferon acts to inhibit virus production at two different stages of protein synthesis. In the presence of interferon, the synthesis of two cellular enzymes is induced. The first is a protein kinase that phosphorylates and thereby inactivates one of the subunits of an elongation factor (eIF-2) necessary for protein synthesis. In some cases, viruses have evolved quite specific mechanisms to prevent the action of this protein kinase. The second is 2′,5′-oligo (adenylate) synthetase, which synthesizes chains of 2′,5′-oligo(A) up to 10 residues in length. The 2′,5′-oligo(A), in turn, activates a constitutive ribonuclease that degrades mRNA molecules. The action of both of these enzymes requires the presence of double-stranded RNA, the intracellular signal that an infection is occurring. This requirement prevents interferon from having an adverse effect on protein synthesis in uninfected cells. Thus, viral infection of a cell that has been exposed to interferon results in a general inhibition of protein synthesis, leading to cell death and no virus production. Therefore a cell that was doomed to die anyway is sacrificed for the good of the whole organism.

Interferons inhibit viral protein synthesis by inducing cellular enzymes that require double-stranded RNA

All protein synthesis is inhibited but only in infected cells

## ADDITIONAL READING

Joklik WK, ed. *Virology*. 3rd ed. Norwalk, CT: Appleton-Century-Crofts; 1988. An excellent overview of medical aspects of virology.

Specter S, Lancz G, eds. *Clinical Virology Manual*. 2nd ed. Norwalk, CT: Appleton and Lange; 1992. An up-to-date text with an emphasis on medical considerations.

Chapter 7

# Viral Genetics

James J. Champoux

In the typical lytic infection considered in Chapter 6, viruses invade a host cell and usurp the machinery of the cell for their own reproduction. The end result is usually cell death with the release of large numbers of new infectious virus particles, most of which are phenotypically identical to the original invading virus. This apparent homogeneity is deceptive, and in this chapter the methods whereby viral genomes change by mutation and recombination are considered, and the medical consequences of some of these changes are examined. The methods used by temperate viruses to enter, maintain, and sometimes leave the latent state are also discussed. Further, the means by which both bacterial and animal cells can be permanently changed by viral latency are examined in some detail.

## MECHANISMS OF GENETIC CHANGE

For DNA bacteriophages, the ratio of infectious particles to total particles usually approaches a value of one. Such is not the case for animal viruses. Typically less than 1% of the particles derived from an infected cell are infectious in other cells. Although some of this discrepancy may be attributable to inefficiencies in the assay procedures, it is clear that many defective particles are being produced. This production of defective particles arises because the mutation rates for animal viruses are unusually high and because many infections occur at high multiplicities, where defective genomes are complemented by nondefective viruses and therefore propagated.

Greater than 99% of animal virus particles from an infected cell are defective

### Mutation

Many DNA viruses use the host DNA synthesis machinery for replicating their genomes and, therefore, benefit from the built-in proofreading and other error-correcting mechanisms used by the cell; however, the largest animal viruses (adenoviruses, herpesviruses, and poxviruses) code for their own DNA polymerases and these enzymes lack efficient proofreading activities. The resulting high error rates in DNA replication endow the viruses with the potential for a high rate of evolution, but are also responsible for the high rate of production of defective viral particles.

Large DNA viruses lack proofreading capability and have high error rates

The replication of RNA viruses is also characterized by very high error rates, because viral RNA polymerases do not possess proofreading capabilities. The result is that error rates for RNA viruses commonly approach one mistake for every 2500 to 10,000 nucleotides polymerized. Such a high misincorporation rate ensures that, even for the smallest RNA viruses, virtually every round of replication introduces one or more nucleotide changes somewhere in the genome. If it is assumed that errors are introduced at random, most of the

Similar high error rates for RNA viruses produce genetically heterogeneous populations

members of a clone (eg, in a plaque) are different genetically from all other members of the clone. Because of the redundancy in the genetic code, some mutations are silent and are not reflected in changes at the protein level, but many occur in essential genes and contribute to the large number of defective particles found with RNA animal viruses. The concept of genetic stability takes on a new meaning in view of these considerations, and the virus population as a whole maintains some degree of homogeneity only because of the high degree of fitness exhibited by a small subset of the possible genome sequences. Thus, strong selective forces continually operate on a population to eliminate most mutants that fail to compete with the few very successful members of the population.

High mutation rates permit adaptation to changed conditions

The high mutation rates found for RNA viruses endow them with a genetic plasticity that leads readily to the occurrence of genetic variants and permits rapid adaptation to new environmental conditions. The large number of serotypes of the rhinoviruses causing the common cold, for instance, may reflect the potential to vary by mutation. Although rapid genetic change occurs for most if not all viruses, no RNA virus has exhibited this phenomenon as conspicuously as influenza virus. Point mutations accumulate in the influenza genes coding for the two envelope proteins (hemagglutinin and neuraminidase), resulting in changes in the antigenic structure of the virions. These changes lead to new variants not recognized by the immune system of previously infected individuals. This phenomenon is called **antigenic drift** (see Chapter 32). Apparently, those domains of the two envelope proteins that are most important for immune recognition are not essential for virus reproduction and, as a result, can tolerate amino acid changes leading to antigenic variation. This feature may distinguish influenza from other human RNA viruses that possess the same high mutation rates, but do not exhibit such high rates of antigenic drift. Antigenic drift in epidemic influenza viruses from year to year requires continual updating of the strains used to produce immunizing vaccines.

Mutations produce a diversity of rhinoviruses and antigenic drift in influenza viruses

Retroviruses use two error-prone polymerases for replication

The retroviruses likewise show high rates of variation because they depend for their replication on two different polymerases, both of which are error prone. In the first step of the replication cycle, the reverse transcriptase that copies the RNA genome into double-stranded DNA lacks a proofreading capability. Once the proviral DNA has integrated into the chromosome of the host cell, the DNA is transcribed by the host RNA polymerase II, which similarly is incapable of proofreading. As expected, these viruses exhibit a high rate of mutation in vitro and in vivo.

HIV-1 antigenic variation makes vaccine development difficult

Retroviruses that exhibit high rates of antigenic variation, such as human immunodeficiency virus type 1 (HIV-1), the causative agent of acquired immunodeficiency syndrome (AIDS), pose particularly difficult problems for the development of effective vaccines. Attempts are being made to identify conserved, and therefore presumably essential, domains of the envelope proteins for these viruses, which might be useful in developing a genetically engineered vaccine. Success will depend on finding regions that are common to all virulent strains and are capable of eliciting a neutralizing immune response.

## Von Magnus Phenomenon and Defective Interfering Particles

Defective interfering particles cause a decline in infectious titer

In early studies with influenza virus, it was noted that serial passage of virus stocks at high multiplicities of infection led to a steady decline of infectious titer with each passage. At the same time, the titer of noninfectious particles increased. As is discussed later, the noninfectious genomes interfere with the replication of the infectious virus and so are called **defective interfering (DI) particles**. Later, these observations were extended to include virtually all DNA as well as RNA animal viruses. The phenomenon is now named after von Magnus, who described the initial observations with influenza virus.

Deletion mutations result from mistakes in replication, recombination, or the dissociation of replicases

A combination of two separate events lead to this phenomenon. First, deletion mutations occur at a significant frequency for all viruses. For DNA viruses, the mechanisms are not well understood, but deletions presumably occur as a result of mistakes in replication or by nonhomologous recombination. The basis for the occurrence of deletions in RNA viruses is better understood. All RNA replicases have a tendency to dissociate from the template RNA, but remain bound to the end of the growing RNA chain. By reassociating with the same or a different template at a different location, the replicase can "finish" replication, but in the process create a shorter or longer RNA molecule. A subset of these variants possess the proper signals for initiating RNA synthesis and continue replicating. Because the deletion variants in the population require less time to complete a replication cycle, they eventually predominate and constitute the DI particles.

Second, as their name implies, the DI particles interfere with the replication of nondefective particles. Interference occurs because the DI particles successfully compete with the nondefective genomes for the limited supply of replication enzymes. The virions released at the end of the infection are therefore enriched for the DI particles. With each successive infection, the DI particles can predominate over the normal particles as long as the multiplicity of infection is high enough so that every cell is infected with at least one normal infectious particle. If this condition is met, then the normal particle can complement any defects in the DI particles and provide all of the viral proteins required for the infection. Eventually, however, as serial passage is continued, the multiplicity of infectious particles drops below one and the majority of the cells are infected only with DI particles. When this happens the proportion of DI particles in the progeny virus decreases.

Defective interfering particles produced by deletion mutations compete successfully for replication enzymes

In good laboratory practice, virus stocks are passaged at high dilutions to avoid the problem of the emergence of high titers of DI particles. Nevertheless, the presence of DI particles is a major contributor to the low fraction of infectious virus found in all virus stocks.

In principle, the emergence of high titers of DI particles during infections in humans could form the basis for a long-term viral infection that is hidden from the immune system and results in the gradual release of infectious virus. Whether this form of latency actually occurs and is a contributing factor to slow viral diseases remains to be seen.

## Recombination

Besides mutation, genetic recombination between related viruses is a major source of genomic variation. Bacterial cells as well as the nuclei of animal cells contain the enzymes necessary for homologous recombination of DNA. Thus, it is not surprising that recombinants arise from mixed infections involving two different strains of the same type of DNA virus. The larger bacteriophages such as λ and T4 code for their own recombination enzymes, a fact that attests to the importance of recombination in the life cycles of these viruses. The fact that recombination has also been observed for cytoplasmic poxviruses suggests that they too code for their own recombination enzymes.

Homologous recombination in DNA viruses

As far as is known, cells do not possess the machinery to recombine RNA molecules. Recombination among at least some RNA viruses has, however, been observed by two different mechanisms. The first is unique to the viruses with segmented genomes (orthomyxoviruses and reoviruses) and involves reassortment of segments rather than true recombination. A mixed infection of two different influenza viruses yields progeny virus different from either of the parents. The "recombinants" can be accounted for by the formation of new combinations of the genomic segments that are free to mix with each other at some time during the infection. Reassortment during mixed infections of human and certain animal influenza viruses is believed to account for the occasional drastic change in the antigenicity of the human virus. These dramatic changes, called **antigenic shifts**, produce strains to which much of the human population lacks immunity and, thus, can have enormous epidemiological and clinical consequences (see Chapter 32).

Genetic exchange between segmented genome RNA viruses involves reassortment of segments

Genomic reassortment probably accounts for antigenic shifts in influenza virus

Genetic recombination between different forms of poliovirus has also been observed. Because the poliovirus RNA genome is not segmented, reassortment cannot be invoked as the basis for the observed recombinants. In this case, it appears that recombination occurs during replication by a "copy choice" type of mechanism. During RNA synthesis, the replicase dissociates from one template and resumes copying a second template at the exact place where it left off on the first. The end result is a progeny RNA genome containing information from two different input RNA molecules. Strand switching during replication, therefore, generates a recombinant virus. Although this is not frequently observed, it is likely that most of the RNA animal viruses are capable of this kind of recombination.

Poliovirus replicase copies from two templates with strand switching to generate recombinants

A copy choice mechanism has also been invoked to explain a high rate of recombination observed with retroviruses. Early after infection, the reverse transcriptase within the virion synthesizes a DNA copy of the RNA genome in the cytoplasm of the infected cell. The process of reverse transcription requires the enzyme to "jump" between two sites on

The diploid nature of retroviruses permits template switching and recombination during DNA synthesis

the RNA genome (see Chapter 41). The propensity to switch templates apparently explains why the enzyme generates recombinant viruses. Because reverse transcription takes place in subviral particles, free mixing of RNA templates brought into the cell in different virus particles is not permitted. However, retroviruses are diploid since each particle carries two copies of the genome. This arrangement appears to be a situation ready-made for template switching during DNA synthesis and most likely accounts for retroviral recombination.

Occasional incorporation of host mRNA into retroviral particles may produce oncogenic virus

Occasionally, retroviruses package a cellular mRNA into the virion instead of a second RNA genome. This arrangement can lead to copy choice recombination between the viral genome and a cellular mRNA. The end result is sometimes the incorporation of a cellular gene into the viral genome. This mechanism is believed to account for the production of highly oncogenic retroviruses containing modified cellular genes (see below).

## THE LATENT STATE

The latent state involves infection of the cell with little or no virus production

Latent genomes can exist extrachromosomally or can be integrated

Latent virus may be silent, change cell phenotype, or reactivate to the lytic cycle

Temperate viruses can infect a cell and enter a latent state that is characterized by little or no virus production. The viral DNA genome is replicated and segregated along with the cellular DNA when the cell divides. There exist two possible states for the latent viral genome. It can exist extrachromosomally like a bacterial plasmid, or it can become integrated into the chromosome like the bacterial F factor in the formation of a high-frequency recombination (HFR) strain (see Chapter 4). Because the latent genome is usually capable of reactivation and entry into the lytic cycle, it is called a **provirus** or, in the case of bacteriophages, a **prophage.** In many cases, viral latency goes undetected; however, limited expression of proviral genes can occasionally endow the cell with a new set of properties. For instance, lysogeny can lead to the production of virulence-determining toxins in some bacteria (lysogenic conversion). Latency by an animal virus may produce oncogenic transformation.

## LYSOGENY

*E. coli* phage λ may be lytic or latent

Infection of an *Escherichia coli* cell by bacteriophage λ can have two possible outcomes. A fraction of the cells (ranging up to 90%) enters the lytic cycle and produces more phage. The remainder of the cells enter the latent state by forming stable lysogens. The proportion of the population that lyses depends on as yet undefined factors including the nutritional and physiologic state of the bacteria. In the lysogenic state, the phage DNA is physically inserted into the bacterial chromosome (see below) and thus replicates when the bacterial DNA replicates. Lambda can replicate either extrachromosomally as in the lytic cycle or as a part of the bacterial chromosome in lysogeny. The only phage gene that remains active in a lysogen is the gene that codes for a repressor protein that turns off expression of all of the prophage genes except its own. This means that the lysogenic state can persist as long as the bacterial strain survives. Because the lysogen contains more repressor proteins than are required to occupy the prophage operators, and because the repressor binds to the operators of any λ DNA entering the cell, the lysogen is resistant to reinfection by λ. This phenomenon is called **superinfection immunity.** Environmental insults, most notably exposure to ultraviolet light, cause inactivation of the repressor, resulting in loss of repression and induction of the bacteria to proceed through the lytic cycle.

When integrated silently, the only active gene encodes repressor for other phage genes

Loss of repressor causes induction and virus production

Once established, perpetuation of the lysogenic state requires a mechanism to ensure that copies of the phage genes are faithfully passed on to both daughter cells during cell division. In the lysogenic state, bacteriophage P1 exists extrachromosomally as an autonomous single-copy plasmid. Its replication is tightly coupled to chromosomal replication and the two replicated copies are precisely partitioned to daughter cells. Bacteriophage λ integrates into the *E. coli* chromosome to guarantee its replication and successful segregation during cell division.

Latent phage P1 exists as an extrachromosomal plasmid

Because of its mechanistic importance and relevance to lysogenic conversion and phage transduction (see Chapter 4), λ integration and the reverse reaction called **excision** are described in some detail. Bacteriophage λ integrates by a site-specific, reciprocal recombination event as outlined in Figure 7–1. There exist unique attachment sites on both the phage and bacterial chromosomes where the crossover occurs. The phage attachment site is called *attP* and the bacterial site, which is found on the *E. coli* chromosome between

Phage λ integrates by site-specific recombination

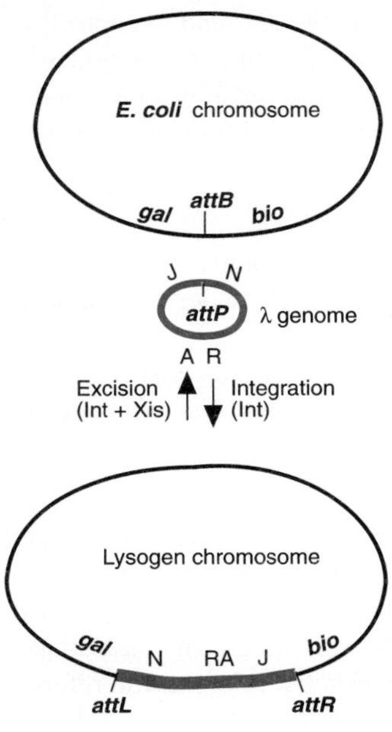


**Figure 7–1.** λ integration and excision. A, J, N, and R show the locations of some λ genes on the λ genome; *gal* and *bio* represent the *Escherichia coli* galactose and biotin operons, respectively.

the galactose and biotin operons, is called *attB*. The recombination reaction is catalyzed by the phage-encoded integrase protein (Int) in conjunction with two host proteins and occurs by a highly concerted reaction that requires no new DNA synthesis.

Excision after induction involves recombination at junctions between host DNA and prophage

Excision of the phage genome after induction of a lysogen by ultraviolet light is just the reverse of integration, except that excision requires, in addition to the Int protein, a second phage protein called Xis. In this case the combined activities of these two proteins catalyze site-specific recombination between the two attachment sites that flank the prophage DNA, *attL* and *attR* (see Fig 7–1). Early after infection, when integration is to occur in some fraction of the infected cells, synthesis of the Xis protein is blocked. Otherwise, the integrated prophage DNA would excise soon after integration and stable lysogeny would be impossible. After induction of a lysogen, however, both the integrase and the Xis proteins are synthesized and catalyze the excision event that releases the prophage DNA from the chromosome.

Specialized transduction occurs because excision can involve genes adjacent to the phage genome

At a very low frequency, excision involves sites other than the *attL* and *attR* borders of the prophage and results in the linking of bacterial genes to the phage genome. Thus, if a site to the left of the bacterial *gal* genes recombines with a site within the λ genome (to the left of the J gene, otherwise the excised genome is too large to be packaged), then the resulting phage can transduce the genes for galactose metabolism to another cell (see Chapter 4). Similarly, transducing particles can be formed that carry the genes involved in biotin biosynthesis. Because only those cellular genes adjacent to the attachment site can be picked up by an aberrant excision event, this process is called **specialized transduction** to distinguish it from generalized transduction, in which virtually any bacterial gene can be transferred by headful packaging (see Chapters 4 and 6).

Lysogenic conversion results from expression of a prophage gene that alters cell phenotype

Several bacterial exotoxins are encoded in temperate phages

Occasionally, one or more phage genes, in addition to the gene coding for the repressor protein, are expressed in the lysogenic state. If the expressed protein confers a new phenotypic property on the cell, then it is said that lysogenic conversion has occurred. Diphtheria, scarlet fever, and botulism are all caused by toxins produced by bacteria that have been "converted" by a temperate bacteriophage. In each case, the gene that codes for the toxin protein resides in the phage DNA and is expressed along with the repressor gene in the lysogenic state. It remains a mystery as to how these toxin genes were acquired by the phage; it is speculated that they may have been picked up by a mechanism similar to specialized transduction.

## MALIGNANT TRANSFORMATION

A tumor is an abnormal growth of cells. Tumors are classified as benign or malignant, depending on whether they remain localized or have a tendency to invade or spread by metas-

Malignant cells fail to respond to signals controlling the growth and location of normal cells

tasis. A malignant cell, therefore, has at least two defects. It fails to respond to controlling signals that normally limit the growth of nonmalignant cells, and it fails to recognize its neighbors and remain in its proper location. Malignant tumor cells, when grown in tissue culture in the laboratory, exhibit a series of properties that correlate with the uncontrolled growth potential associated with the tumor in the organism:

1. Their cell morphology is altered.
2. They fail to grow in the organized patterns found for normal cells.
3. They grow to much higher cell densities than do normal cells under conditions of unlimited nutrients.
4. They have lower nutritional and serum requirements than normal cells.
5. They have the capacity to divide in suspension, whereas normal cells require an anchoring substrate and grow only on surfaces (eg, on glass or plastic).
6. They are able to grow indefinitely in cell culture.

Malignant transformation of cells in culture can be accomplished by DNA viruses and some retroviruses

Oncogenic viruses cause tumors in their host species

Many DNA animal viruses and some representatives of the retroviruses can convert normal cultured cells into cells that possess the properties listed above. This process is called **malignant transformation.** In addition to the listed properties, viral transformation usually, but not always, endows the cells with the capacity to form a tumor when introduced into the appropriate animal. Although the original use of the term **transformation** referred to the changes occurring in cells grown in the laboratory, current usage often includes the initial events in the animal that lead to the development of a tumor. In recent years, it has become increasingly clear that some but not all of these viruses also cause cancers in the host species from which they were isolated. The oncogenic potential of animal DNA viruses is summarized in Table 7–1.

All known DNA animal viruses with the exception of the parvoviruses are capable of causing aberrant cell proliferation under some conditions. For some viruses, transformation or tumor formation has been observed only in species other than the natural host. Apparently infections of cells from the natural host are so cytocidal that no survivors remain to be transformed. In addition, some viruses have been implicated in human or animal tumors without any indication that they can transform cells in culture.

Transformation is analogous to lysogenic conversion but recombination is nonhomologous

In nearly all cases that have been characterized, viral transformation is the result of the continual expression of one or more viral genes (see Chapter 6). In many respects, transformation is analogous to lysogenic conversion and requires that the viral genes be incorporated into the cell as inheritable elements. Incorporation usually involves integration into the chromosome (eg, papovaviruses, the adenoviruses, and the retroviruses), although some papillomavirus DNAs and some herpesvirus DNAs are found in transformed cells as extrachromosomal plasmids. Unlike many temperate bacteriophages that code for the enzymes necessary for integration, papovaviruses and adenoviruses integrate by nonhomologous recombination using enzymes present in the host cell. The recombination event is therefore nonspecific, both with respect to the viral DNA and with respect to the chromosomal locus

**TABLE 7–1. ONCOGENICITY OF DNA VIRUSES**

| Virus or Virus Group | Tumors in Natural Host[a] | Tumors in Other Species[b] | Transform Cells in Tissue Culture |
|---|---|---|---|
| Parvoviruses (rat, mouse, human) | No | No | No |
| Animal polyomaviruses (polyoma, simian virus 40) | No | Yes | Yes |
| Human polyomaviruses (JC, BK) | No | Yes | Yes |
| Papillomaviruses (human, rabbit) | Yes, often benign | ? | Yes |
| Human hepatitis B virus | Yes | ? | No |
| Human adenoviruses | No | Yes | Yes |
| Human herpesviruses | Yes | Yes | Yes |
| Poxviruses (human, rabbit) | Occasionally, usually benign | Yes | No |

[a] "Yes" means that at least one member of the group is oncogenic.
[b] Test usually done in newborns or immunosuppressed hosts.

at which insertion occurs. It follows that for transformation to be successful, the insertional recombination must not occur within any viral gene required for transformation. Furthermore, in many cases only that portion of the viral genome that carries these genes is found integrated into the transformed cell DNA and the complete genome is not recoverable. In summary, two events appear to be necessary for viral transformation: a persistent association of viral genes with the cell and the expression of certain viral "transforming" proteins.

Only part of a transforming viral genome may be integrated; the complete genome is not recoverable

## Transformation by Retroviruses

Two features of the replicative cycle of retroviruses are related to the oncogenic potential of this class of viruses. First, most retroviruses do not kill the host cell, but instead set up a permanent infection with continual virus production. Second, the DNA copy of the RNA genome is integrated into the host cell DNA by a virally encoded integrase (IN); however, unlike bacteriophage λ integration, a linear form of the viral DNA, rather than a circular form, is the substrate for integration. Furthermore, unlike λ, there does not appear to be a specific site in the cell DNA where integration occurs.

Retroviral continuous production proceeds without host cell death

A DNA copy of the viral genome is integrated, but not at a specific site

Retroviruses are known to transform cells by three different mechanisms. First, many animal retroviruses have acquired transforming genes called **oncogenes.** More than 25 such oncogenes have now been found since the original gene *src* was identified in Rous sarcoma virus. Because normal cells possess homologs of these genes (called **protooncogenes**) it is generally assumed that viral oncogenes originated from host DNA. It is possible they were picked up by copy choice recombination involving packaged cellular mRNAs as described earlier. Most viral oncogenes have suffered one or more mutations that make them different from the cellular protooncogenes. These changes presumably alter the protein products so that they cause transformation. Although the mechanisms of oncogenesis are not well understood, it appears that transformation results from inappropriate production of an abnormal protein that interferes with normal signaling processes within the cell. Uncontrolled cell proliferation is the result. Because tumor formation by retroviruses carrying an oncogene is efficient and rapid, these viruses are often referred to as **acute transforming viruses.** Although common in some animal species, this mechanism has not yet been recognized as a cause of any human cancers.

Retroviruses may carry transforming oncogenes

Oncogenes encode a protein that interferes with cell signaling

The second mechanism is called **insertional mutagenesis** and is not dependent on continued production of a viral gene product. Instead, the presence of the viral promoter or enhancer is sufficient to cause the inappropriate expression of a cellular gene residing in the immediate vicinity of the integrated provirus. This mechanism was first recognized in avian B-cell lymphomas caused by an avian leukosis virus, a disease characterized by a very long latent period. Tumor cells from different individuals were found to have a copy of the provirus integrated at the same place in the cellular DNA. The site of the provirus insertion was found to be next to a cellular protooncogene called c-*myc*, where the c stands for cellular. The *myc* gene had previously been identified as a viral oncogene called v-*myc*. In this case, transformation occurs not because the c-*myc* gene is altered by mutation, but because the gene is turned on continuously and the gene product is overproduced. The disease has a long latent period, because, although the birds are viremic from early life, the probability of an integration occurring next to the c-*myc* gene is very low. Once such an integration event does occur, however, cell proliferation is rapid and a tumor develops. No human tumors are known to result from insertional mutagenesis caused by a retrovirus; however, human cancers are known where a chromosome translocation has placed an active cellular promoter next to a cellular protooncogene (Burkitt's lymphoma and chronic myelogenous leukemia).

Insertional mutagenesis causes inappropriate expression of a protooncogene adjacent to integrated viral genome

The third mechanism was revealed by the discovery of the first human retrovirus. The virus, human T-cell lymphotropic virus type 1 (HTLV-1), is the causative agent of adult T-cell leukemia. HTLV-1 is found integrated in the DNA of the leukemic cells, and all the tumor cells from a particular individual have the proviral DNA in the same location. This observation implies that the tumor is a clone derived from a single cell; however, the sites of integration in tumors from different individuals are found to be different. Thus, HTLV-1 does not cause malignancy by promoter insertion near a particular cellular gene. Instead, the virus codes for a protein that acts in trans (ie, on other genes in the same cell) to pro-

Human T-cell leukemia is caused by transactivating factor encoded in integrated HTLV-1

Transactivating factor turns on cellular genes, causing cell proliferation

mote maximal transcription of the proviral DNA and also turns on one or more cellular genes to cause cell proliferation. The viral gene coding for this protein is called *tax* for transactivating factor. The *tax* gene is therefore different from the oncogenes of the acute transforming retroviruses in that it is a viral gene rather than a gene derived from a cellular protooncogene.

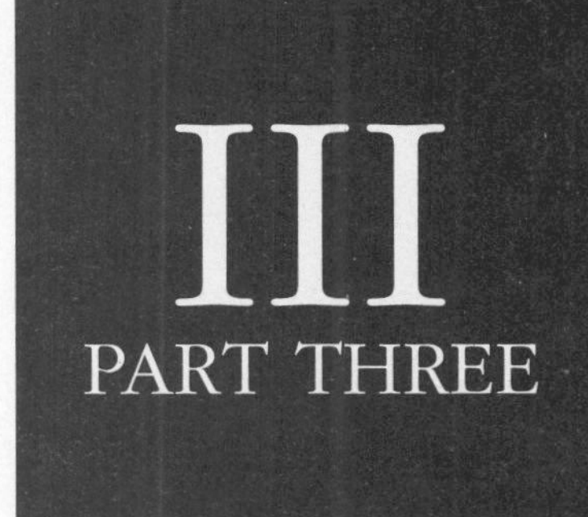


# Host–Parasite Interactions

Chapter

8

# A Survey of Immunologic Principles

*John J. Marchalonis*

There are many innate defenses that protect us from potential pathogens, including structural barriers, phagocytes, and others that are considered in Chapter 10. The immune response of vertebrates differs from these in that it is a specific, inducible, and anticipatory defense mechanism that allows the discrimination between self and nonself. The concept of immunity on which the science of immunology is built begins with ancient observations, such as Thucydides' description of the plague of Athens in 430 BC in which individuals who were infected and survived were not attacked again. A specific contemporary definition of the immune response is that it is a complex and precisely regulated inducible defense mechanism that allows the specific discrimination between self and nonself. The immune system requires for its function the presence of antigen-specific lymphocytes of two major types, thymus-derived lymphocytes (T cells) and bone-marrow derived lymphocytes (B cells), and builds on the more primitive defense mechanisms such as phagocytosis while using mediators of cell communication termed **cytokines** to facilitate regulation of the complex system. Another characteristic that defines the immune response of mammals is that it is anticipatory in that a process of gene rearrangement produces an array of T and B cells of millions of different specificities in advance of any challenge. Those in turn produce circulating antibodies that respond to the foreign challenge as well as to generate the T-cell receptors that allow the initiation of the specific immune process as well as the means for specific recognition by the effector T lymphocytes.

Immunity discriminates between self and nonself

Specific mechanisms are inducible

One of the major successes of immunology has been eradication by vaccination of historic scourges such as smallpox. In addition to defense against infection the immune system is important in normal developmental processes, aging, maintenance of internal homeostasis, and surveillance against neoplasms. This chapter presents an overview of major features of the immune system that are relevant to medical microbiology and infectious diseases. It is also intended to allow readers who have not yet studied immunology to understand the details of host–parasite interactions and immune responses to specific infections that are given elsewhere in the text. A listing of current immunology texts is provided at the end of the chapter.

Important for developmental processes and defense against infectious disease

The immune response differs from the innate or constitutive mechanisms in two major respects. The first is that the response is inducible; that is, the challenge to a healthy individual by a bacterium, virus, or other foreign (nonself) matter initiates a process leading to the production of circulating proteins called **antibodies** that recognize and bind the invading pathogen in a specific manner. A second challenge by the same pathogen results in an accelerated immune response (secondary or anamnestic) that can confer greater protection on the host.

Antibodies are inducible proteins that recognize and bind to invaders

Enormous capacity for diversity in recognition

The second major definitive characteristic of the human immune response is that it is anticipatory; that is, it has the potential to respond to pathogens not yet encountered in evolutionary history. This striking feature of the immune response results from the large number of genes specifying individual antibody combining sites for antigen and from a genetic recombination mechanism that allows us to form millions of potential antibody combining

**TABLE 8–1. CELLS INVOLVED IN THE IMMUNE SYSTEM**

| Cell | Function | Specific Receptors for Antigen | Characteristic Cell Surface Marker | Special Characteristics |
|---|---|---|---|---|
| B cells | Production of antibody<br>Present antigen to T cells | Surface immunoglobulin ($IgM_m$, $IgD_m$) | Fc and complement C3d receptors; MHC class II | Differentiate into plasma cells (major antibody producers) |
| T cells<br>Helpers ($T_H$) | Stimulate B cells by providing specific and nonspecific (cytokine) signals for activation and differentiation | α/β Tcr | CD3+, CD4+, CD8– | Activation is restricted by MHC class II |
| | Activate macrophages by cytokines | | | Can be classified into two types: $T_H1$ activates macrophages, makes interferon γ; $T_H2$ activates B cells, makes IL-4 |
| Cytotoxic ($T_c$) | Lyse antigen-expressing cells such as virally infected cells or allografts | α/β Tcr | CD3+, CD4–, CD8+ | Restricted by MHC class I |
| Suppressors ($T_s$) | Downregulate cellular or humoral immunity | α/β Tcr; other variant Tcr | Can be CD3+ or CD3–; usually CD4–, CD8+ | |
| Natural killer (NK) cells | Spontaneous lysis of tumor cells, antibody-dependent cellular cytotoxicity | Unknown | Fc receptor for IgG | |
| Macrophages (monocytes) | Phagocytosis, secretion of cytokines to activate T cells (eg, IL-1) or other accessory cells such as neutrophils | None but can be "armed" by antibodies binding to Fc receptors | Macrophage surface antigens | Express surface receptors for the activated third component of complement (C3), kill ingested bacteria by oxidative bursts |
| Polymorphonuclear leukocytes (neutrophils, eosinophils) | Phagocytosis killing | None but can be "armed" by antibodies | | Protective in parasitic infections, but adverse side effects such as granuloma formation can occur |

*Abbreviations:* Tcr, T-cell receptor; MHC, major histocompatibility complex.

sites. The system is also endowed with the property of memory, so that reexposure to the inciting agent in the future usually brings about an enhanced response.

## THE IMMUNORESPONSIVE CELLS

The function of the immune system requires antigen-specific lymphocytes of two major types (Table 8–1) and cytokines. **T cells** are thymus-derived lymphocytes and **B cells** are bone marrow-derived lymphocytes. **Cytokines** are secreted polypeptides that modulate the functions of cells (Table 8–2). Those produced by mononuclear cells (ie, lymphocytes and mononuclear phagocytic cells) are called **interleukins.** These (see later discussion) regulate the growth and differentiation of lymphocytes and hematopoietic stem cells.

T cells initiate and modulate immune responses and act directly

T cells are responsible for (1) the initiation and modulation of immune responses (including B-cell responses), (2) cell-mediated immune processes that involve direct damage to antigen-bearing tissue or blood cells (eg, virally infected host cells), and (3) stimulation and enhancement of the nonspecific immune functions of the host (eg, the inflammatory reaction and antimicrobial activity of phagocytes). T cells are classified by the presence of the surface molecules called **CD4** and **CD8**, which in turn are related to functional activities classified as helper, suppressor, or cytotoxic.

B cells responsible for humoral immunity

B cells are responsible for humoral immunity through antibody production. Individual B cells have antibody of a single specificity on their surface that can bind directly to foreign antigens. B cells can also differentiate into plasma cells which produce a soluble antibody that can circulate in blood and body fluids independent of cells.

T and B cells are found throughout the body, particularly in the bone marrow, specialized areas of the lymph nodes and spleen, lymphoid structures adjacent to the alimentary and respiratory tracts (eg, Peyer's patches and adenoids), and subepithelial tissues of the internal organs. They are continually replaced, and there is considerable circulation of B and T cells between the different areas of the body through the lymphatic and blood vascular circulations.

## ANTIGENS AND EPITOPES

Antigens stimulate and react with antibody

An **antigen** is a substance (usually foreign) that reacts with antibody and may stimulate an immune response when presented in an effective fashion. A large structure such as a protein, virus, or bacterium contains many subregions that are the actual antigenic determinants, or **epitopes.** These epitopes can consist of peptides, carbohydrates, or particular lipids

**TABLE 8–2. BIOLOGICAL PROPERTIES OF SOME CHARACTERIZED CYTOKINES**

| Property | IFN-α | IFN-β | IFN-γ | IL-1α | IL-1β | IL-2 | IL-3 | IL-4 | IL-5 | IL-10 |
|---|---|---|---|---|---|---|---|---|---|---|
| Mitogenesis | | | + | + | + | + | + | + | + | + |
| Effect on macrophages | + | + | + | | | + | | + | | + |
| B-cell activation | | | + | + | + | | | + | + | |
| B-cell proliferation | + | + | + | + | + | + | + | + | ? | |
| B-cell differentiation | + | | + | + | + | + | + | + | ? | + |
| Ig isotype selection | | | | | | | | IgE: IgG1 | IgA | + |
| T-cell activation | | | | + | + | + | | + | | |
| T-cell proliferation | + | | | + | + | + | | + | | + |
| T-cell differentiation | | | | | | + | | + | | |
| Pyrogenic | + | + | + | + | + | + | | | | |

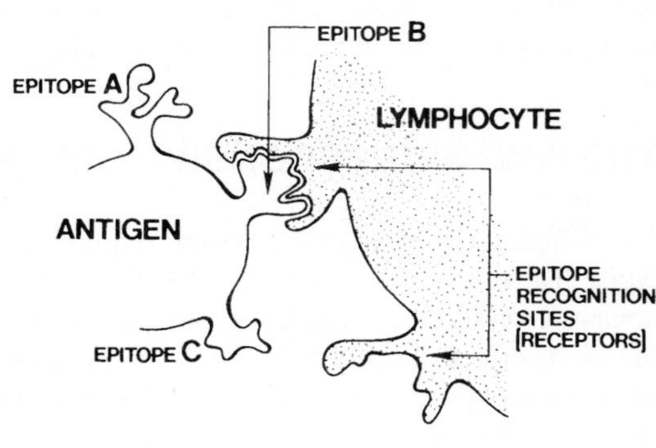


**Figure 8–1.** Schematic of epitope recognition by an immunoresponsive lymphocyte. Epitope B on the antigen binds to a complementary recognition site on the surface of the immunoresponsive cell. Antigens may have multiple different epitopes, but an immunoresponsive lymphocyte has receptors of only one specificity. In most cases, epitopes are recognized on the surface of macrophages that have processed the antigen. The receptor for antigens on B cells is the combining site of the surface immunoglobulin

Epitopes fit to the combining site of T-cell receptors

of the correct size and three-dimensional configuration to fill the combining site of an antibody molecule or a T-cell receptor (Fig 8–1). Approximately six amino acids or monosaccharide units provide a correctly sized epitope. Much of our knowledge of the combining sites of antibodies and their specificities was determined by immunizing animals experimentally with small organic molecules called **haptens.** Some of the best examples of these are substituted phenols, such as 2,4-dinitrophenol, which themselves do not induce the production of antibodies but must be coupled to a **carrier molecule** to be immunogenic. The term **immunogen** is a synonym for antigen, but is sometimes restricted to those antigens able to elicit an immune response as distinguished from the ability to react only with antibodies and with T-cell receptors.

B cells multiply and produce antibody

A foreign antigen entering a human host may by chance encounter a B cell whose surface antibody is able to bind it. This interaction stimulates the B cell to multiply, differentiate, and produce more surface and soluble antibody of the same specificity. Eventually, the process leads to production of enough antibody to bind more of the antigen. This mechanism is most likely to operate with antigens such as polysaccharides which have repeating subunits, thus improving the chance that exposed epitopes are recognized.

Some antigens must be processed first

Large, complex antigens such as proteins and viruses must be processed before their epitopes can be effectively recognized by the immune system. This processing takes place in macrophages or specialized epithelial cells found in the skin and lymphoid organs, where they are adjacent to other immunoresponsive cells. The ingested antigen is degraded to peptides of 10 to 20 amino acids that are presented by MHC products on the host cell surface to be recognized by T cells.

## BASIS OF IMMUNOLOGIC SPECIFICITY

Clonal selection provides diversity

The intellectual framework for understanding the mechanisms of immunologic specificity was laid down by the theory of **clonal selection** developed by Sir Macfarlane Burnet in 1959. It is now generally accepted that our lymphocyte populations, both B and T cells, show a great heterogeneity inasmuch as different cells possess surface receptors, which differ from each other with respect to combining site. This is shown in Figure 8–2 for B cells. In the actual process, great heterogeneity in the immune response even to particular antigens is observed. There are particular portions of the variable domains termed **complementarity-determining** or **hypervariable regions** that provide the actual amino acid residues that confer individual specificity. In the role of B cells in antibody production, there would be a differentiation from the lymphocytes to the plasma cells, and dependent on secondary stimulation and regulatory cytokines, shifts of types of antibody would occur.

Memory cells provide recall ability

With the elimination of antigen, the majority of the clone of immunoreactive lymphocytes is lost over time by normal cell replacement. The speed with which antigen is lost is, however, very variable and depends on such factors as excretion and enzymatic breakdown. Some polysaccharide antigens and bacterial cell wall peptidoglycans are so resistant to host enzymatic breakdown that they can persist for years, whereas many protein antigens are rapidly metabolized. Fortunately, the immune system has a recall ability in the case of protein antigens, because certain cells in the clone, termed **memory cells,** survive long periods and probably slowly replicate to maintain a core population with the capacity to ex-

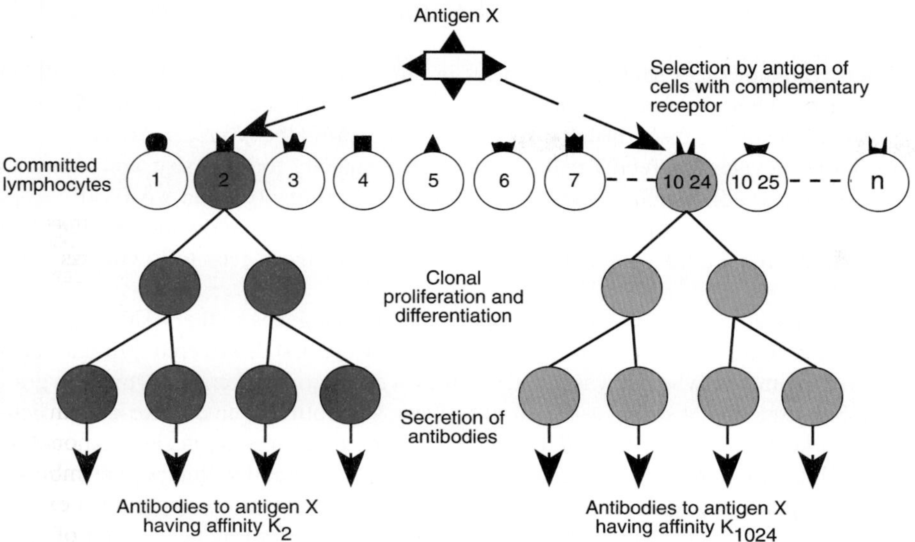


**Figure 8–2.** Diagram of the cellular events involved in the clonal selection of specifically reactive B lymphocytes by antigen. Clonal selection of T lymphocytes could be depicted by a comparable scheme but T cells do not secrete antibodies and the antigen would be presented in association with molecules of the major histocompatibility complex. Each B cell is numbered to show that it represents an individual clone. The schematic representation of the surface immunoglobulin receptors indicates that these have distinct combining sites. The combining sites are formed by interaction of $V_H$ and $V_L$ domains, and the cell-to-cell distinction in receptor specificity results from essentially a random genetic process. If a particular antigen, designated X here, enters the system, it can bind specifically, albeit with different affinities, to two of the cells shown here. If there are proper antigen presentation and interplay of cytokines involved in activation in differentiation, the recognition of antigen by the surface immunoglobulin receptor results in clonal proliferation and differentiation of those cells recognizing the antigen. In this case, antibodies representing two types of combining sites are generated.

pand very rapidly if the antigen (or the same epitope on another antigen) is encountered again.

Secondary response is rapid and greater than primary response

Memory cells may be either T or B cells and are probably variants within the original clone having recognition sites with higher specific affinity for the relevant antigenic determinant and, thus, greater immunologic efficiency. As a consequence, the response to a second encounter with an antigen is more rapid than the first and quantitatively greater in its effect. It is referred to as a secondary response, in contrast to the initial primary response. Memory cells and the secondary response phenomenon account for the prolonged or lifelong immunity that follows many infections (such as measles), and the secondary response is exploited in scheduling doses of various vaccines to obtain the maximum and most long-lived immunity.

## THE T-CELL RESPONSE

The major roles of T cells in the immune response are:

T cell functions

1. Recognition of epitopes presented with major histocompatibility complex (MHC) molecules on cell surfaces. This is followed by activation and clonal expansion of T cells in the case of epitopes associated with class II MHC molecules.
2. Production of lymphokines that act as intercellular signals and mediate the activation and modulation of various aspects of the immune response and of nonspecific host defenses.
3. Direct killing of foreign cells, of host cells bearing foreign surface antigens along with class I MHC molecules (eg, some virally infected cells), and of some immunologically recognized tumor cells.

## Antigen-Specific Receptors of T Cells

$\alpha/\beta$ and $\gamma/\delta$ T-cell receptors associated with CD3 complex

There are two major types of T-cell receptors in humans. Greater than 90% of T cells in adult spleen, lymph nodes, and peripheral blood express the $\alpha/\beta$ receptor, which is depicted in Figure 8–3. A small subset (usually 5%) of T cells express the $\gamma/\delta$ receptor. The $\gamma/\delta$ receptor is more prevalent on fetal T cells, has a limited capacity for diversity, and shows an association with responses to mycobacterial infections. Both the $\alpha/\beta$ and $\gamma/\delta$ T-cell receptors occur in association with the CD3 complex, a set of at least five distinct proteins that is necessary for signal transduction and allows activation of the T cells following recognition of antigen.

MHC presents processed peptides to the T-cell receptor

A particular set of cell surface proteins specified by the genes of the MHC play a major role in the recognition of antigens by T cells. These were first discovered through transplantation experiments, where it was found that they were major markers recognized in graft rejection. Subsequently, a strong association between susceptibility to disease and particular MHC markers was found. The MHC contains sets of genes that are designated as class I and class II determinants. These loci are highly polymorphic, and within populations, association with particular MHC markers correlates with the capacity to respond to particular antigens. Recent studies have shown that peptide determinants produced by proteolytic degradation of proteins by antigen-presenting accessory cells bind to MHC products, which then present the peptide antigen to the $\alpha/\beta$ T-cell receptor. Human class I molecules (HLA-A, HLA-B, and HLA-C) are expressed on virtually all cells of the body, whereas class II molecules (HLA-DR) are restricted to lymphocytes and macrophages.

CD4 and CD8 surface markers vary on T cells

Cytotoxic T cells ($T_c$) recognize antigen on MHC class I molecules and express the CD8 marker. By contrast, cells bearing the $\gamma/\delta$ antigen-specific T-cell receptor (Tcr) lack both CD4 and CD8. Figure 8–3 shows a membrane form of antibody expressed on B cells as a comparison with the $\alpha/\beta$ antigen-specific receptor of T cells. $\alpha/\beta$ T-cell receptors have not been found to any degree in serum and exist predominantly as cell surface recognition molecules. The affinity of T-cell receptors for antigen is low, and the role of MHC presentation of antigen is most probably to compensate for the low affinity.

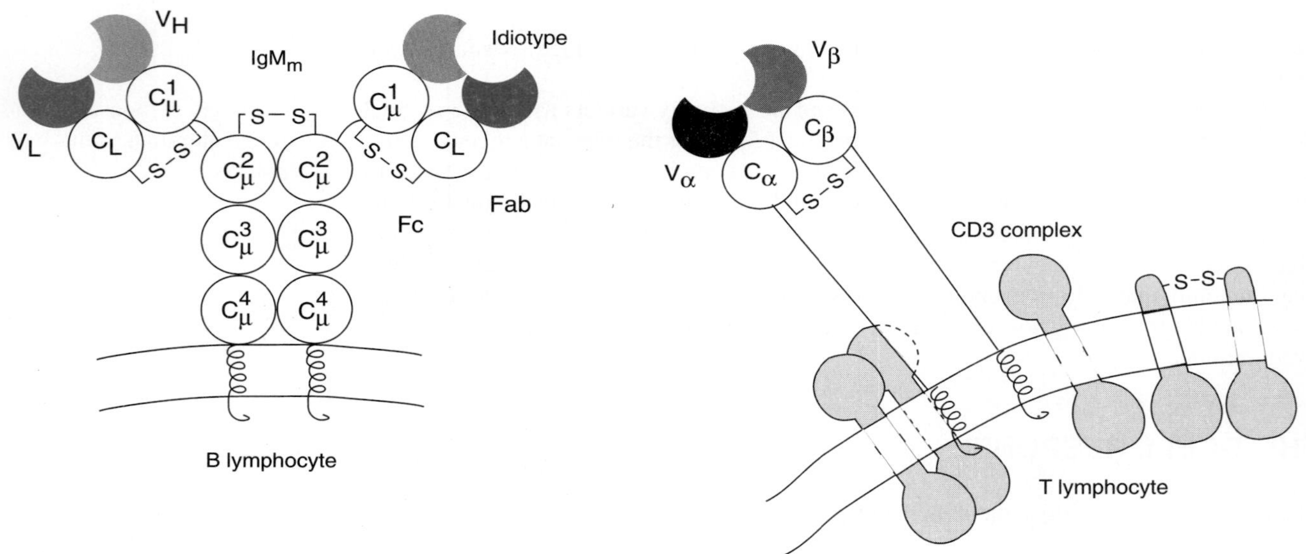


**Figure 8–3.** Comparison of the membrane IgM receptor of primary B cells with the $\alpha/\beta$ T-cell receptor of helper, cytolytic, and delayed-type hypersensitivity T cells. The $IgM_m$ molecule is a monomer consisting of two $\mu$ chains and two light chains, in contrast with the pentamer shown in Figure 8–6. The locations of the combining sites for antigen and the idiotypic marker are depicted. An additional difference between the serum form and the membrane form is the presence of a helical transmembrane region at the C-terminal end of the membrane receptor. In overall form, the $\alpha/\beta$ T-cell receptor is a disulfide-bonded heterodimer that resembles a single Fab fragment of immunoglobulin. In addition, it has an elongated stretch comparable to a hinge that terminates in a membrane-spanning helical region.

Specific T-cell help is initiated by the binding of α/β Tcr to antigen presented by MHC class II molecules. Most of the details of antigen presentation have been established using protein antigens, with an emphasis on virally infected cells so that the general principles apply to specific cytolytic cells as well. These proteins are digested into peptides by phagocytic cells (sometimes referred to as accessory cells), with certain peptides bound in a peptide-binding cleft within the MHC molecules intracellularly. These peptide–MHC complexes are then expressed on the cell surface, where the peptide epitope can be presented to the low-affinity antigen combining site of the α/β Tcr on T cells of compatible MHC type.

The initial specificity of cytotoxic T cells is, likewise, impacted by the α/β Tcr, but the MHC restriction involves class I molecules. In humans, the vast majority of circulating T cells bear the α/β Tcr. The CD3 surface marker comprises at least five distinct proteins involved in forming a membrane activation complex in association with the Tcr. The γ/δ Tcr is the first to appear in fetal development, but constitutes less than 5% of T cells in the adult. Like the α/β Tcr, it occurs in association with CD3. γ/δ Tcr-bearing T cells are cytotoxic, but do not show MHC restriction.

Recognition by T cells involves restriction by MHC molecules

There are other cellular phenomena that can be nonspecific in the sense that neither antigen-specific antibodies nor T-cell receptors are involved. These include natural killer cells, specific cytotoxic killer cells, and delayed-type hypersensitive cells. Natural killer cells are cells that are present in the absence of antigenic stimulation that recognize and kill particular types of tumor cells. The nature of the receptors on these cells is not clear, but it is thought they are a form of thymus-derived lymphocyte. Antigen-specific sensitized killer cells are induced by specific sensitization with the target antigen. They are activated by the presence of processed antigen and cytokines by a MHC-compatible antigen-presenting cell and show a subsequent MHC restriction in their capacity to destroy target cells. Delayed-type hypersensitive cells also are antigen-specific T cells that can be generated in the absence of circulating antibodies. An example of delayed-type hypersensitivity (DTH) is skin sensitization with small organic molecules, such as the quinone produced by poison ivy.

## CD4+ Helper T Lymphocytes

Helper T cells ($T_H$ cells) are stimulated by antigen in the context of MHC class II presentation and are further marked by the presence of the CD4 cell surface antigen. If T cells are of the proper MHC background to recognize the antigen specifically, T-cell activation occurs in the presence of interleukin 1 (IL-1, Table 8–2). The antigen–MHC complex presented to a specific T cell by the macrophage is the specific signal that induces the T cell to become activated and divide. The secretion of IL-2, following stimulation by IL-1, promotes the division of T cells following contact with antigens. The activated helper T cell presents both antigen and regulatory cytokines to the B cells, orchestrating the scheme of B cell differentiation from small lymphocytes to plasma cells producing antibodies of various types. The ability of particular B cells or T cells to respond to stimulation by individual cytokines is dependent on the presence of surface receptors for those cytokines.

Helper T cells present antigen and cytokines to B cells

Cytokines important in cell/cell interactions

Table 8–2 outlines the biological properties of some characterized cytokines. Cytokines can be involved in general physiologic or aphysiologic processes such as the induction of fever, mitogenesis or division of lymphocytes, and the stimulation of phagocytic cells. Other cytokines are involved in regulating activation of specific subsets of lymphocytes, and some have an extremely specific function in regulating the immunoglobulin isotypes expressed. The immune response is a complex but precisely regulated defense system in which specific recognition is imparted by antibodies, B-cell immunoglobulin receptors, and T-cell receptors, and activation and differentiation are dependent on a regulatory cascade of cell/cell communication molecules.

The critical significance of CD4+ helper cells to the body is shown by the catastrophic effects of AIDS in which the human immunodeficiency virus (HIV) binds to the CD4 molecule, enters the cell, and interferes with its function or destroys it. As a result, the body becomes susceptible to a wide variety of bacterial, viral, protozoal, and fungal infections, both through loss of preexisting immunity and through failure to mount an effective immune response to newly acquired pathogens.

HIV binds to CD4 molecule

## CD8+ Cytotoxic T Lymphocytes

Cytotoxic T cells kill virally infected and other cells

CD8+ cytotoxic T lymphocytes are a second class of effector T cells. They are lethal to cells expressing the epitope against which they are directed when the epitope is in conjunction with class I MHC molecules. They too have specific epitope recognition sites, but are characterized by the CD8 cell surface marker and are thus referred to as CD8+ cytotoxic T cells.

These cells recognize the association of antigenic epitopes with class I MHC molecules on a wide variety of cells of the body. This recognition, however, does not itself lead to the necessary clonal expansion of CD8 cells, which also requires the lymphokine IL-2 to be produced by activated CD4+ lymphocytes. In the case of virally infected cells, cytotoxic CD8+ cells prevent viral production and release by eliminating the host cell before viral synthesis or assembly is complete.

## CD8+ Suppressor T Cells

Suppressor T cells modulate T and B cell activities

Suppressor T lymphocytes also carrying the CD8 marker and epitope recognition sites are involved in modulating and terminating the immunologic activities of both T and B cells, thus avoiding excessive or needlessly prolonged responses that could interfere with other immunologic activities. It is known that the suppression they produce may be antigen specific or it may be polyclonal (ie, affecting general immunologic responses irrespective of the inciting antigen). The mechanisms of suppression and control are less well defined than are the activities of CD4+ helper cells. In AIDS, the proportion of CD8+ suppressor cells relative to CD4+ helper T cells is substantially increased because CD8+ lymphocytes are not attacked by HIV. This imbalance, in addition to the depletion of CD4+ helper cells, may contribute to the immunosuppression that is characteristic of the disease.

## Response to Superantigens

Superantigens bind directly to MHC proteins and Tcr Vβ region

A group of antigens have been termed **superantigens** because they stimulate a much larger number of T cells than would be predicted based on the generation of combining site diversity through clonal selection. Superantigens activate between 3 and 30% of T cells in unstimulated animals. The action of superantigens is based on their ability to bind directly to MHC proteins and to particular Vβ regions of the T-cell receptor (see Figure 8–3) without involving the antigen combining site. Individual superantigens recognize exposed portions defined by framework residues that are common to the structure of one or more Vβ regions. Any T cells bearing those Vβ sites may be directly stimulated. A variety of microbial products have been identified as superantigens. An example in which the pyrogenic exotoxins of *Staphylococcus aureus* act as superantigens in **toxic shock syndrome** is presented in Chapter 15.

# CELL-MEDIATED IMMUNITY

Complex system involving T cells and cytokines

Cell-mediated immunity is most dramatically expressed as a response to obligate or facultative intracellular pathogens. These include certain slow-growing bacteria, such as the mycobacteria, against which antibody responses are ineffective. In experimental infections, cell-mediated immunity can be passively transferred from one animal to another by T lymphocytes, but not by serum. (In contrast, short-term, antibody-mediated [B-cell] immunity can be passively transferred with serum.) The mechanisms of cell-mediated immunity are complex and involve a number of cytokines with amplifying feedback mechanisms for their production. The initial processing of antigen is accompanied by sufficient IL-1 production by the macrophages to stimulate activation of the antigen-recognizing CD4+ (helper) cell. Lymphokine feedback from the CD4+ T cells to macrophages further increases IL-1 production. IL-2 produced by the CD4+ T cells facilitates their clonal expansion and activates CD8+ (cytotoxic) T lymphocytes. Other lymphokines from CD4+ T cells chemotactically attract macrophages to the site of infection, hold them there, and activate them to greatly enhanced microbicidal activity. The sum of the individual and collaborative activities of T cells, macrophages, and their products is a progressive mobilization of a range of nonspecific host defenses to the site of infection and greatly enhanced macrophage activity. In the case of viruses, interferon gamma inhibits replication, and CD8+ cytotoxic lymphocytes destroy their cellular habitat, leaving already assembled virions accessible to circulating antibody.

With certain infections in which reaction to protein antigens is particularly strong (eg, tuberculosis), the cell-mediated responses are of such magnitude that they become major deleterious factors in the disease process itself. This is called delayed-type hypersensitivity because reexposure of the host to the antigen that elicited the immune response produces a maximum hypersensitive reaction only after a day or two, when mobilization of immune lymphocytes and of phagocytic macrophages is at its peak.

Cell-mediated response may cause injury

## B CELLS AND ANTIBODY RESPONSES

B lymphocytes are the cells responsible for antibody responses. They develop from precursor cells in the yolk sac and fetal liver before birth and thereafter in the bone marrow before migrating to other lymphoid tissues. Each mature cell of this series carries a specific epitope recognition site on its surface that is the antigen-recognizing (variable) region of antibody that will be produced subsequently by its progeny. In the process of antibody formation, B lymphocytes, following stimulation by antigen, divide and differentiate into plasma cells which are end cells adapted for secretion of large amounts of antibodies. In addition to their essential role in antibody production, B cells can present antigen to T cells.

B cells carry epitope recognition sites on their surface

There are two broad types of antigens. T-independent antigens are those that do not require help by T cells to stimulate B-cell antibody production, and T-dependent antigens are those that are dependent on collaboration between helper T cells and B cells to initiate the process of antibody production. T-independent antigens are generally limited to large polymeric molecules such as carbohydrates with repeating sugar epitopes. Immunologic reactivity to such polysaccharides usually develops much more slowly after birth than do the T-dependent responses, and memory cells do not result from the clonal B-cell expansion. This delay in responsiveness probably contributes to the increased susceptibility to some bacterial infections in early life. Most common antigens, particularly proteins, require T-cell help for antibody production to occur. Following stimulation by antigen processed and presented by macrophages, T cells can become helper cells collaborating with B cells, antigen-specific cytotoxic T cells capable of killing tumor cells, suppressor T cells downregulating the immune system, or T cells mediating delayed-type hypersensitivity. Table 8–1 lists major cells in the immune response and their antigen-specific and nonspecific functions.

T cell dependent and T cell independent responses are possible

T-dependent responses develop more slowly from birth

Following challenge with foreign antigen, there is a lag period of 4 to 6 days before antibody can be detected in serum. This period reflects the events involved in the recognition of the antigen, its processing, and the specific activation of the cells of the immune system. The first event is the clearance of antigen from the circulation by what is essentially a metabolic process in which the antigen is recognized in a nonspecific sense and ingested. The vast preponderance of antigen ends up in circulating phagocytes or in stationary macrophages such as the Kupffer cells in the liver. The macrophages process the antigen so that immunogenic moieties can be presented to T cells, as shown in Figure 8–4. Interleukins 4, 5, and 6, in addition to specific presentation of antigen, cause the B cells to produce immunoglobulins and also are involved in class switches.

Processing causes delay in response

The antibody-forming system is a learning system that responds to challenge by foreign molecules by producing large amounts of specific antibody. In addition, the affinity of its binding to the specifically recognized antigen often increases with time or secondary challenge.

### Antibodies

Antibodies belong to the **immunoglobulin** family of proteins which occur in quantity in serum and on the surfaces of B cells. The basic structure of an immunoglobulin is illustrated in Figure 8–5, which depicts an IgG molecule. Immunoglobulins have a basic tetrameric structure consisting of two light polypeptide chains and two heavy chains associated as

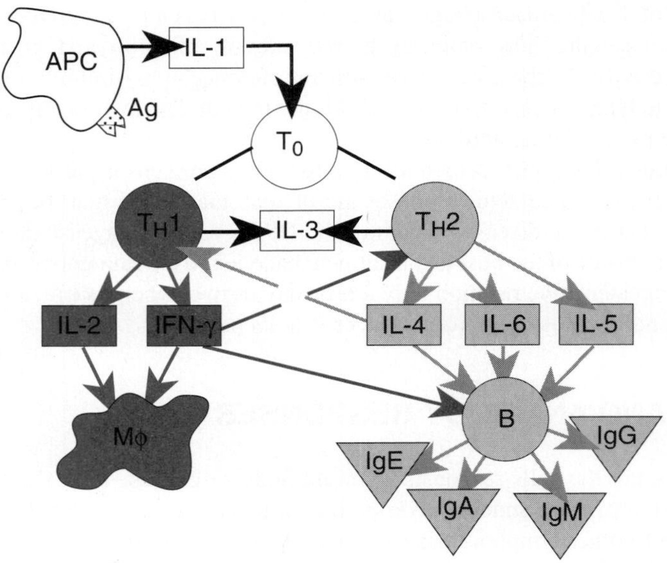


**Figure 8–4.** Simplified diagram illustrating events of helper-T-cell activation leading to either cellular immunity of the delayed-type hypersensitive type ($T_H1$ cells) or antibody production ($T_H2$) involving stimulation of B cells by specific and nonspecific (cytokine) means. The cytokine interleukin 2 plays a major role in causing T-cell mitogenesis and also in the activation of macrophages. This is abbreviated as an antigen-presenting cell (APC), which presents both processed antigen (Ag) to antigen-specific T cells and a stimulatory cytokine (interleukin 1) that causes the stimulated T cell to differentiate into one of two broad types of T cells; termed $T_H1$ and $T_H2$ here. The $T_H1$ cells produce interleukins 2 and 3 and interferon and gamma can stimulate macrophages, $T_H2$ cells, and B cells. The $T_H2$ cells produce interleukins 3, 4, 5, and 6 and carry out a major role as helpers in activating B cells.

Immunoglobulins have tetrameric structure combining light chains and heavy chains

light/heavy pairs by disulfide bonds. The two light/heavy pairs are covalently associated by disulfide bonds to form the tetramer. There are two types of light chains, κ chains and λ chains, which are the products of distinct genetic loci. The class or isotype of the immunoglobulin is defined by the type of heavy chain expressed. In this IgG molecule, the heavy chains are termed γ chains and have characteristic sequences and antigenic markers. IgG immunoglobulins can have either κ or λ chains associated with the γ, but the only type of light chain would be present in the intact molecule; that is, an individual IgG molecule would be either γ2κ2, or γ2λ2, but mixed molecules do not occur. This diagram illustrates other basic structural features of the molecule. The basic building block of immunoglobulins is a domain of approximately 110 amino acids containing an internal disulfide bond stabilizing the structure. **Domains** are compact, tightly folded structures having a characteristic "immunoglobulin fold." The light chains contain two domains: a variable domain and a constant domain. The γ heavy chain contains four domains: $V_H$, $C_\gamma1$, $C_\gamma2$, and $C_\gamma3$.

Antibodies have recognition and effector functions

Antibodies carry out two broad sets of functions: the recognition function is the property of the combining site for antigen, and the effector functions are mediated by the constant regions of the heavy chains. Antibodies combine with foreign antigens, but the actual destruction or removal of antigen requires the interaction of portions of the Fc fragment with other molecules such as complement components or with effector cells which then engulf the recognized cell or particle.

Combining site defines idiotype

The combining site for antigen (antigen binding site) is formed by interaction of the variable domains of the heavy chain and the light chain. The IgG molecule has two such combining sites. Immunoglobulin in the serum of normal individuals occurs as a large pool of individual molecules, each of which has a unique sequence and a defined combining site. The defined combining site of an immunoglobulin has been termed an **idiotype.** The idiotype is a combining site-related antigenic marker that defines individual immunoglobulins. There are other types of antigenic markers of immunoglobulins that define classes or isotypes. These occur on the constant regions of light chains, where they define the κ and λ isotypes. Heavy chains have $C_H$ markers identifying μ, γ, δ, α and ε isotypes. These markers are found in all normal individuals. The third

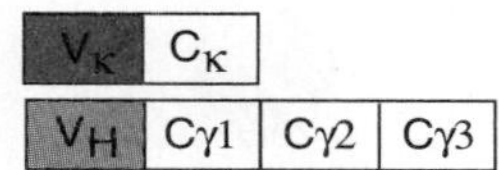


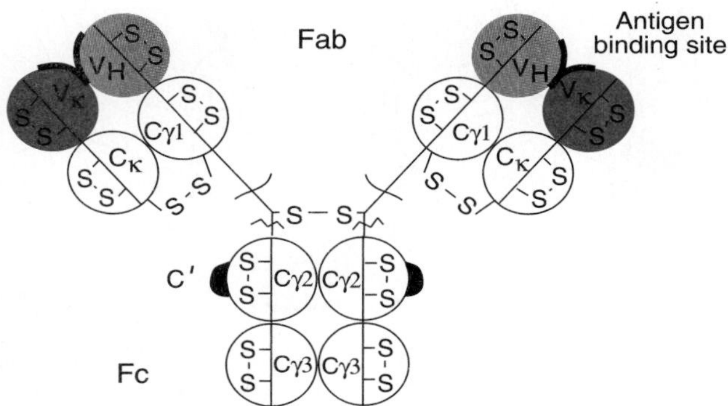


**Figure 8–5.** Schematic representation of an IgG immunoglobulin molecule. This model illustrates the domain structure of immunoglobulin light and heavy chains in a stick model form (top) and as compact, circular domains (bottom). Two combining sites for antigen are present, and these are formed by interaction between the $V_H$ and $V_\kappa$ domains of the molecule. The binding site for complement (C′) is shown to be located in the Cγ2 domain. The region of the heavy chain where no domain structure is shown is the "hinge" region. This region is the site of cleavage of the proteolytic enzymes papain and pepsin. The Fc fragment produced by proteolysis contains the binding site for complement and is crystallizable. The Fab fragment contains the variable regions and binds antigen.

general type of immunoglobulin antigenic determinant is termed **allotypic.** These markers may be found on the light chains (eg, the KM determinant of human κ chains) or heavy chains (eg, the GM markers of human IgG) and define genetic markers that behave as Mendelian alleles in the human population. Allotypic markers are usually associated with constant regions but have been reported for the variable domains of heavy chains as well.

Another structural feature of immunoglobulins that merits consideration is the fact that proteolytic digestion of the IgG molecule by the enzyme papain can cleave the structure into two defined regions. As illustrated in Figure 8–5, two **antigen-binding** or **Fab** fragments are generated and a single **constant** or **Fc** fragment is produced. The cleavage occurs in the so-called hinge region, which is a relatively loose stretch of polypeptide connecting the Fab domains to the $C_\gamma 2$ domain. The tight domain structures themselves are relatively resistant to proteolysis. The positions of the intradomain disulfides are indicated (S-S bonds). The intrachain disulfide bonds connecting the $C_\kappa$ and $C_\gamma 1$ are also indicated, as is the location of the S-S bonds linking the two heavy chains. This basic structure, although using different heavy chains, occurs in all five of the major human immunoglobulin classes, but the number of subunits and the overall arrangement can vary. For example, Figure 8–6 gives a schematic representation of a serum IgM immunoglobulin. This molecule, which was originally called immune macroglobulin because of its large size (approximate mass of 900,000 daltons), consists of five subunits of the form of the typical IgG. The light chains can be either κ or λ, but the type of heavy chain defining the IgM class is termed the μ chain. The molecule occurs as a cyclic pentamer, and a J or joining chain is also associated with the intact structure. When IgM is present on B cells where it serves as a primary receptor for antigen, it is present as a monomer. Other immunoglobulins showing a difference in arrangement from the typical IgG model are the IgA immunoglobulins. In serum these can occur as a monomer, but they can also occur in dimers where the joining chain is required to stabilize the dimer. IgA molecules present in the gut (secretory IgA) occur as dimers where both the J chain and an additional polypeptide, termed the **secretory component,** are present in the complex.

Immunoglobulin domains carry out distinct functions

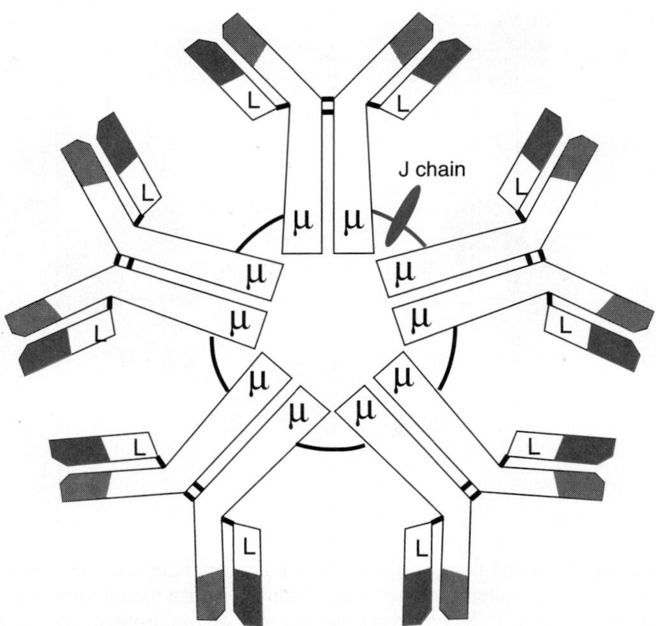


**Figure 8–6.** A planor projection model of serum IgM showing the structure as a cyclic pentamer held together by disulfide bonds. One joining (J) chain is associated with the pentamer. Approximately 10% of the mass of the μ chain consists of carbohydrate which is associated with the constant region of the heavy chain.

## Functional Properties of Immunoglobulins

### Immunoglobulin G Antibody

Immunoglobulin G is the most abundant immunoglobulin in health and provides the most extensive and long-lived antibody response to the various microbial and other antigens that are encountered throughout the life span of the individual. Although at least four subclasses of IgG have been characterized, they are grouped together for the purpose of this chapter. The IgG molecule is bivalent, with two identical and specific combining sites. The rest of the molecule is the constant (Fc) region, which does not vary with differences in specificity of combining sites of different antibody molecules. The constant region has specific sites for binding to phagocytic cells and for reaction with the first component of complement. These sites are made available when the variable region of the antibody molecule has reacted with specific antigen.

Bivalent molecule with specific combining site and constant region

Constant region binds phagocytes

Immunoglobulin G antibody is characteristically formed in large amounts during the secondary response to an antigenic stimulus and usually follows production of IgM (see below) in the course of a viral or bacterial infection. Memory cells are programmed for rapid IgG response when another antigenic stimulus of the same type occurs later.

Neutralizing antibodies slowed during secondary response

Immunoglobulin G antibodies are the most significant antibody class for neutralizing soluble antigens (eg, exotoxins) and viruses. They act by blocking the sites on the antigenic molecule or virus that determine attachment to cell receptors. IgG also enhances phagocytosis of particulate antigens such as bacteria, because the exposed Fc sites of antibody that is bound to the antigen have a specific affinity for receptors on the surface of phagocytic cells. As described later, the third component of complement also mediates attachment to phagocytes. Enhancement of phagocytosis by antibody, complement, or both is referred to as **opsonization.** Accelerated IgG responses from memory cell expansion frequently confer lifelong immunity when directed against microbial antigens that are determinants of virulence. There is active transport of the IgG molecule across the placental barrier, which allows maternal protective antibody to pass and, thus, provides passive immune protection to the fetus and newborn pending development of a mature immune system. It is the only immunoglobulin class known to be placentally transferred. The half-life of passively transferred IgG within the same species is approximately a month, and thus the infant can be protected during a particularly vulnerable period of life.

### Immunoglobulin M Antibody

Monomers of IgM constitute the specific epitope recognition sites on B cells that ultimately give rise to plasma cells producing one or another of the different immunoglobulin classes of antibody. Because of its multiple specific combining sites, IgM is particularly effective in agglutinating particles carrying epitopes against which it is directed. It also contains multiple sites for binding the first component of complement. These sites become available once the IgM molecule has reacted with antigen. IgM is particularly active in bringing about complement-mediated cytolytic damage to foreign antigen-bearing cells. It is not, itself, an opsonizing antibody because its Fc portion is not recognized by phagocytes. Opsonization occurs through its activation of the complement pathway; this process is discussed later in the chapter.

Multiple complement binding sites

Immunoglobulin M is usually the earliest antibody to appear after an antigenic stimulus, but it tends to decline rapidly and is often succeeded by IgG production from the same clone of cells. It is primarily intravascular and does not cross the placental barrier to the fetus (in contrast to IgG). Thus, the presence of specific IgM against a potentially infecting agent in the blood of a neonate is a priori evidence of active infection rather than of passively acquired antibody from the mother. Antibody response to certain antigens, including the lipopolysaccharide O antigen of Gram-negative bacteria, is characteristically IgM. Some universally occurring antibodies (natural antibodies), such as those directed against blood group antigens, are also of the IgM class.

First antibody after antigenic stimulation

### IgA Antibody

Immunoglobulin A has a special role as a major determinant of so-called local immunity in protecting epithelial surfaces from colonization and infection. Certain B cells in lymphoid tissues adjacent to or draining surface epithelia of the intestines, respiratory tract, and genitourinary tract are encoded for specific IgA production. After antigenic stimulus, the clone expands locally and some of the IgA-producing cells also migrate to other viscera and secretory glands. At the epithelia, two IgA molecules combine with another protein, termed the **secretory piece,** which is present on the surface of local epithelial cells. The complex, then termed **secretory IgA** (sIgA), passes through the cells into the mucus layer on the epithelial surface or into glandular secretions where it exerts its protective effect. The secretory piece not only mediates secretion, but also protects the molecule against proteolysis by enzymes such as those present in the intestinal tract.

Secretory antibody produced at mucosal surfaces

The major role of sIgA is to prevent attachment of antigen-carrying particles to receptors on mucous membrane epithelia. Thus, in the case of bacteria and viruses, it reacts with surface antigens that mediate adhesion and colonization and serves to prevent the establishment of local infection or invasion of the subepithelial tissues. It can agglutinate particles, but has no Fc domain for activating the classic complement pathway; however, it can activate the alternative pathway (see below). Reaction of IgA with antigen within the mucous membrane initiates an inflammatory reaction that helps mobilize other immunoglobulin and cellular defenses to the site of invasion. IgA response to an antigen is shorter lived than the IgG response.

Interferes with attachment of microbes

### IgE Antibody

Immunoglobulin E is a monomer consisting of two light chains (either $\kappa$ or $\lambda$) and two heavy chains. It is normally present in very small amounts in serum, and most IgE is bound firmly by its Fc portion to tissue mast cells and basophils, which are major producers of histamine. When IgE bound to mast cells reacts with specific antigen, the mast cells degranulate and release histamine and other factors that mediate an inflammatory reaction with dilatation of the capillaries, exudation of plasma components, and attraction of neutrophils and eosinophils to the site. Thus, IgE contributes to a rapid second line of defense if surface-protective mechanisms are breached. IgE also plays a significant indirect role in the immune response to a number of helminthic (worm) infections because of attraction of eosinophils to the site at which it reacts with antigen. The eosinophils bind to the Fc portions of IgG molecules that have reacted with surface antigens of the parasite and help bring about its destruction.

Bound to mast cells

Important in parasitic infections

Certain types of allergies, to be discussed later in this chapter, are due to excessive production of IgE with specificity for a foreign protein. The pharmacologic effects of histamine and the other vasoactive mediators released from mast cells largely account for the symptoms of the disorder.

### Immunoglobulin D Antibody

Immunoglobulin D antibody consists of two light chains and two heavy chains. It is highly susceptible to proteolytic enzymes in the tissues and is found only in very low concentrations in serum. Its role is not fully understood, although, as indicated earlier, it is present on the surface of unstimulated B cells and may serve as a receptor for antigen.

The chain composition, size, and some major biological properties of the separate classes of immunoglobulins are summarized in Table 8–3.

## Antibody Production

After lag primary response lasts for weeks then declines

The major events characterizing the general phenomenon of antibody production are illustrated in Figure 8–7 and summarized as follows: Initial contact with a new antigen (primary stimulus) evokes the so-called primary response, which is characterized by a lag phase of approximately 1 week between the challenge and the detection of circulating antibodies. In general, the length of the lag phase depends on the immunogenicity of the stimulating antigen and the sensitivity of the detection system for the antibodies produced. **Immunogenicity,** or the capacity to generate an immune response, is contingent on the state of the antigen when injected, the immunologic status of the animal, and the use of adjuvants or nonspecific amplifiers of immune reactivity. Once antibody is detected in serum, the levels rise exponentially to attain a maximal steady state in about 3 weeks. These levels then decline gradually with time if no further antigenic stimulation is given. The major antibodies synthesized in the primary immune response are the immune macroglobulins (IgM class). In the latter phase of the primary response, IgG antibodies arise, and these molecules even-

**TABLE 8–3. STRUCTURAL AND BIOLOGICAL PROPERTIES OF HUMAN IMMUNOGLOBULINS**

| | IgG | IgA | IgM | IgD | IgE |
|---|---|---|---|---|---|
| Heavy chain class | $\gamma$ ($\gamma$1, $\gamma$2, $\gamma$3, $\gamma$4) | $\alpha$ ($\alpha$1, $\alpha$2) | $\mu$ | $\delta$ | $\varepsilon$ |
| Light chain class | $\kappa$ or $\lambda$ | $\kappa$ or $\lambda$ | $\kappa$ or $\lambda$ | $\kappa$ or $\lambda$ | $\kappa$ or $\lambda$ |
| Molecular formula | $\gamma 2\kappa 2$, or $\gamma 2\lambda 2$ | $\alpha 2\kappa 2$ or $\alpha 2\lambda 2$; ($\alpha 2\kappa 2$) SC-J or ($\alpha 2\lambda 2$) SC-J (mucosal form) | ($\mu 2\kappa 2$) $_5$J or ($\mu 2\lambda 2$)$_5$J or $\mu 2\kappa 2_m$ or $\mu 2\lambda 2_m$ (B-cell membrane) | $\delta 2\kappa 2_m$ or $\delta 2\lambda 2_m$ | $\varepsilon 2\kappa 2$ or $\varepsilon 2\lambda 2$ |
| Approximate mass | 150,000 | 160,000 400,000 | 900,000 memb. 180,000 | 180,000 | 190,000 |
| Serum concentration (mg/mL) | 10 | 2 | 1.2 | 0.03 | trace |
| Complement fixation (classic) | + | 0 | +++ | 0 | 0 |
| Placental transfer | + | 0 | 0 | 0 | 0 |
| Reaginic activity | ? | 0 | 0 | 0 | +++ |
| Lysis of bacteria | + | + | +++ | ? | ? |
| Antiviral activity | + | +++ | + | ? | ? |
| B-cell receptor for antigen | + (memory) | + (memory) | + (primary) | + (primary) | + (memory) |

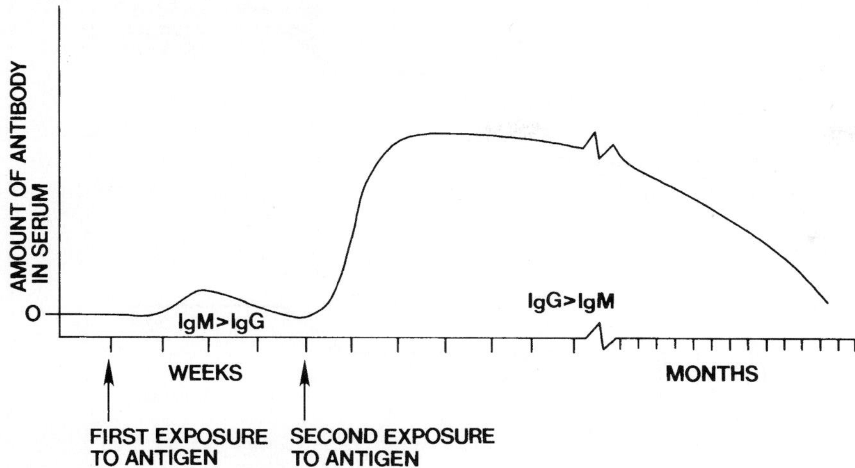


**Figure 8–7.** Primary and secondary immunologic responses. The response to first inoculation of antigen becomes apparent in a week to 10 days. It is small, predominantly of IgM class, and declines rapidly. Activation of memory cells by a second inoculation leads to a much greater, more rapid, and more long-lived IgG response.

tually predominate. This transition is termed the IgM/IgG switch. Following a secondary or booster injection of the same antigen, the lag time between the immunization and the appearance of antibody is shortened, the rate of exponential increase to the maximum steady-state level is more rapid, and the steady-state level itself is higher, representing a larger amount of antibody. Another key factor of the secondary response is that the antibodies formed are predominantly of the IgG class. In addition to higher levels of antibody, the secondary IgG antibodies are often better antibodies in the sense that there has been a maturation in affinity of the combining sites so that the secondary antibodies are more effective at binding the antigen than were the IgM and initial IgG molecules produced. This process of affinity maturation results from a process of somatic mutation ongoing during the response.

IgM response switches to IgG

Secondary response primarily IgG

The preceding description of primary and secondary immune responses represents the idealized case that would be expected in normal individuals. Figure 8–8 illustrates the detailed sequence of IgG, IgM, and IgA antibodies to poliovirus that appears in the serum of a child who was immunized with three doses of attenuated live poliovirus. The inactivated virus was given at monthly intervals to a newborn beginning at 2 months of age. The contributions of serum IgM, IgG, and IgA antibodies are individually depicted. The overall capacity of the serum to neutralize the poliovirus is first detectable about 1 week following the primary immunization and reaches a plateau after the second immunization. The IgM antibody peaks at 1 week and gradually declines during the course of vaccination. Primary IgG plateaus at approximately 2 weeks and increases with the secondary booster injection. IgA appears later than either IgM or IgG and is enhanced by secondary and tertiary boosts. It should be emphasized that in developing vaccines, the quantity or class of antibody produced is secondary to the biological effect. In the polio example, the serum IgA antibody is probably less important than that produced at the mucosal surfaces of the gut where it can block virus attachment.

Multiple responses occur during immunization

## Antibody-Mediated Immunity

Antibodies provide immunity to infection and disease in a variety of ways:

1. They can neutralize the infectivity of a virus, the toxicity of an exotoxin molecule, or the ability of a bacterium to colonize. This is usually brought about by reaction between the antibody and an epitope that is required for attachment of the organism or toxin to a target host cell. IgA and IgG antibodies are particularly significant in neutralizing activity.

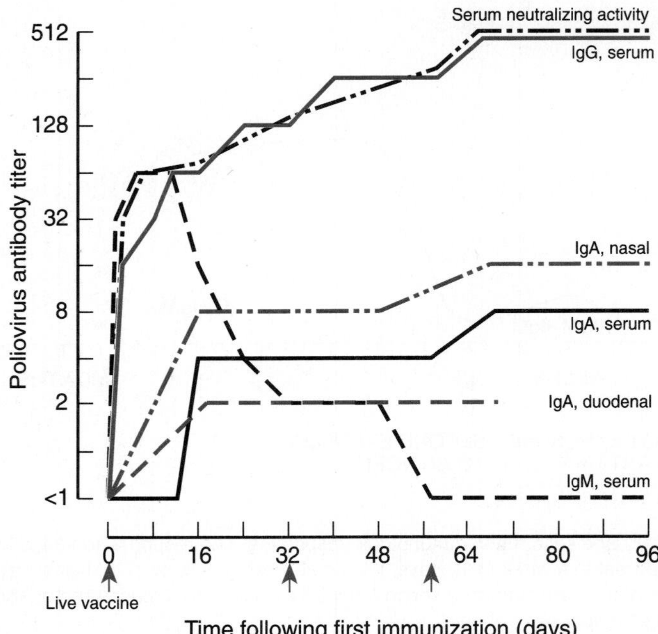


**Figure 8–8.** Detailed sequence of IgG, IgM, and IgA antibodies to poliovirus in serum and secretions of an infant immunized with live attenuated poliovirus. (*Based on Ogra PL, et al.* New Eng. J. Med. *1968;279:893–900.*)

2. Antibodies can inhibit essential nutrient assimilation by some bacteria. This occurs when a specific antigenic site or protein is involved in transport of the essential nutrient into the cell. For example, some iron binding siderophores (see Chapter 3) are antigenic, and antibody against them can prevent assimilation of the iron that is essential for growth.
3. Immunoglobulin G antibody can promote phagocytosis of extracellular bacteria by combining with capsules or other surface antigens that otherwise inhibit ingestion of the organism by phagocytes. When antigen–antibody reactions occur, the attachment sites for phagocytes on the Fc regions of the antibodies are exposed, the organism is bound to the phagocyte, and ingestion occurs. The significance of such opsonization is that many bacteria and some viruses are rapidly destroyed within the phagocytic cell.
4. Antigen–antibody reactions involving IgG and IgM activate the classic pathway of the complement cascade, which is described later. Complement components enhance a wide range of nonspecific host defense mechanisms, synergize antibody-mediated opsonization, and lead to lysis of many Gram-negative bacteria with which antibody has reacted. A similar event occurs with blood and tissue cells carrying surface antigens recognized as foreign.
5. Antibodies that recognize foreign antigens on the surface of a host cell, such as a virally infected cell, react with them and can mediate destruction of the cell by the process of antibody-dependent cell-mediated cytotoxicity (ADCC).

Fc portions bind to cells in ADCC

In ADCC, the antibodies bind to the cells through their Fc portions which attach to cell surface receptors specific for the Fc regions of particular IgG classes. These are termed Fc receptors (FcR). For example, the human monocyte–macrophage has a plasma membrane receptor that recognizes both IgG1 and IgG3 subclasses through a binding site on the $C_\gamma3$ domain. Eosinophils have a low-affinity FcR for IgE, which is much lower than that of mast cells. If the antibody is bound by its Fc piece, the Fab regions are free to bind antigen to initiate ADCC in the case of monocytes or polymorphs or an allergic response when IgE molecules on mast cells are crosslinked by binding to the antigen (allergen).

A variety of clinical problems arise from this antibody-mediated cytotoxicity including transfusion reactions, autoimmune hemolytic anemias, and the autoimmune disease myasthenia gravis, in which antibodies are directed at the acetylcholine receptor in the motor end plate.

## IMMUNOGLOBULIN GENES AND REARRANGEMENT

The genes specifying immunoglobulins are unique because complete genes encoding an immunoglobulin are not found in the genome. Rather, gene segments that provide diversity and commitment by a rearrangement mechanism are inherited in the traditional manner, and the actual genes that are transcribed to form immunoglobulin chains arise from somatic recombination. The immunoglobulin gene clusters have been termed **translocons** because they consist of large numbers of variable gene segments, a smaller number of joining minigenes, sometimes a small number of diversity (D) minigenes, and as few as one constant segment in the case of κ chains to more than 10 for heavy chains. The heavy chains, κ chains, and λ chains are not linked to one another and, in humans, occur on chromosomes 14, 2, and 22, respectively. There are hundreds of variable region genes in each group. Substantial diversity can be generated by the heavy chain translocon, and this is amplified greatly by the presence of the diversity minigene. This capacity of the vertebrate immune system to generate enormous diversity and clonal commitment by gene rearrangement is illustrated in Figures 8–9 and 8–10.

Diversity is achieved by gene rearrangements

Another feature of antibody formation that is related to heavy chain gene arrangement is that of isotype switching. The first immunoglobulin formed following immuniza-

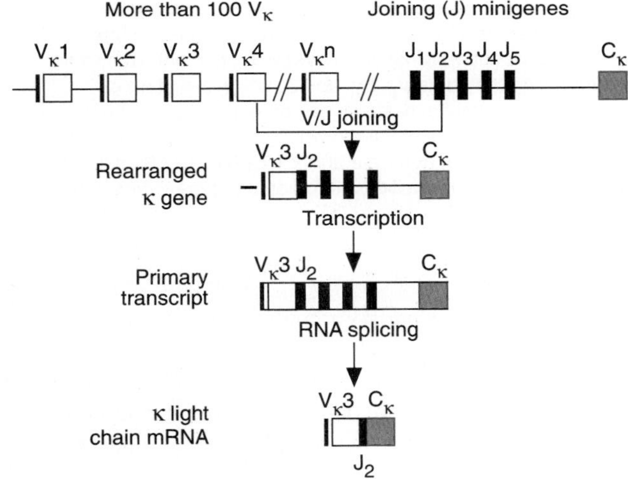


**Figure 8–9.** Light chain rearrangements. The drawings illustrate the arrangement of the κ gene system in the germline (top line) and show the events required for the formation of mRNA specifying a particular κ light chain. There are hundreds of individual $V_\kappa$ genes, each beginning with the leader sequence, that are separated from a small set of J minigenes by a large genetic distance. The $V_\kappa$ segments are spread over a region that spans more than 2 million base pairs of DNA and constitutes approximately 1% of the length of chromosome 2. When a pre-B cell becomes committed to the antigen-specific B-lymphocyte lineage, one of the set of $V_\kappa$ segments and one J segment are fused to form a single continuous exon. This is done via an enzymatic process that deletes the chromosomal region between the 3′ end of the chosen $V_\kappa$ and the 5′ end of the selected J segment. DNA signal sequences are required to allow this fusion to occur. A primary RNA transcript is generated from this fused gene, but this contains intervening unused J segments and the intron lying between the J and 5′ region of the $C_\kappa$ segment. These are removed by RNA splicing and the mRNA formed specifies the leader segment, the selected $V_\kappa$, the selected $J_\kappa$, and the $C_\kappa$. The leader sequence is removed enzymatically following protein synthesis. This rearrangement mechanism illustrates how clonal restriction follows from the selection of one $V_\kappa$ out of a set of hundreds such that the B cell can only make one sequence of κ light chain. If there are 100 $V_\kappa$ genes and 5 $J_\kappa$ segments, 100 × 5 or 500 different V domains can be generated by this combinatorial joining.

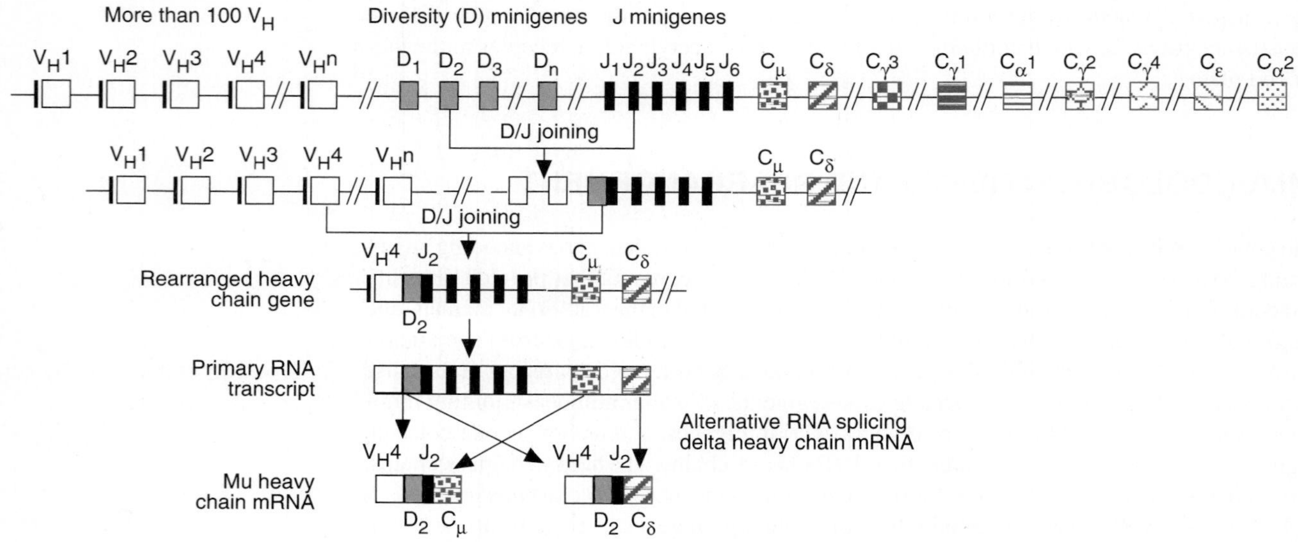


**Figure 8–10.** Heavy chain rearrangements. The drawing illustrates in simplified form the arrangement of the heavy chain gene segments on chromosome 14. One aspect of the simplification is that the heavy chain constant region genes actually consist of a series of exons, each of which specifies a single domain, separated by introns. The constant region genes specifying the heavy chain isotypes are arranged in tandem along the chromosome in the order outlined. There are six $J_H$ minigenes and hundreds of $V_H$ genes. There are at least twenty D minigenes, each of which codes for two or three amino acids. Two separate DNA rearrangements must be completed in the differentiating B lymphocyte to assemble the heavy chain gene. The first rearrangement is between one of the D segments and a joining segment. The second involves the selection of a $V_H$ gene which then joins to the fused D/J segments. The RNA processing events parallel those described for the light chain in Figure 8–9. An interesting feature of heavy chain rearrangement is that the $C_\mu$ and $C_\delta$ genes lie close to one another and are transcribed in the primary RNA transcript. Alternative RNA splicing mechanisms allow the generation of μ chains and δ chains expressing the same $V_H$, $D_H$, and $J_H$ which are often expressed in membrane receptors on early B cells. Substantial diversity can be generated by the heavy chain translocon, and this is amplified greatly by the presence of the diversity minigene. For example, a cluster containing 200 $V_H$, 10 $D_H$, and 6 $J_H$ segments can generate 200 × 10 × 6 or 12,000 different $V_H$ domains. If these are then combined with the 500 $V_\kappa$ possibilities, 6 million antigen-binding sites are possible (500 × 12,000).

Isotype switching related to heavy chain arrangement

tion is IgM, and with time and secondary immunization, there is a switch to production of IgG as the predominant serum antibody. Moreover, different schemes of immunization can predispose to production of IgA (oral immunization) or IgE (anaphylaxis). The V regions for all the heavy chain classes are assembled from a common pool of $V_H$, $D_H$, and $J_H$ segments. Once these are assembled, the complex can be linked to any one of the C region sequences.

## THE COMPLEMENT SYSTEM

Multiple components reacting in cascade fashion when triggered

Non-specific system

The complement system plays a critical adjunctive role to the specific immune system. Complement consists of 20 major distinct components and several other precursors. It is a highly complex system, and focus is on only nine major components for the purposes of this chapter. Some of the components are proenzymes, and all are present in the plasma of healthy individuals. When the complement system is triggered, there occurs a cascade of reactions that activate the different components in a fixed sequence. Several of these activated components have differing and important effects in defense against infection. Components of complement are designated by numbers, which, unfortunately for the student, reflect the order in which they were first described rather than the sequence in which they are activated. There is no immunologic specificity in complement activation or in its effects, although specific antigen–antibody reactions are major initiators of activation, and some complement components enhance the effects of antigen–antibody interactions, for instance, in opsonization.

## Classic Complement Pathway

The classic complement pathway is summarized in Figure 8–11. It is initiated by antigen–antibody reactions involving IgM or IgG. These reactions expose specific sites on the Fc portion of immunoglobulin molecules that bind and activate the C1 component of complement. C1 then activates C4 and C2, and this complex splits C3 into two components, C3a and C3b. C3a liberates histamine and other vasoactive mediators from mast cells and stimulates the respiratory burst of phagocytes, thus increasing their microbicidal power. C3b binds to the membrane of microorganisms or to such cells as tumor cells or red cells and to specific sites on Fc portions of IgM and IgG. Polymorphonuclear leukocytes (PMNs) and macrophages have receptors for C3b, which thus serves as an opsonin for microorganisms. The opsonic process is markedly enhanced when specific antibody has reacted with the organism.

Initiated by antigen antibody reaction

C3b is opsonic

C3b, in association with activated C4 and C2, continues the cascade by splitting C5 into two components, C5a and C5b. C5a stimulates release of histamine and other vasoactive mediators from mast cells, is a chemotactic factor for PMNs, and enhances their metabolic antimicrobial activity. C5b binds to the membrane of cells on which an antigen–antibody reaction has occurred and initiates activation of the terminal components C6 to C9. Insertion of the complex C5b, C6, C7, C8, C9 into the cell membrane produces functional holes and leads to the osmotic lysis of eukaryotic cells against which the antibody was directed. Some Gram-negative bacteria are similarly affected when there is an

C5a is chemotactic for PMNs

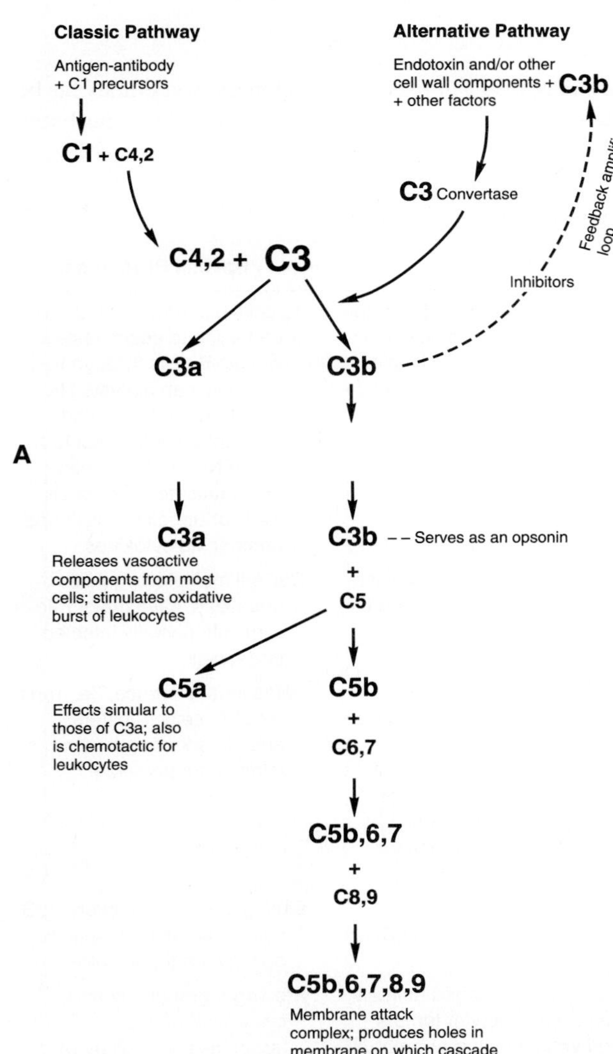


**Figure 8–11.** Schematic of the complement system. **A.** Pathways for activation of C3. (*Note:* Both pathways converge at C3.) **B.** Subsequent cascade and biological effects. Activated components are shown in bold type.

antibody response to accessible sites on the outer membrane. In this case, lysis (bacteriolysis) requires also the activity of lysozyme from phagocytes to break down the peptidoglycan layer of the cell wall.

## Alternative Pathway

Antibody not required

Important early response

The alternative pathway is more primitive than the classic pathway and does not require the presence of antibody. Instead, C3 can be activated by certain nonimmunologic stimuli. These include endotoxin, other bacterial cell wall components, aggregated IgA, and feedback from activation of the classic pathway. The alternative pathway is shown with the classic pathway in Figure 8–11. It produces the same inflammatory mediators (C3a, C5a) and increased phagocytic activity that result from activation of the classic pathway, but is not as efficient in cell lysis, because direction of complement components to the cell membrane by antibody is not involved. This pathway is particularly important in early response to infection.

Inherited deficiencies in complement components are often associated with increased susceptibility to bacterial infections. Most noticeable is the association of recurrent or unusually severe infections due to *Neisseria* (see Chapter 19) and individual complement component deficiencies (usually of C5, C6, C7, or C8).

# ADVERSE EFFECTS OF IMMUNOLOGIC REACTIONS AND HYPERSENSITIVITY

Immunologic reactions in the body may result in excessive responses, sometimes far beyond those needed to remove or neutralize microbial pathogens or molecules contributing

**TABLE 8–4. EFFECTOR CELLS IN CELL-MEDIATED IMMUNITY**

| Cell | Function | Special Properties |
|---|---|---|
| Specific helper T ($T_H$) cells | MHC class II-restricted help to B cells ($T_H2$), or in activation of macrophages ($T_H1$); distinct cytokines are used in the two processes | $T_H$ cells use $\alpha/\beta$ Tcr; $T_H2$ cells can activate eosinophils as well as B cells through IL-5; $T_H1$ cells can activate NK cells through IL-12, and macrophages through IL-2 and IFN-$\gamma$; $T_H2$ cells can communicate either positively or negatively with one another via cytokines |
| Specific cytotoxic T ($T_C$) cells | MHC class I-restricted specific killing; use endogenous $\alpha/\beta$ Tcr | Can kill multiple targets sequentially; have major role in eliminating virally infected target cells |
| Specific suppressor T ($T_S$) cells | Antigen specific; involves "suppressor inducer" T cells (CD4) which generate "suppressor effector"; $T_S$ cells can be antigen specific or idiotype specific; some aspects of the interactions are MHC restricted | "Infectious tolerance," ie, transfer of $T_S$ cells transfers antigen-specific immunosuppression |
| "K cells," macrophages, polymorphonuclear cells | Antibody-dependent cell-mediated cytotoxicity (ADCC) | Bind IgG via Fc receptors; IgG acts as an antigen-specific opsonin on these cells |
| Natural killer (NK) cells | Occur in unchallenged animals; can kill a variety of tumors and virus-infected or embryonic cells in vitro without expression of classic Tcr or bound antibody | Are large, granular lymphocytes; do not phagocytize target cells, but kill by release of toxins |

to disease. Such responses are classified as hypersensitivity reactions if they cause marked physiologic changes or tissue damage or exacerbate disease processes. Four distinct classes of hypersensitivity are recognized, but these do not occur in isolation and injury often results from a combination of the reactions. In each case they represent an extension of a normal defense mechanism. The immune response in practice is very potent and leads to deleterious consequences for the host if it is in operation too long. This is because the antigen-specific portion of the humoral or T-cell reactions constitutes only a small fraction of the overall response and amplification by complement components that can stimulate phagocytic cells and the release of cytokines; these can cause a general recruitment of lymphocytes, monocytes, and polymorphonuclear cells, leading to a cascade of inflammation and prolonged disease. The aspects of hypersensitivity are overexpressions of the beneficial immune responses that act inappropriately. The normal immune basis of the four types of hypersensitivity are described below and included in Tables 8–1 and 8–4. Types I, II, and III hypersensitivity are mediated by antibody; type IV (delayed-type) hypersensitivity is carried out by antigen-specific T cells assisted by macrophages.

Multiple classes of hypersensitivity reactions occur in combinations

## Anaphylactic (Type I) Hypersensitivity

Type I hypersensitivity, also called **anaphylaxis,** is represented by the allergic reactions that occur immediately following contact with the sensitizing antigen (allergen). IgE antibodies are bound to Fc receptors on the surface of mast cells (Fig 8–12). If a multivalent antigen binds to the cell-bound IgE molecules, it crosslinks them, with the result that the mast cell degranulates releasing a variety of pharmacologically active mediators. Among the prominent mediators released following binding of the allergen is histamine, which increases capillary permeability and causes bronchoconstriction. Preformed mediators such as the anticoagulant heparin, complement 3 convertase, and a group of compounds involved in chemotaxis of eosinophils, neutrophils, and platelet activation are also released by degranulation. Slow reactive substances involved in bronchoconstriction and chemotaxis are also produced, as are prostaglandins and thromboxanes, which are implicated in bronchospasm, muscle contraction, and platelet aggregation. Thus, the specific binding of an allergen to the combining site of its antibody can result in a potent release of compounds, leading to painful and life-threatening consequences for the allergic individual. Despite the suffering that hypersensitivity to common allergens such as pollen, bee stings, house dust, and cat dander brings to a large percentage of people, there are possible beneficial conse-

IgE activities liberate vasoactive mediators from mast cells

Anaphylaxis; IgE mediated reaction

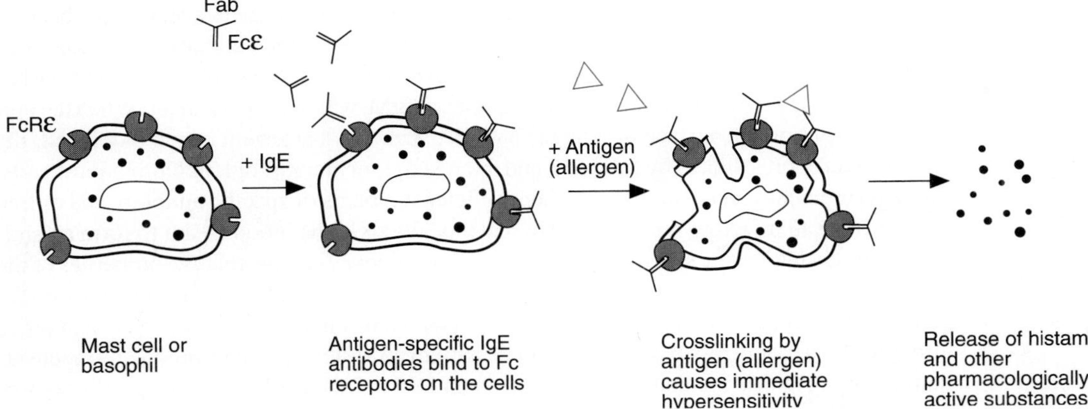


**Figure 8–12.** Diagram outlining the sequence of events in the anaphylactic (allergic) hypersensitive response (type 1) in which IgE antibodies arm mast cells by binding to Fc receptors (FcR) and the response is triggered by crosslinking of these by antigen. Comparable diagrams can be drawn for the arming of macrophages or polymorphonuclear leukocytes by IgG immunoglobulins adhering via their Fc receptors. In these reactions, the Fab arms of the bound antibodies are free to bind antigen specifically, and this binding initiates cellular events leading to sensitized phagocytosis and destruction or, in this case, the release of destructive pharmacologically active substances.

quences of binding of allergen by IgE. These include situations where ADCC by monocytes and eosonophils may provide protection against parasites such as schistosomes (a trematode worm) and trypanosomes (a protozoan).

When hypersensitivity is very marked, or antigen is introduced systemically, mast cells throughout the body degranulate, and systemic anaphylaxis results with constriction of the bronchi, edema of the larynx and other tissues, vascular collapse, and sometimes death. A generalized anaphylactic reaction rarely if ever occurs as a manifestation of an infection, but may occur following parenteral inoculation of an antigen to which the individual has been sensitized (eg, bee sting venom). It may also occur in individuals who have been sensitized to a low-molecular-weight hapten that binds to a tissue protein and becomes antigenic because of the size of the complex. An IgE response to hapten epitopes can then lead to anaphylactic-type hypersensitivity if the epitope is again encountered. A penicillin degradation product has this property, and occasional individuals develop severe anaphylactic reactions to penicillins, although this complication is very rare.

Systemic anaphylaxis occurs from low-molecular-weight haptens

Rapid therapeutic intervention is critical in systemic anaphylaxis. It includes parenteral administration of epinephrine, which reverses the major manifestations of the syndrome by producing bronchodilation, vasoconstriction, and raised blood pressure. Tracheostomy or intubation may be needed to overcome respiratory obstruction due to laryngeal edema.

## Antibody-Mediated (Type II) Hypersensitivity

Type II hypersensitivity is an inappropriate elaboration of antibody-dependent cytotoxicity that occurs when antibody binds to antigens on host cells, leading to phagocytosis, killer cell activity, or complement-mediated lysis. Antibody directed against cell surface or tissue antigens results in the fixation of complement such that a variety of effector cells become involved. The cells to which the antibody is specifically bound, as well as the surrounding tissues, are damaged because of the inflammatory amplification. Such mechanisms appear to be responsible for the tissue damage of rheumatic fever following a streptococcal infection or some clinical manifestations of viral diseases, such as group B coxsackie virus infection (see Chapter 35). These phenomena may involve not only antibodies, but also cytotoxic T cells. It should be recalled that humoral antibodies are required to arm macrophages and polymorphonuclear leukocytes to bind cellular antigens in ADCC and to serve as opsonins that facilitate ingestion with eventual intracellular destruction of target cells by macrophages.

Damage to host cells when antigen is bound to cell surface

## Immune Complex (Type III) Hypersensitivity

When IgG is mixed in appropriate proportions with multivalent antigen molecules (ie, bearing multiple epitopes), aggregates containing a lattice of many antigen and antibody molecules form. With appropriate concentrations of the two reactants, a macroscopic precipitate can develop (see Chapter 14). A similar situation applies to IgM, which is multivalent. When the epitope is present on the surface of a larger particle, such as a bacterium or red blood cell, the particles can be crosslinked by antibody, and microscopic or macroscopic agglutination results. These phenomena can occur in vivo when sufficient amounts of specific antibody and of free antigen from an infecting microorganism react locally or in the bloodstream to form an antigen–antibody lattice; the size of the immune complex depends on the relative properties of the two reactants. Large immune complexes are phagocytosed and usually broken down within the phagocyte. Smaller complexes, however, are deposited in small blood vessels and capillaries through which they do not pass, activate the complement system, and thus produce an acute inflammatory response mediated largely by C3a and C5a. This results in the manifestations of vasculitis. Phagocytes attracted chemotactically to the site release hydrolytic enzymes, and the sum of these effects is tissue damage that is acute and can become chronic depending on the survival of the antigen or on whether it is continually replaced. Acute glomerulonephritis following certain streptococcal infections is an example of an immune complex disease in which glomeruli of the kidney are damaged by the complexes, resulting in various manifestations of

Crosslinking forms lattice of antigen and antibody

Deposit of complexes stimulates inflammation in blood vessels, kidney renal impairment. Inflammatory skin lesions can result from deposition of immune complexes in the cutaneous blood vessels in patients with infective endocarditis. Deposition in joints, the pericardium, or the pleura produces arthritis, pericarditis, and pleuritis or pleurisy, respectively.

A systemic form of immune complex disease, termed **serum sickness,** can follow the injection of foreign antigen. An example is the therapeutic use of diphtheria antitoxin that has been produced in horses. About 10 days after inoculation, sufficient antibody against horse proteins has been produced to form immune complexes made up of human antibody reacting against horse serum protein (including horse immunoglobulins). These complexes are deposited in various organs, resulting in a syndrome of arthritis, nephritis, rash, urticaria, and fever. The disease usually resolves as the foreign antigen concentration decreases through immune clearance and catabolism of the antigen(s).

### Delayed-Type (Type IV) Hypersensitivity

The fourth type of hypersensitivity is termed **delayed type hypersensitivity.** Unlike types I to III, this process cannot be transferred from one animal to another by serum alone. It can, however, be transferred by antigen-specific T lymphocytes. All are initiated by the function of antigen-specific T cells, which then recruit effector cells into the area of recognition of the antigen. Unlike the forms of "immediate" hypersensitivity that can be transferred by antibody, delayed-type hypersensitivity requires days to weeks to express full reactivity. In all of these, the initial reaction is the induction and function of antigen-specific T cells that bear $\alpha/\beta$ T-cell receptors and have been generated in response to antigenic challenge. The time course depends on the involvement of other cells and the properties of the infectious agent involved.

Requires days to weeks to develop

Four major types of delayed-type hypersensitivity are all part of the same process differing in site, mechanism of challenge, and timing. The shortest is the Jones–Mote phenomenon, in which the site of antigen injection is infiltrated by basophils and the skin swelling is maximal 24 hours after antigen injection. This type of hypersensitivity can be raised to soluble antigens, and the reactivity disappears following the appearance of antibody. Contact and tuberculin-type hypersensitivity show maximal reactivity at 48 to 72 hours. Contact sensitivity is observed in response to sensitization with common antigens such as chemicals found in rubber or the small organic compounds produced by poison ivy and poison oak. It is predominantly an epidermal reaction, in contrast to the tuberculin-type hypersensitivity, which is a dermal reaction. The cell that presents antigen for contact sensitization is the Langerhans cell, a dendritic antigen-presenting cell carrying MHC class II antigens. Tuberculin-type hypersensitivity is manifested by individuals who have been sensitized with lipoprotein antigens derived from the tubercle bacillus. Twenty-four hours after intradermal injection of tuberculin, an antigen derived from *Mycobacterium tuberculosis*, there is intense infiltration by lymphocytes, which reaches a maximum in 2 to 3 days.

Four major types of delayed hypersensitivity

Tuberculin hypersensitivity from sensitization by lipoprotein from tubercle bacillus

Probably the most clinically important form of type IV sensitivity is the granuloma, an organized inflammatory lesion that requires at least 14 days to develop. These result from the long-term continuation of the stimulation of effector cells by cytokines produced in initial antigen-specific T-cell response. Granulomatous lesions are a major part of the disease process in chronic diseases caused by bacteria (tuberculosis), fungi (histoplasmosis), and parasites (schistosomiasis).

Long-term stimulation required for granuloma

## TOLERANCE

As discussed earlier, induced cellular and antibody responses follow challenge with antigens that are normally foreign; however, immunization can not only induce the enhanced reactivities described, but can lead to a diminished reactivity known as **tolerance.** When specifically diminished reactivity is induced by treatment with large doses of antigen, the phenomenon is referred to as **immune paralysis.** As the immune system is based on a random generation of combining sites directed against molecular configurations, there is in principle no reason why the immune response cannot react with self components. When it does, autoimmune diseases such as rheumatoid arthritis, systemic lupus erythematosus, and

Tolerance mechanisms prevent pathological reactivity to self antigens

others may result. It is now known, however, that normal healthy individuals express detectable levels of autoantibodies against a variety of self components. A regulatory function for these autoantibodies in the maintenance of homeostasis is suggested by the fact that aged red cells are removed from human circulation by a natural mechanism in which normally occurring IgG autoantibodies specific for a modified membrane component (senescent cell antigen) bind to the cells and lead to their removal by phagocytic cells. Nevertheless, the generation of tolerance or the inability to react against self is a fundamental part of the process of development in vertebrates that results essentially from the removal or inactivation of T cells in the thymus that can react to self antigens.

Autoantibodies may have homeostatic functions

Parallel tolerization procedures for B cells occur, but currently a number of mechanisms now must be proposed for maintenance of nonreactivity to self. Antigen-specific T cells may be either deleted by contact with antigen (clonal abortion) or inactivated without being destroyed. In addition, suppressor T cells that downregulate the specific immune response may be generated that either shut off the antigen-specific helper T cells or are directed toward combining sites of B-cell antibodies. Antigen-specific B cells may be deleted or inactivated or rendered insensitive to secondary stimulation by cytokines. These are central effects that operate at the level of antigen-specific T or B cells.

B cell tolerance also occurs

Both experimentally induced tolerance and innate tolerance can be broken down in two general ways. First, if a large amount of antigen is needed to maintain tolerance, immunity can be generated if the level of antigen falls below the required tolerogenic level. A second way of breaking of tolerance is immunization with a cross-reactive antigen. Two clinically well-known examples of the capacity of cross-reactive antigens to break normal self tolerance are (1) the induction of experimental allergic encephalomyelitis in an animal by the injection of heterologous brain tissue homogenates in emulsified adjuvant and (2) the capacity of infections with group A streptococci to cause rheumatic fever because of a cross-reaction between bacterial antigens and myocardial tissue. The concept of tolerance is critical to much of modern medicine because of increasing interest in autoimmune diseases, which can be considered to result from a failure or breakdown of tolerance.

Tolerance may be disturbed by quantitative or cross-reactive mechanisms

## LABORATORY PRODUCTION OF SPECIFIC ANTIBODIES

Specific antibodies are widely exploited in seroidentification of microorganisms, in basic studies of the immune response, as microchemical reagents in biological research, and as agents in prophylaxis and therapy. Various practical aspects of these uses are described in Chapter 14, but some principles of specific antibody production need to be described here.

Seroidentification procedures use antibodies to detect specific antigenic epitopes on microorganisms and thus aid in their identification. Antisera for this purpose are produced by inoculating one or more animals (usually rabbits, goats, or horses) with a known organism or purified antigens derived from it. The inoculation schedule is designed to produce a maximum antibody response. When this is reached the animal is bled, the serum separated, and its antibody quantitated by testing the ability of increasing dilutions of serum (titration) to react with the inciting antigen in a particular test system (agglutination, neutralization, etc). It is important to recognize that such antisera are usually polyclonal and contain antibodies of many different specificities. These can be against different molecules of the material injected into the animal and against different epitopes on the same molecule. Even when a single epitope is involved, antibodies of varying affinity are produced.

Antibodies prepared by immunizing animals

Antisera are polyclonal

In many cases, when the immunizing antigen is an organism of complex antigenic structure, such as a bacterium, some of the antibodies produced cross-react with the same, or closely similar, antigens on taxonomically distinct organisms. These antibodies can be removed by treating the antisera in vitro with cross-reacting organisms until all antibody to common antigens has reacted with them. The cross-reacting organisms and antibodies that have reacted with them are then removed by centrifugation, and the absorbed serum that remains has become a more specific seroidentification reagent. This is a very simplified account of what may be a complex process. Distinction between the hundreds of different *Salmonella* bacteria, for example, involves discrimination of many different antigenic epitopes represented on flagella, capsules, and cell surface polysaccharide antigens. It requires dozens of absorbed antisera made specific for the different epitopes that exist in many dif-

Cross-reacting antibodies may be removed by absorption

ferent combinations. Obviously, the process is simplified when purified antigen is available for immunizing the animals, but this is often impossible because the precise nature of the antigen is unknown or it has not been separated from others.

## Monoclonal Antibodies

The heterogeneity of antibody responses in terms of specificity and affinity introduces problems in their use as precise tools for identifying specific epitopes. This has been overcome by the development of procedures that allow the almost unlimited production of antibodies that were encoded in a single B cell. The process involves in vitro fusion of antigen-stimulated B cells with cells of a B-cell malignant tumor (myeloma) that synthesizes large amounts of a nonspecific immunoglobulin. The myeloma cell is capable of unrestricted growth in cell culture or in the animal from which it was derived. Genetic reassembly within the fused cells yields some that have the growth characteristics (immortality) and Ig synthesizing capability of the tumor but produce antibody with the specificity encoded in the nonmalignant B cell and thus for a single epitope. These cells are termed **hybridoma cells.**

Antigen stimulated B cells fused with immortal myeloma cells

Hybridoma cells produce homogenous antibody

Techniques have been developed that allow selection of clones of hybridoma cells that produce the desired antibody, and these cells can be grown continually in vitro or in vivo. The concept is outlined in Figure 8–13. Monoclonal antibody is homogeneous and highly specific for a single epitope and can be produced in almost limitless quantities. These antibodies are being used increasingly in seroidentification procedures and have the potential for use as therapeutic agents in instances in which critical antigens of a microorganism or a tumor cell are not recognized by the immune system of the host. The monoclonal antibody can also be combined with a substance that is lethal to the cell or organism carrying the antigen against which it is directed.

Monoclonal antibodies can be produced from hybridoma cells grown in vivo in the peritoneal cavity of mice or from in vitro cultures. Human monoclonal antibody production can result from fusion between human B cells and mouse myeloma cells, but the hybrids are less stable than when antigenically stimulated B cells of mice are used. A variety of ap-

Human B cells can be used

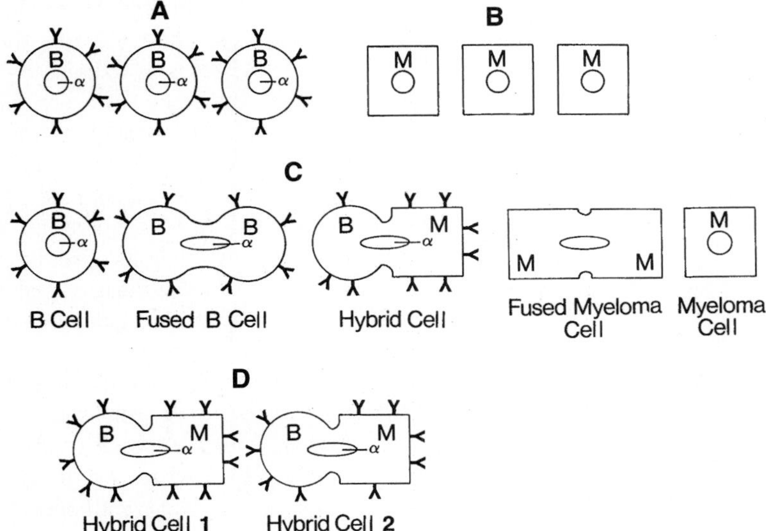


**Figure 8–13.** Concept of monoclonal antibody production. **A.** B cells are each producing Ig against different epitopes and carrying gene α for production of enzyme A. B cells cannot be maintained in culture. **B.** Mutant myeloma cells lack gene α and do not produce specific Ig. Myeloma cells can be propagated indefinitely. **C.** Cell fusion is enhanced with polyethylene glycol. **D.** Incubation is in selective medium that allows growth only of immortal (M) cells that produce enzyme A. These are antibody-producing hybridoma cells. Individual hybrid cells are cloned, expanded in culture, and tested for production of antibody of desired specificity, and that clone is propagated as an epitope-specific hybridoma.

proaches are being explored to facilitate the safe production of human monoclonal antibodies for therapeutic purposes.

## Antigen Surrogates

A recently developed approach has the potential to allow the use of antibodies as antigen surrogates in immunization. Antibodies are themselves antigenic in animal species to which they are foreign. The anti-antibodies that can be produced include some with specificity for unique epitope-reacting portions of the Fab variable region of the antibody against which they are directed as well as for epitope-recognizing sites on immunoresponsive B cells. These are termed **anti-idiotypic antibodies** and have the same three-dimensional geometry as would the epitope molecule. Monoclonal antibodies that have this structure can be selected and produced in large amounts and may then act as antigens for the production of specific antibodies against the epitope of interest. Immunization with such anti-idiotype antibodies has promise for producing specific immunity against critical antigens that are impossible or uneconomical to produce in bulk. At present there are many problems to overcome before such procedures could begin to be applied to humans.

## ADDITIONAL READING

Abbas AK, Lichtman AH, Pober JS. *Cellular and Molecular Immunology*. Philadelphia: WB Saunders; 1991. A detailed survey of immunological mechanisms.

Benjamini E, Leskowitz S. *Immunology. A Short Course*. 2nd ed. New York: Wiley–Liss; 1991. A basic and readily understandable text for use by medical students.

Eisen HN. *General Immunology*. Philadelphia: JB Lippincott; 1990. A comprehensive presentation of cellular and molecular immunologic mechanisms.

Marchalonis JJ. *The Lymphocyte. Structure and Function*. 2nd ed. New York: Marcel Dekker; 1988. Detailed, advanced analysis of lymphocytes, their functions, and their regulation.

Paul WE. *Fundamental Immunology*. 2nd ed. New York: Raven Press; 1989. A comprehensive, detailed, multiauthored volume.

Roitt I. *Essential Immunology*. 7th ed. London: Blackwell; 1991. A basic introductory text.

Roitt IM, Delves PJ, eds. *Encyclopedia of Immunology*. New York: Academic Press; 1992. Extremely useful for concise summaries of most of the major areas of immunology.

Stites DP, Terr AI. *Basic and Clinical Immunology*. 7th ed. Norwalk, CT: Appleton and Lange; 1991. Extremely useful for its presentation of clinical aspects of immunology.

Chapter 9

# Normal Microbial Flora

*Kenneth J. Ryan*

The term **normal flora** or **indigenous flora** is used to describe microorganisms that are frequently found in particular sites in normal, healthy individuals. The constituents and numbers of the flora vary in different areas of the body and sometimes at different ages. They comprise microorganisms whose morphologic, physiologic, and genetic properties allow them to colonize and multiply under the conditions that exist in particular sites, to coexist with other colonizing organisms, and to inhibit competing intruders. Thus, each accessible area of the body presents a particular ecologic niche, colonization of which requires a particular set of properties of the invading microbe.

Organisms of the normal flora may have a symbiotic relationship that benefits the host or may simply live as commensals with a neutral relationship to the host. A parasitic relationship that injures the host would not be considered "normal," but in most instances not enough is known about the organism–host interactions to make such distinctions. Like houseguests the members of the normal flora may stay for highly variable periods. **Residents** are present invariably or for months in a particular site, and **transients** establish themselves briefly but tend to be excluded by competition from residents or by the host's innate or immune defense mechanisms. The term **carrier state** is often used when potentially pathogenic organisms are involved, although its implication of risk is usually not justified. For example, *Streptococcus pneumoniae*, a cause of pneumonia, and *Neisseria meningitidis*, a cause of meningitis, may be isolated from the throat of many healthy people. Whether this represents transient normal flora, resident normal flora, or carrier state is largely semantic. The possibility that it could represent the prelude to disease is impossible to determine simply by culture of a normal flora site.

Flora may stay for short or extended periods

If pathogens are involved the relationship is called the carrier state

It is important for students of medical microbiology and infectious disease to understand the role of the normal flora, because of its significance both as a defense mechanism against infection and as a source of potentially pathogenic organisms. The desired state of balance between host and microbial flora was understood by British poet W. H. Auden when he wrote:

Balance is the desired state, at least for the host

Build colonies: I will supply
adequate warmth and moisture,
the sebum and lipids you need,
on condition you never
do me annoy with your presence,
but behave as good guests should,
not rioting into acne
or athlete's-foot or a boil.

From Auden WH,
*Epistle to a Godson*

It is also important to know its sites and composition to avoid interpretive confusion between normal flora species and pathogens when interpreting laboratory culture results.

## ORIGIN OF THE NORMAL FLORA

Initial flora is acquired during and immediately after birth

The healthy fetus is sterile until the birth membranes rupture. During and after birth, the infant is exposed to the flora of the mother's genital tract, to the skin and respiratory flora of those handling it, and to organisms in the environment. During the infant's first few days of life, the flora reflects chance exposure to organisms that can colonize particular sites in the absence of competitors. Subsequently, as the infant is exposed to a broader range of organisms, those best adapted to colonize particular sites become predominant. Thereafter, the flora generally resembles that of other individuals in the same age group and cultural milieu.

## FACTORS DETERMINING THE NATURE OF THE NORMAL FLORA

Physiologic conditions such as local pH influence colonization

Adherence factors counteract mechanical flushing

Ability to compete for nutrients is an advantage

Local physiologic and ecologic conditions determine the nature of the flora. These conditions are sometimes highly complex, differing from site to site, and sometimes vary with age. Conditions include the amounts and types of nutrients available, pH, oxidation–reduction potentials, and resistance to local antibacterial substances such as bile and lysozyme. Many bacteria have adhesin-mediated affinity for receptors on specific types of epithelial cells which facilitates colonization and multiplication while avoiding removal by the flushing effects of surface fluids and peristalsis. Various microbial interactions also determine their relative prevalence in the flora. These interactions include competition for nutrients, inhibition by the metabolic products of other organisms (eg, by hydrogen peroxide or volatile fatty acids), and production of antibiotics and bacteriocins.

## NORMAL FLORA OF DIFFERENT SITES

The total normal flora of the body probably contains more than 100 distinct species of microorganisms. The major members known to be important in preventing or causing disease as well as those that may be confused with etiologic agents of local infections are summarized in Table 9–1, and most are described in greater detail in subsequent chapters. The student should not attempt to memorize unfamiliar names at this point.

### Blood, Body Fluids, and Tissues

Tissues and body fluids such as blood are normally sterile in health

Transient bacteremia can result from trauma

In health, the blood, body fluids, and tissues are normally sterile. Occasional organisms may be displaced across epithelial barriers as a result of trauma (including physiologic trauma such as heavy chewing) or during childbirth; they may be briefly recoverable from the bloodstream before they are filtered out in the pulmonary capillaries or removed by cells of the reticuloendothelial system. Such transient bacteremia may be the source of infection when structures such as damaged heart valves and foreign bodies (prostheses) are in the bloodstream.

### Skin

Skin flora varies at different sites

Propionibacteria grow in pilosebaceous units

The skin plays host to an abundant flora that varies somewhat according to the number and activity of sebaceous and sweat glands. The flora is most abundant on moist skin areas (axillae, perineum, and between toes). *Staphylococcus epidermidis*, other staphylococci, and members of the genus *Propionibacterium* occur all over the skin, and facultative diphtheroids (corynebacteria) are found in moist areas. Propionibacteria are slim, anaerobic, or microaerophilic Gram-positive rods that grow in subsurface sebum and break down skin lipids to fatty acids. They are thus most numerous in the ducts of hair follicles and of the

**TABLE 9–1. PREDOMINANT AND IMPORTANT FLORA OF VARIOUS BODY SITES IN HEALTH**

| | Flora | |
|---|---|---|
| **Body Site** | ***Potential Pathogens*** | ***Low Virulence Organisms*** |
| Blood | None | None[a] |
| Tissues | None | None |
| Skin, distal urethra, external ear, anterior nares | *Staphylococcus aureus* | *Propionobacterium acnes*, diphtheroids, coagulase-negative staphylococci |
| Mouth | *Candida albicans* | Viridans streptococci, *Neisseria* species, *Moraxella,* anaerobes |
| Nasopharynx | *Streptococcus pneumoniae, Neisseria meningitidis, Haemophilus influenzae,* | Viridans streptococci, *Neisseria* species, *Moraxella,* anaerobes |
| Esophagus/stomach | None | Transient mouth flora |
| Small intestine | None | Scanty, variable |
| Colon | | |
| Breast feeding | None | *Bifidobacterium, Lactobacillus*, streptococci |
| After weaning | *Bacteroides, Clostridium, E. coli*, pseudomonas, *Candida* | *Bifidobacterium*, streptococci anaerobes |
| Vagina | | |
| Prepubertal and postmenopausal | *Candida albicans* | Skin and colonic flora |
| Childbearing | *Candida albicans* | *Lactobacillus*, streptococci |

[a] Organisms such as viridans streptococci may be transiently present following trauma.

sebaceous glands that drain into them (pilosebaceous units). They cannot be completely removed from skin sites bearing pilosebaceous units and small numbers are often isolated from biopsy materials despite the most vigorous washing or application of antiseptics. Organisms of the skin flora are resistant to the bactericidal effects of skin lipids and fatty acids, which inhibit or kill many extraneous bacteria.

Skin flora is not easily removed

## Conjunctival Sac

In health, the conjunctivae have a very scanty flora of nonpathogenic corynebacteria and *S. epidermidis*. The low bacterial count is maintained by the high lysozyme content of lacrimal secretions and by the flushing effect of tears.

## Intestinal Tract

The mouth and pharynx contain large numbers of facultative and strict anaerobes. Different species of streptococci predominate on the buccal and tongue mucosa because of different specific adherence characteristics; one species, *Streptococcus mutans*, shows specific adherence to teeth and plays an etiologic role in caries. Gram-negative diplococci of the genera *Neisseria* and *Moraxella* make up the balance of the facultative organisms most commonly isolated. Strict anaerobes and microaerophilic organisms of the oral cavity have their niches in the depths of the gingival crevices surrounding the teeth and in sites such as tonsillar crypts, where anaerobic conditions can develop readily. Anaerobic members of the normal flora are major contributors to the etiology of periodontal disease (see Chapter 62).

Oropharynx has abundant flora including streptococci

Although it varies from site to site, the total number of organisms in the oral cavity is very high. Saliva usually contains a mixed flora of about $10^8$ organisms per milliliter, derived mostly from the various epithelial colonization sites. The stomach contains few, if any, resident organisms in health because of the lethal action of gastric hydrochloric acid

Stomach has few residents

Small intestinal flora is scanty but increases toward lower ileum

and peptic enzymes on bacteria. The small intestine has a scanty resident flora, except in the lower ileum, where it begins to resemble that of the colon.

Adult colonic flora is abundant and predominantly anaerobic

The colon carries the most prolific flora in the body (Fig 9–1). In the adult, feces are 25% or more bacteria by weight (about $10^{10}$ organisms per gram). More than 90% are anaerobes, predominantly members of the genera *Bacteroides* and *Fusobacterium*, although *Clostridium perfringens*, a major etiologic agent of gas gangrene, is invariably present. The remainder of the flora is composed of facultative organisms such as *Escherichia coli*, enterococci, yeasts, and numerous other species. There are considerable differences in adult flora depending on the diet of the host. Those whose diets include substantial amounts of meat have more *Bacteroides* and other anaerobic Gram-negative rods in their stools than those on a predominantly vegetable or fish diet.

Bifidobacteria are predominant flora of breastfed infants

Bottle-fed infants have a flora similar to that of weaned infants.

The fecal flora of breastfed infants differs from that of adults; up to 99% comprises anaerobic Gram-positive rods of the genus *Bifidobacterium*. Human milk is high in lactose and low in protein and phosphate, and its buffering capacity is poor compared with that of cow's milk. These conditions select for bifidobacteria, which ferment lactose to yield acetic acid and grow optimally under the acidic conditions (pH 5–5.5) that they produce in the stool. Infants fed cow's milk, which has a greater buffering capacity, tend to have less acidic stools and a flora more similar to that found in the colon of the weaned infant or the adult. These findings also apply to infants fed some artificial formulas.

## Respiratory Tract

*S. aureus* is carried in anterior nares

Nasopharynx is often a site of carriage of potential pathogens

The external 1 cm of the anterior nares is lined with squamous epithelium. The nares have a flora similar to that of the skin except that it is the primary site of carriage of a pathogen, *Staphylococcus aureus*. About 25 to 30% of healthy people carry this organism as either resident or transient flora at any given time. The organism may spread to other skin sites or colonize the perineum; it can be disseminated by hand-to-nose contact, by desquamation of the epithelium, or by droplet spread during upper respiratory infection. The nasopharynx has a flora similar to that of the mouth; however, it is often the site of carriage of potentially pathogenic organisms such as pneumococci, meningococci, and *Haemophilus* species.

Lower tract is protected by mucociliary action

The respiratory tract below the level of the larynx is protected in health by the action of the epithelial cilia and by the movement of the mucociliary blanket; thus, only transient

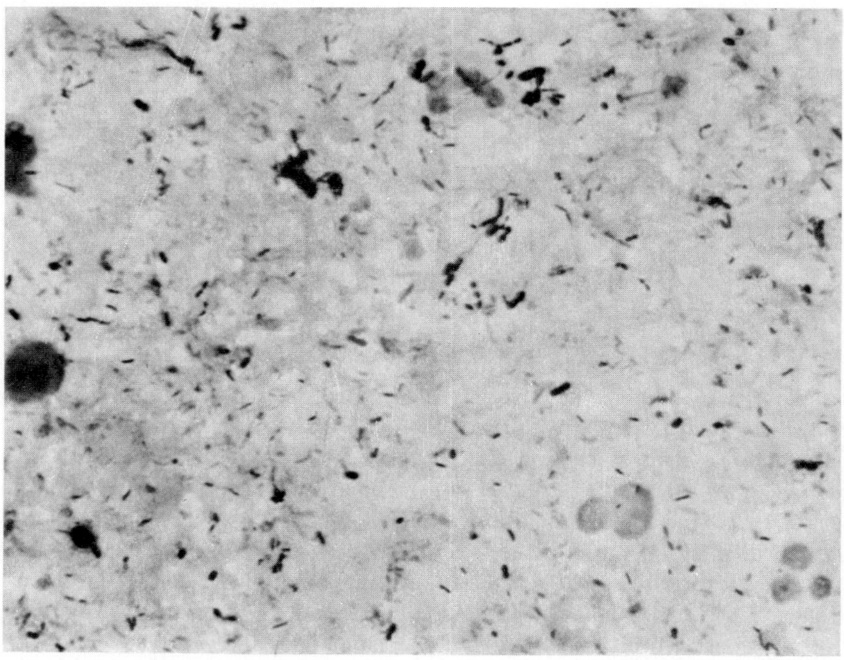

**Figure 9–1.** Smear of feces, showing great diversity of microorganisms.

inhaled organisms are encountered in the trachea and larger bronchi. The accessory sinuses are normally sterile and are protected in a similar fashion, as is the middle ear by the epithelium of the eustachian tubes.

## Genitourinary Tract

The urinary tract is sterile in health above the distal 1 cm of the urethra, which has a scanty flora derived from the perineum. Thus, in health the urine in the bladder, ureters, and renal pelvis is sterile.

Bladder and upper urinary tract are sterile in health

The vagina has a flora that varies according to hormonal influences at different ages. Before puberty and after menopause, it is mixed, nonspecific, relatively scanty, and contains organisms derived from the flora of the skin and colon. During the childbearing years, it is composed predominantly of anaerobic and microaerophilic members of the genus *Lactobacillus*, with smaller numbers of anaerobic Gram-negative rods, Gram-positive cocci, and yeasts that can survive under the acidic conditions produced by the lactobacilli. These conditions develop because glycogen is deposited in vaginal epithelial cells under the influence of estrogenic hormones and metabolized to lactic acid by lactobacilli. This process results in a vaginal pH of 4 to 5, which is optimal for growth and survival of the lactobacilli, but inhibits many other organisms. The consistency of the lactobacillary adult flora is seen in Gram-stained preparations of vaginal smears (Fig 9–2).

Hormonal changes affect the vaginal flora

Use of epithelial glycogen by lactobacilli produces low pH

## ROLE OF THE NORMAL FLORA IN DISEASE

Many species among the normal flora are opportunists in that they can cause infection if they reach protected areas of the body in sufficient numbers or if local or general host defense mechanisms are compromised. For example, certain strains of *E. coli* can reach the urinary bladder by ascending the urethra (see Chapter 66) and cause acute urinary tract infection, usually in sexually active women. Perforation of the colon from a ruptured diverticulum or a penetrating abdominal wound releases feces into the peritoneal cavity; this fecal contamination may be followed by peritonitis, caused primarily by facultative members of the flora, and by intraabdominal abscesses, caused primarily by Gram-negative anaerobes. Viridans streptococci from the oral cavity may reach the bloodstream as a result of physiologic trauma or injury (eg, tooth extraction) and colonize a previously damaged heart valve, initiating bacterial endocarditis (see Chapter 68). These and other diseases, such as actino-

Bacterial flora may gain access to normally sterile sites

Mouth flora may reach heart valves by transient bacteremia

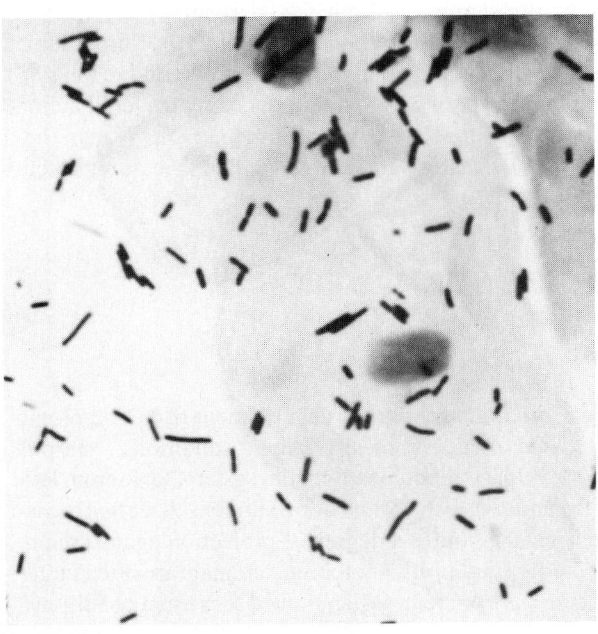

**Figure 9–2.** Smear of normal adult vagina, showing predominant large elongated lactobacilli and squamous epithelial cells.

mycosis (see Chapter 28), result from displacement of normal flora into body cavities or tissues.

Compromised defense systems increase the opportunity for invasion

Reduced specific immunologic responses, defects in phagocytic activity, and weakening of epithelial barriers by vitamin deficiencies can all result in local invasion and disease by normal floral organisms. This source accounts for many infections in patients whose defenses are compromised by disease (eg, diabetes, lymphoma, and leukemia) or by cytotoxic chemotherapy for cancer. One specific local infection of this type is Vincent's angina of the oral mucosa, a local invasion and ulceration apparently caused by the combined action of oral spirochetes and members of the genus *Fusobacterium*. Death after lethal radiation exposure usually results from massive invasion by normal floral organisms, particularly those of the intestinal tract. Caries and periodontal disease are both caused by organisms that are members of the normal flora. They are considered in detail in Chapter 62.

Mouth flora plays a major role in dental caries

Nonspecific "toxic" effects of colonic flora were often postulated in the past

Early in the 20th century, it was widely believed that the normal flora of the large intestine was responsible for many "toxic conditions," including rheumatoid arthritis, degenerative diseases, and a range of conditions now recognized as psychosomatic. Ritualistic purging and colonic lavage flourished, particularly at expensive mineral spas. At the height of this misdirected attack on the normal flora, some London patients were even subjected to colectomy as a cure for thyroid nodules. The concept was given respectability by Elie Metchnikoff, who suggested that the longevity of Georgian peasants in Russia was attributable to their heavy consumption of yogurt, resulting in replacement of their colonic flora with lactobacilli to the general benefit of their health. These concepts fell into disrepute as the etiology of the "toxic" diseases was clarified and when it was found that lactobacillary replacement of flora of the adult colon did not occur under the conditions used. This notion persists today in the alleged benefit of natural (unpasteurized) yogurt, which contains live lactobacilli.

Manipulation of colonic flora with unpasteurized yogurt is futile

Blind-loop overgrowth may cause fat malabsorption and $B_{12}$ deficiency

More recently, however, attention has again been focused on the less specific contributions of the normal flora to health and disease. In patients with large or multiple blind-ended diverticula in the small intestine, heavy colonization by the anaerobic intestinal flora may occur. This colonization results in bacterial deconjugation of bile salts needed for absorption of fat and fat-soluble vitamins and also in competition for vitamin $B_{12}$. Similar situations sometimes occur in the elderly when the small intestine is invaded by colonic flora. If the primary cause cannot be eliminated surgically, these conditions can be ameliorated with antibiotic therapy and fat-soluble vitamin supplements. An analogous situation occurs in tropical sprue, in which secondary colonization of the jejunum by facultative Gram-negative enteric bacteria leads to fat malabsorption and vitamin $B_{12}$ and folic acid deficiencies. It has been postulated that the higher colon cancer rates in those consuming Western as opposed to Oriental diets may be a result of greater production by members of the normal flora of carcinogens such as nitrosamines and bile acid derivatives.

Colonization of jejunum occurs in tropical sprue

Ammonia production and bypass lead to hepatic encephalopathy

Under certain conditions, a "toxemia" can result from the action of the normal colonic flora. In severe hepatic cirrhosis, the portal circulation may be partially diverted to the systemic circulation. The detoxification by the liver of ammonia produced by bacterial action on protein residues is bypassed, and severe dysfunctions of the central nervous system (hepatic encephalopathy) can result. This problem can be ameliorated with a strict low-protein diet.

## BENEFICIAL EFFECTS OF THE NORMAL FLORA

### Priming of Immune System

Sterile animals have little immunity to microbial infection

Organisms of the normal flora play an important role in the development of immunologic competence. Animals delivered and raised under completely aseptic conditions ("sterile" or gnotobiotic, animals) have a poorly developed reticuloendothelial system, low serum levels of immunoglobulins, and none of the antibodies to normal floral antigens that often cross-react with those of pathogenic organisms and confer a degree of protection against them. As long as they are maintained under sterile conditions, gnotobiotic animals are often larger and live longer than those exposed to the environment. When moved to normal conditions, however, they immediately become vulnerable, because many bacteria that are nonpathogenic to normal hosts can be lethal to them, presumably because immunologic priming has not occurred under the protection of maternally derived antibody.

## Exclusionary Effect

The normal flora produces conditions that tend to block the establishment of extraneous pathogens and their ability to infect the host. The bifidobacteria in the colon of the breast-fed infant produce an environment inimical to colonization by enteric pathogens; this protective effect is aided by ingested maternal IgA. Breastfeeding has clearly been shown to help protect the infant from enteric bacterial infection.

Breastfeeding and a bifidobacterial flora have a protective effect

The normal vaginal flora has a similar protective effect. Before the introduction of antibiotic therapy, it was found that institutional outbreaks of fomite-transmitted gonococcal vulvovaginitis in prepubertal girls were controlled by synthetic estrogen therapy. This treatment led to glycogen deposition in the vaginal epithelium and establishment of a protective lactobacillary flora. The possible hazard of such therapy in this age group was not then recognized.

*Lactobacillus* vaginal flora can protect against fomite-transmitted gonorrhea

Antibiotic therapy, particularly with broad-spectrum agents, may so alter the normal flora of the gastrointestinal tract that antibiotic-resistant organisms multiply in the relative ecologic vacuum produced, sometimes causing significant infections, particularly in immunocompromised patients. The pathogenic yeast *Candida albicans*, a minor component of the normal flora, may multiply dramatically and cause superficial fungal infections in the mouth, vagina, or anal area. Pseudomembranous colitis results from overproliferation of a toxin-producing anaerobe, *Clostridium difficile*, which has a selective advantage in the presence of antibiotic therapy. It may be resistant to several antibiotics, that act on other members of the colonic flora, allowing *C. difficile* to increase from a minor to a major component. Its toxins cause diarrhea and direct damage to the colonic epithelium (see Chapter 18).

Antibiotic therapy may provide a competitive advantage for pathogens that are not susceptible

The exclusionary effect of the flora in health has been demonstrated in numerous experiments on gnotobiotic and antibiotic-treated animals. For example, *C. albicans* attaches to oral epithelial cells of germ-free rats; however, prior colonization with certain viridans streptococci that attach to similar epithelial cells prevents establishment of *C. albicans*. In another experiment, the infecting oral dose for mice of streptomycin-resistant *Salmonella* was shown to be approximately $10^5$ organisms in untreated animals. Oral streptomycin treatment, which inhibits many members of the normal flora, reduced the infecting dose by approximately 1000-fold.

Exclusionary effect makes entrance of pathogens more difficult

## Production of Essential Nutrients

In ruminants, the action of the extensive anaerobic flora in the rumen is essential to the nutrition of the animal. The flora digests cellulose to usable form and provides many vitamins, including 70% of the animal's vitamin B requirements. In humans, members of the vitamin B group and vitamin K are produced by the normal flora; however, except for vitamin K the amounts available or absorbed are small compared with those in a well-balanced diet. Bacterial vitamin production is reduced during broad-spectrum antibiotic therapy, and supplementation with vitamin B complex is indicated in malnourished individuals.

Some vitamins are produced by members of the normal flora

# MANIPULATION OF THE NORMAL FLORA

Attempts to manipulate the normal flora have usually been fruitless and have sometimes been dangerous. Exclusion of the normal flora has been effective in patients whose immunologic defenses are massively compromised (eg, following the whole-body irradiation used in bone marrow transplantation). Significant effects require the use of antimicrobics, sterilization of food and supplies, air filtration, and strict aseptic nursing procedures. These conditions substantially reduce the risk of infection during a highly vulnerable period.

Exclusion of normal flora during periods of extreme vulnerability is difficult but effective

Efforts to control which organisms make up the flora have been more problematic.

Adding "benign" flora is hazardous

During nursery outbreaks of *S. aureus* infections in the 1950s deliberate colonization of the infant's nares with *S. aureus* 502A, a strain of low virulence, was attempted as a control measure. This approach was based on the hope that it would exclude more virulent strains of *S. aureus*. Unfortunately, some infections occurred with the 502A strain. Obviously, we need to understand virulence and the extremely complex interactions of the normal flora much better before such fine tuning can be successful.

## ADDITIONAL READING

Noble WC. Skin microbiology: Coming of age. *J Med Microbiol.* 1984;17:1–12.

Rosebury T. *Life on Man.* New York: Berkeley; 1970. A delightful, wry, and instructive paperback. Highly recommended for recreational reading.

Rowland IR, ed. Role of the gut flora in toxicity and cancer. London: Academic Press; 1988. This specialized book contains chapters on the normal intestinal flora and their physiologic host interactions.

Savage DC, Fletcher M, eds. *Bacterial Adhesion: Mechanisms and Physiological Significance.* New York/London: Plenum Press; 1985. A multiauthored book by leading contributors to the field that gives a good account of knowledge of the mechanisms and significance of adherence, including those of members of the normal flora.

Skinner FA, Carr JG, eds. *The Normal Microbial Flora of Man.* Society for Applied Bacteriology Symposium No. 3. London: Academic Press; 1974. This and the Noble reference give excellent coverage of their topics and are good reference sources.

Chapter 10

# Host–Parasite Relationships

*Stanley Falkow*

> Pathogenicity is, in a sense, a highly skilled trade, and only a tiny minority of all the numberless tons of microbes on the earth has ever involved itself in it; most bacteria are busy with their own business, browsing and recycling the rest of life. Indeed, pathogenicity often seems to me a sort of biological accident in which signals are misdirected by the microbe or misinterpreted by the host.
>
> From Lewis Thomas, *The Medusa and the Snail*

The factors that determine the initiation, development, and outcome of an infection involve a series of complex and shifting interactions between the parasite and the host, which can vary with different infecting organisms. These interactions include the following:

1. The host's primary physical barriers against invasion and the ways in which they can be breached
2. The organism's ability to evade destruction by local and tissue host defenses
3. The method the organism uses to spread in the body and cause disease
4. The body's adaptive immunologic ability to control and eliminate invading parasites

Despite the complexity of interactions between different parasites and hosts, several components of pathogenetic processes and principles have broad application to infectious diseases and are described in this chapter with appropriate examples. More details of individual organisms and diseases are given in subsequent chapters. Basic mechanisms of specific immune responses are discussed in Chapter 8 and are not recapitulated here.

In considering this topic, it is essential to bear in mind that the ability of an organism to infect or cause disease depends on the susceptibility of the host. There are remarkable species differences in host susceptibility to many infections. For example, dogs do not get measles, nor do people get canine distemper, although the causative viruses are related.

## WHAT IS A PATHOGEN?

A survival strategy is needed if a pathogen is to produce disease

Infection does not always lead to overt disease

A pathogen is any microorganism having the capacity to cause disease in a particular host. Disease, however, is the end product of an infectious process. The strategy for survival of a pathogen requires infection (persistence, usually by multiplication on or within another living organism). Disease, that is, the overt damage done to a host as a result of its interaction with the infectious agent, may not be an inevitable outcome of the host–parasite interaction. Rather, the requirement for a microbial infection is sufficient multiplication by the pathogen to secure its establishment within the host by transient or long-term colonization or to bring about its successful transmission to a new susceptible host. Indeed, many infections are inapparent and asymptomatic. Symptoms of disease can reflect part of the microbe's strategy for survival within the host. Hence, coughing and sneezing promote the transmission of the tubercle bacillus and influenza virus, and diarrhea spreads enteric viruses and bacteria.

## Degree of Pathogenicity

Primary pathogens have a high probability of producing disease

Certain microorganisms regularly cause infection and disease when they enter a nonimmune host. For example, the bacterium that causes whooping cough, *Bordetella pertussis*, has a very high probability of causing symptomatic disease in susceptible hosts, as does the measles virus. These organisms are **primary pathogens.** In contrast, *Pseudomonas aeruginosa* is ubiquitous in aquatic environments and on vegetation; humans ingest it all the time in salads. This microorganism rarely causes disease in healthy humans, but in a host whose defense systems have been compromised or breached by a burn or instrumentation, *Pseudomonas* causes serious and often fatal disease. Such organisms are called **opportunistic pathogens.**

Opportunistic pathogens require some host compromise

Opportunistic pathogens of increasing importance in aging population

Physicians deal more and more with opportunists because our population is getting older and the practice of medicine keeps individuals alive longer by surgical procedures and powerful drugs that affect the immune status. As a consequence, in the Western world, microorganisms that a scant 30 years ago were considered harmless commensals are now feared opportunistic pathogens. Many of the primary pathogens like measles virus are controlled now by immunization. One view is to believe that we are controlling infectious diseases. Another view is that the host–parasite relationship is still in a dynamic state. Just as many people die of infection as they did 30 years ago; they just die later and because of different infectious agents. It is important to understand that for most of the world, the "classic" pathogens like malaria, the tubercle bacillus and leprosy bacillus, and the cholera vibrio remain leading causes of human misery and death.

Immunization now controls many primary pathogens

Among pathogens there are degrees of virulence

A comparison of pathogenicity in the quantitative sense is called **virulence.** For example, the bacterial species *Haemophilus influenzae* is a common inhabitant of the upper respiratory tract of humans. Members of this species regularly cause middle-ear infection and sinusitis in children and bronchitis in smokers, but one variety of *H. influenzae* (those with capsule type b) can cause systemic disease (meningitis and epiglottitis). All *H. influenzae* are pathogenic, but *H. influenzae* type b are more virulent.

## Toward a Genetic and Molecular Definition of Pathogenicity

Classical study of pathogenesis based on comparison of virulent and avirulent strains

Following on Koch's postulates, the classic investigation of pathogenicity has been based on a linking of natural disease in humans with experimental infection produced by the same organism. The analysis of bacterial virulence determinants was usually the result of the comparative analysis of different clinical isolates of the same species that were either virulent or avirulent in a particular model system. This led to speculation about the potential role of a number of microbial traits as virulence determinants.

Genetic approach focuses on manipulation of single virulence property

This comparative approach has now given way to mutational analysis within a single or limited number of strains of a pathogenic species. The goal is to obtain a single genetic lesion that alters a single virulence property and affects the pathogenesis of infection or the ability of the organism to cause pathology in an appropriate model system. The advances in microbial genetics, DNA biochemistry, and molecular biology now have made it possible to apply a kind of molecular Koch's postulates to the analysis of virulence traits:

Molecular Koch's postulates involve inactivation and restoration of specific genes

1. The phenotype or property under investigation should be associated significantly more often with pathogenic strains of a species than with nonpathogenic strains.
2. Specific inactivation of the gene or genes of interest associated with the suspected virulence trait should lead to a measurable decrease in virulence.
3. Restoration of pathogenicity or full virulence should accompany replacement of the mutated allele with the original "wild-type" gene.

This simplistic goal is not always possible because it is dependent on a suitable infection model in which to test a microorganism. The ideal model can be infected by a natural route using numbers analogous to those seen in human infection and duplicates the relevant pathology observed in the natural host. Except for other primates, such models do not exist for pathogens that are restricted to humans. Thus, for example, it is still difficult to assess the role of IgA1 protease in the pathogenicity of *Neisseria gonorrhoeae* as the enzyme works only on human IgA1 and the microorganism is an exclusive human pathogen.

Animal models greatly aid in the study of microbial virulence factors

Despite these technical limitations there has been a revolution in understanding of the basic pathogenic mechanisms over the past decade and a considerably clearer idea of how microbes bring about infection and disease. The use of transgenic animals, reconstituted human immune systems in rodents, and the extension of cell and organ culture methods to the study of infectious agents will lead to greater understanding of the pathogenesis of infectious diseases. This knowledge will continue to impact how infectious diseases are treated and prevented.

Genetically designed animal systems and organ culture methods aid study

## FIRST-LINE DEFENSES AGAINST MICROBIAL INFECTION

First-line defenses of the healthy individual are those that prevent colonization of certain body surfaces or block access of potentially pathogenic organisms to subepithelial tissues. First-line defenses are summarized in Table 10–1 and are considered below in more detail according to the structures and processes involved.

### Epithelial Barriers

#### Skin, Vaginal, and Conjunctival Epithelium

A simple mechanical barrier to microbial invasion is provided by intact epithelia, the most effective of which is the stratified squamous epithelium of the skin with its superficial cornified anucleate layers. Organisms can gain access to the underlying tissues only by breaks or by way of hair follicles, sebaceous glands, and sweat glands that traverse the stratified layers. The surface of the skin continuously desquamates and thus tends to shed contaminating organisms. It is also inhibitory to the growth of most extraneous microorganisms because of low moisture, low pH, and the presence of substances with antibacterial activity. These include lactic acid from sweat glands, free fatty acids, waxes and alcohols from the secretions of sebaceous glands, and products of metabolic activity of the indigenous microbial flora. Greater moisture (eg, beneath occlusive dressings) can increase the number of potential pathogens on the skin surface. Significant destruction of skin is invariably followed by infection, as in the case of severe burns. The vaginal epithelium, a modified squamous epithelium, is protected during childbearing years by the low pH and exclusionary effects produced by the normal bacterial flora discussed in Chapter 9. The conjunctiva is protected by the flushing effects of the tears, aided by a high concentration of lysozyme, which disrupts the accessible cell wall peptidoglycan of some Gram-positive bacteria, and lactoferrin, which competes for the iron essential to microbial growth.

Stratified squamous epithelium is a formidable barrier

Metabolic products of the skin and its appendages may have antimicrobial activity

Vagina protected by low pH and normal flora

Lysozyme and flushing action of tears protect conjunctiva

#### Respiratory Epithelium

The epithelium of the paranasal sinuses and of the respiratory tract from the level of the larynx to the alveoli is a less effective mechanical barrier. Like most mucous membranes, the respiratory tract is protected by a viscous mucus covering secreted by goblet cells. Microorganisms become trapped in the mucus layer and may be swept away before they reach the epithelial cell surface. This cleansing process is aided by secretory IgA (sIgA) secreted into the mucus and by other secreted antimicrobial substances like lysozyme and lactoferrin. Ciliated epithelial cells constantly move the mucus away from the lower respiratory tract. In the respiratory tract, particles larger than 5 μm are trapped in this fashion, moved upward at a rate of about 1 cm/min to pass through the larynx, and then swallowed and destroyed by the defenses of the alimentary tract. Interference with the action of cilia from toxic substances including alcohol and tobacco smoke or from infections such as influenza and whooping cough can permit colonization and infection of the lower respiratory tract with pathogenic bacteria, leading to the development of bronchitis or pneumonia.

Respiratory epithelium protected by mucus and sIgA

Cilia escalate mucus and particles away from the lung

Injury to cilia increases risk of infection

All of these defense mechanisms, together with the fixed phagocytic cells of the alveoli, keep the lungs essentially sterile. The phagocytic cells are of the macrophage series and

**TABLE 10–1. NONSPECIFIC DEFENSES AGAINST COLONIZATION WITH PATHOGENS**

| Site | Mechanical Barrier | Ciliated Epithelium | Competition by Normal Flora | Mucus | sIgA | Lymphoid Follicles | Low pH | Flushing Effects of Contents | Peristalsis | Special Factors |
|---|---|---|---|---|---|---|---|---|---|---|
| Skin | +++ | – | + | – | – | – | ++ | – | – | Fatty acids from action of normal flora on sebum |
| Conjunctiva | ++ | – | – | – | + | – | – | +++ | – | Lysozyme |
| Oropharynx | +++ | – | +++ | – | + | Yes | – | ++ | – | |
| Upper respiratory tract | ++ | + | +++ | ++ | ++ | Yes | – | + | – | Turbinate baffles |
| Middle ear and paranasal sinuses[a] | ++ | +++ | – | ++ | ? | – | – | + | – | |
| Lower respiratory tract[a] | ++ | +++ | – | ++ | ++ | Yes | – | – | – | Mucociliary escalator, alveolar macrophages; cough reflex |
| Stomach | ++ | – | – | ++ | – | – | +++ | + | + | Production of hydrochloric acid |
| Intestinal tract | ++ | – | +++ | +++ | +++ | Yes | – | + | +++ | Bile; digestive enzymes |
| Vagina | +++ | – | +++ | + | + | – | +++ | – | – | Lactobacillary flora ferments epithelial glycogen |
| Urinary tract[a] | ++ | – | – | – | + | – | + | +++ | – | |

*Abbreviations:* +, ++, +++ = relative importance in defense at each site; – = unimportant.
[a] Sterile in health.

are found free in the alveoli of the lungs. They play a very important role in ingesting and destroying organisms that are inhaled in very small droplet nuclei (less than 5 μm) and escape the mucociliary defenses of the trachea and bronchial tree. Similarly, a few macrophages reach the surface of other mucous membranes, but are less significant in defense.

Alveolar macrophages ingest and destroy inhaled organisms

### Gastrointestinal Epithelium

The epithelium of the intestinal tract below the esophagus is a less efficient mechanical barrier than the skin, but there are other effective defense mechanisms. The high level of hydrochloric acid and gastric enzymes in the normal stomach kill many ingested bacteria, and others are susceptible to pancreatic digestive enzymes or to the detergent effect of bile salts. Like the respiratory tract, the intestinal epithelium is coated with a film of mucus that traps many organisms directly or by reaction with specific sIgA secreted into it. The mucus and attached particles are continuously passed along and out of the alimentary tract by contractile peristaltic waves. Inhibition of these processes decreases the infecting dose of various pathogens or permits colonization of areas, such as the small intestine, that usually have a limited normal flora. The net result is an increased risk of infection. For example, the infecting dose of the cholera vibrio is lowered by several orders of magnitude in patients who have achlorhydria (absence of gastric hydrochloric acid).

Low pH, bile salts, and digestive enzymes protect at various levels

Peristaltic action moves mucus and particles in waves

## Urinary Tract

In addition to the multilayered transitional epithelium of the urinary tract the primary mechanisms of defense are the flushing effect of urine and its relatively low pH, which tend to inhibit microbial growth. Urinary tract infections are much more common in women than men because the shortness of the female urethra allows easier passage of organisms to the bladder; such infections in women are often associated with sexual intercourse. Infections are also common in any situation that produces urinary stasis, such as partial obstruction by an enlarged prostate, or when passage of bacteria into the bladder is facilitated by the use of catheters.

Low pH and flushing action of urine are protective

Stasis predisposes to infection

## Mucosal Immunity

The mucosal surfaces of the human body including the linings of the digestive, respiratory, and urogenital tract have an enormous epithelial surface area that is reinforced by a vast number of antibody-producing cells in mucosal tissue that daily secretes grams of sIgA onto the mucosal surface. The sIgA found in the mucus layer is particularly associated with specific sites in the mucosal lining like Peyer's patches of the small bowel. This gastrointestinal tract-associated lymphoid tissue (GALT) contains specialized surface epithelial cells called M cells (Fig 10–1) which act as antigen-presenting cells. Although GALT is particularly associated with Peyer's patches of the small bowel, similar mucosal lymphoid follicles also are found in the rectum, the tonsils, and the upper respiratory tract. The specialized

Mucosal surfaces contain sIgA-producing cells, particularly at specific sites like Peyer's patches

Specialized M cells act as antigen presenters to organized lymphoid tissue

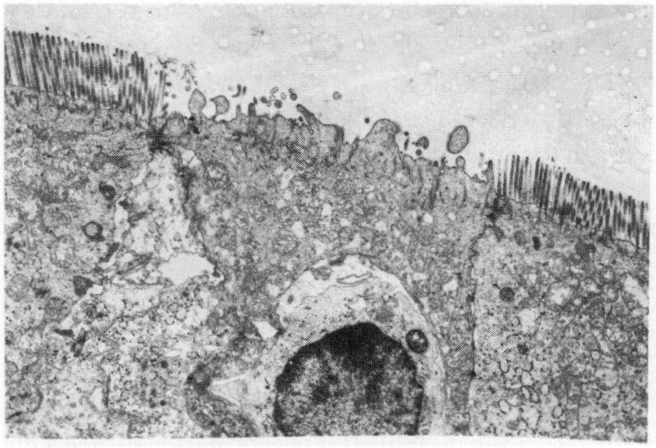

**Figure 10–1.** Intestinal M cell. An M cell in the small intestinal mucosa is shown flanked by two enterocytes. Note the flattened surface in comparison to the microvillus border of the enterocytes. The M cell seems to be making a space for the macrophage sitting immediately below it (magnification of negative 4800X). (*Photograph kindly supplied by Virginia Miller and Jeff Pepe, University of California, Los Angeles.*)

epithelium over these sites delivers small samples of luminal content (including whole bacterial cells and viral particles) into the organized lymphoid tissue below.

Cells committed to sIgA production at one location can migrate to other sites

In response to these imported antigens, cells committed to producing IgA against the transported antigens are generated. These cells migrate systemically and "home" to mucosal tissues and glands throughout the body where they differentiate into IgA-producing plasma cells. The polymeric IgA antibodies produced in subepithelial tissue are bound by polymeric immunoglobulin receptors on the basolateral surface of nearby epithelial cells and are transcytosed into the lumen where they form a barrier with the mucus against invading microbes and the incursion of foreign antigens. In this way, the exposure to an antigen at one location can provide distant mucosal surfaces with immune protection. Thus, secretory IgA plays a special role in protecting epithelial surfaces from colonization and infection, either by direct secretion through mucous membranes or because of its presence in glandular secretions such as breast milk. These antibodies interfere with the first stages of colonization or invasion by preventing attachment of viruses or bacteria to receptors on epithelia. They also block the activity or absorption of soluble antigenic molecules such as toxins that could otherwise contribute to the initiation of infection or disease. Secretory IgA in human milk plays an important role in protecting the infant from intestinal infections. Secreted antimicrobial substances can probably act cooperatively. It has been shown that sIgA can increase the speed of bacterial inactivation by lysozyme.

sIgA can block the initial attachment of pathogens or their secreted toxins

Breast milk contains sIgA

Both within and immediately beneath the epithelial barrier of the several mucosal surfaces lies the complete cellular machinery for a wide range of immunologic responses. The normal microbial flora also acts as a first line of defense by competing with pathogenic intruders for particular ecologic niches (see Chapter 9). Nevertheless, certain pathogenic bacteria and viruses adhere selectively to the epithelium that covers mucosal lymphoid follicles and use them as a portal of entry.

## ATTRIBUTES OF MICROBIAL PATHOGENICITY

### Entry

Pathogens use human environmental contact sites as points of entry

Clearly, human and other animal hosts have various protective mechanisms to prevent microbial entry. At the same time, we and other animals must maintain contact with the environment to exchange air, ingest food, and eliminate wastes. Pathogenic organisms have evolved mechanisms to capitalize on each of the human sites of environmental contact as points of entry. Although the skin is the predominant host barrier that excludes most microorganisms, this organ system can be damaged by trauma of various types that introduce foreign microbes or allow organisms present on the skin to bypass this barrier.

Bite of insects or needle of addicts can bypass skin barrier

One natural mechanism to bypass the skin is direct inoculation by insect bites; several organisms use this route including the plague bacillus *Yersinia pestis* and the malarial parasite. These microorganisms must spend part of their life in a remarkably different environment than the mammalian host and have adapted mechanisms for survival in each accordingly. Another means in the modern world to bypass the skin is through the deliberate inoculation used by drug addicts who suffer from a particular constellation of infectious disease agents as a result.

Pathogens adapt to particular sites by mechanisms counteracting their protecive mechanisms

The other sites of entry into human hosts include the digestive tract, the respiratory tract, the urogenital tracts, and the conjunctiva. As considered earlier, specialized features of these anatomic sites provide mechanical cleansing activities (such as peristalsis and blinking), and the surfaces in contact with the environment are bathed by mucus and antibacterial substances. Take away these normal host–cell functions and we become the victims of opportunists. Moreover, each host surface is the target for different adapted groups of microorganisms that use them as sites of multiplication, as well as the portal for entry into other locations within the host. Pathogens that infect primarily a particular anatomic site have often developed special adherence or enzymatic mechanisms that overcome the constitutive cellular sanitizing activities.

Aerosols can transmit orgnisms from host to host

We still know very little about the microbial factors essential to ensure infectious transmission from host to host. Obviously, microbes adapted to life in humans have evolved to take advantage of existing avenues of contact between their hosts. Dissemination by aerosols is common, but success is more than just random chance; the parasite must design itself for the rigors of atmospheric drying and other environmental factors. The virus of the common cold must exist on inanimate objects (fomites) waiting for a hand to touch and carry them to the conjunctiva or nasopharynx. The burden on an enteric pathogen that follows the fecal–oral route is substantial: (→) feces (→) mouth (→) stomach (→) small bowel (→) large bowel (→) back to the cold cruel world in stool. It is summarily exposed to extremes of temperature, pH, bile salts, digestive enzymes, and a myriad of competing microorganisms. Sexually transmitted pathogens are ordinarily delivered by direct inoculation onto mucosal surfaces. This microbial strategy avoids life in the external environment but is not without its own set of special requirements to overcome changing pH, mucus obstruction, anatomic barriers, local antibody, and phagocytic cells.

Survival in the environment facilitates transmission to a new host

Transmission by direct contact of mucosal surfaces avoids need for environmental survival

Pathogens must move from host to host. Some pathogens can survive outside their host and learn to tolerate different environments. There is considerable evidence that the environmental changes experienced by pathogens are important cues to the organism to elaborate new sets of genes. Thus, a requirement for infectivity is an ability to survive and, if necessary, multiply under conditions that exist on a surface epithelium or in a tissue into which the organisms are deposited. Examples of ability to survive local conditions are the lysozyme indifferent bacteria that cause conjunctivitis and the resistance of pathogens of the lower intestinal tract to the antibacterial effects of bile and the digestive enzymes. The ability of a bacterium to grow in any anatomic site depends on the availability of suitable nutrients and appropriate physicochemical conditions. Ability to grow or replicate at the body temperature of 37°C is also an obvious essential requirement for organisms that infect any area except the skin or nasal mucosal surfaces, which have a lower temperature. Some pathogenic organisms, such as the rhinoviruses of the common cold and the fungi that cause ringworm of the skin, grow poorly, if at all, at 37°C and, thus, cannot invade deeper tissues.

Environmental changes act as cues for organisms to activate new genes

Inability to replicate at 37°C restricts some pathogens to superficial sites

Some pathogens are able to respond to changing conditions. The low level of free $Ca^{2+}$ in the intracellular environment induces the production of new envelope proteins in *Yersinia pestis*, whereas the low level of free oxygen in the bowel lumen signals the typhoid bacillus, *Salmonella typhi*, to synthesize new adherence proteins and to prepare to invade host cells. Indeed, the temperature of the mammalian host is an important environmental signal to virtually all bacteria and fungal pathogens. Viruses cannot respond to environmental signals in the same way bacteria and fungi respond, but their structural proteins are designed to undergo conformational changes in response to the environment, as occurs in the acidic environment of the endocytic vesicle, and the enveloped viruses are considerably more resistant to drying than are the "naked" virions.

Low $Ca^{2+}$ can signal the intracellular environment

Viral structural proteins undergo conformational changes in different environments

All of the factors in the initial encounter of the host with the parasite can be assessed to some degree by measuring the infectious dose of the organism. How many organisms must be given a host to ensure infection in some proportion of the individuals? The measure of the infectious dose-50 ($ID_{50}$) for several pathogens is shown in Table 10–2. It is a simple measurement of a very complex interaction. Moreover, it is somewhat misleading as the endpoint is disease in human volunteers or death (a rigorous endpoint) in animal experiments.

Infecting dose ($ID_{50}$) highly variable

## Adherence: The Search for a Unique Niche

The first major interaction between a pathogenic microorganism and its host entails attachment to a eukaryotic cell surface. In its simplest form, adherence requires the partici-

**TABLE 10–2. DOSE OF MICROORGANISMS REQUIRED TO PRODUCE INFECTION IN HUMAN VOLUNTEERS**

| Microbe | Route | Disease-Producing Dose |
|---|---|---|
| Rhinovirus | Pharynx | 200 |
| *Salmonella typhi* | Oral | $10^5$ |
| *Shigella sp.* | Oral | 10–1000 |
| *Vibrio cholerae* | Oral | $10^8$ |
| *Vibrio cholerae* | Oral + $HCO_3^-$ | $10^4$ |
| *M. tuberculosis* | Inhalation | 1–10 |

Attachment requires an adhesin and a receptor

pation of two factors: a receptor on the host cell and an adhesin on the invading microbe. Most viruses attach specifically to sites on target cells through an envelope protein. For example, the influenza viruses attach specifically to neuraminic acid-containing glycoprotein receptors on the surface of respiratory cells before penetrating to the interior of the cell. Bacteria, like viruses, generally have protein structures on their surface that recognize either a protein or a carbohydrate moiety on the host cell surface. Finding the correct host cell surface in many cases appears to be a probability event related to the infectious dose. Because the mucosal surface is constantly bathed by a moving fluid layer, it is not surprising that many bacteria that infect the bladder or gastrointestinal tract are motile and some (like the typhoid bacillus) may use chemotaxis (see Chapter 3) to home in on the correct host cel! surface. Some bacteria use mucolytic enzymes to help penetrate epithelial surfaces.

Probability of adhesin meeting receptor is related to infecting dose

Multiple classes of pili act as adhesins to glycoprotein or glycolipid receptors

The pili of many Gram-negative bacteria bind directly to sugar residues that are part of glycolipids or glycoproteins on host cells or act as a protein scaffold to which another more specific adhesive protein is affixed. Although many pili look morphologically alike, there are at least four general classes in various Gram-negative bacteria that recognize different entities on the host cell surface. Two of these general classes of pili are distinguished by unusual first amino acids in the pilus structural protein. One has an amino-terminal methionine and the other starts with a methylated phenylalanine as the first residue in the pilus subunit. These latter *N*-methylphenylalanine pili are usually found at the poles of the bacterial cell rather than scattered randomly over the cell surface.

Unusual amino acids characterize some pili

The same organisms produce multiple adhesins

It is important to realize that adhesins like bacterial pili mediate the specific binding of bacteria to particular cell surfaces. For example, the most common adhesin of *Escherichia coli* and many other enteric bacteria recognizes mannose residues commonly found in the mucus overlying mucosal surfaces. Other *E. coli* possess the Pap pilus, which recognizes a digalactoside richly abundant in the genitourinary tract. *Escherichia coli* strains carrying Pap pili are the most commonly isolated organisms from cases of pyelonephritis. Adherence facilitates colonization and subsequent steps in the pathogenesis of infection because it brings the organism into intimate contact with its target and prevents its removal by the flushing effects of host cellular, secretions, or cilia. The activity of bacterial toxins on epithelial cells is enormously enhanced by this juxtaposition. Certain virulent *E. coli* causing traveler's diarrhea synthesize a distinct pilus type that recognizes specific receptors in the small bowel where these bacteria secrete the enterotoxins that lead to the diarrheal illness. Similarly, *Bordetella pertussis* adheres specifically to the cilia of respiratory epithelial cells, and one of its toxins directly inhibits ciliary action. The genes associated with pilus biosynthesis and assembly have often evolved to provide a remarkable degree of antigenic diversity to evade host defenses while still providing the underlying specificity of tissue attachment.

One type of *E. coli* pili binds to common mannose residues, another to digalactosides in urinary epithelium, yet another to intestinal cells

Pilin genes provide antigenic diversity

The pilus model of attachment is the best known means of bacterial attachment to a host cell surface; however, nonpilin adhesins have been demonstrated in a number of bacterial species. A similar class of molecules thought to mediate adherence in the Gram-positive bacteria are surface fibrils composed of proteins and lipoteichoic acid. In the streptococci causing pharyngitis, an M protein–lipoteichoic acid structure is believed to mediate attachment to the prevalent host cell protein, fibronectin.

Surface proteins, lipoteichoic acids, and polysaccharide capsules may act as adhesins

Bacterial capsules, usually an extracellular matrix of polysaccharide, may also mediate adherence to host cells or play an important role in binding layers of bacteria to others immediately adherent to the epithelial surface. These bacterial biofilms not only can coat the mucosal surface but they play an important role in the bacterial colonization of the inert materials used as catheters.

Some organisms excrete an enzyme, IgA protease, that cleaves human IgA1 in the hinge region, to release the Fc portion from the Fab fragment. This enzyme might play an important role in establishing microbial species at the mucosal surface, as bacteria that cleave IgA can bind the antigen binding domain of the immunoglobulin. This is one of several cases of molecular mimicry where bacteria (and probably viruses as well) can coat themselves with a secreted host cell product. This provides a microorganism with two advantages. First, microbes use these secreted products as a bridge to adhere to cell receptors that ordinarily bind these secreted products. Second, by binding a host cell product on its surface, the microbe disguises itself from the host cell immune system.

Bacterial IgA proteases provide a mechanism for molecular mimicry

Unlike bacteria, viruses generally have only one major adhesin that they use to attach to the host cell surface and to gain entry into the cytoplasm. Otherwise, both bacteria and viruses share the same strategy: a protein structure that recognizes a specific receptor. Host cell receptors do not exist for the sole use of infectious agents; they are generally associated with important cellular functions. The adhesive molecule on the microorganism has been selected to take advantage of the importance to its host cell's biological function(s). In this way, the adhesin provides the microbe with a unique niche where the infectious agent has the greatest chance to achieve success (presumably a pathogen's success can be measured by the extent of multiplication subsequent to entry). Adherence is important not only during the initial encounter between the pathogen and its host, but also throughout the infection cycle.

Viruses generally have a single adhesin

Adherence has continuing importance for maintaining the pathogen's niche

## Invasion of Host Cells

### Getting Into Cells

Many pathogenic bacteria are content to fight their way to the mucosal surface, adhere, and multiply. Adherence to a cellular surface may only be the first step in other infections. Host cell invasion is a specialized strategy for survival and multiplication used by a number of pathogens. Organisms may enter either professional phagocytes, such as neutrophils and macrophages, or enter nonprofessional phagocytes, such as epithelial and endothelial cells.

Invader may enter professional or nonprofessional phagocytes

Cell invasion is an essential step for viruses and obligate intracellular bacterial pathogens like *Rickettsia* (typhus) and *Chlamydia* (trachoma). Some bacteria and many parasites are facultative intracellular parasites. These organisms are capable of life both inside and outside host cells. The best known are the enteric bacteria, which cause typhoid (*Salmonella*) and bacillary dysentery (*Shigella*), as well as the tubercle bacillus. These bacteria produce specialized adhesins, sometimes called **invasins,** that bind to host cell receptors (or to a host cell molecule) that induce their uptake by host cells. The binding sites are often members of the integrin family, a family of integral membrane glycoproteins mediating cell–cell and cell–extracellular matrix interactions. Integrins include the receptors for fibronectin, collagen, laminin, vitronectin, and the complement binding receptor of phagocytes. Integrins are linked to the actin microfilament system through a variety of molecules including talin, vinculin, and α-actinin. Thus, the binding of a microbe to an integrin or integrin-like molecule on the host surface may trigger a host cell signal that causes actin filaments to link to the membrane-bound receptor, which then generates the force necessary for parasite uptake. Understanding of the cell biology of microbial invasion is still in its early stages, but it is clear that pathogens gain entry into the host cell by exploiting normal host cell internalization mechanisms. The specificity underlying this initial event should not be underestimated. The precise route of entry into a cell can have a profound influence on host–parasite interactions hours and even days later in the infectious process.

Intracellular pathogens must invade

Invasins induce uptake by host cells

Integrin binding triggers reaction of host cell microfilament system

Some viruses are internalized in much the same way. For example, rhinoviruses of the common cold use membrane-bound glycoprotein intercellular adhesion molecule 1 (ICAM-1) as a receptor. ICAM-1 is also a ligand of certain integrins. More often, as already discussed, virus particles are taken up by the receptor-mediated endocytosis mechanism (see Chapter 6), which is normally responsible for internalizing hormones, growth factors, and some important nutrients.

Viruses are taken in by receptor-mediated endocytosis

### Avoiding Intracellular Pitfalls

Gaining access into the host cell has a number of advantages. Besides avoiding the host immune system, intracellular localization places the pathogen in an environment potentially rich in nutrients and devoid of competing microorganisms. Intracellular life is not, however, free of difficulty. Viruses that enter by fusion are "dumped" directly into the cytoplasm where they may begin the replicative cycle. Bacteria or viruses internalized through the reorganization of the cytoskeleton find themselves within a membrane-bound vesicle in an acidic environment, which may be destined for fusion with potentially degradative lysosomes. Some viruses respond to the acidic environment by changing conformation, binding to the endosomal membrane, and releasing their nucleic acid into the cytoplasm. Bacteria such as Shigella, the cause of bacillary dysentery, and *Listeria monocytogenes*, a causative agent of meningitis and sepsis in the very young or very old, elaborate an enzyme that dissolves away the surrounding membrane and permits the bacterium to replicate within the

Entry may be directly into the cytoplasm or within vesicles

Organism must deal with acidic environment and lysosomal enzymes

Survival strategies include escape to cytoplasm and modification of endosome–lysosome environment

relative safety of the cytoplasm. Other organisms, like the typhoid bacillus and the tubercle bacillus, apparently tolerate the initial endosome–lysosome fusion event; however, most recent evidence suggests that they then modify this intracellular compartment into a privileged niche in which they can replicate optimally. Still other organisms, for example, the protozoan *Toxoplasma gondii*, inhibit the acidification of the endosomal vesicle and this, in turn, inhibits lysosomal fusion. The common theme again is that the microorganism has found a way to circumvent or to exploit host cell factors to suit its own purpose.

## HOST SECOND-LINE DEFENSES AFTER INVASION

Once a microorganism has breached the surface epithelial barrier, it is subject to a series of nonspecific and specific processes designed to remove, inhibit, or destroy it. These defenses are complex, dynamic, and interacting, but are considered under the general headings of the initial environment, the inflammatory response, phagocytic activity, and some general host responses that tend to increase resistance to infection.

### Initial Environment

Tissue fluids are deficient in free iron

Organism must compete with host iron-binding proteins

Microorganisms that reach the subepithelial tissues are immediately exposed to the intercellular tissue fluids, which have some defined properties that act to inhibit multiplication of many bacteria. For example, most tissues contain lysozyme in sufficient concentrations to disrupt the cell wall of some Gram-positive bacteria. Other less well defined inhibitors from leukocytes and platelets have also been described. Tissue fluid itself is a suboptimal growth medium for most bacteria and deficient in free iron. Iron is essential for bacterial growth, but it is sequestered by the body's iron-binding proteins such as transferrin and lactoferrin and is thus inaccessible to organisms that do not themselves produce siderophores (see Chapter 3).

Organism will encounter phagocytic macrophages when past initial barriers

Drainage to lymph nodes presents more macrophages

If an organism proceeds beyond the initial physical and biochemical barriers, it may meet strategically placed phagocytic cells of the monocyte/macrophage lineage whose function it is to engulf, internalize, and destroy large particulate matter, including infectious agents. Examples of such resident phagocytic cells include the alveolar macrophages, liver Kupffer cells, brain microglial cells, lymph node and splenic macrophages, kidney mesangial cells, and synovial A cells. Natural killer (NK) cells recognize cell surface changes occurring on virally and bacterially infected cells and bind to these infected targets and kill them. Furthermore, the natural turnover of tissue fluids from the blood capillary circulation to the lymphatic drainage system serves to move the occasional invading organism to a lymph node, in which the fixed phagocytic cells can remove and destroy it. Hence, most of the myriad of microbes that infect humans and make up their normal flora are held at bay by these mechanisms. Pathogenic bacteria, almost by definition, can overcome these biochemical and cellular shields after they breach the mucosal barrier, but as they begin to multiply, more powerful secondary host defense measures come into play.

### Inflammatory Response

Inflammation with vasodilatation, leukocytes, and complement components is a normal response

Inflammation is a normal host response to a traumatic or infectious injury. When many microorganisms multiply in the tissues, the usual result is an inflammatory response. The blood-carrying capillaries dilate, which leads to local extravasation of fluid containing high levels of protein, including immunoglobulins and complement components. Polymorphonuclear leukocytes are attracted to the infected site and reach the tissue fluids by passing between the capillary endothelial cells. Mediators of the inflammatory response include histamine liberated from mast cells, serotonin from platelets, lysosomal enzymes from damaged leukocytes and tissue cells, and low-molecular-weight peptides termed **kinins** generated from precursor proteins in plasma and tissues. Many of these mediators are cross-activating.

The process of inflammation can be initiated by the alternative complement pathway (or classic pathway when specific IgG or IgM is present) as C5a is tactic for leukocytes, and

C3a and C5a cause mast cells to degranulate and release histamine and other vasoactive mediators. Prostaglandin derivatives of arachidonic acid from damaged host cell membranes are longer acting and serve to maintain the inflammatory response until the infection is controlled. As discussed below, many of these processes are stimulated or enhanced by macrophage-derived interleukin-1 (IL-1) and tumor necrosis factor (TNF). The end results are the classic inflammatory manifestations of **swelling** (tumor), vasodilation of surface vessels with **erythema** (rubor), **heat** (calor) from increased skin temperature, **pain** (dolor) from increased pressure and tissue damage, and **loss of function** because of reflex nerve inhibition or the pain caused by movement.

Classic or alternate complement pathways initiate response

Cytokines modulate responses

The inflammatory response has several immediate defensive effects. It increases tissue fluid flow from the bloodstream to the lymphatic circulation and brings phagocytes, complement, and any existing antibody to the site of infection. Later, the deposition of fibrin may contribute to the walling off of the lesion before the healing process begins. The increased lymphatic drainage serves to bring microbes or their antigens into contact with the cells in the local lymph nodes that mediate the development of specific immune responses.

Increased blood flow brings defensive elements in contact with microbes

A local inflammatory response can also produce important systemic effects largely mediated by IL-1 and TNF. Polymorphonuclear leukocytes (PMNs) are mobilized from the bone marrow pool to increase the numbers of those present at the infected site and to replace those destroyed or at the end of their life span. Thus, polymorphonuclear leukocytosis, involving primarily neutrophils, is a common feature of most bacterial infections and serves to increase the immediately available phagocytic defenses. Fever, a frequent concomitant of inflammation, is mediated primarily by IL-1 and TNF released by macrophages (eg, on exposure to bacterial endotoxin). These act on the hypothalamus and increase the "setting" of the body's thermostatic mechanisms. The value of fever is not completely clear; however, it increases the effectiveness of several processes involved in phagocytosis and microbial killing and frequently reduces the multiplication or replication rate of bacteria or viruses.

Mobilization of PMNs from bone marrow is a common feature of bacterial infections

Fever is mediated by CNS action of IL-1 and TNF

Interleukin-1 has many other effects relating to defense against infection. It enhances release of lactoferrin and lysozyme from neutrophils at the site of infection; stimulates the oxidative antibacterial activity of phagocytes (see next section); enhances chemotaxis of leukocytes to the infected area; increases prostaglandin production by monocytes and macrophages; enhances iron uptake by the liver, which effectively reduces its availability for infecting organisms; and stimulates production of a number of proteins (acute-phase proteins) by the liver that appear to enhance defense against infection. Such acute-phase proteins, exemplified by C-reactive protein (CRP), increase rapidly in concentration in the serum in response to infection. CRP recognizes and binds to molecular groups found on many bacteria and fungi and facilitates their uptake by phagocytes. In short, IL-1 is a major orchestrator of protective responses to infection.

IL-1 has many actions contributing to the inflammatory response and its effects

## Phagocytic Defenses

Phagocytic cells include polymorphonuclear leukocytes (particularly neutrophils), blood monocytes, macrophages, tissue histiocytes, and the fixed phagocytic cells of the reticuloendothelial system. PMNs and macrophages are both descended from bone marrow stem cells. Blood monocytes that reach the tissues assume the characteristics of macrophages when they reach inflammatory sites or, in the absence of infection, become fixed in certain organs like the liver or spleen. The usual order of appearance of cells within an inflammatory exudate is PMNs followed by monocytes and then macrophages. Despite the differences between them, all of these cells share certain common mechanisms for ingesting and attempting to destroy invading microorganisms.

PMNs are followed by monocytes and macrophages that share mechanisms of microbial destructions

### Neutrophils

The PMN is a short-lived (circulating half-life, 7 hours) cell with a multilobed nucleus and numerous cytoplasmic granules containing enzymes and other substances with antimicrobial action. Only a small fraction circulate in the blood; the majority are found loosely adherent to the walls of small blood vessels or within tissues. Hence, they are usually the first phagocytic cells to be mobilized against microbial invaders. PMNs are metabolically ac-

PMNs readily available lining blood vessels

PMNs respond to uniquely prokaryotic elements of the organism

tive and demonstrate marked chemotaxis to the C5a component of complement and to other products of the inflammatory process. They also respond chemotactically to certain peptides released from bacteria like formyl-methionyl-leucyl-phenylalanine (fMet–Leu–Phe) and muramyl dipeptide. It is instructive to see that the phagocytes are positively responding to such compounds, which are uniquely prokaryotic. Presumably this reflects a longstanding broad-spectrum recognition system for microbial components in the evolution of phagocytosis. All of the chemotactic factors attract leukocytes to the sites of microbial invasion.

Like all phagocytes, PMNs have complement receptors that act as binding sites for organisms with complement deposited on their surface by either the classic or alternative pathway. If antibody is present and bound to the bacteria, the phagocytes can often engulf the microorganism through antibody Fc receptors on their surface.

Phagosome produces peroxide and toxic oxygen radicals

Particles, including bacteria, that attach to the proper receptor on the surface of PMNs are internalized within a membrane-bound vacuole called the **phagosome.** Once within the cell there are several mechanisms by which organisms can be killed. These are summarized in Table 10–3. An NADPH oxidase system, which is located in the plasma membrane of the phagocyte and may be in the membrane of the phagosome, produces superoxide anion that reacts spontaneously to produce peroxide, singlet oxygen, and hydroxyl radicals, all of which, although often evanescent, are damaging to many bacteria and viruses. Fusion of the phagosome with one class of granules brings the NADH oxidase into contact with another oxygen-dependent enzyme, myeloperoxidase. Myeloperoxidase uses the peroxide produced by NADH oxidase and halides (eg, chloride) to produce hypochlorous acid, which in turn reacts with primary or secondary amines to form highly microcidal chloramines.

Fusion of the phagosome with granules introduces myeloperoxidase system

Phagolysosome exposes microbe to low pH, lysozyme, phosphatases, and nucleases

Intracellular killing of microorganisms by PMNs also involves equally impressive oxygen-independent mechanisms. When some classes of neutrophil granules fuse with the phagocytic vacuole, they discharge their lysosomal enzymes and other antibacterial substances to form a **phagolysosome.** Any organisms ingested under anaerobic conditions (like those in abscesses) or organisms that have survived the effects of oxygen metabolites are exposed to a pH of 3.0 to 4.0 and to lysozyme, phosphatases, and nuclease. **Defensins** and other cationic proteins also kill certain bacteria, fungi, and even enveloped viruses presumably by membrane damage. Lactoferrin is also released into the phagocytic vacuole to restrict iron. Taken together, these host cell factors serve to produce an environment that is highly hostile to most organisms.

Lysosomal enzymes also damage tissues

Lysosomal enzymes, including collagenase and elastase, are damaging to tissues when released from PMNs and contribute to the enhancement of the inflammatory process; however, failure of the phagocytes to clear bacteria results in continued release of toxic products from the inflammatory exudate, which can be as damaging to the host as released bacterial virulence products.

## Macrophages

Although the earliest inflammatory response involves largely neutrophils, with time the macrophages begin to make their appearance in inflammatory exudates. They play a wider and more continuing role than neutrophils in the continuing evolution of the inflammatory

**TABLE 10–3. MICROBICIDAL RESPONSES OF PHAGOCYTES**

A. Oxygen dependent
   1. Respiratory burst; generation of toxic superoxide, singlet oxygen, and other reactive radicals
   2. Halogenation of critical microbial components by myeloperoxidase system[a] (hydrogen peroxide, myeloperoxide, and halide)

B. Nonoxygen dependent
   Release of antimicrobial lysosomal contents to phagosome including
   1. Cationic proteins[a]
   2. Acid hydrolases
   3. Lysozyme
   4. Lactoferrin[a]
   5. Proteases

[a] Not represented in mature macrophages.

response (including fever), in lymphocyte activation and, subsequently, in the resolution and repair of the tissue.

Macrophages are widely distributed in the tissues, exhibit chemotaxis to C5a and to neutrophil lysates, and phagocytose microorganisms and cellular debris resulting from infection. Like PMNs they are also attracted to fMet–Leu–Phe, muramyl dipeptide, bacterial lipopolysaccharide (LPS), cell wall material from mycobacteria, and fungal wall components. Unlike the shorter-lived neutrophil, the macrophage can resynthesize its lysosomal granules and contained enzymes and repeat the process of phagocytosis and microbial destruction. Also, unlike the neutrophil, macrophages do not possess myeloperoxidase, have a less dramatic respiratory burst, and lack lactoferrin and antimicrobial cationic proteins. Macrophages, however, have a much larger complement of lysosomal enzymes and can be activated by lymphokines to increase their synthesis and antimicrobial effectiveness. The phagocytic and debriding aspects of macrophage function are particularly significant in the later stages of infection and in the control of obligate or facultative intracellular pathogens. The T-cell response is required for the full expression of phagocyte-mediated immunity. Also, host resolution of viral infection and infection by facultative intracellular bacterial parasites, as well as fungal pathogens, requires T-lymphocyte-derived mediators.

Macrophages are attracted by same factors as PMNs

Macrophages can repeat digestion but lack meloperoxidase system

Lymphokine activation increases effectiveness

Other contributions of macrophages to the control of infection are shown in Table 10–4. They include antigen processing and presentation to T cells as described in Chapter 8; synthesis of some complement proteins and precursors; production of tactic factors for neutrophils; synthesis of prostaglandin, transferrin, lysozyme, and interferon; production of proteases, elastase, and collagenase; and synthesis of IL-1 and TNF. Thus, macrophages contribute in a major way to the local and systemic response to infection and to the repair of the damage that ensues, quite apart from their contributions to the immune response.

Macrophage antigen processing and presentation, and other factors are central to cellular immunity

In addition to tissue and alveolar macrophages, cells with similar function and derivation abound in the reticuloendothelial system. They are present particularly in the lymph node sinuses and along small blood vessels and vascular sinuses of the liver, spleen, and bone marrow. Microorganisms that escape from a local lesion into the lymphatic circulation or bloodstream are rapidly cleared by reticuloendothelial cells or arrested in the small pulmonary capillaries and then ingested by phagocytic cells. This process is so efficient that when a million organisms are injected into a vein of a rabbit, few, if any, are usually recoverable in cultures of blood taken 15 minutes after injection, although the ultimate result of such clearance may not be a cure.

Macrophages are distributed throughout the body

## Adaptive Immune Response

When the innate defense system operates to control a microbial infection, one of the usual outcomes is the stimulation of the immune system to proliferate and maturate antibody-producing cells and the longer-lived memory cells, all with the same antigen binding specificity. In subsequent infections by the same microorganism, the host may be able to deal with the pathogen much more efficiently. The microorganism can overcome this by antigenic variation and other tactics (see below). Obviously, the innate and adaptive immune systems do not work in isolation from one another. Lymphocytes are responsible for specific recognition, and they produce antibody and lymphokines that help the phagocytes combat the infection. The antigens processed by the phagocytes are presented to lymphocytes, which can recognize them. The adaptive immune system modulates inflammation through

Specificity of antibody production can be offset by antigenic variation of the microbe

**TABLE 10–4. CONTRIBUTION OF MACROPHAGES AND THEIR PRODUCTS TO CONTROL OF INFECTION**

| |
|---|
| Inflammation and fever |
| IL-1, TNF, prostaglandins, complement factors, clotting factors, $H_2O_2$, acid hydrolases |
| Lymphocyte activation |
| Antigen processing, antigen presentation, IL-1 production |
| Tissue debridement, reorganization, and repair |
| Elastase, collagenase, hyaluronidase, fibroblast-stimulating factor, angiogenesis factor |
| Microbicidal activity |
| Oxygen dependent, oxygen independent |

*Abbreviations:* IL-1 = interleukin-1; TNF = tumor necrosis factor.

the complement system, although complement can be activated directly by the invading microbes. Problems arise when the phagocytes are unable to recognize or deal with an infectious agent, either because they lack a suitable receptor for it or because the microorganism does not activate complement.

Some organisms may not activate complement

Cell-mediated immunity is important for viral, fungal, and parasitic infections

Cell-mediated immune responses are at least as effective as antibody in controlling many infections, particularly those caused by viruses, large parasites, fungi, and bacteria living and multiplying within host cells. Hence, children with congenital B-cell defects, who cannot make antibody but who have T cells, recover normally from the usual childhood viral diseases (mumps, measles) but suffer from recurrent life-threatening infections from pneumococci and staphylococci.

Antibodies can only affect viruses when they are outside their cellular host

The response to viral infection involves different immunologic mechanisms depending on where and how the virus or its antigens are encountered, that is, intracellularly or extracellularly. In a typical viral infection, there is initially local replication at some epithelial site, then one or more viremic (bloodborne) stages, and finally infection and replication in some target organ system. Antibody is capable of binding only to extracellular viruses. IgM and IgG are generally limited to the viremic stages of infection. IgA antibody may protect the epithelial surface. The cell-mediated immune reaction involving cytotoxic T cells and antibody-dependent cytotoxic cells is potentially effective against intracellular viruses, which are recognized by the presence of viral antigens in the membrane of the infected cell.

The granuloma is a feature of faculative intracellular pathogens

When the invading microorganisms (or their surviving antigenic material) cannot be degraded or are resistant to removal or degradation, T cells accumulate and release lymphokines. This leads to the aggregation and proliferation of macrophages and the characteristic appearance of a nodular mass called a **granuloma,** which consists of multinucleate giant cells, epithelioid cells, and activated macrophages. Granulomas are characteristic of infections caused by the tubercle bacillus *Mycobacterium tuberculosis* and other facultative intracellular parasites.

## Phagocytosis

Phagocytosis is facilitated by coating with antibody and C3b

The processes of phagocytosis that can occur when a microbe encounters a phagocyte are enhanced greatly by opsonization with antibodies directed against the infecting organism, as well as by activation of the classic complement pathway. Phagocytic cells have surface receptors for the Fc fraction of IgG and for the C3b derivatives of complement. Thus, bacteria and viruses with attached antibody are brought to the surface of phagocytic cells to facilitate ingestion, and this process is enhanced (or mediated in the case of IgM) by the C3b component of complement. Many bacterial products (particularly endotoxin) and viruses activate the alternative pathway of complement, which can lead to opsonization in the absence of antibody.

Defects in complement or phagocyte receptors lead to pyogenic infections

If there is any question about the importance of complement as an opsonin or the effectiveness of phagocytosis as an essential host defense mechanism, it is dispelled by the observations of the consequences to humans who have inborn deficits in complement cell surface receptors. Thus, patients with a hereditary deficiency in classic pathway components, C3, or a deficiency in CR3 phagocyte receptors suffer from recurrent pyogenic (staphylococcal and streptococcal) infection. Deficiencies in the terminal lytic pathway are associated with recurrent infections by *Neisseria meningitidis* or *Neisseria gonorrhoeae*. Similarly, children with a hereditary defect in making superoxide anion suffer from chronic granulomatous disease characterized by recurrent severe pyogenic infection and early death, even with heroic antimicrobial treatment. An understanding of these hereditary disorders at the genetic and biochemical level provides us with an appreciation of the ways by which our innate immune system functions and also permits us to understand better the pathogenesis of the infectious agents.

Bacteria may evade opsonophagocytosis or grow inside the phagocytes

Ultimately, almost all bacteria are killed by phagocytes. As will be seen in the following sections, some bacteria can avoid opsonization by complement and bacterial capsules and provide many organisms with the means to evade phagocytosis. Other bacteria (eg, the tubercle bacillus) grow perfectly well in ordinary neutrophils or macrophages. In these circumstances, antibody, if present, may enhance opsonization and neutralize the effects of bacterial virulence factors.

Even this brief review of the initial host response to microbial injury leads one to appreciate how well adapted a microorganism must be to sustain a pathogenic lifestyle. Why would any self-respecting organism want to precipitate such a murderous response by the host? As will be seen, microorganisms have evolved several clever ways to avoid just that pitfall.

## ESTABLISHMENT OF PATHOGENS AFTER ENTRY AND THE CONSEQUENCES OF INFECTION

The successful pathogen must gain entry, find a unique niche, and multiply in the face of formidable host defenses. Simply being able to adhere or enter a host cell is not sufficient. Pathogenicity is a multifactorial phenotype and pathogens are typically armed with a number of factors permitting them to overcome, subvert, or nullify the host's nonspecific and specific host defense systems. Not surprisingly, these virulence factors are also the target(s) in the design of vaccines. Some of the microbial factors that permit the establishment of the pathogen in the host environment are essential. That is, if these factors are lost, with them goes the capacity to infect the host or become transmitted successfully. Other virulence factors are nonessential. They contribute to the overall virulence of the pathogen, but loss of the factor may not materially affect the outcome of the host–parasite relationship.

Pathogenicity is multifactorial and includes the ability to nullify the host's response

## TOXINS

### Exotoxins

A number of microorganisms synthesize protein molecules that are toxic to their hosts and are most often secreted into their environment or are found associated with the microbial surface. These exotoxins usually possess some degree of host cell specificity which is dictated by the nature of the binding of one or more toxin components to a specific host cell receptor. The distribution of host cell receptors often dictates the degree and the breadth of the toxicity. Bacterial exotoxins, whether synthesized by Gram-positive or Gram-negative bacteria, fall into two broad classes, each of which represents a general pathogenic theme common to many bacterial species.

Effect of toxins depends on their action and receptor specificialities

#### A–B Exotoxin

The best known theme is represented by the A–B exotoxin. These toxins are divisible into two general domains. One, the B subunit, is associated with the binding specificity of the molecule to the host cell. Generally speaking, the B region binds to a specific host cell surface glycoprotein or glycolipid. The other, subunit A, is the catalytic domain, which enzymatically attacks a susceptible host function or structure. The actual biochemical structure of exotoxins varies. In some cases (diphtheria toxin), the single B subunit of the toxin is linked through a disulfide bond to the A subunit. In other cases (pertussis toxin), multiple B subunits may join with a single A enzymatic subunit. In any event, following attachment of the B domain to the host cell surface, the A domain is transported by direct fusion or by endocytosis into the host cell. Many of the most potent A–B bacterial toxins are ADP-ribosylating enzymes. Some of these affect the protein-synthesizing apparatus of the cell (diphtheria toxin, *Pseudomonas* exotoxin); others affect the cytoskeleton (*Clostridium botulinum* toxin C2) or the normal signal transduction activities of the host (*Bordetella pertussis* and *Vibrio cholerae*). It is notable and not simply fortuitous that the major natural substrates of the toxin ADP-ribosyltransferases are guanine nucleotide-binding proteins (G proteins) involved in signal transduction in eukaryotic cells. In a very simplistic way, one can think that the ADP-ribosylating toxins are all geared to interrupt the biochemical lines of communication within and between host cells. An understanding of bacterial toxins therefore sheds as much light on the intimate details of normal animal cell regulation as it does on bacterial pathogenicity.

B subunits mediate binding to host cell receptor

A subunit catalyses enzymatic reaction affecting host cellular function

ADP-ribosylation is a common enzymatic action of A subunits

Protein synthesis apparatus and signal transducing G proteins are common targets

Several bacterial toxins have been examined in exquisite detail at the biochemical level. The crystal structures of several have been "solved." In many cases, the precise amino acids making up the catalytic site of the toxin are so well appreciated that a single amino acid substitution can be made that is sufficient to detoxify the molecule. These **toxoids** are the ba-

Toxins can be inactivated by substitution of a single amino acid in the catalytic site

sis for new generations of vaccines. Given this level of biochemical sophistication, it is somewhat disconcerting to realize that the actual role of bacterial toxins in microbial pathogenicity has not been clarified. A number of the most fearsome human diseases are the result of intoxication by secreted bacterial toxins. Human disease as a consequence of an accidental contamination of a wound with the tetanus bacillus or the accidental ingestion of food contaminated with botulinum toxin is an individual human disaster, but it does not necessarily reveal the actual role of the toxin in the biology of *Clostridium tetani* or *Clostridium botulinum*. These organisms are not primary pathogens of humans, although their toxins presumably have evolved to play some role in their interaction with other eukaryotic life forms. Nontoxigenic variants of tetanus or the botulinum bacterium are totally avirulent for humans.

Nontoxogenic variants of accidental pathogens are available

Some toxigenic microbes are highly adapted to humans including *Corynebacterium diphtheriae* (diphtheria), *B. pertussis* (whooping cough), and *V. cholerae* (cholera). For these A–B toxins, we understand the biochemical basis for toxigenicity and the indispensability of the toxins for the pathogenicity of the microorganism. We even understand that if we immunize individuals against these toxins, we can prevent disease. What we do not understand is the role of the toxin in the biology of the microorganism. The toxin cannot be so potent that it will rapidly kill all of the hosts that are infected. Toxins may represent the principal determinant of bacterial virulence in some species, but may not be the principal determinant of infectivity; however, it seems likely that toxins play a role in the establishment of the organism in the early phases of infection or they are elaborated only if the organism "senses" danger. Thus, *V. cholerae* devoid of cholera toxin does not colonize susceptible animals as well as toxigenic organisms, nor is it as efficiently transmitted. It is possible that the effects of cholera toxin, the induced net secretion of water and electrolytes into the lumen of the bowel, make conditions right for cholera replication.

The role of toxins in the biology of strict human pathogens is still unclear

Toxin production may be a response to changes sensed in the environment

Currently, molecular cloning techniques, coupled with appropriate infection models, are leading to the elucidation of the roles of some toxins in the pathogenesis of infections. Not all toxins are essential for pathogenicity. For example, *Shigella dysenteriae* produces a very potent cytotoxin called Shiga toxin. Nontoxigenic variants of this organism are still pathogenic, but are not as virulent. The high death rates associated with toxigenic *S. dysenteriae* appear to be associated with damage done to the colonic vasculature by Shiga toxin.

Toxins may be contributory but not essential for pathogenicity

### Membrane-Active Exotoxin

A plethora of other bacterial toxins are described in the medical literature. Most of these are not well characterized, although many of them act directly on the surface of host cells to lyse or to kill them. They may facilitate penetration of host epithelial or endothelial barriers, and some toxins can kill white cells or paralyze the local immune system.

Most bacterial toxins are not well characterized

Many bacteria elaborate substances that cause hemolysis of erythrocytes, and this property has long been postulated to be an important virulence trait. In fact, some bacterial hemolysins are representative of general classes of bacterial exotoxin (the cytotoxins) that kill host cells by disrupting the host cell membrane. Moreover, hemolysins may liberate necessary growth factors, like iron, for the invading microorganisms.

Disruption of erythrocyte and other cell membranes is a common action

Among Gram-negative bacteria, a surprising number of these cytotoxins are members of a single family called the RTX (repeats in toxin) group based on a recurrent theme of a nine-amino-acid tandem duplication. RTX toxins are calcium-dependent proteins that act by creating pores in eukaryotic membranes, which may cause cellular death or at least a perturbation in host cell function. Such toxins are thought to be particularly effective against phagocytic cells. Other exotoxins contribute to the capacity of an organism to invade and spread. The lecithinase α-toxin of *C. perfringens*, for example, disrupts the membranes of a wide variety of host cells, including the leukocytes that might otherwise destroy the organism, and produces the necrotic anaerobic environment in which it can multiply.

RTX cytotoxins create pores in eukaryotic membranes

Lecithinase action disrupts cell membranes

## Hydrolytic Enzymes

Many bacteria produce one or more enzymes that are nontoxic per se, but facilitate tissue invasion or help to protect the organism against the body's defense mechanisms. For example, various bacteria produce collagenase or hyaluronidase or convert serum plasminogen to plasmin, which has fibrinolytic activity. Although the evidence is not conclusive, it is reasonable to assume that these substances facilitate spread of infection. Deoxyribonuclease, elastase, and many other biologically active enzymes are also produced by some bacteria, but their function in the disease process or in providing nutrients for the invaders is uncertain. All are proteins and have most of the characteristics of exotoxin, except specific toxicity. Although many such factors have been thought to be involved in bacterial virulence, formal proof that they may contribute to pathogenicity has not been obtained.

Collagenase and hyaluronidase may facilitate spread in tissues

## Endotoxin

In many infections caused by Gram-negative organisms, the endotoxin (see Chapter 2) of the outer membrane is a significant component of the disease process. Recall that endotoxin is a lipopolysaccharide and that the lipid portion (lipid A) is the toxic portion. The conserved polysaccharide core and the variable O-polysaccharide side chains of endotoxin are responsible for the antigenic diversity seen among enteric bacterial species. The major characteristics of endotoxin are contrasted with those of exotoxin in Table 10–5. As noted earlier, endotoxin is a major cue to the human innate defense system that bacterial multiplication is taking place in the tissues. Endotoxin in nanogram amounts causes fever in humans through release of IL-1 and TNF from macrophages. In larger amounts, whether on intact Gram-negative organisms or cell wall fragments, it produces dramatic physiologic effects associated with inflammation. These include hypotension, lowered polymorphonuclear leukocyte and platelet counts from increased margination of these cells to the walls of the small vessels, hemorrhage, and sometimes disseminated intravascular coagulation from activation of clotting factors. Rapid and irreversible shock may follow passage of endotoxin into the bloodstream. This syndrome is seen when materials that have become heavily contaminated are injected intravenously or when a severe local infection leads to massive bacteremia. The role of endotoxin in more chronic disease processes is less clear, but some manifestations of typhoid fever and meningococcal septicemia, for example, are fully compatible with the known effects of endotoxin in humans. It should be noted that endotoxins are considerably less active than many exotoxins, incompletely neutralized by antibody against their carbohydrate component, and stable even to autoclaving. The latter characteristic is important, because materials for intravenous administration that have become contaminated with Gram-negative organisms are not detoxified by sterilization.

The endotoxin is a part of the Gram-negative outer membrane

Endotoxin lipid A causes fever through cytokine release

Significant endotoxemia leads to shock and intravascular coagulation

Endotoxin is stable to autoclaving

Gram-positive bacteria do not contain endotoxin but they release peptidoglycan fragments and other cell wall determinants that act to "alarm" the host to the presence of bacteria in the tissues. The same cytokines are released and the same physiologic cascade is seen.

Peptidoglycan fragments may cause physiologic effects

**TABLE 10–5. DIFFERENTIAL CHARACTERISTICS OF ENDOTOXINS AND EXOTOXINS**

| Characteristic | Endotoxins | Exotoxins |
|---|---|---|
| Chemical nature | Lipopolysaccharide (lipid A component) | Protein |
| Part of Gram-negative cell outer membrane | Yes | No |
| Most from Gram-positive bacteria | No | Yes |
| Usually extracellular | No | Yes |
| Phage or plasmid coded | No | Many |
| Antigenic | Weakly | Yes |
| Can be converted to toxoid | No | Many |
| Neutralized by antibody | Weakly | Yes |
| Differing pharmacologic specificities | No | Yes |
| Stable to boiling[a] | Yes | No |

[a] Enterotoxin of *Staphylococcus aureus* withstands boiling.

## AVOIDANCE OF THE HOST IMMUNE SYSTEM

The host immune system evolved in large part because of the selective pressure of microbial attack. To be successful, microbial pathogens must escape this system at least long enough to be transmitted to a new susceptible host or to take up residence within the host in a way that is compatible with mutual coexistence.

### Serum Resistance

Some organisms block the lytic action of complement

Many bacteria that come into contact with human complement can be destroyed by opsonization or by direct lysis of the bacterial membrane by complement complexes. Some can avoid this fate by a process called serum resistance. Pathogenic *Salmonella* possess a lipopolysaccharide inhibiting the C5b–9 complement complex from attacking the hydrophobic domains of the bacterial outer membrane. Other bacteria employ different mechanisms, but the end result is the same. These organisms can persist in an environment that is rapidly lethal for nonpathogens.

### Antiphagocytic Activity

A fundamental requirement for many pathogenic bacteria is escape from phagocytosis by macrophages and polymorphonuclear leukocytes. It seems likely that the ability to avoid phagocytosis was an early necessity for microorganisms following the evolution of predatory protozoans. Some bacteria, such as the causative agent of Legionnaire's disease, *Legionella pneumophila*, learned how to replicate in free-living amoebae following phagocytosis and used them as part of their life cycle. *Legionella* uses similar mechanisms to outwit human macrophages. In this one example, it can be seen that pathogenicity in some microorganisms evolved from a very early time in their development.

Capsules are a major means of avoiding phagocytosis

The most common bacterial means to avoid phagocytosis is an antiphagocytic capsule. The significance of the bacterial capsule can hardly be overemphasized. Almost all principal pathogens that cause pneumonia and meningitis have antiphagocytic polysaccharide capsules. Nonencapsulated variants of these organisms are usually avirulent. In many cases, it has been found that the capsule of pathogens prevents complement deposition on the bacterial cell surface. Thus, the capsule prevents nonimmune opsonization and confers resistance to phagocytosis. As noted earlier, along with encapsulation, a common factor of many organisms that cause pneumonia and meningitis is the elaboration of an enzyme that specifically cleaves human IgA1 molecules. IgA proteases are found in the pathogenic *Neisseria, Haemophilus influenzae* type b (Hib), and *Streptococcus pneumoniae*. The combination of a capsule to avoid opsonization with an enzyme that cleaves an important class of secretory antibody is a potent stratagem to avoid phagocytosis.

Capsule prevents complement deposition and nonimmune opsonization

IgA protease cleaves secretary antibody

Fibrinugen binding can sterically hinder complement access to bacterial surface

The group A streptococcal M protein is another example of a bacterial surface product employed by the organism to escape opsonization and phagocytosis. In part, this is a reflection of the ability of M protein to bind fibrinogen and its breakdown product fibrin to the bacterial surface. This sterically hinders complement access and prevents opsonization.

Resisting phagocytosis gives time to multiply

There are many of other examples. The principle, however, is clear. If microorganisms can inhibit phagocytosis, they can often gain the upper hand long enough to replicate sufficiently to establish themselves in the host or become transmitted to a new host. It is important to understand that these encapsulated pathogens are often carried asymptomatically in the normal flora (see Table 9–1). The capsule is important for the organism to establish itself in the nasopharynx.

Anticapsular antibody opsonizes and phagocytosis proceeds

The host responds to its initial encounter with the encapsulated organism by elaborating anticapsular antibodies that opsonize and permit efficient phagocytosis and destruction of the microorganism in subsequent encounters. Thus, the initial interaction between an encapsulated microbe and its host usually has two outcomes. First, the host becomes asymptomatically colonized, and second, the colonization is an immunizing event for the host. The host is protected against serious systemic infection by the organism, but this immunity may not affect the capacity of the organism to live happily on a mucosal surface. Epidemiologic investigations show that serious disease caused by encapsulated pathogens when it occurs does so very shortly after a susceptible individual encounters the microorganism for the first time. This scenario is in contrast to the idea that carriers of microorganisms come down with the disease at some time in the future. If a microorganism meets a host with a compromised immune system or some short-term deficit in its defense systems, then the organism's capacity for replication can overwhelm the host defense mechanisms and cause serious disease. Once colonization and immunity have been established, the steady state is a satisfactory host–parasite relationship. For example, the outcome of encounters with *Neisseria meningitidis* has been demonstrated in military recruits followed for colonization and anticapsular antibody throughout training camp. Disease developed only in those entering the camp lacking both specific antibody and nasopharyngeal colonization with the *N. meningitidis* serogroup responsible for a subsequent meningitis outbreak. Unaffected recruits either had a "successful" encounter followed by development of antibody or already had protective antibody, presumably from a similar experience earlier in life.

Encounter with encapsulated pathogen may be an immunizing event leading to a stable colonization relationship

Some nonimmune individuals progress to disease before antibody appears

## Cutting of Lines of Communication

Pathogens like *Yersinia* have evolved means to neutralize phagocytes directly by using the equivalent of eukaryotic signal transduction molecules. Hence, pathogenic *Yersinia* synthesize tyrosine phosphatase molecules and serine kinase molecules and introduce them into the cytoplasm of macrophages leading to a complete loss in the capacity of these cells either to phagocytose microorganisms or to signal other components of the host immune system by cytokine release. As noted earlier, microbial mimicry can have the same effect by concealing the microorganism under a shroud of host proteins; however, the strategy of directly interfering with host cell function by use of an alternative enzyme is likely to be a more common strategy for the invading microbe than previously realized.

Bacterial phosphatases and kinases can compromise macrophage phagocytic signaling

## Antigenic Variation

Another method by which microorganisms avoid host immune responses is by varying surface antigens. *Neisseria gonorrhoeae* displays an endless array of pili and outer membrane proteins to the host immune system. The organism has learned to preserve its binding specificities, but to vary endlessly the molecular scaffolding on which the functional units are placed. The host sees a bewildering array of new epitopes, whereas the critical regions of the molecule remain hidden from immune surveillance. Of course, among the viruses, antigenic variation is also a common theme; the best known example is the influenza virus. It is instructive that in both the bacterial example and the viral example, recombinational mechanisms act to bring together novel sequences of genetic material. A number of microorganisms known for their antigenic diversity such as those of the genus *Borrelia*, which causes relapsing fever, and the group A streptococci also use homologous recombination of DNA from repeated sequences to generate the diversity in size and sequence observed in their principal immunodominant antigens.

Multiple antigenic types of pili confuse immune surveillance

Bacterial and viral recombination systems generate diversity

# EXOTOXINS THAT INTERFERE WITH THE IMMUNE RESPONSE: THE SUPERANTIGENS

It has become clear in recent years that some microbial exotoxins have a direct effect on cells of the immune system and that this interaction leads to many of the symptoms of disease. Thus, the enterotoxins causing staphylococcal food poisoning, the group A streptococcal exotoxin A responsible for scarlet fever, and the TSST exotoxin responsible for the staphylococcal toxic shock syndrome interact directly with the T-cell receptor. The effect of this interaction is dramatic. Cytokines like IL-1 and TNF are produced leading to their familiar effects systemically and to local skin and gastrointestinal effects (depending on the toxin and its site of action). In addition, after binding to class II major histocompatibility complex (MHC) molecules on antigen-presenting cells, these exotoxin act as polyclonal

Some toxins interact directly with T-cell receptors (superantigens)

Cytokine release may have systemic and immunosuppressive effects

stimulators of T cells so that a significant proportion of all T cells respond by dividing and releasing cytokines. This eventually leads to immunosuppression for reasons that are not totally clear. When trying to assess these findings from the standpoint of bacterial pathogenicity, it is probably important to divorce the disease entity seen in ill patients from the potential role of these toxins in the normal life of the microorganism.

Toxins produced in food may resist boiling and digestive enzymes

For example, staphylococcal food poisoning is an intoxication and does not involve the ingestion of living microbes but rather the ingestion of the products produced in improperly handled food by staphylococci. The toxins that cause such food poisoning are resistant to digestive enzymes. Staphylococcal enterotoxins are also resistant to boiling, so that disease may follow ingestion of contaminated foods in which the organism has already been killed. What then is the role of the toxin in the normal biology of the microbe? Although the complete answer to this question is unknown, it seems likely that the toxins would play a role in the interaction of the microorganism with local host defenses in its preferred human niche, on the skin and the mucosal surface. Here, at the microscopic level, the capacity to neutralize the antigen-presenting cells in the microcosm of the pores of the skin is clearly more important than the induction of vast systemic symptoms. Not all staphylococci carry the enterotoxin genes. Indeed, they may be carried on plasmids or bacterial viruses. Perhaps, the staphylococci that carry such "superantigens" have an advantage over their competing brethren. Such questions need to be answered at the experimental level. Yet, the point is that we must examine the determinants of bacterial pathogenicity with an eye to their role in the biology of the microbe, as well as from the view that they play an essential role in relatively rare cases of overt disease.

Toxins could enhance survival in preferred niche

Superantigens are found in a variety of bacteria and viruses

Superantigens are not restricted simply to bacterial toxins of Gram-positive bacteria. Increasingly, they are reported as potential factors in the pathogenesis of viral infection and in a number of other bacteria. Moreover, polyclonal activation of other immune cells is seen, as in the activation of B cells by Epstein–Barr virus. Hence, the interaction of microbial products directly with cells of the immune system leading to immunosuppression may be a common theme of microbial pathogenicity.

## TISSUE DAMAGE FROM IMMUNE REACTIONS

Antigen–antibody complexes may injure the kidney

Tissue damage and the manifestations of disease may also result from interaction between the host's immune mechanisms and the invading organism or its products. Reactions between high concentrations of antibody, soluble microbial antigens, and complement can deposit immune complexes in tissues and cause acute inflammatory reactions and immune complex disease. In poststreptococcal acute glomerulonephritis, for example, the complexes are sequestered in the glomeruli of the kidney, with serious interference in renal function from the resulting tissue reaction. Sometimes, antibody produced against microbial antigens can cross-react with certain host tissues and initiate an autoimmune process. Such cross-reaction is almost certainly the explanation for poststreptococcal rheumatic fever, and it may be involved in some of the lesions of tertiary syphilis. Some viruses have been shown to have small peptide sequences that are occasionally shared by host tissues. Thus, a virus-induced immune response may also generate antibodies that react with shared determinants on host cells, such as in the heart.

Immune reactions directed at pathogens can cross-react with human tissues

Delayed-type hypersensitivity reactions lead to pathologic manifestation in tuberculosis

In some other infections, the pathologic and clinical features are due largely to delayed-type hypersensitivity reactions to the organism or its products. Such reactions are particularly significant in tuberculosis and other mycobacterial infections. The mycobacteria possess no significant toxins, and in the absence of delayed hypersensitivity, their multiplication elicits little more than a mild inflammatory response. The development of delayed-type, cell-mediated hypersensitivity to their major proteins leads to dramatic pathologic manifestations, which in tuberculosis comprise a chronic granulomatous response around infected foci with massive infiltration of macrophages and lymphocytes followed by central devascularization and necrosis. Rupture of a necrotic area into a bronchus leads to the typical pulmonary cavity of the disease, and rupture into a blood vessel can produce extensive dissemination or massive bleeding from the lung. Injection of tuberculoprotein into an animal with an established tuberculous lesion can lead to acute exacerbation and sometimes death. Thus, the body's defense mechanisms are themselves contributing to the severity of the disease process.

These examples illustrate processes that are probably involved to varying degrees in the pathology and course of most infections. Immune reactions are essential to the control of infectious diseases; however, they are potentially damaging to the host, particularly when large amounts of antigens are involved and the host response is unusually active.

## DISEASE AND TRANSMISSIBILITY

Lethal disease is probably an inadvertent and even unfavorable outcome of infection from a microorganism's standpoint. In many cases, it is to the microbe's advantage to cause some degree of illness that may aid its transmission. In other cases, the interplay between the microbe and the host is subclinical resolution; there may be damage but no disease. Indeed, many of the most severe infectious diseases occur when a microorganism adapted to a nonhuman environment finds itself inadvertently in a human host. The probability of disease is a reflection of the microbial design to live and multiply within a host balanced against the host's capacity to control and limit bacterial proliferation. For certain microorganisms, like *Streptococcus pyogenes*, contact with susceptible hosts that possess normal host defense systems renders a certain proportion clinically ill. In contrast, normal individuals usually shrug off *Proteus* and *Serratia* species. How different the outcome of this interaction when the host is compromised!

It is to the advantage of both the microbe and the host to have a balanced relationship

For microbes exclusively adapted to humans, transmissibility is the key to continued survival. For many organisms this entails microbial persistence in the host and in the environment. A stable pathogen population must retain its viability outside of its preferred niche and still be capable of infection when it next encounters a susceptible host.

Persistence in the host and/or the environment are keys to transmissibility

## COROLLARIES OF MICROBIAL PATHOGENICITY

All parasitic microorganisms need to enter a host, find a unique niche, overcome local defenses, replicate, and be transmitted to a new host. Other factors have become apparent because of these pathogenic attributes. Some are more applicable to bacteria and fungi than to viruses and the larger parasites. The general principles are likely to be true for all pathogens.

1. **Pathogenic microorganisms adapt to changes in the host's biological and social behavior.** Imagine the profound changes in the host–parasite relationship that must have occurred when humanoids began to live in communities and to husband animals. The older diseases such as tuberculosis remained, but the increase in population density meant that "new" epidemic diseases could evolve. In recent times, we have seen new diseases emerge. A material placed in tampons in response to the changing requirements of women in our society enhanced the ability of colonizing staphylococci to produce a toxin. The advent of the birth control pill and the replacement of barrier contraception led to an enormous increase in sexually transmitted diseases. As humans increasingly impinge on other forms of life that have been largely isolated from human populations, one notes an increase in "new" infectious diseases like Lyme disease and quite probably acquired immunodeficiency syndrome (AIDS).

   "New" infectious diseases often reflect changes in human behavior

   Contraception, sexual activity, and sexually transmitted infections are interrelated

   Diseases like toxic shock syndrome, AIDS, Legionnaire's disease, and nosocomial infections are "diseases of human progress" and remind us that we live in a balanced relationship with microorganisms on this planet. Microorganisms will take advantage of any selective advantage that is made available to them to replicate and to establish themselves in a new niche.

   Microorganisms may take advantage of our "progress"

2. **Pathogens are clonal.** Bacteria are haploid as are viruses and some fungi. Consequently, there cannot be a helter-skelter amalgam of genes brought about by promiscuous genetic exchange. If this were so, there would be no bacterial specialization

Genetic mechanisms maximize diversity but preserve useful genes

and they would all possess a consensus chromosomal sequence. Thus, most bacteria (and viruses) have some degree of built-in reproductive isolation, except for members of their own or very closely related species (members of the same gene pool). In this way, diversity within the species through mutation can be maximized (usually by transformation or transduction), while conserving useful gene sequences. The end result of husbanding of important genes during evolution is that at any given time in the world, many bacterial and viral pathogens are representatives of a single or, more often, a relatively few clonal types that have become widespread for the (evolutionary) moment. Thus, all the strains of the typhoid bacillus that have been studied since humans learned to culture them belong to two basic clonal types (Table 10–6). When microbes establish a unique niche, they protect their selective advantage.

Many pathogens are represented by a few virulent clones spread worldwide

The gene pool must be expanded, however. Indeed, how could microorganisms have become pathogens in the first place or adapt to new potential niches? Bacteria have remarkable ways of expanding their genetic diversity, but they do so in a way that is consistent with their haploid lifestyle. From this corollary follows the next.

Carriage of virulence determinants on plasmids and phages preserves chromosomal organization

3. **Pathogens often carry essential virulence determinants on extrachromosomal elements (plasmids) as part of lysogenic phages or on other mobile genetic elements.** It is now well established that many of the essential determinants of pathogenicity are actually replicated as part of an extrachromosomal element or as additions to the bacterial chromosome (see Table 10–7). If haploid organisms must limit their genetic interactions to preserve their individuality, it is not surprising that new genes that bring in important new attributes are found on genetic elements that do not disrupt the organization of the bacterial chromosome. The interchange of plasmids and bacterial viruses among bacteria, coupled with transpositional (illegitimate) recombination between the extrachromosomal element and the chromosome, provides a means for microorganisms to exploit new genes in a haploid world. It is of some note that pathogenic determinants not found associated with a plasmid or a phage are often seen as duplicated genes or associated with transposon-like structures. In a bacterial genus containing both pathogenic and nonpathogenic species, the attributes of pathogenicity are encoded on sequences that do not have any counterpart in the nonpathogen. It seems unlikely that pathogenicity arose as a result of long adaptation of an initially nonpathogenic organism to a more parasitic, host-dependent lifestyle. It is more likely that organisms inherited new gene sequences, often in a large block, that provided them with the capacity to establish themselves more efficiently in a host or to exploit some new niche within the host.

Chromosomal virulence determinants are often duplicated or transposon associated

Probable that virulence is inherited as a large block of new genes

4. **Bacteria and other pathogens use elaborate means to modulate their free-living life from their parasitic life.**

**TABLE 10–6. PROPORTION OF CERTAIN INFECTIOUS DISEASES CAUSED BY COMMON BACTERIAL CLONAL TYPES**

| Species | Total Number of Clonal Types Identified | Number of Clonal Types Commonly Isolated from Cases of Disease | Percentage of Disease Due to Common Clonal Types |
|---|---|---|---|
| *Bordetella pertussis* | 2 | 2 | 100 |
| *Haemophilus influenzae* type b | | | |
| North America | 104 | 6 | 81 |
| Europe | 60 | 3 | 78 |
| *Legionella pneumophila* | | | |
| Global | 50 | 5 | 52 |
| Wadsworth VA Hospital | 10 | 1 | 86 |
| *Shigella sonnei* | 1 | 1 | 100 |

*Modified from Mandell GL, Bennett JE, Dorin E.* Principles and Practice of Infectious Diseases, *4th ed. New York: Churchill Livingstone; 1990, p. 21, with permission.*

**TABLE 10–7. EXAMPLES OF PLASMID AND PHAGE-ENCODED VIRULENCE DETERMINANTS**

| Organism | Virulence Factor | Biological Function |
|---|---|---|
| **Plasmid-encoded** | | |
| Enterotoxigenic *E. coli* | Heat-labile, heat-stable enterotoxins (LT, ST) | Activation of adenyl/guanylcyclase in the small bowel, which leads to diarrhea |
| | CFA/I and CFA/II | Adherence/colonization factors |
| *Salmonella* spp. | Serum resistance and intracellular survival | Invasion of reticuloendothelial system |
| *Shigella* spp. and enteroinvasive *E. coli* | Gene products involved in invasion | Induces internalization by intestinal epithelial cells |
| *Yersinia* spp. | Adherence factors and gene products involved in invasion | Attachment/invasion |
| *Bacillus anthracis* | Edema factor, lethal factor, and protective antigen | Edema factor has adenylcyclase activity |
| *Staphylococcus aureus* | Exfoliative toxin | Causes toxic epidermal necrolysis |
| *Clostridium tetani* | Tetanus neurotoxin | Blocks the release of inhibitory neurotransmitter; which leads to muscle spasms |
| **Phage-encoded** | | |
| *Corynebacterium diphtheriae* | Diphtheria toxin | Inhibition of eukaryotic protein synthesis |
| *Streptococcus pyogenes* | Erythrogenic toxin | Rash of scarlet fever |
| *Clostridium botulinum* | Neurotoxin | Blocks synaptic acetylcholine release, which leads to flaccid paralysis |
| Enterohemorrhagic *E. coli* | Shiga-like toxin | Inhibition of eukaryotic protein synthesis |

*Modified from Mandell GL, Bennett JE, Dorin E.* Principles and Practice of Infectious Diseases, *4th ed. New York: Churchill Livingstone; 1990, p. 22, with permission.*

Bacteria, fungi, and larger parasites have evolved signal transduction networks using environmental clues like temperature, iron concentration, and calcium flux to turn on genes important for pathogenicity (Table 10–8). It was puzzling to consider how a microorganism that makes potent toxins in the laboratory could possibly spare any host it infected. It became clearer when we learned that toxin biosynthesis by the microbe is tightly regulated together with other genes to be activated only in

Microbial signal transduction systems sense environmental cues in order to turn on virulence genes

Toxin genes may be coregulated with other genes

**TABLE 10–8. EXAMPLES OF BACTERIAL VIRULENCE REGULATORY SYSTEMS**

| Organism | Regulatory Gene(s) | Environmental Stimuli | Regulated Functions |
|---|---|---|---|
| *E. coli* | *drd*X<br>*fur* | Temperature<br>Iron concentration | Pyelonephritis-associated pili<br>Shiga-like toxin, siderophores |
| *Bordetella pertussis* | *bvg*AS | Temperature, ionic conditions, nicotinic acid | Pertussis toxin, filamentous hemagglutinin, adenylate cyclase, others |
| *Vibrio cholerae* | *tox*R | Temperature, osmolarity, pH, amino acids | Cholera toxin, pili, outer membrane proteins |
| *Yersinia* spp. | *lcr* loci<br>*vir*F | Temperature, calcium<br>Temperature | Outer membrane proteins<br>Adherence, invasiveness |
| *Shigella* spp. | *vir*R | Temperature | Invasiveness |
| *Salmonella typhimurium* | *pag* genes | pH | Virulence, macrophage survival |
| *Staphylococcus aureus* | *agr* | pH | α-, β-hemolysins; toxic shock syndrome toxin 1, protein A |

*Modified from Mandell GL, Bennett JE, Dorin E.* Principles and Practice of Infectious Diseases, *4th ed. New York: Churchill Livingstone; 1990, p. 23, with permission.*

Host–parasite relationship balanced by selective expression of pathogenic genes

particular sets of circumstances. Only in selective circumstances are genes involved in pathogenicity used and then often sparingly. The organism's reaction to the host need only be sufficient to establish itself and replicate. The host–parasite relationship is delicate.

## MECHANISMS OF VIRAL VIRULENCE AND THE ROLE OF INTERFERONS IN IMMUNITY

Viruses do not directly produce toxins

Disease results from effect on host cell or immune response to it

The pathogenesis of viral diseases differs in a number of respects from that of most bacterial infections because of the totally different modes of replication of viruses and their strict intracellular habitat. No viruses possess lipopolysaccharide (LPS) and animal viruses do not produce exotoxins, although some temperate bacteriophages encode exotoxins that are excreted by their bacterial hosts. Viral diseases result directly or indirectly from the effects of the virus on the cell it infects, and these effects can range from lysis and destruction to subtle changes in cell function. A major component of many viral diseases is the inflammation and tissue damage that results from release of cellular enzymes by viral cytotoxicity or from immunologic attack on the infected cell. Released viral antigens also can be involved in immune complex diseases, initiate autoimmune responses, or mediate delayed-type hypersensitivity reactions. These are considered in more detail in the next section.

Latency is a common feature of viral diseases

Many viral infections can become latent, either by assuming an altered episomal form in the cell or as a result of integration of viral DNA or DNA transcripts into the host genome, and can cause relapses or increased severity of disease when complete virions are resynthesized later. Latency is not a unique characteristic of viruses. It occurs, for instance, with the rickettsia of typhus fever and with the tubercle bacillus; however, it is much more common and often more significant in viral infections. Because of the intimate relationship between virus and cell, the basic mechanisms of these interactions are detailed in Chapters 6 and 7. This section focuses on those aspects directly related to the disease process.

### Initiation of Infection

Routes of infection are similar to other organisms

Blood is an important source of infection

Viruses are acquired by routes similar to those of other pathogenic organisms. Thus, the respiratory, alimentary, and genital tracts, skin, oropharyngeal mucosa, and conjunctiva may all be infected directly with specific viruses. Some viruses, such as many arboviruses, are transmitted by insect bites, and the rabies virus, by bites of infected animals. Other viruses that infect white blood cells or otherwise reach the bloodstream such as cytomegalovirus and hepatitis B virus can be acquired from blood either as a result of inadequate sterilization of needles and syringes or through blood transfusion.

Tissue tropism is related to viral envelope or capsid and cell surface receptors

Viral receptors may have other functions for the cell

The central determinant of the ability of a virus to infect involves contact with a host cell that carries surface receptors for components of the viral envelope or capsid. Such receptors, many of which are glycoproteins, are often restricted to cells of particular tissues and species of animals, and this accounts to a considerable degree for the tissue tropism and host ranges of viruses, although other factors can involve their ability to replicate within a cell. Thus, receptors for the influenza virus occur on ciliated respiratory epithelial cells, those for the human immunodeficiency virus (HIV, the cause of AIDS) occur on CD4+ helper–inducer T lymphocytes and macrophages of humans, whereas receptors for many arboviruses are widely distributed among mammals and mosquitos and thus determine a wider host range. Receptors for viruses are often multifunctional and include hormone receptors and cell surface enzymes, as well as structural surface components. In some cases, receptors are associated with histocompatibility antigens; thus there may be genetic differences in susceptibility to infection among different individuals of the same species.

The mechanisms of receptor-mediated endocytosis and replication of both naked and enveloped DNA and RNA viruses are described in Chapter 6. For a wider infection to develop, replication in the initially infected cell must be followed by spread to other susceptible cells.

## Viral Spread in the Body

Viruses spread in the body by a variety of methods that can influence the duration of the incubation period, the disease syndromes produced, and the ability of the host to control the infection. Some viruses, such as influenza virus, spread directly from cell to cell in the affected epithelium as they are released by cytolysis. Thus, free virus becomes subject to neutralization by antibody when it is produced.

Free virus is released from lipid cells

Many viruses multiply first at a primary site of infection, such as the intestinal or oropharyngeal epithelium, and on release from these cells reach the bloodstream to produce a primary viremia followed by infection of specific target cells in other tissues. An example is the mumps virus, which initially infects the nasopharynx, but causes its major disease manifestations in the salivary glands and sometimes in the central nervous and endocrine systems. In this case, the initial infection and viremia may be subclinical and the incubation period much longer than with the influenza virus.

Spread to bloodstream (viremia) may follow multiplication at primary site

Viruses such as herpes simplex are less prone to cause cytolysis, but pass from cell to cell through syncytial bridges caused by fusion of the membranes of different cells. They tend to produce many chronic and relapsing infections, probably associated with waxing and waning of cell-mediated immune responses and their cytotoxic effector mechanisms. Cell fusion can also allow a virus to enter cells that lack the viral receptor. Herpes simplex and some other viruses have a particular affinity for cells of the nervous system or are able to travel through axons and are thus protected from the host's immune system. The varicella–zoster virus, after causing a childhood attack of chickenpox, may remain latent and protected in dorsal root ganglion cells, but reemerge decades later to produce shingles in the distribution of the affected nerve routes. The rabies virus can pass slowly to its target in the central nervous system by traveling up axons that innervate the area of the original bite and fail to stimulate an immune response during what can be a prolonged incubation period.

Cell-to-cell spread can occur by fusion of membranes

Viruses infecting nervous system can spread through axons

Unlike most bacteria (the spirochete of syphilis being an important exception), several viruses causing infection during pregnancy can traverse the chorionic barrier and chronically infect the developing fetus. Rubella and cytomegalovirus infections are classic examples; both can result in severe developmental abnormalities and noncytolytic alteration of cell function.

Several viruses can pass the coronic barrier to infect the fetus

## Interferons

Interferons (IFNs) are polypeptide cytokines produced by many mammalian cell types. The family includes IFN-$\alpha$ (of which there are several derived from leukocytes), IFN-$\beta$ (derived from fibroblasts and many other cell types), and IFN-$\gamma$ (a product of activated T lymphocytes). IFN-$\alpha$ and IFN-$\beta$ are synthesized when the producing cell is exposed to a variety of stimuli, in particular viral and other infections. Production is also stimulated by endotoxin, some other bacterial products, and natural or synthetic double-stranded RNA. Production of IFN-$\gamma$ by T cells is stimulated by reaction of the cells with the specific antigen to which they are responsive or by some mitogens. The antiviral action of interferon is, however, nonspecific.

Polypeptide cytokines are produced by mammalian cells in response to infection

Interferon action is nonspecific

Interferons inhibit replication of RNA and DNA viruses and some other intracellular pathogens. They do not effect adsorption or endocytosis of viruses, but act by inducing production of proteins within the cell that inhibit viral protein and nucleic acid synthesis and, thus, replication. Their production is blocked by inhibitors of these syntheses. The molecular mechanisms of action of interferon are described in more detail in Chapter 6.

No effect on viral attachment

Interfere with viral replication

In addition to their activity within the infected cell, interferons bind to surface receptors of adjacent uninfected cells, are taken into these cells, and produce what has been termed an antiviral state that prevents replication of any virus that infects the cells. The phenomenon of viral interference (inability of a virus to superinfect during another viral infection) is due largely to interferon produced in response to the first infection.

Interference effect blocks infection by another virus

Interferon clearly play a critical nonspecific role in the early control of many acute viral infections pending the development of humoral and cellular immunity. Interferon gamma

Important prior to immune response

Activates T cell and macrophages

also contributes to resistance to infection by inducing activation and proliferation of natural killer and cytotoxic T cells, by activating macrophages, and by increasing expression of MHC antigens on a variety of cell types and, thus, of antigen presentation to T cells.

Interferon may have negative effects

Not all effects of interferon are beneficial. Interferons inhibit normal cell growth and produce transient suppression of cell-mediated immunity by selective inhibition of protein synthesis, and in some instances IFN-$\gamma$ may excessively enhance inflammatory processes through its action on natural killer and cytotoxic T-cell activity.

Emerging role for recombinant human interferon in therapy

Several interferon genes have been cloned, and their products expressed, in bacteria and yeasts. This has greatly facilitated clinical studies, because interferons are generally specific for each animal species, and human interferons were previously extremely difficult to obtain. The present status of the role of recombinant interferon in the prophylaxis and treatment of viral diseases is considered in Chapter 13.

## Avoidance of Host Defense Mechanisms

Antibody blocks attachment to receptor site

T cells lyse infected cells

Most acute viral infections are controlled to varying extent by the development of neutralizing antibody that blocks attachment of extracellular virus to receptors on susceptible cells and by the action of interferons. Virus may be liberated from its intracellular habitat either by direct cytolysis or by the action on the infected cell of cytotoxic T cells or natural killer cells. Viruses that pass between intercellular bridges, those that are protected within neurons, and those that fail to lyse a cell or express viral antigens on its surface are variably protected from the immune system. Integration of the viral genome into that of the host cell or production only of incomplete virus in the cell may also be totally unrecognized immunologically and result in latency.

Nonlytic and lysogenic viruses are protected from the immune system

Some viruses, like HIV, directly suppress the immune system

Several viral infections are directly immunosuppressive. The receptor for HIV is the CD4 molecule on CD4+ helper–inducer T lymphocytes and on monocytes and other cells of the macrophage series. Infection of CD4+ T lymphocytes directly affects cell-mediated immunity, and nonlethal infection of macrophages leads to reduction of their chemotactic and microbicidal power, as well as providing a reservoir of infectious virus. In addition, the gp120 protein of HIV is homologous to a B-cell-activating lymphokine and produces polyclonal activation of B cells. This leads to excessive but nonspecific immunoglobulin production at the expense of specific antibody responses. Some other viruses, for example, the measles virus, can also infect immunocytes and reduce immune responses, and cytomegalovirus-infected monocytes and macrophages are partially crippled in their microbicidal activities. These viruses, and some others, including influenza viruses, also cause alterations in the functions of polymorphonuclear leukocytes, including chemotactic, oxidative, and bactericidal activity. In each of these cases, the most severe or fatal results of infection are often due to secondary infections with other organisms that develop as a result of the compromised cellular defense mechanisms.

Viruses may reduce monocyte, macrophage, or neutrophil responses

## CONCLUSION

Host–parasite interactions are wonderfully complex and have evolved in a manner that has tended to produce a more balanced state of parasitism between well-established species and the microorganisms with which they frequently come into contact. In this chapter the components of these interactions have been discussed separately, but it is important to recognize the dynamic and shifting nature of their role in determining the course and outcome of an infection. As you review the microbial tactics for survival and the ensuing host response to acute infection and its consequences, it is important to see that systemic symptoms of many viral and bacterial infections—fever, malaise, and anorexia—are the same because they reflect a basic host response to a foreign intruder. The diversity of mechanisms by which a host controls infection can be particularly appreciated if one recognizes that they are all intimately interrelated. Many of the infected patients you will aid during your career will not have inherited defects in their host defense matrix, but they will have disease-associated deficiencies. Increasingly, physician-induced deficits in their innate and adaptive immune systems are brought about by cytotoxic chemotherapy, radiotherapy, and other forms of medical intervention. For example, because of their tumors or treatment, cancer patients often have a variety of interrelated defects and mucosal disruptions increasing the risk of infection. The single most important of these is neutropenia (usually defined as an absolute granulocyte count of 500/mm$^3$ or less). It is no wonder that the presenting symptom in tumors of the bowel may be sepsis or bacterial endocarditis. During the natural progression of malignancy and as a consequence of its current therapy, infection remains as the major cause of morbidity and mortality.

These few examples suffice, but the important point is the importance of normal defense mechanisms. It is more important to preserve and augment the normal host defenses in many circumstances than to use the newest "wonder drug." We can also be fully confident that an understanding of the molecular basis of microbial pathogenesis will provide considerable information about the biology of the pathogens, the host–parasite relationship, human (and other) host-specific defense mechanisms, and, ultimately, ways to prevent infection and disease.

## ADDITIONAL READING

Iglegwski BH, Clark VL (eds). *Molecular Basis of Bacterial Pathogenesis*. San Diego: Academic Press; 1990. This volume collects papers summarizing experimental details related to the pathogenic mechanisms discussed in this chapter using various bacterial systems as models.¡

Salyers A, Whitt D (eds). Microbial Pathogenesis: A Molecular Approach. Washington, DC: American Society for Microbiology (in press).

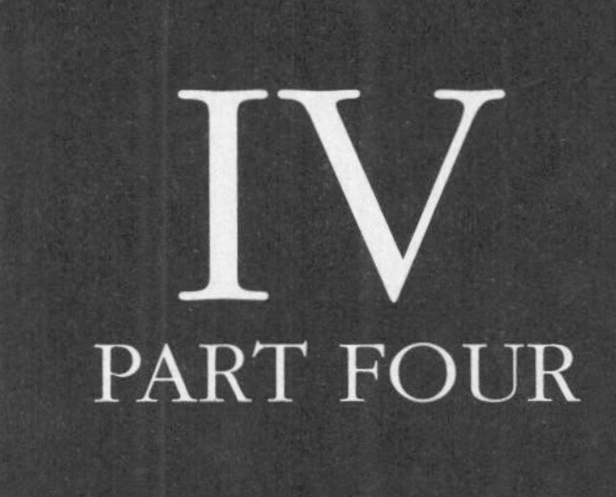


# Spread and Control of Infection

Chapter 11

# Sterilization, Pasteurization, and Disinfection

*Kenneth J. Ryan*

From the time of debates about the germ theory of disease, killing microbes before they reach patients has been a major strategy for preventing infection. In fact, Ignaz Semmelweiss successfully applied disinfection principles decades before bacteria were first isolated (see Chapter 72). This chapter discusses the most important methods used for this purpose in modern medical practice. Understanding how they work is of increasing importance in an environment that includes immunocompromised patients, transplantation, indwelling devices, and acquired immunodeficiency syndrome (AIDS).

## DEFINITIONS

**Death/killing** as it relates to microbial organisms is defined in terms of how we detect them in culture. Operationally it is a loss of ability to multiply under any known conditions. This is complicated by fact that organisms that appear to be irreversibly inactivated may sometimes recover when appropriately treated. For example, ultraviolet (UV) irradiation of bacteria can result in the formation of thymine dimers in the DNA with loss of ability to replicate. A period of exposure to visible light may then activate an enzyme that breaks the dimers and restores viability by a process known as photoreactivation. Mechanisms also exist for repair of the damage without light. Such considerations are of great significance in the preparation of safe vaccines from inactivated virulent organisms.

Absence of growth does not necessarily indicate sterility

**Sterilization** is complete killing, or removal, of all living organisms from a particular location or material. It can be accomplished by incineration, nondestructive heat treatment, certain gases, exposure to ionizing radiation, some liquid chemicals, and filtration.

Sterilization is complete killing

**Pasteurization** is the use of heat at a temperature sufficient to inactivate important pathogenic organisms in liquids such as water or milk, but at a temperature below that needed to ensure sterilization. For example, heating milk at a temperature of 74°C for 3 to 5 seconds or 62°C for 30 minutes kills most pathogenic bacteria that may be present without altering its quality. Obviously, spores are not killed at these temperatures.

Disinfection can be accomplished by heat (pasteurization) or chemical methods

**Disinfection** is the destruction of pathogenic microorganisms by processes that fail to meet the criteria for sterilization. It is most commonly applied to liquid chemical agents known as disinfectants. These agents usually have some degree of selectivity. Bacterial spores, organisms with waxy coats (eg, mycobacteria), and some viruses may show considerable resistance to the common disinfectants. **Antiseptics** are disinfectant agents that can be used on body surfaces, such as the skin or vaginal tract, to reduce the numbers of normal flora and pathogenic contaminants. They have lower toxicity than disinfectants used

Spores are particularly resistant

environmentally, but are usually less active in killing vegetative organisms. **Sanitization** is a less precise term with a meaning somewhere between disinfection and cleanliness. It is used primarily in housekeeping and food preparation contexts.

Asepsis applies sterilization to creating a protective environment

**Asepsis** describes processes designed to prevent microorganisms from reaching a protected environment. It is applied in many procedures used in the operating room, in the preparation of therapeutic agents, and in technical manipulations in the microbiology laboratory. An essential component of aseptic techniques is the sterilization of all materials and equipment used. Asepsis is more fully discussed in Chapter 72.

## MICROBIAL KILLING

Bacterial killing follows exponential kinetics

Killing of bacteria by heat, radiation, or chemicals is usually exponential with time; that is, a fixed proportion of survivors are killed during each time increment. Thus, if 90% of a population of bacteria are killed during each 5 minutes of exposure to a weak solution of a disinfectant, a starting population of $10^6$/mL will be reduced to $10^5$/mL after 5 minutes, to $10^3$/mL after 15 minutes, and theoretically to 1 organism ($10^0$)/mL after 30 minutes. Exponential killing corresponds to a first-order reaction or a "single-hit" hypothesis, in which the lethal change involves a single target in the organism and the probability of this change is constant with time. Thus, plots of the logarithm of the number of survivors against time will be linear (Fig 11–1A); however, the slope of the curve will vary with the effectiveness of the killing process, which is influenced by the nature of the organism, lethal agent, concentration (in the case of disinfectants), and temperature. In general, the rate of killing increases exponentially with arithmetic increases in temperature or in concentrations of disinfectant.

Sterility is not absolute

An important consequence of exponential killing with most sterilization processes is that sterility is not an absolute term, but must be expressed as a probability. Thus, to continue the example given previously, the chance of a single survivor in 1 mL is theoretically $10^{-1}$ after 35 minutes. If a chance of $10^{-9}$ were the maximum acceptable risk for a single

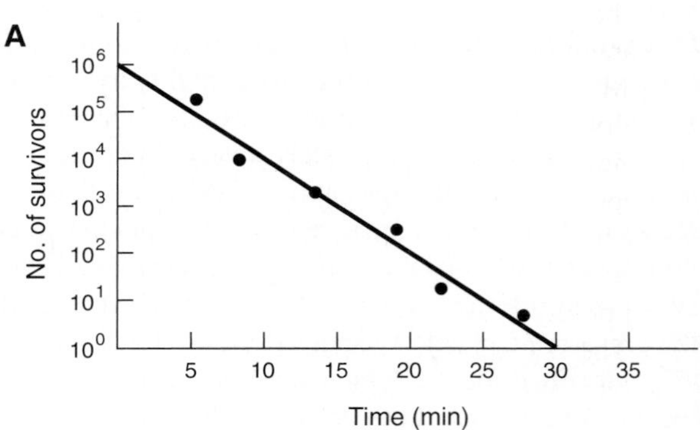


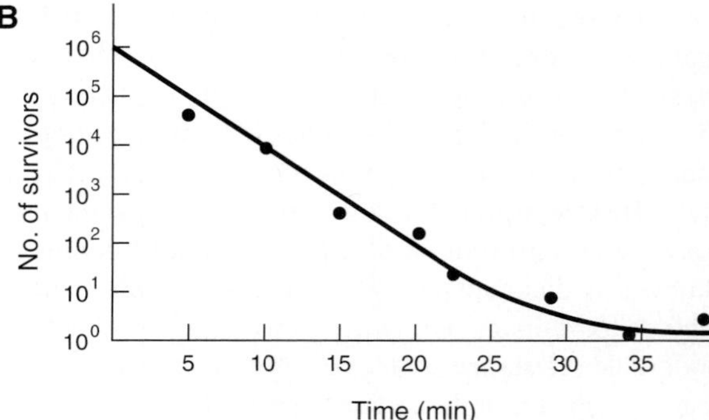


**Figure 11–1.** Kinetics of bacterial killing. **A.** Exponential killing is shown as a function of population size and time. **B.** Deviation from linearity, as with a mixed population, extends the time.

surviving organism in a 1-mL sample (eg, of a therapeutic agent), the procedure would require continuation for a total of 75 minutes.

A simple single-hit curve often does not express the kinetics of killing adequately. In the case of some bacterial endospores, a brief period (activation) may elapse before exponential killing by heat begins. If multiple targets are involved, the experimental curve will deviate from linearity. More significant is the fact that microbial populations may include a small proportion of more resistant mutants or of organisms in a physiologic state that confers greater resistance to inactivation. In these cases, the later stages of the curve are flattened (Fig 11–1B), and extrapolations from the exponential phase of killing may seriously underestimate the time needed for a high probability of achieving complete sterility. In practice, materials that come into contact with tissues are sterilized under conditions that allow a very wide margin of safety, and the effectiveness of inactivation of organisms in vaccines is tested directly with large volumes and multiple samples before a product is made available for use.

Heterogenous microbial populations may not follow simple kinetics

## STERILIZATION

The availability of reliable methods of sterilization has made possible the major developments in surgery and intrusive medical techniques that have helped to revolutionize medicine over the past century. Furthermore, sterilization procedures form the basis of many food preservation procedures, particularly in the canning industry.

### Heat

The simplest method of sterilization is to expose the surface to be sterilized to a naked flame, as is done with the wire loop used in microbiology laboratories. It can be used equally effectively for emergency sterilization of a knife blade or a needle. Disposable material is, of course, rapidly and effectively decontaminated by incineration. Carbonization of organic material and destruction of microorganisms, including spores, occur after exposure to dry heat of 160°C for 2 hours in a sterilizing oven. This method is applicable to metals, glassware, and some heat-resistant oils and waxes that are immiscible in water and cannot, therefore, be sterilized in the autoclave. A major use of the dry heat sterilizing oven is in preparation of laboratory glassware.

Incineration is rapid and effective

Dry heat requires 160° C for 2 hours to kill

Moist heat in the form of water or steam is far more rapid and effective in sterilization than dry heat, because reactive water molecules denature protein irreversibly by disrupting H bonds between peptide groups at relatively low temperatures. Most vegetative bacteria of importance in human disease are killed within a few minutes at 70°C or less, although many bacterial spores (see Chapter 2) can resist boiling for prolonged periods. For applications requiring sterility the use of boiling water has been replaced by the autoclave, which when properly used ensures sterility by killing all forms of microorganisms.

Moist heat is more effective and rapid than dry heat

Boiling water fails to kill bacterial spores

The **autoclave** is, in effect, a sophisticated pressure cooker (Fig 11–2). In its simplest form, it comprises a chamber in which the air can be replaced with pure saturated steam under pressure. Air is removed either by evacuation of the chamber before filling it with steam or by displacement through a valve at the bottom of the autoclave, which remains open until all air has drained out. The latter, which is termed a **downward displacement autoclave,** capitalizes on the heaviness of air compared with saturated steam. When the air has been removed, the temperature in the chamber is proportional to the pressure of the steam; autoclaves are usually operated at 121°C, which is achieved with a pressure of 15 pounds per square inch. Under these conditions, spores directly exposed are killed in less than 5 minutes, although the normal sterilization time is 10 to 15 minutes to account for variation in the ability of steam to penetrate different materials and to allow a wide margin of safety. As the velocity of killing increases logarithmically with arithmetic increases in temperature, a steam temperature of 121°C is vastly more effective than 100°C. For example, the spores of *Clostridium botulinum*, the cause of botulism, may survive 5 hours of boiling, but can be killed in 4 minutes at 121°C in the autoclave.

Autoclave effective because of increased temperature of steam generated under pressure

Steam displaces air from the autoclave

Killing rate increases logarithmically with arithmetic increase in temperature

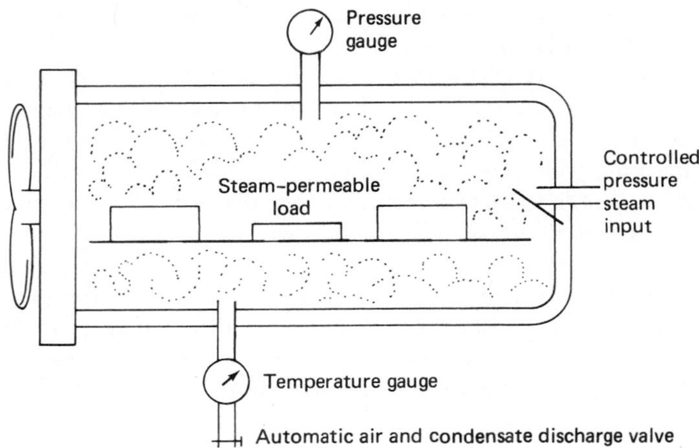


**Figure 11–2.** Simple form of downward displacement autoclave.

Condensation and latent heat increase effectiveness of autoclave

The use of saturated steam in the autoclave has other advantages. Latent heat equivalent to 539 cal/g condensed steam is immediately liberated on condensation on the cooler surfaces of the load to be sterilized. The temperature of the load is thus raised very rapidly to that of the steam. Condensation also permits rapid steam penetration of porous materials such as surgical drapes by producing a relative negative pressure at the surface, which allows more steam to enter immediately. Autoclaves can thus be used for sterilizing any materials that are not damaged by heat and moisture, such as heat-stable liquids, swabs, most instruments, culture media, and rubber gloves.

Access of pure saturated steam is required for sterilization

Impermeable or large volume materials present special problems

It is essential that those who use autoclaves understand the principles involved. Their effectiveness depends on absence of air, pure saturated steam, and access of steam to the material to be sterilized. Pressure per se plays no role in sterilization other than to ensure the raised temperature of the steam. Failure can result from attempting to sterilize the interior of materials that are impermeable to steam or the contents of sealed containers. Under these conditions, a dry heat temperature of 121°C is obtained, which may be insufficient to kill even vegetative organisms. Large volumes of liquids require longer sterilization times than normal loads, because their temperature must reach 121°C before timing begins. When sealed containers of liquids are sterilized, it is essential that the autoclave cool without being opened or evacuated; otherwise, the containers may explode as the external pressure falls in relation to that within.

Flash autoclaves use 134°C for 3 minutes

**"Flash" autoclaves,** which are widely used in operating rooms, often use saturated steam at a temperature of 134°C for 3 minutes. Air and steam are removed mechanically before and after the sterilization cycle so that metal instruments may be available rapidly.

Quality control of autoclaves depends primarily on ensuring that the appropriate temperature for the pressure used is achieved and that packing and timing are correct. Biological and chemical indicators of the correct conditions are available and are inserted from time to time in the loads.

## Gas

Ethylene oxide sterilization is used for heat-labile materials

A number of articles, particularly certain plastics and lensed instruments that are damaged or destroyed by autoclaving, can be sterilized with ethylene oxide. Occasionally, formaldehyde gas is used to decontaminate larger areas such as cabinets or rooms.

Aeration needed after ethylene oxide sterilization

**Ethylene oxide** is an inflammable and potentially explosive gas. It is an alkylating agent that inactivates microorganisms by replacing labile hydrogen atoms on hydroxyl, carboxy, or sulfhydryl groups, particularly of guanine and adenine in DNA. Ethylene oxide sterilizers resemble autoclaves and expose the load to 10% ethylene oxide in carbon dioxide at 50 to 60°C under controlled conditions of humidity. Exposure times are usually about 4 to 6 hours and must be followed by a prolonged period of aeration to allow the gas to diffuse out of substances that have absorbed it. Aeration is essential, because absorbed gas can cause damage to tissues or skin. Ethylene oxide is a mutagen, and special precautions are now taken to ensure that it is properly vented outside of working spaces. Used under properly controlled conditions, ethylene oxide is an effective sterilizing agent for heat-labile devices such as artificial heart valves that cannot be treated at the temperature of the autoclave.

### Ultraviolet Light and Ionizing Radiation

**Ultraviolet light** in the wavelength range 240 to 280 nm is absorbed by nucleic acids and causes genetic damage, including the formation of the thymine dimers discussed previously. The practical value of UV sterilization is limited by its poor ability to penetrate. Apart from its use experimentally as a mutagen, its main application has been in irradiation of air in the vicinity of critical hospital sites and as an aid in the decontamination of laboratory facilities used for handling particularly hazardous organisms. In these situations, single exposed organisms are rapidly inactivated. It must be remembered that UV light can cause skin and eye damage, and workers exposed to it must be appropriately protected.

UV light causes direct damge to DNA

Use of UV light limited by penetration and safety

**Ionizing radiation** carries far greater energy than UV light. It, too, causes direct damage to DNA and produces toxic free radicals and hydrogen peroxide from water within the microbial cells. Cathode rays and gamma rays from cobalt-60 are widely used in industrial processes, including the sterilization of many disposable surgical supplies such as gloves, plastic syringes, specimen containers, some foodstuffs, and the like, because they can be packaged before exposure to the penetrating radiation. Ionizing irradiation does not always result in the physical disintegration of killed microbes. As a result, plasticware sterilized in this way may carry significant numbers of dead but stainable bacteria. This has occasionally caused confusion when it has involved containers used to collect normally sterile body fluids such as cerebrospinal fluid. The dead bacterial bodies may produce a "false-positive" Gram-stained smear and result in inappropriate administration of antibiotics.

Ionizing radiation damages DNA

Industrial use for surgical supplies, food

Killed organisms may remain morphologically intact and stainable

### Filtration

Both live and dead microorganisms can be removed from liquids by positive- or negative-pressure filtration. Membrane filters, usually composed of cellulose esters (eg, cellulose acetate), are available commercially with pore sizes of 0.005 to 1 μm. For removal of bacteria, a pore size of 0.2 μm is effective because filters act not only mechanically but by electrostatic adsorption of particles to their surface. Filtration is used for sterilization of large volumes of fluid, especially those containing heat-labile components such as serum.

Membrane filters remove bacteria by mechanical and electrostatic mechanisms

## PASTEURIZATION

Pasteurization involves exposure of liquids to temperatures in the range 55 to 75°C to remove all vegetative bacteria of significance in human disease. Spores are unaffected by the pasteurization process.

Kills vegetatvie bacteria but not spores

Pasteurization is used commercially to render milk safe and extend its storage quality. To the dismay of some of his compatriots, Pasteur proposed application of the process to winemaking to prevent microbial spoilage and vinegarization. This method has no effect on the quality or bouquet of wine when undertaken properly, but most wines currently available are filter sterilized. Pasteurization in water at 70°C for 30 minutes has also been used to render inhalation therapy equipment free of organisms that may otherwise multiply in mucus and humidifying water and cause respiratory infections.

Used for foods and medical equipment

## DISINFECTION AND DECONTAMINATION

Given access and sufficient time, chemical disinfectants cause the death of pathogenic vegetative bacteria. Most are general protoplasmic poisons and are not currently used in the

Most agents are general protoplasmic poisons

Disinfectants inactivated by organic material

treatment of infections other than very superficial lesions, having been replaced by antimicrobics (see Chapter 13). Some, such as the quaternary ammonium compounds, alcohol, and the iodophors reduce the superficial flora and can eliminate contaminating pathogenic bacteria from the skin surface. Others, such as the phenolics, are valuable only for treating inanimate surfaces or for rendering contaminated materials safe. All are bound and inactivated to varying degrees by protein and dirt and lose considerable activity when applied to other than clean surfaces. Their activity increases exponentially with increases in temperature, but the relationship of increases in concentration to killing effectiveness is more complex and varies for each compound. Optimal in-use concentrations have been established for all available disinfectants. The major groups of compounds currently used are briefly discussed next.

## Alcohols

Alcohols require some water for antibacterial effectiveness

Alcohol action is not rapid

The alcohols are protein denaturants that rapidly kill vegetative bacteria when applied as aqueous solutions in the range 70 to 95% alcohol. They are inactive against bacterial spores and many viruses. Solutions of 100% alcohol dehydrate organisms rapidly but fail to kill, because the lethal process requires water molecules. Ethanol (70–90%) and isopropyl alcohol (90–95%) are widely used as skin decontaminants before simple invasive procedures such as venipuncture. Their effect is not instantaneous, and the traditional alcohol wipe, particularly when followed by a vein-probing finger, is more symbolic than effective, because insufficient time is given for significant killing. Isopropyl alcohol has largely replaced ethanol in hospital use because it is somewhat more active and is not subject to diversion to housestaff parties.

## Halogens

Tincture of iodine in alcohol is most common

Allergenicity may limit use

Iodophors combine iodine with organic detergents

**Iodine** is an effective disinfectant that acts by iodinating or oxidizing essential components of the microbial cell. It is commonly used as a tincture of 2% iodine in 50% alcohol. It kills more rapidly and effectively than alcohol alone, but has the disadvantage of sometimes causing hypersensitivity reactions and of staining materials with which it comes into contact. It is an excellent preparation for use on skin before drawing a blood culture, a procedure in which contamination must be excluded as much as possible. Tincture of iodine is applied and allowed to dry, and the iodine then removed with alcohol swabs. This procedure ensures an application time sufficient for adequate skin disinfection. Other preparations are available in which iodine is combined with organic compounds such as detergents in dissociable complexes. These agents, termed **iodophors,** cause less skin staining and dehydration than tinctures and are widely used in preparation of skin before surgery. Although less allergenic than inorganic iodine preparations, iodophors should not be used on patients with a history of iodine sensitivity.

Chlorine oxidative action is rapid

Activity reduced by organic matter

**Chlorine** is a highly effective oxidizing agent, which accounts for its lethality to microbes. It exists as hypochlorous acid in aqueous solutions that dissociate to yield free chlorine over a wide pH range, particularly under slightly acidic conditions. In concentrations of less than one part per million, chlorine is lethal within seconds to most vegetative bacteria, and it inactivates most viruses; this efficacy accounts for its use in rendering supplies of drinking water safe and in chlorination of water in swimming pools. Chlorine reacts rapidly with protein and many other organic compounds, and its activity is lost quickly in the presence of organic material. This property, combined with its toxicity, renders it ineffective on body surfaces; however, it is the agent of choice for decontaminating surfaces and glassware that have been contaminated with viruses or spores of pathogenic bacteria. For these purposes it is usually applied as a 5% solution of sodium hypochlorite.

## Surface-Active Compounds

Hydrophobic and hydrophilic groups of surfactants solubilize

**Surfactants** are compounds with hydrophobic and hydrophilic groups that attach to and solubilize various compounds or alter their properties. Anionic detergents such as soaps are highly effective cleansers, but have little direct antibacterial effect, probably because their charge is similar to that of most microorganisms. Cationic detergents, particularly the **quaternary ammonium compounds** ("quats") such as benzalkonium chloride, are highly bactericidal in the absence of contaminating organic matter. Their hydrophobic and lipophilic groups react with the lipid of the cell membrane of the bacteria, alter the membrane's surface properties and its permeability, and lead to loss of essential cell components and death. These compounds have little toxicity to skin and mucous membranes and, thus, have been used widely for their antibacterial effects in a concentration of 0.1%. They are inactive against spores and most viruses. Quats in much higher concentrations than those used in medicine (eg, 5–10%) can be used for sanitizing surfaces.

Action on lipid of bacterial cell membrane

The greatest care is needed in the use of quats because they adsorb to most surfaces with which they come into contact, such as cotton, cork, and even dust. As a result, their concentration may be lowered to a point at which certain bacteria, particularly *Pseudomonas aeruginosa*, can grow in the quat solutions and then cause serious infections. Many instances have been recorded of severe infections resulting from contamination of ophthalmic preparations or of solutions used for treating skin before transcutaneous procedures. It should also be remembered that cationic detergents are totally neutralized by anionic compounds. Thus, the antibacterial effect of quaternary ammonium compounds is inactivated by soap. Because of these problems, quats have been replaced by other antiseptics and disinfectants for most purposes.

"Quats" adsorbed to surfaces may become contaminated with bacteria

Cationic detergents neutralized by soaps

## Phenolics

**Phenol**, one of the first effective disinfectants, was the primary agent employed by Lister in his antiseptic surgical procedure, which preceded the development of aseptic surgery. It is a potent protein denaturant and bactericidal agent. Substitutions in the ring structure of phenol have substantially improved activity and have provided a range of phenols and cresols that are the most effective environmental decontaminants available for use in hospital hygiene. Concern about their release into the environment in hospital waste and sewage has created some pressure to limit their use. This is another of the classic environmental dilemmas of our society: a compound that reduces the risk of disease for one group may raise it for another.

Environmental decontamination with phenols and cresols limits use

Phenolics are less deviated by protein than are most other disinfectants, have a detergent-like effect on the cell membrane, and are often formulated with soaps to increase their cleansing property. They are too toxic to skin and tissues to be used as antiseptics although brief exposures can be tolerated. They are the active ingredient in many mouthwash and sore throat preparations.

Relatively stable to protein

Two diphenyl compounds, hexachlorophene and chlorhexidine, have been extensively used as skin disinfectants. **Hexachlorophene** is primarily bacteriostatic. Incorporated into a soap, it builds up on the surface of skin epithelial cells over 1 to 2 days of use to produce a steady inhibitory effect on skin flora and Gram-positive contaminants, as long as its use is continued. It was a major factor in controlling outbreaks of severe staphylococcal infections in nurseries during the 1950s and 1960s, but cutaneous absorption was found to produce neurotoxic effects in some premature babies. When it was applied in excessive concentrations, similar problems occurred in older children. It is now a prescription drug.

Skin decontamination with hexachlorophene effective for staphylococci

Toxicity of hexachlorophene absorbed through skin limits use

**Chlorhexidine** has replaced hexachlorophene as a routine hand and skin disinfectant and for other topical applications. It has greater bactericidal activity than hexachlorophene without its toxicity but shares with hexachlorophene the ability to bind to the skin and produce a persistent antibacterial effect. It acts by altering membrane permeability of both Gram-positive and -negative bacteria. It is cationic and, thus, its action is neutralized by soaps and anionic detergents.

Chlorhexidine less toxic but binds to skin

## Glutaraldehyde and Formaldehyde

Glutaraldehyde and formaldehyde are alkylating agents highly lethal to essentially all microorganisms. Formaldehyde gas is irritative, allergenic, and unpleasant, properties that limit its use as a solution or gas. Glutaraldehyde is an effective sterilizing agent for appa-

Glutaraldehyde useful for decontamination of equipment

ratus that cannot be heat treated, such as some lensed instruments and equipment for respiratory therapy. Formaldehyde vapor, an effective environmental decontaminant under conditions of high humidity, is sometimes used to decontaminate laboratory rooms that have been accidentally and extensively contaminated with pathogenic bacteria, including those, such as the anthrax bacillus, that form resistant spores. Such rooms are sealed for processing and thoroughly aired before reoccupancy.

## Microwave Disinfection

Microwaves can produce moist heat for disinfection

Another method for disinfection is the use of microwaves in the form of microwave ovens or specially designed units. These systems are not under pressure but can achieve temperatures near boiling if moisture is present. In some situations they are being used as a practical alternative to incineration for disinfection of hospital waste. These procedures cannot be considered sterilization only because the most heat-resistant spores may survive the process.

## CLINICAL APPLICATION

There is some risk of infection in all health care settings. Hospitalized patients are particularly vulnerable and the hospital environment is complex. The proper matching of the principles and procedures described here to general and specialized situations together with aseptic practices can markedly reduce the risks. The building of such systems is generally referred to as infection control and is discussed further in Chapter 72.

## ADDITIONAL READING

Favero MS, Bond WW. Sterilization, disinfection and antisepsis in the hospital. In: Balows A, Hausler WJ Jr, Herrmann KL, Isenberg HD, Shadomy HJ, eds. *Manual of Clinical Microbiology*. 5th ed. Washington, DC: American Society for Microbiology; 1991. A good account of the practical use of disinfectants.

Russell AD, Hugo WB, Ayliffe GAJ. *Disinfection, Preservation, and Sterilization*. 2nd ed. London: Blackwell Scientific; 1992. A good, comprehensive reference source.

Chapter 12

# Epidemiology and Prophylaxis of Infectious Diseases

*W. Lawrence Drew*

Epidemiology, the study of the distribution of determinants of disease and injury in human populations, is a discipline that includes both infectious and noninfectious diseases. Most epidemiologic studies of infectious diseases have concentrated on the factors that influence acquisition and spread, because this knowledge is essential for developing methods of prevention and control. Historically, epidemiologic studies and the application of the knowledge gained from them have been central to the control of the great epidemic diseases, such as cholera, plague, smallpox, yellow fever, and typhus.

An understanding of the principles of epidemiology and the spread of disease is essential to all medical personnel, whether their work is with the individual patient or with the community. Most infections must be evaluated in their epidemiologic setting; for example, has the patient recently traveled to an area of special disease prevalence? Is there a possibility of nosocomial infection from recent hospitalization? What is the risk to the patient's family, schoolmates, and work or social contacts?

Epidemiological questions often central to infectious illness

## SOURCES AND COMMUNICABILITY

Infectious diseases of humans may be caused by exclusively human pathogens, such as the measles virus, by environmental organisms, such as *Legionella pneumophila*, or by organisms that have their primary reservoir in animals, such as the plague bacillus. They can generally be classified as noncommunicable or communicable.

**Noncommunicable infections** are those that are not transmitted from human to human and include (1) infections derived from the patient's normal flora, such as peritonitis after rupture of the appendix; (2) infections caused by the ingestion of preformed toxins, such as botulism; and (3) infections caused by certain organisms found in the environment, such as clostridial gas gangrene. Some zoonotic infections (diseases transmitted from animals to humans), such as rabies and brucellosis, are not transmitted between humans, but others such as plague may be at certain stages. Noncommunicable infections may still occur as common-source outbreaks, such as food poisoning from an enterotoxin-producing *Staphylococcus aureus*-contaminated chicken salad or multiple cases of pneumonia from extensive dissemination of *Legionella* through an air-conditioning system. As these diseases are not transmissible to others, they do not lead to secondary spread.

Noncommunicable infections are indigenous, environmental, and zoonotic

Single-source outbreaks of noncommunicable diseases occur but without secondary spread

Endemic, epidemic, and pandemic spread of communicable diseases is a matter of degree

**Communicable infections** are transmissible from person to person. They can be **endemic,** which implies that the disease is present at a low but fairly constant level, or **epidemic,** which involves a level of infection above that usually found in a community or population. Communicable infections may be widespread in a region and sometimes worldwide with high attack rates, in which case they are termed **pandemic.** A communicable infection requires that an organism be able to leave the body in a form that either is directly infectious to others or is able to become so after development in a suitable environment. An example of direct communicability is the respiratory spread of the influenza virus. In contrast, the malarial parasite requires a developmental cycle in a biting mosquito before another human can be infected.

## INFECTION AND DISEASE

Some infections may be subclinical.

Some infections result in carrier state following disease

Subclinical infections and long incubation periods may obscure epidemic spread

An important consideration in the study of the epidemiology of communicable organisms is the distinction between infection and disease. **Infection** involves multiplication of the organism in or on the host and can be inapparent, for example, during the incubation period. **Disease** represents a clinically apparent response by or injury to the host as a result of infection. With many communicable microorganisms, infection is much more common than disease, and apparently healthy infected individuals play an important role in disease propagation. Inapparent infections are termed **subclinical,** and the individual is sometimes referred to as a **carrier.** The latter term is also applied to situations in which an infectious agent establishes itself as part of a patient's flora or causes low-grade chronic disease after an acute infection. For example, the clinically inapparent presence of *S. aureus* in the anterior nares is termed **carriage,** as is a chronic gallbladder infection with *Salmonella typhi* that can follow an attack of typhoid fever and result in fecal excretion of the organism for years. With some infectious diseases, such as measles, infection is invariably accompanied by clinical manifestations of the disease itself. These manifestations facilitate epidemiologic control, because the existence and extent of infection in a community are readily apparent. Organisms associated with long incubation periods or high frequencies of subclinical infection (eg, HIV or hepatitis B virus) may propagate and spread in a population for long periods before the extent of the problem is recognized. This makes epidemiologic control more difficult.

## INCUBATION PERIOD AND COMMUNICABILITY

Determinants of short and long incubation periods relate to replication rate and other factors

Hepatitis B incubation varies from 7 to 200 days

The **incubation period** is the time between exposure to the organism and appearance of the first symptoms of the disease. Generally, organisms that multiply rapidly and produce local infections, such as gonorrhea and influenza, are associated with short incubation periods (eg, 2–4 days). Diseases such as typhoid fever, which depend on hematogenous spread and multiplication of the organism in distant target organs to produce symptoms, often have longer incubation periods (eg, 10 days to 3 weeks). Some diseases have even more prolonged incubation periods because of slow passage of the infecting organism to the target organ, as in rabies, or slow growth of the organism, as in tuberculosis. Incubation periods for one agent may also vary widely depending on route of acquisition and infecting dose; for example, the incubation period of hepatitis B virus infection may vary from 7 to more than 200 days.

Shedding and communicability vary related to disease and immune response

Communicability of a disease in which the organism is shed in secretions may occur primarily during the incubation period. In other infections the disease course is short but the organisms can be excreted from the host for extended periods. In yet other cases, the symptoms are related to host immune response rather than the organism's action, and thus the disease process may extend far beyond the period in which the etiologic agent can be isolated or spread. Some viruses can integrate into the host genome or survive by replicating very slowly in the presence of an immune response. Such dormancy or latency is exemplified by the herpesviruses, and in each case the organism may emerge long after the original infection and potentially infect others.

The inherent infectivity and virulence of a microorganism are also important determinants of attack rates of disease in a community. In general, organisms of high infectivity spread more easily and those of greater virulence are more likely to cause disease than subclinical infection (see Chapter 10). The infecting dose of an organism also varies with different organisms and thus influences the chance of infection and development of disease.

Infectivity and virulence determine attack rates and infecting dose

## ROUTES OF TRANSMISSION

Various transmissible infections may be acquired from others by direct contact, by aerosol transmission of infectious secretions, or indirectly through contaminated inanimate objects or materials. Some, such as malaria, involve an animate insect vector. These routes of spread are often referred to as **horizontal transmission,** in contrast to **vertical transmission** from mother to fetus. The major horizontal routes of transmission of infectious diseases are summarized in Table 12–1 and discussed next.

Horizontal spread is by aerosol and contact vectors Vertical transmission from mother to fetus

### Respiratory Spread

Many infections are transmitted by the respiratory route, often by aerosolization of respiratory secretions with subsequent inhalation by others. The efficiency of this process depends in part on the extent and method of propulsion of discharges from the mouth and nose, the size of the aerosol droplets, and the resistance of the infectious agent to desiccation and inactivation by ultraviolet light. In still air, a particle 100 μm in diameter requires only seconds to fall the height of a room; a 10-μm particle remains airborne for about 20 minutes, smaller particles even longer. When inhaled, particles with a diameter of 6 μm or greater are usually trapped by the mucosa of the nasal turbinates, whereas particles of 0.6 to 6.0 μm attach to mucus sites at various levels along the upper and lower respiratory tract and may initiate infection. Respiratory secretions are often transferred on hands or inanimate objects

Respiratory aerosols and droplet spread related to particle size

**TABLE 12–1. COMMON ROUTES OF TRANSMISSION[a]**

| Route of Exit | Route of Transmission | Example |
|---|---|---|
| Respiratory | Aerosol droplet inhalation | Influenza virus; tuberculosis |
| | Nose or mouth → hand or object → nose | Common cold (rhinovirus) |
| Salivary | Direct salivary transfer (eg, kissing) | Oral-labial herpes; infectious mononucleosis |
| | Animal bite | Rabies |
| Gastrointestinal | Stool → hand → mouth and/or stool → object→ mouth | Enterovirus infection; hepatitis A |
| | Stool → water or food → mouth | Salmonellosis; shigellosis |
| Skin | Skin discharge → air → respiratory tract | Varicella, poxvirus infection |
| | Skin to skin | Human papilloma virus (warts); syphilis |
| Blood | Transfusion or needle prick | Hepatitis B; cytomegalovirus infection; malaria; AIDS |
| | Insect bite | Malaria; relapsing fever |
| Genital secretions | Urethral or cervical secretions | Gonorrhea; herpes simplex; *Chlamydia* infection |
| | Semen | Cytomegalovirus infection |
| Urine | Urine → hand → catheter | Hospital-acquired urinary tract infection |
| Eye | Conjunctival | Adenovirus |
| Zoonotic | Animal bite | Rabies |
| | Contact with carcasses | Tularemia |
| | Arthropod | Plague; Rocky Mountain spotted fever; Lyme disease |

[a] The examples cited are incomplete, and in some cases more than one route of transmission exists.

Manual and fomitic spread of respiratory infections on hands

(fomites) and may reach the respiratory tract of others in this way. For example, spread of the common cold may involve transfer of infectious secretions from nose to hand by the infected individual, with transfer to others by hand-to-hand contact and then from hand to nose by the unsuspecting victim.

## Salivary Spread

Salivary transmission by kissing or in day-care centers

Some infections, such as herpes simplex and infectious mononucleosis, can be transferred directly by contact with infectious saliva through kissing. Salivary transmission of infectious secretions among children in day-care centers through shared toys and utensils often accounts for the rapid dissemination of agents such as respiratory syncytial virus.

## Fecal–Oral Spread

Direct and indirect contamination of food and water related to hygenic practices

Risk of infection greater in achlorhydric host

Fecal–oral spread involves direct or finger-to-mouth spread, the use of night soil as a fertilizer, or fecal contamination of food or water. Food handlers who are infected with an organism transmissible by this route constitute a special hazard, especially when their personal hygienic practices are inadequate. Some viruses disseminated by the fecal–oral route infect and multiply in cells of the oropharynx, then disseminate to other body sites to cause infection. Commonly, however, organisms that are spread in this way multiply in the intestinal tract and may cause intestinal infections. They must therefore be able to resist the acid in the stomach, the bile, and the gastric and small-intestinal enzymes. Many bacteria and enveloped viruses are rapidly killed by these conditions, but Enterobacteriaceae and unenveloped viral intestinal pathogens are more likely to survive. Even with these organisms, the infecting dose in patients with reduced or absent gastric hydrochloric acid is often much smaller than in those with normal stomach acidity.

## Skin-to-Skin Transfer

Direct and fomitic skin-to-skin spread by unnoticed breaks

Skin-to-skin transfer occurs with a variety of infections in which the skin is the portal of exit. Examples are the spirochete of syphilis (*Treponema pallidum*), strains of group A streptococci that can cause impetigo, and the dermatophyte fungi that cause ringworm and athlete's foot. In most cases, an inapparent break in the epithelium is probably involved in infection. Other diseases may be spread through fomites such as shared towels and inadequately cleansed shower and bath floors. Skin-to-skin transfer usually occurs through abrasions of the epidermis, which may be unnoticed.

## Bloodborne Transmission

Blood-to-blood transmission requires needles or insect vectors

Bloodborne transmission through insect vectors requires a period of multiplication or alteration within an insect vector before the organism can infect another human host; such is the case with the mosquito and the malarial parasite. Direct transmission from human to human through blood has become increasingly important in modern medicine because of the use of blood transfusions and blood products and the increased self-administration of illicit drugs by intravenous or subcutaneous routes, using shared unsterile equipment. Hepatitis B and C viruses as well as HIV are frequently transmitted in this way.

## Genital Transmission

Transmission of genital pathogens occurs between sex partners or to infants at birth

Disease transmission through the genital tract has emerged as one of the most common infectious problems in the latter half of the 20th century and reflects changing social and sexual mores. Spread can be between sexual partners or to the infant at birth. A major factor in these infections has been the persistence, high rates of asymptomatic carriage, and frequency of recurrence of organisms such as *Chlamydia trachomatis*, cytomegalovirus, herpes simplex virus, human papilloma viruses, and *Neisseria gonorrhoeae*.

## Eye-to-Eye Transmission

Infections of the conjunctiva may occur in epidemic or endemic form. Epidemics of adenovirus and *Haemophilus* conjunctivitis may occur in institutions and are highly contagious. The major endemic disease is trachoma, caused by *Chlamydia*, which remains a frequent cause of blindness in developing countries. These diseases may be spread by direct contact or by secretions passed manually or through fomites such as towels.

Direct contact or fomites transmit to eye

## Zoonotic Transmission

**Zoonotic infections** are those spread from animals, where they have their natural reservoir, to humans. Some zoonotic infections, such as rabies contracted from the bite of a rabid animal, are blind-ended in humans. Others may be transferred between humans once the disease is established in a population. Plague, for example, has a natural reservoir in rodents. Human infections contracted from the bites of rodent fleas may produce pneumonia, which may then spread to other humans by the respiratory droplet route.

Zoonotic infections may be blind-ended or further transmitted between humans

## Vertical Transmission

Certain diseases can spread from the mother to the fetus through the placental barrier. This mode of transmission involves organisms such as rubella virus that can be present in the mother's bloodstream and may occur at different stages of pregnancy with different organisms. Another form of transmission from mother to infant occurs by contact during birth with organisms such as group B streptococci which colonize the vagina. Cytomegalovirus can spread by both vertical methods as it may be present in blood or may colonize the cervix. This virus may also be transmitted by breast milk, a third mechanism of vertical transmission.

Vertical transmission may be transplacental or by contact during childbirth

# EPIDEMICS

The characterization of epidemics and their recognition in a community involve several quantitative measures and some specific epidemiologic definitions. **Infectivity,** in epidemiologic terms, equates to attack rate and is measured as the frequency with which an infection is transmitted when there is contact between the agent and a susceptible individual. The **disease index** of an infection can be expressed as the number of persons who develop the disease divided by the total number infected. The **virulence** of an agent can be estimated as the number of fatal or severe cases per the total number of cases. **Incidence,** the number of new cases of a disease within a specified period, is most often described as a rate in which the number of cases is the numerator and the number of people in the population under surveillance is the denominator. **Prevalence,** which can also be described as a rate, is the total number of cases existing in a population at risk at a point in time or during a defined period.

Infectivity, disease index, virulence, incidence, and prevalence expressed as quantitative measures

The prerequisites for propagation of an epidemic from person to person are a sufficient degree of infectivity to allow the organism to spread, sufficient virulence for an increased incidence of disease to become apparent, and sufficient level of susceptibility in the host population to permit transmission and amplification of the infecting organism. Thus, the extent of an epidemic and its degree of severity are determined by complex interactions between parasite and host.

Propagated epidemics have multiple requirements

Host factors such as age, genetic predisposition, and immune status can dramatically influence the manifestations of an infectious disease. Together with differences in infecting dose, these factors are largely responsible for the wide spectrum of disease manifestations that may be seen during an epidemic.

Host factors greatly influence manifestations of disease

The effect of age can be quite dramatic. For example, in an epidemic of measles in an isolated population in 1846, the attack rate for all ages averaged 75%; however, mortality was 90 times higher in children less than 1 year of age (28%) than in those 1 to 40 years of age (0.3%). Conversely, in one outbreak of poliomyelitis, the attack rate of paralytic polio was 4% in children 0 to 4 years of age and 20 to 40% in those 5 to 50 years of age. Sex may

Age, race and sex influence attack rates and severity

be a factor in disease manifestations; for example, the likelihood of becoming a chronic carrier of hepatitis B is twice as high for males as for females.

Prior exposure of a population to an organism may alter immune status and the frequency of acquisition, severity of clinical disease, and duration of an epidemic. For example, measles is highly infectious and attacks most susceptible members of an exposed population. Infection, however, gives solid lifelong immunity. Thus, in unimmunized populations in which the disease was maintained in endemic form, epidemics occurred at about 3-year intervals when a sufficient number of nonimmune hosts had been born to permit rapid transmission between them. When a sufficient immune population was reestablished, epidemic spread was blocked and the disease again became endemic. When immunity is short-lived or incomplete, epidemics can continue for decades if the mode of transmission is unchecked, which accounts for the present epidemic of gonorrhea.

Degree and duration of immunity influence epidemic frequency

Prolonged and extensive exposure to a pathogen during previous generations selects for a higher degree of innate genetic immunity in a population. For example, extensive exposure of Western urbanized populations to tuberculosis during the 18th and 19th centuries conferred a degree of resistance greater than that among the progeny of rural or geographically isolated populations. The disease spread rapidly and in severe form, for example, when it was first encountered by Native Americans. An even more dramatic example concerns the resistance to the most serious form of malaria that is conferred on peoples of West African descent by the sickle-celled trait (see Chapter 52). These instances are clear cases of natural selection, a process that accounts for many differences in racial immunity.

Natural selection influences the susceptibility of a population

Occasionally, an epidemic arises from an organism against which immunity is essentially absent in a population and that is either of enhanced virulence or appears to be of enhanced virulence because of the lack of immunity. When such an organism is highly infectious, the disease it causes may become pandemic and worldwide. A prime example of this situation is the appearance of a new major antigenic variant of influenza A virus against which there is little if any cross-immunity from recent epidemics with other strains. The 1918–1919 pandemic of influenza was responsible for more deaths (about 20 million) than World War I. Subsequent but less serious pandemics have occurred at intervals because of the development of strains of influenza virus with major antigenic shifts (see Chapter 32). Another example, AIDS, illustrates the same principles but also reflects changes in human ecologic and social behavior.

Pandemics of infection occur when immunity is low or absent

Cross-immunity may be lost by antigenic shifts of the organism

A major feature of serious epidemic diseases is their frequent association with poverty, malnutrition, disaster, and war. The association is multifactorial and includes overcrowding, contaminated food and water, an increase in arthropods that parasitize humans, and the reduced immunity that can accompany severe malnutrition or certain types of chronic stress. Overcrowding and understaffing in day-care centers or institutes for the mentally impaired can similarly be associated with epidemics of infections.

Social and ecological factors determine aspects of epidemic diseases

In recent years, increasing attention has been given to hospital (nosocomial) epidemics of infection. The hospital is not immune to the epidemic diseases that occur in the community; however, most nosocomial infections involve opportunistic organisms and result from the close association of infected patients with those who are unusually susceptible because of chronic disease, immunosuppressive therapy, or the use of bladder, intratracheal, or intravascular catheters and tubes. Control depends on the techniques of medical personnel, hospital hygiene, and effective surveillance. This topic is considered in greater detail in Chapter 72.

Nosocomial (hospital-associated) epidemics usually involve opportunistic pathogens

## CONTROL OF EPIDEMICS

The first principle of control is recognition of the existence of an epidemic. This recognition is sometimes immediate because of the high incidence of disease, but often the evidence is obtained from ongoing surveillance activities, such as routine disease reports to health departments and records of school and work absenteeism. The causative agent must be identified and characterized antigenically if more than one serotype exists. Studies to determine route of transmission (eg, food poisoning) must be initiated.

Routine surveillance important for recognition

Measures must then be adopted to control the spread and development of further infection. These methods include (1) blocking the route of transmission if possible (eg, improved food hygiene or arthropod control); (2) identifying, treating, and, if necessary, isolating infected individuals and carriers; (3) raising the level of immunity in the uninfected population by immunization; (4) making selective use of chemoprophylaxis for subjects or populations at particular risk of infection, as in epidemics of meningococcal infection; and (5) correcting conditions such as overcrowding or contaminated water supplies that have led to the epidemic or facilitated transfer.

Methods of control include isolation, treatment, and immunization

## GENERAL PRINCIPLES OF IMMUNIZATION

Immunization is the most effective method of specific individual and community protection against many epidemic diseases. Recent developments in molecular biology and protein chemistry have brought greater sophistication to the identification and purification of specific immunizing antigens and epitopes and to the preparation and purification of specific antibodies for passive protection. Thus, immunization is being applied to a broader range of infections.

Immunization can be active, with stimulation of the body's immune mechanisms through administration of a vaccine, or passive, through administration of plasma or globulin containing preformed antibody to the agent desired. Active immunization with living attenuated organisms generally results in a subclinical or mild illness that duplicates to a limited extent the disease to be prevented. Live vaccines generally provide both local and durable humoral immunity. Killed or subunit vaccines such as influenza vaccine and tetanus toxoid provide immunogenicity without infectivity. They generally involve a larger amount of antigen than live vaccines and must be administered parenterally with two or more spaced injections to elicit a satisfactory secondary response. Immunity usually develops more rapidly with live vaccines, but serious overt disease from the vaccine itself can occur in patients whose immune responses are suppressed. Live attenuated virus vaccines are generally contraindicated in pregnancy because of the risk of infection and damage to developing fetus. Current vaccines and their uses are listed in Appendix 12–1 and Appendix 12–2.

Inactivated vaccines administered parenterally

Nonliving vaccines require more antigen and several inoculations

Live vaccines stimulate broader immunity but carry more risk

Prophylaxis or therapy of some infections can be accomplished or aided by passive immunization. This procedure involves administration of preformed antibody obtained from humans, derived from animals actively immunized to the agent, or produced by hybridoma techniques. Animal antisera induce immune responses to their globulins that result in clearance of the passively transferred antibody within about 10 days and carry the risk of hypersensitivity reactions such as serum sickness and anaphylaxis. Human antibodies are less immunogenic and are detectable in the circulation several weeks after administration. Two types of human antibody preparations are generally available. Immune serum globulin (gamma globulin) is the immunoglobulin G fraction of plasma, from a large group of donors, that contains antibody to many infectious agents. Hyperimmune globulins are purified antibody preparations from the blood of subjects (see Appendix 12–3) with high titers of antibody to a specific disease that have resulted from natural exposure or immunization. Hepatitis B immune globulin, rabies immune globulin, and human tetanus immune globulin are examples of the latter. Details of the use of these globulins can be obtained from the chapters that discuss the diseases in question. Appendix 12–3 lists the diseases in which passive immunization has proved to be useful in preventing acquisition of disease. Passive antibody is most effective when given during the incubation period.

Passive immunization provides preformed antibody

Human antibody preparations less immunogenic

## ADDITIONAL READING

Advisory Committee on Immunization Practices. Recommendations for the use of *Haemophilus* b conjugate vaccines and a combined diphtheria, tetanus, pertussis, and *Haemophilus* b vaccine. *Morb Mortal Wkly Rep.* 1993;42:No. RR-13.

Advisory Committee on Immunization Practices. Prevention and control of influenza: Part I, vaccines. *Morb Mortal Wkly Rep.* 1993;42:No. RR-6.

National Vaccine Advisory Committee. Standards for pediatric immunization practices. *Morb Mortal Wkly Rep.* 1993;42:No. RR-5.

Evans AS, ed. *Viral Infections of Humans: Epidemiology and Control.* 3rd ed. New York: Plenum Press; 1989.

McNeill WH. *Plagues and Peoples.* Garden City, NY: Anchor Press/Doubleday; 1976. This interesting book describes the impact of infectious diseases on the evolution of society and on the rise and fall of civilizations.

APPENDIX 12–1. VACCINES FOR USE IN HUMANS[a]

| Disease | Type of Vaccine | Administration and Frequency | Indications and Comments |
|---|---|---|---|
| Adenovirus | Live attenuated bivalent (types 4 and 7) | Oral once | Used only in military recruits |
| Anthrax | Inactivated bacilli | SC primary series + booster each 6 mo | Laboratory or industrial workers with special exposure |
| Cholera | Inactivated bacilli | SC primary series + booster each 6 mo for long-term residence | For travel to cholera endemic areas; 50% effective in preventing disease; not effective in decreasing transmission |
| Diphtheria, tetanus | Toxoids | IM, childhood series, booster at least every 10 y[b] | Routine use in all persons |
| *Haemophilus influenzae* type B | Purified polysaccharide protein conjugate vaccine | IM three dose primary series followed by booster; fewer doses for older toddlers | Routine use in children 2–59 mo of age or older |
| Hepatitis b | Recombinant | IM, three-dose primary series | Infants and groups at high risk for acquisition of hepatitis B (needle-stick and IV exposure, household contacts of hepatitis B patients, patients requiring large volumes of clotting factors, homosexual men, selected medical and dental personnel, infants of infected mothers) |
| Influenza | Inactivated | IM yearly | Directed at reducing morbidity and mortality in those at risk of complications of influenza (ie, chronic heart and pulmonary disease patients, those over 65) |
| Measles | Live attenuated | SC once[b] | Routine use in all children and susceptible adults (born after 1956, unimmunized) |
| Meningococcus (groups A and C) | Purified capsular polysaccharide | SC once | Military recruits; complement-deficient individuals; control of localized epidemics and adjunct to chemoprophylaxis in household contacts; travelers to epidemic areas |
| Mumps | Live attenuated | SC once[b] | Routine use in children; prevention of orchitis in susceptible seronegative male patients |
| Pertussis | Inactivated bacilli | IM, childhood series combined with diphtheria/tetanus toxoid[b] | Routine use in all children |

| | | | |
|---|---|---|---|
| Plague | Inactivated bacilli | SC, primary series, boosters every 1–2 yr | Agricultural workers in endemic areas; laboratory and field personnel with high exposure risk |
| Pneumococcal infection | Purified multivalent polysaccharide | SC or IM once | Same population as influenza vaccination; also, patients with functional or surgical asplenia, cirrhosis, multiple myeloma, nephrotic syndrome, or AIDS |
| Poliomyelitis | Live attenuated trivalent | Oral, primary series of three doses[b] | Preferred for routine use and during epidemics for those <18 yr. non-ICP |
| | Inactivated trivalent | Booster, once<br>SC primary series | Travel to developing country<br>ICP and their household contacts; unimmunized adults |
| Rabies | Inactivated | Dependent on preexposure vs. postexposure | Exposed individual or workers with rabies virus |
| Rubella | Live attenuated | SC once[b] | Routine use in children and in adult women who are antibody (HI) negative if pregnancy can be prevented for 3 mo after vaccination; routine use in control of outbreaks |
| Tetanus (see Diphtheria, tetanus) | | | |
| Tuberculosis | Live attenuated bacille Calmette–Guérin | SC or intradermally once | Considered for use in tuberculin negative subjects persistently exposed to positive sputum or in endemic areas |
| Typhoid | Oral, attenuated | Four doses repeated every other day; repeat series in 5 years | Travellers to endemic areas |
| Varicella | Live attenuated | IM once | For selected children (especially immunosuppressed) at risk of varicella; selective use in nonpregnant susceptible adults[c] |
| Yellow fever | Live attenuated | SC once every 10 y | For travel to yellow fever-endemic areas |

*Abbreviations:* IM, intramuscularly; SC, subcutaneously; HI, hemagglutination inhibition; ICP, immunocompromised patient

[a] These are vaccines available at the time of writing. Most attenuated vaccines are contraindicated in pregnancy and in immunosuppressed individuals. Up-to-date recommendations and package inserts must be consulted before use.

[b] Recommended schedules are listed in Appendix 12–2.

[c] Not approved in United States as of January 1994.

**APPENDIX 12–2. IMMUNIZATION FOR NORMAL INFANTS, CHILDREN AND ADOLESCENTS**

| Recommended Age | Vaccine |
|---|---|
| 2 mo | DPT-1, OPV-1, Hib-1[a] |
| 4 mo | DPT-2, OPV-2, Hib-2[a] |
| 6 mo | DPT-3, Hib-3[ab] |
| 15 mo | MMR, DPT-4, OPV-3, Hib-4 |
| 4–6 y | DPT-5, OPV-4[c] |
| 14–16 y | Td[c] |

*Note:* These recommendations are based on those of the Immunization Practices Advisory Committee of the Public Health Service. For all products used, the recommendations given in the manufacturers product inserts must be followed.

*Abbreviations:* DPT, diphtheria/pertussis/tetanus vaccine; OPV, oral polio vaccine; MMR, mumps/measles/rubella vaccine; Hib, *Haemophilus influenzae* type b conjugate vaccine; Td, adult diphtheria/tetanus toxoid.

[a] A single vaccine (DPT + Hib) may be substituted for the 2 separate vaccines for children <12–15 mo.

[b] May be given with DPT and OPV.

[c] Repeat every 10 years throughout life.

**APPENDIX 12–3. PASSIVE IMMUNIZATION**

| Disease | Preparation | Route | Comment |
|---|---|---|---|
| Cytomegalovirus | CMV immune globulin | IV | Prevention of CMV in seronegative organ transplant recipients; treatment of CMV pneumonia in bone marrow transplant recipients |
| Diphtheria | Equine antiserum | IM or IV | Dose dependent on extent of pharyngeal membrane and degree of toxicity; has also been used to protect unimmunized household contacts |
| Hepatitis A | Human immune serum globulin | IM | Used in household contacts, those who have eaten food suspected to be contaminated, and travelers to areas of poor hygiene |
| Hepatitis B | Human hepatitis B immune globulin (HBIG) | IM | Prophylaxis for direct parenteral exposure (needle-stick) or mucous membrane contact in susceptible hosts, newborns of HBsAg positive mothers |
| | Human immune serum globulin | | May prevent nonparenteral transmission if it contains antibody to hepatitis B surface antigen; HBIG preferable |
| Measles | Human immune serum globulin | IM | Used in exposed susceptible infants and household contacts, exposed susceptible pregnant women, and immunodeficient hosts |
| Rabies | Human rabies immune globulin | Locally and IM | Possibly used for postexposure prophylaxis |
| Rubella | Human immune serum globulin | IM | Used in exposed susceptible pregnant women who will not consider termination of pregnancy |
| Tetanus | Human tetanus immune globulin | IM | For immediate prophylaxis when potentially contaminated wounds in the unimmunized occur; when given with tetanus toxoid, use different syringes and sites |
| Varicella-Zoster | Human zoster immune globulin | IM | Prevention and amelioration of varicella in exposed susceptible immunosuppressed hosts |

Chapter 13

# Antimicrobics and Chemotherapy of Bacterial and Viral Infections

*James J. Plorde*

One of the major revolutions in medicine has been the introduction of a large range of clinically effective antimicrobial agents over the past half century. Natural materials with some activity against microbes were used in folk medicine in earlier times, such as the bark of the cinchona tree (containing quinine) in the treatment of malaria; however, rational approaches to chemotherapy began with Ehrlich's development of arsenical compounds for the treatment of syphilis early in the century. Many years then elapsed before the next major development, which was the discovery of the therapeutic effectiveness of a sulfonamide (prontosil rubrum) by Domagk in 1935. Penicillin, which had been discovered in 1929 by Fleming, could not be adequately purified at that time; however, this was accomplished later, and it was produced in sufficient quantities for its clinical effectiveness to be demonstrated by Florey and his colleagues in the early 1940s. Since then, numerous new antimicrobial agents have been discovered or developed, and many have found their way into clinical practice. These agents have played an important role in the extraordinary decline in morbidity and mortality from bacterial diseases, particularly in developed countries.

## ANTIBACTERIAL AGENTS

### Major Principles and Definitions

Clinically effective antimicrobial agents all exhibit selective toxicity toward the parasite rather than the host, a characteristic that differentiates them from the disinfectants (see Chapter 11). In most cases, selective toxicity is explained by action on microbial processes or structures that differ from those of mammalian cells. For example, some agents act on bacterial cell wall synthesis, and others on functions of the 70 S bacterial ribosome but not the 80 S eukaryotic ribosome. Some antimicrobial agents, such as penicillin, are essentially nontoxic to the host, unless hypersensitivity has developed. Others, such as the aminoglycosides, have a much lower therapeutic index, which is defined as the ratio of the dose toxic to the host to the effective therapeutic dose; as a result, control of dosage and blood levels must be much more precise.

Selective toxicity exploits differences between microbial and host cells

Therapeutic index a ratio of toxic to therapeutic dose

Some antimicrobial agents, such as the penicillins and aminoglycosides, may be able to kill susceptible microorganisms without the intercession of humoral or cellular immune

Bactericidal activity kills the bacterium

defenses. In the case of bacteria, this process is termed **bactericidal activity.** Other agents, such as the sulfonamides and tetracyclines, reversibly inhibit essential metabolic processes, and metabolism can recommence when their level becomes subinhibitory. This process is termed **bacteriostatic activity,** and the ultimate destruction of an infecting organism depends on host defenses. Analogous terms for antifungal agents are **fungicidal activity** and **fungistatic activity,** respectively.

Bacteriostatic action is reversible

The basic measures of the in vitro activity of an antimicrobial agent against an organism are the **minimum inhibitory concentration** (MIC) and the **minimum lethal concentration** (MLC) or, in the specific case of bacteria, **minimum bactericidal concentration** (MBC). The MIC is the least amount that prevents growth of the organism under standardized conditions; the MLC is the least amount required to kill a predetermined portion of an inoculum (usually 99.9%) in a given time. The procedures for determining MICs and MLCs are considered in greater detail later in this chapter. For most clinically effective antimicrobial agents, the MICs for fully susceptible organisms range from 100 to 0.01 μg/mL or less, and successful therapy usually appears to require levels above the MIC at the site of the infection.

MIC and MLC or MBC are in vitro measures of activity

The pharmacologic characteristics of antimicrobial agents are critical in deciding their selection, their dosage, and the routes and frequency of administration. Among such characteristics are whether they are absorbed from the upper gastrointestinal tract, whether they are excreted and concentrated in active form in the urine, whether they can pass into cells, whether and how rapidly they are metabolized, and the duration of effective antimicrobial levels in blood and tissues. Most agents are bound to some extent to serum albumin, and the protein-bound form is usually unavailable for antimicrobial action. The amount of free to bound antibiotic can be described as an equilibrium constant that varies for different antibiotics. In general, high degrees of binding lead to more prolonged but lower serum levels of active antimicrobial agent after a single dose.

Pharmacologic absorption and distribution determine use and dosage

Protein binding may limit available drug

There are three sources of antimicrobial agents. The true antibiotics are of biological origin and probably play an important part in microbial ecology in the natural environment. Penicillin, for example, is produced by several molds of the genus *Penicillium*, and the prototype cephalosporin antibiotics were derived from other molds. The largest source of naturally occurring antibiotics is the genus *Streptomyces*, the members of which are Gram-positive, branching bacteria found in soils and freshwater sediments. Streptomycin, the tetracyclines, chloramphenicol, erythromycin, and many other antibiotics were discovered by screening large numbers of *Streptomyces* isolates from different parts of the world. A few antibiotics, mostly with low therapeutic indices, are derived from soil bacteria of the genus *Bacillus*, but because of their toxicity are now limited mostly to local application rather than systemic use. Antibiotics are mass produced by techniques derived from the procedures of the fermentation industry.

Antibiotics are derived from other organisms

The true chemotherapeutic agents are chemically synthesized antimicrobial agents. Most of the early chemotherapeutics were discovered among compounds synthesized for other purposes and tested for their therapeutic effectiveness in animals. The sulfonamides, for example, were discovered as a result of routine screening of aniline dyes. More recently, active compounds have been synthesized with structures tailored to be effective inhibitors or competitors of known metabolic pathways. Trimethoprim, which inhibits dihydrofolate reductase, is an excellent example.

Chemotherapeutics are synthetic chemicals

The third source of new antimicrobial agents is molecular manipulation of previously discovered antibiotics or chemotherapeutics to broaden their range and degree of activity against microorganisms or to improve their pharmacologic characteristics. This approach has been the major thrust of developments over the past 20 years, particularly with the antibiotics. Examples include the development of penicillinase-resistant and broad-spectrum penicillins, as well as a large range of aminoglycosides and cephalosporins of increasing activity, spectrum, and resistance to inactivating enzymes.

Molecular manipulation of antibiotics and chemotherapeutics lead to new agents

The distinction between antibiotics and chemotherapeutics has become increasingly irrelevant, because some antibiotics, such as chloramphenicol and aztreonam, are now produced synthetically. The terms continue to be used, but the generic terms **antimicrobic** and **antimicrobial agent** are preferable for both classes of compounds. The term **chemotherapy** is used to describe treatment with antimicrobics or antitumor compounds.

Antimicrobic or antimicrobial agent preferred terms

The range of activity of each antimicrobic is called its **spectrum,** a term used to describe the genera and species against which it has been shown to be active. Spectra overlap, but are usually characteristic for each broad class of antimicrobic. Some antibacterial antimicrobics are known as **narrow-spectrum agents**; for example, benzyl penicillin is highly active against many Gram-positive and Gram-negative cocci, but has little activity against enteric Gram-negative bacilli. Chloramphenicol and tetracycline, on the other hand, are **broad-spectrum agents** that inhibit a wide range of Gram-positive and Gram-negative bacteria, including some obligate intracellular organisms. Spectra relate to the general behavior of a genus or species when the antimicrobic is introduced; resistant strains have since been selected within most species, and thus the spectrum of an antimicrobic often does not indicate or predict the behavior of an individual strain. For example, the spectrum of benzyl penicillin is considered to include *Staphylococcus aureus*, although most strains now are penicillin resistant.

Spectrum of antimicrobics describes the range of activity

Narrow-spectrum agents are restricted

Broad-spectrum agents act against multiple unrelated microbes

Bacterial resistance to antimicrobics may be caused by (1) altered antimicrobic uptake secondary to diminished permeability of the cell envelope or active efflux of the antimicrobic agent; (2) diminished affinity to or absence of a specific antimicrobic target site; (3) ability of the organism to bypass a blocked metabolic pathway; (4) synthesis of a substance that binds antimicrobic and protects its target; and (5) production by the organism of an enzyme that inactivates the antimicrobic. Resistance to an antimicrobic may be innate to all members of a species and involve any of the preceding mechanisms, or strains within a susceptible species may develop resistance. Such acquired resistance can be mutational or derived from another organism by one of the mechanisms of genetic exchange described in Chapter 4. Many resistance genes are grouped on plasmids (R plasmids), which can determine resistance to several different antimicrobics. Some of these genes are present on transposable elements that can move from plasmid to plasmid or between plasmid and chromosome. Resistant or multiresistant strains of many previously susceptible species are now encountered, sometimes as the predominant phenotype. Acquired resistance can involve all of the mechanisms responsible for innate resistance, but most often results from production of antimicrobic inactivating enzymes.

There are multiple mechanisms of bacterial resistance to antimicrobics

Innate resistance is inherent to the microbial species

Acquired resistance is usually by mutation or genetic exchange

R plasmid genes can encode resistance to many antimicrobics

Combinations of different classes of antimicrobics may be synergistic, additive, or antagonistic. A combination is **synergistic** if its effect is greater than the sum of the effects of its components. For example, a penicillin and an aminoglycoside may kill an enterococcus far more effectively than would either acting alone, because inhibition of cell wall synthesis by penicillin allows passage of the highly lethal aminoglycoside to its target in the cell. The effect of an **additive** combination is no greater than the sum of the effects of its components. In an **antagonistic** combination, one antimicrobic, usually that with the least important properties, partially prevents the second from expressing its activity. Antagonism occurs with certain combinations of bacteriostatic antimicrobics with a β-lactam antimicrobic, such as penicillin. Penicillin exerts its bacterial effect only on dividing cells, and inhibition of growth by a bacteriostatic antimicrobic may prevent the lethal activity of penicillin.

Antimicrobic combinations may be synergistic, additive or antagonistic

One particular indication for combined therapy with different classes of antimicrobics is a large population of infecting organisms with a relatively high frequency of mutational resistance. If a lesion contains $10^9$ organisms, and the frequency of resistant mutants to two antimicrobics, A and B, is $10^{-6}$ for each, the chance of relapse by selection of a resistant mutant is high with single therapy. The chance of a double mutant, however, is only $10^{-12}$, and combined therapy usually prevents this development. Pulmonary tuberculosis is an example, and established tuberculosis is always treated with two or more effective antimicrobics to reduce the risk of emergence of resistance.

Use of combinations prevents expression of resistant mutants

Double resistance mutants are extremely rare

These aspects of antimicrobics, chemotherapy, and resistance are now considered in more detail with respect to the modes of action and major groups of antimicrobial agents. Principles are stressed using antimicrobics commonly employed as examples. Details on specific antimicrobic use, dosage, and toxicity should be sought in one of the specialized texts or handbooks written for that purpose.

## Antimicrobics Acting Against Cell Wall Synthesis

Synthesis of the murein sac has been considered in some detail in Chapter 3. It will be recalled that an *N*-acetylmuramic (NAM) acid residue bearing its tetrapeptide with an addi-

Synthetic steps of cell wall synthesis are unique to bacteria

tional terminal D-alanine is first synthesized in the cytoplasm. This is attached to a carrier molecule, bactoprenol, in the cell membrane where *N*-acetylglucosamine (NAG) is added. Finally, the NAM–NAG disaccharide with attached peptide is added to the growing glycan chain of the cell wall, and crosslinks are established by transpeptidation using energy derived from release of the terminal "excess" D-alanine. These processes are described in Chapter 2. They are unique to bacteria and offer targets that have been points of attack of two of the most important groups of antimicrobics, the β-lactams and the glycopeptides (vancomycin and teicoplanin).

## β-Lactam Antimicrobics

Activity of all classes of β-lactams depends on intact β-lactam ring

The β-lactam antimicrobics comprise the penicillins, cephalosporins, carbapenems, and monobactams. The first member of this class of antimicrobics, the penicillins, was derived from molds of the genus *Penicillium.* Penicillin and all subsequent natural, semisynthetic, and synthetic β-lactams share possession of a β-lactam ring that is essential to their antibacterial activity.

Pharmacologic properties, activity, and spectra determined by side chains

The basic structural formulas of each of the four major classes of β-lactams are shown in Figure 13–1. Differences in side chains of the basic molecules influence pharmacologic properties and spectra by determining permeability into the bacterial cell, affinity for enzymes involved in cell wall synthesis, and susceptibility or resistance to inactivation by β-lactamase enzymes.

β-Lactams interfere with transpeptidation reactions in cell wall synthesis

The β-lactam antimicrobics interfere primarily with the transpeptidation reactions that seal the peptide crosslinks between glycan chains. Their activity is probably due to stereochemical similarity to the D-analyl-D-analine end of the pentapeptide. β-Lactams thus prevent the completion of the murein sac in growing cells.

Penicillin binding proteins are targets of β-lactam antimicrobics

PBPs have multiple roles in cell wall synthesis

The target enzymes of the β-lactams occur on the cytoplasmic membrane. They are described as penicillin-binding proteins (PBPs) because they were first detected with penicillin, although many of them bind other β-lactam antimicrobics avidly. Several distinct PBPs occur in any one bacterium, are usually species specific, and vary in their ability to react with different β-lactam antimicrobics. There are also functional differences between PBPs. Some appear to be responsible for forging the peptidoglycan linkages that give an organism its shape, and others are particularly involved in synthesizing the cross-walls that separate newly formed cells. Yet others have no known function. A β-lactam that is active primarily on a PBP that determines shape causes susceptible organisms to round up and swell before lysis occurs. One that acts primarily on cell separation and division can produce long cells with multiple nucleoids that can stretch from one side of a microscopic field to the other.

Bacterial action of β-lactams are usually due to cell lysis

β-Lactam antimicrobics are usually highly bactericidal to susceptible bacteria. Killing involves attenuation and disruption of the developing peptidoglycan "corset," liberation or activation of autolytic enzymes that further disrupt weakened areas of the wall, and finally osmotic lysis from passage of water through the cytoplasmic membrane to the hypertonic

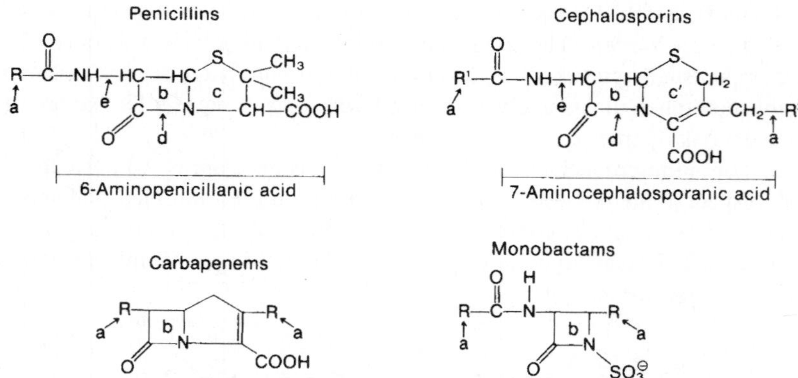


**Figure 13–1.** Basic structure of β-lactam antibiotics. a, Different side chains determine degree of activity, spectrum, pharmacologic properties, resistance to β-lactamases; b, β-lactam ring; c, thiazolidine ring; c′, dihydrothiazine ring; d, site of action of β-lactamases; e, site action of amidase.

interior of the cell. As would be anticipated, cell wall-deficient organisms, such as *Mycoplasma*, are insusceptible to β-lactam antimicrobics, nongrowing cells are not killed, and osmotically stabilized protoplasts remain viable in the presence of the antimicrobic. Mutations that reduce or eliminate the activity of autolytic enzymes result in diminished lysis and killing by β-lactams and can, in effect, change the action of the antimicrobics from bactericidal to bacteriostatic. This phenomenon is termed **tolerance.**

Cell wall-deficient and nongrowing cells not killed by β-lactams

Antimicrobic tolerance related to diminished lysis

Inherent resistance to β-lactam antimicrobics is sometimes due to lack of susceptible PBPs or to failure to traverse outer membrane porin channels of Gram-negative bacteria because of charge, degree of hydrophobicity, or general molecular configuration. In some cases, inherent resistance is due to chromosomally encoded β-lactamases that open the β-lactam ring and inactivate the antimicrobic. Some chromosomal genes encoding β-lactamase production are under repressor control and subject to induction by certain β-lactam antimicrobics. This leads to increased production of β-lactamase, which usually results in resistance to the inducer and to some other β-lactams to which the organism would otherwise be susceptible. Various other chromosomally encoded enzymes with β-lactamase activity are found in very low concentrations in almost all bacterial species, including those highly susceptible to β-lactam antimicrobics. They are believed to be involved in cell wall synthesis and turnover.

Inherent resistance to β-lactams due to lack of PBP target, outer membrane permeability, or β-lactamase

Acquired resistance to β-lactam antimicrobics can be mutational, in which case it usually involves changes in PBPs or alterations in outer membrane proteins and permeability. Because mutations occur at low frequency and are often associated with other effects that are disadvantageous to the cell, strains that are resistant by these mechanisms have tended to evolve slowly. Much more commonly, acquired resistance is due to acquisition of genetic elements encoding β-lactamases. These are often transposable and usually found on plasmids, but may become chromosomal. In nature, they are most frequently acquired by conjugation and sometimes by transduction. Multiple β-lactamases have been described that have different specificities for different antimicrobics. One, the inducible penicillinase of *Staphylococcus aureus*, now predominates among clinical isolates all over the world. Another, termed **TEM,** is encoded in a transposable element and is particularly significant among Gram-negative organisms in mediating resistance to some important β-lactams. It probably originated in Gram-negative rods of the normal intestinal flora, and has transposed to plasmids of a variety of organisms important in human diseases including enteric Gram-negative pathogens, *Haemophilus influenzae*, and *Neisseria gonorrhoeae*. As new β-lactams are developed that are unaffected by most known β-lactamases, genes encoding enzymes with different specificities tend to appear and spread, thus producing further problems of antimicrobic resistance. Recently, point mutations within plasmid or transposon genes encoding TEM and SHV enzymes have led to the appearance of extended-range, broad-spectrum β-lactamases capable of hydrolyzing newer cephalosporins and monobactams.

Mutational resistance due to change in permeability or PBPs

Plasmid-determined β-lactamase resistance is common

Multiple β-lactamases differ in specificity for various β-lactams

Plasmid genes encoding β-lactamases have spread through a wide range of species

Most of the search for new β-lactams has been driven by the need for broader spectra, greater activity, and resistance to commonly occurring β-lactamases. It has, however, also lead to the discovery of β-lactams that inactivate some β-lactamases, but have little or no useful antimicrobic action. Thus, for example, clavulanic acid is a potent inhibitor of some β-lactamases; when used in combination with certain penicillins that are susceptible to these enzymes, it extends their activity to organisms that would otherwise be resistant.

Nonantimicrobic β-lactamase inhibitors useful in combinations

### Penicillins

All penicillins are derivatives of 6-aminopenicillanic acid, the basic structure of which is a β-lactam ring linked to a thiazolidine ring (see Fig 13–1). Side chains of the molecule confer antibacterial activity and determine the pharmacologic properties and spectrum of the penicillin.

6-Aminopenicillanic acid is nucleus

The prototype penicillin is benzyl penicillin (penicillin G), from which earlier semisynthetic penicillins were derived. The action of an enzyme, amidase, breaks the bond between the β-lactam ring and the side chain, allowing replacement with other side chains.

Benzyl penicillin and derivatives differ in side chain

Examples of commonly used penicillins, their side chains, and their major properties are shown in Table 13–1. They can be classified conveniently as narrow-spectrum penicillins, narrow-spectrum penicillins resistant to staphylococcal penicillinase, broad-spectrum penicillins, and extended-spectrum penicillins.

The narrow-spectrum penicillins are active mainly against Gram-positive organisms,

TABLE 13–1. DIFFERENTIAL CHARACTERISTICS OF SOME REPRESENTATIVE PENICILLINS

| Class | Compound | Side Chain | Route of Administration | | Resistance to Staphylococcal β-Lactamase | Activity Against Some Enterobacteriaceae | Activity Against Some Pseudomonas |
|---|---|---|---|---|---|---|---|
| | | | *Parenteral* | *Oral* | | | |
| Narrow spectrum | Benzyl penicillin G | 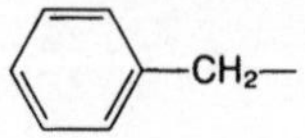 —$CH_2$— | + | – | – | – | – |
| | Penicillin V | —O—$CH_2$— | – | + | – | – | – |
| Narrow spectrum, penicillinase resistant | Nafcillin | 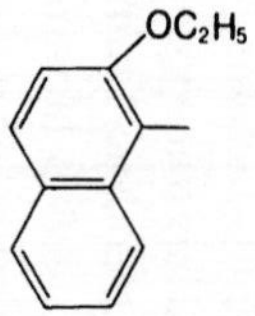 $OC_2H_5$ | + | ± | + | – | – |
| | Dicloxacillin | Cl, Cl, N, O, $CH_3$ | – | + | + | – | – |
| Broader spectrum | Ampicillin | 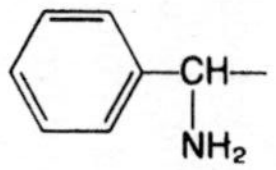 —CH—, $NH_2$ | + | + | – | + | – |
| | Carbenicillin[a] | —CH—, COOH | + | – | – | + | + |
| Extended spectrum | Piperacillin[b] | 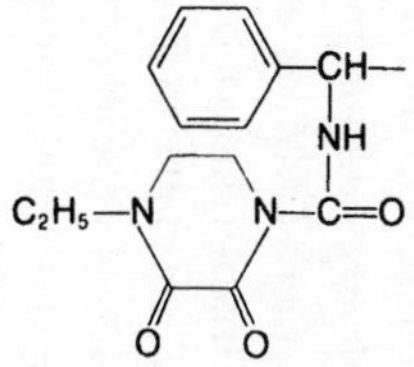 —CH—, NH, $C_2H_5$—N, N—C=O, O, O | + | – | – | + | + |

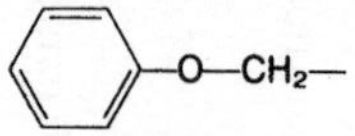

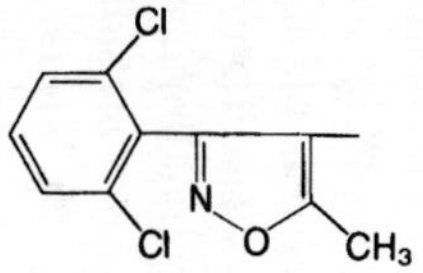

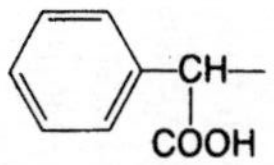

[a] Carbenicillin is used primarily in *Pseudomonas* infections.
[b] Piperacillin combines the advantageous properties of ampicillin and carbenicillin, but with greater activity.

some Gram-negative cocci, and some spirochetes including the spirochete of syphilis. They have little action against most Gram-negative bacilli, because the outer membrane prevents passage of these antibiotics to their sites of action on cell wall synthesis. Penicillin G is the least toxic and least expensive of all the penicillins; however, it is unstable in acid and, when given by mouth, may be largely destroyed by gastric hydrochloric acid. The modification of the molecule in penicillin V confers acid resistance, and this preparation is used orally.

Narrow-spectrum penicillins fail to penetrate envelope of most Gram-negative bacteria

Benzyl penicillin G unstable in acid

The penicillinase-resistant penicillins also have narrow spectra, but are active against β-lactamase-producing *S. aureus*. They appear to owe their insusceptibility to the enzyme to steric hindrance resulting from the configuration of their side chain. They are, however, not resistant to other β-lactamases.

Penicillinase-resistant penicillins active against β-lactamase-producing staphylococci

The broader-spectrum penicillins owe their expanded activity to the ability to traverse the outer membrane of some Gram-negative bacteria. Some, such as ampicillin, have excellent activity against a range of Gram-negative pathogens, but are ineffective against an important opportunistic pathogen, *Pseudomonas aeruginosa*. Others, such as carbenicillin, are active against many *Pseudomonas* strains when given in very high dosage, but are less active than ampicillin against some other Gram-negative organisms. It should be noted that broader-spectrum penicillins are all inactivated by staphylococcal penicillinase.

Broader-spectrum agents add activity against some Gram negatives

Extended-spectrum penicillins, such as the ureido penicillin piperacillin, are more active than ampicillin and carbenicillin against enteric bacteria and *Pseudomonas* and have a wider spectrum of activity against Gram-negative bacteria.

Extended-spectrum penicillins active against *Pseudomonas*

Varying proportions of strains resistant to some or most of the penicillins are now encountered among the majority of species that were originally susceptible. In most cases, resistance involves plasmid-mediated β-lactamases, but PBP mutants of increased resistance have been selected among gonococci and pneumococci and account for resistance of some staphylococci (methicillin-resistant staphylococci) to the penicillinase-resistant penicillins. Likewise, some permeability mutants have occurred among Gram-negative bacteria. Fortunately, some species that were originally susceptible to penicillin, such as the spirochete of syphilis and group A streptococcus, have thus far retained their susceptibility over the more than four decades of use of the antimicrobic.

Mutational and β-lactamase-mediated resistance acquired by many species

Some species (e.g., *Treponema pallidum*) have retained original susceptibility

The penicillins are among the least toxic agents used in therapy. Very high concentrations may be associated with convulsions, but doses on the order of 10 to 30 g a day of benzyl penicillin or carbenicillin are usually well tolerated. Occasionally, hypersensitivity develops to the penicillins. This reaction may manifest as an anaphylactic type of response (which may sometimes be very severe) or more commonly as serum sickness, fever, or skin rash.

Very low toxicity but hypersensitivity occurs

### Cephalosporins

The first cephalosporin antimicrobics were derived from cultures of *Cephalosporium* molds. Some members of the group, obtained from cultures of a genus of branching bacteria related to *Streptomyces*, have been termed the cefamycins. Their basic chemical structure is the same, however, and we refer to all of them as cephalosporins.

The cephalosporins resemble the penicillins in possessing a β-lactam ring, the integrity of which is essential to their activity. They differ from the penicillins in that the five-membered thiazolidine ring is replaced by a six-membered dihydrothiazine ring. The nucleus of the cephalosporins, 7-aminocephalosporanic acid, like 6-aminopenicillanic acid, has little antibacterial action. Activity, pharmacologic properties, and spectra are conferred on the molecule by side chains in the positions indicated in Figure 13–1. The structure of the cephalosporins confers substantial or complete resistance to hydrolysis by staphylococcal penicillinase (β-lactamase), but the β-lactam ring of the earlier members of the group was opened by β-lactamases of many Gram-negative bacilli. The more recently introduced cephalosporins are much more resistant to such enzymatic inactivation, which accounts in part for their wider spectrum.

Cephalosporins have β-Lactam ring

7-aminocephalosporanic acid nucleus differs from penicillin

Resistance to staphylococcal β-lactamase

Later cephalosporins resist many Gram-negative β-lactamases

As with the penicillins, many semisynthetically produced cephalosporins are now available with extended spectra, varying pharmacologic properties, and increased resistance to β-lactamases. New compounds continue to be introduced, while others decline in popularity. It would thus be quite unrewarding for the student to attempt to learn the specific details of those currently available. Even for the clinician, it is best to become familiar with two or three cephalosporins and learn to use them well. For these reasons, we consider only

Number and diversity of cephalosporins is great

a few representatives of the group, ranging from those with the narrowest to those with the broadest spectrum.

First-generation cephalosporins similar to penicillinase-resistant penicillins plus some Gram-negative activity

Six cephalosporins are considered in Table 13–2. Those designated first-generation agents have a more restricted spectrum than those developed subsequently. Their spectrum against Gram-positive organisms resembles that of the penicillinase-resistant penicillins, but they are also active against some Gram-negative bacilli (Appendix 13–1). They continue to have therapeutic value because of their high activity against Gram-positive organisms and because a broader spectrum may be unnecessary and is more likely to predispose the patient to the problem of superinfection. Of the two first-generation cephalosporins listed in Table 13–2, cefazolin must be given parenterally, but the side chains of cephalexin confer acid stability and absorbability and make it an effective oral preparation.

Second-generation cephalosporins extend spectrum to anaerobes and more Gram-negatives

Second-generation cephalosporins are resistant to chromosomally or plasmid-determined β-lactamases of some Gram-negative organisms that inactivate first-generation compounds. For example, cefotetan is active against many strains of *Bacteroides fragilis* and *Serratia* species that are resistant to first-generation compounds and also resists breakdown by the TEM-type β-lactamase.

Third-generation cephalosporins have extended Gram-negative spectrum

Third-generation cephalosporins, such as ceftriaxone, have an even wider spectrum and are active against Gram-negative organisms in extremely low concentrations. They are resistant to many β-lactamases. Both second- and third-generation cephalosporins are generally less active against Gram-positive cocci than those of the first generation or the penicillins.

Resistance mechanisms include permeability and cephalosporinases

As with the penicillins, resistance to cephalosporins may result from failure to permeate the cell membrane, absence of high-affinity PBPs, lack of cell wall, or plasmid- or chromosomally determined β-lactamases. Many chromosomal β-lactamases of Gram-negative bacilli are cephalosporinases, which inactivate all first-generation compounds. The newer agents are progressively more resistant to such attack, as well as to enzymes that are plasmid encoded; however, with their increased use, mutant TEM and SHV plasmid-encoded beta β-lactamases are being encountered that attack even the more resistant third-generation compounds. Chromosomal mutations conferring resistance to several cephalosporins occur at relatively high frequency ($10^{-6}$ to $10^{-8}$), particularly among *Enterobacter*, *Citrobacter*, *Ser-*

**TABLE 13–2. CEPHALOSPORINS**

| Class | Compound | Route of Administration: *Parenteral* | Route of Administration: *Oral* | Spectrum |
|---|---|---|---|---|
| First generation | Cefazolin | + | – | *Staphylococcus aureus* (penicillinase producing and nonproducing) and streptococci (other than enterococci); *Escherichia coli; Klebsiella* species; *Proteus mirabilis* |
| | Cephalexin | – | + | |
| Second generation[a] | Cefuroxime | + | – | First-generation spectrum moderately expanded to include additional Gram-negative species, including *Haemophilus* |
| | Cefotetan | + | – | Similar to cefuroxime, plus *Proteus* and many Gram-negative anaerobes |
| Third generation[a] | Ceftriaxone | + | – | Expanded spectrum against enteric and other Gram-negative rods. |
| | Ceftazidime | + | – | High activity against *Haemophilus influenzae* and *Neisseria gonorrhoeae*, including β-lactamase-producing strains; active against *Pseudomonas aeruginosa* and many Gram-negative anaerobes |

[a] Second- and third-generation cephalosporins have less activity than first-generation agents against Gram-positive organisms. Each agent has specific advantages in activity against particular organisms.

*ratia*, and *Pseudomonas* species. Resistance results from mutational derepression of a chromosomally encoded cephalosporinase.

The cephalosporins now in use are of low toxicity and can be given in large doses for complex infections. Hypersensitivity may develop, but cross-sensitivity to the penicillins is unusual.

Hypersensitivity may not cross with penicillins

### Carbapenems

Like the penicillins, carbapenems have a β-lactam ring fused with a second five-membered ring; their name (carbapen-) derives from the substitution of a carbon atom for the sulfur atom of the thiazolidine ring of the penicillins (see Fig 13–1). Thienamycin, the parent compound of this category of β-lactam antibiotics, was derived from a species of *Streptomyces*, but is not in use clinically because it is chemically unstable. The only carbapenem currently available in the United States, imipenem, is a stable semisynthetic amidine derivative. Imipenem is rapidly hydrolyzed by a renal tubular dehydropeptidase and is, therefore, coadministered with an inhibitor of this enzyme (cilastatin), which greatly improves its urine levels and other pharmacokinetic characteristics.

Imipenem is administered with inhibitor of renal dehydropeptidase

The mode of action of the carbapenems is similar to that of other β-lactams. They readily penetrate bacterial cells, including Gram-negative bacilli, and the conformation of their side chains renders them highly resistant to β-lactamases of staphylococci and most Gram-negative bacilli except *Xanthomonas maltophilia* and *Pseudomonas cepacia*. Accordingly, carbapenems have the broadest spectrum of all β-lactam antibiotics. They are active against streptococci, more active than cephalosporins against staphylococci, highly active against both β-lactamase-positive and -negative strains of gonococci and *H. influenzae*, as active as third-generation cephalosporins against Gram-negative rods, and effective against obligate anaerobes. Carbapenems are potent inducers of chromosomal β-lactamases of Gram-negative bacilli, even though they are unaffected by the enzymes. Combinations of carbapenems with other β-lactams may thus render the latter inactive.

Carbapenems are highly resistent to most β-lactamases

Very wide spectrum of activity

Strains of *P. aeruginosa* frequently develop mutational resistance to imipenem during the course of therapy, probably because of mutational loss of an outer membrane porin leading to impaired penetration. No cross-resistance has been demonstrated with other β-lactam agents. Adverse reactions are uncommon and similar to those of the other β-lactams: cross-hypersensitivity to the penicillins can occur.

*Pseudomonas aeruginosa* may develop resistance during therapy

### Monobactams

Monobactams are naturally occurring substances produced by a variety of soil bacteria. Aztreonam, the first monobactam licensed in the United States, is a natural product of *Chromobacterium violaceum*, but the commercial preparation is produced synthetically.

As their name suggests, monobactams are monocyclic compounds (see Fig 13–1), a feature that distinguishes them from the other β-lactams. A sulfonic acid group, instead of a fused ring, serves to activate the β-lactam ring. Side chains identical to those found in third-generation cephalosporins impart stability and enhanced activity against Gram-negative bacilli, including *P. aeruginosa*. The mode of action is similar to that of other β-lactam agents, but the spectrum of aztreonam is limited to aerobic and facultatively anaerobic Gram-negative bacteria including Enterobacteriaceae, *P. aeruginosa*, *Haemophilus*, and *Neisseria*.

Monocyclic β-lactams action similar to other β-lactams

Monobactams have poor affinity for the PBPs of Gram-positive organisms and anaerobes and thus little activity against them. They are highly resistant to hydrolysis by most plasmid- and chromosomally mediated β-lactamases of Gram-negative bacilli and do not induce production of chromosomally encoded enzymes, suggesting they can be used effectively in combination with other β-lactams. Emergence of resistant bacteria has been uncommon, although both chromosomally mediated resistance and plasmid-determined β-lactamases with activity against monobactams have now been encountered. Cross-resistance with other antimicrobial agents is rare. Untoward effects have been similar to those of other β-lactam antimicrobial agents; although hypersensitivity reactions, including anaphylaxis, have been reported, there appears to be little cross-sensitivity with penicillins and cephalosporins. Anaerobic superinfections and major distortions of the bowel flora are less common with aztreonam therapy than with other broad-spectrum β-lactam antimicrobics, presumably because aztreonam does not produce a general suppression of gut anaerobes.

Little activity against Gram-positive organisms and anaerobes

Resistant to action of most β-lactamases

Bowel superinfections uncommon with aztreonam

**Suicide inhibitors of β-lactamases**

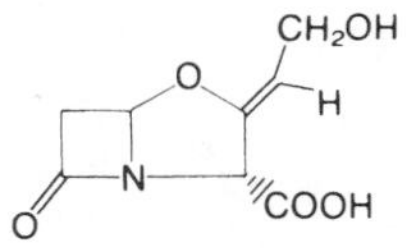

Clavulanic acid

Combinations with some penicillins extend their spectra

Little or no activity against cephalosporinases

β-LACTAMASE INHIBITORS

A number of β-lactams with little or no antimicrobic activity are capable of binding irreversibly to β-lactamase enzymes and, in the process, rendering them inactive. Two such compounds, clavulanic acid (a clavam) and sulbactam (a penicillanic acid sulfone), are referred to as suicide inhibitors, because they must first be hydrolyzed by a β-lactamase before becoming effective inactivators of the enzyme. Both are highly effective against staphylococcal penicillinases and TEM-type broad-spectrum β-lactamases; their capacity to inhibit cephalosporinases is significantly less. Combinations of one of these inhibitors with an appropriate β-lactam antimicrobic protects the therapeutic agent from destruction by many β-lactamases and significantly enhances its spectrum. Three such combinations are now available in the United States: amoxicillin/clavulanate, ticarcillin/clavulanate, and ampicillin/sulbactam. They all expand the spectrum of their contained penicillin to one roughly approximating that of the second-generation cephalosporins. Bacteria producing chromosomally encoded inducible cephalosporinases are not susceptible to the combinations. Whether these three combinations offer therapeutic or economic advantages compared with the β-lactamase-stable antibiotics now available remains to be determined.

Agents of choice for susceptible infections due to bactericidal activity and low toxicity

CLINICAL USE

The β-lactam antibiotics are usually the drugs of choice for infections by susceptible organisms because of their very high therapeutic index and bactericidal action. They have also proved of great value in the prophylaxis of many infections. They are excreted by the kidney and achieve very high urinary levels. Penicillins reach the cerebrospinal fluid when the meninges are inflamed and are used in the treatment of meningitis due to susceptible organisms. First- and most second-generation cephalosporins show poor penetration even with inflammation and are not appropriate for the treatment of meningitis. In contrast, the third-generation cephalosporins, carbapenems and monobactams, penetrate much better, and their marked activity makes them agents of choice in the treatment of meningitis caused by some Gram-negative organisms.

### Glycopeptide Antimicrobics

Bactericidal activity against Gram-positives

Used against β-lactam resistant strains

Resistance although rare, can occur

Two agents, vancomycin and teicoplanin, fall into this group. Each of these antimicrobics inhibits the use of lipid-linked cell wall intermediates in the assembly of the linear peptidoglycan molecule. Both agents are primarily bactericidal and active against Gram-positive organisms. They are particularly useful against strains of *S. aureus* and coagulase-negative staphylococci that are resistant to the penicillinase-resistant penicillins and cephalosporins. They are also useful in the treatment of penicillin-resistant enterococcal endocarditis when used in combination with an aminoglycoside. Neither agent is absorbed by mouth, although both have been used orally to treat *Clostridium difficile* infections of the bowel (see Chapter 18). Their main use has been against multiresistant Gram-positive infections and infections involving prosthetic devices. Vancomycin is administered intravenously because it is toxic to tissues on local injection. Teicoplanin can also be administered intramuscularly.

Initially, it appeared that resistance to these agents did not occur or was very rare. It has now been shown that mutational resistance in one species of coagulase-negative staphylococci can occur during therapy, and plasmid-encoded resistance has been increasingly encountered in enterococci. These agents have been of great value when held in reserve for use in infections that are not responsive to β-lactam antimicrobics.

## Antimicrobics Acting on the Outer and Cytoplasmic Membranes: The Polymyxins

Activity against *P. aeruginosa*

A number of polypeptide antimicrobics are produced by bacteria of the genus *Bacillus*, which are aerobic, Gram-positive, spore-forming rods living primarily in soil. All the polypeptide antimicrobics are relatively toxic, but two, polymyxin B and polymyxin E (colistin), were used parenterally in the past largely because of activity against *P. aeruginosa* and other Gram-negative rods that were resistant to the antimicrobics then available.

The polymyxins have a cationic detergent-like effect. They bind to the cell membranes of susceptible Gram-negative organisms and alter their permeability, resulting in loss of essential cytoplasmic components and bacterial death. They react to a lesser extent with cell membranes of the host, resulting in nephrotoxicity and neurotoxicity. These agents are now essentially limited to topical applications and have the advantage that resistance to them rarely develops.

Detergentlike effect on cell membranes

## Inhibitors of Protein Synthesis at the Ribosomal Level

### Aminoglycoside–Aminocyclitol Antibiotics

The aminoglycoside–aminocyclitol antibiotics are a group of bactericidal agents characterized by combinations of six-membered aminocyclitol rings with varying side chains that determine their spectra and degrees of resistance to inactivating enzymes. The structure of tobramycin is shown in the margin. Streptomycin and other earlier members of the group were produced from species of *Streptomyces.* The newer members are semisynthetic derivatives.

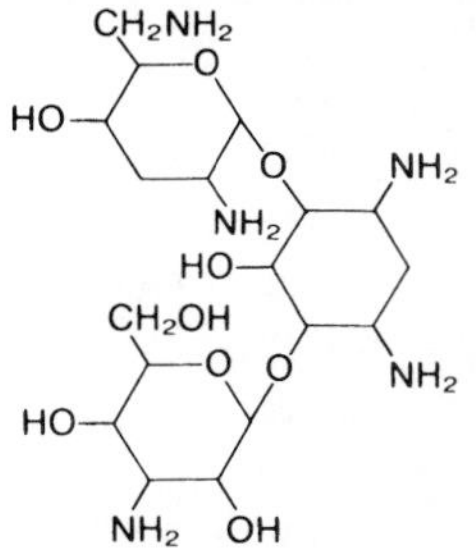

**Family of bactericidal agents**



Tobramycin

The most important and commonly used members of the group are listed in Table 13–3, together with some key properties. Streptomycin is now rarely used, except in combination therapy for tuberculosis or in combination with a β-lactam for treatment of bacterial endocarditis, because high-level and stable resistant mutants are frequently selected during therapy. Similarly, kanamycin use has declined in relationship to the newer agents. Neomycin, the most toxic aminoglycoside, is used as an oral preparation to reduce the facultative flora of the large intestine before certain types of intestinal surgery. It is very poorly absorbed, and most of its activity is expressed in the bowel. Gentamicin, tobramycin, amikacin, and netilmicin have extended spectra that include activity against many strains of *P. aeruginosa.* Of these, amikacin is the most resistant to aminoglycoside-inactivating enzymes and may thus act on some gentamicin- and tobramycin-resistant strains.

Susceptibility to inactivating enzyme varies

Streptomycin inhibits protein synthesis by combining with the bacterial ribosomal protein designated S12 of the 30 S ribosomal subunit. With the newer and more active aminoglycosides, a similar process involves other binding sites on both 30 S and 50 S subunits, resulting in a broader spectrum of activity that includes many streptomycin-resistant strains. In sufficient concentrations, aminoglycosides bind to the ribosome irreversibly, block initiation complexes, and prevent elongation of polypeptide chains, resulting in a rapid bactericidal effect. Lower concentrations lead to distortion of the site of attachment of messenger (m)RNA, misreading of the message, and failure to produce the correct proteins with dramatic effects on growth and bacterial structure.

Irreversible inhibition of protein synthesis at ribosomal level

The aminoglycosides are actively transported into the bacterial cell by a mechanism that involves oxidative phosphorylation. Thus, they have little or no activity against strict anaerobes or facultative organisms that metabolize only fermentatively (eg, streptococci). It appears highly probable that aminoglycoside activity against facultative organisms is similarly reduced in vivo when the oxidation–reduction potential is low.

Actively transported into cells by oxidative phospory-lation

Inactive under anaerobic conditions

Eukaryotic ribosomes are resistant to aminoglycosides, and the antimicrobics are not actively transported into eukaryotic cells. These properties account for their selective toxicity and also explain their ineffectiveness against intracellular bacteria such as *Rickettsia* and *Chlamydia*.

**TABLE 13–3. CHARACTERISTICS OF COMMONLY USED AMINOGLYCOSIDES**

| Compound | Single-Step High Mutational Resistance | Anti-Pseudomonas Activity | Susceptibility to Aminoglycoside-Inactivating Enzymes[a] |
|---|---|---|---|
| Streptomycin | + | – | +++ |
| Neomycin | + | – | +++ |
| Kanamycin | ± | – | ++ |
| Gentamicin | – | + | + |
| Tobramycin | – | + | + |
| Amikacin | – | + | ± |

[a] Number of plus signs indicates degree of susceptibility to enzymatic attack.

Broad spectra other than against anaerobes

The newer aminoglycosides, gentamicin, tobramycin, amikacin, and netilmicin, have a broad spectrum of bactericidal action against many aerobic and facultative Gram-positive and Gram-negative rods, including *P. aeruginosa*. Their detailed spectrum is given in Appendix 13–1. It merits restressing that all anaerobes are resistant to their action and that they have little activity against streptococci, except when cell penetrability is increased by simultaneous action of a β-lactam antibiotic.

Mutational resistance limited by multiple active sites

High-level mutational resistance to streptomycin can occur in a single step because of its single target protein. With more than one molecular target, mutational resistance to the newer aminoglycosides is much less common and of lower level. When it does occur, it usually involves permeability changes across the outer membrane, thus leading to increased resistance to all aminoglycosides.

Plasmid-determined enzymatic resistance by multiple mechanisms

Newer compounds increasingly resistant to enzymatic inactivation

The most common cause of bacterial resistance involves production of one or more of a range of enzymes that can acetylate, adenylate, or phosphorylate various critical groups on the aminoglycoside molecule. This mechanism abrogates or greatly reduces antibacterial activity. Production of these enzymes is determined by transposable genes that are usually borne by plasmids. Aminoglycosides have been successively developed with fewer sites susceptible to such inactivation, and amikacin and netilmicin are currently among the most resistant. In many hospitals, plasmids encoding resistance to gentamicin and tobramycin have been selected and have spread to a number of Gram-negative pathogens under the pressure of antimicrobic use. Nevertheless, these antimicrobics have retained a broad range of clinical usefulness.

Toxic to auditory and vestibular functions of eighth cranial nerve

Blood level monitoring needed

All of the aminoglycoside antimicrobics are toxic to varying degrees to the vestibular and auditory branches of the eighth cranial nerve. Kanamycin and amikacin affect primarily hearing, whereas streptomycin and gentamicin are most toxic to vestibular function. The damage can lead to complete and irreversible loss of hearing and balance. These agents may also be toxic to the kidneys. Toxicity to the eighth cranial nerve greatly limits dosage, and even the most recent aminoglycosides have a very low therapeutic index for infections with *P. aeruginosa*. For example, the maximum safe blood level for gentamicin is approximately 9 μg/mL, whereas its MIC for many strains of *P. aeruginosa* is 2 to 4 μg/mL. Monitoring blood levels during therapy is often essential to ensure adequate, yet nontoxic dosage, especially when renal impairment diminishes excretion of the antimicrobic. The mechanism of toxicity appears to involve concentration of the antimicrobic in the inner ear fluids and destruction of the critical sensory cells mediating hearing and balance.

Limited disruption of normal flora

Synergistic activity with β-lactam antimicrobics

The clinical value of the aminoglycosides resides in their rapid bactericidal effect, their broad spectrum, the slow development of resistance to the agents now most often used, and their action against *Pseudomonas* strains that resist many other antimicrobics. They cause fewer disturbances of the normal flora than most other broad-spectrum antimicrobics, probably because of their lack of activity against the predominantly anaerobic flora of the bowel, and because they are only used parenterally for systemic infections. The β-lactam antibiotics often act synergistically with the aminoglycosides, probably because they facilitate aminoglycoside penetration into the bacterial cell. This effect has been exploited in treatment of bacterial endocarditis using combinations of penicillins and aminoglycosides and in treatment of severe *P. aeruginosa* infections using piperacillin or a related analog and one of the aminoglycosides. Synergism has been demonstrated by in vitro bactericidal studies and in clinical trials. Unexpectedly, it has been found that piperacillin and other extended-spectrum penicillins can slowly inactivate gentamicin in solution. Therefore, these agents are never mixed in the same intravenous bottle.

The aminoglycosides are often used in combination with a β-lactam antibiotic in the initial treatment of life-threatening infections of unknown etiology until the results of cultures are available to allow more specific therapy. Their use has, however, declined with the advent of β-lactams of increasing activity, spectrum, and resistance to β-lactamases.

Orally absorbed broad spectrum agents

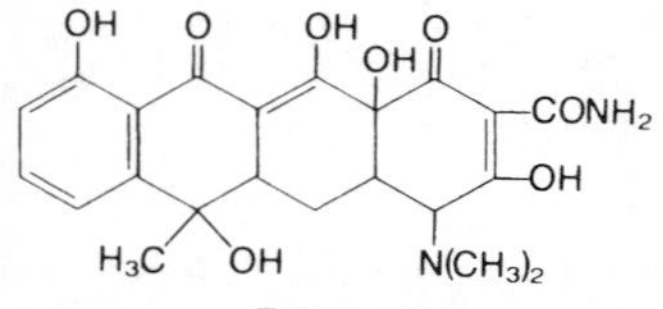

OH O OH OH O CONH$_2$ OH $H_3C$ OH $N(CH_3)_2$

Tetracycline

## Tetracyclines

The tetracyclines are a group of antimicrobics of which the prototype, chlortetracycline, was derived from a species of *Streptomyces*. The newest agents are produced semisynthetically. All are absorbed orally and have similar and broad spectra (see Appendix 13–1), with relatively inconsequential differences in ranges of activity. Acquired resistance to one generally confers resistance to all. Chemically, the tetracyclines are polycyclic compounds that differ from each other in their side groups.

Two classes of compounds are now in common use: tetracycline, which produces relatively short therapeutic levels after single doses and is about 65% protein bound, and longer-acting tetracyclines, which are more highly protein bound but are better absorbed and give higher and more prolonged blood levels. In general, they also have a slightly expanded spectrum. Minocycline and doxycycline are examples of longer-acting agents.

Longer-acting tetracyclines in more general use

Like the aminoglycosides, the tetracyclines are inhibitors of protein synthesis. They are taken into the cell by an energy-dependent process, bind to the 30 S subunit of the ribosome, and block attachment of aminoacyl transfer (t)RNA to the mRNA–ribosome complex. Unlike the aminoglycosides, their effect is reversed on dilution; thus, they are bacteriostatic rather than bactericidal.

Reversible inhibition of protein synthesis: bacteriostatic activity

The tetracyclines are broad-spectrum agents with a range of activity that encompasses most common pathogenic species, including Gram-positive and -negative rods and cocci and both aerobes and anaerobes. They are active against cell wall-deficient organisms, such as *Mycoplasma* and spheroplasts, and against some obligate intracellular bacteria, including members of the genera *Rickettsia* and *Chlamydia*. There are a few minor differences in spectrum between members of the group. For example, doxycycline has some activity against tetracycline-resistant anaerobic Gram-negative rods of the genus *Bacteroides*, and minocycline has greater activity than tetracycline against meningococci and *Nocardia*.

Active against obligate intracellular bacteria

Tetracycline resistance, whether innate, mutational, or plasmid determined, involves energy-dependent efflux of the antimicrobic from the cell or synthesis of a protein that binds antimicrobic and protects the ribosomes. Inactivating enzymes do not appear to play a role. Resistant strains of most pathogenic species are now common and have been selected by the extensive use of these antimicrobics.

Resistance involves efflux from cell or protein binding

The tetracyclines are chelated by divalent cations, and their absorption and activity are reduced. Thus, they should not be taken with dairy products or many antacid preparations. Tetracyclines are excreted in the bile and urine in active form.

Chelated by dairy products and antacids

The tetracyclines have a strong affinity for developing bone and teeth, to which they give a yellowish color, and are avoided in children up to 8 years of age. Common complications of tetracycline therapy are gastrointestinal disturbance due to alteration of the normal flora and superinfection with tetracycline-resistant organisms and vaginal or oral candidiasis (thrush) due to the opportunistic yeast *Candida albicans*.

Discolor developing teeth

Because of their broad spectrum, the tetracyclines have been used extensively in the treatment of polymicrobial infections or infections of unknown etiology derived from the respiratory or gastrointestinal tracts. They have been widely used in the treatment of otitis media and sinusitis, because the most common etiologic agents are usually susceptible. In many cases, however, they have been used in the treatment of viral infections, against which they are quite inactive.

Tetracyclines are agents of choice in the treatment of infections caused by the obligate intracellular parasites *Rickettsia* and *Chlamydia* and by *Mycoplasma*. They have been used as alternates to penicillin in the treatment of syphilis and gonorrhea, although many strains of gonococci are now resistant. They were used in the past as primary agents in the treatment of infections caused by intestinal anaerobes, but many are now resistant. Probably no group of antimicrobics has been more overprescribed and, thus, has contributed significantly to the overall problem of resistance.

## Chloramphenicol

Chloramphenicol is a broad-spectrum, orally adsorbed antimicrobic originally derived from a culture of *Streptomyces*. Its relatively simple structure allowed its chemical synthesis, and it has since been produced commercially in this way.

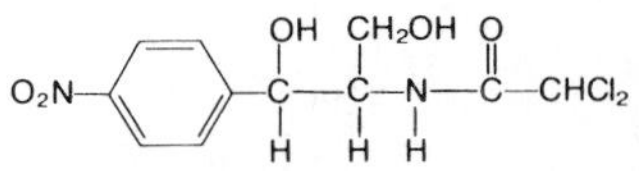

Chloramphenicol

Chloramphenicol acts at the level of the 50 S ribosomal subunit by inhibiting peptidyl transferase and thus prevents protein synthesis. Its action is reversed by dilution, and it is thus bacteriostatic. It has little effect on eukaryotic ribosomes, which explains its selective toxicity. Chloramphenicol is a broad-spectrum antibiotic that, like tetracycline, has a wide range of activity against both aerobic and anaerobic species (see Appendix 13–1). It permeates readily into mammalian cells and is active against *Rickettsia* and *Chlamydia*. It diffuses readily across the blood–brain barrier and attains excellent levels in the cerebrospinal fluid. Its use is restricted, however, by its occasional severe toxicity.

Bacteriostatic protein synthesis inhibitor

Good permeability across blood–brain barrier

Resistance by plasmid-encoded chloramphenicol acetylase

Acquired resistance to chloramphenicol is usually determined by plasmid genes encoding production of the enzyme chloramphenicol acetyltransferase. This enzyme acetylates and inactivates the antimicrobic. It is of interest that chloramphenicol resistance is much less common than tetracycline resistance, which probably reflects the less frequent use of chloramphenicol because of its toxicity.

Metabolized in liver, urine levels low

Chloramphenicol is readily adsorbed from the upper gastrointestinal tract. It is conjugated in the liver to the glucuronide form, which has no antimicrobial activity. Little of the dose is excreted in the bile or urine. Unlike those of most antimicrobics, urine levels of chloramphenicol are low, and it is not useful in urinary tract infections.

Bone marrow hypoplasia is dose related and reversible

Aplastic anemia and agranulocytosis rare but irreversible

Neonatal gray syndrome related to hepatic immaturity

High and prolonged doses of chloramphenicol result in some inhibition of blood-forming cells in the bone marrow (marrow hypoplasia). This inhibition is reversed on cessation of therapy and probably results from the action of the antimicrobic on host mitochondrial ribosomes. Occasionally, and probably by a different mechanism, progressive bone marrow aplasia with aplastic anemia and agranulocytosis develops even after low dosages and it is often fatal. The development of this complication in about 1 in 50,000 patients has restricted the use of chloramphenicol to a limited number of highly specific indications. Chloramphenicol may also produce **gray syndrome** in the neonate, with abdominal, circulatory, and respiratory dysfunction. This syndrome, which can be fatal, results when excessive levels of active antibiotic accumulate because of failure of the infant liver to conjugate chloramphenicol to the glucuronide. Use of the drug is avoided in infants less than 1 month of age.

Chloramphenicol is now largely restricted to treatment of severe infections for which its spectrum and diffusibility make it particularly valuable. These infections include typhoid fever, ampicillin-resistant *H. influenzae* meningitis, meningitis due to pyogenic cocci when the penicillins are contraindicated, intraabdominal anaerobic Gram-negative infections, and some cases of cerebral abscess. It is also an alternative to tetracycline in the treatment of *Rickettsia* infections. As with the tetracyclines, it is now much less used because of the availability of new β-lactams with equivalent spectra.

## Macrolide and Lincosamide Antibiotics

The first agents in these groups, erythromycin and lincomycin, are derived from different species of *Streptomyces*. Erythromycin is still the most commonly used macrolide, but two recently introduced macrolides, azithromycin and clarithromycin, significantly expand the spectrum of this group of antimicrobic agents. The lincosamides, lincomycin and clindamycin (7-chlorolincomycin), are chemically unrelated to the macrolides but have similar modes of action and spectra and are thus considered with them.

Protein synthesis inhibitors with predominantly bacteriostatic effect

Macrolides and lincosamides both act on protein synthesis at the ribosomal level by binding to the 50 S subunit and blocking the translocation reaction. The effect on sensitive bacteria is primarily bacteriostatic, but a higher proportion of the population is killed than is the case with chloramphenicol. These agents are concentrated within phagocytes and other cells, and are effective against some intracellular pathogens.

Spectrum of erythromycin similar to penicillin

Erythromycin has a spectrum of activity that is close to that of benzyl penicillin, but also includes penicillinase-producing *S. aureus*, *Legionella pneumophila*, *Mycoplasma pneumoniae*, *Campylobacter jejuni*, *Chlamydia pneumoniae*, and *Chlamydia trachomatis*. Lincomycin has a generally similar spectrum. Clindamycin, a more active compound, is highly effective against many Gram-negative and Gram-positive anaerobic bacteria (see Appendix 13–1).

Mutational and plasmid-determined resistance involves permeability or ribosomal mechanisms

Mutational and plasmid-determined resistance occurs against both groups of antimicrobics. The former sometimes develops during therapy and may decrease permeability or affect the ribosomes so that the antimicrobics are not bound. Plasmid-determined resistance involves methylation of ribosomal RNA, which is induced by erythromycin and prevents its binding. Interestingly, induction with erythromycin leads to clindamycin resistance, although the reverse is unusual.

Oral and intravenous preparations of both erythromycin and the lincosamides are available. Both classes of antimicrobics are eliminated by the liver, in the bile, and, to a much lesser extent, through the kidney.

Erythromycin in the estolate form can cause a reversible hepatitis, but is otherwise of low toxicity. Clindamycin can also be mildly hepatotoxic, but the most serious complication of clindamycin treatment is pseudomembranous enterocolitis as a result of inhibition of most of the anaerobic flora of the bowel and overgrowth by the clindamycin-resistant *Clostridium difficile*, which elaborates both a cytotoxin and enterotoxin. These toxins are discussed in more detail in Chapter 18.

Low toxicity except for clindamycin-associated pseudomembranous enterocolitis

Erythromycin is a drug of choice in treating Legionnaires' disease and, in the event treatment is needed, *Campylobacter* intestinal infections. It is effective in some *Chlamydia* and *Mycoplasma* infections. Clindamycin has displaced lincomycin in therapy, and its major role is in treating serious anaerobic Gram-negative infections.

The two recently introduced macrolides, azithromycin and clarithromycin, are active against all organisms inhibited by erythromycin; Gram-positive cocci resistant to the older agent are resistant to the new drugs as well. Azithromycin, however, is four to eight times more active than erythromycin against *H. influenzae*, and both agents inhibit *Moraxella catarrhalis*, *M. pneumoniae*, *Legionella* species, and *Chlamydia* species at lower concentrations than erythromycin. Most interesting, however, is their efficacy against unusual pathogens. Both are active against the agent of Lyme disease as well as the rapidly growing mycobacteria. Moreover, clarithromycin inhibits *Mycobacterium avium* at concentrations readily achieved in pulmonary macrophages, whereas azithromycin demonstrates activity against the protozoan parasite *Toxoplasma gondii*. These two microorganisms are responsible for difficult-to-treat superinfections in patients with acquired immunodeficiency syndrome (AIDS).

Newer macrolides have higher activity against same organisms

Added spectrum includes Mycobacteria, Lyme spirochete, and protozoa

Both azithromycin and clarithromycin are taken orally, producing less gastric distress than erythromycin. Moreover, they are better absorbed from the gastrointestinal tract and reach significantly higher tissue and intracellular concentrations. Food decreases the bioavailability of azithromycin, requiring each dose be taken on an empty stomach. Its extremely long serum half-life (68 hours), however, permits once-a-day dosing.

## Inhibitors of Nucleic Acid Synthesis and Replication: The Quinolones

The quinolones (Fig 13–2) have a nucleus of two fused six-membered rings and are produced synthetically. The first antimicrobic of this class was nalidixic acid, which had limited clinical value because therapeutic levels were attained only in the urine, and high-level, single-step mutational resistance developed rapidly. More recently, a series of fluoroquinolones have been developed that give excellent levels of bactericidal activity against a wide range of organisms, have low protein binding, can be administered orally, and are much less prone to the development of resistance.

Broad-spectrum bactericidal activity of fluoroquinolones

The fluoroquinolones differ from nalidixic acid in the presence of fluorine and piper-

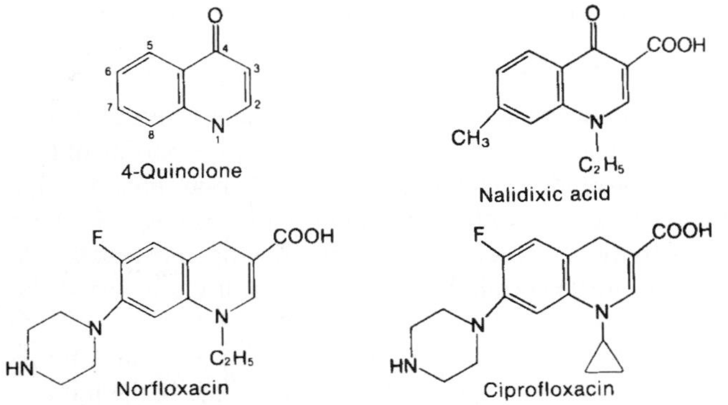

**Figure 13–2.** Examples of structures of quinolones and fluoroquinolones.

Fluorine atom enhances Gram-negative activity and adds Gram-positive spectrum

azine substitutes at the 6- and 7-positions, respectively. Fluorine enhances activity against Gram-negative organisms and adds activity against Gram-positive organisms. Piperazine improves tissue concentrations and provides activity against *P. aeruginosa*. Four fluoroquinolones—norfloxacin, ciprofloxacin, ofloxacin, and lomefloxacin—have been approved for use in the United States at the time of writing; the formulas for the first two are shown in Figure 13–2 with that of nalidixic acid.

Inhibit DNA gyrase

Like nalidixic acid, the primary target of the fluoroquinolones appears to be bacterial DNA gyrase, which is the enzyme responsible for supercoiling, nicking, and sealing bacterial DNA. Four genes encode four subunits of the enzymes, only one of which is the target of nalidixic acid. This explains the occurrence of high-level, single-step mutations to resistance to this agent. It appears that the fluoroquinolones have more than one target on the enzyme, which greatly reduces the chance of mutational resistance. Resistant strains can, however, be selected in vitro. A significant minority of hospital-acquired isolates of *S. aureus*, *P. aeruginosa*, *Proteus*, and *Serratia* are now resistant to ciprofloxacin; most appear to be permeability mutants. Neither enzymatic inactivation of fluoroquinolones nor plasmid-mediated resistance has been observed.

Most resistant strains are permeability mutants

Wide spectrum includes *P. aeruginosa,* little or no activity against anaerobes

The fluoroquinolones are highly active and bactericidal against a wide range of aerobes and facultative anaerobes; however, streptococci and *Mycoplasma* are only marginally susceptible, and anaerobes are generally resistant. Ofloxacin demonstrates significant activity against *Chlamydia*, whereas ciprofloxacin is particularly useful against *P. aeruginosa*.

Oral administration and excellent pharmacologic properties

In addition to their broad spectrum, fluoroquinolones possess a number of favorable pharmacologic properties. These include oral administration, low protein binding, good distribution to all body compartments, penetration of phagocytes, and a prolonged serum half-life that allows once- or twice-a-day dosing. Blood levels with accepted dosage are lower than those achieved with most antimicrobics, but this is offset by much lower MICs against most susceptible organisms. Norfloxacin, ciprofloxacin, and lomefloxacin are excreted by hepatic and renal routes, resulting in high drug concentrations in the bile and urine; ofloxacin is excreted primarily by the kidney.

Adverse effects with the fluoroquinolones are relatively uncommon with recommended dosage. These antimicrobics concentrate in and damage cartilage of young animals and consequently are not recommended for use in children and in pregnant or nursing women.

## Metabolic Inhibitors (Folate Inhibitors)

Many bacteria must synthesize folate; mammalian cells use dietary folate

The use of metabolic inhibitors as antimicrobics must exploit pathways that are present in microorganisms, but not in the host. The major successes in this field have been with agents that interfere with synthesis of folic acid by bacteria, because mammalian cells are unable to accomplish this feat and use preformed folate from dietary sources.

Folic acid is derived from *para*-aminobenzoic acid (PABA), glutamate, and a pteridine unit. In its reduced form it is an essential coenzyme for the transport of one-carbon compounds in the synthesis of purines, thymidine, some amino acids, and, thus, indirectly of nucleic acids and proteins. The major inhibitors of the folate pathway are the sulfonamides, trimethoprim, *para*-aminosalicylic acid, and the sulfones. The latter two are of significance only in mycobacterial infections and are considered in Chapter 27.

$NH_2$ $NH_2$

$SO_2NHR$ $COOH$

Sulfonamides p-Aminobenzoic acid

### SULFONAMIDES

Shortly after Domagk demonstrated the chemotherapeutic effectiveness of Prontosil Rubrum in 1935, the Trefouels in Paris showed that the active portion of the molecule was *para*-aminobenzenesulfonamide, which was termed **sulfanilamide.** Subsequently, numerous compounds were synthesized with substitutions of the amide group. These compounds provided increased activity and special pharmacologic properties, such as higher or more prolonged blood levels, greater solubility in urine, or failure to be absorbed from the intestinal tract.

Competitive inhibitors or PABA metabolism

Sulfonamides are structural analogs of PABA and compete with it for the enzyme (dihydropteroate synthetase) that combines PABA and pteridine in the initial stage of folate synthesis. Differences in the activity of the various sulfonamides largely reflect their ability to compete with PABA for this enzyme system. The effect of sulfonamides is exclusively bacteriostatic, and addition of PABA to a medium that contains them neutralizes the inhibitory effect and allows growth to resume.

Sulfonamides are bacteriostatic

Originally, the more active sulfonamides had a very broad spectrum that included pathogenic streptococci, pneumococci, a number of enteric Gram-negative rods (especially *Escherichia coli*), gonococci, meningococci, and *Chlamydia*. They also had some activity against pathogenic staphylococci and anaerobes. Unfortunately, resistance developed and spread quickly, and their activity is now unpredictable without laboratory tests for measuring susceptibility.

Spectrum is broad but limited by mutational and plasmid-determined resistance

Both mutational resistance and R-plasmid-mediated resistance are common in susceptible species. Resistance encoded in R plasmids usually involves decreased permeability to sulfonamides. Mutational resistance can involve decreased affinity for sulfonamides of the enzyme handling PABA, decreased permeability, or occasionally enhanced PABA production.

Sulfonamides are well absorbed by the oral route, except those specifically designed to act only within the intestinal tract. They penetrate readily into host cells and across the blood–brain barrier. They are excreted in the urine, predominantly in active form, and very high urine levels are achieved.

Oral absorption distribution good

Most toxic effects of the sulfonamides are hypersensitivity phenomena. They include fever, rashes, a serum sickness-like syndrome, and a rare, but highly lethal, bullous skin reaction known as the Stevens–Johnson syndrome. Occasionally, bone marrow depression occurs, which may progress to agranulocytosis or aplastic anemia.

Sulfonamides, alone or combined with trimethoprim, are still among the agents of choice for treatment of uncomplicated primary urinary tract infections, because most strains of *E. coli* encountered in the community have retained their susceptibility. Sulfonamides are also used in the treatment of some *Chlamydia* infections, in prophylaxis of meningococcal infections during epidemics caused by susceptible strains, and in the treatment of *Nocardia* infections (see Chapter 28). They have little or no activity in abscesses or markedly purulent exudates, because disintegrating inflammatory cells provide many of the end products of folate activity that, like PABA, can neutralize the effects of sulfonamides. They have limited clinical value compared with the more powerful antibiotics, but their range of utility is considerably extended when combined with trimethoprim.

Indicated for urinary tract infections

### TRIMETHOPRIM

Trimethoprim is a synthetic structural analog of the pteridine portion of the folic acid molecule. It competitively inhibits the activity of bacterial dihydrofolate reductase, which catalyzes the conversion of folate to its reduced active coenzyme form. Trimethoprim has little activity against the mammalian enzyme. As would be expected, this effect is not neutralized by PABA, but can be reversed by end products of essential reactions for which tetrahydrofolate serves as a coenzyme, particularly by thymidine. Trimethoprim is primarily bacteriostatic. When combined with a sulfonamide, the sequential blockade of the pathway leading to production of tetrahydrofolate often results in synergistic bacteriostatic or bactericidal effects. This quality is exploited in therapeutic preparations combining both agents in concentrations designed to give optimum synergy in vivo.

Competitive inhibitor of bacterial dihydrofolate reductase

Synergism and bactericidal effects result from combination with sulfonamides

Trimethoprim inhibits a considerable range of Gram-positive and Gram-negative facultative bacteria (see Appendix 13–1), including those causing enteric and urinary tract infections. It is also active against some eukaryotic pathogens, including the malarial parasite and *Pneumocystis carinii* (see Chapter 50).

Acquired resistance can be mutational or plasmid mediated. The latter involves production of large amounts of a plasmid-encoded tetrahydrofolate reductase for which trimethoprim has a lower affinity.

Mutational and plasmid-determined resistance related to new dihydrofolate reductase

Trimethoprim is readily absorbed by mouth and is excreted in the urine, yielding very high levels. Combinations with sulfonamides have a range of toxic effects similar to that of the sulfonamides themselves. The most important potential side effect of trimethoprim is folate deficiency. Despite its poor affinity for mammalian dihydrofolate reductase, those on the verge of folate deficiency may become deficient during trimethoprim therapy. For this reason, trimethoprim is avoided in the newborn and during pregnancy.

The trimethoprim–sulfonamide combination is widely and effectively used in the treatment of many urinary tract infections and in the treatment of otitis media and sinusitis (partly because of activity against *H. influenzae*), prostatitis, typhoid fever, and bacillary dysentery. It is the agent of choice in the treatment of *P. carinii* pneumonia.

The major characteristics of the antimicrobics just discussed are summarized in Table 13–4.

## Other Clinically Valuable Antibacterial Agents

Several other effective antimicrobics are in use for special types of infections such as tuberculosis, urinary tract infections, and anaerobic infections. It is beyond the scope and intent of this book to provide comprehensive coverage of all available agents, if only because the field is rapidly changing. Table 13–5 lists a number of the commonly used agents that are not discussed herein, together with their more important properties and uses.

## Laboratory Tests in Chemotherapy

Laboratory tests involve both the infecting organism and the antimicrobic

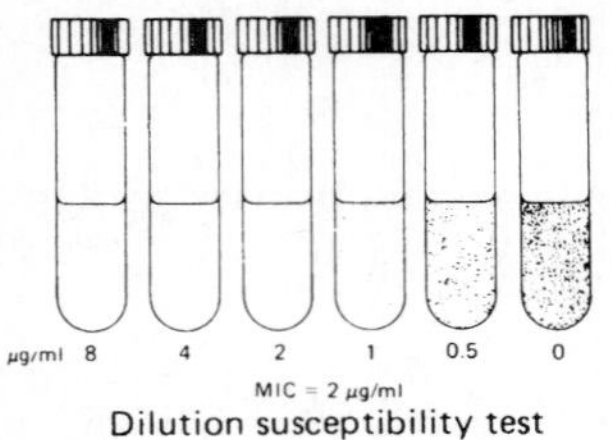

Dilution susceptibility test

The discovery of the great majority of effective antimicrobics and the characterization of their spectra were based on in vitro tests in the laboratory, and similar tests have become increasingly important in clinical work. Susceptibility tests to determine the responsiveness of individual strains of a species are often needed when resistance has become common through widespread use of the antimicrobic. Tests to determine bactericidal activity are sometimes used because infections in immunocompromised patients may be controlled by agents or combinations that will kill the infecting strain only in the absence of host defense factors. Measurements of levels of antimicrobics in blood or other fluids have become routine with agents such as the aminoglycosides for which the toxic and therapeutic levels are relatively close. It is therefore important to understand the principles underlying these tests.

### Susceptibility Tests

Susceptibility methods test the organism against varying concentrations of the antimicrobic

Antimicrobic susceptibility tests, used to determine the inhibitory activity of an antimicrobic against a particular strain, are divided into two broad classes: **dilution tests** and **diffusion tests.** Dilution susceptibility tests are the most direct. In a typical manual dilution test, twofold dilutions of the antimicrobic are prepared in broth in test tubes or microdilution wells to span a clinically significant range of concentrations. A control tube without antimicrobial is included. Equal volumes of broth containing $10^5$ to $10^6$ bacteria to be tested are then added, thus diluting the original antimicrobic concentration in half. The tubes are incubated overnight and examined for turbidity from bacterial growth. The least amount of antimicrobic to prevent any visible growth is taken as the minimum inhibitory concentration (MIC) of the organism.

Automated procedures can determine MICs rapidly

Automated instruments are now available that measure bacterial growth turbidimetrically or fluorometrically and indirectly determine MICs to individual antimicrobial agents by comparing the differences in the growth of the organism in control and antimicrobic-containing compartments. Results are based on computer-analyzed algorithms and are usually available within 4 to 6 hours.

Results of susceptibility test procedures are influenced by a variety of methodologic factors; however, reference procedures and standard control strains of defined performance have allowed the different procedures to give reasonably comparable results. With certain defined exceptions, results of automated early-read procedures correlate well with those of overnight dilution tests. In most clinical situations, successful treatment requires that the MIC of an antimicrobic for an organism should be substantially below the level achieved at the site of infection.

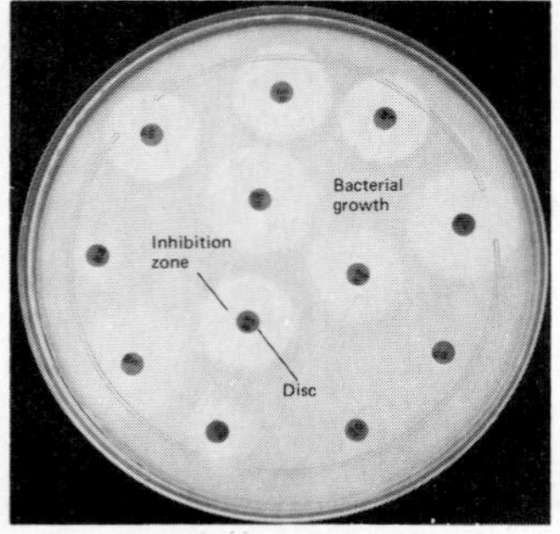

Diffusion test

Disk diffusion susceptibility tests are less direct, but are simple, economic, and flexible for routine use. A standardized inoculum of the organism to be tested is seeded onto the surface of an agar plate, and filter paper disks containing defined amounts of antimicrobics are applied. The plates are then incubated overnight. The antimicrobic diffuses from each disk into the medium at a rate dependent on its chemical and physical characteristics. Zones of inhibition of growth of the organism develop, the diameter of which is determined by the susceptibility (MIC) of the organism, its growth rate, and the diffusibility

**TABLE 13–4. SUMMARY OF ACTIVITY OF SOME ANTIBACTERIAL ANTIMICROBICS**

| Agent | Mode of Action | Basis of Selective Toxicity | Major Mechanisms of Acquired Resistance[a] | Spectrum[a] | Effect |
|---|---|---|---|---|---|
| **Cell Wall-Active Compounds** | | | | | |
| β-Lactams (penicillins, cephalosporins, etc) | Inhibit final transpeptidation reaction in crosslinking peptidoglycan (third stage of murein synthesis) | Absence of peptidoglycan in mammalian cells | β-Lactamase production (P, M); permeability alteration (M); alteration of penicillin-binding proteins (M) | G+,G– | Cidal |
| Vancomycin | Inhibits use of lipid-linked intermediate (second stage of murein synthesis) | Absence of peptidoglycan in mammalian cells | Very rare (M, P) | G+ | Cidal |
| Cycloserine | Structural analog of D-analine; inhibits alanine racemase, preventing formation of pentapeptide (first stage of murein synthesis) | Absence of peptidoglycan in mammalian cells | ? | G+,G–, primarily mycobacteria | Cidal |
| **Outer and Cytoplasmic Membrane-Active Compounds** | | | | | |
| Polymyxins | Cationic surfactants bind to and disrupt outer and cytoplasmic membranes | Lower toxicity to mammalian cell membranes | None | G– | Cidal |
| **Inhibitors of Protein Synthesis at Ribosomal Level** | | | | | |
| Streptomycin | Binds to 30 S subunit; causes misreading and irreversible inhibition of protein synthesis | Differences between bacterial (70 S) and mammalian (80 S) ribosomes | Ribosomal and permeability alterations (M); antibiotic-modifying enzymes (P) | G+,G– | Cidal |
| Other aminoglycosides | Similar to streptomycin but other targets on 30 S and 50 S subunits | Differences between bacterial (70 S) and mammalian (80 S) ribosomes | Ribosomal and permeability alterations (M); antibiotic-modifying enzymes (P) | G+,G– | Cidal |
| Tetracyclines | Reversibly bind to 30 S subunit, inhibit binding of aminoacyl tRNA | Differences between bacterial (70 S) and mammalian (80 S) ribosomes | Permeability and uptake change (P) | G+,G– | Static |
| Chloramphenicol | μReversibly binds to 50 S subunit; inhibits peptidyl transferase and peptide bond formation | Differences between bacterial (70 S) and mammalian (80 S) ribosomes | Antibiotic-modifying enzyme (P) | G+,G– | Static |
| Erythromycin and clindamycin | Bind to 50 S subunit; inhibit peptidyl transferase and translocation reactions | Differences between bacterial (70 S) and mammalian (80 S) ribosomes | Inducible methylation of ribosomal RNA (P); alteration of 50 S binding site (M) | G+ (G– and G+ anaerobes in case of clindamycin) | Static in most cases |
| **Nucleic Acid Synthesis and Replication** | | | | | |
| Quinolones (derivatives of nalidixic acid) | Inhibit DNA gyrase and thus replication | Analogous mammalian enzymes insensitive | Target alteration (M) | G–,G+ | Cidal |
| Rifampin | Inhibits DNA-dependent RNA polymerase (transcription) | Mammalian enzyme insensitive | Target alteration (M) | G+ and mycobacteria | Cidal |
| **Metabolic Inhibitory** | | | | | |
| Sulfonamides | Competitive inhibitors of enzyme handling PABA in folate synthesis pathway | Mammalian cells require preformed folate | Altered enzyme with poor affinity for sulfas (P, M); decreased permeability (P, M) | G+,G– | Static |
| Trimethoprim | Competitive inhibitor of dihydrofolate reductase | Mammalian enzyme essentially unaffected | Altered enzyme with poor affinity for trimethoprim (P) | G+,G– | Static |

*Abbreviations:* P, usually plasmid or transposon coded; M, mutational; G+, Gram-positive; G–, Gram-negative; PABA, para-Aminobenzoic acid.

[a] Not all species in these classes are inhibited by an agent.

TABLE 13–5. SOME OTHER ANTIBACTERIAL ANTIMICROBICS

| Compound | Route of Administration | | Mechanism | Major Spectrum | Clinical Usage | Special Properties |
|---|---|---|---|---|---|---|
| | Parenteral | Oral | | | | |
| Nitrofurantoin | – | + | ? | Enteric Gram-negative rods and enterococci | Urinary tract infections | Absent blood levels |
| Spectinomycin | + | – | Protein synthesis inhibition | Gonococcus | Penicillin-resistant gonorrhea | Unique aminoglycoside |
| Rifampin | – | + | Blocks initiation of transcription | Gram-positive bacteria, *Neisseria*, and mycobacteria | Tuberculosis, meningococcal carriage | High mutation rate to resistance |
| *para*-Aminosalicylic acid | – | + | PABA antagonist | Mycobacteria | Tuberculosis | Gastrointestinal disturbances |
| Isoniazid | – | + | ? Inhibition of lipid synthesis | Mycobacteria | Tuberculosis | Neurotoxicity and nephrotoxicity |
| Ethambutol | – | + | ? | Mycobacteria | Tuberculosis | Visual disturbances |
| Sulfones | – | + | PABA antagonists | *Mycobacterium leprae;* some protozoa | Leprosy | Anemia; hypersensitivity reactions |
| Metronidazole | – | + | Interference with anaerobic metabolism | Anaerobic Gram-negative rods; some protozoa | Anaerobic infections | ? Teratogenic |

*Abbreviations:* PABA, *para*-Aminobenzoic acid; ?, Mechanisms yet to be fully determined.

of the antimicrobic. For common pathogenic bacteria such as the Enterobacteriaceae, *Pseudomonas*, staphylococci, and enterococci, differences in growth rate are relatively unimportant, and there is an inverse linear relationship between log MIC of such organisms and zone diameter. Thus, semiquantitative susceptibilities can be determined by a standardized procedure. The National Committee for Clinical Laboratory Standards (Kirby–Bauer) method used in the United States is such a standardized diffusion procedure. The diameters of the zones of inhibition obtained with the various antibiotics are measured and converted to "sensitive," "moderately sensitive," and "resistant" categories by reference to a table. **Sensitive** implies that the organism is readily inhibited by the concentration of antibiotic attainable in the blood (or urine, in the case of those agents active only in the urinary tract) with doses appropriate for treatment of uncomplicated systemic infections caused by the infecting organism. **Resistant** implies that the organism is not inhibited by normally attainable levels. Organisms in the moderately sensitive (intermediate) range should be specially studied if therapy with that agent is to be used. The categories were developed by comparisons of zone diameter, MIC, and blood level data and from studies on the distribution of zone diameters (susceptibilities) of many species of known clinical responsiveness.

Diffusion zone sizes inversely related to MIC

Interpretive categories of susceptibility relate to relation of MIC to achievable blood/urine levels

Intermediate results may require further study

Resistance and sensitivity are not always absolute. For example, relatively nontoxic antimicrobial agents, such as the penicillins and cephalosporins, can be administered in massive doses and may thereby inhibit some pathogens that would normally be considered resistant in vitro. Furthermore, in urinary infections, urine levels of some antimicrobics may be very high, and organisms that are seemingly resistant in vitro may be eliminated. When such therapy is considered, dilution tests are often needed for guidance. Diffusion tests with slow-growing organisms and with very poorly diffusing antimicrobics such as the polymyxins must be interpreted with caution. Resistance is significant, but sensitivity may need checking by a dilution test if systemic infections are to be treated. Obviously, diffusion tests do not measure bactericidal effects.

Susceptibility categories and results are not absolute

Recently, a commercially developed quantitative diffusion susceptibility test has been introduced that permits determination of direct MIC values of the nonfastidious Gram-negative and Gram-positive aerobic bacteria, as well as the anaerobes and *Haemophilus* species. This "E test" is inoculated in the same manner as the disk diffusion test; however, thin plastic antimicrobic strips (5 × 50 mm), rather than filter paper disks, are placed on the inoculated agar surface. Each strip contains an exponential antimicrobic gradient along its length; the top side of the strip is marked with a MIC reading scale in μg/mL. After incubation, bacterial growth outlines an elliptic zone of inhibition centered along the strip. The MIC is read directly from the strip at the point where the edge of the zone intersects the strip. The procedure combines the simplicity and flexibility of the disk diffusion test with the quantitative results of dilution tests. The results are reproducible and correlate well with those obtained by doubling dilution and disk diffusion methods.

E tests allow determination of MIC by diffusion procedure

## Tests of Bactericidal Activity

Broth dilution tests can be adapted to determine the bactericidal or bacteriostatic effects of the antimicrobic on the organism tested. The number of viable organisms in the inoculum is measured, and samples are removed at intervals from tubes containing antimicrobic for viable counts (see Chapter 3). Such counts can indicate the rate of killing if precautions are taken to ensure that the entire inoculum is exposed to antimicrobic and that antimicrobic carried over to the counting medium is either sufficiently diluted or neutralized to prevent any inhibition on the agar plate. A more commonly used procedure is simple measurement of the minimum bactericidal concentration (MBC), which is usually defined as the least amount of antimicrobic needed to kill 99.9% of an inoculum under standardized conditions after overnight incubation. Unfortunately, this measurement is subject to a series of technical problems that make it considerably less valuable than the more complex study of the rate of killing.

Determining rate of killing by antimicrobics quantitates bactericidal effect

MBC is a measure of killing in overnight test

## Limits of Sensitivity Tests

In selecting therapy, the results of laboratory tests cannot be taken alone, but must be considered with information about the clinical pharmacology of the agent, the cause of the disease, the site of infection, and the pathology of the lesion. All of these factors must be taken into account in selecting the appropriate antimicrobic from those to which the organism has

Other factors influence effectiveness and selection of antimicrobics been reported as sensitive. Obviously, if the agent cannot reach the site of infection, it will be ineffective. For example, the agent must reach the subarachnoid space and cerebrospinal fluid in the case of meningitis. Similarly, therapy may be ineffective for an infection that has resulted in abscess formation unless the abscess is surgically drained. In some instances (eg, bacterial endocarditis and agranulocytosis), it is necessary to use an agent that is bactericidal, and a routine susceptibility test does not indicate this property. Previous clinical experience is also critical. In typhoid fever, for instance, chloramphenicol is effective and aminoglycosides are not, even though the typhoid bacillus may be sensitive to both in vitro. This finding appears to result from the failure of aminoglycosides to achieve adequate concentrations inside infected cells.

In vitro tests must be validated by clinical experience

### Antimicrobic Assays

Chemical and immunoassays replacing microbiologic methods

Levels of antimicrobics in blood and body fluids may be measured biologically, but, physical, chemical, and immunologic techniques, such as high-pressure liquid chromatography and immunoassays, are increasingly being used. Most bioassays use diffusion techniques in which inhibition of a standard assay strain by test samples is compared with that of standards of known concentration. When biologic assays are used it is important for the laboratory to know whether more than one antimicrobic is being used to treat a patient, so that steps are taken to ensure that only the activity of the agent under consideration is being measured.

### Other Tests

Tests of serum activity against infecting strain expressed as a dilution

Sometimes it is desirable to determine directly the effectiveness of antimicrobic levels in the patient's serum against the infecting organism. Dilutions of the patient's serum can be made in normal serum and equal amounts of broth containing $10^5$/mL of the infecting organism added. After incubation, the inhibitory activity and the lethal activity are measured as in MIC and MBC tests and expressed according to effective dilutions of the patient's serum. Tests of the activity of combinations of antimicrobial agents are sometimes important. These tests are made by inoculating the infecting organism into broth containing clinically relevant amounts of the antibiotics being studied, both alone and in combination. The tubes are incubated and quantitative counts made at intervals. This approach indicates whether the effects of the combinations are synergistic, additive, or antagonistic.

## Selection and Administration of Antibacterial Antimicrobics

This topic is largely beyond the scope of the book, but a few principles merit stressing. Most bacterial infections are now potentially curable by chemotherapy alone or as an adjunct to surgical or other treatment, but the plethora of antimicrobics available to the physician makes the selection of the most appropriate agent(s) a particular challenge. Ideally the cause of the infection and its susceptibility to relevant antimicrobics would be known before treatment is initiated. This may be possible in subacute or chronic infections or in localized infections in which delay will not jeopardize the patient. In most cases of serious infection, however, the time required to obtain these data is unacceptable and a decision must be made as to which agents to use pending more specific information. The factors involved in this decision include the following:

Treatment must often begin empirically

1. Clinical signs and tests that indicate the most probable infection and infectious agent(s): In some cases these may be diagnostic, for example, when the clinical picture and cerebrospinal fluid cytology indicate bacterial meningitis and the direct Gram smear shows an organism resembling a meningococcus. In other cases they are less specific, as when a computed tomographic scan indicates an abscess derived from the colon suggesting an infection with aerobes and anaerobes derived from the intestinal flora. In yet other cases a very wide range of etiologic possibilities may exist, for example, when clinical findings suggest the development of bacteremia in a patient with agranulocytosis.
2. Previous experience from the literature as to the effectiveness of particular agents against the range of etiologic possibilities. For example, penicillin may be expected to be effective in the case of group A streptococcal cellulitis, whereas antimicro-

Site of infection evaluated by clinical and laboratory criteria

Published experience with antimicrobic(s) important

bial therapy covering both aerobic and anaerobic intestinal flora is needed for a paraintestinal abscess. In the case of possible bacteremia in agranulocytosis, broad-spectrum bactericidal antimicrobics covering the most common organisms shown to be associated with this condition are needed.

3. Recent data concerning the proportions of susceptible and resistant organisms among each species that may be etiologically involved: This is particularly important in hospital-acquired infections, and most clinical laboratories make updated information available at regular intervals.

Local susceptibility data is helpful

In all serious or potentially serious infections, it is essential that the appropriate specimens be obtained from the patient before the initiation of therapy so that a specific diagnosis may be made and the susceptibility of the etiologic agent(s) definitively established as soon as possible. This will allow appropriate changes in treatment to be made if the patient is not responding to the initial empiric therapy; change to an agent with a narrower spectrum and lesser potential for superinfection; or replacement with an equally effective but less costly agent.

Specimens must be taken before initiating treatment

In many common community-acquired bacterial infections, treatment is based on extensive studies of different therapies, and bacteriologic diagnosis1 may not be sought. Examples include first attacks of cystitis in young women, early middle ear infection in a child, or "walking pneumonia" in a teenager with radiologic evidence compatible with a *Mycoplasma* infection. This approach is clinically justified as long as immediate steps are taken to obtain a specific diagnosis in the absence of a prompt response. What is unacceptable is the use of broad-spectrum antimicrobics for infections that have a high probability of a viral etiology in an otherwise healthy individual. This practice is sometimes based on the assumption that it prevents bacterial superinfection, but is more often simply the result of a desire to let the patient feel that something is being done. Any needless or inappropriate antimicrobic therapy contributes to the resistance problem, to unpleasant superinfections, and to the cost of medical care. Furthermore, it may obscure the diagnosis of a really serious infection by interfering with recovery of the etiologic agent in culture without curing the infection.

Specific bacteriologic diagnosis may not be sought in some situations

Needless antimicrobic therapy must be avoided

## ANTIVIRAL AGENTS

Because the method of replication of viruses is so intimately associated with the metabolism of the host cell (see Chapter 6), there is less opportunity for the development of nontoxic agents that attack the processes of viral synthesis than for the development of agents that inhibit bacterial or fungal growth. Nevertheless, viral attachment, penetration, replication, and assembly are rather unique processes that offer potential sites of attack, and a number of antiviral agents are available that exploit these possibilities. The principal agents in current use are considered next according to their modes of action.

Viral attachment, penetration, replication, and assembly points of antiviral attack

### Inhibitors of Attachment

Attachment of a virus to a cell receptor is a specific event, and blocking this process is the mechanism of viral neutralization by antibody. Until now, no clinically effective antiviral agent has been found that acts in this way, although the use of a recombinant CD4 molecule alone or linked to antibody has been shown to block attachment of HIV to CD4+ T lymphocytes and macrophages under experimental conditions. Similar approaches are being explored with other viruses.

Antibody blocks attachment

### Inhibitors of Cell Penetration and Uncoating

Two related synthetic amines, amantadine and rimantadine, are believed to act similarly at an early stage of infection by certain RNA viruses, by preventing viral uncoating after cell entry, inhibiting initial viral RNA transcription, or both. Low concentrations of the drugs may also inhibit viral assembly. They are active against influenza A viruses, but influenza B viruses are uniformly resistant. Naturally occurring influenza A viruses that are resistant to both agents have been shown to emerge during treatment and could become an increasing problem in the future. Development of resistance appears to require only a single amino acid change in the transmembrane portion of the viral M2 matrix protein. Amantadine and rimantadine are taken by mouth, have low toxicity, and have been used to provide temporary protection to particularly susceptible subjects, such as nursing home residents during acute epidemics. The agents also reduce the severity of the disease if given within the first few hours of development of symptoms.

Resistance by change of single amino acid

## Inhibitors of Nucleic Acid Synthesis

At present, most antiviral agents are nucleoside analogs that either interfere with viral DNA and RNA synthesis or serve as chain terminators after incorporation into nucleic acids. Those that are most effective act on virus-specified nucleic acid polymerases or transcriptases and have much less activity against host nucleic acid synthesis. One investigational agent with this category of activity, trisodium phosphonoformate, is not a nucleotide.

Most antivirals interfere with synthesis of, or are incorporated in, viral nucleic acid

### Idoxuridine and Trifluorothymidine

Idoxuridine (5-iodo-2′-deoxyuridine, IUdR) is a halogenated pyrimidine that blocks nucleic acid synthesis through incorporation into DNA in place of thymidine to produce a nonfunctional molecule. When given systemically, it is phosphorylated by thymidine kinase to active derivatives that inhibit both viral and cellular DNA synthesis. The resulting host toxicity precludes systemic administration in humans; it can be used topically for the effective treatment of herpetic infection of the cornea (keratitis). Trifluorothymidine is a related pyrimidine analog that is also effective in treating herpetic corneal infections, including those caused by some strains that fail to respond to IUdR.

Idoxuridine is a halogenated pyrimidine

Blocks viral and cellular DNA synthesis

### Adenine Arabinoside

Adenine arabinoside (vidarabine) is a purine that inhibits DNA polymerase. It is phosphorylated intracellularly to its active derivative like the preceding two agents, but it has some selective action, in that herpes group viral polymerases are about 15 to 30 times more susceptible than the host cell enzyme. Thus, systemic toxicity is less than with IUdR and trifluorothymidine, but destruction of blood-forming elements in the bone marrow can occur with high dosages. When given intravenously, adenine arabinoside reduces the mortality of herpes encephalitis and has been useful in the treatment of neonatal herpes simplex infection and herpes zoster in immunocompromised patients. It is used topically for treatment of herpetic infections of the eye, in which it has approximately the same effectiveness as IUdR.

Adenine arabinoside purine inhibitor of DNA polymerase

### Acyclovir

Acyclovir (acycloguanosine) is very active against replicating herpes simplex virus (HSV), but progressively less so against the varicella–zoster virus (VZV) and Epstein–Barr virus. It is first phosphorylated to its monophosphate by virally specified thymidine kinase (but not cellular kinases), limiting the presence of the derivative to virus-infected cells. It is then further phosphorylated by cellular kinases to its triphosphate form, which selectively binds and inhibits viral DNA polymerase. Because of its mode of action, acyclovir has little toxicity for host cells. Cytomegalovirus (CMV) does not encode a viral thymidine kinase and is thus resistant to this agent. Acyclovir is available in topical, oral, and intravenous preparations. Oral therapy is effective in reducing the severity and duration of primary genital herpes simplex attacks. Prophylactic use is helpful in suppressing frequent recurrences of genital herpes in normal hosts and herpes simplex recurrences in the immunosuppressed. Given in high doses it also shortens the severity and duration of localized herpes zoster lesions. Intravenous acyclovir is used to manage severe genital herpes and disseminated herpes simplex in normal hosts and for VZV infections in immunocompromised and burn patients. It is the drug of choice in the treatment of disseminated neonatal herpes infections and adult herpes encephalitis.

Acyclovir phosphorylated form inhibits DNA polymerase

Active against herpes simplex but not CMV

Resistant isolates of HSV and VZV sometimes emerge after long-term administration. This is usually the result of development of thymidine kinase-deficient mutants; other mechanisms include alterations in viral DNA polymerase or the substrate specificity of thymi-

Resistance related to thymidine kinase mutants

dine kinase. The resistant mutants are generally sensitive to foscarnet and vidarabine, agents that do not require viral thymidine kinase for activation. Adverse effects are uncommon and generally mild, although more serious central nervous system dysfunctions may occur.

### Ganciclovir

Ganciclovir (DHPG) is an acyclovir analog that inhibits growth of all human herpesviruses including CMV. It is phosphorylated to the active form by host cell thymidine kinase, and it possesses significant toxicity for uninfected host cells, producing suppression of spermatogenesis, bone marrow precursors, and gut mucosal cells. It has been used to treat severe CMV infections in immunodeficient patients including those with AIDS. It seems to be most effective in treating CMV retinitis and appears to be somewhat useful in CMV pneumonia and enteritis; however, elimination of the virus often does not occur, relapses of infection are common when the drug is stopped, and resistant strains can develop.

Ganciclovir is more toxic than acyclovir, but active against CMV

### Foscarnet

Foscarnet (trisodium phosphonoformate) is a pyrophosphate analog that directly inhibits DNA polymerase of all herpesviruses, RNA polymerase of influenza viruses, and reverse transcriptase of retroviruses. Unlike acyclovir, it does not require activation by viral-specified thymidine kinase and, thus, is highly active against CMV and acyclovir-resistant herpes simplex. Although it lacks the hematologic toxicity of ganciclovir, it is nephrotoxic and must be administered by continuous intravenous infusion. Like ganciclovir, it is most useful for the treatment of severe CMV infections in immunodeficient patients, particularly those with AIDS. Treatment with either agent results in stabilization or improvement of clinical manifestations in 80 to 100% of patients. Resistance develops to both over time with subsequent relapses; sequential or concurrent therapy with the two agents appears helpful in their management.

Foscarnet is a pyrophosphate analog that inhibits DNA and RNA polymerases and reverse transcriptase

### Ribavirin

Ribavirin is a synthetic triazole nucleoside that is active in vitro and in vivo in experimental animals against a range of DNA and RNA viruses. The exact mechanism of the antiviral effect is unclear, but it inhibits the synthesis of guanosine 5′-phosphate, which is required for synthesis of viral nucleic acid. It shows some promise for use as an aerosol in prevention and treatment of some respiratory viral infections, especially influenza A and B, and respiratory syncytial viral infection. Oral and intravenous preparations have been effective in treatment of Lassa fever, a serious infection caused by an arenavirus, and should be useful for postexposure prophylaxis. Ribavirin also suppresses HIV in vitro and appears to delay progression of AIDS-related complex (ARC) to AIDS. Unfortunately, it interferes with the action of zidovudine (see next) in vitro and should probably not be used in this combination.

Ribavirin active against multiple respiratory viruses

Used as an aerosol

### Zidovudine

Zidovudine (azidothymidine, AZT) is a thymidine analog that inhibits HIV replication in vitro. It is phosphorylated in vivo by cellular enzymes to the 5′-triphosphate form, which inhibits viral reverse transcriptase and terminates viral DNA elongation. Controlled studies in patients with AIDS and ARC have demonstrated that the drug reduces the frequency of opportunistic infections, and transiently increases CD4+ T lymphocyte counts. There is also some evidence that it may reverse AIDS-related neuropsychiatric dysfunction, at least temporarily. In low doses, it has been found to delay onset of ARC and AIDS in asymptomatic HIV-infected patients with low CD4+ T lymphocyte counts for 1 year on average, at which time the virus demonstrates resistance to the drug. It appears to prolong life only briefly, if at all. It has significant toxicity for the bone marrow, producing severe anemia in 80% of patients. Severe headaches, myalgia, insomnia, seizures, and encephalopathy have all complicated treatment. Toxicity is significantly less when AZT is given in low doses to asymptomatically infected patients.

AZT inhibits reverse transcriptase

Delays onset of HIV infections

Toxic to bone marrow

### Didanosine and Zalcitabine

Didanosine (ddI, dideoxyinosine) and zalcitabine (ddC, dideoxycytidine) are more recently released agents capable of inhibiting HIV replication. Following intracellular phosphorylation to their active triphospate form, they, like zidovudine, block viral DNA by inhibiting

ddI and ddC inhibit reverse transcriptase

viral reverse transcriptase. Neither agent is curative and neither appears to prolong survival. Their use, however, is commonly associated with a rise in the CD4+ T lymphocyte count, a decrease in HIV p24 antigen levels, an improved clinical status, a delay in the onset of the first AIDS-defining infection, or all of these benefits. Serious side effects of treatment include peripheral neuropathy and pancreatitis, both dose related. The neuropathy is seen in approximately one third of treated patients and is probably secondary to inhibition of mitochondrial DNA synthesis. The condition is slowly reversible with discontinuation of treatment. A smaller percentage of patients develop pancreatitis. Hematologic abnormalities are uncommon. Didanosine is currently approved for patients with advanced HIV infection who are deteriorating on zidovudine therapy. Zalcitabine has been approved for use in combination with zidovudine in adults with advanced HIV infection who show deterioration.

Toxic neuropathy is reversible

## Inhibitors of Viral Assembly and Release

Although clearly a potential target, no antiviral agent that acts on viral assembly and release is in clinical use, although one, **methisazone,** acts as a specific inhibitor of poxvirus infections by blocking late viral protein synthesis. It thus leads to production of incomplete virus. It has been proven effective in the prophylaxis of poxvirus infections, but because of the elimination of smallpox from the world, it now is only of historic interest in human medicine.

Methisazone inhibits poxvirus protein synthesis

## Interferons

The human interferons and their role in defense against viral infections are considered in Chapters 6 and 10. Definition of their place in the therapy and prophylaxis of viral infections has become feasible now that recombinant DNA techniques have allowed relatively inexpensive large-scale production of interferons by some bacteria and yeasts.

Recombinant alpha-interferon used in treatment and prophylaxis of herpes zoster, CMV, hepatitis B, hepatitis C and HIV infections

Interferon alpha has been shown to have a definite role in the prophylaxis and treatment of herpes zoster and CMV infections, particularly in immunocompromised patients. It has also proved beneficial in the treatment of chronic active hepatitis B and hepatitis C liver infection. It is active against HIV in vitro and is synergistic with zidovudine. It has induced remissions in some patients with Kaposi's sarcoma.

Topical use in herpes keratitis and papillomavirus

Topical interferon application has been shown to be beneficial in the treatment of herpes keratitis and180 human papillomavirus infections. Under experimental conditions, it has shown some effect in preventing colds caused by at least one type of rhinovirus, but it is still unclear whether this approach has practical clinical application.

Unfortunately, the interferon preparations that have been tested clinically all show some toxicity at the doses used, partly because of their effect on host cell protein synthesis. It remains to be determined whether other interferons will prove more effective and less toxic for therapy and prophylaxis.

# EPIDEMIOLOGY OF ANTIMICROBIC RESISTANCE

## Development of Increased Resistance

Response predictable when antimicrobics first introduced

When each antimicrobic was first introduced, its activity against individual isolates of a species was almost completely predictable from studies of its spectrum of activity. Some species were uniformly naturally resistant, and others were susceptible with few, if any, exceptions. With the use of most antimicrobics, resistant strains of many previously susceptible species became increasingly common, sometimes very rapidly, with serious clinical and epidemiologic consequences. For example, most strains of *S. aureus* were fully susceptible to penicillin when it was first introduced in 1944. By 1950, only about 30% of hospital isolates remained susceptible; the current figure is about 15%, and many isolates are multiresistant to several previously active antimicrobics. Similarly, many enteric Gram-negative rods developed resistance to antimicrobics such as ampicillin, cephalosporins, tetracycline, chloramphenicol, and aminoglycosides, with many strains becoming multi-

Resistance and multiresistance developed later

resistant to as many as 15 agents. Fortunately, these developments have not been universal, and the spirochete of syphilis and the group A streptococcus, for example, have thus far retained their susceptibility to penicillin. Even this list may change, however, because 15 years ago it would have included the pneumococcus, but resistant strains of this organism have now been isolated in many countries. Resistance to antiviral agents may develop during the course of therapy, and this has been seen with both acyclovir and zidovudine.

Some species retain predictable susceptibility

## Origin of Resistant Strains

Resistant strains were occasionally found in a very small proportion of members of a species before introduction of an antimicrobic, and their frequency was greatly increased by its use. This situation was unusual, but partly explains the origin of penicillinase-producing *S. aureus*. In other cases, resistance involved the mutational or recombinational events discussed in Chapter 4. Many resistant mutants are genetically unstable in the absence of the selecting agent, but some, such as low-level penicillin-resistant gonococci and pneumococci and isoniazid-resistant mycobacteria, retain their virulence and can undergo epidemiologic spread. More important, plasmids carrying resistance genes have little, if any, adverse influence on the capacity of most organisms to survive, infect, and spread, and they frequently confer multiresistance. Transposable resistance genes introduce considerable genetic plasticity, and resistance determinants to new antimicrobics can be added to plasmids very quickly.

Preexisting resistant strains selected

Some resistant mutants are genetically stable

Plasmid- and transposon-determined resistance can spread rapidly

The origin of plasmid-carried determinants of resistance remains somewhat obscure. Some known to have preexisted the clinical use of the antimicrobic may have played a role in nature by protecting an organism against another that produced the agent. Some may have been derived from antibiotic-producing *Streptomyces*, in which they served to protect the cell from its own antibiotic. Some have almost certainly been chromosomal genes transposed to plasmids, and some may have been plasmid genes that mutated to provide altered specificity.

Origin of plasmid resistance genes obscure

## Enhancement and Spread of Resistance

The central factors involved in the increasing incidence of resistance are the selective effect of the use of antimicrobics, the spread of infection in human populations, and the ability of plasmids to cross species and even generic lines. Therapeutic or prophylactic use of antimicrobics, particularly those with a broad spectrum of activity, produces a relative ecologic vacuum in sites with a normal flora or on lesions prone to infection and allows resistant organisms to colonize or infect with less competition from others. Treatment with a single antimicrobic may select for strains that are also resistant to many other agents. Thus, chemotherapy can both enhance the opportunity for acquiring resistant strains from other sources and increase their numbers in the body. The amplifying effect of antimicrobic therapy on resistance is also apparent with the transfer of resistance plasmids to previously susceptible strains. This effect occurs primarily in the lower intestinal tract, where the antimicrobic may reduce the flora and also produce an increased oxidation–reduction potential that favors plasmid transfer to the same or other species.

Antimicrobics affect susceptibility to infection with resistant strains

Ecologic vacuum created by broad spectrum agents

Resistance amplified with R plasmid transfer

As an example, consider a patient harboring a strain of *E. coli* carrying a plasmid with genes encoding resistance to tetracycline, ampicillin, chloramphenicol, and the sulfonamides as a very small part of his facultative intestinal flora. He develops an infection with a *Shigella dysenteriae* bacillus susceptible to all of these antimicrobics and is treated with tetracycline. Most of the normal flora and the *Shigella* are inhibited, but the resistant *E. coli* increases because its multiplication is not impeded and competition is removed. Plasmid transfer occurs between the resistant *E. coli* and some surviving *Shigella;* the latter then multiply, causing a relapse of the disease with a strain that is now multiresistant. Any endemic or epidemic spread of dysentery from this patient to others will now be with the multiresistant *Shigella* strain, and its ability to infect will be enhanced if the recipient is on prophylaxis or therapy with any of the four antimicrobics to which it is resistant.

Example of acquisition and spread of plasmid-borne resistance determinants

Spread of R plasmids and transposable elements can be traced

Such occurrences are commonplace and involve both virulent organisms and members of the normal flora, especially enteric Gram-negative rods. They account for the much higher incidence of resistance and multiresistance that characterizes hospital-acquired as opposed to community-acquired strains. The procedures described in Chapter 4 allow resistance plasmids or even individual transposable elements to be "fingerprinted." It has thus been possible to trace their "epidemic" spread through different species and genera of bacteria.

## Major Selective Factors

Hospitals' central role in antimicrobic resistance

Community-acquired resistance also occurs

The hospital remains the major source and reservoir of resistant organisms that affect humans, although similar selection and spread occur in the community. Isolates of group A β-hemolytic streptococci and pneumococci are frequently resistant to tetracycline and reflect what was widespread and often inappropriate community use of that agent. Most strains of gonococci now show substantially higher resistance to penicillin than was the case when the antibiotic was introduced, largely because of extensive suboptimal therapy.

Environmental contamination and animal feed supplementation

There are selective factors other than use of antimicrobics in human therapy and prophylaxis. Contamination of the hospital environment, with antimicrobic from aerosols produced during administration or from high concentrations in urine, may be sufficient to inhibit the susceptible normal flora of the anterior nares of personnel and increase the carriage rate of resistant *S. aureus*. Such contamination has been shown to occur in human and veterinary hospitals and in an antibiotic processing plant; its significance merits further study. Much attention has been paid to the use of antimicrobics added to animal feeds for prophylaxis against infection or for their growth-promoting effects, which are economically important but involve mechanisms not yet fully characterized. Cattle or poultry that consume feed supplemented with antimicrobics rapidly develop a resistant enteric flora that spreads throughout the herd. Resistance is largely plasmid determined and has been shown capable of spreading to the flora of farm workers and of those living in close proximity to cattle-rearing farms. *Salmonella* species, which commonly infect intensively raised cattle and poultry, usually acquire the resistance plasmids, and multiplication of the bacteria in contaminated food products can result in individual infections or epidemics of food poisoning caused by multiresistant *Salmonella*. Patients on treatment with antibiotics to which the organisms are resistant may become clinically infected by numbers of *Salmonella* well below those that will usually cause disease in healthy individuals. As a consequence, many countries have banned or controlled addition to animal feeds of antimicrobics that are useful for systemic therapy in humans. Important theoretic concerns are that stabilization of plasmids may occur under intensive antimicrobic pressure and may then persist and spread in the absence of the selective agents and acquire other undesirable genetic traits, such an enhanced virulence.

Resistant zoonotic Salmonella infections

Stabilization of R plasmids a concern

Despite these various sources of resistant strains, by far the most significant contributors to the problem in medicine remain the large-scale use of antimicrobics for treating or preventing actual or assumed infections and epidemiologic spread of resistant strains in hospitals and the community under the selective pressure of antimicrobic use.

## Control of Resistance

Resistance lost on withdrawal of selective agent

In the past, numerous examples in the literature showed that the extent of resistance in a hospital directly reflects the extent of usage of an antimicrobic, and that withdrawal or control can lead to rapid reduction of the incidence of resistance. Obviously such measures have little impact on levels of resistance in the community, and they have rarely been applied effectively. Furthermore, some resistance determinants have now become so stabilized that they are less likely to be lost in the absence of the selective agent; however, experience and our understanding of the mechanisms and spread of resistance indicate that certain principles can help to keep the problem under control, can sometimes reverse it, and are compatible with good therapeutic practice:

1. Use antimicrobics conservatively and specifically in therapy.
2. Use an adequate dosage and duration of therapy to eliminate the infecting organism and reduce the risk of selecting resistant variants.

3. Whenever possible, select antimicrobics according to the proved or anticipated known susceptibility of the infecting strain.
4. Use, when possible, narrow-spectrum rather than broad-spectrum antimicrobics when the specific etiology of an infection is known.
5. Use antimicrobic combinations when they are known to prevent emergence of resistant mutants.
6. Use antimicrobics prophylactically only in situations in which it has been proven valuable and for the shortest possible time to avoid selection of a resistant flora.
7. Avoid environmental contamination with antimicrobics.
8. Rigidly apply careful, aseptic and hand-washing procedures to help prevent spread of resistant organisms.
9. Use containment isolation procedures for patients infected with resistant organisms that pose a threat to others, and use protective precautions for those who are highly susceptible.
10. Epidemiologically monitor resistant organisms or resistance determinants in an institution and apply enhanced control measures if a problem develops.
11. Restrict the use of therapeutically valuable antimicrobics for nonmedical purposes.

The problem of antimicrobic resistance and its spread has a considerable behavioral component. Needless and excessive therapy, failure to observe basic rules for preventing spread of infection to others, and lack of understanding of the process all serve to increase the problem. Conversely, intelligent, conservative, and specific use of chemotherapy with adequate precautions to prevent cross-infection provides the best chance of retaining the value of many of the agents we now possess (see Appendix 13–1 and Appendix 13–2).

Problem of antimicrobic resistance has behavioral aspects

## ADDITIONAL READING

Connolly KJ, Hammer SM. Antiretroviral therapy. *Antimicrob Agents Chemother.* 1992;36:245–254, 509–520. These two concise reviews with superb bibliographies cover the tremendous progress made in retroviral therapy over the past 5 years. They cover both the reverse transcriptase inhibitors and some of the newer therapeutic modalities currently being explored.

Gilman AG, Rall TW, Nies AS, Taylor P, eds. *Goodman and Gilman's The Pharmacological Basis of Therapeutics.* 8th ed. New York: Pergamon Press; 1990. A standard reference text with excellent sections on antibiotics and chemotherapy.

Jacoby GA, Archer GL. New mechanisms of bacterial resistance to antimicrobial agents. *N Engl J Med.* 1991;324:601–612. A brief, recent discussion of resistant mechanisms.

Knight V, Gilbert BE. Antiviral chemotherapy. *Infect Dis Clin North Am.* 1987;1(2). An excellent series of articles by experts in the field.

Kunin CM. Resistance to antimicrobial drugs—A worldwide calamity. *Ann Intern Med.* 1993;118:557–561. The urgent need for more appropriate selection and use of antimicrobial agents is described.

Peterson PK, Verhoef J, eds. *The Antimicrobial Agents Annual 2.* Amsterdam/New York: Elsevier; 1987. An up-to-date series of chapters emphasizing particularly the clinical pharmacology and application of antimicrobials.

Pratt WB, Fekety R. *The Antimicrobial Drugs.* New York: Oxford University Press; 1986. An exceptionally informative account of the basis of antibacterial and antiviral chemotherapy, the characteristics of antimicrobics, and their clinical application.

Sanders CC, Sanders WE Jr. β-Lactam resistance in Gram-negative bacteria: Global trends and clinical impact. *Clin Infect Dis.* 1992;15:824–839. The authors trace the increase in multiple β-lactam resistance among a number of organisms including Enterobacteriaceae, *Pseudomonas aeruginosa*, and *Xanthomonas maltophilia* that has been associated with increased use of newer cephalosporins.

Tyrell DAJ. Interferons and their clinical value. *Rev Infect Dis.* 1987;9:243–249. An excellent overview of the use of interferons in medicine.

## APPENDIX 13–1. USUAL SUSCEPTIBILITY PATTERNS OF COMMON BACTERIA TO SOME COMMONLY USED BACTERIOSTATIC AND BACTERICIDAL ANTIMICROBIAL AGENTS

| Antimicrobic | Bactericidal | Bacteriostatic | *Staphylococcus aureus* | Enterococci | Other Streptococci | *Neisseria* | *Haemophilus* | *Legionella* | *Mycoplasma* | *Escherichia coli* | *Proteus mirabilis* | Other *Proteus* spp | *Klebsiella* | *Enterobacter* | *Serratia* | *Pseudomonas aeruginosa* | *Bacteroides fragilis* | Other Gram-negative Anaerobes | *Clostridium* | *Rickettsia* | *Chlamydia* | |
|---|---|---|---|---|---|---|---|---|---|---|---|---|---|---|---|---|---|---|---|---|---|---|
| Benzyl penicillin | + | | 1 ◕ | C ◍ | 1 ◔ | 1 ◔ | ◍ | ● | ● | ● | ◍ | ● | ● | ● | ● | ● | ● | 1 ◔ | 1 ○ | ● | ● | Narrow-spectrum agents |
| Penicillinase-resistant penicillins | + | | 1 ◔ | ● | 2 ◔ | ● | ● | ● | ● | ● | ● | ● | ● | ● | ● | ● | ● | ● | ● | ● | ● | |
| Erythromycin | ± | + | 2 ◔ | 2 ◔ | 2 ◔ | ◔ | | 1 ○ | 1 ○ | ● | ● | ● | ● | ● | ● | ● | – | – | – | – | 2 ○ | |
| Clindamycin | ± | + | 2 ◔ | – | ◔ | ● | ● | – | – | ● | ● | ● | ● | ● | ● | ● | ◔ | ◔ | ◔ | – | – | |
| Vancomycin | + | | 2 ○ | 1 ○ | 2 ○ | ● | ● | ● | ● | ● | ● | ● | ● | ● | ● | ● | – | – | 1 ○ | – | – | |
| Ampicillin | + | | 2 ◕ | 1 ◔ | 2 ◔ | 1 ◔ | 1 ◔ | ● | ● | 1 ◔ | 1 ◔ | ● | ● | ● | ● | ● | ● | – | 1 ○ | ● | ● | Broad-spectrum agents |
| Piperacillin | + | | – | ○ | ○ | – | ◔ | ● | ● | – | 1 ○ | 1 ◔ | 1 ◔ | 1 ◔ | 1 ◔ | 1 ◔ | 2 ◔ | 1 ○ | – | ● | ● | |
| Cephalothin | + | | 2 ◔ | ● | 2 ◔ | – | ● | ● | ● | ◔ | ○ | ● | ◔ | ● | ● | ● | ● | ◔ | ◔ | ● | ● | |
| Cefotetan | + | | – | ● | 1 ○ | 1 ○ | – | ● | ● | 1 ○ | 1 ○ | 1 ○ | 1 ○ | ● | ◔ | ● | 2 ◔ | ○ | – | ● | ● | |
| Ceftazidime | + | | – | – | – | – | ○ | ● | ● | 1 ○ | 1 ○ | 1 ○ | 1 ○ | 2 ◔ | 2 ◔ | ◔ | ◔ | – | – | ● | ● | |
| Imipenem | + | | 2 ○ | 2 ○ | 2 ○ | 1 ○ | 1 ○ | – | ● | 1 ○ | 1 ○ | 1 ○ | 1 ○ | 1 ○ | 1 ○ | 1 ◔ | 1 ○ | 1 ○ | 1 ○ | – | – | |
| Aztreonam | + | | ● | ● | ● | 1 ○ | 1 ○ | – | ● | 1 ◔ | 1 ◔ | 1 ○ | 1 ○ | ◔ | 1 ◔ | 1 ◔ | ● | ● | ● | – | – | |
| Gentamicin | + | | ◔ | C ● | ● | – | – | ● | – | 1 ◔ | 1 ○ | 1 ○ | 1 ◔ | 1 ◔ | 1 ◔ | 1 ◔ | ● | ● | ● | – | – | |
| Amikacin | + | | ◔ | C ● | ● | – | – | ● | – | 1 ◔ | 1 ○ | 1 ○ | 1 ◔ | 1 ◔ | 1 ◔ | 1 ◔ | ● | ● | ● | – | – | |
| Tetracycline | | + | ◔ | ● | ◕ | ◔ | ○ | 2 ○ | 1 ○ | ◔ | ● | ● | ◔ | ◔ | ◕ | ● | ◕ | ◔ | ◔ | 1 ○ | 1 ○ | |
| Chloramphenicol | | + | ◔ | ◔ | ◔ | ◔ | ◔ | 2 ● | – | ◔ | ◔ | ◔ | ◔ | ◔ | ◕ | ● | 1 ◔ | 2 ○ | – | 1 ○ | – | |
| Ciprofloxacin | + | | ◔ | ◍ | ◍ | 2 ○ | – | – | ● | 1 ◔ | 1 ○ | 1 ○ | 1 ○ | 1 ○ | 1 ○ | 2 ◔ | ● | ● | – | – | ◍ | |
| Sulfamethoxazole + trimethoprim | ± | + | – | – | – | – | 1 ◔ | – | – | 1 ◔ | ◔ | ◔ | ◔ | ◔ | ◔ | ● | ◔ | – | – | – | 3 – | |

Proportions of susceptible and resistant strains: ○, 100% susceptible ◔, 25% resistant ●, 100% resistant ◍, intermediate susceptibility.

**APPENDIX 13–2. SUGGESTED ANTIMICROBIC THERAPY**

| Organism | Antimicrobic |
|---|---|
| **Gram-positive cocci** | |
| Staphylococci | |
| *S. aureus* | Nafcillin (± gentamicin)<br>Cephalothin<br>Vancomycin |
| *S. epidermidis* | Vancomycin |
| Streptococci | |
| Enterococci | Ampicillin (± gentamicin)<br>Vancomycin (± gentamicin) |
| Other streptococci | Penicillin |
| **Gram-negative cocci** | |
| Gonococci | Ceftriaxone |
| Meningococci | Penicillin |
| *Moraxella catharrhalis* | Amoxycillin/clavulanate<br>Trimethoprim/sulfamethoxazole, erythromycin<br>2nd or 3rd generation cephalosporin |
| **Gram-negative rods** | |
| Enterobacteriaceae | |
| *E. coli* | Any cephalosporin |
| *Klebsiella* | Any cephalosporin |
| *Proteus mirabilis* | Any cephalosporin, ampicillin |
| *Enterobacter* | Imipenem, ciprofloxacin, 3GC |
| *Proteus* (not mirabilis) | 3rd generation cephalosporin |
| *Providencia* | 3rd generation cephalosporin |
| *Salmonella* | 3rd generation cephalosporin |
| *Serratia* | 3rd generation cephalosporin |
| *Shigella* | Ciprofloxacin, Trimethoprim/sulfamethoxazole |
| *Pseudomonas aeruginosa* | Mezlocillin or Piperacillin plus aminoglycoside or ceftazadime |
| *Haemophilus influenzae* | 2nd or 3rd generation cephalosporin<br>Ampicillin[a] for UTI, bronchitis |
| **Anaerobes** | |
| *Peptostreptococcus* | Penicillin G, clindamycin, metronidazole |
| *Clostridium* | Penicillin G, clindamycin, metronidazole |
| *Bacteroides* | Clindamycin, metronidazole |

[a] If β lactamase negative.

Chapter 14

# Principles of Laboratory Diagnosis of Infectious Diseases

*Kenneth J. Ryan and C. George Ray*

The diagnosis of a microbial infection begins with an assessment of clinical and epidemiologic features, leading to the formulation of a diagnostic hypothesis. Anatomic localization of the infection with the aid of physical and radiologic findings (for example, right lower lobe pneumonia, subphrenic abscess) is usually included. This clinical diagnosis suggests a number of possible etiologic agents based on knowledge of infectious syndromes and their courses (Chapters 59 through 72). The specific cause is then established by the application of methods described in this chapter. A combination of science and art on the part of both the clinician and laboratory worker is required: The clinician must select the appropriate tests and specimens to be processed and, where appropriate, suggest the suspected etiologic agents to the laboratory. The laboratory worker must design a battery of methods that will demonstrate the probable agents, and be prepared to explore other possibilities suggested by the clinical situation or findings of the laboratory examinations. The best results are obtained when communication between the clinic and laboratory is maximal.

## THE SPECIMEN

Specimen selection and collection crucial

The primary connection between the clinical encounter and diagnostic laboratory is the specimen submitted for processing. If it is not appropriately chosen and/or collected, no degree of laboratory skill will rectify the error. Failure at the level of specimen collection is the most common reason for failure to establish an etiologic diagnosis, or worse, for suggesting a wrong diagnosis. In the case of bacterial infections, the primary problem lies in distinguishing resident or contaminating normal floral organisms from those causing the infection. The three specimen categories illustrated in Figure 14–1 and discussed below are covered more specifically in Chapters 59 to 72.

Normal flora complicates the problem

### Direct Tissue or Fluid Samples

Direct specimens easily interpreted

**Direct specimens** (Fig 14–1A) are collected from normally sterile tissues (lung, liver) and body fluids (cerebrospinal fluid, blood). The methods range from needle aspiration of an abscess to surgical biopsy. In general, such collections require the direct involvement of a

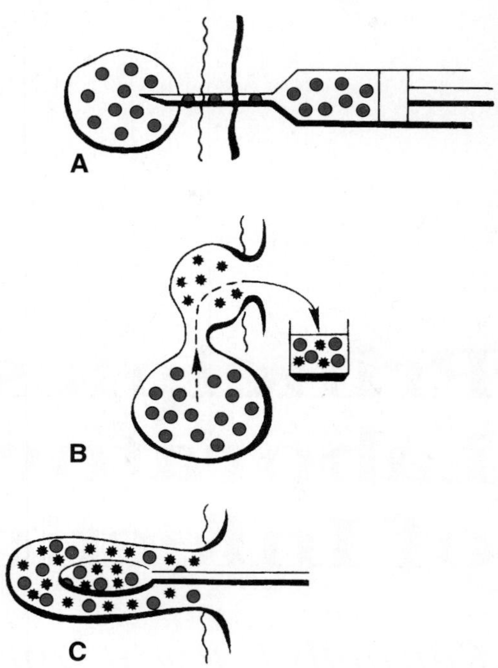


**Figure 14–1.** Specimens for the diagnosis of infection. **A.** Direct specimen. The pathogen (●) is localized in an otherwise sterile site, and a barrier such as the skin must be passed to sample it. This may be done surgically or by needle aspiration as shown. The specimen collected contains only the pathogen. Examples: deep abscess, cerebrospinal fluid. **B.** Indirect sample. The pathogen is localized as in A, but must pass through a site containing normal flora (*) in order to be collected. The specimen contains the pathogen, but is contaminated with the nonpathogenic flora. The degree of contamination is often related to the skill with which the normal floral site was "bypassed" in specimen collection. Examples: expectorated sputum, voided urine. **C.** Sample from site with normal flora. The pathogen and nonpathogenic flora are mixed at the site of infection. Both are collected and the nonpathogen is either inhibited by the use of selective culture methods or discounted in interpretation of culture results. Examples: throat, stool.

physician and may carry some risk for the patient. The results are always useful, because positive findings are diagnostic and negative findings can exclude infection at the suspected site.

## Indirect Samples

Indirect samples attempt to bypass a normal flora site

**Indirect samples** (Fig 14–1B) are specimens of inflammatory exudates (expectorated sputum, voided urine) that have passed through sites known to be colonized with normal flora. The site of origin is usually sterile in healthy persons; however, some assessment of the probability of contamination with normal flora during collection is necessary before these specimens can be reliably interpreted. This assessment requires knowledge of the potential contaminating flora (Chapter 9) as well as the probable pathogens to be sought. Indirect samples are usually more convenient for both physician and patient, but carry a higher risk of misinterpretation. For some specimens, such as expectorated sputum, guidelines to assess specimen quality have been developed by correlation of clinical and microbiologic findings (Chapter 64).

Collection is easy but interpretation is more difficult

## Samples from Sites With a Normal Flora

May not be possible to exlude normal flora

Frequently the primary site of infection is in an area known to be colonized with many organisms (pharynx and large intestine) (Fig 14–1C). In such instances, examinations are selectively made for organisms known to cause infection that are not normally found at the infected site. For example, Salmonella, Shigella, and Campylobacter may be specifically sought in a stool specimen because they are known to cause diarrhea. It is neither practical nor relevant to describe the other stool flora.

## Specimens for Viral Diagnosis

Viral normal flora nil

The selection of specimens for viral diagnosis is easier because there is essentially little normal viral flora to confuse interpretation. This allows selection guided by knowledge of which sites are most likely to yield the suspected etiologic agent. For example, mumps and enteroviruses are among the more common viruses involved in acute infection of the central nervous system. Specimens that might be expected to yield these agents on culture would include throat, stool, and cerebrospinal fluid. Examples for the most common viral infections are shown in Table 14–1.

Selection dictated by common replication sites

## Specimen Collection and Transport

The **sterile swab** is the most convenient and most commonly used tool for specimen collection; however, it provides the poorest conditions for survival, and can only absorb a small volume of inflammatory exudate. The worst possible specimen is a dried-out swab; the best is a collection of 5 to 10 mL or more of the infected fluid or tissue. The volume is important because infecting organisms present in small numbers maynot be detected in a small sample.

Swabs convenient but not ideal for survival of microbe

Fluid or tissue best specimens

Specimens should be transported to the laboratory as soon after collection as possible, because some microorganisms survive only briefly outside the body. For example, unless special **transport media** are used, isolation rates of the organism that causes gonorrhea (*Neisseria gonorrhoeae*) are decreased when processing is delayed beyond a few minutes. Likewise, many respiratory viruses survive poorly outside the body. On the other hand, some bacteria survive well and may even multiply after the specimen is collected. The growth of enteric Gram-negative rods in specimens awaiting culture may in fact compromise specimen interpretation and interfere with the isolation of more fastidious organisms. Significant changes are associated with delays of more than 3 to 4 hours.

Viability may be lost if specimen is delayed

Various transport media have been developed to minimize the effects of the delay between specimen collection and laboratory processing. In general, they are buffered fluid or semisolid media containing minimal nutrients and are designed to prevent drying, maintain a neutral pH, and minimize bacterial growth. Other features may be required to meet special requirements, such as an oxygen-free atmosphere for obligate anaerobes.

Transport media stabilize conditions and prevent drying

**TABLE 14–1. SOME APPROPRIATE SPECIMENS FOR VIRAL ISOLATION[a]**

| | Specimen | | | | | |
|---|---|---|---|---|---|---|
| **Agent** | ***Throat*** | ***Stool*** | ***Cerebrospinal Fluid*** | ***Urine*** | ***Vesicle Fluid*** | ***Other*** |
| Meningitis and encephalitis | | | | | | |
| Mumps | ++++ | – | ++ | + | – | – |
| Enteroviruses | +++ | ++++ | ++ | – | – | – |
| Herpes simplex | ± | – | ± | – | + | ++++ (Brain biopsy) |
| Arboviruses[b] | – | – | + | – | – | ++ (Brain) + (Blood) |
| Respiratory diseases | | | | | | |
| Influenza and parainfluenza viruses | ++++ | – | – | – | – | |
| Adenoviruses | ++++ | ++++ | – | – | – | |
| Exanthems | | | | | | |
| Measles | ++++ | – | – | + | – | |
| Rubella[b] | ++++ | – | – | + | – | |
| Varicella | – | – | – | – | ++++ | |
| Herpes simplex | ++ | – | – | – | ++++ | |
| Cytomegalovirus | ++ | – | – | ++++ | – | + (Leukocyte tissue biopsy) |

*Abbreviations:* – = no yield; ± to ++++ = relatative yield (low to high).

[a] In general, it should be remembered that virus shedding often diminishes rapidly after onset of acute illness; it is therefore important to attempt specimen collection as early as possible.

[b] Because it is frequently very difficult to isolate these agents from the disease in question, it is emphasized that serologic tests are particularly important to ensure a diagnosis.

# DIAGNOSTIC METHODS

The general approaches to laboratory diagnosis vary with different microorganisms and infectious diseases. The types of methods, however, will usually be some combination of direct examinations, culture, antigen detection, and antibody detection (serology). Newer approaches involving direct detection of genomic components are also important, although few have become practical enough for routine use. In this chapter, we shall consider these principles, emphasizing their application to the diagnosis of diseases caused by bacteria and viruses. Most of the approaches to be described can also be applied, with certain variations, to the diagnosis of diseases caused by fungi and parasites.

## Direct Examination

Of the infectious agents discussed in this book, only some of the parasites are large enough to be seen with the naked eye. Bacteria can be seen clearly with the light microscope when appropriate methods are used; individual viruses can be seen only with the electron microscope, although aggregates of viral particles in cells (viral inclusions) may be seen by light microscopy. Various stains are used to visualize and differentiate microorganisms in smears and histologic sections.

### Light Microscopy

Direct examination of stained or unstained preparations by **light (bright field) microscopy** (Fig 14–2A) is particularly useful for detection of bacteria. Even the smallest bacteria (0.15

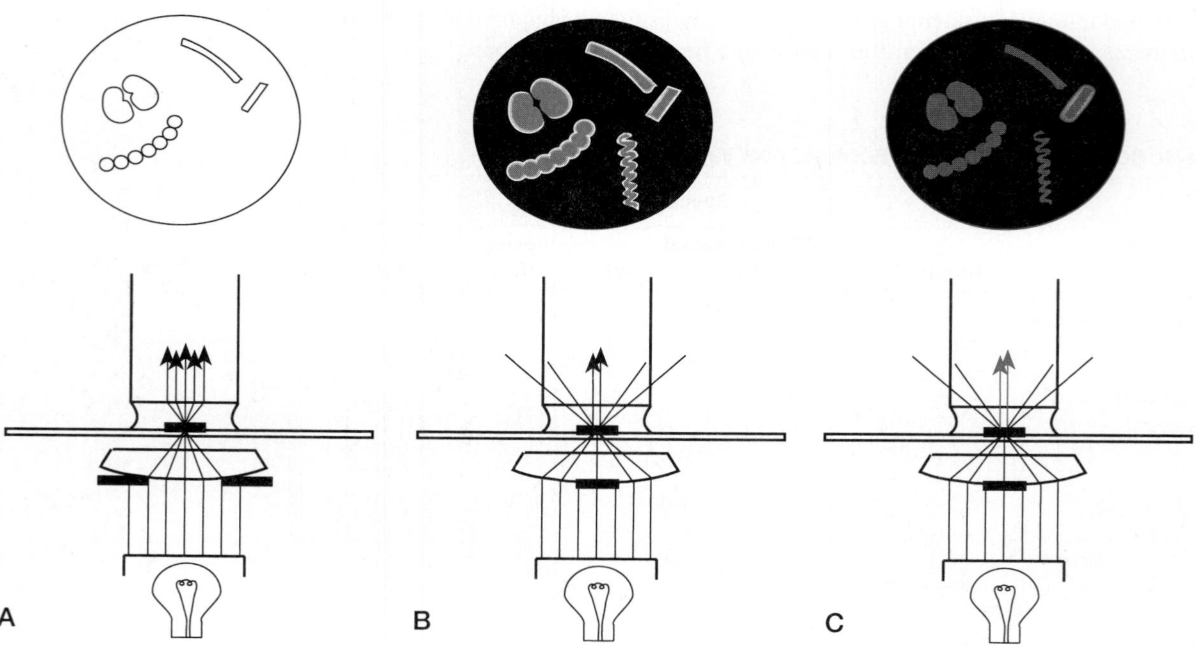


**Figure 14–2.** Bright-field, dark-field, and fluorescence microscopy. **A.** Bright-field illumination properly aligned. The purpose is to focus light directly on the preparation for optimal visualization against a bright background. **B.** In dark-field illumination, a black background is created by blocking the central light. Peripheral light is focused so that it will be collected by the objective only when it is reflected from the surfaces of particles (for example, bacteria). The microscopic field shows bright halos around some bacteria and reveals a spirochete too thin to be seen with bright-field illumination. **C.** Fluorescence microscopy is similar to dark-field microscopy, except the light source is ultraviolet and the organisms are stained with fluorescent compounds. The incident light generates light of a different wavelength, which is seen as a halo (red in this illustration) around only the organism tagged with fluorescent compounds. For the most common fluorescent compound the light is green.

μm wide) can be visualized, although some require special lighting techniques. As the resolution limit of the light microscope is near 0.2 μm, the optics must be ideal if organisms are to be seen clearly by direct microscopy. These conditions may be achieved with a 100× oil immersion objective, a 5 to 10× eyepiece, and optimal lighting. Unstained bacteria are too transparent to see directly, although their presence can be indicated by the voids they create when suspended in particulate matter such as India ink.

All bacteria visible if optics are maximized

Bacteria may be stained by a wide variety of dyes, including methylene blue, crystal violet, carbol-fuchsin (red), and safranin (red). The two most important methods, the Gram and acid-fast techniques, employ staining, decolorization, and counterstaining in a manner that helps to classify as well as stain the organism.

### The Gram Stain

The differential staining procedure described in 1884 by the Danish physician Hans Christian Gram has proved one of the most useful in microbiology and medicine. The procedure (Fig 14–3) involves the application of a solution of iodine in potassium iodide to cells previously stained with an acridine dye such as crystal violet. This treatment produces a mordanting action in which purple insoluble complexes are formed with the cell's ribonucleic acid. The difference between Gram-positive and Gram-negative bacteria is in the permeability of the cell wall to these complexes upon treatment with mixtures of acetone and alcohol solvents. This extracts the purple iodine–dye complexes from Gram-negative cells, whereas Gram-positive bacteria retain them. An intact cell wall is necessary for a positive reaction, and Gram-positive bacteria may fail to retain the stain if the organisms are old, dead, or damaged by antimicrobial agents. No similar conditions cause a Gram-negative organism to appear Gram positive. The stain is completed by the addition of red counterstain such as safranin, which is taken up by bacteria that have been decolorized. Thus, cells stained purple are Gram positive, and those stained red are Gram negative. As indicated in Chapter 2, Gram positivity and negativity correspond to major structural differences in the cell wall.

Gram-positive bacteria retain purple iodine-dye complexes

Gram-negative bacteria do not retain complexes when decolorized

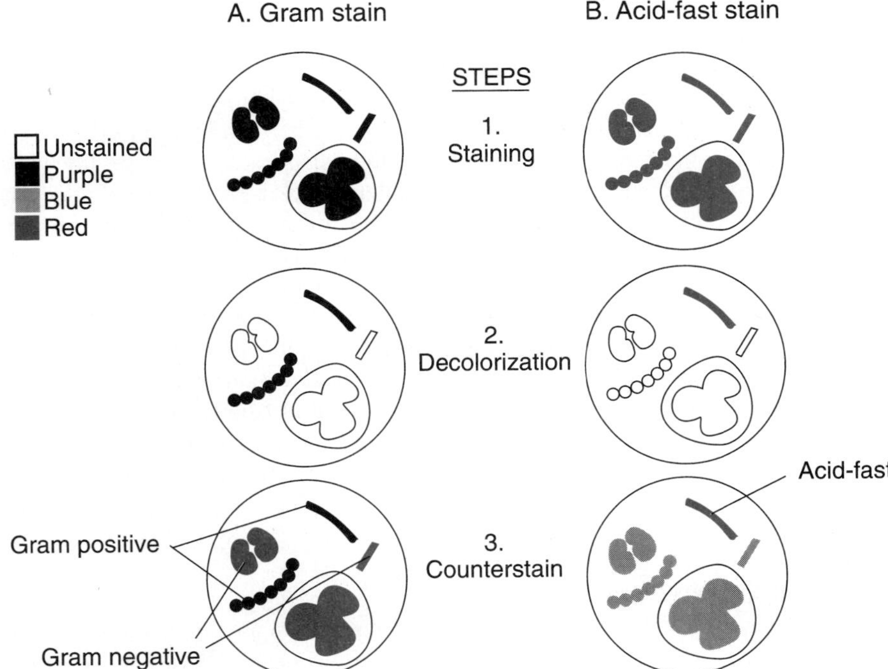


**Figure 14–3.** The Gram and acid-fast stains. Four bacteria and a PMN are shown at each stage. All are initially stained purple by the crystal violet and iodine of the Gram stain (A1) and red by the carbol fuchsin of the acid-fast stain (B1). Following decolorization, Gram-positive and acid-fast organisms retain their original stain. Others are unstained (A2, B2). The safranin of the Gram counterstain stains the Gram-negative bacteria and the background red (A3), and the methylene blue leaves a blue background for the contrasting red acid-fast bacillus (B3).

Properly decolorized background should be red

When the Gram stain is applied to clinical specimens, the purple or red bacteria are seen against a Gram-negative (red) background of leukocytes, exudate, and debris. Retention of the purple dye in tissue or fluid elements, such as the nuclei of polymorphonuclear leukocytes, is an indication that the smear has been inadequately decolorized. In smears of uneven thickness, judgments on the Gram reaction can be made only in well-decolorized areas.

Gram reaction plus morphology guide clinical decisions

In many bacterial infections, the etiologic agents are readily seen on stained Gram smears of pus or fluids. This information, combined with the clinical findings, may guide the management of infection before culture results are available. Interpretation requires considerable experience and knowledge of probable causes, of their morphology and Gram reaction, and of any organisms normally present in health at the infected site.

#### The Acid-fast Stain

Acid fastness is a property of the mycobacteria (for example, *Mycobacterium tuberculosis*) and related organisms. Acid-fast organisms generally stain very poorly with dyes, including those used in the Gram stain. They can, however, be stained by prolonged application of more concentrated dyes, and staining is facilitated by heat treatment. Their unique feature is that once stained, acid-fast bacteria resist decolorization by concentrations of mineral acids and ethanol that remove the same dyes from other bacteria. This combination of weak initial staining and strong retention once stained is probably related to the high lipid content of the mycobacterial cell wall. Acid-fast stains are completed with a counterstain to provide a contrasting background for viewing the stained bacteria (Fig 14–3).

Acid-fast bacteria take stains poorly

Once stained retain it strongly

The classic acid-fast procedure is the **Ziehl–Neelsen stain,** in which the slide is flooded with carbol-fuchsin (red), heated, and then decolorized with a 3% solution of hydrochloric acid in alcohol. When counterstained with methylene blue, acid-fast organisms appear red against a blue background. A variant of this method is the **Ponder–Kinyoun (cold) acid-fast stain,** in which a more concentrated fuchsin is used and heating is omitted. Another variant is the **fluorochrome stain,** which uses a fluorescent dye, auramine, or an auramine–rhodamine mixture followed by decolorization with acid–alcohol. Acid-fast organisms retain the fluorescent stain, which allows their visualization by fluorescence microscopy.

There are multiple variants of the acid-fast stain

### Darkfield and Fluorescence Microscopy

Some bacteria, such as *Treponema pallidum*, the cause of syphilis, are too thin to be visualized with the usual bright-field illumination. They can be seen by use of the dark-field technique. With this method, a condenser focuses light diagonally on the specimen in such a way that only light reflected from particulate matter such as bacteria reaches the eyepiece (Fig 14–2B). The angles of incident and reflected light are such that the organisms are surrounded by a bright halo against a black background. This type of illumination is also used in other microscopic techniques, in which a high light contrast is desired, and for observation of fluorescence. Fluorescent compounds, when excited by incident light of one wavelength, emit light of a longer wavelength and thus a different color. When the fluorescent compound is conjugated with an antibody as a probe for detection of a specific antigen, the technique is called **immunofluorescence,** or **fluorescent antibody microscopy.** The appearance is the same as in dark-field microscopy except that the halo is the emitted color of the fluorescent compound (Fig 14–2C). For improved safety, most modern fluorescence microscopy systems direct the incident light through the objective from above **(epifluorescence).**

Darkfieled creates a halo around organisms too thin to see by brightfield

Fluorescent stains convert darkfield to fluorescence microscopy

### Phase-contrast Microscopy

Phase-contrast is a form of microscopy in which differences in refractive index in the specimen are converted to differences in intensity of light in the image. This allows better visualization of structures in unstained specimens (eg, within eukaryotic cells) than is possible with bright- or dark-field illumination. It is primarily used to view host cells, fungi, and parasites.

Phase contrast allows visualization without stains

### Electron Microscopy

Electron microscopy demonstrates structures by transmission of an electron beam and has 10 to 1000 times the resolving powerful of light-microscopic methods. For practical reasons its diagnostic application is limited to virology, where due to the resolution possible at high magnification it offers results not possible by any other method. Using negative staining techniques, direct examination of fluids and tissues from affected body sites enables visualization of viral particles. In some instances electron microscopy has been the primary means of discovery of viruses that do not grow in the usual cell culture systems.

Viruses visible only by electron microscopy

## Culture

Growth and identification of the infecting agent in vitro is usually the most sensitive and specific means of diagnosis and is thus the method most commonly used. Most bacteria and fungi can be grown in a variety of artificial media, but strict intracellular microorganisms (eg, *Chlamydia*, *Rickettsia*, and human and animal viruses) can be isolated only in cultures of living eukaryotic cells.

### Isolation and Identification of Bacteria

#### Bacteriologic Culture

Almost all medically important bacteria can be cultivated outside the host in artificial culture media. Usually, a single bacterium placed in the proper culture medium and environment will multiply to numbers that are sufficient to cause changes detectable by the naked eye. Bacteriologic media are essentially souplike recipes prepared from digests of animal or vegetable protein supplemented with substances such as glucose, yeast extract, serum, or blood, to meet the metabolic requirements of the organism. Their chemical composition is therefore complex, and their success depends on the similar nutritional requirements of most heterotrophic living things.

Bacteria will grow in souplike media

Media are initially prepared in the fluid state (broths) to which bacteria or clinical specimens may be added directly. The presence of bacteria in broth medium will not be apparent to the naked eye until they grow to numbers sufficient to produce turbidity or macroscopic clumps. Turbidity results from reflection of transmitted light by the bacteria; depending on the size of the organism, more than $10^6$ bacteria per milliliter of broth are usually required. Some strictly aerobic bacteria may grow as a film on the surface of stationary cultures; other bacteria grow as a sediment.

Large numbers of bacteria in broth produce turbidity

The addition of a gelling agent to a broth medium allows its preparation in solid form as plates in petri dishes. The universal gelling agent for diagnostic bacteriology is **agar,** a polysaccharide extracted from certain types of seaweed. Agar has the convenient property of becoming liquid at about 95°C but not returning to the solid state as a gel until cooled to less than 50°C. This allows the addition of a heat-labile substance, such as blood, to the medium before it sets. At the temperatures used in the diagnostic laboratory (37°C or lower), broth–agar exists as a smooth, solid, nutrient gel. This medium, usually termed "agar," may be qualified with a description of any supplement (eg, blood agar).

Agar is a convienient gelling agent

Separation of bacteria may be accomplished by using a sterile wire loop to spread a small sample over the surface of an agar plate in a structured pattern called **plate streaking.** Bacteria well separated from others grow as isolated colonies, often reaching 2 to 3 mm in diameter after overnight incubation. For diagnostic work, growth of bacteria on solid media has advantages over the use of broth cultures. It allows isolation of bacteria in pure culture (Fig 14–4), because a colony well separated from others can be assumed to arise from a single organism or an organism cluster (colony-forming unit). Colonies vary greatly in size, shape, texture, color, and other features. For example, colonies of organisms possessing large polysaccharide capsules are usually mucoid; those of organisms that fail to separate after division are frequently granular. Colonies from different species or genera often differ substantially, whereas those derived from the same strain are usually consistent. Differences in **colonial morphology** are very useful for separating bacteria in mixtures and as clues to their identity. Some examples of colonial morphology are shown in Figure 14–5.

Bacteria may be separated in isolated colinies on agar plates

Colonies may have consistent and characterisitic features

New methods that do not depend on visual changes in the growth medium or colony formation are also used to detect bacterial growth in culture. These techniques include optical, chemical, and electrical changes in the medium, produced by the growing numbers of bacterial cells or their metabolic products. Many of these methods are more sensitive than classical techniques and thus can detect growth hours, or even days, earlier than clas-

Optical, chemical, and electrical methods can detect growth

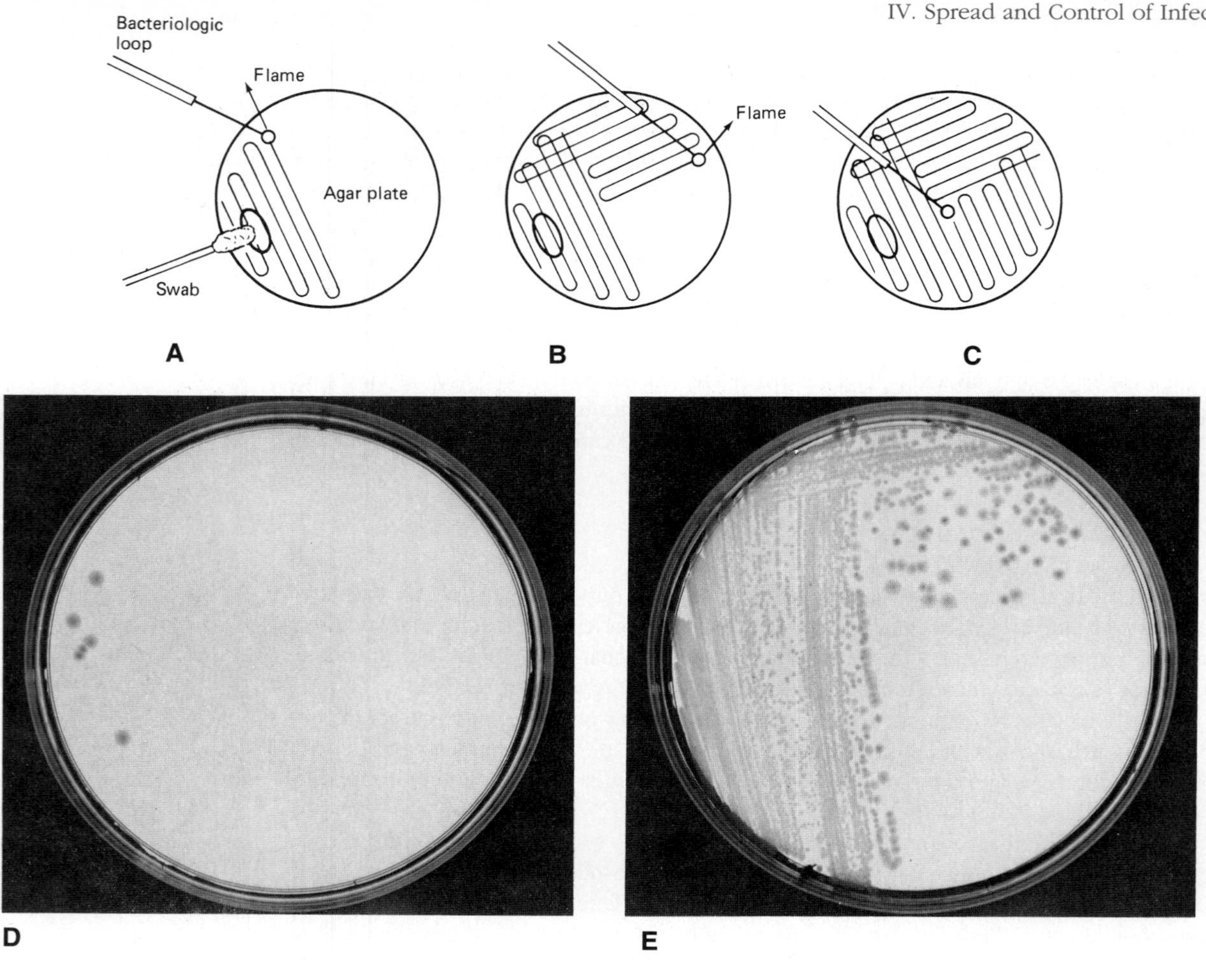


**Figure 14–4.** Bacteriologic plate streaking. Plate streaking is essentially a dilution procedure. **A.** The specimen is placed on the plate with a swab, loop, or pipette, and evenly spread over approximately one-fourth of the plate surface with a sterilized bacteriologic loop. **B.** The loop is flamed to remove residual bacteria. A secondary streak is made, overlapping the primary streak initially but finishing independently. **C.** The process is repeated in a tertiary streak. **D.** and **E.** Two plates streaked in a similar manner. **D.** Only a few bacteria grew. **E.** A large number of bacteria grew. In each case, however, isolated colonies were produced for further study.

sical methods. Some have also been engineered for instrumentation and automation. For example, one fully automated system that detects bacterial metabolism fluorometrically can complete a bacterial identification and antimicrobial susceptibility test in 2 to 4 hours.

Bacteriologic Media. Over the past 100 years, countless media have been developed by bacteriologists to aid in the isolation and identification of medically important bacteria. Only a few have found their way into routine use in clinical laboratories. These may be classified as nutrient, selective, or indicator media.

Media to grow the widest range of bacteria prepared from animal or plant products

- **Nutrient media.** The nutrient component of a medium is designed to satisfy the growth requirements of bacteria to permit isolation and propagation. For medical purposes, the ideal medium would allow rapid growth of all bacteria. No such medium exists; however, several suffice for good growth of most medically important bacteria. These media are prepared with enzymatic or acid digests of animal or plant products such as muscle, milk, or beans. The digest reduces the native protein to a mixture of polypeptides and amino acids that also includes trace metals, coenzymes, and various undefined growth factors. For example, one common broth contains a pancreatic digest of casein (milk curd) and a papaic digest of soybean meal. To this nutrient base, salts, vitamins, or body fluids such as serum may be added to provide pathogens with the conditions needed for optimum growth.

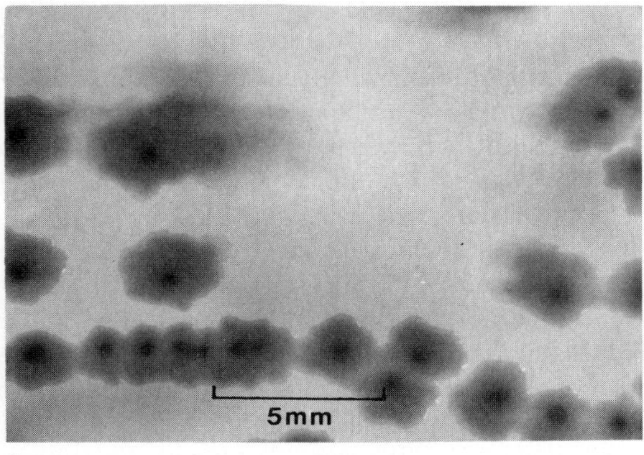


A

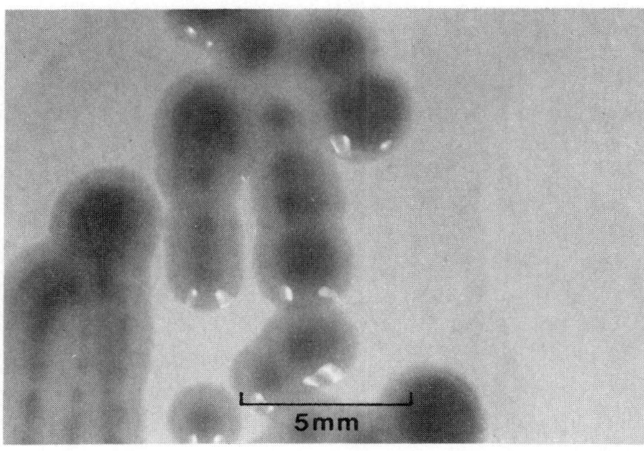


B

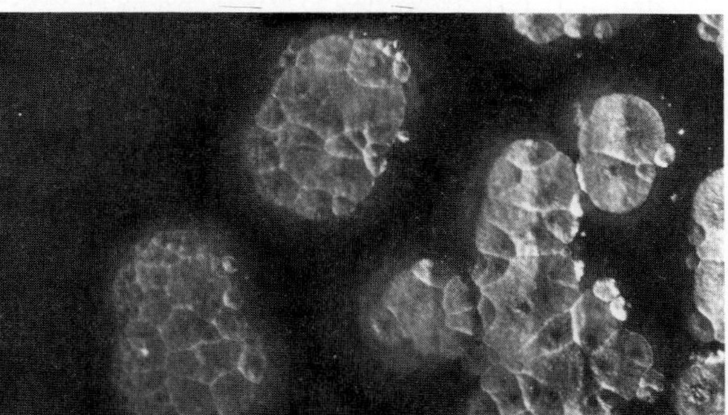


C

**Figure 14–5.** Bacterial colonial morphology. The colonies formed on agar plates by three different Gram-negative bacilli are shown at the same magnification. Each is typical for its species but variations are common. **A.** *Escherichia coli* colonies are flat with an irregular scalloped edge. **B.** *Klebsiella pneumoniae* colonies with a smooth entire edge and a raised glistening surface. **C.** *Pseudomonas aeruginosa* colonies with an irregular reflective surface suggesting hammered metal.

- **Selective media.** Selective media are used when specific pathogenic organisms are sought in sites with an extensive normal flora (for example, *N. gonorrhoeae* in specimens from the uterine cervix or rectum). In these cases, other bacteria may overgrow the suspected etiologic species in simple nutrient media, either because the pathogen grows more slowly or because it is present in much smaller numbers. Selective media usually contain dyes, other chemical additives, or antimicrobics at concentrations designed to inhibit to contaminating flora but not the suspected pathogen.

Unwanted organisms can be inhibited with chemicals or antimicrobics

- **Indicator media.** Indicator media contain substances designed to demonstrate biochemical or other features characteristic of specific pathogens or organism groups. The addition to the medium of one or more carbohydrates and a **pH indicator** is frequently employed. A color change in a colony indicates the presence of acid products and thus of fermentation or oxidation of the carbohydrate by the organism. Other indicator media may enhance the production of a **pigment** or other changes useful for early recognition of certain bacteria. The addition of red blood cells to plates allows the **hemolysis** produced by some organisms to be used as a differential feature (see Chapter 16). In practice, nutrient, selective, and indicator properties are often combined to various degrees in the same medium. It is possible to include an indicator system in a highly nutrient medium and also make it selective by adding appropriate antibimicrobics. Some examples of culture media commonly used in diagnostic bacteriology are listed in Appendix 14–1, and more details of their constitution and application are provided in Appendix 14–2.

Selected properties of bacteria demonstrated by incorporation of substrate in medium

Cultural Conditions. Once inoculated, most cultures are placed in an incubator with temperature maintained at 35 to 37°C. Slightly higher or lower temperatures are used occasionally to selectively favor a certain organism or organism group. For example, **Listeria**

**monocytogenes** (Chapter 17) is able to grow in the cold and will outgrow most competitors at 4°C. Most bacteria that are not obligate anaerobes will grow in air; however, $CO_2$ is required by some and enhances the growth of others. Incubators that maintain a 2 to 5% concentration of $CO_2$ in air are frequently used for primary isolation, because this level is not harmful to any bacteria and improves isolation of some. A simpler method is the candle jar, in which a lighted candle is allowed to burn to extinction in a sealed jar containing plates. This method adds 1 to 2% $CO_2$ to the atmosphere.

Incubation temperature and atmosphere can be selective

**Anaerobic incubation** is a special case: Strictly anaerobic bacteria will not grow under the conditions described previously, and many will die if exposed to atmospheric oxygen or high oxidation-reduction potentials. Most medically important anaerobes will grow in the depths of liquid or semisolid media containing any of a variety of **reducing agents,** such as cysteine, thioglycollate, ascorbic acid, or even iron filings. An anaerobic environment for incubation of plates can be achieved by replacing air with a gas mixture containing hydrogen, $CO_2$, and nitrogen and allowing the hydrogen to react with residual oxygen on a catalyst to form water. A convenient commercial system accomplishes this chemically in a packet to which water is added before the jar is sealed. Specimens suspected to contain significant anaerobes need to be processed under conditions designed to minimize exposure to atmospheric oxygen at all stages.

Anaerobes require reducing conditions and protection from oxygen

Routine laboratory systems for processing specimens from various sites are needed because no single medium or atmosphere is ideal for all bacteria. Combinations of broth and solid-plated media and aerobic, $CO_2$, and anaerobic incubation must be matched to the organisms expected at any particular site or clinical circumstance. Examples of such routines are shown in Table 14–2. In general, it is not practical to routinely include specialized media for isolation of rare organisms such as *Corynebacterium diphtheriae.* For detection of these and other uncommon organisms, the laboratory must be informed by the physician in advance of their possibility. Appropriate media and procedures can then be included.

Routine systems designed for the most common organisms

### Bacterial Identification

Once growth is detected in any medium, the process of identification begins. Identification involves the use of methods to obtain pure cultures from single colonies, followed by tests designed to characterize and identify the isolate. The exact tests and their sequences vary with different groups of organisms, and the taxonomic level (genus, species, subspecies, and so on) of identification needed varies according to the medical usefulness of the information. In some cases, only a general description or the exclusion of particular organisms is important. For example, a report of "mixed oral flora" in a sputum spec-

**TABLE 14–2. ROUTINE USE OF GRAM SMEAR AND ISOLATION SYSTEMS FOR SELECTED CLINICAL SPECIMENS[a]**

| Medium (Incubation) | Specimen | | | | | | | |
|---|---|---|---|---|---|---|---|---|
| | *Blood* | *Cerebrospinal Fluid* | *Wound, Pus* | *Genital, Cervix* | *Throat* | *Sputum* | *Urine* | *Stool* |
| Gram smear | | X | X | X | | X | X | |
| Soybean–Casein digest broth ($CO_2$) | X | X | X | | | | | |
| Selenite F broth (air) | | | | | | | | X |
| Blood agar ($CO_2$) | | X | X | X | | X | X | |
| Blood agar (anaerobic) | | | X | | X[b] | | | |
| MacConkey agar (air) | | | X | X | | X | X | X |
| Chocolate agar ($CO_2$) | | X | X | X | | X | | |
| Martin–Lewis agar ($CO_2$) | | | | X | | | | |
| Hektoen agar (air) | | | | | | | | X |
| Campylobacter agar ($CO_2$, 42°C)[c] | | | | | | | | X |

[a] The added sensitivity of a nutrient broth is used only when contamination by normal flora is unlikely. Exact media and isolation systems may vary between laboratories.
[b] Anaerobic incubation used to enhance hemolysis by β-hemolytic streptococci.
[c] Incubation in a reduced oxygen atmosphere.

imen or "no *Neisseria gonorrhoeae*" in a cervical specimen may provide all of the information needed.

### Features Used to Classify Bacteria

- **Cultural characteristics.** Cultural characteristics include the demonstration of properties such as unique nutritional requirements, pigment production, and the ability to grow in the presence of certain substances (sodium chloride, bile) or on certain media (MacConkey, nutrient agar). Demonstration of the ability to grow at a particular temperature or to cause hemolysis on blood agar plates is also used.

Growth under various conditions has differential value

- **Biochemical characteristics.** The ability to attack various substrates or to produce particular metabolic products has broad application to the identification of bacteria. The most common properties examined are listed in Appendix 14–3. Biochemical and cultural tests for bacterial identification are analyzed by reference to tables that show the reaction patterns characteristic for individual species. In fact, advances in computer analysis have now been applied to identification of many bacterial and fungal groups. These systems employ the same biochemical principles, but use computerized databases to determine the most probable identification from the observed test pattern.

Biochemical reactions analysed by tables and computers give identification probability

- **Demonstrations of toxin production and pathogenicity.** Direct evidence of virulence in laboratory animals is rarely needed to confirm a clinical diagnosis. In some diseases caused by production of a specific toxin, the toxin may be detected in vitro through cell cultures or immunologic methods. Neutralization of the toxic effect with specific antitoxin is the usual approach to identify the toxin.

Detection of specific toxin may define disease

- **Antigenic structure.** As discussed in Chapter 2, bacteria possess many antigens, such as capsular polysaccharides, flagellar proteins, and several cell wall components. Serology involves the use of antibodies of known specificity to detect antigens present on whole bacteria or free in bacterial extracts (soluble antigens). The methods used for demonstrating antigen–antibody reactions are discussed in a later section.

Antigenic structures of organism detected with antisera

- **Genomic structure.** Nucleic acid sequence relatedness as determined by homology comparisons have become a primary determinant of taxonomic decisions. They are discussed later in the section on nucleic acid methods.

## Isolation and Identification of Viruses

### Cell and Organ Culture

Living cell cultures that can support their replication are the primary means of isolating pathogenic viruses. The cells are derived from a tissue source by outgrowth of cells from a tissue fragment (explant) or by dispersal with proteolytic agents such as trypsin. They are allowed to grow in nutrient media on a glass or plastic surface until a confluent layer one cell thick (monolayer) is achieved. In some circumstances, a tissue fragment with a specialized function (for example, fetal trachea with ciliated epithelial cells) is cultivated in vitro and used for viral detection. This procedure is known as organ culture.

Cell cultures derived from human or animal tissues used to isolate viruses

Three basic types of cell culture monolayers are used in diagnostic virology. The **primary cell culture,** in which all cells have a normal chromosome count (diploid), is derived from the initial growth of cells from a tissue source. Redispersal and regrowth produces a **secondary cell culture,** which usually retains characteristics similar to those of the primary culture (diploid chromosome count and virus susceptibility). Monkey and human embryonic kidney cell cultures are examples of commonly used primary and secondary cell cultures.

Monkey kidney used in primary and secondary culture

Further dispersal and regrowth of secondary cell cultures usually leads to one of two outcomes: the cells eventually die, or they undergo spontaneous transformation, in which the growth characteristics change, the chromosome count varies (haploid or heteroploid), and the susceptibility to virus infection differs from that of the original. These cell cultures have characteristics of "immortality"; that is, they can be redispersed and regrown many times (serial cell culture passage). They can also be derived from cancerous tissue cells or produced by exposure to mutagenic agents in vitro. Such cultures are commonly called **cell lines.** A common cell line in diagnostic use is the *Hep*-2, derived from a human epithelial carcinoma.

Primary cultures either die out or transform

Cells from cancerous tissue may grow continuously

A third type of culture is often termed a **cell strain.** This culture comprises diploid

Cell strains regrow a limited number of times

cells, commonly fibroblastic, that can be redispersed and regrown a finite number of times; usually 30 to 40 cell culture passages can be made before the strain dies out or spontaneously transforms. Human embryonic tonsil and lung fibroblasts are common cell strains in routine diagnostic use.

#### Detection of Viral Growth

Viral CPE due to morphologic changes or cell death

CPE characteristic for virus

Viral growth in susceptible cell cultures can be detected in several ways. The most common effect is seen with lytic or cytopathic viruses; as they replicate in cells, they produce alterations in cellular morphology (or cell death) that can be observed directly by light microscopy under low magnification (×30 or ×100). This **cytopathic effect (CPE)** varies with different viruses in different cell cultures. For example, enteroviruses often produce cell rounding, pleomorphism, and eventual cell death in various culture systems, whereas measles and respiratory syncytial viruses cause fusion of cells to produce multinucleated giant cells (syncytia). The microscopic appearance of some normal cell cultures and the CPE produced in them by different viruses are illustrated in Figure 14–6.

Hemadsorption or interference mark cells that may not show CPE

Other viruses may be detected in cell culture by their ability to produce **hemagglutinins.** These hemagglutinins may be present on the infected cell membranes, as well as in the culture media, as a result of release of free, hemagglutinating virions from the cells. Addition of erythrocytes to the infected cell culture will result in their adherence to the cell surfaces, a phenomenon known as **hemadsorption.** Another method of viral detection in cell culture is by **interference.** In this situation, the virus that infects the susceptible cell culture produces no CPE or hemagglutinin, but can be detected by "challenging" the cell culture with a different virus that normally produces a characteristic CPE. The second, or challenge, virus fails to infect the cell culture because of interference by the first virus, which is thus detected. This method is obviously cumbersome, but has been applied to the detection of rubella virus in certain cell cultures.

Immunologic or genomic probes detect some viruses

For some agents, such as Epstein–Barr virus (EBV) or human immunodeficiency virus (HIV), even more novel approaches may be applied. Both EBV and HIV can replicate in vitro in suspension cultures of normal human lymphocytes such as those derived from neonatal cord blood. Their presence may be determined in several ways; for example, EBV-infected B lymphocytes and HIV-infected T lymphocytes will express virus-specified antigens and viral DNA, which can be detected with immunologic or genomic probes. In addition, HIV reverse transcriptase can be detected in cell culture by specific assay methods.

Immunologic and nucleic acid probes (see below) can also be used to detect virus in clinical specimens or in situations where only incomplete, noninfective virus replication has occurred in vivo or in vitro. An example is the use of in situ cytohybridization, whereby specific labeled nucleic acid probes are used to detect and localize papillomavirus genomes in tissues where neither infectious virus nor its antigens can be detected.

#### In Vivo Isolation Methods

*In vivo* methods for isolation are also sometimes necessary. The embryonated hen's egg is still used for the initial isolation and propagation of influenza A virus. It is also required for isolation of influenza C virus, which grows poorly in cell cultures. Virus-containing material is inoculated on the appropriate egg membrane, and the egg is incubated to permit viral replication and recognition.

Embryonated eggs and animals required for isolation of some viruses

Animal inoculation is still used for detecting some viruses. The usual animal host for viral isolation is the mouse; suckling mice in the first 48 hours of life are especially susceptible to many viruses. Evidence for viral replication is based on the development of illness, manifested by such signs as paralysis, convulsions, poor feeding, or death. The nature of the infecting virus can be further elucidated by histologic and immunofluorescent examination of tissues or by detection of specific antibody responses. Many arboviruses and rabies virus are detected in this system.

Specimen preparation required

Viral isolation from a suspect case involves a number of steps. First, the viruses believed most likely to be involved in the illness are considered, and appropriate specimens are collected. Centrifugation or filtration and addition of antimicrobics are frequently required with respiratory or fecal specimens to remove organic matter, cellular debris, bacteria, and fungi, which can interfere with viral isolation. The specimens are then inoculated

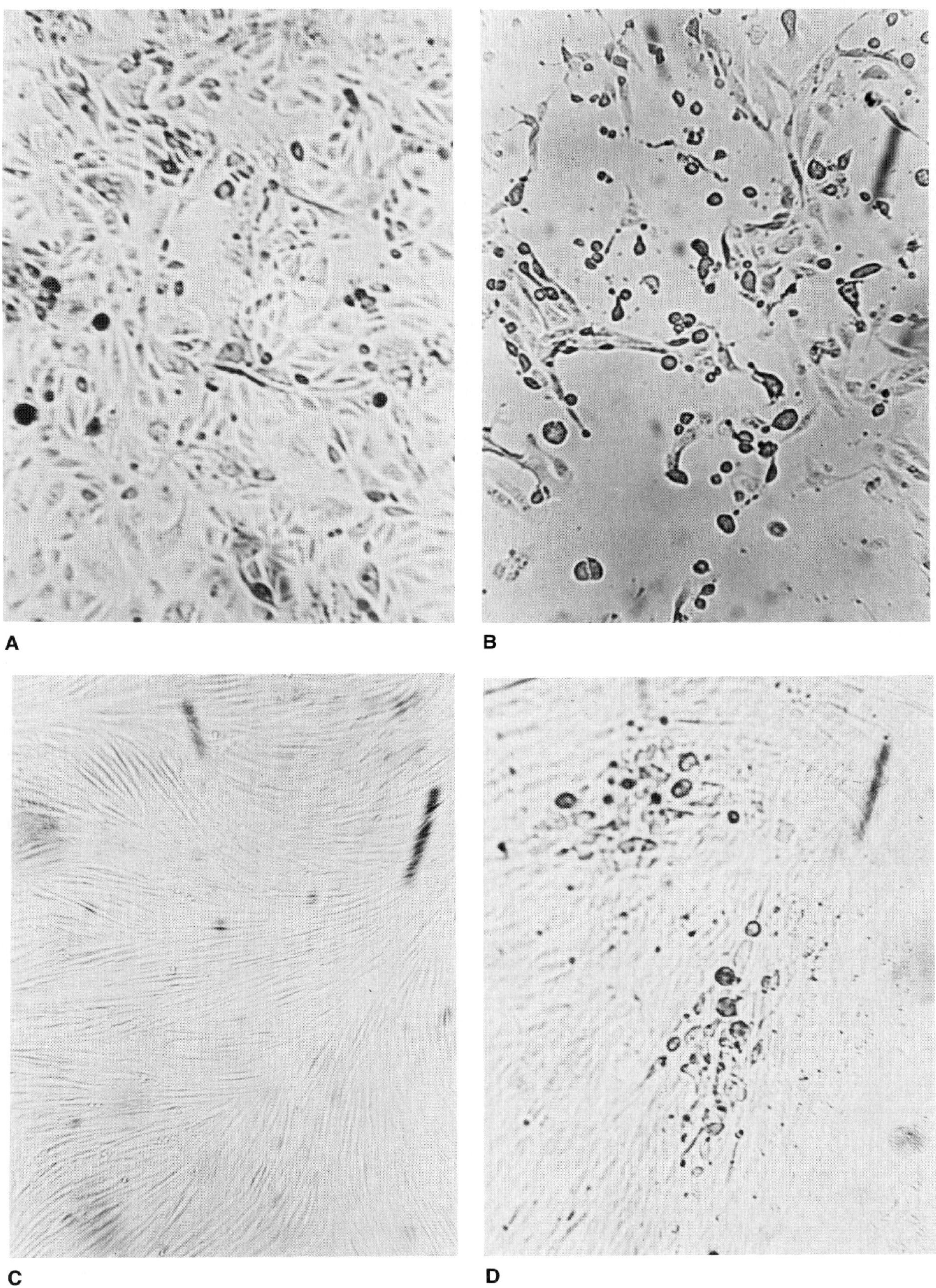


**Figure 14–6. A.** Normal monkey kidney cell culture monolayer. **B.** Enterovirus cytopathic effect in a monkey kidney cell monolayer. Note cell lysis and monolayer destruction. **C.** Normal human diploid fibroblast cell monolayer. **D.** Cytomegalovirus cytopathic effect in human diploid cell monolayer. Note rounded, swollen cells in a focal area. (A–D × 40.)

into the appropriate cell culture systems. The time between inoculation and initial detection of viral effects varies; for most viruses, however, positive cultures are usually apparent within 5 days of collection. With proper collection methods and application of the diagnostic tools discussed later, many infections can even be detected within hours. On the other hand, some viruses may require culture for a month or more before they can be detected.

### Viral Identification

Nature of CPE and cell cultures affected may suggest virus

**Effect on Cell Cultures.** Upon isolation, a virus can usually be tentatively identified to the family or genus level by its cultural characteristics (for example, type of CPE produced). Confirmation and further identification may require enhancement of viral growth to produce adequate quantities for testing. This result may be achieved by inoculation of the original isolate into fresh culture systems (viral passage) to amplify replication of the virus, as well as improve its adaptation to growth in the in vitro system.

Neutralization of biologic effect with specific antisera confirms identification

**Neutralization and Serologic Detection.** Of the several ways to identify the isolate, the most common is to neutralize its infectivity by mixing it with specific antibody to known viruses before inoculation into cultures. The inhibition of the expected viral effects on the cell culture such as CPE or hemagglutination is then evidence for that virus. As in bacteriology, demonstration of specific viral antigens is an important parameter for identifying the agent. In fact, it assumes even greater importance in virology, because viruses have a more limited number of parameters on which to base their identification. Immunofluorescence and enzyme immunoassay (EIA) are the most common methods.

Inclusions and giant cells suggestive

- **Cytology and histology.** In some instances, viruses will produce specific cytologic changes in infected host tissues that aid in diagnosis. Examples include specific intranuclear inclusions (herpes, Fig 14–7); cytoplasmic inclusions; and cell fusion, which results in multinucleated epithelial giant cells (chickenpox, Fig 14–8). Although such findings are useful when seen, their overall diagnostic sensitivity and specificity are usually considerably less than those of the other methods discussed.

Immune electron microscopy shows agglutination of viral particles

- **Electron microscopy.** When virions are present in sufficient numbers, they may be further characterized by specific agglutination of viral particles upon mixture with type-specific antiserum. This technique, immune electron microscopy, can be used to identify viral antigens specifically or to detect antibody in serum using viral particles of known antigenicity.

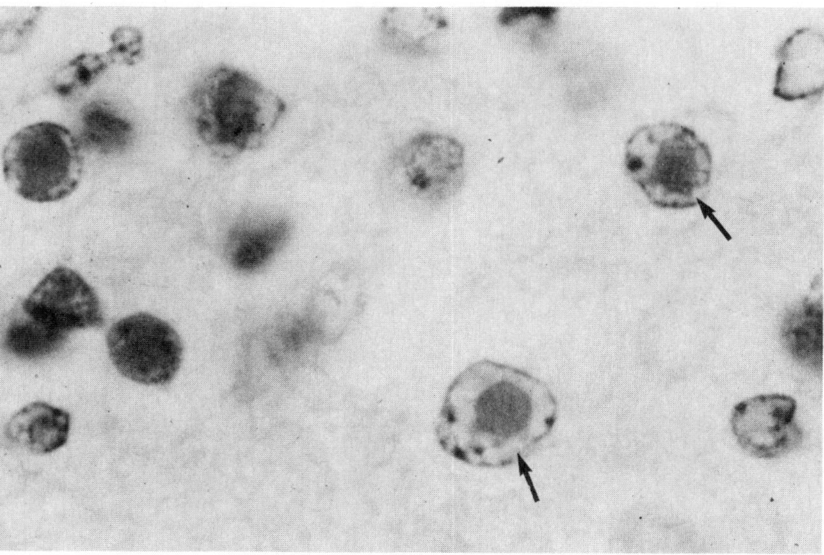

**Figure 14–7.** Brain biopsy from a patient with herpes simplex encephalitis. Arrows indicate infected neuronal nuclei with marginated chromatin and typical intranuclear inclusions. The cytoplasmic membranes are not clearly seen in this preparation (hematoxylin–eosin stain; × 400).

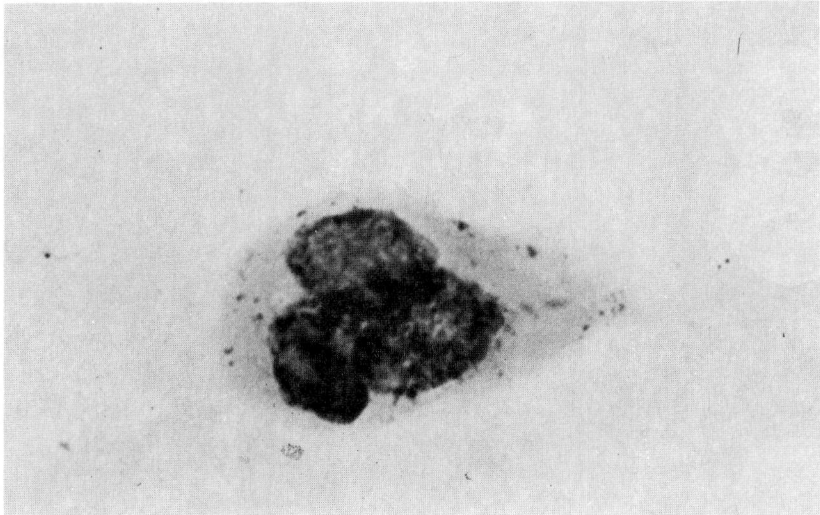

**Figure 14–8.** Multinucleated epithelial cells from a vesicle scraping of a patient with chickenpox. Cell fusion of this type can be seen with both varicella-zoster and herpes simplex infections (Wright's stain; × 400).

Some viruses (for example, human rotaviruses, hepatitis A and B viruses) grow poorly or not at all in the laboratory culture systems currently available. These viruses have been demonstrated in some instances by inoculation of susceptible volunteers, and some will replicate and cause disease in subhuman primates such as chimpanzees. Obviously, such methods of cultivation cannot be used in routine diagnosis.

## Antigen and Antibody Detection in Diagnostic Microbiology

Diagnostic microbiology makes great use of the specificity of the binding between antigen and antibody. Antisera of known specificity are used to detect their homologous antigen in cultures, or more recently, directly in body fluids. Conversely, known antigen preparations are used to detect circulating antibodies as evidence of a current or previous infection with that agent. Many methods are in use to demonstrate the antigen–antibody binding. The greatly improved specificity of **monoclonal antibodies** has had a major impact on the quality of methods where they have been applied. Before discussing their application to diagnosis, the principles involved in the most important methods will now be discussed.

### Direct Methods

#### Precipitin Tests

Antigen–antibody precipitates demonstrated by immunodiffusion and CIE

When antigen and antibody combine in the proper proportions, a visible precipitate is formed (Fig 14–9A). Optimum antigen–antibody ratios can be produced by allowing one to diffuse into the other, most commonly through an agar matrix **(immunodiffusion).** In the immunodiffusion procedure, wells are cut in the agar and filled with antigen and antibody. One or more precipitin lines may be formed between the antigen and antibody wells; depending on the number of different antigen–antibody reactions occurring. **Counterimmunoelectrophoresis** (CIE) is immunodiffusion carried out in an electrophoretic field. The net effect is that antigen and antibody are rapidly brought together in the space between the wells to form a precipitin line. Both the speed and the sensitivity of immunodiffusion are improved by CIE.

#### Agglutination

RBCs and latex particles coated with antigen or antibody

The amount of antigen or antibody necessary to produce a visible immunologic reaction can be reduced if either is on the surface of a relatively large particle. This condition can be produced by fixing soluble antigens or antibody onto the surface of red blood cells or micro-

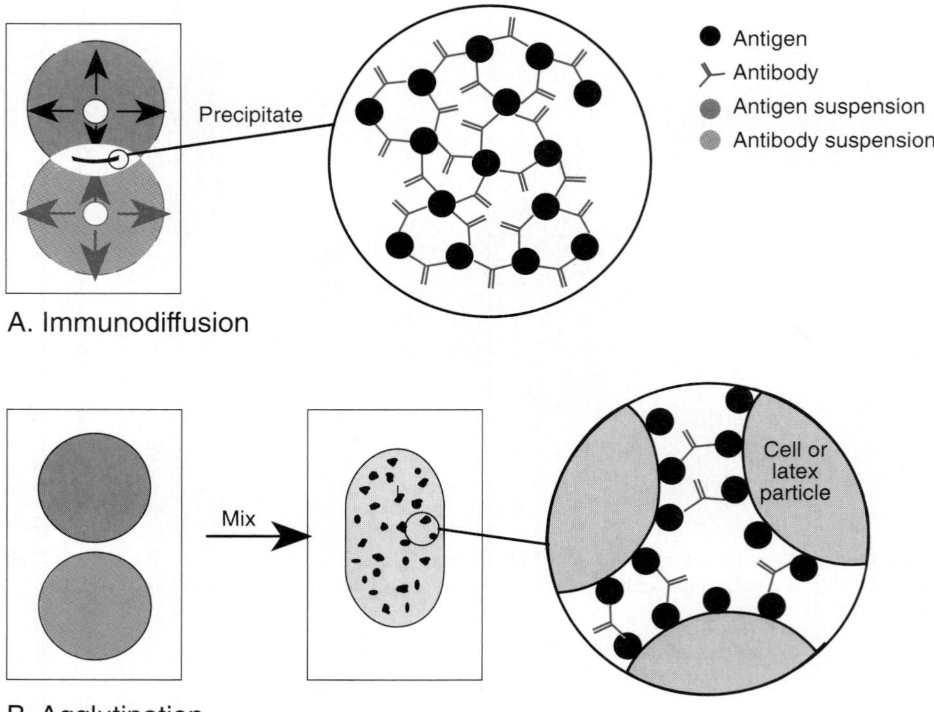


**Figure 14–9.** Immunodiffusion and agglutination. **A.** In immunodiffusion the antigen and antibody diffuse through a support matrix (eg, agarose). Where they reach optimal proportions a precipitin line is formed by the antigen–antibody complex. **B.** In agglutination the antigen–antibody reaction can be seen because one is on the surface of a relatively large particle. In the figure the antigen is bound to the particle, but the reaction could be reversed.

Simple mixing on slide causes agglutination

scopic latex particles (Fig 14–9B). Whole bacteria are large enough to serve as the particle if the antigen is present on the microbial surface. The relative proportions of antigen and antibody thus become less critical, and antigen–antibody reactions are detectable by agglutination when immune serum and particulate antigen, or particle-associated antibody and soluble antigen, are mixed on a slide. The process is termed bacterial agglutination, passive hemagglutination, or latex agglutination depending on the nature of the sensitized particle. A variant of this procedure, coagglutination, uses the unique ability of staphylococcal protein A on the surface of killed *Staphylococcus aureus* cells to bind the *Fc* fragment of IgG, leaving the *Fab* portions free to react with homologous antigen.

### Neutralization

Bacterium, virus, toxin mixed with antibody prior to addition to test system

Neutralization as commonly employed takes some observable function of the agent, such as cytopathic effect of viruses or the action of a bacterial toxin, and neutralizes it. This is usually done by first reacting the agent with antibody, and then placing the antigen–antibody mixture into the test system. The steps involved are illustrated in Figure 14–10. In viral neutralization, a single antibody molecule can bind to surface components of the extracellular virus and interfere with one of the initial events of the viral multiplication cycle (adsorption, penetration, or uncoating). Some bacterial and viral agents directly bind to red blood cells (hemagglutination). Neutralization of this reaction by antibody blocking the receptor is called hemagglutination inhibition (Fig 14–11).

### Complement Fixation

Action of complement or RBCs used as indicator system

Complement fixation assays depend on two properties of complement. The first is fixation (inactivation) of complement upon formation of antigen–antibody complexes. The second is the ability of bound complement to cause hemolysis of sheep red blood cells (RBCs) coated with anti-sheep RBC antibody (sensitized RBCs). Complement fixation assays are performed in two stages: The test system reacts the antigen and antibody in the presence of

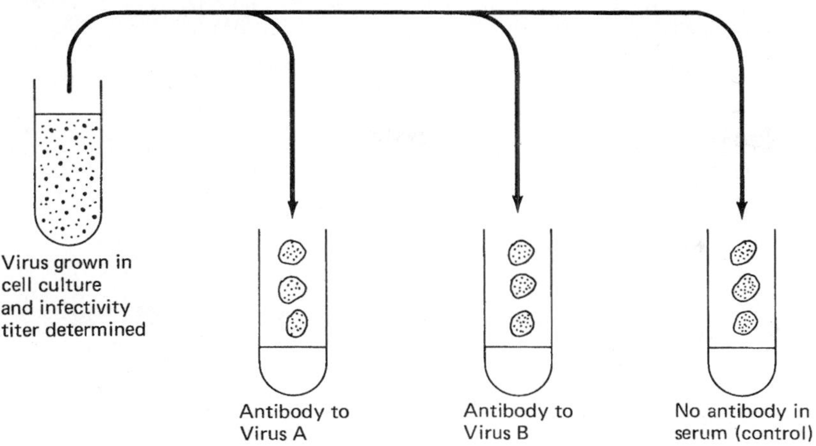


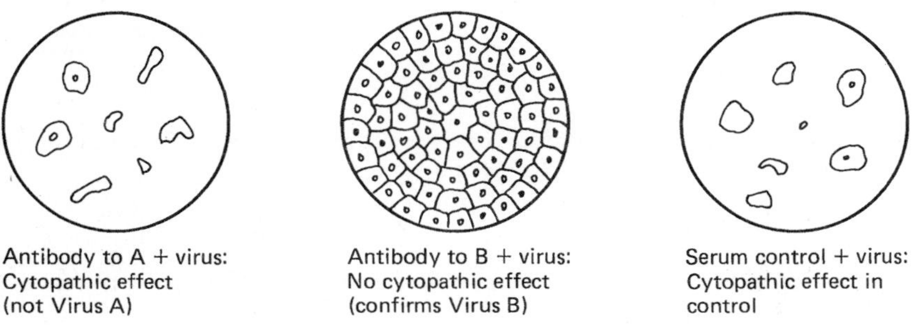


**Figure 14–10.** Identification of a virus isolate (cytopathic virus) as "Virus B."

complement; the indicator system, which contains the sensitized RBCs, detects residual complement. Hemolysis indicates that complement was present in the indicator system and therefore that antigen–antibody complexes were not formed in the test system. Primarily used to detect and quantitate antibody, complement fixation is gradually being replaced by simpler methods.

Complement fixation being replaced

## Labeling Methods

Detection of antigen–antibody binding may be enhanced by attaching a label to one (usually the antibody) and detecting the label after removal of unbound reagents. The label may be a fluorescent dye (immunofluorescence), a radioisotope **(radioimmunoassay,** or **RIA),** or an enzyme **(enzyme immunoassay,** or **EIA)**. The presence or quantitation of antigen–antibody binding is measured by fluorescence, radioactivity, or the chemical reaction catalysed by the enzyme.

### Immunofluorescence

The most common labeling method in diagnostic microbiology is immunofluorescence (Fig 14–12), in which antibody labeled with a fluorescent dye, usually **fluorescein isothiocyanate (FITC)**, is applied to a slide of material that may contain the antigen sought. Under fluorescence microscopy, binding of the labeled antibody can be detected as a bright green halo surrounding bacterium, or in the case of viruses, as a fluorescent clump in an infected cell. The method is called "direct" if the FITC is conjugated directly to the antibody with the desired specificity. In "indirect" immunofluorescence the specific antibody is not labeled, but its binding to an antigen is detected in an additional step using an FITC-labeled

Labeled antibody binding to antigen viewed by fluorescence microscopy

Use of direct vs. indirect methods purely technical

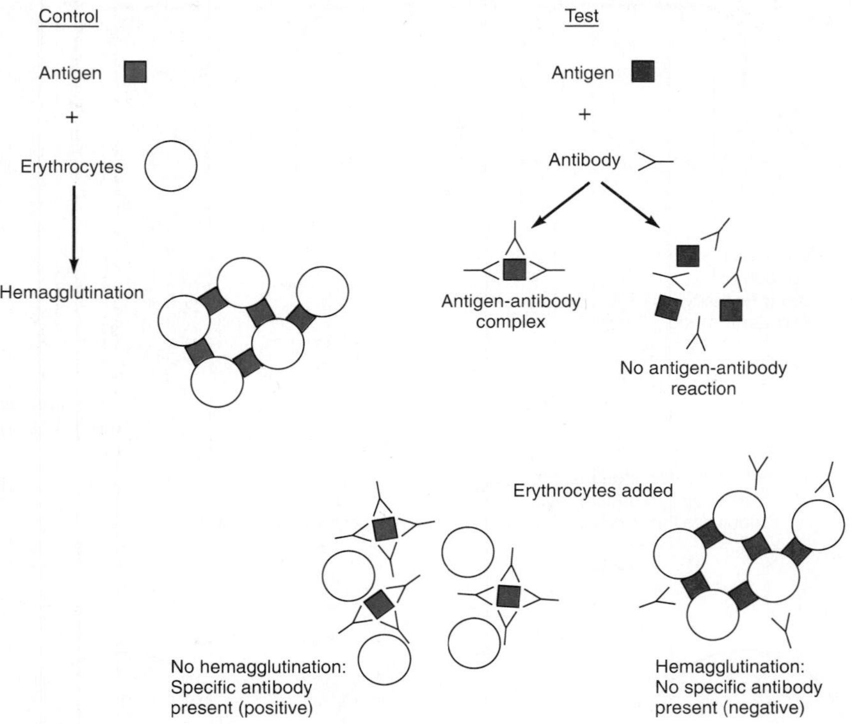


**Figure 14–11.** Hemagglutination inhibition for antibody detection (used when antigen agglutinates erythrocytes).

anti-immunoglobulin antibody of appropriate specificity. Choice between the two approaches involves purely technical considerations.

### Radioimmunoassay (RIA) and Enzyme Immunoassay (EIA)

Liquid phase RIA and EIA methods have many vairants

The labels used in RIA and EIA are more suitable for liquid phase assays and are particularly used in virology. They are also used in direct and indirect methods and many other ingenious variations such as the "sandwich" methods, so called because the antigen of interest is "trapped" between two antibodies (Fig 14–12C). These extremely sensitive techniques will be discussed further with regard to antibody detection.

Antigenic systems must be worked out before diagnostics can be applied

Before these techniques can be applied to the diagnosis of specific infectious diseases, considerable study of the causative agent(s) is required. Antigen–antibody systems may vary in complexity from a single epitope to scores of epitopes on several macromolecular antigens whose chemical nature may or may not be known. The cause of the original 1976 outbreak of Legionnaire's disease (*Legionella pneumophila*, Chapter 25) was proven through the development of immune reagents that detected the bacteria in tissue and antibodies directed against the bacteria in the serum of patients. Now, almost 20 years later, there are more than a dozen serotypes and many additional species, each requiring specific immunologic reagents for antigen or antibody detection for diagnosis. Each infectious agent has its own state of knowledge (or ignorance) of antigenic composition.

### Antigen Detection in Culture Isolates

Serologic classification primarily of epidemiologic value

For most important antigens of diagnostic significance, antisera are commercially available. The most common test methods for bacteria are agglutination and immunofluorescence; and for viruses, neutralization. In most cases these methods serve to subclassify organisms below the species level, and thus are primarily of value for epidemiologic and research pur-

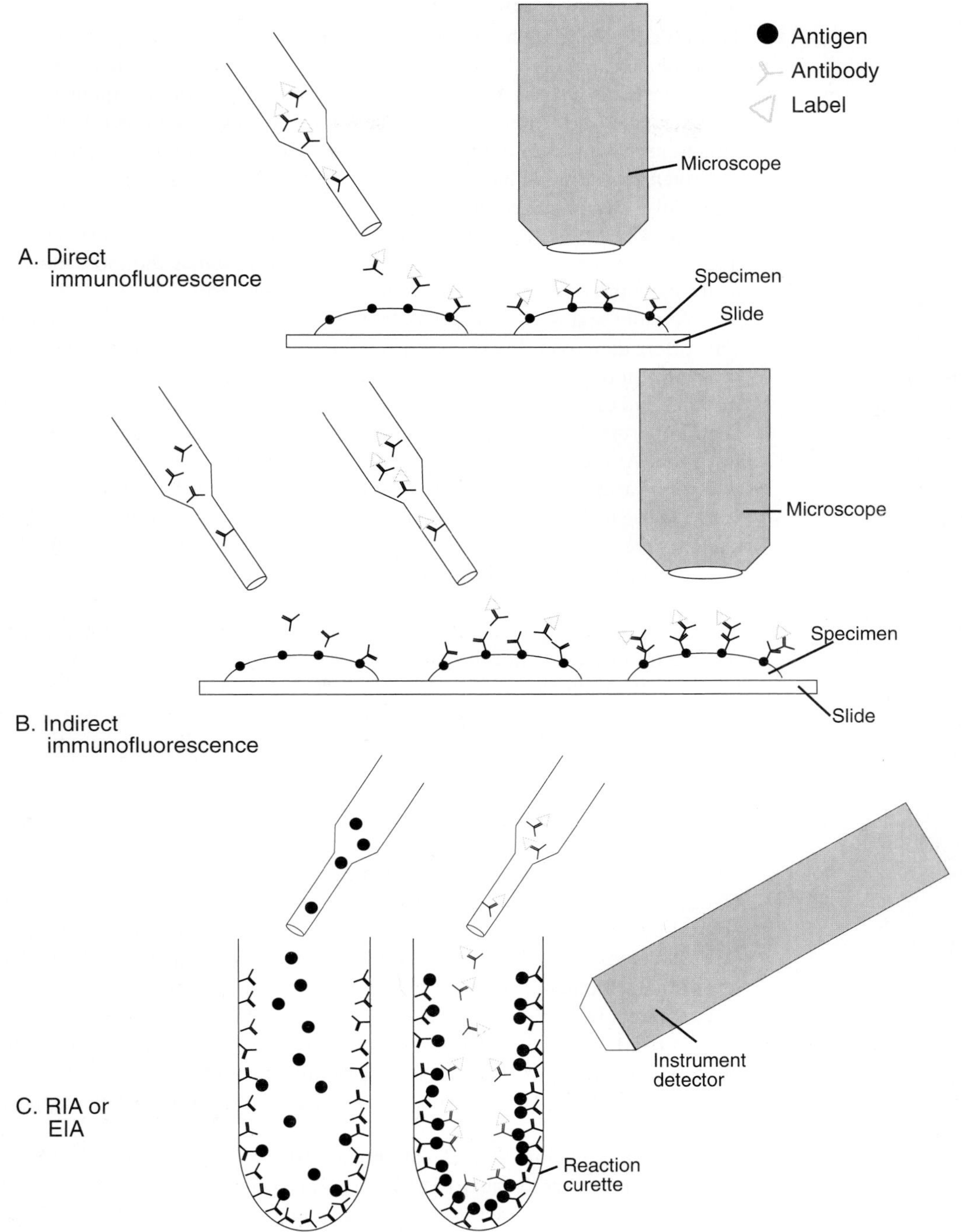


**Figure 14–12.** Labeling methods. **A.** In direct immunofluorescence the fluorescent compound is bound to the specific antibody and can be visualized as shown in Figure 14–2C. **B.** Indirect immunofluorescence has an extra step because the specific antibody is unlabeled. Its binding is detected by a second labeled antiglobulin antibody. **C.** A liquid phase immunoassay is shown. The antigen is "sandwiched" between an antibody bound to the tube and the labeled antibody. If the label is radioactive this is called radioimmunoassay (RIA), and if it is an enzyme it is called enzyme immunoassay (EIA). Many variations are possible.

poses. The terms "serotype" or "serogroup" are used together with numbers, letters, or Roman numerals with no apparent logic other than historical precedent. For a few genera the most fundamental taxonomic differentiation is serologic. This is the case with the streptococci (Chapter 16), where an existing classification based on biochemical and cultural characteristics was superseded because a serologic classification scheme developed by Rebecca Lancefield correlated better with disease.

Serologic classification of primary importance with Streptococci

Antigen Detection in Body Fluids or Tissues

Immunofluorescence allows direct detection of agents in clinical specimens

Generally less sensitive than culture

Theoretically, any of the methods described for detecting antigen–antibody interactions could be applied directly to clinical specimens. The most common of these is immunofluorescence, in which antigen is detected on the surface of the organism or in cells present in the infected secretion. The greatest success with this approach has been in respiratory infections where a nasopharyngeal, throat washing, sputum, or bronchoalveolar lavage specimen may contain bacteria or viral aggregates in sufficient amount to be seen microscopically. Although the fluorescent tag makes it easier to find organisms, these methods are generally not as sensitive as culture. With some genera and species, the immunofluorescent detection of antigens in clinical material provides the most rapid means of diagnosis, as with Legionella and respiratory syncytial virus.

Polysaccharide antigens released into body fluids detectable by agglutination

Another approach is to detect free antigen released by the organism into body fluids. This offers the possibility of bypassing direct examination, culture, and identification tests to achieve a diagnosis. Success requires a highly specific antibody, a sensitive detection method, and the presence of the homologous antigen in an accessible body fluid. The latter is an important limitation, because not all organisms release free antigen in the course of infection. At present, diagnosis by antigen detection is limited to some bacteria and fungi with polysaccharide capsules (eg, *Haemophilus influenzae*), *Chlamydia*, and to certain viruses. The techniques of agglutination with antibody bound to latex particles, CIE, RIA, and EIA are used to detect free antigen in serum, urine, cerebrospinal fluid, and joint fluid.

Antigen detection not affected by therapy

Live organisms are not required for antigen detection, and these tests may still be positive when the causative organism has been eliminated by antimicrobial therapy. The procedures can yield results within an hour or two, sometimes within a few minutes. This feature is attractive for office practice, because it allows diagnostic decisions to be made during the patient's visit. A number of commercial products detect group A streptococci in sore throats with over 90% sensitivity; however, because these tests are less sensitive than culture, negative results must be confirmed by culture.

Antibody Detection in Serum (Serologic Diagnosis)

Antibodies formed in response to infection

Antibodies may indicate current, recent, or past infection

During infection—whether viral, bacterial, fungal, or parasitic—the host usually responds with the formation of antibodies, which can be detected by modification of any of the methods used for antigen detection. The formation of antibodies and their time course depends on the antigenic stimulation provided by the infection. The precise patterns vary depending on the antigens used, classes of antibody detected, and method. An example of temporal patterns of development and increase and decline in specific antiviral antibodies measured by different tests is illustrated in Figure 14–13. These responses can be used to detect evidence of recent or past infection. The test methods do not inherently indicate immunoglobulin class but can be modified to do so, usually by pretreatment of the serum to remove IgG to differentiate the IgM and IgG responses. Several basic principles must be emphasized:

Paired specimens compared

1. In an acute infection, the antibodies usually appear early in the illness, and then rise sharply over the next 10 to 21 days. Thus, a serum sample collected shortly after the onset of illness (acute serum) and another collected 2 to 3 weeks later (convalescent serum) can be compared quantitatively for changes in specific antibody content.

Titer is the highest serum dilution demonstrating activity

2. Antibodies can be quantitated by several means. The most common method is to dilute the serum serially in appropriate media and determine the maximal dilution that will still yield detectable antibody in the test system (for example, serum dilutions of 1:4, 1:8, and 1:16). The highest dilution that retains specific activity is called the antibody titer.

Seroconversion or fourfold rise in titer most conclusive

3. The interpretation of significant antibody responses (evidence of specific, recent infection) is most reliable when definite evidence of seroconversion is demonstrated; that is, detectable specific antibody is absent from the acute serum (or pre-illness serum, if available) but present in the convalescent serum. Alternatively, a fourfold or greater increase in antibody titer supports a diagnosis of recent infection; for example, an acute serum titer of 1:4 and a convalescent serum titer of 1:16 or greater would be considered significant.
4. In instances in which the average antibody titers of a population to a specific agent

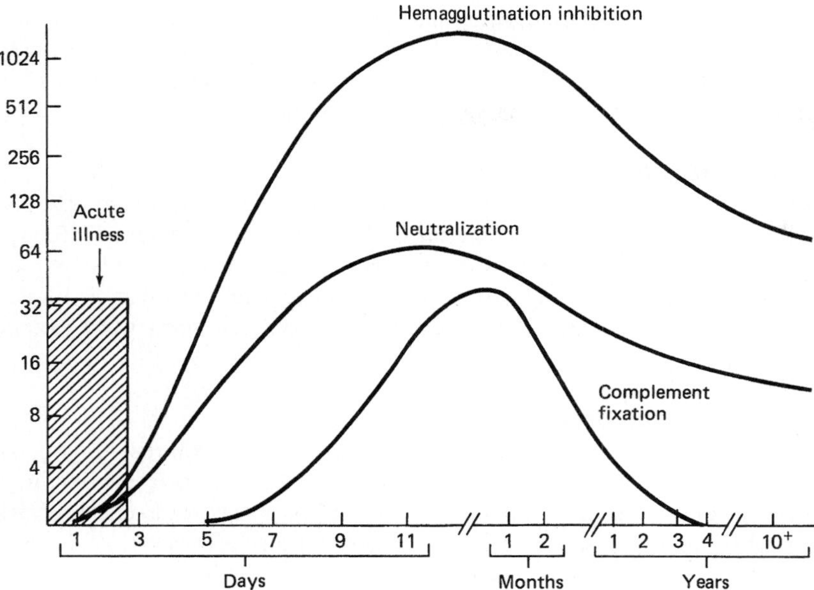


**Figure 14–13.** Examples of patterns of antibody responses to an acute infection, measured by three different methods.

are known, a single convalescent antibody titer significantly greater than the expected mean may be used as supportive or presumptive evidence of recent infection. This finding, however, is considerably less valuable than those obtained by comparing responses of acute and convalescent serum samples. An alternative and somewhat more complex method of serodiagnosis is to determine which major immunoglobulin subclass constitutes the major proportion of the specific antibodies. In primary infections, the IgM-specific response is often dominant during the first days or weeks after onset, but is replaced progressively by IgG-specific antibodies; thus, by 1 to 6 months after infection, the predominant antibodies belong to the IgG subclass. Consequently, serum containing a high titer of antibodies of the IgM subclass would suggest a recent, primary infection.

Single titers may be useful in some circumstances

IgM responses indicate acute infection

The immunologic methods used to identify bacterial or viral antigens are applied to serologic diagnosis by simply reversing the detection system: that is, using a known rather than an unknown antigen to detect the presence of an antibody. The methods of serologic diagnosis to be employed are selected on the basis of their convenience and applicability to the antigen in question. As shown in Figure 14–13, the temporal relationships of antibody response to infection vary according to the method used. Of the methods for measuring antigen–antibody interaction discussed previously, those now used most frequently for serologic diagnosis are agglutination, RIA, and EIA (Figs 14–9 and 14–11).

Western Blot. The Western blot immunoassay is another technique that is now commonly employed to detect and confirm the specificity of antibodies to a variety of epitopes. Its greatest use has been in the diagnosis of human immunodeficiency virus infections (see Chapter 41), in which virions are electrophoresed in a polyacrylamide gel to separate the protein and glycoprotein components and then transferred onto nitrocellulose. This is then incubated with patient serum and antibody to the different viral components detected by using an antihuman globulin IgG antibody conjugated with an enzyme label.

Western blot confirms specificity of antibodies for protein components of the agent (eg, HIV)

## Nucleic Acid Analysis

Analysis of the DNA or RNA of microorganisms is the basis of newer taxonomic studies, and increasingly applied to diagnostic and epidemiologic work. It is also possible to use cloned or synthesized nucleic acid probes to detect genes or smaller nucleotide sequences specific for a variety of bacterial, viral, and other infectious agents. As with antigen–antibody reactions, a variety of methods have been developed for analysis of nucleic acids. Those relevant to the study of infectious diseases are briefly summarized below. The student is referred to textbooks of molecular biology for more complete coverage.

### Nucleic Acid Extraction

DNA readily extracted from microbial cells

DNA is a hardy molecule that will withstand fairly harsh chemical treatment. RNA is more fragile primarily because it is readily digested by RNAse enzymes commonly found in biologic systems. The extraction process for bacteria and fungi involves breaking open the cells, precipitating the protein, and extracting the nucleic acid with ethanol. Viral procedures are similar except that much of the separation and concentration may be accomplished by ultracentrifugation.

### Agarose Gel Electrophoresis

Agarose gel electrophoresis separates DNA fragments or plasmids based on size

Nucleic acids may be separated in an electrophoretic field in an **agarose** (highly purified agar) gel. The speed of migration depends on size, with the smaller molecules moving faster and appearing at the bottom (end) of the gel. This method is able to separate DNA fragments in the range of 0.1 to 50 kilobases, which is far below the size of bacterial genomes but includes some naturally occurring genetic elements such as bacterial plasmids (Fig 14–14). A variant of agarose gel electrophoresis, pulsed field electrophoresis, alternates the orientation of electrical field in a fashion that allows resolution of much larger DNA fragments.

### Restriction Endonuclease Digestion

Restriction endonuclease digestion refines electrophoretic analysis of DNA

Restriction endonucleases are enzymes that recognize specific nucleotide sequences in DNA molecules and digest (cut) them at all sites at which the sequence appears. A large number of these enzymes have been isolated from bacterial strains and are commercially available together with information on the sequences they recognize. While the four- to eight-base pair sequences recognized by these endonucleases are not unique to any one organism, their spacing along the chromosome or other genomic structure may be. The size of fragments generated by endonuclease digestion of DNA molecules may be compared by agarose gel electrophoresis (Fig 14–14).

### DNA Hybridization

DNA hybridization methods allow DNA from different sources to combine

If the DNA double helix is opened, leaving single-stranded (denatured) DNA, the nucleotide bases are exposed and thus available to interact with other single-stranded nucleic acid molecules. If complementary sequences of a second DNA molecule are brought into physical contact with the first, they will hybridize to it, forming a new double-stranded molecule in that area. A variety of methods are in use that allow hybridization to take place between two or more nucleic acid molecules. The reaction mixtures vary from tiny probes to the entire genome of an organism. Most immobilize the single-stranded target DNA on a membrane to prevent it from rehybridizing with its own complementary strand, but liquid phase assays have also been developed. A variant in which the DNA is separated by agarose gel electrophoresis before binding to the membrane is called **Southern hybridization.**

### Polymerase Chain Reaction

PCR amplifies targeted segments of the genome

The polymerase chain reaction (PCR) is an amplification technique that allows the detection and selective replication of a targeted portion of the genome. The technique uses special DNA polymerases that through alternate changes in test conditions (such as temperature) can be manipulated to initiate replication in either the 3′ or 5′ direction. The specificity is provided by primers that recognize a pair of unique sites on the chromosome so that the DNA between them can be replicated by repetitive cycling of the test conditions. Because each newly synthesized fragment can serve as the template for its own replication, the amount of DNA doubles with each cycle (Fig 14–16).

### Nucleic Acid Sequence Analysis

For some time it has been possible to chemically determine the exact nucleotide sequence of genomic segments or cloned genes. Published sequences are systematically entered into

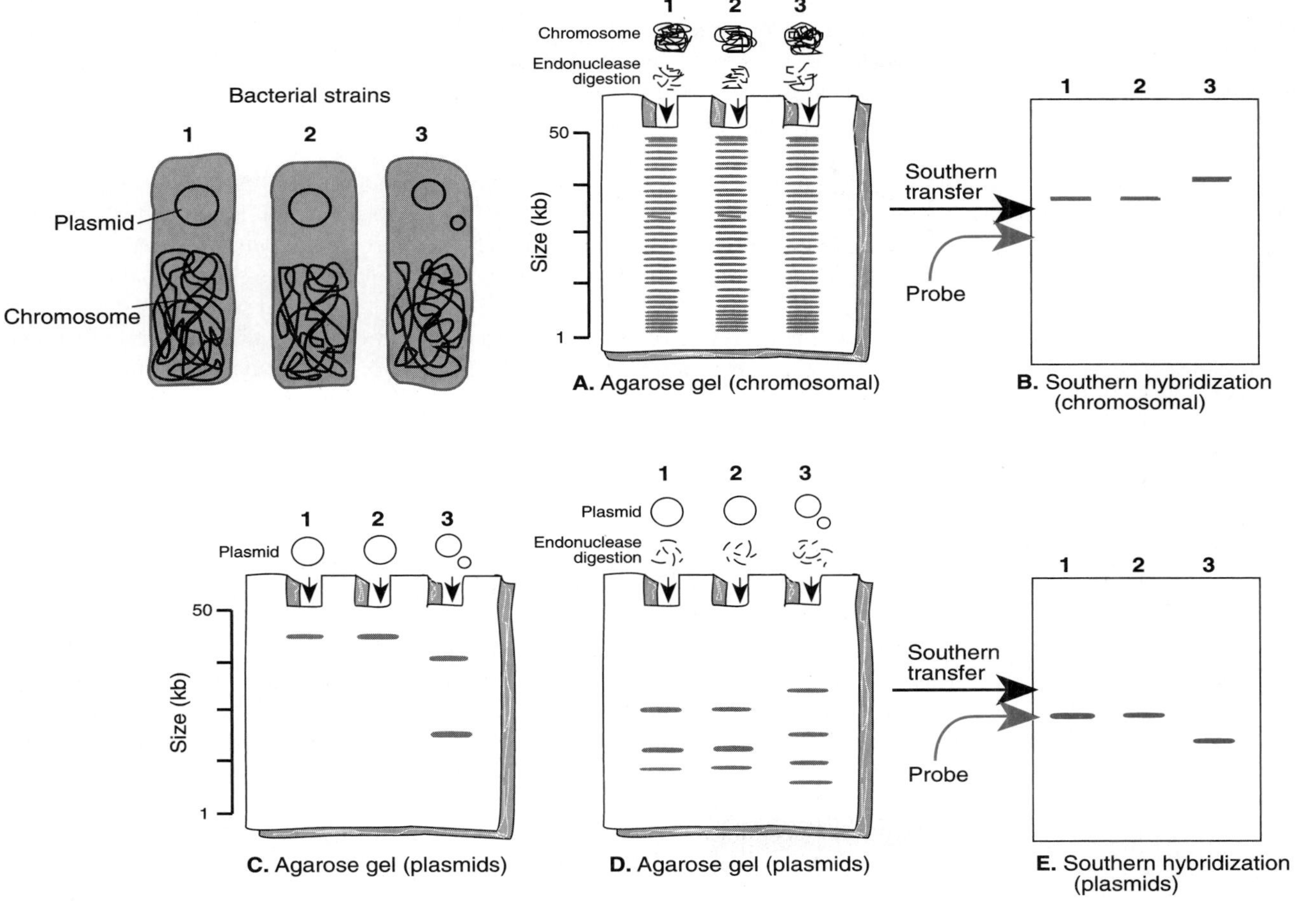


**Figure 14–14.** Molecular diagnostic methods. Three bacterial strains of the same species are shown each with chromosome and plasmid(s). **A.** The chromosomal DNA of each strain is isolated, digested with a restriction endonuclease, and separated by agarose gel eletrophoresis. An almost continuous range of fragment sizes is generated for each strain, making them difficult to distinguish. **B.** The restriction fragments in A are transferred to a membrane (Southern transfer) and hybridized with a probe. The probe binds to a single fragment from each strain, but the larger size of the fragment from strain 3 indicates variation in restriction sites and thus a genomic difference between it and strains 1 and 2. **C.** Plasmids from each strain are isolated and separated in the same manner as A. The results show a plasmid of the same size from 1 and 2. Strain 3 has two plasmids each of a different size than strains 1 and 2. **D.** The same plasmids are restriction digested prior to electrophoresis. The plasmids from 1 and 2 show three fragments of identical size, proving they are identical. Strain 3's plasmids appear unrelated. **E.** The fragments in D are transferred and reacted with a probe. The positive result with the largest of the stain 1 and 2 fragments confirms their relatedness. The positive hybridization with one of the strain 3 fragment suggests it contains at least some DNA that is homologous to the plasmid from strains 1 and 2.

computer databases such as GenBank and are widely available for analysis by computer software designed to solve a wide variety of problems. Conversely, given the known sequence, short segments of DNA can be synthesized for use as probes or primers. It is even possible to compare a sequenced gene or putative probe against all known sequences using the computer, an "experiment" that would be impossible in the laboratory.

Nucleic acid sequence data available in powerful computerized formats

## Application of Nucleic Acid Methods to Infectious Diseases

### Bacterial and Viral Genomic Sizing

The only intact genetic elements of infectious agents that are small enough to be directly detected and sized by agarose gel electrophoresis are bacterial plasmids. Not all bacterial species typically harbor plasmids, but those that do may carry one or a number of plasmids ranging in size from less than 1 to over 50 kilobases. This diversity makes the presence or absence, number, and sizes of plasmids of considerable value in differentiating strains for epidemiologic purposes. Because plasmids are not stable components of the bacterial genome, plasmid analysis also has the element of a timely "snapshot" of the circumstances of a disease outbreak. The specificity of these results can be improved by digesting the plasmids with restriction endonucleases prior to electrophoresis. Two plasmids of the same size from different strains may not be the same, but if an identical pattern of fragments is generated from the digestion, they almost certainly are. These principles are illustrated Figure 14–14 and their application to an outbreak is shown in Figures 4–12 and 4–13.

Number and size of plasmids differentiates strains

Endouclease digestion of plasmids refines their composition

Due to their larger size, the primary genomes of bacteria must be digested with endonucleases in order to resolve them on gels. For viruses the outcome is much like that with plasmids, depending on the genomic size and the endonuclease used. Digested bacterial chromosomes can be compared in this manner, but the number of fragments is very large and the patterns complex. The combined use of endonucleases, which make infrequent cuts, and pulsed-field electrophoresis can produce a comparison comparable to that possible with plasmids. This approach is also used for analysis of the multiple chromosomes of fungi and parasites.

Bacterial chromosomes must be digested prior to electrophoresis

## DNA Probes

A "probe" is a fragment of DNA that has been cloned or otherwise recovered from a genomic or plasmid source. It may contain a gene of known function or simply sequences empirically found to be useful for the application in question. In some cases the probe is synthesized as a single chain of nucelotides (oligonucleotide probe) from known sequence data. The probes are labeled with a radioisotope or other marker and used in hybridization reactions either to detect the homologous sequences in unknown specimens (Fig 14–15) or to further refine gel electrophoresis findings (Fig 14–14). In the latter instance, Southern hybridizations are used in order to retain knowledge of the size of fragments involved. For example, the information that the same gene is present in each of two strains but in different size restriction fragments is evidence for a genomic difference between the two strains (Fig 14–14B).

DNA probes may be cloned or synthesized from known sequences

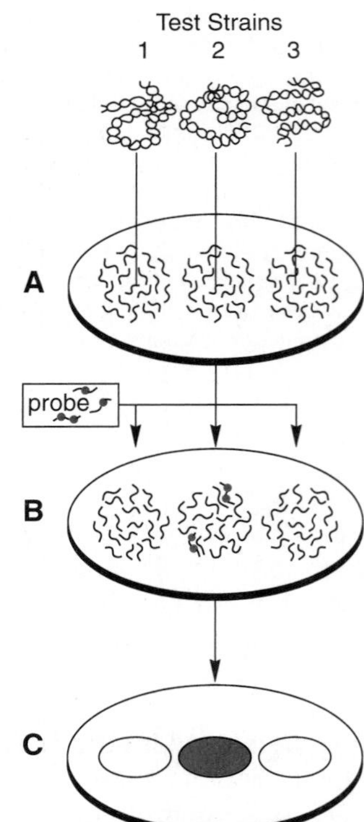


**Figure 14–15.** DNA probe detection. **A.** Chromosomal and/or plasmid DNA from three unknown strains is fragmented, denatured, and bound to filters. **B.** The probe (—•—) is a small DNA fragment labeled with a radioactive or other marker. It is allowed to react with the single-stranded test DNAs on the filter and binds wherever homologous sequences are found. **C.** Probe that has hybridized with test DNA is detected on the filter by an appropriate test for the marker. Test strain 2 contained sequences homologous to the probe and thus gives a positive reaction.

The diagnostic use of DNA probes is to detect or identify microorganisms by hybridization of the probe to homologous sequences in DNA extracted from the entire organism. A number of probes have been developed that will quickly and reliably identify organisms already isolated in culture. The application of probes for detection of infectious agents directly in clinical specimens such as blood, urine, and sputum is more difficult, because most of the systems developed to date are not as sensitive as culture and are more expensive. This approach offers the potential, however, for rapid diagnosis and the detection of characteristics not possible by routine methods. For example, a bacterial toxin gene probe can demonstrate both the presence of the related organism and its toxigenicity without the need for culture.

DNA probes can detect DNA of pathogen directly in clinical specimens

### Polymerase Chain Reaction Applications

The amplification power of the polymerase chain reaction (PCR) offers a solution for the sensitivity problems inherent in the direct application of probes (Fig 14–16). Although the nucleic acid segment amplified by PCR can be seen directly on a gel, the greatest sensitivity and specificity are achieved when probe hybridization is carried out following PCR. This approach has been successful for a wide range of infectious agents and awaits only further resolution of practical problems for wider use.

PCR combined with probes gives the greatest sensitivity

Another creative use of PCR has been in the study of infectious agents seen in tissue but not grown in culture. PCR primers derived from sequences known to be highly conserved among bacteria, such as ribosomal RNA, have been applied to tissue specimens. The amplification produces enough DNA to clone and sequence. This sequence can then be compared with sequences published for other organisms using computers. Thus, taxonomic relationships can be inferred for an organism that has never been isolated.

PCR from tissue allows study of organisms that connot be cultured

### Ribotyping

Ribotyping also makes use of the conserved nature of bacterial ribosomal RNA and of the ability of RNA to hybridize to DNA under certain conditions. Labeled ribosomal NA of one organism can be hybridized with restriction-endonuclease-digested chromosomal DNA of another. In this case ribosomal RNA is being used as a massive probe of restriction fragments separated by electrophoresis. Hybridization to multiple fragments is common, but if the organisms are genetically different, the restriction fragments, which contain the ribosomal RNA sequences, will vary in size. The pattern of bands produced by epidemiologically related strains can then be compared side by side.

Ribotyping refines comparison of chromosomal endonuclease digestion patterns

### DNA–DNA Homology

DNA homology techniques hybridize the total genomic DNA of one organism to that of another in a manner demonstrated in Figure 14–17. The relatedness of strains can be expressed as a percent homology. Strains related at the species level should show homology in the 60 to 90% range, whereas strains with increasing taxonomic divergence show progressively less homology. These findings are now a major factor in decisions on the taxonomic classification of all microorganisms, allowing species, genus, and higher taxonomic groupings to be assessed by means that are not subject to the phenotypic variation inherent with classical methods.

Percent DNA homology now a primary tool for taxonomic assignments

## SUMMARY

The application of some combination of the principles described in this chapter is appropriate to the diagnosis of any infectious disease. The usefulness of any individual method differs among infectious agents due to biologic variation and uneven study. In general, for agents that can be grown in vitro, culture remains the "gold standard" as both the most sensitive and specific method. Molecular methods have the potential to replace culture once they are more fully evaluated and cost effective.

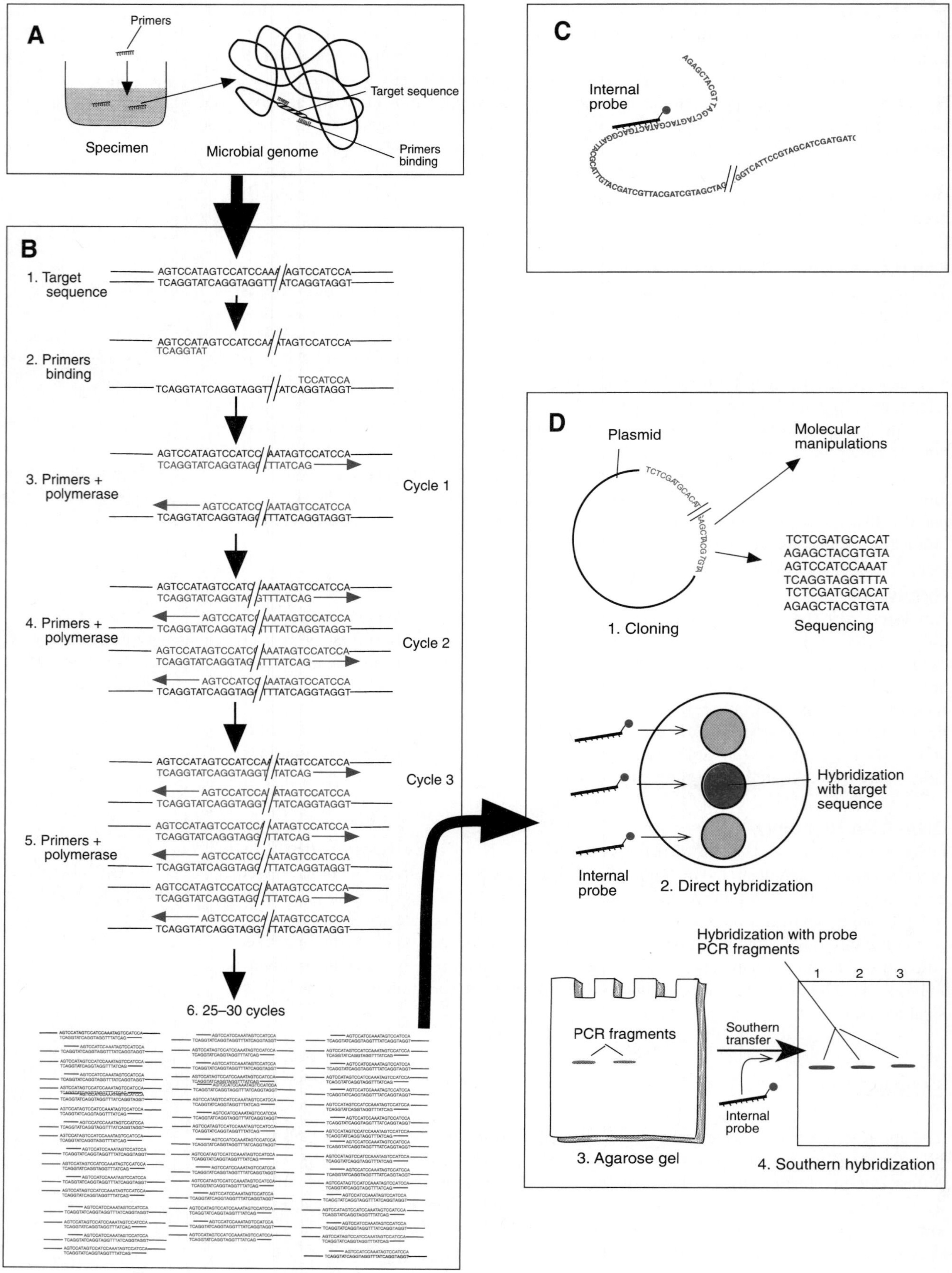

**A**

Primers

Target sequence

Specimen

Microbial genome

Primers binding

**B**

1. Target sequence

AGTCCATAGTCCATCCAAA // AGTCCATCCA
TCAGGTATCAGGTAGGTTT // ATCAGGTAGGT

2. Primers binding

AGTCCATAGTCCATCCAA // TAGTCCATCCA
TCAGGTAT

TCCATCCA
TCAGGTATCAGGTAGGT // ATCAGGTAGGT

3. Primers + polymerase

Cycle 1

AGTCCATAGTCCATCC // AATAGTCCATCCA
TCAGGTATCAGGTAG // TTATCAG

AGTCCATCC // AATAGTCCATCCA
TCAGGTATCAGGTAG // TTATCAGGTAGGT

4. Primers + polymerase

Cycle 2

AGTCCATAGTCCATC // AAATAGTCCATCCA
TCAGGTATCAGGTA // GTTTATCAG

AGTCCATC // AATAGTCCATCCA
TCAGGTATCAGGTAG // TTTATCAGGTAGGT

AGTCCATAGTCCATC // AATAGTCCATCCA
TCAGGTATCAGGTAG // TTTATCAG

AGTCCATC // AATAGTCCATCCA
TCAGGTATCAGGTAG // TTTATCAGGTAGGT

5. Primers + polymerase

Cycle 3

AGTCCATAGTCCATCCA // TAGTCCATCCA
TCAGGTATCAGGTAGGT // TATCAG

AGTCCATCCA // ATAGTCCATCCA
TCAGGTATCAGGTAGGT // TATCAGGTAGGT

AGTCCATAGTCCATCC // AATAGTCCATCCA
TCAGGTATCAGGTAGG // TTATCAG

AGTCCATCC // AATAGTCCATCCA
TCAGGTATCAGGTAGG // TTATCAGGTAGGT

AGTCCATAGTCCATCC // AATAGTCCATCCA
TCAGGTATCAGGTAGG // TTATCAG

AGTCCATCCA // ATAGTCCATCCA
TCAGGTATCAGGTAGG // TTATCAGGTAGGT

6. 25–30 cycles

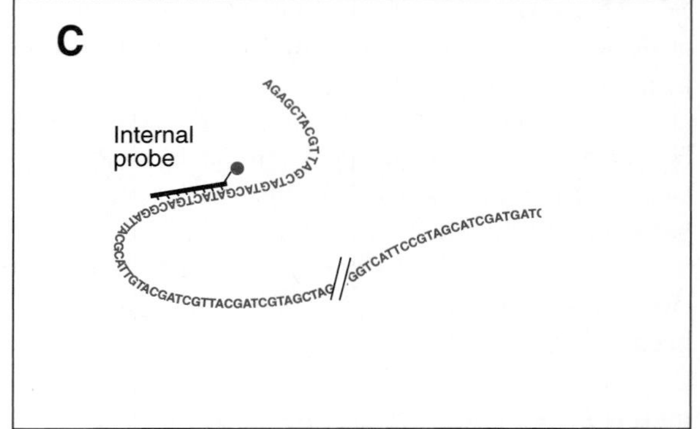


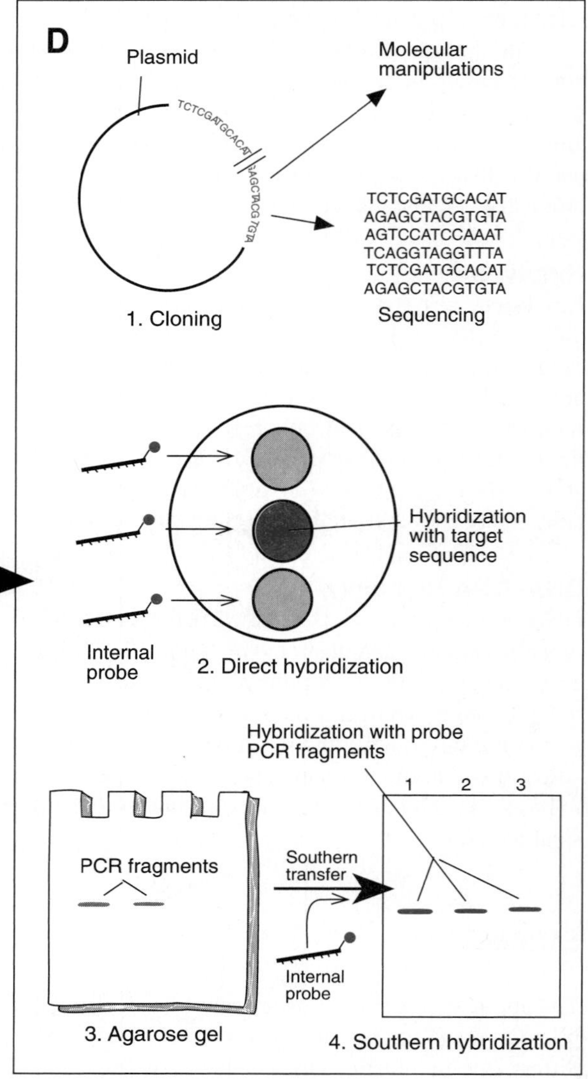

**Figure 14–16.** Diagnostic applications of the polymerase chain reaction (PCR). **A.** A clinical specimen (pus, tissue, etc.) contains DNA from many sources as well as the chromosome of the organism of interest. If the DNA strands are separated (denatured), the PCR primers can bind to their target sequences in the specimen itself. **B.** Amplification of the target sequence by PCR. (1) The target sequence is shown in its native state. (2) The DNA is denatured, allowing the primers to bind where they find the homologous sequence. (3) In the presence of the special DNA polymerase new DNA is synthesized from both strands in the region between the primers. (4 to 6) Additional cycles are added by temperature control of the polymerase with each new sequence acting as the template for another. The DNA doubles with each cycle. After 25 to 30 cycles enough DNA is present to analyse diagnostically. **C.** Internal probe. The amplified target sequence is shown. A probe can be designed to bind to a sequence located between (internal to) the primers. **D.** Analysis of PCR amplified DNA. (1) The amplified sequence can be cloned into a plasmid vector. In this form a variety of molecular manipulations or sequencing may be carried out. (2) Direct hybridizations usually make use of an internal probe. The example shows three specimens each of which went through steps **A** and **B**. Following amplification each was bound to a separate spot on a filter (dot blot). The filter is then reacted with the internal probe to detect the PCR amplified DNA. The result shows that only the middle specimen contained the target sequence. (3) The amplified DNA may be detected directly by agarose gel electrophoresis. The example shows detection of amplified fragments in two of three lanes on the gel. (4) The sensitivity of detection may be increased by use of the internal probe following Southern transfer. The example shows detection of a third fragment of the same size that was not seen on the original gel because the amount of DNA was too small.

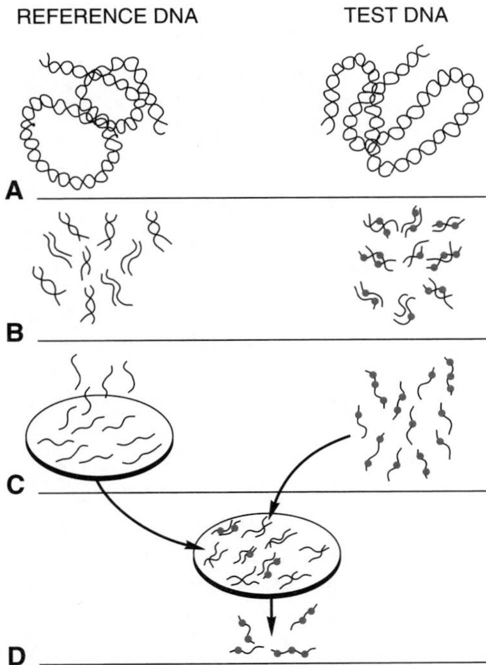


**Figure 14–17.** DNA–DNA homology. **A.** Double-stranded chromosomal DNA from a test strain is to be compared with a reference strain of the same or another species. **B.** Both DNAs are fragmented and denatured. The test DNA is labeled (—●—) with a radioisotope or some other marker. **C.** The denatured (single-stranded) reference DNA is bound to a support matrix such as a nitrocellulose or nylon filter, thus leaving the nucleotide bases available for pairing. **D.** The labeled test DNA is reacted with the material on the filter allowing homologous sequences to pair (hybridize) with the reference DNA. Nonhomologous DNA is washed away, and the amount of bound label measured. The percentage homology of the test to the reference DNA is determined from the ratio of bound to unbound label.

## ADDITIONAL READING

Balows A, Hausler WJ, Jr, Herrmann KL, et al, eds: *Manual of Clinical Microbiology*, 5th ed. Washington, DC, American Society for Microbiology, 1991. A widely used comprehensive text for clinical microbiology and virology.

The *CUMITECH* series. Washington, DC, American Society for Microbiology. *Cumulative Techniques and Procedures in Clinical Microbiology* (CUMITECH) is a series of 10- to 25-page pamphlets, each of which covers important topics related to diagnostic microbiology (blood cultures, urinary tract infections, antimicrobial susceptibility testing, and the like). Each pamphlet is jointly written by at least three authors representing the clinical as well as the laboratory viewpoint, and includes clinical, specimen collection, isolation, and identification recommendations for all agents pertinent to the topic.

Relman DA, Schmidt TM, MacDermott RP, Falkow S: Identification of the uncultured bacillus of Whipple's disease. *N Engl J Med* 1992;327:293–301. A wonderful example of taxonomy by molecular methods alone.

Tompkins LS: The use of molecular methods in infectious disease. *N Engl J Med* 1992;327:1290–1296. A complete and readable discussion of all the molecular methods discussed here, with clinical examples and excellent illustrations.

### APPENDIX 14–1. SOME MEDIA USED FOR ISOLATION OF BACTERIAL PATHOGENS

| Medium | Uses |
|---|---|
| **General-purpose Media** | |
| Nutrient broths (eg, Soybean–Casein digest broth) | Most bacteria, particularly when used for blood culture |
| Thioglycolate broth | Anaerobes, facultative bacteria |
| Blood agar | Most bacteria (demonstrates hemolysis) |
| Chocolate agar | Most bacteria, including fastidious species (eg, *Haemophilus*) |
| **Selective Media** | |
| MacConkey agar | Nonfastidious Gram-negative rods |
| Hektoen-enteric agar | *Salmonella* and *Shigella* |
| Selenite F broth | *Salmonella* enrichment |
| **Special-purpose media** | |
| Löwenstein–Jensen medium, Middlebrook agar | *Mycobacterium tuberculosis* and other mycobacteria (selective) |
| Martin–Lewis medium | *Neisseria gonorrhoeae* and *N. meningitidis* (selective) |
| Fletcher medium (semisolid) | Leptospira (nonselective) |
| Tinsdale agar | *Corynebacterium diphtheriae* (selective) |
| Charcoal agar | *Bordetella pertussis* (selective) |
| Buffered charcoal–yeast extract agar | Legionella species (nonselective) |
| *Campylobacter* blood agar | *Campylobacter jejuni* (selective) |
| Thiosulfate-citrate-bile-sucrose agar (TCBS) | *Vibrio cholerae* and *V. parahemolyticus* (selective) |

## APPENDIX 14–2. CHARACTERISTICS OF COMMONLY USED BACTERIOLOGIC MEDIA

1. **Nutrient broths.** Some form of nutrient broth is used for culture of all direct tissue or fluid samples from sites that are normally sterile to obtain the maximum culture sensitivity. Selective or indicator agents are omitted to prevent inhibition of more fastidious organisms.
2. **Blood agar.** The addition of defibrinated blood to a nutrient agar base enhances the growth of some bacteria, such as streptococci. It often yields distinctive colonies and provides an indicator system for hemolysis. Two major types of hemolysis are seen: β-hemolysis, a complete clearing of red cells from a zone surrounding the colony; and α-hemolysis, which is incomplete (that is, intact red cells are still present in the hemolytic zone), but shows a green color caused by hemoglobin breakdown products. The net effect is a hazy green zone extending 1 to 2 mm beyond the colony. A third type, α′-hemolysis, produces a hazy, incomplete hemolytic zone similar to that caused by α-hemolysis, but without the green coloration.
3. **Chocolate agar.** If blood is added to molten nutrient agar at about 80°C and maintained at this temperature, the red cells are gently lysed, hemoglobin products are released, and the medium turns a chocolate brown color. The nutrients released permit the growth of some fastidious organisms, such as *H. influenzae,* that fail to grow on blood or nutrient agars. This quality is particularly pronounced when the medium is further enriched with vitamin supplements. Given the same incubation conditions, any organism that grows on blood agar will also grow on chocolate agar.
4. **Martin–Lewis medium.** A variant of chocolate agar, Martin–Lewis medium is a solid medium selective for the pathogenic *Neisseria* (*N. gonorrhoeae* and *N. meningitidis*). Growth of most other bacteria and fungi in the genital or respiratory flora is inhibited by the addition of antimicrobics. A current formulation includes vancomycin, colistin, trimethoprim, and anisomycin.
5. **MacConkey agar.** MacConkey agar is both a selective and an indicator medium for Gram-negative rods, particularly members of the family Enterobacteriaceae and the genus *Pseudomonas.* In addition to a peptone base, the medium contains bile salts, crystal violet, lactose, and neutral red as a pH indicator. The bile salts and crystal violet inhibit Gram-positive bacteria and the more fastidious Gram-negative organisms, such as *Neisseria* and *Pasteurella.* Gram-negative rods that grow and ferment lactose produce a red (acid) colony often with a distinctive colonial morphology.
6. **Hektoen enteric agar.** The Hektoen medium is one of many high selective media developed for the isolation of *Salmonella* and *Shigella* species from stool specimens. It has both selective and indicator properties. The medium contains a mixture of bile, thiosulfate, and citrate salts that inhibits not only Gram-positive bacteria, but members of the Enterobacteriaceae other than *Salmonella* and *Shigella* that appear among the normal flora of the colon. The inhibition is not absolute; recovery of *E. coli* is reduced 1000- to 10,000-fold relative to that on nonselective media, but there is little effect on growth of *Salmonella* and *Shigella.* Carbohydrates and a pH indicator are also included to help to differentiate colonies of *Salmonella* and *Shigella* from those of other enteric Gram-negative rods.
7. **Anaerobic media.** In addition to meeting atmospheric requirements, isolation of some strictly anaerobic bacteria on blood agar is enhanced by reducing agents such as L-cysteine and by vitamin enrichment. Sodium thioglycolate, another reducing agent, is often used in broth media. Plate media are made selective for anaerobes by the addition of aminoglycoside antibiotics, which are active against many aerobic and facultative organisms but not against anaerobic bacteria. The use of selective media is particularly important with anaerobes because they grow slowly and are commonly mixed with facultative bacteria in infections.
8. **Highly selective media.** Media specific to the isolation of almost every important pathogen have been developed. Many will allow only a single species to grow from specimens with a rich normal flora (for example, stool). The most common of these media are listed in Appendix 14–1; they are discussed in greater detail in following chapters.

## APPENDIX 14–3. COMMON BIOCHEMICAL TESTS FOR MICROBIAL IDENTIFICATION

1. **Carbohydrate breakdown.** The ability to produce acidic metabolic products, fermentatively or oxidatively, from a range of carbohydrates (eg, glucose, sucrose, and lactose) has been applied to the identification of most groups of bacteria. Such tests are crude and imperfect in defining mechanisms, but have proved useful for taxonomic purposes. More recently, gas chromatographic identification of specific short-chain fatty acids produced by fermentation of glucose has proved useful in classifying many anaerobic bacteria.
2. **Catalase production.** The enzyme catalase catalyzes the conversion of hydrogen peroxide to water and oxygen. When a colony is placed in hydrogen peroxide, liberation of oxygen as gas bubbles can be seen. The test is particularly useful in differentiation of staphylococci (positive) from streptococci (negative), but also has taxonomic application to Gram-negative bacteria.
3. **Citrate utilization.** An agar medium that contains sodium citrate as the sole carbon source may be used to determine ability to use citrate. Bacteria that grow on this medium are termed **citrate positive.**
4. **Coagulase.** The enzyme coagulase acts with a plasma factor to convert fibrinogen to a fibrin clot. It is used to differentiate *S. aureus* from other, less pathogenic staphylococci.
5. **Decarboxylases and deaminases.** The decarboxylation or deamination of the amino acids lysine, ornithine, and arginine is detected by the effect of the amino products on the pH of the reaction mixture or by the formation of colored products. These tests are used primarily with Gram-negative rods.
6. **Hydrogen sulfide.** The ability of some bacteria to produce $H_2S$ from amino acids or other sulfur-containing compounds is helpful in taxonomic classification. The black color of the sulfide salts formed with heavy metals such as iron is the usual means of detection.
7. **Indole.** The indole reaction tests the ability of the organism to produce indole, a benzopyrrole, from tryptophan. Indole is detected by the formation of a red dye after addition of a benzaldehyde reagent. A spot test can be done in seconds using isolated colonies.
8. **Nitrate reduction.** Bacteria may reduce nitrates by several mechanisms. This ability is demonstrated by detection of the nitrites and/or nitrogen gas formed in the process.
9. **O-Nitrophenyl-β-D-galactoside (ONPG) breakdown.** The ONPG test is related to lactose fermentation. Organisms that possess the β-galactoside necessary for lactose fermentation but lack a permease necessary for lactose to enter the cell are ONPG positive and lactose negative.
10. **Oxidase production.** The oxidase tests detect the *c* component of the cytochrome-oxidase complex. The reagents used change from clear to colored when converted from the reduced to the oxidized state. The oxidase reaction is commonly demonstrated in a spot test, which can be done quickly from isolated colonies.
11. **Proteinase production.** Proteolytic activity is detected by growing the organism in the presence of substrates such as gelatin or coagulated egg.
12. **Urease production.** Urease hydrolyzes urea to yield two molecules of ammonia and one of $CO_2$. This reaction can be detected by the increase in medium pH caused by ammonia production. Urease-positive species vary in the amount of enzyme produced; bacteria can thus be designated as positive, weakly positive, or negative.
13. **Voges–Proskauer test.** The Voges–Proskauer test detects acetylmethylcarbinol (acetoin), an intermediate product in the butene glycol pathway of glucose fermentation.

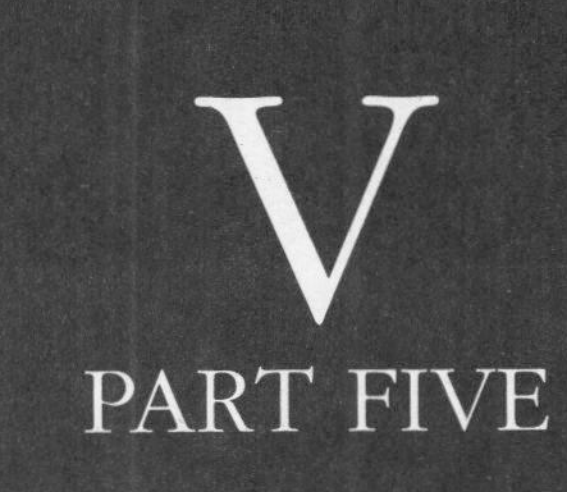


# Pathogenic Bacteria

# Staphylococci

*Kenneth J. Ryan*

Members of the genus *Staphylococcus* (staphylococci) are round, Gram-positive cocci that can divide in any plane and tend to be arranged in grapelike clusters (from the Greek staphyle, bunch of grapes). They are readily grown on common bacteriologic media and many species are indigenous to the normal flora of the skin. The type species, *Staphylococcus aureus*, has remained one of the most common and virulent of bacterial pathogens from the preantibiotic era to the present, and is a common colonizer of the human anterior nares. The other species are common in the skin flora, but disease produced by them is less aggressive and usually requires some form of compromise of the host defense mechanisms.

## THE STAPHYLOCOCCI: GROUP CHARACTERISTICS

Although staphylococci have a marked tendency to form clusters, some single cells, pairs, and short chains are also seen. Staphylococci have a typical Gram-positive cell wall structure. Like all medically important cocci, they are nonflagellate, nonmotile, and non-spore-forming. Staphylococci grow best aerobically, but are facultatively anaerobic. They can oxidize or ferment various carbohydrates. In contrast to streptococci, staphylococci produce catalase. There are more than a dozen species of staphylococci that colonize humans. Of these, three are of major medical importance: *Staphylococcus aureus, S. epidermidis*, and *S. saprophyticus* (Table 15–1). The ability of *S. aureus* to form coagulase separates it from the other, less virulent species.

All form clusters

Catalase positive

Coagulase separates *S. Aureus* from other species

## STAPHYLOCOCCUS AUREUS

### ■ The Organism: *Staphylococcus aureus*

#### Morphology and Staining

In cultures the cells of *S. aureus* are regular in size, fitting together in clusters with the precision of a collection of pool balls. They are uniformly Gram positive. In older cultures, in resolving lesions, and in the presence of some antibiotics the cells often become more variable in size, and many lose the Gram positivity.

#### Cell Wall and Other Surface Structures

The cell wall of *S. aureus* consists of a typical Gram-positive peptidoglycan (Chapter 2). The peptidoglycan is interspersed with molecules of a ribitol-teichoic acid, which is antigenic and relatively specific for *S. aureus*. In most strains, the peptidoglycan of the cell wall is overlaid with surface proteins; one protein, protein A, is unique in that it binds the *Fc*

Protein A binds *Fc* portion of IgG

**TABLE 15–1. FEATURES OF HUMAN STAPHYLOCOCCI**

| | | | Pathogenic Features | | |
|---|---|---|---|---|---|
| *Species* | Coagulase | Common Habitat | *Catheter Colonization* | *Furuncles* | *Exotoxin Production* |
| *S. aureus* | + | Anterior nares, perineum | + | + | +[b] |
| *S. epidermidis* | – | Anterior nares, skin | +[a] | – | – |
| *S. saphrophyticus* | – | Urinary tract | + | – | – |
| Others | – | various | +[a] | – | – |

[a] Some strains produce surface slime.
[b] Including exfoliatin, TSST-1, pyrogenic exotoxins.

portion of IgG molecules, leaving the antigen-reacting *Fab* portion directed externally. This phenomenon has been exploited in test systems for detecting free antigens (see Chapter 14). It probably contributes to the virulence of *S. aureus* by interfering with opsonization. Occasional strains have a polysaccharide capsule of unknown significance.

## Cultural Characteristics

Grows rapidly forming white to golden colonies

Often hemolytic

Under aerobic conditions, *S. aureus* grows rapidly and diffusely in liquid medium. After overnight incubation on blood agar, it produces soft, regular, low, convex colonies approximately 2 to 3 mm in diameter. Most, but not all, strains show a rim of clear beta-hemolysis surrounding the colony. The colonies are initially off-white, but the tendency of many to turn a buff-golden color with time is the basis of the species epithet *aureus* (golden). Occasional strains require the addition of 2 to 10% carbon dioxide to the atmosphere for growth. The ability of *S. aureus* to grow in the presence of 7.5% sodium chloride and to ferment mannitol has been exploited in a selective/indicator medium, mannitol salt agar. This medium is used in environmental and public health studies when it is necessary to detect potential *S. aureus* colonies among those of contaminating organisms.

## Tests for Identification and Subtyping

Coagulase action results in fibrin clot

Slide clumping factor correlates with coagulase

The single most important test used to distinguish *S. aureus* from other staphylococci is the production of coagulase. Coagulase is demonstrated by inoculating staphylococci into diluted mammalian plasma and incubating at 35 to 37°C. Coagulase production results in development of a fibrin clot, usually within 4 hours. Coagulase nonenzymatically binds to prothrombin to form a complex that initiates the polymerization of fibrin. A dense emulsion of staphylococcal cells in water will also clump immediately upon mixing with undiluted plasma due to direct binding of fibrinogen to a factor on the cell surface (clumping factor). This is the basis of a very useful laboratory test called the slide coagulase or clumping test. Despite its high correlation (95%) with the standard coagulase method, it appears the clumping factor is distinct from coagulase. Commercial agglutination tests that correlate well with the coagulase test are also in use.

Bacteriophage typing fingerprints useful in epidemiologic investigations

Some phage groups have links to pathogenesis

Strains of *S. aureus* can be subdivided by bacteriophage typing and thus "fingerprinted" for epidemiologic purposes. The procedure depends on differing susceptibilities to lysis of different strains by bacteriophages. It employs an international set of more than 20 bacteriophages derived originally from lysogenic strains of *S. aureus*. The phages are dropped onto a plate seeded with the strain to be tested. Lysis in the area of a drop read after overnight incubation indicates susceptibility to that phage (Fig 15–1). The phage type "fingerprint" is a listing of the positive reactions, for example, 52/52A/80/81. Mutation or lysogenization during the course of an epidemic may occasionally change the reaction of a staphylococcus to particular phages. Thus, interpretation of phage typing results in the epidemiologic setting requires experience and familiarity with the test. Phage typing patterns have been grouped together to reflect some common characteristics; four such groups (I, II, III, and IV) are recognized. Such grouping has been helpful in suggesting pathogenic associations (for example, bullous impetigo is linked with phage group II strains).

Like all bacteria, *S. aureus* has many antigenically active components. Although a

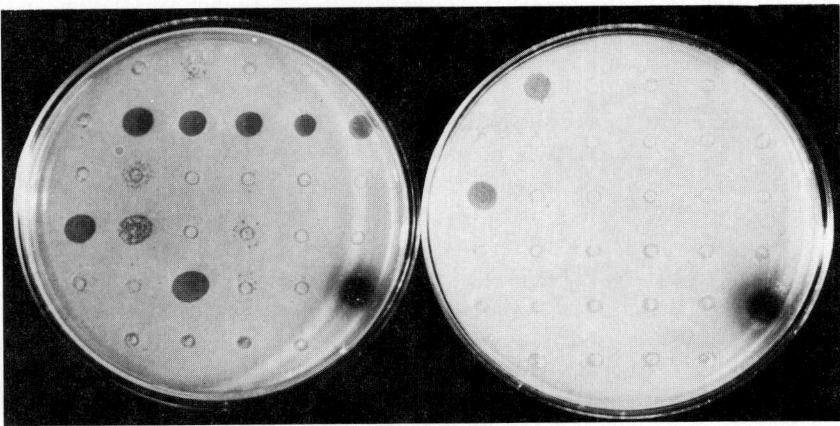

**Figure 15–1.** Bacteriophage typing of two strains of *S. aureus:* results after overnight incubation. Lysis is indicated by absence of growth at the site of deposition of individual phages to which the strain is susceptible. The test shows that the two strains are not of common origin.

number of surface protein and cell wall structural antigens have been described, none are of crucial pathogenic significance or in general use for epidemiologic studies.

## Staphylococcal Disease

### Epidemiology

The central epidemiologic problem with *S. aureus* is that the organism is commonly found colonizing healthy persons yet some strains clearly have enhanced potential to produce disease. We currently have no way to define the more virulent strains in advance of disease production. The basic human habitat of *S. aureus* is the anterior nares. About 30% of individuals in the community carry the organism in this site at any given time. Nasal carrier rates among hospital personnel and patients may be much higher when staphylococcal infections both result from and contribute to the staphylococcal environmental load. Some individuals have extensive colonization of the perineum. They, and some nasal carriers, may disseminate the organism extensively with desquamated epithelial cells, and thus constitute a source of infection to others.

Anterior nares colonization common in healthy people

No way to distinguish strains of increased virulence

Most *S. aureus* infections acquired in the community are autoinfections with strains that the subject has been carrying in the anterior nares, on the skin, or both. Community outbreaks of bullous impetigo in children are usually associated with poor hygiene and fomite transmission from case to case. Unlike many pathogenic vegetative organisms, *S. aureus* can survive long periods of drying; for example, recurrent skin infections can result from use of uncleaned clothing contaminated with pus from a previous infection.

Most community infections endogenous

*S. aureus* survives drying

Hospital epidemics caused by a single strain of *S. aureus* are a continuing and recurrent problem. Outbreaks are usually associated with patients who have undergone surgical or other invasive procedures or with nurseries. The initial source of the outbreak may be a patient with an overt or inapparent (for example, decubitus ulcer) staphylococcal infection; spread to other patients can occur through fomites, occasionally through air transmission, but is usually through the hands of personnel. A nasal or perineal carrier among medical, nursing, or other hospital staff may be the source of an outbreak, especially if carriage is heavy and numerous organisms are disseminated. A more serious source is the medical attendant with a staphylococcal lesion (for example, a furuncle on the wrist), whose hands may become heavily contaminated with *S. aureus* of proved pathogenicity.

Hospital spread primarily on the hands of medical personnel

Outbreaks involve nasal carrier or worker with lesion

Hospital outbreaks of *S. aureus* infection can be self-perpetuating: infected patients and those who attend them frequently become carriers, and the total environmental load of the causative staphylococcus is increased. The principles of control of epidemics in general and of hospital outbreaks are described in Chapters 12 and 72.

In *S. aureus* outbreaks, it is critical to define the extent of infection with the responsible strain and to detect carriers who may have initiated or contributed to continuation of the outbreak. For these purposes, phage typing and determination of patterns of resistance to antimicrobics (antibiograms) are critical epidemiologic tools.

## Toxins and Biologically Active Extracellular Enzymes

Strains of *S. aureus* produce a wide range of substances that contribute, or may possibly contribute, to their virulence. The most important appear to be the following.

### Alpha-toxin (Alpha-hemolysin)

α–toxin inserts in lipid bilayer to form transmembrane pores

Alpha-toxin is a chromosomally encoded, antigenic protein of low molecular weight secreted by almost all strains of *S. aureus* and not by coagulase negative staphylococci. It has long been known to cause lysis of erythrocytes, leukocytes, and platelets, and to cause necrosis on local injection or death systemically in experimental animals. The toxin has lipid-binding domains and acts by direct insertion into the lipid bilayer of mammalian cells to form transmembrane pores (Fig 15–2). The resultant egress of vital molecules leads to death. This action is similar to other biologically active cytolysins such as streptolysin O (Chapter 16), complement, and the effector proteins of cytotoxic T lymphocytes. Although other locally acting toxins (hemolysins) have been described, alpha-toxin has the only clear links to virulence. It substantially accounts for the dramatic destructive nature of lesions found at all sites where *S. aureus* is multiplying.

### Pyrogenic Exotoxins

Multiple pyrogenic exotoxins are similar to those of group A streptococci

The pyrogenic exotoxins are a family of secreted proteins produced by certain strains of *S. aureus* that are able to produce a wide variety of toxic effects at sites remote from the live staphylococci. They include the staphylococcal enterotoxins and the toxic shock syndrome toxin (TSST-1). Individual strains may produce one or more pyrogenic exotoxin. These toxins share physiochemical and biologic activity similarities with each other and with the pyrogenic exotoxins of the group A streptococcus (Chapter 16). All have been recently determined to act as superantigens (Chapters 8 and 10); that is, they are able to stimulate enhanced T-lymphocyte responses by direct interaction with surface T cell and class II MHC receptors. The resultant release of cytokines, such as tumor necrosis factor (TNF) and interleukin-1 (IL-1), from monocytes has the potential for widespread effects.

Act as superantigens

Once formed enterotoxins stable to boiling and digestive enzymes

Stimulate vomiting by central mechanism

**Staphylococcal Enterotoxins.** Certain strains of *S. aureus* produce exotoxins that cause acute gastrointestinal symptoms within 2 to 5 hours of ingestion and are thus termed enterotoxins. Ingestion of sufficient preformed toxin in food results in staphylococcal food poisoning. There are several antigenically distinct low-molecular-weight proteins in this class, which have been classified by letters (eg, staphylococcal enterotoxin A, B). Production of some has been shown to be encoded in temperate bacteriophages. An important feature in their ability to produce food poisoning is that once formed, these toxins retain activity even after 30 minutes of boiling and are resistant to gastric and jejunal enzymes. In addition to the superantigen-mediated actions, the toxin appears to act directly on neural receptors in the upper gastrointestinal tract, leading to stimulation of the vomiting center in the brain.

**Toxic Shock Syndrome Toxin.** It is now clear that the major cause of staphylococcal toxic shock syndrome is the pyrogenic exotoxin termed toxic shock syndrome toxin 1 (TSST-1).

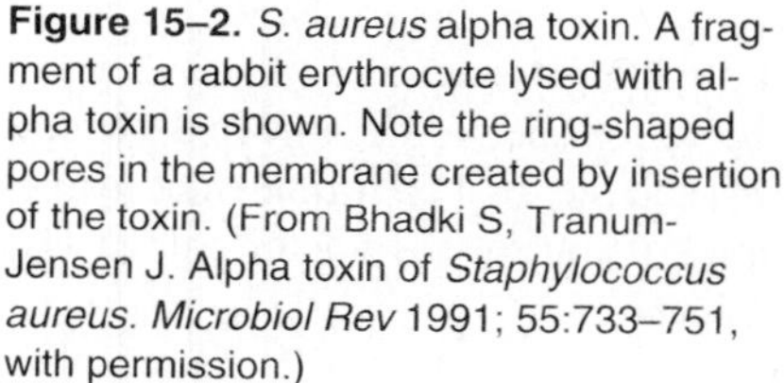

**Figure 15–2.** *S. aureus* alpha toxin. A fragment of a rabbit erythrocyte lysed with alpha toxin is shown. Note the ring-shaped pores in the membrane created by insertion of the toxin. (From Bhadki S, Tranum-Jensen J. Alpha toxin of *Staphylococcus aureus. Microbiol Rev* 1991; 55:733–751, with permission.)

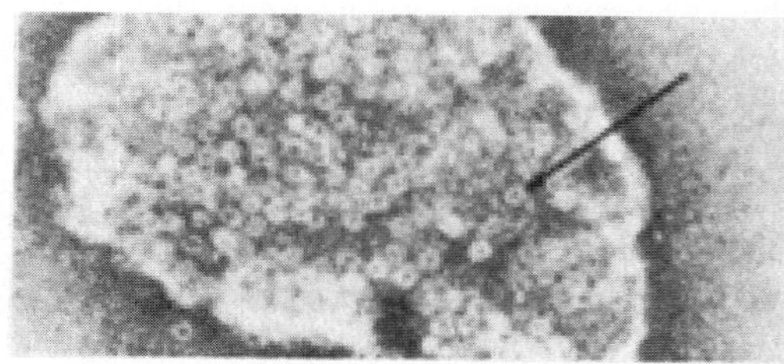

(TSST-1). This toxin is produced in vivo during the course of a staphylococcal infection with systemic disease as a result of absorption of toxin from the local site. Production and release of the toxin is influenced by many factors, including growth conditions such as pH, $Pco_2$, and degree of aeration. TSST-1 can stimulate the release of cytokines through the superantigen mechanism, but may also have direct toxic effects on endothelial cells. The latter action may lead to capillary leakage, hypotension, and shock.

TSST-1 produces systemic disease through absorption from site of infection

#### Exfoliatins

Certain strains of *S. aureus* belonging to phage group II produce exfoliatin, an exotoxin that leads to intercellular splitting of the epidermis between the stratum spinosum and stratum granulosum, presumably by disruption of intercellular junctions. Two distinct exfoliatins, one chromosomally and the other plasmid mediated, have been described. Individual strains of staphylococci can produce one, both, or neither. Sufficient toxin may be produced at a local site of infection to cause marked epithelial desquamation at remote sites of the body (staphylococcal scalded skin syndrome). The toxins are antigenic, and circulating antibody confers immunity to their effects.

Exfoliation splits intercellular junctions

#### Coagulase

Although coagulase is not a toxin, it probably plays some role in the pathogenesis of staphylococcal infections and in determining their nature. Staphylococci coated with fibrin are resistant to phagocytosis, and fibrin deposition in the area of a staphylococcal infectious focus may help to localize the lesion.

#### Other Extracellular Products

Strains of *S. aureus* produce many other extracellular, biologically active substances, including hemolysins, hyaluronidase, nuclease, lipase, protease, and a plasminogen activator. Their roles in the pathogenesis of staphylococcal infection remain obscure.

### Other Probable Contributors to Virulence

Staphylococcal teichoic acid binds specifically to fibronectin on the surface of host cells and to subendothelial tissues and clots. Clumping factor may also mediate adherence of the organism and contribute to the initiation of infection. Surface protein A is a potent antiphagocytic factor. It binds the *Fc* portion of IgG, making it unavailable to its receptor site on the phagocyte. If strains of *S. aureus* reach the bloodstream, exposed peptidoglycan may produce massive complement activation, leukopenia, thrombocytopenia, and a clinical syndrome of septic shock.

Many candidate virulence factors

Once phagocytosed, *S. aureus* strains are much more resistant to lysosomal killing than are coagulase-negative staphylococci, and they may multiply within and kill the phagocyte. Furthermore, *S. aureus* can multiply in fresh human serum, whereas the growth of many coagulase-negative strains is partially or completely inhibited.

Although *S. aureus* has a variety of characteristics and products that may contribute to its virulence, no single factor can be singled out as the primary contributor to its ability to multiply and cause lesions in tissues. A single candidate for an effective immunizing vaccine appears unlikely.

Virulence of *S. aureus* is multifactorial

### Infectivity, Pathogenesis, and Immunity

In general, strains of *S. aureus* are of quite low infectivity unless trauma, foreign matter, or other local conditions provide special opportunities for initiation of infection. In experimental infections, intradermal injection of approximately $10^5$ to $10^6$ organisms is required to initiate a small, local lesion. In the presence of a suture or talcum powder, less than $10^2$ organisms are required.

Foreign matter lowers infecting dose

Once beyond the mucosal or skin barrier, the early stages of staphylococcal disease are poorly understood. Various mechanisms, including surface protein A and production of coagulase, may serve to protect the organisms from phagocytosis long enough for alpha toxin to initiate local injury. There is an acute inflammatory response to the microbial products and to the tissue and leukocyte damage some of them cause. The developing lesion tends to be localized, perhaps due to the local injury and to coagulase-mediated fibrin deposition.

Early survival allows $\alpha$-toxin production

Lesions tend to be localized

Focal lesions tend to drain spontaneously

The resolution of staphylococcal infection in the absence of medical intervention usually results from an abscess "pointing" to the skin, with superficial necrosis followed by drainage of pus and healing by granulation and fibrosis. This process can occur with a small lesion, such as a furuncle, or with a large subcutaneous abscess. Immune mechanisms are undoubtedly involved; however, the relative roles of humoral and cellular immune mechanisms are uncertain, and attempts to induce immunity artificially with various staphylococcal products have been disappointing at best. The natural history of staphylococcal infections indicates that immunity is of short duration and incomplete. Chronic furunculosis, for example, can recur over many years.

Immunity poorly understood

It seems likely that the imprecision of our understanding of staphylococcal infection and immunity reflects its multifactorial nature, in which different toxins, biologically active enzymes, antigens, and immune responses have a different constellation of roles in different cases.

## Staphylococcal Infections: Clinical Aspects

Staphylococcal infections are characterized by intense suppuration, necrosis of local tissues, and a tendency for the infected area to become walled off with the formation of a pus-filled local abscess.

### Furuncle and Carbuncle

Boils develop in hair follicles

The prototypic, and most common, infection is the furuncle or boil. This is a superficial skin infection that develops in a hair follicle, sebaceous gland, or sweat gland. Blockage of the gland duct with inspissation of its contents causes predisposition to infection. Furunculosis is often a complication of acne vulgaris. Infection at the base of the eyelash gives rise to the common stye. The infected patient is often a carrier of the offending *Staphylococcus*, usually in the anterior nares. The course of the infection is usually benign, and the infection resolves upon spontaneous drainage of pus. No surgical or antimicrobic treatment is needed.

Multiple lesions form carbuncle

Infection can spread from a furuncle with the development of one or more abscesses in adjacent subcutaneous tissues. This lesion known as a carbuncle occurs most often on the back of the neck, but may involve other skin sites. Carbuncles are serious lesions that may result in bloodstream invasion (bacteremia).

### Chronic Furunculosis

Relapsing infections show little evidence of immunity

Some individuals are subject to chronic furunculosis, in which repeated attacks of boils are caused by the same strain of *S. aureus*. There is little, if any, evidence of acquired immunity to the disease; indeed, delayed-type hypersensitivity to staphylococcal products appears responsible for much of the inflammation and necrosis that develops. Chronic staphylococcal disease may be associated with factors that depress host immunity, especially in patients with diabetes or congenital defects of polymorphonuclear leukocyte function. In most instances, however, predisposing disease other than acne is not present.

### Impetigo

Exfoliation producing strains cause bullous impetigo

*S. aureus* is found together with group A streptococci in up to 30% of cases of typical pustular impetigo (Chapter 16). Whether it is a primary pathogen or secondary invader is unsettled. It is clear that strains of *S. aureus* that produce exfoliatin can cause bullous impetigo, a highly communicable superficial skin infection characterized by large blisters containing many staphylococci in the superficial layers of the skin. Bullous impetigo is seen most often in infants and children under conditions in which spread by direct contact can occur (for example, sharing of contaminated towels). Bullous impetigo can be considered a localized form of scalded skin syndrome.

### Deep Lesions

Acute osteomyelitis primarily a *S. aureus* disease

*S. aureus* can cause a wide variety of infections of deep tissues, by bacteremic spread from a skin lesion that may be unnoticed. These include infections of bones, joints, deep organs, and soft tissues. More than 90% of the cases of acute osteomyelitis in children are caused by *S. aureus*. Staphylococcal pneumonia is always secondary to some other insult to the lung, such as influenza, aspiration, or pulmonary edema. At deep sites the organism has the same tendency to produce localized, destructive abscesses that it does in the skin. All too often the containment is less effective, and spread with multiple metastatic lesions occurs. Bacteremia and endocarditis can develop. All are serious infections that constitute acute medical emergencies. In all of these situations, diabetes, leukocyte defects, or general reduction of host defenses by alcoholism, malignancy, old age, or steroid or cytotoxic therapy can be a predisposing factor. Severe *S. aureus* infections, including endocarditis, are particularly common in drug abusers using injection methods.

Preumonia and deep tissue lesions highly destructive

Bacteremic spread, endocarditis most common in drug abusers

## Wound Infections

The organism is also a major cause of wound infection. The source may be the patient's own carrier state, other carriers (for example, physicians or nurses), or other infected patients. Cross-infection of the umbilical stump of the newborn infant can lead to extensive contamination of the infant and its environment. Spread to other infants and mothers in the hospital can result in a variety of staphylococcal infections, such as furuncles, conjunctivitis, breast abscess, and other deep infections. Surgical wound infections can be very severe, and infections at the site of intravenous lines can result in bacteremia and metastatic infection.

Leading cause of infection of wounds of all types

## Diseases Caused by Staphylococcal Toxins

### Scalded Skin Syndrome

Staphylococcal scalded skin syndrome results from the production of exfoliatin in a staphylococcal lesion, which can be quite minor (for example, conjunctivitis). The toxin is absorbed into the bloodstream, and erythema and intraepidermal desquamation may occur at remote sites from which *S. aureus* cannot be isolated (Fig 15–3). The disease is most common in neonates and children less than 5 years old. The face, axilla, and groin tend to be affected first, but the erythema, bullous formation, and subsequent desquamation of epithelial sheets can spread to all parts of the body. The disease occasionally occurs in adults, particularly those who are immunocompromised.

Widespread desquamation in neonates caused by exfoliatin producing strains

Milder versions of what is probably the same disease are staphylococcal scarlet fever, in which erythema occurs without desquamation, and bullous impetigo, in which local desquamation occurs.

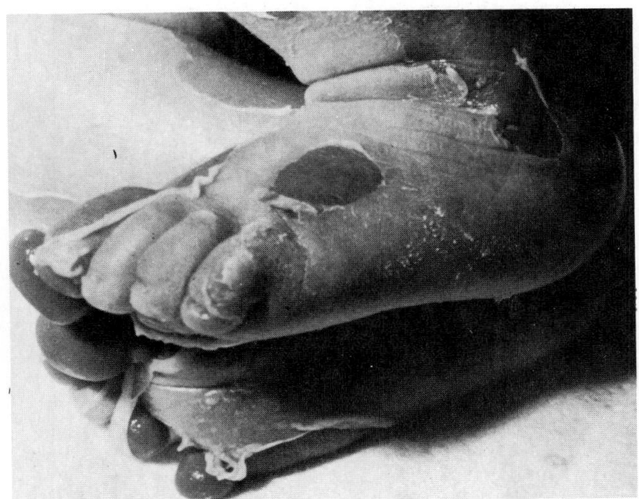

**Figure 15–3.** Staphylococcal scalded skin syndrome in a neonate. The staphylococcal infection was a breast abscess in the infant.

Fever, vomiting, and diarrhea leading to shock

Associated with highly adsorbent tampons

Menstrual conditions favor TSST-1 production

### Toxic Shock Syndrome

Toxic shock syndrome is a life-threatening disease associated with *S. aureus*. It was first described in children but came to public attention during the early 1980s when hundreds of cases were reported in young women using intravaginal tampons. The disease is characterized by the development of high fever, vomiting, diarrhea, sore throat, and muscle pain. Within 48 hours, it may progress to severe shock with evidence of renal and hepatic damage. A skin rash may develop, followed by desquamation at a deeper level than in scalded skin syndrome. Blood cultures are usually negative. The outbreak receded with the withdrawal of certain brands of highly adsorbent tampons. Following these events, cases were increasingly recognized that were not associated with menstruation but were related to a variety of staphylococcal infections.

The pathogenesis of toxic shock syndrome was clarified by the discovery of a new toxin, TSST-1, and its association with this disease. Less than 5% of women carry *S. aureus* in their vaginal flora, and only one in five of these staphylococci have the potential to produce TSST-1. The combination of menstruation and high-absorbancy tampon usage provides conditions that enhance the production of toxin, which is then absorbed from the local site (Fig 15–4). The relative role the superantigen-mediated and direct effects of the circulating toxin play in the multiple manifestations of disease are unknown.

Some cases of full-blown staphylococcal toxic shock syndrome are associated with strains that do not produce TSST-1. This is particularly true of the nonmenstrual cases.

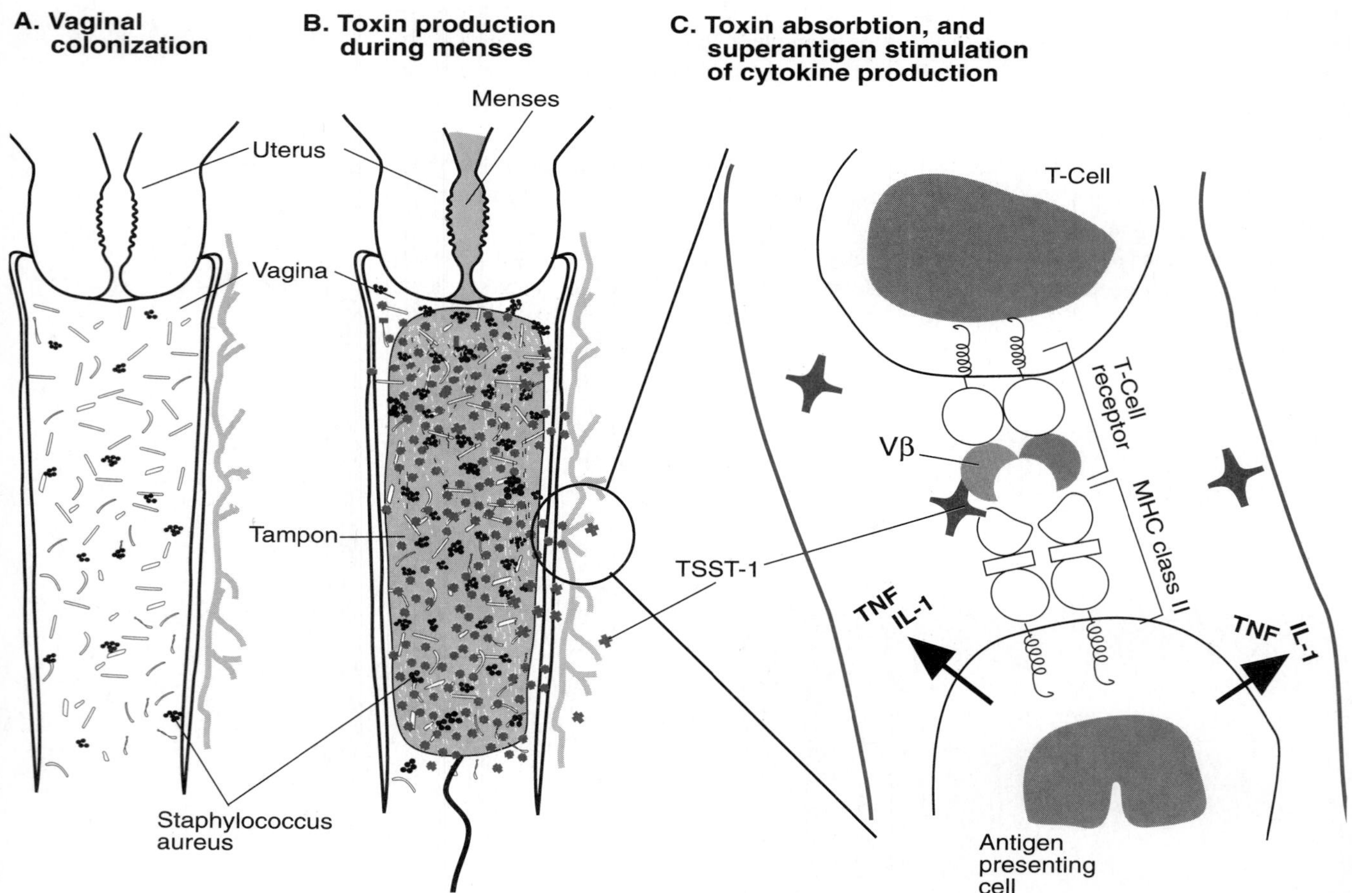


**Figure 15–4.** Pathogenesis of staphylococcal toxic shock syndrome. **A.** The vagina is colonized with normal flora and a strain of *S. aureus* containing the TSST-1 gene. **B.** The conditions with tampon usage facilitate growth of the *S. aureus* and TSST-1 production. **C.** The toxin is absorbed from the vagina and circulates. The systemic effects may be due to the direct effect of the toxin or via cytokines released by the superantigen mechanism. The toxin is shown binding directly with the Vβ portion of the T cell receptor and the class II MHC receptor. This Vβ stimulation signals the production of cytokines such as IL-1 and TNF.

Staphylococcal enterotoxins have been detected in these strains and have been shown to produce experimental toxic shock. Recent evidence indicates that toxic shock syndrome may be the result of in vivo production of any of the staphylococcal pyrogenic exotoxins, with TSST-1 simply the most common offender.

Nonmenstrual cases may not have TSST-1 producing strain

In contrast to others in the same age group, most of those who develop menstruation-associated toxic shock syndrome have low or absent antibody levels to TSST-1, and often fail to mount significant antibody response during the disease. Repeated attacks have been recorded and also suggest a genetic predisposition. These observations need to be evaluated in light of the possibility that other toxins are involved.

#### Staphylococcal Food Poisoning

Staphylococcal food poisoning results from production of a staphylococcal enterotoxin in food before ingestion. It is an intoxication, not an infection. Characteristically, the food is moist and highly nutritious to *S. aureus*, as well as to people. Potato salads and creamy dishes are often involved. The food is contaminated by a carrier or, more often, by a preparer with a staphylococcal lesion. If the food is not refrigerated or refrigeration is inadequate, staphylococcal multiplication can result in $10^5$ or more *S. aureus* per gram. If the strain produces enterotoxin, the food becomes toxic. Because of the heat resistance of the toxin, toxicity persists even if the food is subsequently heated to boiling.

Toxin preformed in food is digested

Ingestion of the food results in acute vomiting and diarrhea within 1 to 5 hours. There is prostration, but usually no fever. Recovery is rapid, except sometimes in the elderly and in those with another disease. Staphylococcal food poisoning has been an unhappy and embarrassing sequel to innumerable group picnics and wedding receptions in which gastronomic delicacies have been exposed to temperatures that allow bacterial multiplication.

Incubation period short and vomiting prominent

### Laboratory Diagnosis

In general, laboratory procedures to assist in diagnosis of staphylococcal infections are quite simple. Most acute lesions contain numerous polymorphonuclear leukocytes and large numbers of *S. aureus*. Infections with coagulase-negative staphylococci usually contain large numbers but in association with a medical device. These findings are readily demonstrated by a direct Gram smear of pus unless the patient has been treated with antibiotics. Deep staphylococcal infections, such as osteomyelitis or perirenal abscess, present special diagnostic problems when the lesion cannot be aspirated or surgically sampled. Blood cultures are usually positive in acute staphylococcal arthritis, osteomyelitis, and endocarditis, but less often in localized infection such as deep abscesses.

Gram stain and culture are primary diagnostic methods

The organism can usually be grown aerobically on blood agar, and typical colonies develop overnight. Coagulase tests can be performed directly from these colonies. Antibiotic susceptibility tests are usually indicated because of the unpredictability of staphylococcal susceptibility patterns.

### Treatment

When penicillin was first introduced, most strains of *S. aureus* were highly susceptible to it. Now, because of penicillinase production encoded by plasmid genes, most isolates from the community as well as from hospitals are penicillin resistant. Most penicillin-resistant strains of *S. aureus* are still fully susceptible to the penicillinase-resistant penicillins and cephalosporins, but resistance to other antistaphylococcal antimicrobics is common, particularly in hospitals. Vancomycin is the exception, and resistance to it is very rare.

Most *S. aureus* penicillin resistant

Most staphylococcal resistance is plasmid determined, and strains may carry several R plasmids. Resistance may be acquired by transduction between strains of *S. aureus* or by conjugative transfer from other strains of *S. aureus*, coagulase-negative staphylococci, or even enterococci. Conjugative transfer does not involve sex pili and appears to be facilitated by conditions on the surface of the skin. It should be noted that transduction may be accompanied by lysogenization with a new bacteriophage, and this can lead to alteration of the phage type of the lysogenized strain.

Penicillinase plasmid medicated

Some multiresistant strains are resistant to the penicillinase-resistant penicillins and cephalosporins and have caused epidemics of hospital infection in many parts of the world. These strains have been widely referred to as methicillin-resistant *S. aureus* (MRSA), despite the fact that resistance applies also to other beta-lactam antimicrobics. The most im-

Methicillin-resistant strains produce new PBP

portant mechanism for this resistance is chromosomal acquisition of a gene (*mecA*) encoding a new peptidoglycan transpeptidase (penicillin-binding protein, PBP-2′) with a low affinity for beta-lactam antimicrobics. This transpeptidase is able to effectively substitute for the other staphylococcal transpeptidases to carry out cell wall synthesis in the presence of beta-lactams. The clinical significance of methicillin resistance has been clearly established.

MRSA-detection requires special conditions

There are some problems in detecting MRSA due to the fact that in most strains the resistant cells represent only a small portion of the total population (heteroresistance). Tests must be done with selected beta-lactams under special conditions that facilitate detection of the resistant subpopulation, and the results extrapolated to other agents. For example, an oxacillin-resistant strain is considered resistant to all other penicillinase-resistant penicillins and cephalosporins, irrespective of the results of susceptibility tests made under other conditions. Most American hospitals report MRSA rates of 1 to 5%, but outbreaks are increasing and resistance rates over 30% have been reported in other countries. Fortunately vancomycin remains effective against almost all MRSA.

MRSA rates are increasing

Superficial lesions resolve spontaneously

Simple drainage usually suffices for superficial staphylococcal lesions and is also an important component of treatment of chronic lesions. Acute, serious staphylococcal infections (for example, pneumonia or bacteremia) require immediate antibiotic therapy. A penicillinase-resistant penicillin or cephalosporin would normally be used pending the results of a susceptibility test. Infections proved to be caused by strains susceptible to benzyl-penicillin are thus best treated with that antibiotic. Severe infections caused by MRSA strains are usually treated with vancomycin.

Penicillinase-resistant used pending susceptibility tests

Vancomycin for MRSA

There is synergy between cell-wall-active antibiotics and the aminoglycosides when the staphylococcus is sensitive to both. Such combinations are often used in severe systemic infection, particularly in the compromised host, when effective and rapid bactericidal action is needed.

Some chronic or recurrent infections of the compromised host can be controlled by administration over months or years of an oral preparation of one of the penicillinase-resistant penicillins.

### Prevention

Antistaphylococal soaps block infection

In patients subject to recurrent infection, such as chronic furunculosis, preventive measures are aimed at controlling reinfection and, if possible, eliminating the carrier state. Clothes and bedding that may cause reinfection should be washed at a sufficiently high temperature to destroy staphylococci (70°C or higher) or dry-cleaned. In adults, the use of chlorhexidine or hexachlorophene soaps in showering and washing increases the bactericidal activity of the skin (see Chapter 11). In such individuals, or in medical personnel found to be a source of infection to patients, anterior nasal carriage can be reduced and often eliminated with nasal creams containing antimicrobics not used for systemic infections (eg, mupirocin, neomycin, and bacitracin) used in conjunction with oral therapy with antimicrobics that are concentrated within phagocytes and nasal secretions (eg, rifampin or ciprofloxacin). Attempts to reduce nasal carriage more generally among medical personnel in an institution are usually fruitless and encourage replacement of susceptible strains with those that are multiresistant.

Elimination of nasal carriage difficult

Chemoprophylaxis during high risk surgery effective

Chemoprophylaxis is effective in surgical procedures such as hip and cardiac valve replacements, in which infection with *S. aureus* or coagulase-negative staphylococci can have devastating consequences for the prosthesis and thus the patient. Brief high-dose chemoprophylaxis is given around the time of surgery with the intention of preventing the superinfections that often complicate longer periods of antibiotic administration.

## COAGULASE-NEGATIVE STAPHYLOCOCCI

Common colonizers of the skin

*S. epidermidis* and a number of other species of coagulase-negative staphylococci are normal commensals of the skin, anterior nares, and ear canals of humans. Their large numbers and ubiquitous distribution result in frequent contamination of specimens collected from or through the skin, making these organisms among the most frequently isolated in the clinical laboratory. In the past, they were rarely the cause of significant infections, but with the increasing use of implanted catheters and prosthetic devices, they have emerged as important agents of hospital-acquired infections. Immunosuppressed or neutropenic patients have been particularly affected.

Organisms may contaminate prosthetic devices during implantation, seed the device during a subsequent bacteremia, or gain access to the lumina of shunts and catheters when they are temporarily disconnected or manipulated. The outcome of the bacterial contamination is determined by the microbe's capacity to attach to the surface of the foreign body and to multiply there. Initial adherence is facilitated by the hydrophobic nature of the synthetic polymers used in medical devices and the natural hydrophobic nature of many coagulase-negative staphylococci. Following attachment, some strains produce a viscous extracellular polysaccharide **slime** or biofilm. This biofilm provides additional adhesion, completely covers the bacteria, and serves as a mechanical barrier to antimicrobial agents and host defense mechanisms; it is also believed to enhance nutrition of the microbes by functioning as an ion-exchange resin. Strains able to produce the polysaccharide biofilm are more likely to colonize intravenous catheters but have no known advantage in adherence to human tissues such as heart valves. The resistance of many coagulase-negative staphylococci to multiple antimicrobic agents contributes further to their persistence in the body. Infections are generally low grade, but unless controlled, they can proceed to serious tissue damage or a fatal outcome.

Commonly infect implanted medical devices

Polysaccharide slime production enhances attachment and survival

The interpretation of blood cultures that grow coagulase-negative staphylococci is fraught with difficulty. In most cases, the finding is attributable to skin contamination, although it can indicate infection when a patient has implanted devices, or has defenses that are otherwise compromised. The repeated isolation of organisms with similar antibiograms and biochemical characteristics strongly indicates the presence of an infection. Unfortunately, there is at present no standardized phage-typing procedure for coagulase-negative staphylococci that can establish the identity of repeated isolates. A number of molecular procedures, including plasmid pattern analysis, restriction endonuclease analysis of plasmid or chromosomal DNA, and DNA hybridization techniques, can compare isolates but are not yet generally available in clinical laboratories.

Most common skin contaminant in blood cultures

Repeated positives suggest infection

*S. saprophyticus*, which is widely dispersed in the environment, has a similar, but restricted ability to cause opportunistic infection in the compromised host. It is, however, a uropathogen, and is the etiologic agent in 10 to 20% of primary urinary tract infections in young women.

*S. saprophyticus* associated with urinary infection

Most coagulase-negative staphylococci now encountered are resistant to penicillin, either because of penicillinase production or because of intrinsic resistance. Many are also resistant to the penicillinase-resistant penicillins (such as oxacillin and cloxacillin), as well as to other antimicrobics with spectra of activity that include many Gram-positive cocci. Vancomycin resistance is also being encountered. Many resistance determinants are plasmid encoded. As with *S. aureus,* strains resistant to the penicillinase-resistant penicillins are considered resistant to the cephalosporins as well. Treatment of coagulase-negative staphylococcal infections of prosthetic devices frequently requires removal of the device, as well as chemotherapy to prevent recurrence.

Multiple antimicrobic resistance common

## MICROCOCCI

A genus related to *Staphylococcus* is *Micrococcus*. The micrococci comprise commensal, free-living, Gram-positive cocci that are often larger than *S. aureus* and often arranged in regular packets of four or eight, depending on whether they divide in two or three planes before separation. They are coagulase negative and, like the staphylococci, produce catalase. In contrast to the staphylococci, micrococci metabolize oxidatively only and cannot grow anaerobically. Their pathogenic significance is similar to that of the coagulase-negative staphylococci.

## ADDITIONAL READING

Bhakdi S, Tranum-Jensen J: Alpha-toxin of *Staphylococcus aureus*. *Microbiol Rev* 1991;55:733–751. A detailed comprehensive review of this important toxin.

Bohach GA, Fast DJ, Nelson RD, Schlivert PM: Staphylococcal and streptococcal pyrogenic exotoxins involved in toxic shock syndrome and related illnesses. *CRC Crit Rev Microbiol* 1990;17:251–272. This review begins to bring together the pathogenic basis for the toxic syndromes.

Elek SD, Conan PE: The virulence of Staphylococcus pyogenes for man. A study of the problems of wound infections. *Br J Exp Pathol* 1957;38:573–586. A classic study of the factors influencing the development of staphylococcal wound infections in humans.

Pfaller MA, Herwaldt LA: Laboratory, clinical and epidemiological aspects of coagulase-negative staphylococci. *Clin Microb Rev* 1988;1:281–299. Reviews the epidemiologic and pathogenetic factors influencing the emergence of coagulase-negative staphylococci as important nosocomial pathogens.

See RH, Kum WWS, Chang AH, et al: Induction of tumor necrosis factor and interleukin-1 by purified staphylococcal toxic shock syndrome toxin 1 requires the presence of both monocytes and T lymphocytes. *Infect Immun* 1992;60:2612–2618. A study that defines the superantigen characteristics of TSST-1.

Chapter

16

# Streptococci and Enterococci

*Kenneth J. Ryan and Stanley Falkow*

The genus *Streptococcus* comprises species of Gram-positive spherical or oval cocci that tend to be arranged in chains. Most grow best in enriched bacteriologic media. Streptococci form a significant portion of the indigenous microflora of humans and animals; most of these species are found in the oral cavity and nasopharynx but some inhabit the intestinal tract. Although most species rarely cause disease, the genus includes three of the most important pathogens of humans: *S. pyogenes*, the group A streptococcus, causes a variety of acute infections and can stimulate the poststreptococcal sequelae of rheumatic fever and acute glomerulonephritis. *S. agalactiae*, the group B streptococcus, is the most important cause of neonatal sepsis and meningeal infection. *S. pneumoniae* is a major cause of both acute bacterial pneumonia and acute purulent meningitis.

## THE STREPTOCOCCI: GROUP CHARACTERISTICS

### Morphology

Streptococci stain readily with common dyes, demonstrating coccal cells 0.5 to 1 μm in diameter. In contrast to staphylococci, streptococcal cells are generally smaller and ovoid in shape. They are usually arranged in chains with oval cells touching end to end, because they divide in one plane and tend to remain attached. Length may vary from a single pair to continuous chains of over 30 cells, depending on the species and growth conditions. Medically important streptococci are not acid fast, do not form spores, and are nonmotile. Some members form capsules composed of polysaccharide complexes or hyaluronic acid.

Oval cocci chain end to end

### Cultural and Biochemical Characteristics

Streptococci grow best in media enriched with digests of animal tissues, serum, or defibrinated blood. The plating medium most commonly used is blood agar, which consists of a simple nutrient broth to which agar and animal blood are added. Sheep blood is preferred because of its clear demonstration of streptococcal hemolytic patterns. Medically important species grow best at temperatures of 35 to 37°C. Streptococci metabolize carbohydrates fermentatively, fail to produce catalase, but can grow under atmospheric conditions ranging from aerobic to strictly anaerobic. Growth of many strains is enhanced by the presence of 2 to 10% carbon dioxide. Strictly anaerobic strains, previously called anaerobic streptococci, are now classified in the genus *Peptostreptococcus* (Chapter 18).

Blood agar demonstrates hemolytic patterns

Catalase negative

After incubation for 18 to 24 hours on blood agar plates, small colonies ranging from pinpoint size to 0.5 to 2 mm in diameter are produced. A distinctive feature of streptococ-

α or β hemolysis produced

cal growth on blood agar is the production by many species of alpha (green) or beta (clear) hemolysis of the erythrocytes suspended in the agar (Chapter 14). Hemolysis is dependent on several cultural features and nonhemolytic variants of inherently hemolytic species may be seen. Streptococci are biochemically active, attacking a variety of carbohydrates, proteins, and amino acids. Glucose fermentation yields mostly lactic acid.

## Classification

Lancefield carbohydrate antigens define important subgroup more than hemolysis

Initially, streptococci were classified on the basis of the hemolysis and certain biochemical tests. It was known that hemolytic strains were often, but not always, associated with important infections in humans and animals. This taxonomy was put on a sounder basis by the studies of Rebecca Lancefield. Among the beta-hemolytic streptococci she demonstrated carbohydrate antigens in cell-wall extracts that allowed classification into groups correlating well with known bacteriologic, epidemiologic, and pathogenic features. Later, it was shown that some nonhemolytic streptococci had the same cell wall antigens and pathogenic significance as the beta-hemolytic strains. Thus, presence or absence of a Lancefield antigen is more fundamental for classification of streptococci than hemolysis.

Hemolysis remains important in diagnostic laboratories

From a practical point of view, type of hemolysis and certain biochemical reactions remain valuable for the initial recognition and presumptive classification of streptococci, and as an indication of what subsequent taxonomic tests to perform. Thus, beta-hemolysis indicates that the strain has one of the Lancefield group antigens, but strains of some Lancefield groups may be alpha-hemolytic or nonhemolytic. The streptococci will be considered as follows: (1) pyogenic streptococci (Lancefield groups); (2) pneumococcus; (3) viridans streptococci; and (4) other, principally nonhemolytic, streptococci (Table 16–1).

### Pyogenic Streptococci

Lancefield antigen positive defined as pyogenic Streptococci

Groups A and B most common causes of disease

Streptococci with cell-wall antigens of Lancefield (Table 16–1) frequently cause purulent infections in humans or animals and are thus termed pyogenic streptococci. The primary characteristic of pyogenic streptococci is the presence of one of the Lancefield antigens, designated as groups A through T. The most common Lancefield groups of streptococci isolated from humans are A, B, C, F, and G, and of these, groups A and B are of greatest pathogenic significance. Some of these group designations correlate with species names previously assigned on the basis of cultural, biochemical, and pathogenic features, such as *S. pyogenes* (group A) and *S. agalactiae* (group B). To recapitulate, most but not all streptococci possessing Lancefield group antigens are beta-hemolytic; however, all that are beta-hemolytic are included among the pyogenic streptococci.

### Pneumococci

Pneumococci defined by polysaccharide capsule

This category contains a single species, *S. pneumoniae* (pneumococcus). Its distinctive feature is the presence of a polysaccharide capsule. Differences in the polysaccharide polymer composition, and thus the antigenic specificity, of the capsules of different pneumococci has defined more than 80 immunotypes. Although the pneumococcal cell wall shares some common antigens with other streptococci, it does not possess any of the Lancefield group antigens. The pneumococcus is alpha-hemolytic.

### Viridans and Nonhemolytic Streptococci

Viridans streptococci are alpha-hemolytic and lack both the group carbohydrate antigens of the pyogenic streptococci and the capsular antigens of the pneumococcus. The term encompasses several species, including *S. salivarius* and *S. mitis*. Viridans streptococci comprise members of the normal oral flora of humans. They almost never demonstrate invasive qualities.

Other streptococci lack Lancefield antigens or capsules

A variety of other streptococci may be encountered that lack the features of the pyogenic streptococci or pneumococci; they would be classified with the viridans group, except they are not alpha-hemolytic. Such strains are usually assigned descriptive terms such as nonhemolytic streptococci or microaerophilic streptococci. They have been less thor-

TABLE 16–1. CLASSIFICATION OF STREPTOCOCCI AND ENTEROCOCCI BY HEMOLYTIC AND SEROLOGIC REACTIONS

| Group | Common Terms | Hemolysis | Taxonomically Useful Antigens | | | Disease Associations |
|---|---|---|---|---|---|---|
| | | | *Lancefield Cell Wall* | *Surface Protein* | *Surface Polysaccharide* | |
| **Streptococci** | | | | | | |
| Pyogenic | | | | | | |
| *S. pyogenes* | Group A streptococcus | β | A | 70 + M protein | — | Pyogenic, scarlet fever, rheumatic fever, glomerulonephritis |
| *S. agalactiae* | Group B streptococcus | β, occasionally α or nonhemolytic | B | — | Ia, Ib, III, III, IV | Pyogenic, neonatal sepsis, meningitis |
| *S. bovis* | Nonenterococcal group D | α or nonhemolytic | D | — | — | Low virulence, endocarditis |
| *S. equi*<br>*S. anginosus* (milleri)<br>Other species | | β, occasionally α or nonhemolytic | C, E–T | — | — | Pyogenic |
| Pneumococcus (*S. pneumoniae*) | Pneumococcus | α | — | — | 80+ | Pneumonia, meningitis |
| Viridans and nonhemolytic<br>*S. sanguis*<br>*S. salivarius*<br>*S. mitis*<br>*S. mutans*<br>Other species | Viridans streptococci or nonhemolytic streptococci (depending on hemolytic reaction) | α or nonhemolytic | — | — | — | Low virulence, endocarditis; *S. mutans* associated with dental caries |
| **Enterococci** | | | | | | |
| *E. faecalis*<br>*E. faecium*<br>*E. durans* | Enterocci | α or nonhemolytic (rarely β) | D | — | — | Pyogenic, urinary infection |

oughly studied, but generally have the same biologic behavior as the viridans streptococci. The usual hemolytic biochemical and cultural reactions of commonly encountered streptococci are summarized in Table 16–2.

## Group A Streptococci (*Streptococcus pyogenes*)

### Morphology and Growth

Clear, sharp β-hemolysis

Group A streptococci typically appear in purulent lesions or broth cultures as spherical or ovoid cells in chains of short to medium length (4 to 10 cells). On blood agar plates, colonies are usually compact, small, and surrounded by a 2- to 3-mm zone of beta-hemolysis that is easily seen and sharply demarcated. Beta-hemolysis is caused by two hemolysins, **streptolysin S** and the oxygen-labile **streptolysin O,** both of which are produced by most group A strains. Occasional strains lack streptolysin S, and beta-hemolysis by streptolysin O then occurs only under anaerobic conditions. This feature is of practical importance, because such strains would be missed if incubated only under the usual aerobic conditions.

Strains lacking streptolysin S β-hemolytic only anaerobically

### Structure

The structure of group A streptococci is illustrated in Figure 16–1. The cell wall is built upon a peptidoglycan matrix that provides rigidity, as in other Gram-positive bacteria. Within this matrix lies the group-specific antigen, which is composed of rhamnose and *N*-acetylglucosamine. By definition all group A streptococci possess this antigen. *S. pyogenes* produces adhesive projections, hairlike pili that contain a protein component, M protein, and lipoteichoic acid (LTA; Fig 16–2). Group A streptococci are divided into more than 80 serotypes based on antigenic differences in epitopes of the M protein. Some strains have an overlying nonantigenic hyaluronic acid capsule.

Group A antigen in cell wall

Pili, M protein, LTA on surface

#### M Protein

The M protein itself is a fibrillar molecule with its carboxy terminal rooted in the peptidoglycan of the cell wall and the amino-terminal regions extending toward the surface. There is evidence that the antigenic specificity of M protein lies in the amino-terminal portion because it is the most variable part of the molecule and the most available to immune surveillance. There is currently great effort being directed toward assigning specific biologic functions such as attachment, phagocytosis resistance, and stimulation of heart cross-reactive immune reactions to precise regions and epitopes of the molecule.

Amino-terminal M protein external and highly variable

**TABLE 16–2. USUAL HEMOLYTIC, BIOCHEMICAL, AND CULTURAL REACTIONS OF COMMON STREPTOCOCCI AND ENTEROCOCCI**[a]

| | Susceptibility to | | | | |
|---|---|---|---|---|---|
| | *Bacitracin* | *Optochin* | Bile Solubility | Bile/Esculin Reaction[b] | PYR[c] |
| **Streptococci** | | | | | |
| β-Hemolytic | | | | | |
| Lancefield group A | + | – | – | – | + |
| Lancefield groups B, C, F, G | – | – | – | – | – |
| α-Hemolytic | | | | | |
| *S. pneumoniae* | – | + | + | – | – |
| Viridans group | – | – | – | – | – |
| Nonhemolytic | – | – | – | – | – |
| **Enterococci** | – | – | – | + | + |

[a] All are tests commonly substituted for serological identification in clinical laboratories.
[b] Tests for the ability to grow in bile and reduce esculin.
[c] PYR = pyrrolidonyl arylamidase test.

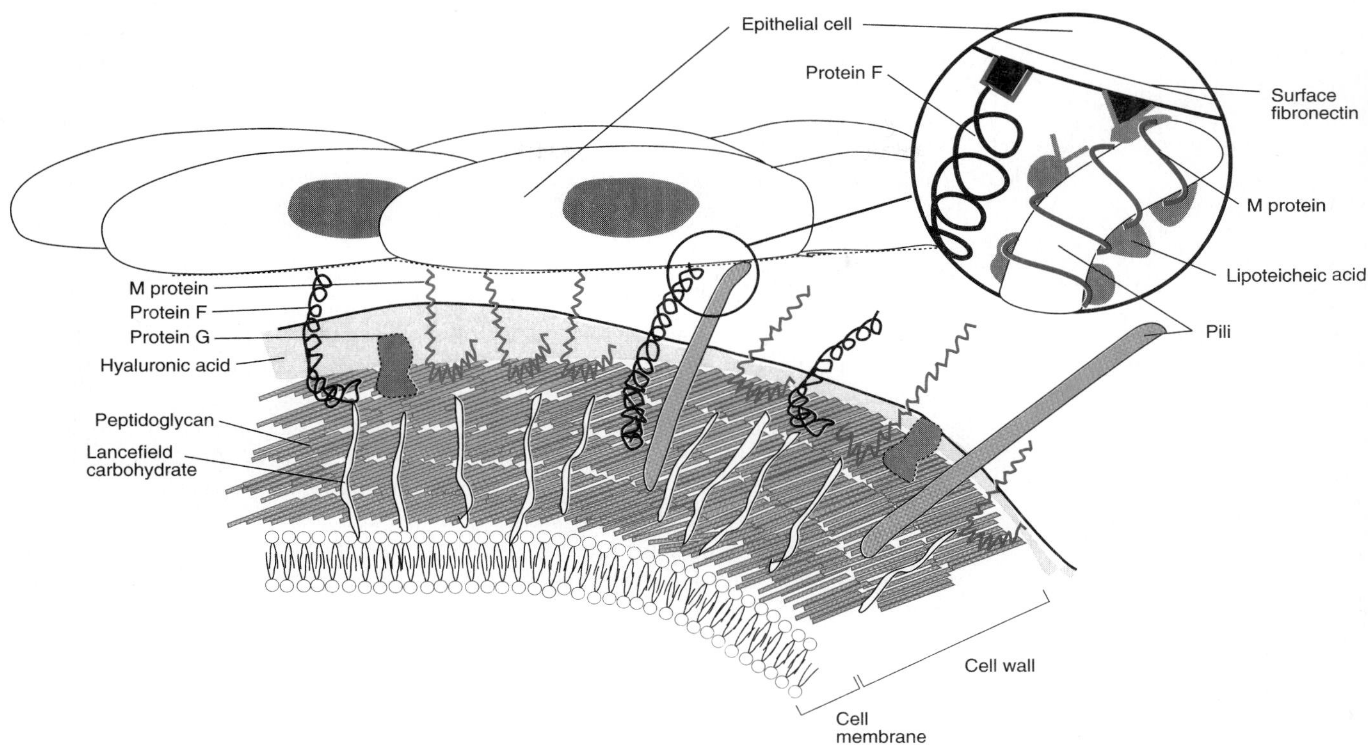


**Figure 16–1.** Antigenic structure of *S. pyogenes*, and adhesion to an epithelial cell. The location of peptidoglycan and Lancefield carbohydrate antigen in the cell wall is shown in the diagram. M protein and lipoteichoic acid are associated with the cell surface and the pili. Lipoteichoic acid and protein F mediate binding to fibronectin on the host surface.

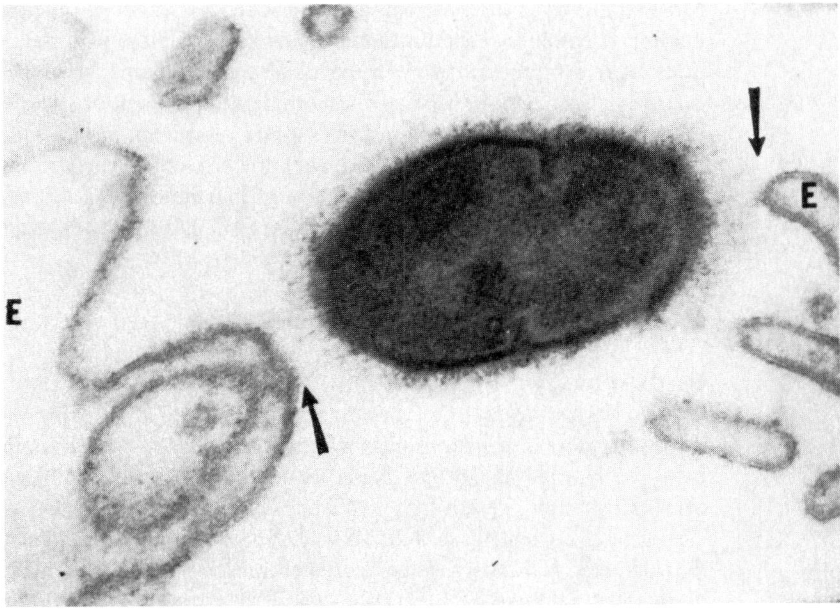


**Figure 16–2.** A group A β-hemolytic streptococcus is shown attaching to the cell membrane of a human oral epithelial cell (E). Note the hairlike pili (*arrows*), which mediate the attachment. As in Figure 16–1, both M protein and lipoteichoic acid are associated with the pili. (*Reproduced with permission from Beachey EH, Ofek I. J Exp Med 1976;143:764. Figure 2.*)

Protein F binds fibronectin

Protein G binds *Fc* fragments

PROTEIN F AND PROTEIN G

Fibronectin binding is mediated by a polypeptide, protein F, exposed on the streptococcal surface (Fig 16–1). Another cell-surface protein called protein G binds the *Fc* portion of antibodies. In principle this could lead to a covering of antibody molecules on the streptococcal surface that are facing the "wrong way." This could lend a cloak of invisibility to the host immune system and/or interfere with the complement activation at the bacterial surface in tandem with M protein.

### Toxins, Hemolysins, and Biologically Active Extracellular Products

STREPTOLYSINS O AND S

Streptolysin O pore-forming toxin similar to staphylococcal α-toxin

Streptolysin O oxygen labile and antigenic

The two hemolysins responsible for beta hemolysis are streptolysin O (oxygen labile) and streptolysin S. Streptolysin O is a general sulfhydral-activated cytotoxin, lysing leukocytes, tissue cells, and platelets. The toxin inserts directly into the cell membrane of a variety of host cells, forming circular transmembrane pores similar to those produced by complement and by staphylococcal alpha-toxin (Chapter 15). Antibodies against streptolysin O are often formed as a result of *S. pyogenes* infection, and inhibition of hemolysis by these antibodies is the basis of the antistreptolysin O diagnostic test.

Streptolysin S is a nonantigenic low-molecular-weight peptide. It is oxygen stable and is responsible for the hemolysis seen around colonies of group A streptococci on blood agar plates incubated aerobically.

PYROGENIC EXOTOXINS

SPEs have multiple effects including scarlet fever

SPEs are superantigens

Gene in lysogenic phage

A minority of group A strains form pyrogenic exotoxins that have long been associated with classic **scarlet fever** under the name **erythrogenic toxin.** They are now known to share biological activity and sequence similarity with other pyrogenic exotoxins such as those produced by *Staphylococcus aureus* (Chapter 15). This activity includes stimulation of cytokine release through the superantigen mechanism (Chapter 8). The **streptococcal pyrogenic exotoxins (SPE)** produce multiple effects including fever, rash (scarlet fever), T-cell proliferation, B-lymphocyte suppression, and heightened sensitivity to endotoxin. The SPEs occur in three antigenic forms, which differ considerably in geographic distribution. Only strains lysogenized with a temperate bacteriophage that contains the toxin gene produce pyrogenic exotoxins.

OTHER EXTRACELLULAR PRODUCTS

Other products may aid spread or injury

Most strains of group A streptococci produce a number of other extracellular products including streptokinase, hyaluronidase, nucleases, **C5a peptidase,** and others. The C5a peptidase is an extracellular enzyme that degrades complement component C5a, the main factor that attracts phagocytes to sites of complement deposition. The enzymatic actions of the others likely play some role in tissue injury or spread, but no specific roles have been defined. Some are antigenic and have been the basis of serologic tests. **Streptokinase** causes lysis of fibrin clots through conversion of plasminogen in normal plasma to the protease plasmin; this activity is now used in the treatment of acute myocardial infarction.

## ■ Group A Streptococcal Disease

### Epidemiology

GROUP A STREPTOCOCCAL PHARYNGITIS

Spread over short distances from throat and nasal sites

Acute streptococcal pharyingitis is the most common bacterial infection of the throat seen by physicians and its correct diagnosis and treatment are important. Without treatment, the organism is often present for 1 to 4 weeks after symptoms have disappeared. Asymptomatic carrier rates are usually less than 5%. Carriage may be both pharyngeal and nasal and occasionally anal. Nasal carriers have greater infectivity than those who carry *S. pyogenes* in the throat only. Spread is by direct contact with the mucosa or secretions or through large droplets produced by coughing, sneezing, or even conversation. Droplet transmission is most efficient at the short distances (2 to 5 feet) at which interaction is common in families and institutions such as schools and military barracks. Environmental sources and fomites are not important means of spread, although group A streptococci survive for some time in dried secretions.

Recurrent infections are sometimes seen in families when prompt antimicrobial therapy has prevented the development of type-specific immunity. This situation allows reinfection from other infected or colonized siblings when antimicrobic treatment is stopped. Such "ping-pong" infection–reinfection cycles sometimes require simultaneous treatment of the entire family to prevent continued transmission.

Incomplete immunity linked to reinfection

### Impetigo

Impetigo caused by *S. pyogenes* has an earlier peak age incidence (2 to 5 years) than streptococcal pharyngitis. Clinical impetigo is often preceded by skin colonization, which is favored by poor hygiene. Minor trauma of colonized skin (for example, insect bites) then leads to development of the lesions. Transmission involves direct contact or shared fomites such as towels. Impetigo is most common among lower socioeconomic groups, in hot climates, and at times when insect bites are frequent. The M protein types of *S. pyogenes* most commonly associated with impetigo are different from those causing respiratory infection, and some are nephritogenic. Multiple cases of acute glomerulonephritis have occurred in association with epidemics of impetigo.

Skin colonization plus trauma leads to impetigo

Nephritogenic strains cause glomerulonephritis

### Nosocomial Wound and Puerperal Infections

Group A streptococci were once a leading cause of nosocomial postoperative wound and puerperal infections (Chapter 72). The primary mode of transmission from patient to patient was by the hands of physicians or other medical attendants and through poor hygienic practices. The potential for hospital spread, however, is still present. Infections may be derived from staff or patients ill with pharyngitis or carrying the organism in the pharynx or nose. Contaminated particles or epithelial cells from nonrespiratory carriage sites can also be a source of infection. For example, some nosocomial outbreaks of group A streptococcal infections have been traced to anal carriers who disseminated the organisms widely in operating rooms.

Hospital outbreaks linked to carriers

## Pathogenesis

*S. pyogenes* has evolved the ability to adhere to epithelial cells of the nasopharynx and skin. Until recently, M protein and LTA complexes were thought to be the major adhesive factors through mediating binding by LTA to the glycoprotein fibronectin on the cell surface. Recent advances in streptococcal genetics have permitted a better understanding of how the surface protein repertory of group A streptococci controls its cellular tropism. The case for the fibronectin-binding **protein F** is supported by experiments that show that when its gene is inactivated, group A streptococci are no longer capable of adhering to nasopharyngeal epithelial cells; but intestinal inhabitant, *Enterococcus faecalis*, expressing the same gene acquires the ability to bind to respiratory epithelial cells.

Surface molecules binding to fibronectin important first step

Protein F crucial for nasopharyngeal cell adherance

On the other hand, M protein appears to be dominant in binding to the epidermis through its ability to interact with keratinocytes, the most numerous cell type in cutaneous tissue. M-protein-deficient cells still adhere to the cutaneous epithelium but only to epidermal Langerhans cells, while mutants unable to produce either M protein or protein F are not capable of adhering to any cutaneous cell. Thus, both bacterial factors contribute to adherence of these pyogenic cocci to the cutaneous epithelium but each directs adherence to a specific population of epithelial cells.

M protein dominant in epidermis binding

Expression of M protein and protein F is environmentally regulated in response to changing concentrations of $O_2$ and $CO_2$. Experimental evidence suggests that a high $O_2$ environment favors protein F and adherence to Langerhans cells, while an environment richer in $CO_2$ favors M-protein synthesis and interaction with keratinocytes. This environmentally controlled sequential interaction of *S. pyogenes* with different types of host cells should play some mitigating role either in establishing the microbe or in altering the development of a normally protective host response. In this vein it is interesting to note that Langerhans cells are important antigen-presenting cells whereas keratinocytes are initiators of cutaneous inflammation.

M protein and protein F expressed in response to $O_2$ and $CO_2$ environmental cues

After the initial events of attachment and multiplication, it appears that the concerted activity of the M protein, immunoglobulin-binding proteins, and the C5a peptidase play the key roles in allowing the streptococcal infection to continue. M protein plays an essential role in group A streptococcal resistance to phagocytosis. Mutants lacking this factor are avirulent. The antiphagocytic activity of M protein is thought to be related to its capacity

Multiple factors allow continuation of infection

M protein antiphagocytic

M protein interferes with alternate pathway opsonization

to bind serum factor H leading to a diminished availability of alternate pathway generated complement component C3b for opsonization (Fig 16–3). In the presence of M-type-specific antibody, classical pathway opsonophagocytosis proceeds, and the streptococci are rapidly killed. It has long been known that antibody directed against a particular M type is protective only for subsequent infection with other strains of the same type **(type-specific immunity).** Unfortunately there are many M types, so repeated infections with other M types can occur.

Type-specific antibody reverses phagocytie resistance

The precise role of other bacterial factors in the pathogenesis of infection is uncertain, but the combined effect of streptokinase, DNAase, and hyaluronidase may prevent effective localization of the infection, while the streptolysins produce tissue injury and are toxic to phagocytic cells. Antibodies against these components are formed in the course of streptococcal infection, but are not known to be protective.

Virulence factors may be organized together on chromosome

The genes for the M protein, C5a peptidase, and the IgG-binding protein G, are all located in the same region of the bacterial chromosome. A regulatory locus in this gene cluster acts possibly as a transcriptional activator of multiple genes and responds to environmental cues including $CO_2$. Thus, multifaceted aspects of streptococcal pathogenesis show evidence that the microbe responds to host signals by targeting different cell types. The organism appears able to respond to these signals by producing specific virulence factors and turning others off.

## Poststreptococcal Sequelae

### Rheumatic Fever

**Acute rheumatic fever (ARF)** is a nonsuppurative inflammatory disease characterized by fever, carditis, subcutaneous nodules, chorea, and migratory polyarthritis. The most serious

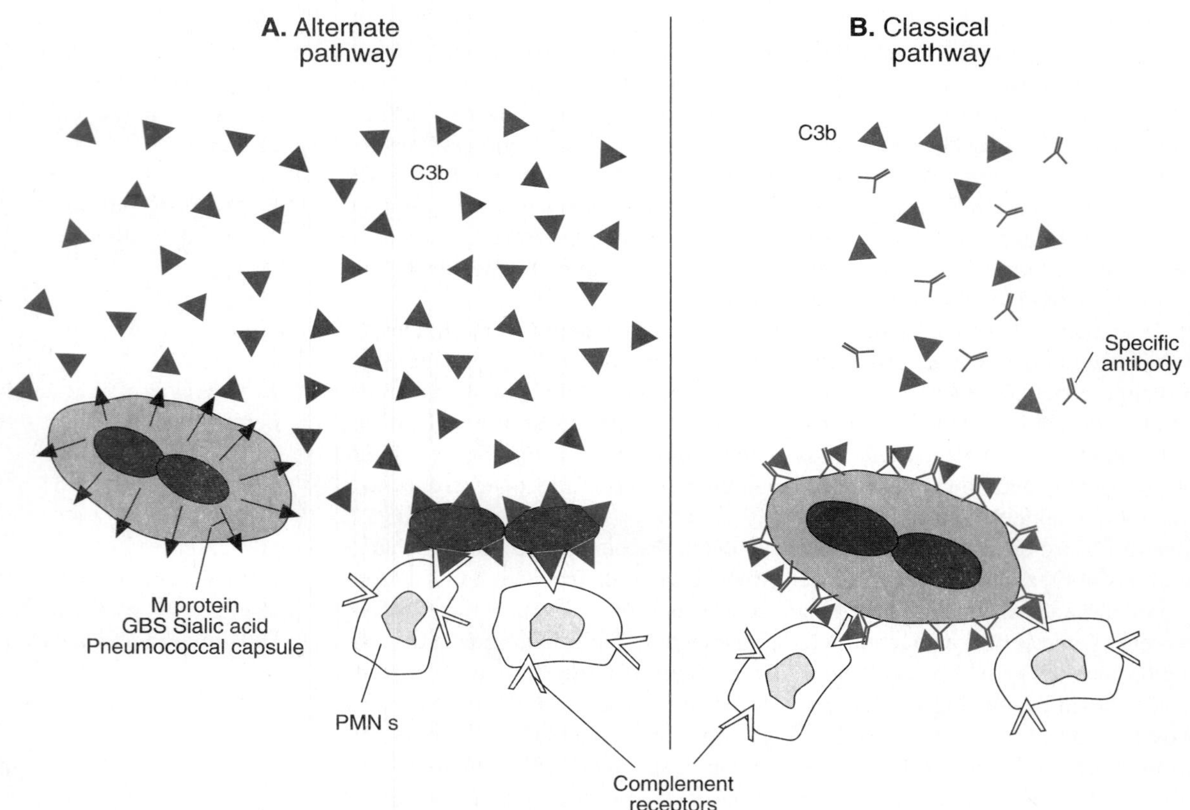


**Figure 16–3.** Streptococcal resistance to opsonophagocytosis. **A.** Streptococci with surface molecules that interfere with alternate pathway complement activation are protected from phagocyte recognition. Group A streptococcal M protein, group B streptococcal capsular sialic acid, and pneumococcal capsular polysaccharides act in this manner. **B.** In the presence of specific antibody to the surface antigen, classical pathway mechanisms operate and phagocytes recognize the organism.

of these involve the connective tissue and the endocardium, particularly of the heart valves. Cardiac enlargement, valvular murmurs, and effusions are seen clinically and reflect endocardial, myocardial, and epicardial damage, which can lead to heart failure. Attacks typically begin 3 weeks (range, 1 to 5 weeks) after a group A streptococcal pharyngitis, and in the absence of antiinflammatory therapy last 2 to 3 months. ARF also has a predilection for recurrence with subsequent streptococcal infections as new M types are encountered. The first attack usually occurs between the ages of 5 and 15 years. The risk of recurrent attacks after subsequent group A streptococcal infections continues into adult life and then decreases. Repeated attacks lead to progressive damage to the endocardium and heart valves, with scarring and valvular stenosis or incompetence (rheumatic heart disease).

ARF causes inflammation of connective tissue, endocardium

New M types trigger recurrences

Recurrences lead to permanent damage to heart valves

The association between group A streptococci and ARF is based on epidemiologic studies linking group A streptococcal pharyngitis and heightened immune responses to streptococcal products. ARF does not follow nonrespiratory infections or infections with streptococci other than group A. Although some "rheumatogenic" M types appear to be more likely to cause initial attacks, it is not known if recurrences are triggered by a few or many M protein types. The use of continuous prophylactic penicillin for prevention of recurrence assumes protection against all subsequent group A streptococcal infections is required.

ARF only follows respiratory infection

Prophylactic penicillin preventative

Of the many theories advanced to explain the role of group A streptococci in rheumatic fever, an autoimmune mechanism related to antigenic similarities between streptococci and human tissue antigens has the most experimental support. Patients with rheumatic fever have higher levels of antistreptococcal antibodies than those with streptococcal infections who do not develop ARF. Some of these antibodies have been shown to react with both heart tissues and streptococcal antigens. For example, antibodies directed against streptococcal cell wall and cell membrane components cross-react with cardiac sarcolemmal sheaths, smooth muscle of vessel walls, and cells of the endocardium. Just which of the many group A streptococcal antigens stimulate these antibodies presents a unique dilemma if the eventual goal is prevention by immunization. A poorly crafted vaccine could cause the very disease it is designed to prevent.

Antistreptococcal antibodies also react with heart sarcolemma

A number of interesting cross-reactions have been investigated such as one between the group A polysaccharide and a glycoprotein isolated from heart valves, but the most promising are those involving M protein. M protein fragments from a serotype strongly associated with ARF have been shown to stimulate antibodies that cross-react with human heart sarcolemma membranes. Immunochemical and genetic studies of M proteins from different M types are now directed at defining the epitopes responsible and the extent to which they are shared between strains. Evidence is increasing that certain conserved domains of the M protein molecule may be responsible for the heart cross-reactivity, while other domains confer the factor H and fibrinogen binding responsible for its antiphagocytic properties. Identifying and separating the epitopes responsible is crucial both to understanding rheumatic fever and to approaches to its prevention through immunization.

Cross-reactive epitopes are located in M protein

Cross-reactive domains may be separable from other function of M protein molecule

ARF patients also show enhanced cell-mediated immune responses to streptococcal antigens. A cellular reaction pattern consisting of lymphocytes and macrophages aggregated around fibrinoid deposits is found in human hearts. This lesion, called the **Aschoff body,** is considered characteristic of rheumatic carditis. Recent suggestion that M protein has superantigen properties must still be reconciled with the prolonged nature of the illness.

Genetic factors are probably also important in ARF because only a small proportion of individuals infected with group A streptococci develop the disease. Attack rates have been highest among those of lower socioeconomic status and vary among those of different racial origins. ARF declined dramatically in the United States during the 1960s and 1970s, but a resurgence in the form of several outbreaks began in the 1980s. In contrast to earlier experience, some of these outbreaks have primarily affected children of higher socioeconomic status. The gene for an alloantigen found on the surface of B lymphocytes occurs among rheumatic fever patients at a frequency fourfold to fivefold greater than the general population. This further suggests a genetic predisposition to hyperreactivity to streptococcal products.

Genetic factors associated with hyperreactivity to streptococci

Recent outbreaks of ARF

## Acute Glomerulonephritis

Poststreptococcal glomerulonephritis is primarily a disease of childhood, characterized clinically by edema, hypertension, hematuria, and proteinuria, and pathologically by diffuse proliferative lesions of the glomeruli. The clinical course is usually benign, with spon-

Glomerulonephritis follows respiratory or skin infection

taneous healing over weeks to months. Occasionally a progressive course leads to renal failure and death. The disease may follow either respiratory or cutaneous group A streptococcal infection, and involves only certain "nephritogenic" strains. The average latent period between infection and glomerulonephritis is 10 days from a respiratory infection, but generally about 3 weeks from a skin infection. Nephritogenic strains are limited to a few M types.

Only nephritogenic strains

Glomerular injury related to desposition of antigen-antibody complexes

The pathogenesis of acute glomerulonephritis appears to involve immunologic mechanisms. Immunoglobulins, complement components, and antigens that react with antibodies against group A streptococci have been identified in the diseased glomerulus. The renal injury may be caused by deposition in the glomerulus of antigen–antibody complexes with complement activation and consequent inflammation. The M proteins of some nephritogenic strain have been shown to share antigenic determinants with glomeruli, which suggests an autoimmune mechanism similar to rheumatic fever.

## Group A Streptococcal Infections: Clinical Aspects

### Clinical Manifestations

#### Streptococcal Pharyngitis

One of the most common bacterial infections is streptococcal pharyngitis. Although it may occur at any age, it is most frequent between 5 and 15 years. The illness is characterized by acute sore throat, malaise, fever (38.9 to 40°C), and headache. Infection typically involves the tonsillar pillars, uvula, and soft palate, which become red, swollen, and covered with a yellow-white exudate. The cervical lymph nodes that drain this area may also become swollen and tender. Although these clinical features are typical, there is enough overlap with viral pharyngitis that culture is required for diagnosis.

Strep throat syndrome overlaps with viral pharyngitis

Group A streptococcal pharyngitis is usually self-limiting. Typically, the fever is gone by the third to fifth day, and other manifestations subside within a week. Occasionally the infection may spread beyond the pharynx to produce peritonsillar or retropharyngeal abscesses, otitis media, suppurative cervical adenitis, and acute sinusitis. Rarely, more extensive spread occurs, producing meningitis, pneumonia, or bacteremia with metastatic infection in distant organs. In the preantibiotic era, these suppurative complications were responsible for a mortality of 1 to 3% from acute streptococcal pharyngitis. Such complications are much less common now, and fatal infections are rare.

Spread beyond the pharynx uncommon

#### Impetigo

Group A streptococcal infection of healthy skin usually produces a localized skin disease known as impetigo. Invasion is through minor trauma, such as skin abrasions or insect bites. The primary lesion of streptococcal impetigo is a small (up to 1 cm) vesicle surrounded by an area of erythema. The vesicle enlarges over a period of days, becomes pustular, and eventually breaks to form a yellow crust. The lesions usually appear in 2- to 5-year-old children on exposed body surfaces, typically the face and lower extremities. Multiple lesions may coalesce to form deeper ulcerated areas. Although *Staphylococcus aureus* produces a clinically distinct bullous form of impetigo (Chapter 15), it can also cause vesicular lesions resembling streptococcal impetigo. Both pathogens are isolated from some cases.

Exposed skin of 2- to 5-year-old children

Tiny pustules may combine to form ulcers

#### Erysipelas

Erysipelas is a distinct form of streptococcal infection of the skin and subcutaneous tissues, primarily affecting the dermis. It is characterized by a spreading area of erythema and edema with rapidly advancing, well-demarcated edges, pain, and systemic manifestations, including fever and lymphadenopathy. Infection usually occurs on the face, and a previous history of streptococcal sore throat is common. Erysipelas is a serious disease that requires immediate antimicrobial therapy.

Spreading erythema of deeper tissues

#### Wound and Burn Infections

Although less common than in the past, group A streptococcal infections of wounds and burns can develop and spread rapidly to adjacent tissues, with the risk of sepsis and bacteremia. Burn infections are associated with failure of skin grafts. Burn and wound infections in hospitalized patients carry a substantial risk of cross-infection to other patients with similar conditions.

PUERPERAL INFECTION

Infection of the endometrium at or near delivery is a life-threatening form of group A streptococcal infection. Fortunately, it is now relatively rare, but in the 19th century the clinical findings of "childbed fever" were characteristic and common enough to provide the first clues to the transmission of bacterial infections in hospitals (see Chapter 72). Spread to other pelvic organs and the bloodstream via the lymphatic vessels produces a rapidly progressive infection. Special precautions may be needed to prevent its spread to other hospitalized patients.

Classic puerperal (childbed) fever by group A Streptococci

DISEASE ASSOCIATED WITH STREPTOCOCCAL PYROGENIC EXOTOXINS

**Scarlet Fever.** Infection with strains that elaborate any of the pyrogenic exotoxins may superimpose the signs of scarlet fever on a streptococcal pharyngitis. In scarlet fever, the buccal mucosa, temples, and cheeks are deep red, except for a pale area around the mouth and nose (circumoral pallor). Punctate hemorrhages appear on the hard and soft palates, and the tongue becomes covered with a yellow-white exudate through which the red papillae are prominent (strawberry tongue). A diffuse red "sandpaper" rash appears on the second day of illness, spreading from the upper chest to the trunk and extremities. Circulating antibody to the toxin neutralizes these effects. For unknown reasons, scarlet fever is both less frequent and less severe than earlier in the century.

Scarlet fever is strep throat with a characterisitic rash

**Toxic Shock-like Syndrome.** In the late 1980s an increased frequency and severity of group A streptococcal infections was noted in the United States and other countries. Rapid progression to death in only a few days was seen in previously healthy persons, including Sesame Street Muppet creator Jim Henson. Although group A streptococcal infections have long been known to be life-threatening when spread beyond the common pharyngeal and skin sites, a number of similarities to staphylococcal toxic shock syndrome (TSS) have caused these cases to be tentatively called toxic shock-like syndrome (TSLS). The clinical findings of shock, renal impairment, rash, respiratory failure, and diarrhea suggest the multiple organ system involvement characteristic of systemic toxins. A high proportion of these cases have been caused by strains producing one or more of the streptococcal pyrogenic exotoxins, particularly SPE A. As indicated above, these toxins have actions similar to TSST-1 and the other staphylococcal pyrogenic exotoxins. Many of the clinical features are consistent with cytokine action triggered by the superantigenicity of these pyrogenic exotoxins. A significant difference from staphylococcal TSS is that most of these patients have obvious progressive infection, usually with bacteremia. This syndrome may represent bacteriophage-mediated horizontal transfer of the SPE genes among recently emerged clones of enhanced invasive potential, a deadly combination.

Streptococcal TSLS is a rapidly progressive multisystem disease

Strains producing SPEs linked to TSLS

SPE superantigen action may contribute

TSLS patients often bacteriemic

### Treatment and Prevention

Group A streptococci are highly susceptible to penicillin G, the antimicrobic of choice. Concentrations as low as 0.01 μg/mL have a bactericidal effect, and penicillin resistance is so far unknown. Numerous other antimicrobics are also active, including other penicillins, cephalosporins, tetracyclines, chloramphenicol, and erythromycin, but not aminoglycosides. Tetracycline resistance has been found in 5 to 10% of strains, and erythromycin resistance also occurs when that agent is widely used.

Group A streptococci remain susceptible to penicillin

Patients allergic to penicillin are usually treated with erythromycin if the organisms are susceptible. Impetigo is often treated with erythromycin to cover the prospect of *Staphylococcus aureus* involvement. Adequate treatment of streptococcal pharyngitis within 10 days of onset will prevent rheumatic fever by removing the antigenic stimulus; its effect on the duration of the pharyngitis is less, because of the short course of the natural infection. Penicillin does not prevent the development of acute glomerulonephritis.

Treatment of pharyngitis within 10 days prevents ARF

Penicillin prophylaxis with long-acting preparations is used to prevent recurrences of rheumatic fever during the most susceptible ages (5 to 15 years). Patients with a history of rheumatic fever or known rheumatic heart disease receive antimicrobial prophylaxis while undergoing procedures known to cause transient bacteremia, such as dental extraction.

### Laboratory Diagnosis

In pharyngitis, a swab of the posterior pharynx and tonsils is taken to include all inflamed areas. A direct Gram-stained smear is unhelpful because of the many other streptococci in the normal pharyngeal flora, but smears from normally sterile sites will usually demonstrate streptococci. Blood agar plates incubated anaerobically give the best yield because they favor the demonstration of beta-hemolysis (see streptolysins, above). Beta-hemolytic colonies are identified by Lancefield grouping using immunofluorescence or agglutination methods. Direct detection of group A antigen extracted from throat swabs is now available in a wide variety of kits marketed for physicians' offices. These methods are rapid and have high specificity, but in many studies are only 90 to 95% sensitive compared to culture. Given the importance of detection of group A streptococci in prevention of ARF (it is the reason for doing throat cultures), these negatives must be confirmed by culture before withholding treatment.

Anaerobic blood agar plates best for demonstrating β hemolysis

Direct antigen detection methods miss 5–10% of cases

In smaller laboratories an indirect method, the bacitracin test, may be used for identification of isolates. It is based on the exquisite susceptibility of group A strains to bacitracin and the relative resistance of strains of other groups (Table 16–2). When a disc containing a small amount of bacitracin (0.02 U) is placed on a plate streaked from an isolated colony, more than 99% of group-A strains show a zone of inhibition, whereas 90 to 95% of non-group-A strains do not. The low rate of false-negative results has made this method a practical but only presumptive test.

Bacitracin susceptibility presumptive test for group A

Several serologic tests have been developed to aid in the diagnosis of poststreptococcal sequelae. They include the antistreptolysin O, anti-DNAase B, and some combination tests. High titers of antistreptolysin O are usually found in sera of patients with rheumatic fever, so that test is used most widely.

## Group B Streptococci (Streptococcus agalactiae)

Group B streptococci (GBS) are the leading cause of neonatal sepsis and meningitis. Surveillance estimates suggest that over 15,000 cases and 1300 deaths occur in the United States each year. The organism is acquired by neonates from the mother's vaginal flora at or shortly before birth.

### Bacteriology

GBS produce short chains and diplococcal pairs of spherical or ovoid Gram-positive cells. Colonies are larger and beta-hemolysis is less distinct than with group A streptococci. Hemolysis may be completely absent, particularly under aerobic conditions. In addition to the Lancefield antigen, GBS produce polysaccharide capsules that form the basis of a serologic typing system for strains within the group. The major type antigens are designated Ia, Ib, II, III, and IV. All five capsular polysaccharides contain sialic acid in the form of terminal side chain residues. Type III GBS is by far the most common type found in infections.

GBS have polysaccharide capsules containing sialic acid

## Group B Streptococcal Disease

### Pathogenesis and Immunity

Exposure to GBS during childbirth is common as vaginal colonization rates between 10 and 30% have been repeatedly demonstrated in pregnant and nonpregnant women. Disease appears to require a combination of GBS resistance to antibody-independent opsonophagocytosis and the absence of type-specific anticapsular maternal, and thus transplacental, IgG. The sialic acid moiety of the GBS capsule has been shown to prevent C3 deposition on the organism, and inhibits alternate pathway activation of complement (Fig 16–3). In the presence of specific antibody, classical opsonization, phagocyte recognition, and killing proceed normally. GBS have also been shown to produce a peptidase that inactivates C5a, the major chemoattractant for PMNs. This may correlate with the observation that serious neonatal infections often show a paucity of infiltrating PMNs.

GBS capsule interferes with alternate pathway complement deposition

### Epidemiology and Clinical Manifestations

The incidence of neonatal GBS infections has been estimated at 1 to 3 cases per 1000 births, and the mortality is between 30 and 60% of infected cases. Prematurity and rupture of membranes more than 12 hours prior to birth increase the risk of disease. The clinical findings are similar to those found in sepsis, meningitis, and other serious infections in the neonatal period (Chapter 69). Respiratory distress, fever, lethargy, and hypotension are common. Although most cases begin in the first few days of life, a "late-onset" syndrome may also occur 3 to 8 weeks after birth. It is not known to what extent these cases represent nursery cross-infection or acquisition of the organisms from the mother after leaving the hospital.

High mortality rate in high-risk neonates

GBS also colonize the respiratory tract of children and adults, and have been associated with a variety of pyogenic infections at nonrespiratory sites. The most common are puerperal fevers and infections associated with gynecologic manipulations or surgery. Group B streptococci are not associated with rheumatic fever or acute glomerulonephritis.

GBS causes a variety of other acute infections

### Diagnosis

The laboratory diagnosis of GBS infection is by culture of cerebrospinal fluid, blood, or other appropriate specimen. Definitive identification involves serologic determination of the Lancefield group by the same methods used for group A streptococci. Rapid methods for direct detection of GBS antigen in vaginal specimens are available, but their sensitivity is significantly worse than the group A/throat procedures. Simple biochemical and cultural identification tests have been used with GBS in a manner similar to the bacitracin test (above), but have generally been eclipsed by the latex agglutination procedures for the group B antigen.

Standard methods used for diagnosis

### Treatment and Prevention

Group B streptococci are susceptible to the same antimicrobics as group A organisms; however, they are less susceptible to penicillin G (MIC, 0.2 to 1.0 μg/mL) and less readily killed by the antibiotic. For this reason GBS infections are often treated with combinations of penicillin and an aminoglycoside. Intrapartum antimicrobial prophylaxis has been shown to prevent transmission and disease in high-risk populations known to be colonized with GBS. Because this approach requires screening all pregnant women for GBS colonization prior to onset of labor, obstetricians and pediatricians do not agree on its practicality. Prevention by immunization with purified GBS capsular polysaccharide has been shown to be feasible, and considerable effort is now being directed at development of a vaccine.

Penicillin plus aminoglycoside frequently used

Intrapartum prophylaxis can prevent transmission

## Other Pyogenic Streptococci

The other pyogenic streptococci occasionally produce various respiratory, skin, wound, soft tissue, and genital infections, which may resemble those caused by group A and B streptococci. None has been clearly associated with poststreptococcal sequelae. Bacteremia with *S. bovis* has been associated with colonic cancer. The role of pyogenic streptococci other than those of group A in acute pharyngitis is unestablished. A few case reports of food-borne outbreaks have shown some strains of groups C and G streptococci to cause pharyngitis, but the evidence is not yet strong enough to be able to make this diagnosis in individual cases, as they are commonly found in healthy persons. The organisms are susceptible to penicillin, and infections are managed in a manner similar to deep tissue infections caused by group A and B streptococci.

Infections similar but less frequent than groups A or B

## Streptococcus pneumoniae

### Morphology and Growth

*S. pneumoniae* (pneumococci) are Gram-positive, oval diplococci with their axes end to end (Fig 16–4), giving the individual cell a bullet or lancet shape. Virulent strains are encapsulated. Growth requirements are the same as for other streptococci. $CO_2$ may be required by some strains. On blood agar, encapsulated pneumococci produce round, glistening 0.5 to 2.0-mm colonies surrounded by a zone of alpha-hemolysis. One unique feature is their tendency to spontaneously lyse after initial rapid growth. Turbid broths may clear and colonies

Lancet-shaped diplocci

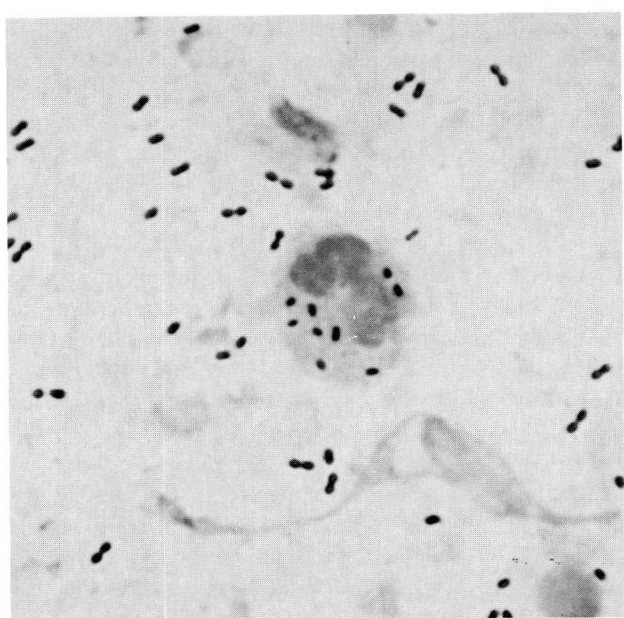

**Figure 16–4.** *S. pneumoniae* in sputum of patient with pneumonia. Note the marked tendency to form oval diplococci.

Bile salts enhance autolytic tendency

begin to lyse in the center developing a craterlike appearance. This behavior is due to their susceptibility to autolytic enzymes and to peroxides produced during growth. Autolysis can be hastened with surfactants such as detergents and bile. This characteristic is the basis of the bile solubility test that distinguishes them from the alpha-hemolytic viridans streptococci.

## Pneumococcal Disease

### Epidemiology

Pneumococci most common cause of bacterial pneumonia

*S. pneumoniae* is by far the most common cause of bacterial pneumonia. As with other bacterial pneumonias, viral respiratory infection and underlying chronic disease are important predisposing factors. Although infection may occur at any age, the incidence and mortality of pneumococcal pneumonia increase sharply after 50 years. Alcoholism, diabetes mellitus, chronic renal disease, and some malignancies are all associated with more frequent and serious pneumococcal pneumonias. In the preantibiotic era, the mortality in hospitalized patients was 20 to 30%; it has now been reduced to 5 to 10%. Although these mortality estimates are probably higher than those for cases in the community, the disease remains an important cause of death.

### Pathogenesis and Immunity

THE PNEUMOCOCCAL CAPSULE

Polysaccharide capsules comprise over 80 distinct polymers and serotypes

The structural features of pneumococci are similar to those of other streptococci; the important exception is their surface capsules, which are high-molecular-weight complex polysaccharide polymers that include sugars, choline, acetyl, and phosphoryl groups, and other components. They are antigenic comprising a system of more than 80 distinct serotypes. The chemical structure of the polysaccharide has been determined for a number of serotypes and shows unique features for each. Given the complexity of pneumococcal polysaccharide, it is not surprising that antibodies against capsules of certain serotypes are known to cross-react with polysaccharide produced by other bacteria (*Haemophilus, Klebsiella*) and even with human blood group isoantigens.

Pneumococcal capsule required for virulence

The polysaccharide capsule of the pneumococcus inhibits its engulfment by phagocytes and is the major determinant of virulence. Unencapsulated mutants are avirulent in experimental infections. Type-specific anticapsular antibody opsonizes capsulate strains and confers immunity to infection. The antiphagocytic effect of the capsule has long been attributed to its physical size and electrostatic charge, but recent studies suggest that mechanisms similar to the antiphagocytic effects of M protein or GBS sialic acid are more important. As with the other two it is the ability to prevent antibody independent opsonization via the alternate pathway that allows the organisms to survive. In the case of pneumococci it appears the capsular polysaccharide either interferes with C3b deposition directly or covers C3 fragments that are deposited on the cell wall. In either case the complement fragments recognized by phagocyte receptors are not available (Fig 16–3). When antibody binds to the capsular polysaccharide C3b generated by the classical pathway binds and opsonophagocytosis proceeds efficiently.

Capsule interferes with C3b deposition

Type-specific antibody allows opsonophagocytosis to proceed

#### Pneumolysin

Some of the clinical features seen in the course of pneumococcal infections are not explainable by the capsule alone. These include the dramatic abrupt onset, toxicity, fulminant course and disseminated intravascular coagulation seen in some cases. All pneumococci produce pneumolysin, which is a member of the thiol-activated cytolysin family of toxins. This protein is related to liseriolysin and *S. pyogenes* streptolysin O. These toxins interact with their target cell membrane possibly through cholesterol followed by oligomerization of toxin molecules to form transmembrane pores, resulting in cell lysis. Pneumolysin has a variety of documented deleterious effects on human cells. It can slow ciliary beating and disrupt the surface integrity of cultured human respiratory epithelium. Pneumolysin is toxic for pulmonary endothelial cells, a property that might contribute to disruption of the endothelial barrier and the spread of pneumococci from the alveoli into the bloodstream. Indeed, the injection of purified pneumolysin into the lung of experimental rats caused all of the salient histological hallmarks of pneumococcal pneumonia.

Pneumolysin pore-forming action similar to streptolysin O

Injury to cilia and endothelial cells may aid spread

Pneumolysin deficient pneumococci are clearly less virulent than their identical toxin-producing counterparts. Genetic studies have led to the cloning of the pneumolysin gene and the demonstration its inactivation leads to about a 100-fold reduction in the lethal $dose_{50}$. Most patients with pneumococcal disease exhibit an antibody response to pneumolysin and pneumolysin immunization is protective in animals.

Loss of pneumolysin reduces virulence

#### Other Determinants of Virulence

Pneumococcal surface protein A (PspA) is found on all pneumococci and is highly variable both immunologically and in molecular mass. Passive immunization with anti-PspA is protective and genetic inactivation of the PspA structural gene results in a significantly less virulent strain. Yet, the precise function of this surface protein in the pathogenesis of infection remains unclear. The search for a pneumococcal adhesin has been unrewarding even though it seems logical that at some point adherence to host epithelial cells should be a requirement for establishment of the bacteria in the host.

No adherence molecule has been identified

Pneumococci produce a neuraminidase that, like pneumolysin, is released upon autolysis. Despite the involvement of neuraminidase in the colonization by other bacteria, there is simply no proven role in pneumococcal virulence. All pneumococci also produce an sIga protease, a property shared with other species causing pneumonia and meningitis. This enzyme could play a part in establishment of the microorganism in the nasopharynx, but no definitive role for this enzyme in virulence has been proven.

Other cell components have unclear role

Another feature of pneumococcal infection is the heightened acute inflammatory response that may itself be destructive to the host. Peptidoglycan and teichoic acid components of the cell wall have been shown to stimulate inflammation and cerebral edema in experimental meningitis and may do so at other stages of infection.

#### Pneumococcal Pneumonia

Pneumococcal pneumonia begins with aspiration of respiratory secretions containing pneumococci. This event must be common, as 10 to 30% of normal people carry one or more serologic types of *S. pneumoniae* in the throat. Aspirated organisms are normally cleared rapidly by the defense mechanisms of the lower respiratory tract, including the cough and epiglottic reflexes, the mucocilliary "blanket," and phagocytosis by alveolar macrophages. Events that impair the combined efficiency of these defenses can allow pneumococci to reach and multiply in the alveoli. They include the chronic illnesses mentioned previously, damage to bronchial epithelium from smoking or air pollution, and respiratory dysfunction from alcoholic intoxication, narcotics and other drugs, anesthesia, and trauma.

Aspirated pneumococci must be cleared from lower respiratory tract

In absence of specific antibody, pneumococci reaching alveoli may multiply

In immune individuals with a sufficient level of circulating antibody against the capsular polysaccharide of organisms that reach the alveoli, the infection is controlled rapidly; in nonimmune individuals, however, continued alveolar multiplication is followed by a profuse outpouring of serous edema fluid, which facilitates growth and spread of pneumococci to adjacent alveoli and interferes with gas exchange. The fluid outpouring is quickly followed by an influx of polymorphonuclear leukocytes and erythrocytes, the latter as a result of capillary fragility. By the second or third day of illness, the lung segment has increased three- to fourfold in weight through accumulation of this cellular, hemorrhagic fluid. By the fourth or fifth day, neutrophils predominate in the consolidated alveoli, which usually affect a single lobe of the lung.

Effective immune response leads to recovery with no lung damage

In the absence of opsonizing antibody, multiplication of the organism continues and bacteremia is common. Even when formation of anticapsular antibody begins, it may be ineffective due to binding by free soluble capsular polysaccharide in the exudate and bloodstream. Once antibody reaches the pneumococci they are readily phagocytosed and destroyed. When actively growing pneumococci are no longer present, macrophages replace the granulocytes and resolution of the lesion ensues. A remarkable feature of pneumococcal pneumonia is the lack of structural damage to the lung, which usually leads to complete resolution on recovery.

## Pneumococcal Disease: Clinical Aspects

### Clinical Manifestations

#### Pneumococcal Pneumonia

Onset of fever, shaking, chill, and blood sputum

Lobar or bronchial pneumonia

Clinically, pneumococcal pneumonia begins abruptly with a shaking chill and high fever. Cough with production of sputum pink to rusty in color (indicating the presence of red blood cells) and pleuritic chest pain are common. Physical findings usually indicate pulmonary consolidation. Children and young adults typically demonstrate a lobar consolidation on chest radiography, whereas older patients may show a less localized bronchial distribution of the infiltrates. Without therapy, sustained fever, pleuritic pain, and productive cough continue until, in patients who recover, a "crisis" occurs 5 to 10 days after onset of the disease. The crisis involves a sudden decrease in temperature and of improvement in the patient's condition. It is associated with effective levels of opsonizing antibody reaching the lesion.

#### Pneumococcal meningitis

Most common bacterial meningitis at advanced ages

With *Neisseria meningitidis* and *Haemophilus influenzae*, *S. pneumoniae* is one of the three leading causes of bacterial meningitis. The signs and symptoms are similar to those produced by other bacteria (Chapter 67). Acute purulent meningitis may follow pneumococcal pneumonia, infection at another site, or appear with no apparent antecedent infection. It may also develop after trauma involving the skull. All ages are affected; however, in later life, pneumococcal meningitis is the most common form of the disease. The mortality and frequency of sequelae are slightly higher with pneumococcal meningitis than with other forms of pyogenic meningitis. This is generally attributed to injury caused by the inflammatory response.

#### Other Infections

Pneumococci are common causes of sinusitis and otitis media. The latter frequently occurs in children in association with viral infection. Chronic infection of the mastoid or respiratory sinus sometimes extends to the subarachnoid space to cause meningitis. Pneumococci may also cause endocarditis, arthritis, and peritonitis, usually in association with bacteremia. Patients with ascites caused by diseases such as cirrhosis and nephritis may develop spontaneous pneumococcal peritonitis. Pneumococci do not cause pharyngitis or tonsillitis.

### Treatment and Prevention

Pneumococci are usually highly susceptible to penicillin and other beta-lactam agents. In recent years pneumococci with decreased susceptibility to beta-lactams have emerged. These strains require penicillin concentrations of 0.12 to 8.0 μg/mL for inhibition, whereas fully susceptible strains are inhibited by 0.01 to 0.05 μg/mL. Patients with pneumonia and meningitis caused by these strains respond poorly or not at all to penicillin therapy. The mechanism of resistance appears to be mutational and involves the production of cell wall transpeptidases with altered penicillin-binding properties. Penicillinase is not produced. Resistance to erythromycin or chloramphenicol are uncommon but more likely with penicillin-resistant strains. Tetracycline resistance is common and aminoglycosides are not effective.

Pneumococcal resistance to penicillin increasing

Altered penicillin binding proteins produced by resistant strains

Penicillin is still the antimicrobic of choice unless local susceptibility data indicate a higher frequency of resistance than seen in most parts of the world (1 to 5%). Penicillin-resistant strains require treatment with erythromycin, chloramphenicol, or vancomycin if multiresistant. The therapeutic response to treatment of pneumococcal pneumonia is often (but not always) dramatic. Reduction in fever, respiratory rate, and cough can occur in 12 to 24 hours, but may occur gradually over several days. Chest radiography may yield normal results only after several weeks.

A vaccine has been prepared from capsular polysaccharide extracted from the 23 types of *S. pneumoniae* most commonly encountered. This vaccine, which is protective against these 23 types, is presently recommended for patients particularly susceptible to pneumococcal infection because of age, underlying disease, or immune status.

Polysaccharide vaccine protects against 23 common types

### Laboratory Diagnosis

Gram smears of material from sites of pneumococcal infection usually show typical Gram-positive, lancet-shaped diplococci (Fig 16–4). A properly collected sputum sample comprising inflammatory exudate from the affected lung segment will usually reveal the typical appearance. Sputum collection may be difficult, however, and specimens contaminated with respiratory flora are useless for diagnosis. Other types of lower respiratory specimens may be needed for diagnosis (Chapters 14 and 64).

*S. pneumoniae* grows well overnight on blood agar medium incubated aerobically. The pneumococcal capsule can be demonstrated by mixing the cells with type-specific antisera. The opsonized capsule absorbs water, and becomes increasingly refractile and thus visible under the light microscope. This quellung (capsular swelling) test is not done routinely due to the cost of the polyvalent antiserum (80 types) required. Instead the pneumococcus is usually distinguished from viridans streptococci by susceptibility to the synthetic chemical ethylhydrocupreine (Optochin) or by a bile solubility (see Table 16–2). Bacteremia is common in pneumococcal pneumonia and meningitis, and blood cultures are valuable supplements to cultures of local fluids or exudates.

Optochin susceptibility or bile solubility commonly used for identification

Blood cultures useful

Pneumococcal capsular antigen can be demonstrated in body fluids, serum, and urine using latex agglutination or other antigen detection methods (Chapter 14). This is valuable primarily when cultures are negative due to previous antimicrobic therapy.

Polysaccharide antigen detectable in body fluids

## ■ Viridans Streptococci

The viridans group comprises all alpha-hemolytic streptococci that remain after the criteria for defining pyogenic streptococci and pneumococci have been applied. Characteristically members of the normal flora of the oral and nasopharyngeal cavities, they have the basic bacteriologic features of streptococci, but lack the specific antigens, toxins, and virulence of the other groups. Although the viridans group includes several species (see Table 16–2), they are usually not characterized in clinical practice because there is little difference among them in medical significance. Viridans streptococci generally produce small (0.5- to 1.0-mm) colonies surrounded by a zone of alpha-hemolysis. They lack the autolytic properties of pneumococci, even in the presence of surface-active agents such as bile salts.

Species usually not separated

Although their virulence is very low, viridans strains can cause disease when they are protected from host defenses. The prime example is subacute bacterial endocarditis. In this disease, viridans streptococci reach previously damaged heart valves as a result of transient bacteremia associated with manipulations, such as tooth extraction, that disturb their usual habitat. Protected by fibrin and platelets, they multiply on the valve, causing local and systemic disease that is fatal if untreated. Extracellular production of glucans, complex polysaccharide polymers, may enhance their attachment to cardiac valves in a manner similar to the pathogenesis of dental caries by *S. mutans* (Chapter 62). The clinical course of viri-

Transient bacteremia may lead to endocarditis on damaged heart valve

Glucan polymers may aid attachment to valves

dans streptococcal endocarditis is subacute, with slow progression over weeks or months (Chapter 68). It is effectively treated with penicillin, but uniformly fatal if untreated. The disease is particularly associated with valves damaged by recurrent rheumatic fever. The decline in the occurrence of rheumatic heart disease has reduced the incidence of this particular type of endocarditis.

## ENTEROCOCCI

Enterococci have Lancefield group D antigen

Until DNA homology studies dictated their separation into the genus Enterococcus, the enterococci were classified as streptococci. Indeed, they share most of the bacteriologic characteristics described above for streptococci, including presence of the Lancefield group D antigen. The term enterococcus derives from their presence in the intestinal tract and the many biochemical and cultural features that reflect that habitat. These include the ability to grow in the presence of high concentrations of bile salts and sodium chloride. Some enterococci are beta-hemolytic, but most produce nonhemolytic or alpha-hemolytic colonies that are larger than those of streptococci. Several species are recognized based on biochemical and cultural reactions, but they are generally not separated in the clinical laboratory.

Relatively resistant to penicillin

β–lactimase producers have emerged recently

The enterococci are generally more resistant to antimicrobics than the streptococci. They require 4 to 16 μg/mL penicillin for inhibition and much higher concentrations for bactericidal effect. Recently beta-lactamase-producing strains have been isolated with increasing frequency, particularly from *E. faecalis*. The beta-lactamase genes have been linked to transposons derived from *Staphylococcus aureus*. Vancomycin resistance is often linked to beta-lactamase production. Enterococci are consistently resistant to sulfonamides, often resistant to tetracycline, and occasionally resistant to erythromycin and chloramphenicol. Ampicillin is the antimicrobial agent most consistently active.

Penicillins aminoglycoside combinations may be synergistic

Enterococci share with streptococci a relative resistance to aminoglycosides based on failure of the antimicrobic to be actively transported into the cell. Despite this, many strains of enterococci are inhibited and rapidly killed by combinations of low concentrations of penicillin and aminoglycosides. Under these conditions, the action of penicillin on the cell wall allows the aminoglycoside to enter the cell, and act at its ribosomal site. Some strains show high level resistance to aminoglycosides based on ribosomal resistance or the presence of aminoglycoside-inactivating enzymes. These strains do not demonstrate synergistic effects with penicillin.

### Enterococcal Diseases

Diseases similar to enteric organisms

Enterococci cause opportunistic urinary tract infections, and occasionally wound and soft tissue infections, in much the same fashion as members of the Enterobacteriaceae family. Infections are often associated with urinary tract manipulations, malignancies, biliary tract disease, and gastrointestinal disorders. There is often an associated bacteremia, which can result in the development of endocarditis on previously damaged cardiac valves.

Treatment of enterococcal infection depends on its site and severity. Ampicillin is effective in most urinary tract and minor soft tissue infections. More severe infections, particularly endocarditis, are usually treated with combinations of a penicillin and aminoglycoside. If the strain fails to demonstrate penicillin/aminoglycoside synergism and/or is vancomycin resistant, some other combination guided by susceptibility testing must be selected.

## ADDITIONAL READING

Fischetti VA: Streptococcal M protein: Molecular design and biologic behavior. *Clin Microbiol Rev* 1989; 2:285–314. This in-depth review addresses aspects of M-protein structure, immunochemistry, and genetics which are important for designing a vaccine to prevent group A streptococcal disease.

Hanski E, Caparon M: Protein F, a fibronectin-binding protein is an adhesin of the group A streptococcus, *Streptococcus pyogenes*. *Proc Natl Acad Sci USA* 1992;89:6172–6176. The evidence for the most recently discovered streptococcal adhesin is presented.

Hoge CW, Schwartz B, Talkington DF, et al: The changing epidemiology of invasive group A streptococcal infections and the emergence of streptococcal toxic shock-like syndrome. *JAMA* 1993;269:384–389. The epidemiologic basis for a new view of acute streptococcal infections is presented.

Lancefield RC: A serological differentiation of human and other groups of hemolytic streptococci. *J Exp Med* 1933;57:571–595. The classic study that changed streptococcal classification.

Larsen JW, Dooley SL: Group B streptococcal infections: An obstetrical viewpoint. *Pediatrics* 1993;91:148–149. The issues involved in screening for and preventing neonatal GBS disease are discussed.

Paton JC. Pathogenesis of pneumococcal disease. 1993. Curr Opin Infect Dis. 1993;6:363-368. The current views on the role of the pneumococcal virulence factors is discussed.

Chapter 17

# Corynebacteria, *Listeria*, *Bacillus*, and Other Aerobic and Facultative Gram-positive Rods

*Kenneth J. Ryan and Stanley Falkow*

This chapter includes a variety of Gram-positive rods, some of which are highly pathogenic, but none of which are currently common causes of human disease in the United States. Their importance to the student lies in the lessons in pathogenesis, epidemiology, and prevention learned when they were more common, and in the continued threat that their existence poses. *Corynebacterium diphtheriae,* the cause of diphtheria, is a prototype for toxigenic disease, and *Bacillus anthracis,* the cause of anthrax, has virulence and environmental survival characteristics that still cause concern about its potential use in biological warfare. *Listeria monocytogenes* has long been recognized as a sporadic cause of meningitis and other infections in the fetus and immunocompromised host, and has now been shown to cause epidemic foodborne disease.

## CORYNEBACTERIA

### Group Characteristics

The genus *Corynebacterium* includes many species of aerobic and facultative gram-positive rods. Corynebacteria (from the Greek koryne, club) are small and pleomorphic. The cells tend to have clubbed ends, and often remain attached after division, forming "Chinese letter" or palisade arrangements. Spores are not formed. Growth is generally best under aerobic conditions, but many strains will grow under microaerophilic or anaerobic conditions on media enriched with blood or other animal products.

Small club-shaped Gram positive rods

Colonies on blood agar are usually small (1 to 2 mm) and most are nonhemolytic. Catalase is produced, and many strains form acid (usually lactic acid) through carbohydrate fermentation. *C. diphtheriae* produces a powerful exotoxin that is responsible for the disease diphtheria. Other corynebacteria are nonpathogenic commensal inhabitants of the pharynx, nasopharynx, distal urethra, and skin; they are collectively referred to as "diphtheroids."

*C. diphtheria* produces exotoxin

Other corynebacteria called diphtheroids

## The Organism: Corynebacterium diphtheriae

### Bacteriology

Special media designed to demonstrate *C. diphtheriae*

Because it is important to distinguish *C. diphtheriae* rapidly from members of the pharyngeal flora, several selective media have been developed to isolate this organism. Most contain potassium tellurite, which inhibits members of the normal oral flora. *C. diphtheriae* also reduces the potassium tellurite to produce gray or black colonies, the morphology of which differs with each of three types of the organism: gravis, mitis, and intermedius. Differentiation of *C. diphtheriae* from other corynebacteria is by biochemical reactions.

## Diphtheria

### Epidemiology

Most cases in unimmunized transients

*C. diphtheriae* is transmitted by droplet spread, by direct contact with cutaneous infections, and, to a lesser extent, by fomites. Some subjects become convalescent pharyngeal or nasal carriers and continue to harbor the organism for weeks to months or even for a lifetime. Diphtheria still occurs in developing countries, but is rare where immunization is widely used. In the United States, for example, less than 10 cases are now reported each year. These are usually small outbreaks in populations that have not received adequate immunization, such as migratory workers, transients, and those who refuse immunization on religious grounds.

### Pathogenesis

Diphtheria is caused by the local and systemic effects of diphtheria toxin (Fig 17–1), a protein exotoxin with potent cytotoxic features. It inhibits protein synthesis in cell-free extracts

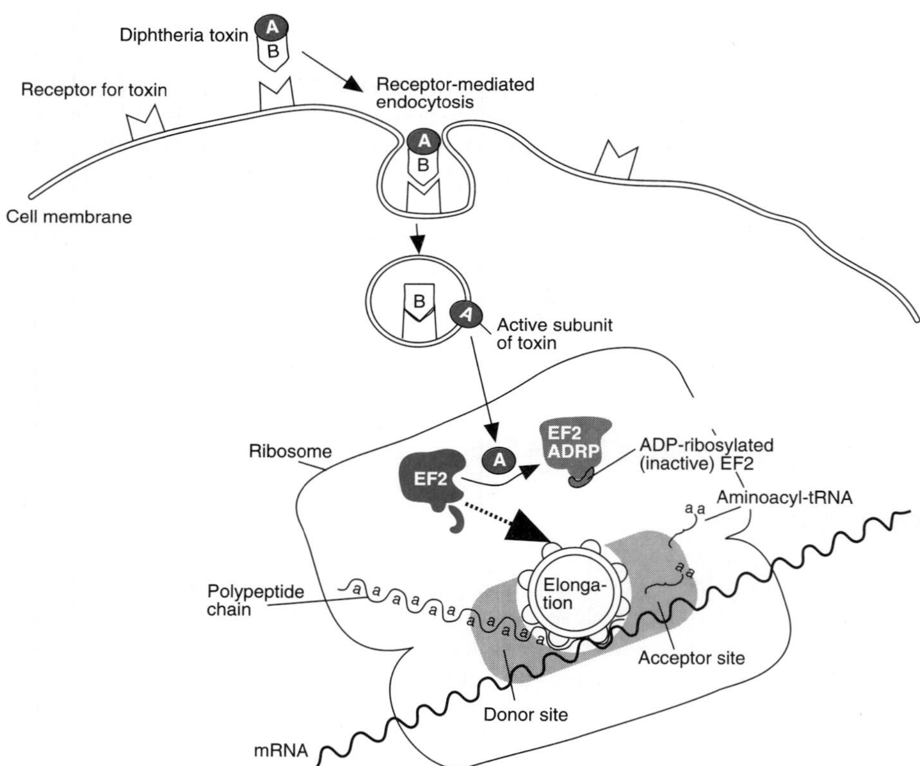


**Figure 17–1.** Action of diphtheria toxin. The toxin-binding (B) portion attaches to the cell membrane, and the complete molecule enters the cell. In the cell, the A subunit dissociates and catalyzes a reaction that ADP-ribosylates and thus inactivates elongation factor 2 (EF-2). This factor is essential for ribosomal reactions at the acceptor and donor sites, which transfer triplet code from messenger RNA (mRNA) to amino acid sequences via transfer RNA (tRNA). Inactivation of EF-2 stops building of the polypeptide chain.

of virtually all eukaryotic cells, from protozoa and yeasts to higher plants and humans. Its toxicity for intact cells varies among mammals and organs primarily due to differences in toxin binding and uptake. The diphtheria toxin molecule contains both an active subunit A, which catalyzes the toxic activity, and a subunit B, which mediates receptor binding and membrane translocation. Recently, the receptor for diphtheria toxin was cloned by transfection of a toxin-resistant cell with the genes from a toxin-sensitive cell line. The gene encoding susceptibility was found to be identical to a heparin-biding epidermal growth factor, a member of a common family of eukaryotic receptors found in the cell membrane that regulate cell growth and differentiation. The common pathogenic theme of exploiting a common host mechanism is again demonstrated for one of the best-known determinants of bacterial pathogenicity.

*Diphtheria* exotoxin is protein synthesis inhibitor

B subunit of toxin binds to cell receptor

Toxin receptor gene related to those binding eukaryotic growth factors

At some point the subunits separate and the B fragment facilitates translocation of the A subunit from the phagosome to the cytosol. Separation is required for full activity of the A subunit on its target protein elongation factor 2 (EF-2), which transfers polypeptidyl-transfer RNA from acceptor to donor sites on the ribosome of the host cell. The specific action of the A subunit is to catalyze the transfer of the adenine ribose phosphate portion of nicotinamide adenine dinucleotide (NAD) to EF-2, an enzymatic reaction called **ADP-ribosylation.** Covalent attachment of the ADP-ribosyl group occurs at an unusual derivative of histidine, called diphthamide. This inactivates EF-2 and shuts off protein synthesis. The ADP-ribosylation leaves the toxin itself free to catalyze another reaction, making it possible for a single DT molecule to inhibit protein synthesis in a cell within a few hours. ADP-ribosylation is now known to be the enzymatic mechanism of action for a number of toxins including those that act on EF-2 (diphtheria toxin, *Pseudomonas aeruginosa* exotoxin A) and those with other target proteins (cholera toxin, *Escherichia coli* LT, pertussis toxin). *C. diphtheriae* itself is unaffected because it does not have EF-2.

A subunit catalyses ADP-ribosylation of EF-2 to inactive form

The structural gene for the diphtheria toxin molecule is contained in a bacteriophage genome (β phage), and only strains of *C. diphtheriae* that are lysogenic for these phages produce toxin. Nontoxigenic strains of *C. diphtheriae* can produce pharyngitis, but not the toxic manifestations of diphtheria. They can be converted to toxigenicity by lysogenization in vitro with phage, and this process can probably occur in vivo. The **tox gene** of the bacteriophage is regulated by a chromosomally encoded repressor protein DtxR in response to iron limitation. Toxin biosynthesis is greatest when the bacteria are grown in low iron. DtxR also regulates a corynebacterial siderophore system under iron-limiting conditions, and therefore iron seems to play a central role in the expression of virulence.

Toxin gene contained in temperate phage

Iron concentration modulates toxin and other correclates of virulence

It is extraordinary that while *C. diphtheriae* is one of the best-studied pathogens, little is known about determinants that permit it to colonize the skin and nasopharynx. There has been some speculation that toxin biosynthesis aids in this capacity, but its precise role remains obscure.

### Immunity

Diphtheria toxin is antigenic, stimulating the production of antitoxin antibodies during natural infection. Formalin treatment of toxin produces **toxoid,** which retains the antigenicity but not the toxicity of native toxin and is used in immunization against the disease. It is clear that this process functionally inactivates fragment B. Whether it also inactivates fragment A or prevents its ability to dissociate from fragment B is not known. Molecular studies of the A subunit structure and action suggest that another approach to immunization may be through genetic engineering. For example, substitution of a single amino acid located in the NAD-binding site of the A subunit of DT can completely detoxify, but retain the immunogenic specificity of the toxin. The membrane-translocation properties of the B subunit have also been used to transport other proteins into the cytosol by linking them to DT.

Toxin is antigenic and neutralized by antibody

Toxoid is formalin inactivated toxin

Single amino acid substitution in binding site can inactivate toxin

## ■ Diphtheria: Clinical Aspects

### Clinical Manifestations

After an incubation period of 2 to 4 days, diphtheria usually presents as pharyngitis or tonsillitis. Typically, malaise, sore throat, and fever are present, and a patch of exudate or membrane develops on the tonsils, uvula, soft palate, or pharyngeal wall. The gray-white

Usually localized pharyngeal or upper respiratory infection

Diphtheritic "membrane" composed of fibrin and leukocytes

membrane, composed of a coagulum of fibrin, leukocytes, and cellular debris, is caused by local cytotoxicity of the toxin. It adheres to the mucous membrane, and may extend from the oropharyngeal area down to the larynx and into the trachea. Associated cervical adenitis is common, and in severe cases cervical adenitis and edema produce a "bullneck" appearance. In uncomplicated cases, the infection gradually resolves and the membrane is coughed up after 5 to 10 days.

Cervical lymphadentitis plus edema produce "Bullneck"

Respiratory obstruction may block airway

Circulating toxin acts on heart to produce myocarditis

Neurologic manifestations appear late

The complications and lethal effects of diphtheria are caused by respiratory obstruction or by the systemic effect of DT absorbed at the site of infection. Mechanical obstruction of the airway produced by the membrane, edema, and hemorrhage can be sudden and complete and can lead to suffocation, particularly if large sections of the membrane separate from the tracheal or laryngeal epithelial surface. Diphtheria toxin absorbed into the circulation causes injury to various organs, the most serious of which is to the heart. Diphtheritic myocarditis appears during the second or third week in severe cases of respiratory diphtheria. It is manifested by cardiac enlargement and weakness, arrhythmia, and congestive heart failure with dyspnea. Nervous system involvement appears later in the course of disease, most often involving paralysis of the soft palate, oculomotor (eye) muscles, or select muscle groups. The paralysis is reversible and is generally not serious unless the diaphragm is involved.

Cutaneous diphtheria produces ulcerative lesion

*C. diphtheriae* may produce nonrespiratory infections, particularly of the skin. The characteristic lesion ranges from a simple pustule to a chronic, nonhealing ulcer and is most common in tropical and hot, arid regions. Cardiac and neurologic complications from these infections are infrequent, suggesting that the efficiency of toxin production or absorption is low compared to that in respiratory infections.

*C. diphtheriae* has little invasive capacity

Thus, the manifestations of diphtheria are produced by multiplication of the organism and toxin production at the local site of infection. *C. diphtheriae* itself has little invasive capacity, but the toxin causes tissue damage at both local and distant sites. The disease resolves with the formation of antitoxin antibody.

## Diagnosis

Primary diagnosis is clinical

Direct smears of throat or membrane unreliable guides

Culture requires special medium

The initial diagnosis of diphtheria is entirely clinical. There are presently no rapid laboratory tests of sufficient value to influence the decision regarding antitoxin administration. Direct smears of infected areas of the throat are not reliable diagnostic tools. Definitive diagnosis is accomplished by isolating and identifying *C. diphtheriae* from the infected site and demonstrating its toxigenicity. Isolation is usually achieved with a selective medium containing potassium tellurite (eg, Tinsdale medium). The toxigenicity (virulence) tests classically performed in animals are now usually done by immunodiffusion methods.

Laboratory must be notified of suspicion in advance

It should be acknowledged that while this diagnosis could be made and confirmed with great confidence in the past, it is now more difficult because experience with the disease is rare. Most physicians have never seen a case of diphtheria, and most laboratories have never isolated the organism. Because routine throat culture procedures will not isolate *C. diphtheriae*, the physician must advise the laboratory in advance of the suspicion of diphtheria. Generally, 2 days are required to exclude *C. diphtheriae* (that is, no colonies isolated on Tinsdale agar); however, more time is needed to complete identification and toxigenicity testing of a positive culture.

## Treatment

Antitoxin therapy aimed at neutralizing free toxin

Erythromycin most effective antimicrobic therapy

Treatment of diphtheria is directed at neutralization of the toxin with concurrent elimination of the organism. The former is most critical and is accomplished by administering a diphtheria antitoxin that neutralizes free toxin but has no effect on toxin already fixed to cells. *C. diphtheriae* is susceptible to a variety of antimicrobics, including penicillins, cephalosporins, erythromycin, and tetracycline. Of these, erythromycin has been the most effective. The complications of diphtheria are managed primarily by supportive measures.

## Prevention

Toxoid immunization prevents disease

The mainstay of diphtheria prevention is immunization. Three to four doses of diphtheria toxoid produce immunity by stimulating antitoxin production. The initial series is begun in the first year of life (Chapter 12). Booster immunizations at 10-year intervals will maintain immunity. This vaccine is highly effective. Fully immunized individuals may become infected with *C. diphtheriae*, because the antibodies are directed only against the toxin, but the disease is mild. Serious infection and death occur only in unimmunized or incompletely immunized individuals.

## Other Corynebacteria

Corynebacteria other than *C. diphtheriae* are often called diphtheroids; some are commonly found in the normal flora of the skin and other body sites. The term actually encompasses several well-defined species, some of which have definite but unusual disease associations. Some species, such as *C. ulcerans*, may carry the beta-phage, produce a small amount of diphtheria toxin, and cause infections with mild toxic manifestations. *C. jeikeium* has been increasingly associated with nosocomial infections in immunosuppressed patients. They include bacteremia, which is often associated with intravascular devices such as catheters and prosthetic heart valves. A striking feature of this corynebacterium is the extent of its antimicrobic resistance, which typically includes all common agents except vancomycin.

*C. ulcerans* produces small amount of diphtheria toxin

*C. jeikeium* strains important cause of bacteremia in immunosuppressed patients

Diphtheroids are not usually speciated in clinical laboratories, because the vast majority of isolates represent colonization or contamination rather than disease. When circumstances suggest that a diphtheroid isolate may be significant, further identification can be accomplished with several standard bacteriologic tests.

# LISTERIA

## ■ The Organism: Listeria monocytogenes

*Listeria monocytogenes* is a Gram-positive rod with some bacteriologic features that resemble those of both corynebacteria and streptococci. In stained smears of clinical and laboratory material, the organisms resemble diphtheroids. In culture, a small, smooth colony surrounded by a narrow rim of beta-hemolysis is produced. *Listeria* species are catalase positive, which distinguishes them from streptococci, and produce a characteristic tumbling motility in fluid media at 25°C that distinguishes them from corynebacteria. Eleven serotypes based on cell wall and flagellar antigens are recognized, but the majority of human cases are limited to only three serotypes. Molecular methods have been useful in investigating outbreaks.

Gram-positive rod morphologically resembling corynebacteria
Produce beta hemolysis

## ■ Listeriosis

### Epidemiology

Members of *Listeria* are widespread among animals in nature, including those associated with our food supply (fowl, ungulates). The human reservoir appears to be intestinal colonization which various studies have shown at rates between 2% and 12%. In the United States there are up to 2000 cases and 450 deaths each year. It has only recently become clear that foodborne transmission is important in listeriosis. A widely publicized 1985 California outbreak involved Mexican-style soft cheese and included 86 cases and 29 deaths. Fifty-eight of the cases were among mother–infant pairs. An important feature of some epidemics has been the ability of *L. monocytogenes* to grow at refrigerator temperatures, a long-known characteristic of the organism. Initial concern that *L. monocytogenes* might be relatively resistant to pasteurization has not been confirmed. The dairy product outbreaks probably relate to postpasteurization contamination or deviation from recommended time and temperature guidelines.

Reservoir in intestinal flora

Foodborne transmission important
*L. monocytogenes* can grow at refrigerator temperatures

### Pathogenesis and Immunity

*L. monocytogenes* animal models have long been used for the study of cell-mediated immunity because of the organism's ability to grow in nonimmune macrophages. An activated macrophage is needed to clear the infection, and in fact the concept of the activated macrophage that appears throughout this book owes much to the study of experimental *Lis-*

Grows in nonimmune macrophages

*teria* infection. More recently, *Listeria* has generated great interest because of its ability to reorganize host cell actin and use this to spread in macrophages as well as nonprofessional phagocyes such as epithelial cells.

Surface internalin starts epithelial cell invasion

*L. monocytogenes* attaches to and invades animal cells. Bacterial internalization into undifferentiated epithelial cells, M cells, intestinal crypt cells, and macrophages is mediated by a protein called internalin, which bears some similarity to streptococcal M protein. *Listeria* enters the cell in a membrane-bound vacuole, but rapidly escapes into the host cell cytosol by elaborating listeriolysin O (LLO), a sulfhydryl-activated, pore-forming cytolysin that shares amino acid homology with streptolysin O and pneumococcal pneumolysin (see Chapter 16). LLO-defective mutants exhibit greatly reduced virulence for experimental animals, indicating the prime importance of this toxin. *L. monocytogenes* produces at least two other hemolysins, which act as phospholipases, hydrolyzing host cell membranes rather than by forming pores. They may be important in the initial encounter of the bacteria with PMN. LLO, the phospholipases, a metalloprotease, and several other genes involved in actin rearrangement are all part of a virulence regulon controlled by a genetic locus that may be sensing temperature as a regulatory cue.

Enters cell in vacuole

LLO aids escape to cytosol

Once in the cytosol, *L. monocytogenes* is able to stimulate nucleation and rearrangement of host cell actin, forming a comet-like "tail" structure composed of short actin filaments and actin-binding proteins (Fig 17–2). This arrangement appears to facilitate rapid movement through the cell and the formation of pseudopods that extend into adjacent host cells. It may be here that the phospholipases play a role in dissolving the double set of host cell membranes encasing the invading microbe. Once the double-membrane vacuole is digested, LLO is elaborated again and the process begins anew. This complex strategy allows *L. monocytogenes* to spread with minimal contact with the immune system. This strategy is not unique to *Listeria*; it is also employed by *Shigella* (Chapter 20) and recently established for the *Rickettsia* (Chapter 30).

Rearranges cellular actin as transit to adjacent cell

Immunity to *Listeria* infection owes little to humoral and much to cell-mediated mechanisms. Neutrophils may play some role in early stages, but it is cytokine-activated macrophages that reverse the intracellular growth in macrophages. This is emphasized by the increased frequency of listeriosis in those with compromised cellular immune function due to disease (AIDS), immunosupressive therapy, age, or pregnancy.

Cytokine activated macrophages most important immune mechanism

## Listeriosis: Clinical Aspects

Meningitis, bacteremia, and peurperal infection most common

The most common human infections are meningitis and bacteremia without an obvious focus. Neonatal and puerperal infections, associated with vaginal colonization by *Listeria,* appear in settings similar to those of infections with group B streptococci. Rarely, intrauterine

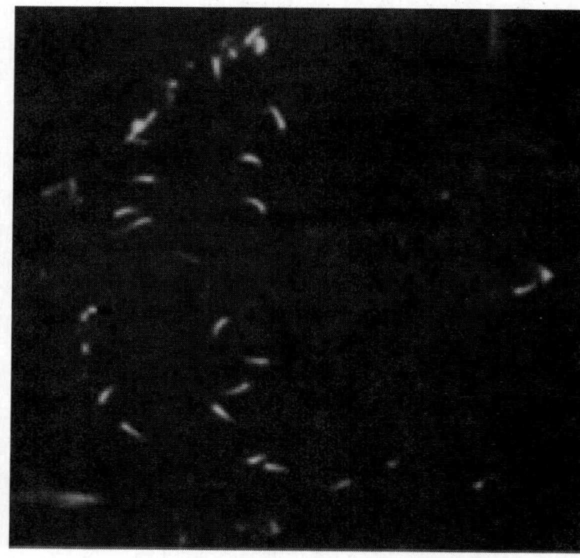

**Figure 17–2.** Intracellular movement of *Listeria monocytogenes. L. monocytogenes* cells are shown within infected cells in culture. The immunofluorescent stain used an antibody that binds to actin demon strating the comet-like actin "tails," which trail the bacteria as they move through the cell. (*From Niebuhr K, Chakraborty T, Rohde M, et al:* Infect Immun. *1993;61:2793–2802, figure 4a, with permission.*)

infection results in the clinical syndrome of granulomatosis infantiseptica, in which the fetus is often stillborn with disseminated abscesses and/or granulomas. The elderly and immunocompromised have an increased risk of disease. The number of cases in AIDS patients has been estimated at 300 times the general population.

Greatly increased incidence in AIDS patients

Diagnosis of listeriosis is usually by culture of blood, cerebrospinal fluid, or focal lesions. *L. monocytogenes* is susceptible to penicillin G, ampicillin, erythromycin, and chloramphenicol, all of which have been used effectively.

## ERYSIPELOTHRIX

*Erysipelothrix rhusiopathiae* is a Gram-positive rod with features similar to those of both corynebacteria and *Listeria*. This organism is widely distributed among animals and in decaying organic matter. Traumatic inoculation of *E. rhusiopathiae* into the skin produces erysipeloid, an occupational disease of fishermen, butchers, veterinarians, and others who handle animal products. Erysipeloid is a painful, slow-spreading, erythematous swelling of the skin. Penicillin is the treatment of choice, although the organism is also susceptible to erythromycin and tetracycline.

Erysipeloid an erythematous spreading lesion following trauma

## LACTOBACILLUS

Lactobacilli are Gram-positive, non-spore-forming rods. They are typically nonmotile and nonacid fast. The cells, which are usually long and slender with squared ends, are often arranged to form chains. They are aerobic and facultatively anaerobic and grow optimally at about pH 6. Lactobacilli actively ferment carbohydrates, forming lactic acid as the primary metabolic product. Numerous species have been described, of which the most commonly occurring in humans is *Lactobacillus acidophilus*.

Acidophilic Gram-positive non-spore forming rods

Lactobacilli are important members of the normal human oral, gastrointestinal, and vaginal flora. Their reputation as beneficial members of the intestinal flora is responsible for the popularity of certain "natural" foods, such as yogurt, that contain lactobacilli and their fermentation products (Chapter 9). Lactobacilli are not pathogenic for humans or animals, although *L. acidophilus* may play a role in the pathogenesis of dental caries (Chapter 62).

Member of the normal intestinal and vaginal flora

## PROPIONIBACTERIUM

Bacteria of the genus *Propionibacterium* resemble corynebacteria morphologically. Members are anaerobes or microaerophiles and are a major and significant part of the normal skin flora (Chapter 9). Like most normal floral organisms, propionibacteria can be an occasional cause of bacterial endocarditis or of other infections in the severely immunocompromised.

## BACILLUS

The genus *Bacillus* includes many species of aerobic or facultative, spore-forming, Gram-positive rods. With the exception of one species, *B. anthracis,* they are low-virulence saprophytes widespread in air, soil, water, dust, and animal products. *B. anthracis* causes the zoonosis anthrax, a disease of animals that is occasionally transmitted to humans.

Gram-positive spore-forming rods

### Group Characteristics

The genus comprises rod-shaped organisms that can vary from coccobacillary to rather long-chained filaments. Motile strains have peritrichous flagella. Formation of round or oval spores, which may be central, subterminal, or terminal depending on the species, is char-

Gram positivity often lost in older cultures

acteristic of the genus. *Bacillus* species are Gram positive; however, positivity is often lost, depending on the species and the age of the culture.

Aerobic conditions required for growth

Heat resistant spores survive boiling

Growth is obtained with ordinary media incubated in air and is reduced or absent under anaerobic conditions. They are catalase positive and metabolically active. The spores survive boiling for varying periods and are sufficiently resistant to heat that those of one species are used as a biologic indicator of autoclave efficiency. Spores of *B. anthracis* survive in soil for decades.

## Bacillus anthracis

### Bacteriology

Capsule and Medusa head colonies typical for *B. anthracis*

*B. anthracis* has a tendency to form very long chains of rods with elliptic central spores. This appearance has sometimes been likened to that of bamboo rods. In infected tissues, chains are shorter and capsules are prominent, but spores do not develop. Colonies, which consist of parallel interlacing chains of bacilli, are characterized by a rough, uneven surface with multiple curled extensions at the edge resembling a "Medusa head." *B. anthracis* is nonmotile and nonhemolytic; these characteristics combined with other important bacteriologic features, help to differentiate the organism from other *Bacillus* species (Table 17–1).

### Anthrax

Pasteur produced vaccine with attenuated anthrax strain

The isolation of *B. anthracis,* the proof of its relationship to anthrax infection, and the demonstration of immunity to the disease are among the most important events in the history of science and medicine. Robert Koch rose to fame in 1877 by growing the organism in artificial culture using pure culture techniques. He defined the stringent criteria needed to prove that the organism caused anthrax (Koch's postulates), then met them experimentally. Louis Pasteur made a convincing field demonstration at Pouilly-le-Fort to show that vaccination of sheep, goats, and cows with an attenuated strain of *B. anthracis* prevented anthrax. He was cheered and carried on the shoulders of the grateful farmers of the district, an experience now, unhappily, largely restricted to successful football coaches.

#### Epidemiology

Infection through spores gaining access to small epithelial lesions

Disease spread among herbivores and occasionally to humans

Anthrax is usually acquired through unrecognized breaks in skin or mucous membranes to which spores of *B. anthracis* gain access. The spores germinate to yield vegetative cells, which multiply and produce either localized or systemic infection depending on the animal species infected and the site inoculated. Herbivores such as horses, sheep, and cattle are most commonly affected and develop fatal septicemic disease. The disease is spread by spores in pastures contaminated with exudates of infected animals. Humans are usually infected by contact with infected animals or animal products. Because of the long survival of the spores, infection may result from contaminated hides, wool, bone, and even imported

**TABLE 17–1. SOME CHARACTERISTICS OF BACILLUS SPECIES**

| | Bacteriologic Features | | | | |
|---|---|---|---|---|---|
| **Organism** | ***Capsule*** | ***Motility*** | **Toxin Production** | **Distribution** | **Human Disease** |
| *B. anthracis* | + | – | Exotoxin (EF, PA, LF) | Animals and contaminated soil where disease is enzootic | Anthrax |
| *B. cereus* | – | + | Enterotoxin; pyogenic toxin | Ubiquitous | Food poisoning; opportunistic infections (rare) |
| Other species | – | + | — | Ubiquitous | Opportunistic infections (rare) |

*Abbreviations:* EF = edema factor; PA = protective antigen; LF = lethal factor.

processed items such as fertilizer containing bone meal. The disease is now rare in developed countries, although animal anthrax persists in the southern United States. The incidence in humans in the United States has decreased from more than 100 cases annually in the 1920s to only a few reported cases each year. In the past, farmers, veterinarians, and meat handlers were infected most frequently. With control of animal anthrax the rare case in the United States is now usually related to contaminated imported materials. More ominously, aerosolizing anthrax spores has been considered as a means of biological warfare. An episode with over 50 anthrax deaths in the former Soviet Union is now attributed to an explosion at a biological warfare research facility involving over 20 pounds of anthrax spores.

Most cases related to materials from countries with animal anthrax

Use for biological warfare a continuing threat

PATHOGENESIS

The prime *B. anthracis* virulence factors are its capsule and production of exotoxins. The capsule is a D-glutamic acid polypeptide of a single antigenic specificity. It has antiphagocytic properties and is required for full virulence. The exotoxin(s) produces extensive edema and death in a variety of animals. This activity has been separated into at least three components: edema factor, protective antigen, and lethal factor. These factors are proteins or protein–carbohydrate complexes. The edema factor has adenylate cyclase activity similar to that seen in *Bordetella pertussis* (Chapter 23). Strains repeatedly subcultured at 42°C become avirulent. This characteristic was the basis of Pasteur's attenuated vaccine, and has been shown to be due to loss of a plasmid-encoding toxin production.

Antiphagocytic effect of D-glutamic acid capsule required for virulence

Exotoxin has multiple activities

Attenuation due to loss of toxin plasmid

IMMUNITY

The specific mechanisms of immunity against *B. anthracis* are not known. Experimental evidence favors antibody directed against the toxin complex, but the relative role of the three toxin components is not clear. The capsular glutamic acid is not immunogenic.

### ■ Anthrax: Clinical Aspects

Cutaneous anthrax usually begins 2 to 5 days after inoculation of spores in an exposed part of the body, typically the forearm or hand. The initial lesion is an erythematous papule, which may be mistaken for an insect bite. This papule usually progresses through vesicular and ulcerative stages over 7 to 10 days to form a black eschar (scab) surrounded by edema. This complex is known as the malignant pustule, although it is neither malignant nor a pustule. Associated systemic symptoms are usually mild, and the lesion typically heals after the eschar separates. Less commonly, the disease progresses with massive local edema, toxemia and bacteremia, and a fatal outcome if untreated.

Initial papule becomes "malignant pustule"

Pulmonary anthrax (wool-sorter's disease) is contracted by inhalation of spores. It can develop when contaminated hides, hair, wool, and the like are handled in a confined space or following laboratory accidents. After 1 to 5 days of nonspecific malaise, mild fever, and nonproductive cough, progressive respiratory distress and cyanosis ensue with massive edema of the neck, chest, and mediastinum. If untreated, progression to a fatal outcome is usually very rapid once edema has developed. Enormous numbers of organisms are found in the lungs, blood, and all organs. A gastrointestinal form of anthrax results from ingestion of raw or inadequately cooked meat containing *B. anthracis* spores.

Woolsorters disease is the pulmonary form of anthrax

## Other Bacillus Species

As spores are widespread in the environment, isolation of one of the more than 20 *Bacillus* species other than *B. anthracis* from clinical material usually represents contamination of the specimen. Occasionally *B. cereus, B. subtilis,* and some other species produce genuine infections, including infections of the eye, soft tissues, and lung. Infection is usually associated with immunosuppression, trauma, an indwelling catheter, or contamination of complex equipment such as an artificial kidney. The relative resistance of *Bacillus* spores to disinfectants aids their survival in medical devices that cannot be heat sterilized.

Isolation of *Bacillus* species usually represents environmental contamination

Spores enhance survival in medical devices

*B. cereus* deserves special mention. It is the species most likely to cause opportunistic infection, which suggests a virulence intermediate between that of *B. anthracis* and the other species. A strain isolated from an abscess has been shown to produce a destructive

*B. cereus* most common opportunist

Pygenic toxin and enterotoxin detected

pyogenic toxin. *B. cereus* can also cause food poisoning by means of enterotoxins. One enterotoxin acts by stimulating adenyl cyclase production and fluid excretion in the same manner as toxigenic *E. coli* and *Vibrio cholerae* (Chapters 20 and 21).

## Diagnosis

Diagnosis of *Bacillus* infections follows the principles outlined in Chapter 14. The organisms are readily grown on a variety of media. *B. anthracis* may be distinguished from other species by the characteristics listed in Table 17–1, by its virulence to experimental animals, and by other biochemical and cultural features. The appropriate tests may not be performed unless the suspicion of anthrax is communicated to the clinical laboratory. Isolates of other *Bacillus* species are usually contaminants; the rare situation in which they play a pathogenic role is suggested by multiple isolations, large numbers of organisms in fresh specimens, and the special circumstances of the case.

## Treatment

Penicillin most common treatment

Because *B. anthracis* is susceptible to penicillin, anthrax is treated with this agent. Antimicrobial therapy for other species must be guided by in vitro testing, because susceptibilities to penicillins, cephalosporins, aminoglycosides, tetracycline, and chloramphenicol are not predictable. Other modes of management of opportunistic *Bacillus* infections, such as removal of indwelling catheters, may be equally important.

## ADDITIONAL READING


Farber J, Peterkin P: *Listeria monocytogenes*, a food-borne pathogen. *Microbiol Rev* 1991;55:476–511.

McCloskey RV, Eller JJ, Green M, et al: The 1970 epidemic of diphtheria in San Antonio. *Ann Intern Med* 1970;75:495–503. A clear and informative description of a diphtheria outbreak is provided. The clinical features are given in detail, including color photographs of diphtheritic membranes.

Mikesell P, Ivins BE, Ristroph JD, Dreier TM: Evidence for plasmid-mediated toxin production in *Bacillus anthracis. Infect Immun* 1983;39:371–376. These investigators repeated Louis Pasteur's attenuation experiments but with molecular studies to explain why his strains lost virulence.

Portnoy DA, Chakraborty T, Goebel W, Cossart P. Molecular determinants of *Listeria monocytogenes* pathogenesis. *Infect Immun* 1992;60:1263–1267. This minireview concisely updates current research on the correlates between listerial structures and products and their role in disease.

Schlech WF, Lavigne PM, Bortolussi RA, et al: Epidemic listeriosis-evidence for transmission by food. *N Engl J Med* 1983;308:203–206. This epidemiological study nicely traces events beginning on a Halifax farm to 34 cases of listeriosis. This outbreak was the first evidence that *Listeria* was a food-borne pathogen.

Schuchat A, Swaminathan B, Broome CV: Epidemiology of human listeriosis. *Clin Microbiol Rev* 1991; 4:169–183. This review covers clinical as well as epidemiological aspects of the recent upsurge in listeriosis.

Tilney LG, DeRosier DJ, Weber A, Tilney MS: How *Listeria* exploits host cell actin to form its own cytoskeleton. *J Cell Biol* 1992;118:71–93.

Chapter 18

# Clostridia, Gram-negative Anaerobes, and Anaerobic Cocci

*James J. Plorde*

The bacteria discussed in this chapter do not require oxygen for growth or reproduction. Although correctly known as obligate anaerobes, they are more commonly referred to simply as anaerobes. They generate energy solely by fermentation (see Chapter 3), and not only lack the capacity to use oxygen as an electron acceptor, but are damaged by it to varying degrees. Some are sensitive to oxygen concentrations as low as 0.5% and are killed by even brief exposures to air. Most can survive in 3 to 5% oxygen. A few actually grow, although poorly, in the presence of air, and are often referred to as aerotolerant anaerobes.

Energy generated by fermentation

Anaerobes inhibited or killed by oxygen

## THE NATURE OF ANAEROBIASIS

Several explanations have been proposed for obligate anaerobiosis and oxygen toxicity. Anaerobes lack the cytochromes required to use oxygen as a terminal electron acceptor in energy-yielding reactions. Most, but not all, lack catalase and peroxidase enzymes, but possess flavoproteins; thus, in the presence of oxygen they may produce hydrogen peroxide, which is toxic to many of them. Some anaerobes, which lack or only produce low concentrations of the enzyme superoxide dismutase, may be inhibited or killed by other peroxides and toxic oxygen radicals. Certain critical enzymes (for example, fumarate reductase) of some anaerobes must be in the reduced state to be active; thus, aerobic conditions create a metabolic block. It therefore seems probable that no single characteristic is responsible for obligate anaerobic requirements or oxygen toxicity; some of those indicated previously, rather than being its cause, may have been selected because of the anaerobic nature of the organism.

Anaerobiosis not explained by any single factor

Despite our constant immersion in air, anaerobes are able to colonize the many oxygen-deficient or oxygen-free microenvironments of the body. Often these are created by the presence of facultative organisms whose growth reduces oxygen and decreases the local oxidation-reduction potential. Such sites include the sebaceous glands of the skin, the gingival crevices of the gums, the lymphoid tissue of the throat, and the lumina of the intestinal and urogenital tracts (Table 18–1). The anaerobic flora of these sites normally live in harmless commensal relationships with the host. However, they may cause life-threatening infections when introduced into tissues devitalized by trauma, malignancy, inflammation, or impaired blood supply.

Anaerobes are common members of the normal flora

Infections can result when anaerobes are displaced into tissues

TABLE 18–1. USUAL LOCATIONS OF OPPORTUNISTIC ANAEROBES IN THE HUMAN BODY

| | Location | | | |
|---|---|---|---|---|
| Organism | *Mouth or Pharynx* | *Intestine* | *Urogenital Tract* | *Skin* |
| *Bacteroides fragilis* group | – | + | – | – |
| *Prevotella melaninogenica* | + | + | + | – |
| Clostridia | – | + | – | – |
| *Fusobacterium* | + | + | – | – |
| Peptostreptococci | + | + | + | – |
| *Propionibacterium* | – | – | – | + |

Infections are often polymicrobial

Anaerobic infections are frequently polymicrobic, containing a number of different anaerobic and facultative species. Exquisitely oxygen-sensitive anaerobes are seldom involved, probably because they are inactivated by even the small amounts of oxygen dissolved in tissue fluids. Except for infections with some environmental clostridia, the organisms are almost always derived from the patient's normal flora. Person-to-person transfer is very rare except with some hospital-acquired *Clostridium difficile* infections.

The major groups of clinically significant anaerobes are as follows:

Gram-positive spore formers found in soil and intestinal flora

- **Clostridia.** The clostridia are Gram-positive, spore-forming motile or nonmotile bacilli. Some species are potentially highly pathogenic to humans or animals and produce potent exotoxins associated with particular disease syndromes. Others are nonpathogenic. Clostridia are found in soil (particularly soil fertilized with animal excreta) and in the lower intestinal tract of humans and animals. They are generally highly susceptible to penicillin.

Gram-negative rods present in the oral and intestinal flora

- ***Bacteroides.*** Members of the genus *Bacteroides* are Gram-negative, non-spore-forming rods. Although organisms previously known as pigmented, bile-sensitive bacteroides have been recently reclassified into the genera *Porphyromonas* and *Prevotella,* they will, for the sake of clarity, be considered with the bacteroides in this chapter. Some species within this grouping are markedly pleomorphic, but others are quite uniform. They are distinguished from *Fusobacterium* by the organic acids that constitute their metabolic end products. *Bacteroides* species occur among the normal flora of the oral cavity and colon in humans and animals. *Porphyromonas* and *Prevotella* species are found principally in the mouth, particularly in the gingival crevices.

Fusiform Gram-negative rods similar to *Bacteroides*

- **Fusobacteria.** Fusobacteria are also Gram-negative, non-spore-forming rods. Their morphology is fusiform with pointed ends, and they are distinguished from *Bacteroides* by metabolic end-product analysis. Their habitat is the same as that of *Bacteroides.*

Gram-positive cocci present in alimentary and respiratory flora but are seldom pathogenic

- **Peptostreptococci.** Peptostreptococci, commonly but erroneously known as anaerobic streptococci, are Gram-positive, nonmotile organisms that generally occur in chains. They are part of the normal flora of the upper alimentary and respiratory tracts and lower intestinal tract in humans and animals. Anaerobic Gram-positive cocci forming clusters rather than chains were previously referred to as peptococci. Recent studies of their DNA content has revealed a close taxonomic relationship to peptostreptococci, and they have now been reassigned to that genus. They rarely play a pathogenic role.

Some other genera and species of anaerobic organisms (for example, *Actinomyces israelii*) are considered elsewhere in this text. Many others are not included in this chapter because they rarely cause disease, and because those discussed herein serve as satisfactory models for both specific and mixed anaerobic infections.

## CLOSTRIDIA

Many clostridia are of great significance as causes of disease in livestock and wildlife; however, these organisms are beyond the scope of this text. Discussion is limited to those that cause disease in humans. They may be categorized as follows:

1. The gas gangrene group, of which the most important is *Clostridium perfringens.* In addition to its role in gas gangrene, *C. perfringens* can cause anaerobic cellulitis, anaerobic puerperal sepsis, food poisoning, and antibiotic-induced diarrhea.
2. *C. tetani,* the cause of tetanus.
3. *C. botulinum,* the cause of botulism.
4. *C. difficile,* cause of toxic enterocolitis.

## Clostridium perfringens

*C. perfringens* produces four major (α, β, ε, ι) and eight or nine minor exotoxins including θ-toxin and enterotoxin. The species has been subdivided on the basis of the major toxins into five types (A to E), which have different pathogenic significance in different animal species. Type A is by far the most important in humans and is found consistently in the colon and often in soil.

Subtypes are based on toxin production

### Bacteriologic Features

MORPHOLOGIC, CULTURAL, AND METABOLIC CHARACTERISTICS

*C. perfringens* is a large, Gram-positive, nonmotile encapsulated rod with squarish ends. Spores are rarely seen in culture or during infection, but develop in the natural habitat. The organism grows very rapidly overnight on blood agar medium or in broth under anaerobic conditions. Its mean generation time can be as short as 7 minutes. Incubation overnight on sheep blood agar (usually used in diagnostic laboratories) produces round, smooth colonies about 2 to 3 mm in diameter; they are surrounded by a zone of complete hemolysis caused by θ-toxin and a wider zone of incomplete hemolysis caused by α-toxin (Fig 18–1). If the plate is refrigerated and rewarmed, the outer zone of hemolysis becomes complete. In broth containing fermentable carbohydrate, growth of *C. perfringens* is accompanied by the production of large amounts of hydrogen and carbon dioxide, which can result in markedly increased pressure in a sealed container. Much gas is also produced in vivo in necrotic tissues; hence the term gas gangrene.

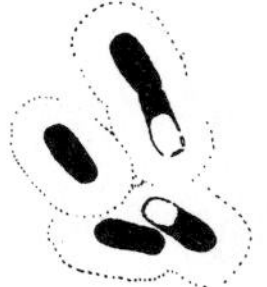

*Clostridium perfringens*

Hemolytic activity caused by alpha- and theta-toxins

Gas produced from carbohydrates in culture and in tissue

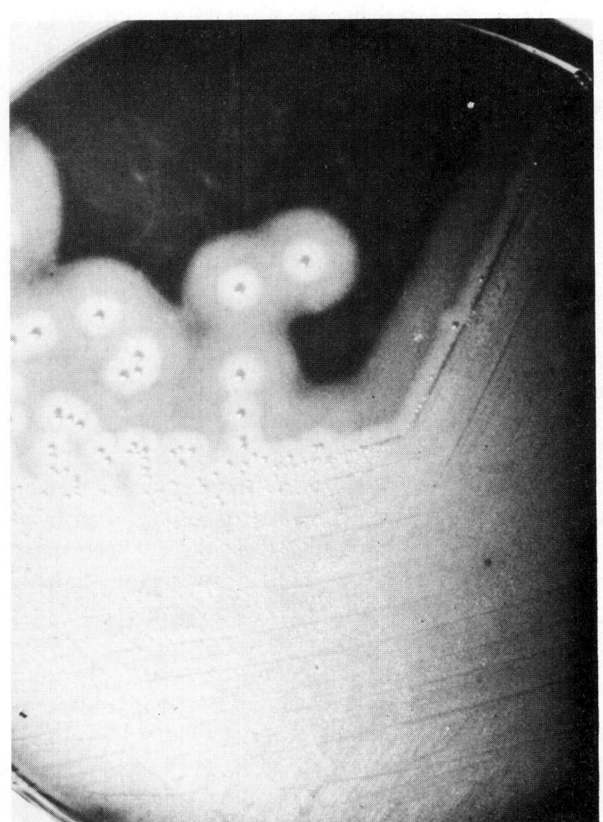

**Figure 18–1.** *C. perfringens* colonies on a blood agar plate showing double zone of hemolysis.

Heat-resistant spores correlated with food poisoning

RESISTANCE

Spores of *C. perfringens* are resistant to all disinfectants and to boiling for brief periods. The spores of some strains that cause food poisoning are often more heat resistant: they can withstand temperatures of 100°C for an hour or more, which accounts for their survival in cooked food. The vegetative cells are readily killed by disinfectants. They are susceptible to penicillin and many other antimicrobics, except the aminoglycosides.

α-toxin has lecithinase and cytotoxic activity

θ-toxin alters capillary permeability; related to streptolysin O

Exterotoxin of *C. perfringens* type A inserts into intestinal cell membranes

TOXINS AND BIOLOGICALLY ACTIVE EXTRACELLULAR ENZYMES

Several of the exotoxins contribute to virulence. The most important is the α-toxin, a phospholipase C that hydrolyzes lecithin and sphingomyelin and thus disrupts the cell membranes of various host cells, including erythrocytes, leukocytes, and muscle cells. The median lethal dose (LD50) of the toxin for experimental animals is approximately 5 μg/kg.

θ-Toxin is an oxygen-labile hemolysin that also alters capillary permeability and is toxic for heart muscle. It is closely related to streptolysin O (Chapter 16) and is responsible for the complete beta-hemolysis seen after overnight incubation on blood agar plates.

The enterotoxin, a heat-labile protein produced by some strains of *C. perfringens* type A, is responsible for a common and benign form of bacterial food poisoning. This low-molecular-weight protein is released into the upper gastrointestinal tract after ingestion of vegetative forms of the organism. Following attachment to protein receptor sites on the epithelial surface, it inserts into the cell membrane. An increase in intracellular calcium, altered membrane permeability, and loss of cellular fluid and macromolecules quickly follow. The ileum is most severely involved.

Other biologically active extracellular products include a collagenase, a deoxyribonuclease, a hyaluronidase, and proteases. All may contribute to invasive pathologic processes, but none shares the central role of the α-toxin.

## Diseases Caused by C. perfringens

GAS GANGRENE

Open wounds with muscle damage predispose to gas gangrene

Other clostridia may cause the disease

Gas gangrene can develop in severe traumatic open lesions, such as compound fractures or bullet wounds, when there is muscle damage, contamination with dirt, clothing, or other foreign material, and if *C. perfringens* or, less commonly, one of the other gas-gangrene-causing clostridia (for example, *C. novyi* or *C. septicum*) is introduced. The disease is most often seen in war wounds, but occasionally follows severe trauma in civilian life. It can develop within a few hours of wounding. Because *C. perfringens* is sometimes present in bile in cholecystitis, gas gangrene of the abdominal muscles is an occasional complication of gallbladder or bile duct surgery, particularly when bile is spilled.

Low oxidation reduction potential required in tissue

α-toxin production kills cells locally

Further multiplication causes muscle necrosis and gas production

θ-toxin and oxygen deprivation contribute to shock

If the oxidation-reduction potential in a wound is sufficiently low, *C. perfringens* spores can germinate and the organism can multiply very rapidly. Infections are always mixed; the presence of numerous facultative species contributes to the reducing conditions. *C. perfringens* elaborates its α-toxin, which passes along the muscle bundles killing all cells, including inflammatory cells, and producing additional necrotic areas into which the organism can grow. Fermentation of muscle carbohydrate by *C. perfringens* produces gas in the subcutaneous tissues that can be felt when palpated (crepitation) and seen on radiography. As the disease progresses, increased vascular permeability and shock cause severe systemic disease. θ-Toxin and oxygen deprivation due to the metabolic activities of *C. perfringens* are probable contributors. Ultimately, *C. perfringens* bacteremia develops. Untreated gas gangrene is always fatal.

α-toxin plays crucial role in disease

The critical role of anaerobiosis and of α-toxin production in the development of the infection has been clearly demonstrated in animal experiments. *C. perfringens* cells washed free of toxin and inoculated intramuscularly into guinea pigs cause no lesion. When substances causing muscle necrosis or actively metabolizing aerobic organisms are introduced, however, gas gangrene develops. Active immunization with α-toxin or passive immunization with anti-α-toxin antibody will prevent the disease.

Early surgical debridement of dead tissue needed

Treatment must be initiated immediately. Excision of all devitalized tissue is of paramount importance because it denies the organism the anaerobic conditions required for further multiplication and toxin production. This often entails wide resection of muscle groups, hysterectomy, and even amputation of limbs. Administration of massive doses of penicillin is an important adjunctive procedure. Recent animal studies have indicated that antimicrobics that inhibit protein synthesis may be equally or more effective, possibly due to their ability to directly suppress toxin formation. As non-clostridial anaerobes and *Enterobacteriaceae* frequently contaminate injury sites, clindamycin and broad spectrum cephalosporins are often added to the antibiotic regimen. Placing the patient in a hyperbaric oxygen chamber increases the tissue level of dissolved oxygen and has been shown to slow the spread of disease, probably by inhibiting bacterial growth and toxin production and by neutralizing the activity of θ-toxin. This measure also appears to reduce the "toxicity" of the patient. In the past, gas gangrene polyvalent antitoxin was administered intravenously in large amounts to neutralize free toxin. It may have helped prevent hemolysis, but was of doubtful benefit in halting the gangrene; its use is no longer recommended and production of this biologic agent has been discontinued.

Hyperbaric oxygen may have direct effect on toxins

The single most effective method for preventing gas gangrene is the surgical debridement of traumatic injuries as soon after wounding as possible. Thorough cleansing, removal of dead tissue and foreign bodies, and drainage of hematoma will limit organism multiplication and toxin production. In heavily contaminated wounds, this is supplemented with antimicrobic therapy in an attempt to inhibit accessible clostridia and delay infection with other organisms that may promote clostridial disease. Antimicrobic prophylaxis cannot replace surgical debridement, and the disease may develop in cases receiving such treatment because the antimicrobics fail to reach the organism in devascularized tissues.

Surgical debridement primary treatment

Antimicrobial therapy adjunctive

### Anaerobic Cellulitis

Anaerobic cellulitis is a clostridial infection of wounds and surrounding subcutaneous tissue in which there is marked gas formation (more than that in gas gangrene), but in which the pain, swelling, and toxicity of gas gangrene are absent. It is much less serious than gas gangrene and can be controlled with less rigorous methods.

### Clostridial Endometritis

If *C. perfringens* gains access to necrotic products of conception retained in the uterus, it may multiply and infect the endometrium. Necrosis of uterine tissue and septicemia with massive intravascular hemolysis due to α-toxin may then follow. Clostridial uterine infection was seen more commonly in the past, usually after an incomplete illegal abortion with inadequately sterilized instruments. The disease is extremely serious and may require emergency hysterectomy and hemodialysis for renal shutdown resulting from hemoglobinemia.

Septicemia and intravascular hemolysis associated with nonsterile abortions

### Clostridial Food Poisoning

*C. perfringens* can cause food poisoning if large numbers of an enterotoxin-producing strain are ingested. The incubation period of 8 to 24 hours is followed by nausea, abdominal pain, and diarrhea. There is no fever, and vomiting is rare. Recovery is usual within 24 hours. The disease is caused by the enterotoxin, which is liberated from ingested vegetative organisms in the small intestine. Outbreaks of the disease usually involve meat dishes such as stews, soups, or gravy. Heat-resistant spores of *C. perfringens* may survive the initial cooking and the organism multiplies rapidly if cooling and storage at room temperature are prolonged or if the food is rewarmed. Prevention involves good cooking hygiene and adequate refrigeration. There is growing evidence that enterotoxin-producing strains of *C. perfringens* may also be responsible for some cases of antimicrobic-induced diarrhea.

After incubation period 8–24 hours; diarrhea without fever

*C. perfringens* spores survive brief heating then grow rapidly at warm temperatures

### Diagnosis of *C. perfringens* Infections

Diagnosis is based ultimately on clinical observations. Bacteriologic studies are adjunctive. It is quite common, for example, to isolate *C. perfringens* from contaminated wounds without evidence of clostridial disease. The organism can also be isolated from the postpartum uterine cervix of healthy women or from those with only mild fever. Occasionally, *C. perfringens* is even isolated from blood cultures of patients who do not develop serious clostridial infection.

Isolation of *C. perfringens* may not mean disease

Gram smears from cases of gas gangrene show many clostridia and other organisms (for example, *Enterobacteriaciae*) that multiply in the necrotic tissue. Pieces of necrotic muscle may be seen, and the absence of inflammatory cells is noteworthy. The appearance of smears from the endometrium in clostridial endometritis or of aspirates from skin blebs

Inflammatory cells commonly absent in gas gangrene and clostridial endometritis

surrounding gas gangrene lesions is similar, although in these cases *C. perfringens* is usually the only organism present.

In clostridial food poisoning, isolation of more than $10^5$ *C. perfringens* per gram of the ingested food in the absence of any other cause is usually sufficient to confirm the etiology of a characteristic food poisoning outbreak.

## Clostridium tetani

*C. tetani* spores exist in many soils, especially if they are manured. The organism is sometimes found in the lower intestinal tract of humans and animals.

### Bacteriologic Features

Primary reservoir in soil

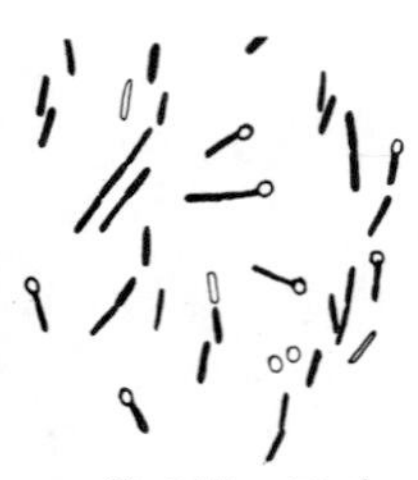
*Clostridium tetani*

Terminal spores are highly resistant

MORPHOLOGY AND CULTURAL CHARACTERISTICS

*C. tetani* is a slim, Gram-positive rod; it may be predominantly Gram negative in very young or old cultures. It forms spores readily in nature and in culture, yielding a typical round terminal spore that gives the organism a drumstick appearance before the residual vegetative cell disintegrates. The organism is flagellate and motile. *C. tetani* requires strict anaerobic conditions. Because of its motility, it spreads over the surface of anaerobic blood agar plates in a thin veil of growth. Its identity is suggested by cultural and biochemical characteristics, but definite identification depends on demonstrating its neurotoxic exotoxin. *C. tetani* spores remain viable in soil or culture for many years. They are resistant to most disinfectants and withstand boiling for several minutes. They are killed by autoclaving at 121°C for 15 minutes.

Tetanospasmin is a neurotoxic exotoxin

Toxin is convertible to toxoid

TOXIN PRODUCTION

The most important product of *C. tetani* is its neurotoxic exotoxin, tetanospasmin, a large, extracellular protein encoded by a plasmid-carried gene. It is heat labile, antigenic, readily neutralized by antitoxin, and rapidly destroyed at 65°C and by intestinal proteases. Treatment with formaldehyde yields a nontoxic product, toxoid, that retains the antigenicity of toxin and thus stimulates production of antitoxin. The LD50 of the toxin for mice is on the order of $10^{-4}$ μg; less than 1 μg would probably be lethal to humans.

## Tetanus

EPIDEMIOLOGY

Tetanus may result from small contaminated wounds or splinters

Neonatal and postpartum tetanus common in developing countries

Spores of *C. tetani* may be introduced into wounds with contaminated soil or foreign bodies. The predisposing wounds are often quite small, for example, a puncture wound containing a splinter. In contrast to those in gas gangrene, infected wounds often do not extend below the subcutaneous tissues. Occasionally, the disease may follow severe burns; it has also occurred as a complication of chronic otitis media, probably when the organism gains access to the middle ear through a perforated eardrum. In many less developed countries, the majority of tetanus cases occur in recently delivered babies and their mothers. The uterus of the new mother may be infected by inexpert removal of the placenta. The neonate suffers infection when the umbilical cord is severed or bandaged in an uncleanly manner. Similarly, tetanus may follow an unskilled abortion, scarification rituals, female circumcision, and even surgery performed with unsterile instruments or dressings.

PATHOGENESIS

Low Eh in wound allows spores to germinate

The usual predisposing factor for tetanus is an area of very low oxidation-reduction potential in which tetanus spores can germinate. This can be provided by a large splinter, an area of necrosis from introduction of soil, or necrosis after injection of contaminated illicit drugs. Infection with facultative or other anaerobic organisms can contribute to the development of an appropriate anaerobic nidus for spore germination.

Toxin produced locally ascends motor nerves to anterior horn cells

Tetanus bacilli multiply locally and neither damage nor invade adjacent tissues. Tetanospasmin is elaborated at the site of infection and reaches the central nervous system mainly by ascending the motor nerves. In the spinal cord, it acts at the level of the anterior horn cells by blocking postsynaptic inhibition of spinal motor reflexes. Thus, an afferent stimulus produces spasmodic contractions of both protagonist and antagonist muscles, initially in the area of the causative lesion. In the more serious forms of the disease toxin extends up and down the spinal cord, and generalized spasms can result from minor stimuli, such as a sound or a draft.

## Tetanus: Clinical Aspects

### Clinical Manifestations

The incubation period of the disease is from 4 days to several weeks. The shorter incubation period is usually associated with wounds in areas supplied by the cranial motor nerves, probably because of a shorter transmission route for the toxin to the central nervous system. In general, shorter incubation periods are associated with more severe disease.

Incubation period depends on location of wound

Although tetanus may be localized to muscles innervated by nerves in the region of the infection, it is usually more generalized. The masseter muscles are often the first to be affected, resulting in inability to open the mouth properly **(trismus);** this effect accounts for the use of the term **lockjaw** to describe the disease. As other muscles become affected, intermittent spasms can become generalized to include muscles of respiration and swallowing. In extreme cases, generalized convulsions produce opisthotonos, caused by massive contractions of the back muscles. Risus sardonicus (sardonic smile) is a late sign in which trismus combined with facial spasm leads to separation of the lips over clenched teeth. Untreated patients with tetanus retain consciousness and are aware of their plight, in which small stimuli can trigger massive contractions. In fatal cases, death results from exhaustion and respiratory failure. All of these results are attributable to very small amounts of tetanospasmin produced at the site of what is often a small, sometimes unrecognized local lesion. The amount of toxin is so small that unimmunized patients often do not have an antibody response. Untreated, the mortality caused by the generalized disease varies from 15 to more than 60%, according to the lesion, incubation period, and age of the patient. Mortality is highest in the neonate and in the elderly.

Masseter muscle involvement causes lockjaw

Severe tetanus has generalized muscle spasms

Spasms may be triggered by minor stimuli

### Treatment

Specific treatment of the disease involves neutralization of any unbound toxin with large doses of human tetanus immune globulin (TIG), which is derived from the blood of volunteers hyperimmunized with toxoid. In countries where TIG is unavailable, horse antitoxin is still used. Most important in treatment are nonspecific supportive measures, including maintenance of a quiet dark environment, sedation, and provision of an adequate airway. In severe cases, curarelike drugs are used to block nerve impulses at the neuromuscular junctions. These patients require artificial ventilation to maintain oxygenation because of respiratory paralysis. Such measures have resulted in a substantially reduced mortality.

Tetanus immune globulin given to neutralize unbound toxin

Supportive measures include airway and curarelike drugs

### Prevention

Routine active immunization with tetanus toxoid, combined with diphtheria toxoid and pertussis vaccine (DPT) for primary immunization in childhood, can completely prevent the disease. It has reduced the incidence of tetanus in the United States to less than 50 reported cases per year. Five doses of DPT are now recommended, to be given at the ages of 2, 4, 6, and 18 months, and once again between the ages of 4 and 6 years. Thereafter a booster of adult-type tetanus diphtheria toxoid should be given every 10 years. Unfortunately, routine childhood immunization is not administratively and economically feasible in many less well-developed countries, where as many as a million cases of tetanus occur annually. In such settings, immunization efforts have been focused on the pregnant woman, because transplacental transfer of antibodies to the fetus also prevents the highly lethal neonatal tetanus.

Disease preventable by active immunization with tetanus toxoid

Active immunization of a pregnant woman protects the infant

Unimmunized subjects with tetanus-prone wounds should be given passive immunity with a prophylactic dose of TIG as soon as possible. This immunization provides immediate protection. Those who have had a full primary series of immunizations, and appropriate boosters, are given toxoid for tetanus-prone wounds if they have not been immunized within the previous 10 years in the case of clean minor wounds or 5 years for more contaminated wounds. If immunization is incomplete or the wound has been neglected and poses a serious risk of disease, TIG is also given.

Passive immunization used for exposed unimmunized subjects

Penicillin therapy is a prophylactic adjunct in serious or neglected wounds, but in no way alters the need for specific prophylaxis. All those who have not been actively immunized should be given a first dose of toxoid as soon as possible and followed up for a complete immunization series. If toxoid and TIG are given in opposite arms with different syringes there is no significant interference between them. Recommended immunization schedules change from time to time, and those responsible for their administration should be familiar with current recommendations.

## Clostridium botulinum

Environmental habitat is widespread

Spores of *C. botulinum* are found in soil, pond, and lake sediments in many parts of the world, including the United States. The major characteristic of medical importance is that strains of *C. botulinum* elaborate one of seven antigenically distinct neurotoxins of extraordinary toxicity: the estimated lethal dose for humans is less than 1 μg. The organism is classified into types A through G, based on the antigenic specificity of these toxins. Metabolic characteristics allow division of *C. botulinum* into four physiologic groups, distinguishable by DNA relatedness studies; it has been suggested that each should be accorded independent species status. Unfortunately, the correlation between physiologic groups and toxin types is incomplete.

Type differentiation by antigenic differences in neurotoxins

Toxins heat labile but resistant to digestive enzymes

Production of toxin is determined by carriage of temperate phage in *C. botulinum* types C and D, a plasmid in type G organisms, and probably by chromosomal genes in types A, B, E, and F. All of the toxins are heat labile and destroyed rapidly at 100°C. They are resistant to the enzymes of the gastrointestinal tract and are readily absorbed by this route. They act on neuromuscular junctions by inhibiting release of acetylcholine, resulting in muscular paralysis. Both the voluntary and autonomic cholinergic nervous systems are affected.

Paralysis produced by blocking acetylcholine release

Heat-resistant spores germinate and cells multiply in alkaline and neutral foods

Spores of *C. botulinum* resist boiling for long periods, but are rapidly destroyed by moist heat at a temperature of 121°C. Germination of spores and growth of *C. botulinum* can occur in a variety of alkaline or neutral foodstuffs when conditions are sufficiently anaerobic. Occasionally, under the same conditions, the organism can multiply in wounds or in the lower intestinal tract of infants.

Toxin detected and typed by neutralization studies

*C. botulinum* is identified by its morphologic, cultural, and biochemical characteristics, particularly its toxin production. Toxin is detected by injecting culture supernatants into unprotected mice and into mice protected with antitoxins against the different serotypes of toxin. Unprotected mice and mice given heterologous antitoxin die of paralytic disease within 3 days. Mice protected against the specific serotype of toxin survive.

### Botulism

EPIDEMIOLOGY AND PATHOGENESIS

Home canning of alkaline foods greatest risk

Human botulism is almost always caused by *C. botulinum* types A, B, or E. In the continental United States the causative agent is most commonly type A or B, the former dominating in the western part of the country and the latter in the eastern states. Disease typically follows ingestion of home-canned alkaline vegetables, such as green beans or mushrooms, that have not been heated at temperatures sufficient to kill *C. botulinum* spores. The organism multiples on storage, often with no change in food taste or odor, and elaborates its toxin. If the food is ingested without cooking, botulism will result. In Alaska, type E food-borne disease is more common and follows ingestion of home-preserved fish or, occasionally, inadequately sterilized or canned commercial fish products. Acidic foods such as canned fruit do not support the growth of *C. botulinum*. The disease often occurs in small epidemics among those who have eaten the toxic food uncooked.

### Botulism: Clinical Aspects

CLINICAL MANIFESTATIONS

Muscular paralysis first sign of disease

After an incubation period of 18 to 96 hours, signs of paralysis develop, first involving the ocular, pharyngeal, laryngeal, and respiratory muscles. There may be extensive paralysis of voluntary muscles. Dry mouth, constipation, and urinary retention occur through the action of the toxin on the autonomic cholinergic nervous system. The mortality caused by the disease is 10 to 20%.

TREATMENT

The availability of intensive supportive measures, particularly mechanical ventilation, is the single most important determinant of clinical outcome; with proper ventilatory support, mortality should be less then 10%. The administration of large doses of trivalent (A, B, C) horse *C. botulinum* antitoxin is thought to be useful in neutralizing free toxin. Frequent hypersensitivity reactions related to the equine origin of this preparation makes it unsuitable for use in infants; an antitoxin of human origin is currently undergoing evaluation in this latter population. Antimicrobic agents are given only to patients with wound botulism (see below).

Antitoxin treatment and support determine outcome

Human antitoxin under evaluation

PREVENTION

Adequate pressure cooking or autoclaving in the canning process will kill spores. Heating food at 100°C for 10 min before eating will destroy the toxin. Food from damaged cans or those that present evidence of positive inside pressure should not even be tasted because of the extreme toxicity of the *C. botulinum* toxin.

Adequate cooking inactivates toxin

INFANT BOTULISM

In recent years, a syndrome associated with *C. botulinum* has been recognized in infants between the ages of 3 weeks and 8 months. It is now the most commonly diagnosed form of botulism. The organism is apparently introduced on weaning or with dietary supplements, especially honey, and multiplies in the infant's colon, with absorption of small amounts of toxin. The infant shows constipation, poor muscle tone, lethargy, and feeding problems and may have ophthalmic and other paralyses similar to those in adult botulism. Infant botulism may contribute to the sudden infant death syndrome. The benefits of antitoxin and antimicrobic agents have not been clearly established for this form of disease.

Toxin can be produced in infant's colon

WOUND BOTULISM

Very rarely, wounds infected with other organisms may allow *C. botulinum* to grow. Recently, wound botulism has been reported in parenteral cocaine users, and maxillary sinus botulism in intranasal users of this same agent. Disease similar to that from food poisoning can develop. Botulism without an obvious food or wound source is occasionally reported in individuals beyond infancy. It is possible that some such cases result from ingestion of spores of *C. botulinum* with subsequent in vivo production of toxin in a manner similar to that in infant botulism.

Toxin production may occur in wounds of drug users

LABORATORY DIAGNOSIS

Toxin can frequently be demonstrated in blood, intestinal contents, or remaining food, by inoculation into mice. Unprotected mice die, whereas those protected with specific antitoxin survive. *C. botulinum* may also be isolated from stool or from foodstuffs apparently responsible for botulism.

Diagnosis is by toxin detection

## Clostridium difficile

*C. difficile* was first isolated from the stools of healthy newborn children over three decades ago, but its role as an enteric pathogen was more recently documented. The organism appears to be widespread in the environment and occurs in the intestinal flora of 2 to 4% of healthy adults. Asymptomatic carriage in the stools of hospital-delivered neonates and outbreaks of *C. difficile*-induced diarrhea in hospitalized adults suggests that many hospitals are heavily contaminated with the spores of this organism. Once in this environment, they may persist for many months and be passed from patient to patient on the hands of hospital personnel.

Formed in the environment, in healthy individuals, and in hospitals

Medically important strains produce two distinct large polypeptide toxins, A and B, which are encoded in linked chromosomal genes and released during stationary or poststationary growth phases of the vegetative organism, perhaps at the time of cell lysis. Highly virulent strains produce up to a million times as much toxin as weakly virulent members of the species.

Two toxins produced

Toxin A primarily enterotoxin

Toxin A is primarily an enterotoxin that stimulates infiltration of neutrophils and release of inflammatory mediators, causing fluid secretion, altered membrane permeability, and hemorrhagic necrosis. Cytotoxic activity can also be demonstrated in vitro. It is thought to be primarily responsible for the clinical colitis associated with this organism.

Toxin B, a cytotoxin, disrupts microfilaments and inhibits protein synthesis

Toxin B is a highly potent cytotoxin, which disrupts the microfilament system of cells and decreases cellular protein synthesis and in a fashion similar to that of diphtheria toxin (see Chapter 17). Animal studies suggest that toxin-A-induced mucosal damage allows absorption of toxin B from the gut lumen.

### ■ C. difficile and Antimicrobic-associated Diarrhea

Antibiotic associated diarrhea may progress to PMC

Diarrhea is a frequent side effect of antimicrobic treatment. In some patients, it may progress to a severe, occasionally lethal inflammation of the colon. When this is accompanied by the formation of an overlying "pseudomembrane" composed of fibrin, leukocytes, and necrotic colonic cells, the clinical syndrome is referred to as pseudomembranous colitis (PMC). It is now known that *C. difficile* is responsible for most PMC and perhaps many of the milder cases of antimicrobic-associated diarrhea (AAD).

Newborns are colonized without disease

Antimicrobics alter flora followed by increase in *C. difficile*

Toxin production causes watery or bloody diarrhea

The fastidious *C. difficile* is seldom able to establish itself in the colon of individuals with normal gut flora, although newborn children, who lack the complex flora of adults, frequently become colonized during their brief stay in a hospital nursery. Newborns rarely suffer clinical consequences, possibly because toxin receptors within their gut are immature or unavailable. On the other hand, alteration of the colonic flora of the adult with antimicrobics (particularly with ampicillin, cephalosporins, and clindamycin) or antineoplastic agents can result in overgrowth of the organism with diarrhea or PMC. The diarrhea may be mild and watery or bloody and accompanied by abdominal cramping, leukocytosis, and fever. It is estimated that *C. difficile* is responsible for 25% of all reported cases of AAD and for the overwhelming majority of those with PMC. Interestingly, the rate of colonization of newborns within a hospital nursery closely parallels the incidence of clinically manifested *C. difficile* disease in adult patients, suggesting newborn colonization rates reflect the level of environmental contamination with *C. difficile* within a hospital.

#### Diagnosis

Detection of toxin in stool by tissue culture or immunoassay

Endoscopic examination of the colon is the most definitive procedure for establishing the presence of a pseudomembrane. The organism can be isolated using a selective medium and identified on the basis of its morphologic and biochemical characteristics. Both toxins may be detected in stool, toxin B by tissue culture assays, and both toxin A and B with recently introduced enzyme immunoassays.

#### Treatment

Discontinuation of antimicrobic usually suffices; oral vancomycin or metronidazole therapy

Usually, discontinuing the implicated antimicrobic will result in the resolution of clinical symptoms. If patients are severely ill or fail to respond to drug withdrawal, they are treated with oral antimicrobics, such as vancomycin or metronidazole. Relapses or reinfections requiring retreatment occur in as many as 20% of patients. *C. difficile* is susceptible to the penicillins and cephalosporins in vitro, but they are ineffective and may predispose to the disease, because they are destroyed by beta-lactamases produced by other intestinal organisms.

## ANAEROBIC GRAM-NEGATIVE RODS AND ANAEROBIC COCCI

Two large and important groups of organisms, anaerobic Gram-negative rods and anaerobic cocci, are considered together because they share many features in terms of habitat, diseases produced, and methods used in identification. They are more common causes of disease than the clostridia; those associated with human infections are opportunists, however, and their determinants of pathogenicity are more obscure. All are members of the normal flora of the upper alimentary and respiratory tracts, the female genital tract, and the colon. The most commonly isolated genera, species, and subspecies of these organisms and the sites of infections with which they are usually associated are listed in Table 18–2. The student should not attempt to commit the names of the individual species to memory.

**TABLE 18–2. ANAEROBIC GRAM-NEGATIVE RODS AND ANAEROBIC COCCI**

| Organism Groups | Percentage of All Anaerobic Isolates | Frequency Within Group | Isolation Site | | | | |
|---|---|---|---|---|---|---|---|
| | | | *Ororespiratory* | *Intestinal* | *Genital* | *Soft Tissue* | *Bone* |
| *Bacteroides fragilis* complex | 35 | | ± | ++++ | ++ | ++ | + |
| *B. fragilis* | | Common | | | | | |
| *B. thetaiotaomicron* | | Occasional | | | | | |
| *B. vulgatus* | | Rare | | | | | |
| *B. distasonis* | | Rare | | | | | |
| *B. uniformis* | | Rare | | | | | |
| *B. ovatus* | | Rare | | | | | |
| *Prevotella/Porphyromonas* complex | 10 | | ++++ | − | ++ | + | ++ |
| *P. asaccharolytica* | | Common | | | | | |
| *Pr. intermedius* | | Occasional | | | | | |
| *Pr. melaninogenica* | | Rare | | | | | |
| *P. gingivalis* | | Rare | | | | | |
| *Fusobacterium* spp. | 5 | | +++ | ++ | ++ | − | + |
| *F. nucleatum* | | Common | | | | | |
| *F. necrophorum* | | Rare | | | | | |
| *F. mortiferum* | | Rare | | | | | |
| *F. varium* | | Rare | | | | | |
| *Peptostreptococcus* spp. | 25 | | +++ | +++ | +++ | +++ | + |
| *P. magnus* | | Common | | | | | |
| *P. anaerobius* | | Common | | | | | |
| *P. asaccharolyticus* | | Common | | | | | |

Numbers of + signs indicate frequency of occurrence.

## Gram-negative Anaerobic Disease: General Features

### Pathogenesis

Diseases caused by these organisms are almost invariably examples of autoinfection: the normal flora transgress epithelial barriers through trauma or pathologic conditions (for example, a ruptured appendix or colonic diverticulum) or because of compromised immune defenses. The result is usually abscess formation. The great majority of infections are mixed; that is, two or more anaerobes are isolated, often in combination with facultative bacteria such as *Escherichia coli* (Fig 18–2). In some cases the components of these mixtures syn-

Autoinfection results from transgression of epithelial barriers

Most infections mixed, including other anaerobes and facultative bacteria

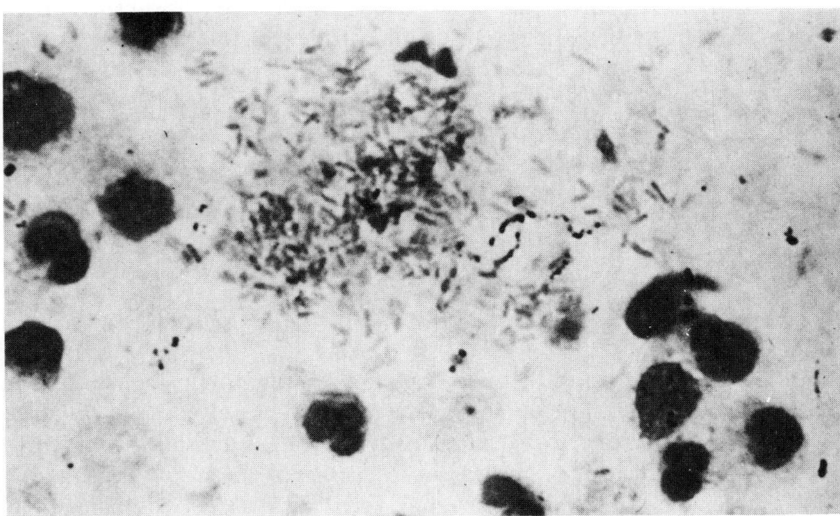

**Figure 18–2.** Gram smear of pus from an abdominal abscess showing polymorphonuclear leucocytes and large numbers of Gram-negative anaerobes and some peptostreptococci. (*Reproduced with permission of Schering Corporation, Kenilworth, NJ, the copyright owner. All rights reserved.*)

ergize each other's growth. Multiplication of these opportunistic pathogens in abscesses is facilitated by inhibition of oxygen-dependent leukocyte bactericidal functions under the anaerobic conditions in the lesions. Those with the greatest virulence are selected out and multiply under conditions of sufficiently low oxidation-reduction potential (Eh). The more aerotolerant anaerobes may occasionally cause endocarditis.

Abscess conditions facilitate low oxidation-reduction potential, leukocyte inhibition

### Clinical Manifestations

*Bacteroides, Fusobacterium,* and peptostreptococci alone or together with other facultative or obligate anaerobes, are responsible for the overwhelming majority of localized abscesses or empyemas within the cranium, periodontium, thorax, peritoneum, liver, and female genital tract. In addition, they appear to play major causal roles in chronic sinusitis, chronic otitis media, aspiration and necrotizing pneumonia, bronchiectasis, cholecystitis, septic arthritis, osteomyelitis, decubitus ulcers, and soft tissue infections of patients with diabetes mellitus. Many, but not all, anaerobic infections are associated with foul-smelling lesions, and thrombophlebitis is a common complication. They account for approximately 2 to 8% of positive blood cultures; the mortality rate of bacteremias arising from nongenital sources is 20 to 40%, which is equivalent to the rates with bacteremias due to staphylococci or Enterobacteriaceae.

Localized abscess most common finding

Sometimes associated with foul-smelling lesions

### Laboratory Diagnosis

The key to detection and identification of anaerobes is a good specimen, preferably pus or fluid exudate directly from the infected site. It should be collected in special anaerobic transport tubes or a syringe from which all air is excluded to minimize contact with atmospheric oxygen. Specimens should be taken quickly to the microbiology laboratory for prompt placement in culture.

Special transport needed to exclude oxygen

A direct Gram-stained smear of clinical material is often helpful. Numerous pale-staining Gram-negative rods are usually seen in anaerobic Gram-negative infections. They are often slim or fusiform and are frequently associated with some Gram-positive bacteria. Numerous polymorphonuclear leukocytes are usually seen (Fig 18–2). These findings are highly suggestive of anaerobic Gram-negative infection, especially if little or no growth occurs on overnight aerobic culture.

Gram smear often suggestive

Identification often requires special procedures. Media maintained under reduced or anaerobic conditions are used throughout, and exposure to atmospheric oxygen is kept to a minimum. Specific identification procedures include morphology, biochemical characterization, and metabolic end-product detection by gas chromatography.

Specific identification may be time-consuming

### Treatment

In most cases, treatment requires detection of abscesses and drainage of the purulent material, in addition to appropriate chemotherapy. Frequently, chemotherapy alone is ineffective because of failure to penetrate the site of infection. Anaerobic organisms derived from the oral flora are usually susceptible to penicillin and are the most common cause of infection above the diaphragm. Fecal anaerobes, particularly *B. fragilis,* are usually resistant to penicillin and are the etiologic agents of most abdominal infections. They are most likely to respond to chloramphenicol, clindamycin, metronidazole, or an appropriate third-generation cephalosporin. It merits further emphasis, however, that surgical drainage is often essential to therapeutic success.

Drainage needed for prompt recovery

Oral anaerobes penicillin susceptible

Fecal *B. fragilis* typically penicillin-resistant

## Features of Anaerobe Groups

### Bacteroides Group

The *B. fragilis* group comprises the most common opportunistic pathogens of the genus *Bacteroides*. They are slim, pale-staining, capsulate, Gram-negative rods that form colonies overnight on blood agar medium and are relatively tolerant to atmospheric oxygen. The implication of fragility in the name is misleading, because they are actually among the hardier and more easily grown anaerobes. Although *B. fragilis* constitutes less than 10% of *Bacteroides* species in the normal colon, it predominates among Gram-negative infections in the abdominal cavity. Its polysaccharide capsule confers resistance to phagocytosis, stimulates abscess formation when injected into experimental animals, and may inhibit mac-

*B. fragilis* group most commonly pathogens derived from colonic flora

*B. fragilis* capsule is antiphagocytic

rophage migration. *Bacteroides* species produce a number of extracellular enzymes that may contribute to pathogenicity including collagenase, IgA protease, heparinase, and DNase. Bacteroides fragilis is almost always resistant to penicillin and many other beta-lactams in part because of chromosomally encoded beta-lactamase. Resistance to tetracycline is common, but most strains are susceptible to chloramphenicol, clindamycin, and metronidazole, although increasing resistance has been reported. Plasmids carrying resistance determinants have been demonstrated in *B. fragilis*.

*B. fragilis* produces chromosomal β-lactamase

The pigmented, bile-sensitive anaerobic Gram-negative rods previously known as the *B. melaninogenicus–asaccharolyticus* complex have recently been reassigned to the *Porphyromonas* and *Prevotella* genera. They comprise the second most common cause of human infection caused by anaerobic Gram-negative bacilli. *Prevotella melaninogenica* derives its name from the characteristic black colonies it forms as a result of production of a black pigment from hemoglobin derivatives. Organisms of this group are found in the oral cavity, upper alimentary and respiratory tracts, and colon. In contrast to that of the *B. fragilis* complex, the cell wall has powerful endotoxic properties, and the organisms are usually susceptible to penicillin. Infections with *P. melaninogenica* are usually derived from the oral flora; they include dental and sinus infections, pulmonary infections and abscesses, and infections of human bites. The latter tend to be serious and refractory unless treated adequately with debridement and antibiotics. This group of organisms is also encountered in abdominal and pelvic lesions.

*P. melaninogenicus* found in mouth, upper alimentary, and respiratory tracts

Penicillin-sensitive organisms that possess potent endotoxin

Several other designated species of *Bacteroides* comprise the predominant organisms in the adult colon. Their pathogenic potential is less than that of the groups discussed above.

### Fusobacterium

*Fusobacterium nucleatum* is the most common species of the genus in human infection. It is a spindle-shaped, slow-growing, Gram-negative, anaerobic rod that inhabits the oral cavity, the colon, and sometimes the female genital tract. It is less virulent than the species of *Bacteroides* discussed previously and usually appears in mixed infections. It is sensitive to penicillin. Other fusobacteria contribute to chronic ulcerative lesions of the gums, to abscesses deriving from the oral cavity and pharynx, and to a necrotic ulcerative lesion of the pharynx called Vincent's angina (Chapters 26 and 62).

Contributes to oral infections including Vincent's angina

### Peptostreptococcus and Microaerophilic Streptococci

The taxonomy of this group of organisms has been shifting and has thus been a source of considerable confusion. Some clinically important species, previously designated as peptostreptococci, although primarily anaerobic can grow slowly in reduced oxygen or increased $CO_2$ concentrations and have been reassigned to the genus *Streptococcus*. They have pathogenic potential similar to that of the peptostreptococci and will be considered here as microaerophilic streptococci.

Some species similar to streptococci

These organisms are usually small, Gram-positive cocci that tend to occur in long chains in clinical material and to lose their Gram positivity easily. They are members of the normal flora of the oral cavity, colon, and female genital tract. They are opportunists and are often found in lesions with other anaerobic and facultative organisms. Sometimes peptostreptococci or microaerophilic streptococci are the sole etiologic agents in cerebral and other abscesses and in puerperal infections and pelvic peritonitis. They can cause anaerobic cellulitis and are often associated with septic thrombophlebitis, which may result in metastatic abscesses. Peptostreptococcal lesions tend to be foul smelling and to show gas production.

Causes of some abscesses, puerperal infections, and thrombophlebitis

Microaerophilic streptococci can cause a form of spreading, synergistic, subcutaneous gangrene (Meleney's ulcer) in association with *Staphylococcus aureus,* usually after serious abdominal surgery. The infection arises in a suture line. Peptostreptococci and microaerophilic streptococci are sensitive to penicillin and usually to other antimicrobics active against Gram-positive cocci, with the exception of the aminoglycosides.

Subcutaneous tissue infections and synergistic gangrene

## OTHER ANAEROBIC ORGANISMS

Many other anaerobic species of Gram-negative and non-spore-forming Gram-positive rods have been described. Their role in infection is usually only subsidiary, so they will not be

*Veillonella* are Gram-negative cocci

discussed here. It is important to remember, however, that they probably play an important adjunctive role in lesions such as periodontal disease, the single major cause of tooth loss and oral sepsis. The genus *Veillonella*, which comprises small anaerobic Gram-negative cocci, merits special mention, because it may be confused with *Neisseria* on Gram staining. It is often present in anaerobic lesions, but plays little role in infection.

## ADDITIONAL READING

Clabots CR, Johnson S, Olson MM, et al: Acquisition of *Clostridium difficile* by hospitalized patients: Evidence for colonized new admissions as a source of infection. *J Infect Dis* 1992;166:561–567. An interesting study that suggests that the spread of *C. difficile* and the persistence of the organism in the hospital is propagated by readmission of previously hospitalized and largely asymptomatic patients who harbor the bacterium.

Finegold SM: *Anaerobic Infections in Human Disease*. San Diego, Academic Press, 1989. A comprehensive text with particular emphasis on clinical syndromes, significance, and therapy.

Hatheway CL: Toxigenic clostridia. *Clin Microbiol Rev* 1990;3:66–98. A comprehensive review of the historical aspects, organism characteristics, clinical diseases, and toxins of 13 species of clostridia.

Kasper DL, Onderdonk AB: Introduction: International symposium on anaerobic bacteria and bacterial infections. *Rev Infect Dis* 1990;12:S121–S252. This supplemental issue is devoted to the scientific papers given at an international symposium held in Monte Carlo. It is a comprehensive and timely presentation of the microbiologic and structural aspects, pathogenesis, immune mechanisms, susceptibility testing, and management of infections caused by the obligate anaerobes.

Lombardi DP, Englebery NC: Anaerobic bacteremia: Incidence, patient characteristics, and clinical significance. *Am J Med* 1992;92:53–60. This retrospective study documents a much lower rate of positive bloods cultures for anaerobes (2 to 3%) than older studies. This probably reflects a real decline in incidence.

Lyerly DM, Krivan HC, Wilkins TD: *Clostridium difficile:* Its disease and toxins. *Clin Microbiol Rev* 1988;1:1–18. An excellent review of the pathogenesis of *C. difficile* infections and of its toxins.

Schofield F: Selective primary health care: Strategies for control of disease in the developing world, XXII. Tetanus. A preventable problem. *Rev Infect Dis* 1986;8:144–156. A very important review with particular emphasis on prevention of neonatal tetanus.

Schreiner MS, Field E, Ruddy R: Infant botulism: A review of 12 years' experience at the Children's Hospital of Philadelphia. *Pediatrics* 1991;87:159–165. A well-referenced update of knowledge of this disease.

Stevens DL, Maier KA, Mitten JE. Effects of antibiotics on toxin production and viability of *Clostridium perfringens. Antimicrob Ag Chemother* 1987;31:213–218. Evidence is presented that protein-synthesis-inhibiting antimicrobics may be more effective than penicillin in inhibiting toxin production.

Weber JT, Hibbs RG Jr, Darwish A, et al: A massive outbreak of type E botulism associated with traditional salted fish in Cairo. *J Infect Dis* 1993;167:451–454.

Chapter 19

# *Neisseria*

*Kenneth J. Ryan and Stanley Falkow*

*Neisseria* are Gram-negative diplococci. The genus contains two pathogenic and many commensal species, most of which are normal inhabitants of the upper respiratory and alimentary tracts. The pathogenic species are *Neisseria meningitidis* (meningococcus), a major cause of meningitis and bacteremia, and *Neisseria gonorrhoeae* (gonococcus), the cause of gonorrhea.

## GENERAL FEATURES

### Morphology and Structure

Gram-negative bean-shaped diplococci

The organisms are Gram-negative cocci that typically appear in pairs with the opposing sides flattened, imparting a "kidney bean" appearance. Both gonococci and meningococci are readily phagocytosed by polymorphonuclear leukocytes (PMNs); cells containing 10 or more pairs of gonococci may be seen in Gram smears of pus. *Neisseria* are nonmotile, nonspore forming, and non-acid fast. Their cell walls are typical of Gram-negative bacteria with a peptidoglycan backbone and endotoxic lipopolysaccharide (LPS) complexed with protein in an outer membrane. Capsules and pili may be demonstrated by ultrastructure or by immunologic techniques.

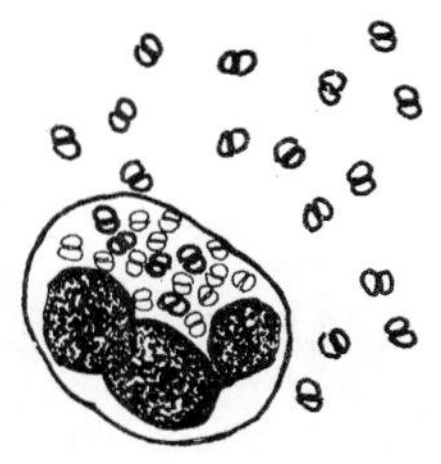

*Neisseria gonorrhoeae* in WBC

### Cultural Characteristics

Gonococcus more fastidious than meningococcus

The gonococcus and the meningococcus require an aerobic atmosphere with added carbon dioxide and enriched medium for optimal growth. The gonococcus grows more slowly and is more fastidious than the meningococcus, which can grow on routine blood agar. Both grow only at 30 to 37°C. Other *Neisseria* are generally less fastidious and can also grow at temperatures as low as 22 to 25°C.

### Classification

All *Neisseria* are oxidase positive

All *Neisseria* are oxidase positive. Some of the bacteriologic and biochemical features used to distinguish the various species are illustrated in Table 19–1. Gonococci and meningococci may also be differentiated from the other *Neisseria* by immunologic methods such as slide agglutination and immunofluorescence. There is increasing use of monoclonal antibodies in such tests.

TABLE 19–1. DIFFERENTIAL BACTERIOLOGIC FEATURES OF NEISSERIA

| | Growth | | | Acid Production From Carbohydrates | | | |
|---|---|---|---|---|---|---|---|
| Organism | *Blood Agar* | *Room Temperature* | *Special Medium*[a] | *Glucose* | *Sucrose* | *Maltose* | *Lactose* |
| *N. gonorrhoeae* | –[b] | – | + | + | – | – | – |
| *N. meningitidis* | + | – | + | + | – | + | – |
| Other *Neisseria* | + | + | –[d] | V[c] | V | V | V |

[a] Thayer–Lewis or similar selective medium.
[b] Poor growth may occur with some strains.
[c] Reaction varies with different strains and species.
[d] *N. lactamica* is an exception.

# NEISSERIA MENINGITIDIS

## Bacteriologic Features

### Growth and Structure

Growth enhanced by $CO_2$

Meningococci grow on most nonselective routine laboratory media and produce about 1.5-mm-diameter colonies after overnight incubation on blood agar. Carbon dioxide enhances growth, but is not required. A small polysaccharide capsule is generally not seen by routine microscopic methods.

### Antigenic Structure

Serogroups based on capsular polysaccharide

Group B polysaccharide differs in immunogenicity

Meningococci are divided into nine serogroups, largely on the basis of their polysaccharide capsules. The most important serogroups are A, B, C, W-135, and Y. The chemical structure of the group-specific polysaccharide has been identified for most serogroups. Purified polysaccharides of all except group B are immunogenic and available as vaccines. The immunogenicity of the group B polysaccharide differs from that of the other groups, although the reasons for this are not clear. In addition to the group antigens, several serotypes have been identified based on differences in outer membrane proteins. These outer membrane proteins, when linked to capsular polysaccharide, are also candidate immunogens for vaccine preparations.

## Meningococcal Disease

### Epidemiology

Most endemic disease now due to groups B, C, Y, and W-135

Group A meningococci have epidemic potential

The incidence of meningococcal infections in the United States varies between 1.0 and 2.0 cases per 100,000 population. B and C are the major serogroups involved, with the remainder of infections caused primarily by serogroup Y, and serogroup W-135, which has emerged as an important cause of disease since 1975. All occur primarily as isolated cases, as sporadic small epidemics, or in small family or closed-population (school or day-care center) outbreaks. Group A strains are more ominous and have the potential to cause widespread epidemics, which in the past have appeared in 8- to 12-year cycles. At other times only 1 to 2% of reported cases of meningococcal infection are due to this group. It has been more than 40 years since a group A epidemic has occurred in the United States, although serious group A epidemics have occurred in recent years in Brazil, the Sudan, Kenya, and South Africa.

Transmission by close contact, respiratory droplets

High risk for family contacts lacking antibody

Transmission of meningococci is by respiratory droplets and requires both close contact and susceptibility (lack of antibody). This combination is most likely to occur in family members of an index case, particularly children. The attack rate of meningococcal infections among family members is 1000-fold higher than in the general population; prophylactic chemotherapy is indicated. Despite their contact with meningococcal infections, hospital employees have not shown an increased frequency of infection, probably because of the lack of prolonged close contact in a largely immune adult population.

### Pathogenesis

The meningococcus is an exclusively human parasite; it can either exist as an apparently harmless member of the normal flora or produce acute disease. Carrier rates of meningococci in the upper respiratory tract vary between 5 and 15% in healthy adults and children, higher colonization rates are found occasionally in closed populations such as military recruit camps and boarding schools. The carrier state is associated with the development of group-specific antibodies and immunity, but before immunity develops, meningococci may sometimes spread from the nasopharynx to produce bacteremia, endotoxemia, and meningitis. The initial events of infection have been studied using human nasopharyngeal organ cultures. The meningococci attach selectively to the microvilli of the nonciliated columnar epithelium, entering within a membrane-bound vesicle and passing through these cells to the submucosa. In the process they damage the ciliated cells, possibly by direct action of the meningococcal lipopolysaccharide. The specific attachment mechanisms are not clear, although piliated meningococci adhere more readily than nonpiliated strains. Like the other principal agents of bacterial meningitis, the meningococcus produces a potent human IgA1 protease that is thought to help it survive on the mucosal surface.

High carrier rates in healthy people

Contact may lead to immunity or disease

Attachment to microvilli of nonciliated epithelium

Enter and pass through cell to submucosa

If the meningococci gain access to the bloodstream it is likely that their survival is enhanced by the polysaccharide capsule which resists neutrophil phagocytosis as well as complement-mediated bactericidal activity. At the same time the potent endotoxic activity of the cell wall is responsible for some of the clinical manifestations of meningococcal disease. Endotoxin activates the complement cascade. Patients with deficiencies in the terminal complement components are particularly susceptible to infection with the pathogenic *Neisseria* but usually with a favorable outcome; prognosis is worse in untreated patients with an intact complement system. *Neisseria meningitidis* and gonococci have been shown to readily release endotoxin-containing blebs from the cell surface (Fig 19–1).

Polysaccharide capsule aids survival

Potent endotoxin produces disease manifestations

Complement activity linked to clinical outcome

The exact mechanism of central nervous system (CNS) invasion by the meningococcus is unclear, but it is probably related to the age of the host and the level of the bacteremia. Most experimental data suggest that the choroid plexus with its exceptionally high rate of blood flow is the site of bacterial entry into the CNS. After CNS invasion, an intense subarachnoid space inflammatory response is generated, induced by the release of cell wall peptidoglycan, LPS, and possibly other virulence factors causing the release of inflammatory cytokines (interleukin-1 [IL-1] and tumor necrosis factor [TNF]). Experimental studies and several clinical trials suggest that the administration of anti-inflammatory agents may reduce the pathophysiologic consequences of bacterial meningitis. Hence, the host response as much as the products of the invading microbe may be responsible for the injury caused by meningococcal disease. We still know relatively little about the virulence determinants

CNS invasion mechanism unclear

Injury related to inflammatory response

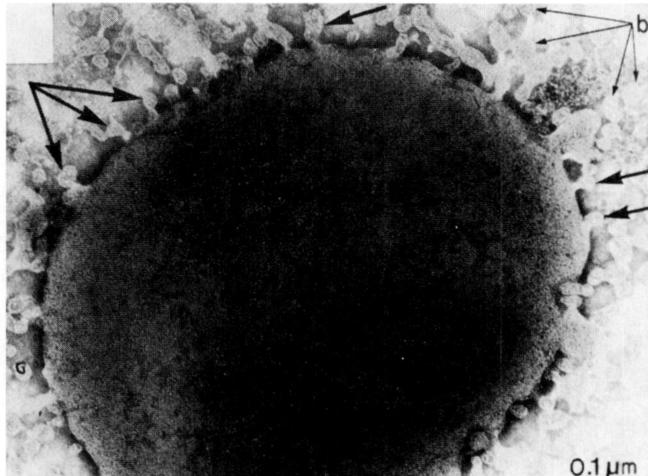


**Figure 19–1.** *Neisseria meningitidis.* Cell wall is shown shedding multiple "blebs" (*arrows*) containing lipopolysaccharide–endotoxin. Note the typical trilamellar Gram-negative cell wall structure in the wall and the blebs. (*Reprinted with permission from Devoe IW, Gilcrist JE.* J Exp Med. *1973;138:1160, Figure 3.*)

of meningococci and their regulation, but given the close genetic relationship between the gonococcus and meningococcus it is likely they share common strategies for survival within the human host.

### Immunity

Group-specific anticapsular antibody is protective

Most common age of infection is 6–24 months

Immunity to meningococcal infections is related to circulating group-specific opsonizing and bactericidal antibody; antibody against endemic serogroups is present in many but not all adults. The peak incidence of serious infection is between 6 months and 2 years of age, which corresponds to the time between loss of transplacental antibody and the appearance of naturally acquired antibody (Fig 19–2). Infections later in life appear when populations carrying virulent strains mix with susceptible individuals lacking specific antibody. Examples include outbreaks of meningococcal disease among children and young adults in schools and in military recruit camps. In these outbreaks, *N. meningitidis* spreads among the newly exposed readily, but disease develops only among those lacking group-specific antibody.

Outbreaks related to mixing susceptible populations

Protective antibody apparently acquired through carrier state

Protective antibody is usually acquired through subclinical or overt infection and through the carrier state, which produces immunity within a few weeks; however, natural immunization may not require infection or colonization with every serogroup or even with *N. meningitidis*, because antibody may be produced in response to cross-reacting antigens from other *Neisseria* groups or species and even other genera. For example, the surface polysaccharide of *Escherichia coli* K1 strains is chemically and immunologically identical to the group B meningococcal polysaccharide.

## Meningococcal Disease: Clinical Aspects

### Clinical Manifestations

Meningitis most frequent infection

The most frequent form of meningococcal infection is acute purulent meningitis, with clinical and laboratory features similar to those of meningitis from other causes (see Chapter

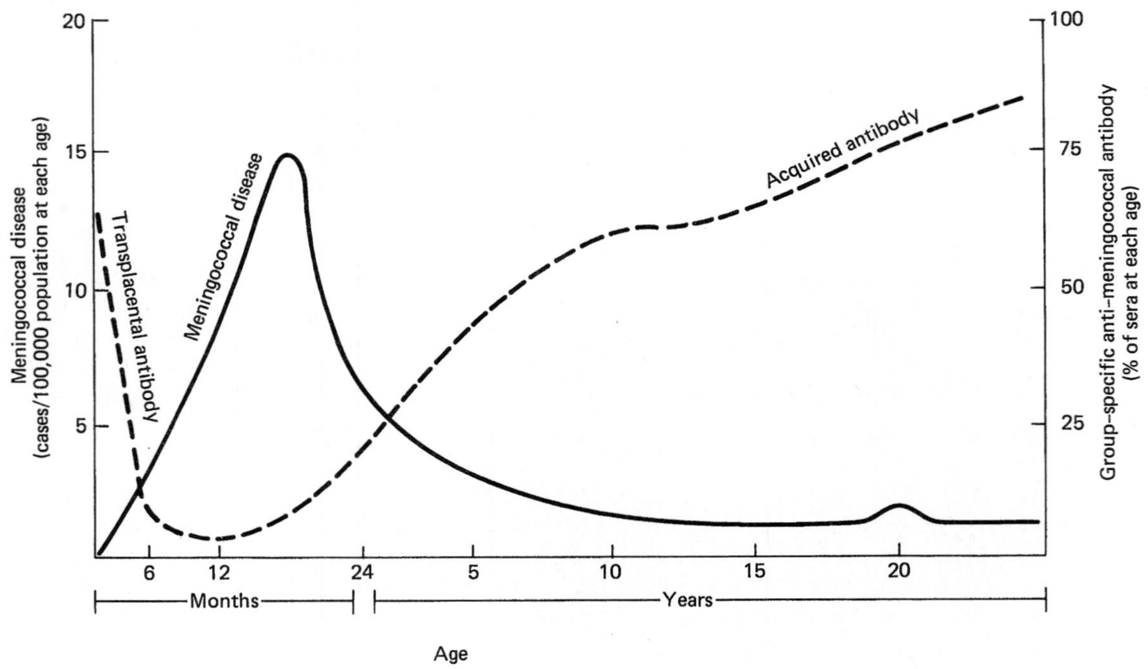


**Figure 19–2.** Immunity to the meningococcus. The inverse relationship between bactericidal meningococcal antibody and meningococcal disease is demonstrated. The "blip" in the disease curve around age 20 is attributable in part to military and other closed-population outbreaks. (*Adapted with permission from Goldschneider I, Gotschlich EC, Liu TY, Artenstein MS. Human immunity to the meningococcus I-V.* J Exp Med. *1969;129:1307–1395.*)

67). A distinguishing feature of meningococcal meningitis is the appearance of scattered skin petechiae, which may evolve into ecchymoses or a diffuse petechial rash. These features are manifestations of meningococcal bacteremia (meningococcemia) and thrombocytopenia which develops with evolution of the disseminated intravascular coagulation (DIC) syndrome. Many of these features are similar to those of experimental endotoxic shock. Meningococcemia sometimes occurs without meningitis, and may progress to fulminant DIC and shock with bilateral hemorrhagic destruction of the adrenal glands (Waterhouse–Friderichsen syndrome). It is not always fulminant, however, and some patients have only low-grade fever, arthritis, and skin lesions that develop slowly over a period of days to weeks. The finding of *N. meningitidis* in the blood or even the cerebrospinal fluid (CSF) of patients with chronic meningococcemia is often unexpected from the clinical severity of the illness. Meningococci may also cause pneumonia, but this disease is uncommon and is not associated with the more common manifestations of meningococcal infection.

Meningococcemia and rash may progress to DIC

Systemic features resemble endotoxic shock

Chronic meningococcal bacteremia may be mild

## Diagnosis

Direct Gram smears of CSF in meningitis usually demonstrate the typical bean-shaped, Gram-negative diplococci. Definitive diagnosis is by culture of CSF, blood, or skin lesions. Although reputed to be somewhat fragile, the organism requires no special handling for isolation from presumptively sterile sites such as blood and CSF; *N. gonorrhoeae*, in contrast, is more fragile and fastidious. Growth is good on blood or chocolate agar after 18 hours of incubation. If sufficient growth is present, confirmation and serogrouping may be done directly from the primary plates by slide agglutination methods. Speciation is based on carbohydrate degradation patterns (see Table 19–1).

Direct CSF Gram smears diagnostic

Culture requires only blood agar

For rapid diagnosis and in cases in which cultures are negative because of previous antimicrobical therapy, meningococcal polysaccharide antigen may be detected in CSF, blood, and urine by latex agglutination procedures (see Chapter 14). False-negative results are common, however, particularly in serogroup B infections.

Antigen detection in blood, CSF, and urine by latex agglutination

## Treatment

Penicillin is the treatment of choice for meningococcal infections because of its antimeningococcal activity and because it can penetrate inflamed meninges. Resistance mediated by both β-lactamase and altered penicillin-binding proteins has been reported but is rare. Newer cephalosporins such as cefotaxime are effective alternatives to penicillin, as is chloramphenicol.

Penicillin is primary treatment

## Prevention

Until the development and spread of sulfonamide resistance in the 1960s chemoprophylaxis with these agents was the primary means of preventing spread of meningococcal infections. Sulfonamides are now little used because of the time required to document susceptibility. Rifampin is the primary chemoprophylactic agent but ciprofloxacin has also been highly effective. Penicillin is not effective as a prophylactic agent, probably because of inadequate penetration to the surface of the uninflamed nasopharyngeal mucosa. Selection of cases to receive prophylaxis is based on epidemiologic assessment of risk. Typically, family members are given prophylaxis but hospital employees are not, unless unusually close contact such as mouth-to-mouth resuscitation has occurred. Culture findings play no role in these decisions, because they do not accurately predict the risk of disease.

Rifampin primary antimicrobic for chemoprophylaxis

Close contact with case is indication for prophylaxis

Purified polysaccharide meningococcal vaccines have been shown to prevent group A and C disease in military and civilian populations, and a quadrivalent vaccine containing A, C, Y, and W-135 polysaccharides is now licensed for use in the United States. These vaccines comprise T-independent polysaccharide antigens that stimulate immunity, which may not last more than a few years in adults, and elicit a poor antibody response in the first year of life. Meningococcal vaccines are currently used in populations at particular risk, such as in military recruit camps and in the control of epidemics. Routine immunization of children is not recommended unless there are predisposing factors such as deficiencies of the terminal complement components or asplenia. Polysaccharide–protein conjugate vaccines, such as those developed for *Haemophilus influenzae*, are under investigation. The lack of an effective serogroup B vaccine remains a problem.

Meningococcal vaccines prepared from purified polysaccharides

Vaccines useful in high risk populations

Protein conjugate vaccines may expand usefulness to children

# NEISSERIA GONORRHOEAE

## Bacteriologic Features

### Growth

Gonococci grow only on chocolate agar or special medium

*Neisseria gonorrhoeae* grows well only on chocolate agar and on specialized medium enriched to ensure its growth. It requires carbon dioxide supplementation. Small colonies appear after 18 to 24 hours of incubation and are well developed (2 to 4 mm) after 48 hours. The colonies are smooth and nonpigmented. The ability to grow on defined medium lacking specific nutrients has been used to develop an auxotyping scheme for gonococci. More than 30 types, some of which have been associated with particular clinical or epidemiologic features, can be separated with these procedures.

Different auxotypes useful for epidemiology

### Structure

In addition to the typical Gram-negative cell wall structure, gonococci possess numerous pili that extend through and beyond the peptidoglycan and outer membrane (Fig 19–3). More than thirty years ago it was demonstrated that only gonococci expressing pili (or a cofactor expressed with pili) were able to establish infection in male volunteers. The pili are polymers of repeating protein subunits that are antigenically diverse between strains. They belong to the family of *N*-methylphenylalanine-type pili similar to those seen for *Pseudomonas aeruginosa*, *Moraxella*, and *Vibrio cholerae*. In general, only fresh virulent isolates have pili.

Pili of N-methylphenylalanine type

The gonococcal outer membrane is composed of phospholipids, lipopolysaccharide, and several distinct outer membrane proteins (OMPs). Of the outer membrane protein classes, the principal structural protein of the outer membrane (OMP I) and the opacity or Opa proteins have the most importance in vivo. OMP I is also the major antigen used in serotyping gonococci. Opa proteins are actually members of a set of as many as 11 closely related outer membrane proteins, most of which confer an opaque appearance to colonies as a result of increased adherence between gonococcal cells. Only a few (or none) of the Opa proteins are expressed at any one time. Gonococcal strains have been shown to possess surface polysaccharide and capsules, but the pathogenic significance of these structures is not yet known.

OMP I principle structural outer membrane protein

Multiple Opa proteins also in outer membrane

### Antigenic Variation

*Neisseria gonorrhoeae* is one of several microorganisms under intensive study to determine the occurrence, mechanism, and significance of antigenic variation within the same strain. The structures of major interest in gonococci are the surface pili and Opa proteins as well

Pili, Opa proteins, and LOS undergo antigenic variation

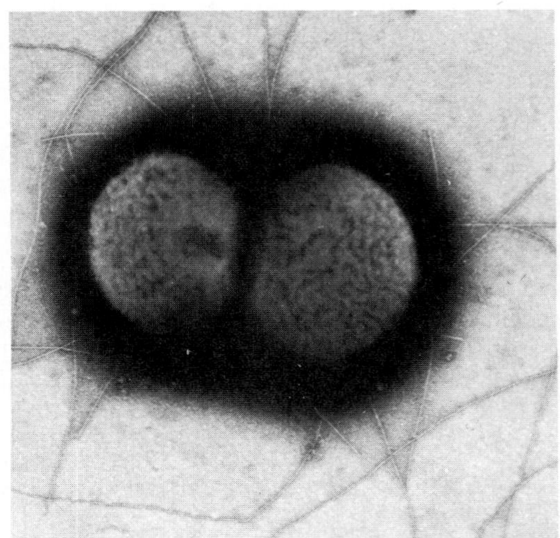

**Figure 19–3.** *Neisseria gonorrhoeae*. Surface pili are shown. These structures are associated with virulence and may mediate initial attachment to epithelial surfaces. (*Courtesy of Dr. John Swanson.*)

Gonococcal pili are variable to an extraordinary extent. The mechanism of this variation appears to be recombinational exchange that occurs within a pilin expression locus, *pilE*, and involves the transfer of variable sequences from a repertoire of incomplete, nonexpressed, or silent loci (*pilS*) to the expression locus. As gonococci naturally take up species-specific DNA by transformation, the variation could be generated by intragenic recombination or through the uptake of exogenous pilin sequences. Whatever the mechanism, there are more than a million possible sequence combinations leading to the production of antigenically variant pili as well as revertible nonpiliated phase variants. PilC is another phase-variable gonococcal protein that plays a role in the assembly of pili and cellular adhesion. The PilC protein that is expressed determines the type of pili assembled and whether or not the bacteria adhere to epithelial cells.

Antigenic variation of pili genetic recombination between silent and expression loci

Transformation could provide mechanism for exogenous DNA

Genes encoding gonococcal Opa proteins exist in multiple copies scattered around the genome. Variation or "switching" between different Opa proteins occurs at a high rate per cell per generation. Control of Opa expression occurs by means of variations in the length of a five-nucleotide DNA repeat, $(CTCTT)^n$, within the signal sequence-encoding region of Opa genes. Variations in numbers of the $(CTCTT)^n$ repeat result in translational frame shifts and, therefore, control of expression at the level of translation.

Opa genes switch by translational frame shift mechanism

Variation in gonococcal LOS has been observed in volunteer subjects challenged with intraurethral *N. gonorrhoeae*. This variation reflects high-frequency variation produced by an unknown mechanism in expression of certain core sugars. In addition, the LOS can be sialylated using cytidine monophosphate–*N*-acetylneuraminic acid (CMP–NANA) as substrate. This sialyation confers serum resistance on the bacteria, but it has also been noted that highly sialylated gonococci are no longer invasive for epithelial cells; however, spontaneous LOS variants binding decreased amounts of sialic acid can still invade cells even in the presence of CMP–NANA. This complex, high-frequency, multifactorial, antigenic variation of the gonococci seems to serve the dual purposes of escape from immune surveillance and provision of specific ligands for different cell receptors.

LOS varies by unknown mechanism

Surface sialyation affects invasiveness

Evasion of immune surveillance is multifactorial

## Gonorrhea

### Epidemiology

Gonorrhea is a major worldwide public health problem. In 1992, the reported cases in the United States exceeded 200 per 100,000 population, and the rates for adolescents are much higher. Each year more than one case of gonorrhea is reported for every 100 females between the ages of 15 and 19 years. No truly effective means of control is yet in sight. The reasons for our inability to control gonorrhea are complex and include changed sexual mores and practices, lack of an effective means to detect asymptomatic cases, decreased susceptibility of *N. gonorrhoeae* to penicillin (see Treatment), and, to some extent, lack of appreciation of the importance of this disease. The latter is evidenced by failure of patients to seek medical care and of physicians to report cases to public health authorities to protect the privacy of their patients. In the minds of many, syphilis is dreaded and "unclean," whereas gonorrhea is only "the clap" ("clap" is from the archaic French clapoir, "a rabbit warren"; later, "a brothel").

Highest rates of gonorrhea among adolescents

No means to detect asymptomatic cases

The major reservoir for continued spread of gonorrhea is the asymptomatic patient. Screening programs and case contact studies have shown that almost 50% of infected women are asymptomatic or at least do not have symptoms usually associated with venereal infection. Most men (95%) have acute symptoms with infection. Many who are not treated become asymptomatic but remain infectious. Asymptomatic male and female patients can remain infectious for months. The attack rates for those engaging in genital intercourse with an infected patient are not known, but are estimated to be 20 to 50%. The organism may also be transmitted by oral–genital contact or by rectal intercourse. When all of these factors operate in a sexually active population, it is easy to explain the high prevalence of gonorrhea. Although gonococci can survive for brief periods on the proverbial toilet seat, nonsexual transmission is extremely rare. Fomite transmission of a purulent vulvovaginitis in prepubescent girls has been reported, but currently most gonococci isolated from children can be traced to sexual abuse by an infected adult.

Asymptomatic infections occur in 50% of women and 5% of men

Transmission is by sexual activity

Nonsexual tranmission rare

## Pathogenesis and Immunity

Pili and Opa mediate attachment at various sites

Gonococci are not normal inhabitants of the respiratory or genital flora. When introduced onto a mucosal surface by sexual contact with an infected individual, adherence ligands such as pili and one or more Opa proteins allow initial attachment of the bacteria to epithelial cells. Pili are the primary mediators of adherence to urethral and vaginal epithelium, nonciliated fallopian tube cells, sperm, and neutrophils. Opa is involved in cervical and urethral epithelial cell adherence and in adhesion between gonococcal cells, contributing to the formation of large clusters of gonococci. These "sticky" clusters could be the primary infectious unit for transmission of gonorrhea. Variation in both Pil and Opa have been demonstrated in human infection presumably using the mechanisms described earlier for antigenic variation. There is considerable evidence that other variations, largely phenotypic, occur in response to environmental changes in the urethra, endocervix, fallopian tube, and nasopharynx of the host. For example, there is increased synthesis of iron-repressed gonococcal OMPs, some of which are necessary for binding the human iron transport proteins transferrin and lactoferrin. Gonococci also seem to adapt to anaerobic microenvironments both in vitro and in vivo.

Antigenic variation occurs during human infection

Environmental factors can regulate virulence factors

OMP I facilitates invasion

Gonococcal invasion of epithelial cells has been demonstrated in vitro but it is not clear if this represents a normal part of uncomplicated mucosal infection. Certain OMPs facilitate invasion, including OMP I and some other Opa proteins. There is evidence to suggest that in deeper, more complicated infections, such as salpingitis and disseminated gonococcal infection (DGI), cellular invasion is an important factor in the pathogenesis of disease. The most critical interactions between gonococci and the human host occur at the mucosal surface through attachment and subsequent multiplication. To accomplish this the organism must resist innate host defenses as well as defenses that may have been acquired from previous infection. Gonococci have multiple mechanisms that protect them against serum complement and antibody including LOS sialylation, which may limit or alter complement binding. Another mechanism for phenotypic serum resistance is the binding of "blocking" antibodies to an outer membrane protein (Rmp) that interferes with the binding of antibodies against OMP I. Blocking antibodies have been found in patients with repeated gonococcal infection. Gonococci also produce large amounts of human-specific IgA1 protease that may inactivate the high concentrations of IgA found at the mucosal surface.

Surface sialylation and blocking antibodies may block immune responses

A hallmark of gonococcal infection is the presence of a painful purulent exudate. The brisk granulocyte response seen in gonorrhoea is likely responsible for the most of the mucosal damage and scarring seen in this disease. Gonococci associate intimately with phagocytes and urethral exudates contain intracellular as well as extracellular gonococci. Some mechanisms have been demonstrated that may enhance the ability of gonococci to survive exposure to neutrophils, even in the absence of specific antibody. For example, some Opa$^+$ gonococci adhere to granulocytes and thus bypass phagocytosis and killing. Gonococci express surface factors such as pili which are antiphagocytic, and the organisms are also able to defend against oxidative killing inside the phagocyte by upregulation of catalase production. The binding of neutrophil-secreted lactoferrin to receptors on the gonococcal surface enables the organism to scavenge iron needed for growth. Although all mechanisms explaining gonococcal survival during neutrophil attack are still speculative, the evidence indicates that killing by neutrophils is sufficiently retarded to allow prolonged survival of gonococci in mucosal and submucosal locations.

Gonococci may escape phagocytic killing

As indicated earlier not all gonococcal infection is symptomatic. The gonococci that remain in the cervix and the urethra for long periods without producing symptomatic disease often have unique nutritional requirements and a limited capacity to activate the complement cascade or attract neutrophils.

Pili aid spread to fallopian tubes

Gonococci invade through cells

LOS and peptidoglycan fragments cause injury

Infection may spread to deeper structures by progressive extension to adjacent mucosal and glandular epithelial cells. These include the prostate and epididymis in men and, in women, the paracervical glands and the fallopian tubes. Spread to the fallopian tubes may be facilitated by pilus-mediated attachment to sperm and then to the microvilli of nonciliated fallopian tube cells. The gonococci are then able to enter and pass through these cells in a manner similar to *N. meningitidis* in nasopharyngeal epithelium. Injury to the fallopian epithelium seems to be mediated by lipopolysaccharide and peptidoglycan fragments. Gonococci are known to turn over their peptidoglycan rapidly during exponential growth, releasing peptidoglycan fragments into the local environment. Injury by this mechanism has been demonstrated in fallopian tube organ cultures and presumably may also operate at other sites.

Further extension can lead to seeding of the pelvic cavity or, in a small proportion of cases, the DGI syndrome with bacteremia and hematogenous spread. The strains involved in cases of DGI differ from other gonococci in possessing a greater resistance to the bactericidal effects of normal human serum and commonly belong to a limited number of clonal types of gonococci. Both DGI and salpingitis tend to begin during or shortly after completion of menses. This may relate to changes in the cervical mucus and reflux into the fallopian tubes during menses.

DGI strains differ

Spread linked to menses

The apparent lack of immunity to gonococcal infection has long been a mystery. Among sexually active persons with multiple partners, repeated infections are the rule rather than the exception. Gonococcal antigenic variation now seems certain to be the prime mechanism by which the gonococcus avoids immune surveillance. Antigenic variation of pili, Opa, and LOS is particularly likely to be important. Outbreaks have been traced to a single strain that demonstrated multiple pilin variations and Opa types in repeated isolates from the same person or from sexual partners. In experimental models, passive administration of antibody directed against one pilin type has been followed by emergence of new pilin variants. Changes in Opa may also occur as suggested by differences in its expression in mucosal versus tubal isolates. The emerging pattern is that immunity to gonococcal infection is present, but its effectiveness is compromised by the ability of the organism to change key structures during the course of infection.

Gonococcus varies multiple structures to avoid immune surveillance

## Gonorrhea: Clinical Aspects

### Clinical Manifestations

#### Genital Gonorrhea

In men, the primary site of infection is the urethra. Symptoms begin 2 to 7 days after infection and consist primarily of purulent urethral discharge and dysuria. Although uncommon, local extension can lead to epididymitis or prostatitis. The endocervix is the primary site in women, in whom symptoms include increased vaginal discharge, urinary frequency, dysuria, abdominal pain, and menstrual abnormalities. As mentioned previously, symptoms may be mild or absent in either sex, particularly women.

Urethritis and endocervicitis primary infections

#### Other Local Infections

Rectal gonorrhea occurs after rectal intercourse or, in women, after contamination with infected vaginal secretions. It is generally asymptomatic but may cause tenesmus, discharge, and rectal bleeding. Pharyngeal gonorrhea is transmitted by orogenital sex and, again, is usually asymptomatic. Sore throat and cervical adenitis may occur. Infection of other structures near primary infection sites, such as Bartholin's glands in women, may lead to abscess formation.

Rectal and pharyngeal infection related to sexual practices

Inoculation of gonococci into the conjunctiva produces a severe, acute, purulent conjunctivitis. Although this infection may occur at any age, the most serious form is gonococcal ophthalmia neonatorum, acquired by a newborn from an infected mother. The disease was formerly a common cause of blindness, and for this reason eye prophylaxis is used at birth. Gonococcal ophthalmia neonatorum had all but disappeared in the United States in the 1950s, but with the increase in gonococcal infections and antimicrobic resistance, it is now being encountered again.

Conjunctivitis and ophthalmia neonatorum transmitted at birth

#### Pelvic Inflammatory Disease

The clinical syndrome of pelvic inflammatory disease (PID) includes fever, lower abdominal pain, adnexal tenderness, and leukocytosis with or without signs of local infection. These features are caused by spread of organisms along the fallopian tubes to produce salpingitis and into the pelvic cavity to produce pelvic peritonitis and abscesses. PID is now known to develop when other genital pathogens ascend by the same route. These organisms include anaerobes and *Chlamydia trachomatis*, which may appear alone or mixed with gonococci. The most serious complications of PID are infertility and ectopic pregnancy secondary to scarring of the fallopian tubes.

Salpingitis and pelvic peritonitis cause scaring and infertility

DISSEMINATED GONOCOCCAL INFECTION (DGI)

Skin rash, arthralgia, and arthritis associated with bacteremia

Purulent arthritis involves large joints

Any of the local forms of gonorrhea or their extensions such as PID may lead to bacteremia. In the bacteremic phase the primary features are fever, migratory polyarthralgia, and a petechial, maculopapular, or pustular rash. These features may be immunologically mediated, as gonococci are infrequently isolated from the skin or joints at this stage despite their presence in the blood. The bacteremia may lead to metastatic infections such as endocarditis and meningitis, but the most common is purulent arthritis. The arthritis typically follows the bacteremia and involves large joints such as elbows and knees. Gonococci are readily cultured from the pus.

## Diagnosis

GRAM SMEAR

Direct smear requires experience

Social and legal implications must be considered

The presence of multiple pairs of bean-shaped, Gram-negative diplococci within a neutrophil is highly characteristic of gonorrhea when the smear is from a genital site (Fig 19–4). The direct Gram smear is more than 95% sensitive and specific in symptomatic men. Unfortunately, it is only 50 to 70% sensitive in women and its specificity is complicated by the presence of other bacteria in the female genital flora that may have a similar morphology. Experience is required in reading smears and they cannot be relied on for diagnosis of cases in which the findings are unexpected or may have social (divorce) or legal (rape, child abuse) implications.

CULTURE

Urethra and cervix are preferred culture sites

Attention to detail is necessary for isolation of the gonococcus, as it is a fragile organism often mixed with hardier members of the normal flora. Success requires proper selection of culture sites, protection of specimens from environmental exposure, culture on appropriate media, and definitive laboratory identification. In men the best specimen is urethral exudate or urethral scrapings (obtained with a loop or special swab). In women cervical swabs are preferred over urethral or vaginal specimens. The highest diagnostic yield in women is with the combination of a cervical and an anal canal culture, because some patients with rectal gonorrhea have negative cervical cultures. Throat or rectal cultures in men are needed only if indicated by the patient's sexual practices.

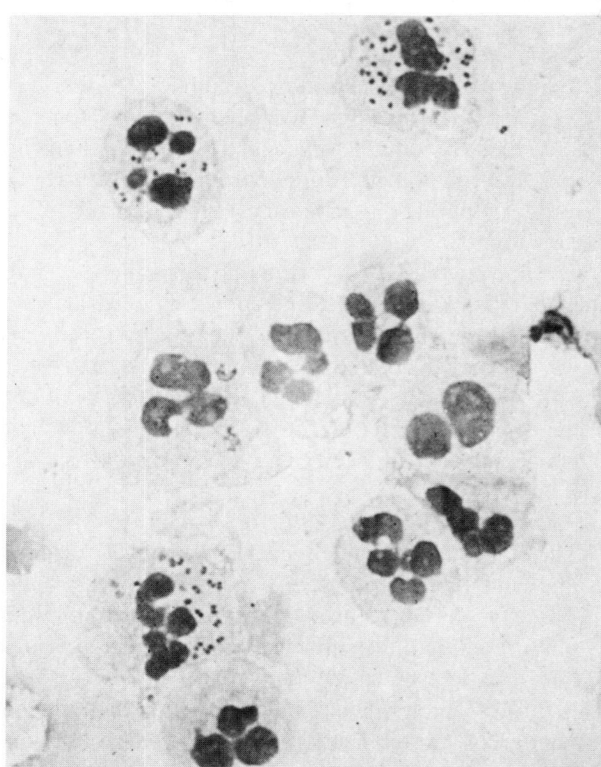

**Figure 19–4.** Gram smear of urethral exudate of an acute case of gonorrhea in a male. Note typical intracellular diplococci in polymorphonuclear leukocytes. The gonococci are Gram negative.

Swabs may be streaked directly onto culture medium or transmitted to the laboratory in a suitable transport medium if the delay is not more than 4 hours. Laboratory requests must specify the suspicion of gonorrhea, so that selective media that satisfy the nutritional requirements of the gonococcus and inhibit competing normal flora can be seeded. The most common is Martin–Lewis agar, an enriched selective chocolate agar. The exact formulation has changed over the years, but includes antimicrobics active against Gram-positive bacteria (vancomycin), Gram-negative bacteria (colistin, trimethoprim), and fungi (nystatin, anisomycin) at concentrations that do not inhibit *N. gonorrhoeae*.

Transport media required unless plating is immediate

Selective medium inhibits competing flora

Colonies appear after 1 to 2 days of incubation in carbon dioxide at 35°C. They may be identified as *Neisseria* by demonstration of typical Gram stain morphology and a positive oxidase test. Classically, speciation is by carbohydrate degradation pattern (see Table 19–1), but this approach is being replaced by immunologic procedures (immunofluorescence, coagglutination, enzyme immunoassay) some of which use monoclonal antibodies to OMP I. A DNA probe test is also available. *Neisseria* other than *N. gonorrhoeae* are unusual in genital specimens, but speciation is the only way to be certain of the diagnosis.

Identification of *Neisseria* isolates by fermentation, immunoassay or DNA probe

#### Direct Detection

Much effort has been directed at developing methods that detect gonococci in clinical specimens without culture. Such methods could have particular importance for screening populations where culture is impractical. Enzyme immunoassay (EIA) and DNA–rRNA hybridization methods show promise in this regard. Another method based on the ability of gonococcal DNA in a dried specimen to transform a reference strain has shown good sensitivity compared with culture.

Direct detection under development

#### Serology

Attempts to develop a serologic test for gonorrhea have not yet achieved the needed sensitivity and specificity. A test that would detect the disease in asymptomatic patients would be very useful in control of this disease.

No serologic test

### Treatment

Penicillin is no longer the antimicrobic of choice for the primary treatment of gonorrhea because of the development of resistance involving multiple mechanisms. The first resistance to be recognized was a decreased susceptibility based on penicillin-binding protein (PBP) changes which in retrospect began as far back as the 1950s. These strains initially had only modestly decreased susceptibility which could be overcome with increased penicillin dosage. In recent years strains with minimum inhibitory concentrations (MICs) greater than 1.0 μg/mL have become more frequent and are associated with treatment failures. In the late 1970s, penicillinase-producing *N. gonorrhoeae* (PPNG) appeared in the Far East and by the mid-1980s were endemic in the United States. These strains produce a plasmid encoded TEM-type β-lactamase identical to that of members of the Enterobacteriaceae and have MICs that far exceed achievable therapeutic levels. This situation has caused a shift to third-generation cephalosporins such as ceftriaxone because of their high activity and resistance to β-lactamases. Other agents proven effective against the gonococcus include erythromycin, tetracycline, and spectinomycin, but resistance is also limiting their usefulness. Newer quinolones are promising and can be taken orally.

Increasing mutational resistance due to PBP changes

Plasmid-coded penicillinase production limits use

Ceftriaxone now first-line therapy

### Prevention

Methods to block direct mucosal contact (condoms) or inhibit the gonococcus (vaginal foams, douches) have not been studied extensively, but it is likely that they provide protection against gonorrhea if used regularly. The classic public health methods of case–contact tracing and treatment have become more difficult with the increasing size of the primary reservoir. The availability of a good serologic test would greatly aid control, as it has for syphilis. The development of a gonococcal vaccine awaits further understanding of the immunology and epidemiology of gonorrhea. Vaccines using pili or OMP I failed to confer clinically useful immunity to gonococcal infection. Even though the gonococci are masters of disguise, the development of a vaccine coupled with educational strategies leading to a reduction in risky sexual practices could reduce the appalling morbidity associated with this infectious disease.

Condoms should block transmission

Vaccine strategies require more understanding of gonococcal disguise

## OTHER NEISSERIA SPECIES

Other *Neisseria* are oral and upper respiratory tract commensals

Many other *Neisseria* species exist primarily as normal inhabitants of the oral cavity and upper respiratory tract. Some are rare causes of mild to serious infections, including meningitis. With the exception of *Neisseria lactamica*, these other *Neisseria* generally fail to grow on Martin–Lewis agar (see Table 19–1). They are distinguished from *N. gonorrhoeae* and *N. meningitidis* by biochemical and serologic tests. They can grow at 22 to 25°C and frequently produce dry, wrinkled, or pigmented colonies, which are readily distinguished from those of pathogenic species.

## ADDITIONAL READING

Cohen MS, Sparling PF. Mucosal infection with *Neisseria gonorrhoeae*: Bacterial adaptation and mucosal defenses. *J Clin Invest*. 1992;89:1699–1705. An excellent perspective on gonococcal pathogenesis.

Goldschneider I, Gotschlich EC, Liu TY, Artenstein MS. Human immunity to the meningococcus I-V. *J Exp Med* 1969;129:1307–1395. This series of five papers defines the basis of immunity to *Neisseria meningitidis* and the development of vaccines from the polysaccharide capsule.

McGee ZA, Stephens DS, Hoffman LH. Mechanisms of mucosal invasion by pathogenic *Neisseria*. *Rev Infect Dis* 1983;5:S708–S714. An electron microscope study demonstrating the attachment and invasive properties of gonococci and meningococci using human organ cultures.

Roberts M, Elwell LP, Falkow S. Molecular characterization of two beta-lactamase-specifying plasmids isolated from *Neisseria gonorrhoeae*. *J Bacteriol*. 1977;131:557–562. This molecular study shows the mechanism of penicillinase production by gonococci and the relation of these plasmids to others, such as those found in *Haemophilus influenzae*.

Robertson BD, Meyer TF. Genetic variation in pathogenic bacteria. *Trends Genet*. 1992;8:422–427. A contemporary review of the mechanisms that bring about genetic variation in pathogens and its consequences for the host and the microbe with special emphasis on the gonococcus.

Seifert HS, So M. Genetic mechanisms of antigenic variation. *Microbiol Rev* 1988;52:327–366. The genetics of antigenic variation are nicely explained and the evidence for the importance of these changes in clinical gonorrhea is discussed.

Swanson J, Belland RJ, Hill SA. Neisserial surface variation: How and why? *Curr Opin Genet Dev*. 1992; 2:805–811. A very good overview of the striking variability of the gonococcal pili, Opa, and LOS determinants in vitro and in vivo.

Tunkel AR, Scheld WM. Pathogenesis and pathophysiology of bacterial meningitis. *Annu Rev Med*. 1993; 44:103–120. A very readable overview of bacterial meningitis with comparative descriptions of streptococcal, *Haemophilus*, *Escherichia coli*, and meningococcal meningitis.

Chapter 20

# Enterobacteriaceae

*Kenneth J. Ryan and Stanley Falkow*

The Enterobacteriaceae are a large and diverse family of Gram-negative rods, members of which are found free living in nature and as part of the indigenous flora of humans and animals. They grow rapidly under aerobic and anaerobic conditions and are metabolically active, attacking a variety of substrates. Many species are motile, but none forms spores or demonstrates acid fastness. Enterobacteriaceae are the most common cause of urinary tract infection and some of the species are important etiologic agents of diarrhea throughout the world. Spread of Enterobacteriaceae to the bloodstream leads to Gram-negative sepsis, a dreaded complication of hospitalized patients.

## ENTEROBACTERIACEAE: GENERAL FEATURES

### Morphology

The Enterobacteriaceae are among the larger bacteria that colonize humans. They are usually 2 to 4 μm in length and 0.4 to 0.6 μm in width, with parallel sides and rounded ends; the length is variable, however, producing forms that range from large coccobacilli to an elongated, filamentous appearance. Motile strains have peritrichous flagella, which extend 1 to 5 μm beyond the cell wall. Many also have surface pili. Some species (for example, *Klebsiella*) are typically encapsulated. Most have extracellular surface slime layers, which are often poorly circumscribed. The cell wall, cell membrane, and internal structure, which are morphologically similar for all Enterobacteriaceae, are as described in Chapter 2 for Gram-negative bacteria.

Large Gram-negative rods

May be motile or encapsulated

### Growth

Enterobacteriaceae grow readily on simple media, often with only a single carbon energy source. Growth is rapid under both aerobic and anaerobic conditions, producing 2- to 5-mm colonies on agar media and diffuse turbidity in broth after 12 to 18 hours of incubation. Their simple growth requirements and relative resistance to many substances, such as bile salts and some bacteriostatic dyes, are exploited in selective media and in identification methods. Conversely, their ability to grow under almost all cultural conditions may interfere with the isolation of more fastidious bacteria.

Rapid growth on simple media under aerobic or anaerobic conditions

## Antigenic Structure

Cell wall LPS=O antigen

Multiple serotypes based on O antigen side chains

Surface polysaccharide=K antigen

Flagella=H antigen

The cell wall, capsular slime layer, and flagellar antigens are valuable in identification and in subtyping for epidemiologic purposes. The cell wall lipopolysaccharide (LPS) is called the **O antigen.** The antigenic specificity of the O antigen is determined by the composition and linkage of the sugars that form the polysaccharide side chains. The remaining portion of the LPS is a conserved core polysaccharide backbone linked to **lipid A** (see Chapter 2 for details). Passive immunization using antisera directed against the LPS core antigen from one strain of *Escherichia coli* has been explored in an effort to achieve broad-spectrum protection against Gram-negative endotoxemia. This approach shows promise but is not yet proven to be efficacious. Cell-surface antigens are generally polysaccharides and are termed **K antigens** (from the Danish Kapsel, capsule) regardless of whether or not they form a well-defined capsule. Flagellar proteins are called **H antigens.** The pilin proteins are antigenic but not yet part of any formal typing scheme.

## Habitat

Found in intestine and environment

May increase in respiratory tract of debilitated

Most Enterobacteriaceae are primarily inhabitants of the lower gastrointestinal tract of humans and animals. Many survive readily in nature, and many are found living free where water and minimal energy sources are available. In humans they are the main facultative portion of the bacterial content of the colon. They are also found in the female genital tract and as transient colonizers of the skin. Enterobacteriaceae are scant in the respiratory tract of healthy persons; however, their numbers may increase in hospitalized patients with chronic debilitating diseases. *E. coli* is the most common species of Enterobacteriaceae found among the indigenous flora, followed by *Klebsiella, Proteus,* and *Enterobacter* species. *Salmonella, Shigella,* and *Yersinia* species are intestinal pathogens and not considered part of the normal flora.

## Classification

Genera classified by differences in cultural and biochemical characteristics

Species identified by battery of biochemical tests

Lactose fermentation useful for screening

Subspecies classified by antigenic structure

The Enterobacteriaceae are classified to the species level on the basis of their many cultural and biochemical characteristics together with DNA homology data. All are facultative, all ferment glucose and reduce nitrates to nitrites, and are oxidase negative. In clinical laboratories, genus and species designations are based primarily on batteries of physiologic characteristics, including most of those discussed in Chapter 14. They include the ability to ferment various carbohydrates, indole production from tryptophan, citrate utilization, amino acid breakdown, and hydrogen sulfide production from sulfur-containing amino acids. These and many other characteristics are used to construct probability tables for assignment of individual isolates to genera and species. The currently recognized genera and species of significant medical importance and their major characteristics are shown in Appendix 20–1.

Rapid fermentation of lactose, as demonstrated by acid (pink) colonies on MacConkey agar, is a useful characteristic for initial screening of Enterobacteriaceae. The most common members of the intestinal flora, *E. coli*, *Klebsiella*, and *Enterobacter*, ferment lactose promptly in more than 90% of cases, whereas many other genera, including the intestinal pathogens *Salmonella, Shigella,* and *Yersinia,* are rarely positive.

Within species, differences in O, H, and K antigens are used for further subdivision into serotypes. For some species, panels of bacteriocins or bacteriophages have been used to establish typing systems in place of, or in addition to, serotyping systems.

## Toxins

Endotoxin present in all species

All Enterobacteriaceae possess the LPS endotoxin, the structure and functional effects of which are discussed in Chapters 2, 10, and 68. Many of the effects of endotoxin such as fever, leukopenia, and activation of blood coagulation factors are seen in human infections, particularly when organisms enter the bloodstream to produce bacteremia. In addition to

LPS endotoxin, some Enterobacteriaceae also produce exotoxins, including enterotoxins and cytotoxins. These toxins will be discussed with the individual species, although it is now clear the same toxin may be found in more than one species. The genes for many are coded on plasmids that may be exchanged among the various genera. These toxins are discussed in relation to particular species below and summarized in Appendix 20–2.

Some species produce enterotoxins and cytotoxins

## Diseases Caused by Enterobacteriaceae

The Enterobacteriaceae produce the widest variety of infections of any microbial agents. This family includes species that are the leading causes of two of the most common infectious states, urinary tract infection and acute diarrhea, and virtually any species can cause opportunistic infections. The bacteriologic, pathogenic, immunologic, and clinical features of these infections will be discussed below in relation to the individual genera and species most commonly causing them. Greater detail of the clinical aspects may be found in the syndromic chapters at the end of the book, particularly Chapters 65 (diarrhea), 66 (urinary tract infections), and 68 (septic shock).

Urinary infection and other specific diseases produced

Most act as opportunists

## ESCHERICHIA COLI

### ■ Bacteriology

*Escherichia coli* is the most commonly encountered member of the Enterobacteriaceae in the normal colonic flora and a leading cause of opportunistic infections. Most strains ferment lactose rapidly and produce indole. Biochemical reactions are sufficient to identify the species, although there are many biotypes. Serotyping systems have been established based on O, K, and H antigens. There are over 150 somatic O antigens (for example, 055, 0111, 0144). The *E. coli* K and H antigens are also designated by number. Thus, the antigenic structure of individual strains is described by designations such as 0111:H7 or 018:K76.

Typically rapid lactose fermentor

Serotypes involve O, K, and H antigens

A number of *E. coli* products are found more frequently in strains isolated from human infections than in normal floral or environmental isolates. These include a pore-forming cytolytic protein called alpha-hemolysin, which disrupts plasma membranes leading to cell death; and iron-chelating proteins called siderophores, which enhance survival of *E. coli* in the iron-poor environment of human body fluids. **Aerobactin,** the most efficient of these siderophores, is able to bind iron with high affinity, making it available for the organism's nutritional needs. Capsular polysaccharide is associated with blocking activation of the alternate complement pathway, thus reducing the efficiency of opsonophagocytosis.

α-hemolysin a pore-forming toxin

Siderophores chelate iron from tissue fluids

#### E. coli Pili

Pili (also called fimbriae) are frequently present on the surface of *E. coli* strains and play a role in virulence as mediators of attachment to human epithelial surfaces. The pili present on most *E. coli* are called **type 1,** and bind to the D-mannose residues present on the surface of a wide variety of cells. Other more specialized pili are found in subpopulations of *E. coli*. The most important of these are the **pyelonephritis associated** pili (P or Pap) and the intestinal **colonization factor antigens** (CFA). The P pili bind to digalactoside (Gal–Gal) moieties present on certain mammalian cell and in the P blood group antigen. The specific binding receptor for the CFAs is not known. At least five other pilin and pilin-like adhesins have been identified in *E. coli* strains.

Type 1 pili bind to mannose

P and CFA pili are specialized

The terms mannose sensitive (MS) and mannose resistant (MR) have been used to indicate whether binding of pili to epithelial cells is blocked by the addition of mannose to the system. Although useful for experimental purposes, this only separates type 1 pili (MS) from all the rest. The relationships of *E. coli* pili are summarized in Table 20–1.

The genetics of pilin expression is complex. The genes are organized into multicistronic clusters that encode structural pilin subunits and regulatory functions. Pili of different types may coexist on the same bacterium, and their expression may vary under different environmental conditions. Type 1 pilin expression can be turned on or off by in-

Multiple pilins may be present in same strain

TABLE 20–1. ADHERENCE CHARACTERISTICS OF ESCHERICHIA COLI STRAINS

| Strain | Epithelial Cell Type | Pili | Epithelial Cell Receptor | Genetic Control |
|---|---|---|---|---|
| General (common) | Various | Type 1 | D-Mannose | Chromosomal |
| Uropathic | Bladder, kidney | P (Gal–Gal) | Galactopyranosyl–galactopyranoside (P blood group) | Chromosomal |
| ETEC (human) | Enterocyte (human) | CFA | Unknown | Plasmid |
| ETEC (animal) | Enterocyte (pigs, calves) | K88, K99 | Unknown | Plasmid |

*Abbreviations:* ETEC = enterotoxigenic *E. coli;* CFA = colonizing factor antigens, CFA I, CFA II, others (see text).

Type 1 pilin switch by inversion of promoter

version of a chromosomal DNA sequence containing the promoter responsible for initiating transcription of the pilin gene. Other genes control the on/off orientation of the "switch."

# E. coli Infections

## Urinary Tract Infection

Most common cause of UTI

Trauma allows bladder access

Certain serotypes more common in UTI

*Escherichia coli* accounts for more than 90% of cystitis (bladder) and pyelonephritis (renal pelvis and kidney) infections, known as urinary tract infection (UTI), that develop in otherwise healthy persons. The most common symptoms are dysuria and urinary frequency. In pyelonephritis, fever and flank pain are common and bacteremia may develop. The attack rate is highest in sexually active women. These findings are explained in part by intestinal *E. coli* contaminating the perineal and urethral area. Relatively minor trauma or the mechanical effect of sexual intercourse have been shown to allow bacteria access to the bladder. Factors that violate bladder integrity (urinary catheters) or that obstruct urine outflow (enlarged prostate) are also associated with infection. This cannot be the whole story, however, because fewer than 10 *E. coli* serotypes account for the majority of UTI cases, and these UTI serotypes are much less prevalent in the fecal flora.

P pili strongly associated with pyelonephritis

P pili bind to digalactoside on urinary epithelium

The ability of certain strains of *E. coli* to produce UTI is related to general virulence factors such as alpha hemolysin, together with pili-mediated adherence to uroepithelial cells. The percentage of *E. coli* with P pili increases from 20% in the fecal flora to 70% in pyelonephritis isolates. Asymptomatic bacteriuria and cystitis isolates fall in between. The digalactoside receptor for P pili is present on uroepithelial cells, to which the bacteria bind avidly, particularly in the upper urinary tract. Type 1 pili may be important in periurethral colonization and attachment to bladder epithelium by strains that lack P pili. Antibody against P pili blocks adherence in experimental systems, suggesting that immunization could be an approach to UTI prevention.

## Intestinal Infections

Multiple mechanisms of diarrhea

All must adhere to bowel epithelium

Diarrhea-causing *E. coli* are classified according to their virulence properties as **enterotoxigenic (ETEC), enteropathogenic (EPEC), enteroinvasive (EIEC), enterohemorrhagic (EHEC),** or **enteroaggregative (EAEC).** Remarkably, all of these enteropathogens share the property of plasmid-mediated adherence to the epithelium of the small and/or large bowel as a first step in infection. The replicative features of the plasmids found in these *E. coli* are often related, but the encoded specificity of adherence is quite distinct. Toxins that are often phage or plasmid-mediated with many of these strains play an important role in infection and disease.

EHEC reservoir in cattle

Each group causes disease by a different mechanism, and the resulting syndromes usually differ clinically and epidemiologically. For example, human ETEC and EIEC strains infect only humans. Food and water contaminated with human waste, as well as person-to-person contact, are the principal means of infection. In contrast, the principal reservoir of EHEC is cattle, so that consumption of undercooked contaminated beef or raw milk are more important causes of infection. A summary of the pathogenesis of infection, clinical syndromes, and epidemiology of infection for each enteropathogen is shown in Table 20–2.

ENTEROTOXIGENIC *E. COLI* (ETEC)

ETEC are an important cause of diarrhea in infants and in travelers to less developed countries. The disease in infants is a leading cause of morbidity and mortality during the first 2 years of life in developing countries. It is rarely contracted by infants or others in industrialized nations. Transmission is generally through contaminated food and water. In travelers, the disease, like that seen in children, ranges from minor discomfort to a severe cholera-like illness.

ETEC seen mostly in developing countries and travellers to them

Plasmid-encoded pili are essential virulence factors that have evolved to permit colonization of the small bowel of a specific animal species. Some termed colonization factors (CFA I, CFA II, CFA III, etc) are specific for humans. Others bind preferentially to pig intestine (K88), or to the small bowel of calves and lambs (K99). Because animal ETEC do not normally cause disease in humans, humans acquire the infection only from other humans by the fecal–oral route. The CFA pili permit tight adherence to the microvilli, and this alone can cause mild diarrheal disease. However, classically, ETEC produce one or more plasmid-encoded enterotoxins: a **heat-labile toxin, LT,** highly related to cholera toxin, and/or a low-molecular-weight **heat-stable enterotoxin, ST.**

CFA pili mediate specific binding in small bowel

Adherence allows delivery of toxin

LT is a classic AB bacterial toxin. The active unit ADP-ribosylates a regulatory protein, leading to the activation of adenylate cyclase and a cascade of events resulting in the net secretion of fluid and electrolytes into the bowel lumen. This explains the profuse, watery, noninflammatory diarrhea seen in patients. The mechanism is the same as cholera toxin and is described in more detail in Chapter 21. ST toxins are small (17 to 18 amino acid) peptides that bind to a glycoprotein receptor, resulting in the activation of a membrane-bound guanylate cyclase. The resulting increase in cyclic GMP concentration causes the net secretion of fluid and electrolytes into the bowel lumen, and LT-like watery diarrhea. At least one-half of ETEC elaborate only one type of toxin, but strains that elaborate both LT and ST cause the most severe illness. The genes encoding the ST and LT pili in ETEC may be on separate plasmids or carried on a common plasmid. There are several variant forms of both ST and LT as well as CFAs.

LT action is like cholera toxin

ST similar but acts on guanylate cyclase

Toxin and pilin genes carried on plasmid

**TABLE 20–2. FEATURES OF INTESTINAL INFECTION BY ESCHERICHIA COLI**

| Feature | ETEC | EIEC | EHEC | EPEC | EAEC |
|---|---|---|---|---|---|
| Primary pathogenic mechanism | Enterotoxin LT and/or ST | Invasion of enterocytes | Shigalike cytotoxin | Adherence to enterocytes | Adherence to enterocytes |
| Primary site | Small intestine | Large intestine | Large intestine | Small intestine[a] | ? |
| Mucosal pathology | Intact, hyperemia | Necrosis, ulceration, inflammation | Effacement of microvilli, cell death | Effacement of microvilli | ? |
| Epidemiology | Traveler's diarrhea, childhood diarrhea[b] | Sporadic, uncommon | Hemorrhagic colitis; hemolytic uremic syndrome | Infantile and childhood diarrhea[b] | ? |
| Fever | Absent | Common | Absent | Common | Occasional |
| Stools | | | | | |
| Nature | Copious, watery | Scanty, purulent | Copious, bloody | Copious, watery | Watery |
| Blood | Absent | Common | Prominent | Absent | Absent |
| Pus (WBCs) | Absent | Prominent | Absent | Minimal | Absent |

*Abbreviations:* ETEC = enterotoxigenic *E. coli*; EIEC = enteroinvasive *E. coli*; EHEC = enterohemorrhagic *E. coli*; EPEC = enteropathogenic *E. coli*; EAEC = enteroaggregative *E. coli*; LT = heat-labile toxin; ST = heat-stable toxins; WBCs = white blood cells.

[a] In experimental animals EPEC strains produce lesions in the large intestine as well.

[b] These are much more common in developing countries. ETEC strains are rare in the United States.

LT immunogenic, ST is not

ETEC leading cause of traveler's diarrhea

Although there can be more than one episode of the disease, infections with ETEC can result in immunity presumably mediated by sIgA specific for LT and CFAs. The small ST peptides are nonimmunogenic. Adults living in endemic areas have much lower attack rates than do nonimmune travelers from industrialized nations who visit the area. Consequently, ETEC are the leading cause of traveler's diarrhea, accounting for well over one-half of the cases. Repeated bouts of diarrhea caused by ETEC and other infectious agents are an important cause of growth retardation, malnutrition, and developmental delay in third world countries where ETEC are important causative agents of dehydrating diarrhea. It is instructive to note that the disease is of very low incidence in breast-fed infants, underscoring the protective effect of maternal antibody and the epidemiologic fact that the disease is transmitted by contaminated food and water.

### Enteropathogenic *E. coli* (EPEC)

EPEC originally seen in nursery outbreaks

Significant cause of childhood diarrhea in developing world

EPEC strains were first identified as the cause of outbreaks of diarrhea in hospital nurseries in the United States and Great Britain during the 1950s. The disease has all but disappeared in the industrialized nations except for sporadic cases. It has now been recognized that EPEC account for a significant proportion (about 20%) of diarrhea in bottle-fed infants below 1 year of age in less developed parts of the world, particularly among the urban poor of South America, Africa, and Southeast Asia.

Special pilus mediates tight attachment

Effacement of microvilli leads to cytoskeleton rearrangement

The interaction of EPEC with the host is seen initially as the formation of small clumps or microcolonies tightly adherent to the enterocytes of the small bowel. This event is dependent upon factors encoded by a plasmid present in EPEC strains; it is likely that a plasmid-encoded **bundle-forming pilus (BFP)** is responsible for this attachment. After initial attachment, factors encoded on the bacterial chromosome mediate a more intimate adherence, leading to an increase in calcium ions in host cell protein phosphorylation, and to other pathophysiologic alterations within the epithelial cell. The resulting loss of microvilli (effacement) results from cytoskeletal rearrangement with the formation of dense "pedestals" of filamentous actin under the site of microbial attachment (Fig 20–1). Occasionally, bacteria are seen entering the epithelial cell within membrane-bound vesicles. A 94-kd bacterial protein, **intimin**, necessary for intimate attachment and entry is encoded by a chromosomal gene of EPEC. Homologs of this protein are found in pathogenic *Yersinia*, EHEC (see below), and other enteropathogens.

Effacing lesions cause watery diarrhea

The attaching and effacing (AE) lesions seen in EPEC infection give rise clinically to watery diarrhea sometimes associated with fever. The occasional entry of EPEC into the mucosa may be responsible for the mild inflammatory infiltrate seen in this infection. The diarrheal illness is usually self-limiting, but occasionally EPEC causes chronic diarrhea in infants. It is one of the few bacterial-mediated chronic diarrheal syndromes, and typical AE lesions can be seen in duodenal biopsies. The course of acute EPEC illness can be shortened by antibiotic therapy and treatment is curative in chronic disease.

The reservoir of EPEC is not well defined. EPEC-like organisms are seen in animal

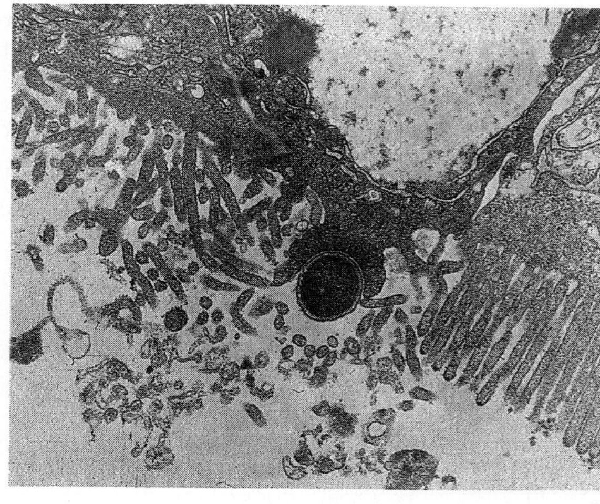

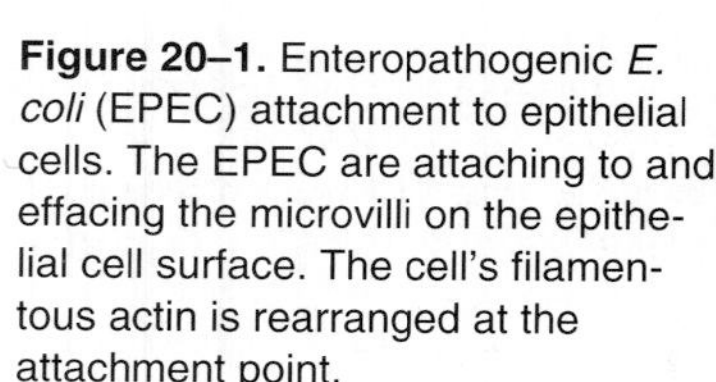

**Figure 20–1.** Enteropathogenic *E. coli* (EPEC) attachment to epithelial cells. The EPEC are attaching to and effacing the microvilli on the epithelial cell surface. The cell's filamentous actin is rearranged at the attachment point.

disease, but it has not been unequivocally determined if these ever cause human disease. In endemic areas, EPEC can be isolated often from the stool of asymptomatic adults, indicating that acquired immunity to infection is widespread and that humans may be the crucial reservoir.

### Enterohemorrhagic *E. coli* (EHEC)

It has been known for decades that certain *E. coli* serotypes produced a powerful cytotoxin similar to the classical Shiga toxin of *Shigella dysenteriae*. This observation took on new dimensions when in 1982 there was a multistate outbreak of hemorrhagic colitis traced to a strain of *E. coli* O157:H7. Subsequently, this syndrome has been seen with increasing frequency, usually involving the same serotype.

Multistate outbreak of hemorrhagic colitis caused by serotype O157:H7

EHEC cause the same AE lesions as EPEC. However, they colonize the cecum and large bowel as well as the distal ileum. Initial adherence requires a plasmid-mediated factor but it is probably different from the BFP seen in classical EPEC infection. EHEC elaborate one or more related Shiga-like toxins of the AB type consisting of five B subunits and a 30-kDA toxic A subunit. The B units bind to a membrane glycolipid. After internalization of the holotoxin by endocytosis into a membrane-bound vesicle, the A subunit crosses the vacuolar membrane in the trans-Golgi network and enzymatically modifies 28S ribosomal RNA of the 60s-ribosomal subunit by removing an adenine base. This prevents elongation-factor-1-dependent binding of amino acyl t-RNA to the ribosome-blocking protein synthesis, leading to cell death.

Effacing lesions similar to EPEC produced

Shiga-like toxin acts on rRNA to block protein synthesis

Experiments in animals with Shiga toxin, as well as purified toxin(s) from EHEC strains, indicate that they cause capillary thrombosis and associated inflammation of the colonic mucosa leading to the hemorrhagic colitis seen in patients. It is also believed that these toxins play a central role in the pathogenesis of the hemolytic uremic syndrome (HUS) either by causing direct renal endothelial damage or by causing damage in other vascular beds or altering platelet function.

Systemic circulation of toxin causes hemolytic uremic syndrome

The epidemiology and clinical manifestations of the disease are striking. Serotype O157:H7 causes diarrhea that may be hemorrhagic in calves and is commonly isolated from asymptomatic dairy cows. The organism is generally transmitted to humans in contaminated raw milk or in undercooked ground beef in which surface contamination has been distributed throughout by the grinding process. Disease outbreaks have been associated with the consumption of ground beef products from fast food restaurants. However, it is important to understand that many sporadic cases are associated with the consumption of undercooked beef products in the home, particularly in the warm summer months. It is also clear from outbreaks that there is an important component of person-to-person transmission of EHEC as seen by secondary cases in families. The increased prevalence of EHEC may be related to modern methods of animal husbandry and "advances" in the food processing industry that provide fresher meat (and bacteria) from farm to hamburger. This infection is essentially absent in third world countries.

Transmission to humans by undercooked beef in fast food restaurants

Person-to-person transmission seen in families

Symptomatic EHEC disease develops about 4 days after exposure as a watery diarrhea associated with intense abdominal pain. This is followed 1 to 2 days later by bloody diarrhea. Unlike bacillary dysentery caused by *Shigella* species (see below), fever is not prominent, and although pus cells may be seen in the EHEC stool, the frank muco-pus seen in shigellosis is absent. Colonoscopy reveals edema, hemorrhage, and pseudomembrane formation. Yet, resolution of the disease usually takes place over a 3- to 10-day period, and there are few residual effects on the bowel mucosa.

Diarrhea is bloody but fever absent

HUS develops as a complication in 8 to 11% of EHEC cases, primarily in children under 5 years. This disease is characterized by microangiopathic hemolytic anemia, thrombocytopenia, and thrombosis of the glomerular capillaries. The systemic effects are often life-threatening, requiring transfusion and hemodialysis for survival.

HUS complications may require dialysis

### Enteroinvasive *E. coli* (EIEC)

The clinical features and pathogenesis of EIEC disease are indistinguishable from shigellosis (see below), but generally less severe. This similarity underscores that members of the *Shigella* and *Escherichia* genera are highly related. Infections with this organism are essentially restricted to children under 5 years of age living in developing nations. It is an un-

EIEC disease similar but less severe than of shigellosis

common cause of infection in industrialized nations, although one outbreak in the United States was traced to contaminated imported cheese. Humans are the only known reservoir.

ENTEROAGGREGATIVE *E. COLI* (EAEC)

Adherence primary virulence factor

EAEC strains were first defined on the basis of their adherence pattern to cultured mammalian cells. They are associated with watery diarrhea on epidemiologic grounds, and one strain caused disease in volunteer studies. There is some evidence that EAEC cause prolonged diarrhea in certain populations in developing countries. The pathogenesis of infection is not clearly understood, but a plasmid conferring BFP pili has been implicated as mediating adherence. Some investigators have reported an ST-like molecule that is distinct from that seen in ETEC.

TREATMENT AND PREVENTION

Hydration primary treatment

Antimicrobics may reduce duration of diarrhea in ETEC, ETIC, and EPEC

Like all infectious diarrheal disease, the proper treatment of human and animal sewage and the availability of potable water is essential. As noted, EHEC can be prevented by sensible cooking and food-handling practices. In cases of disease, regardless of the causative agent, oral rehydration is the mainstay of therapy. Antimicrobic treatment with trimethoprim/sulfamethoxazole (TMP-SMX) or quinolones reduces the duration of diarrhea in ETEC, EIEC, and EPEC infection, although many physicians feel that treatment is unnecessary. Antimotility agents are clearly contraindicated in children or others in which an invasive pathogen might be the etiologic agent of the disease. Neither the course of hemorrhagic colitis nor the risk of HUS are altered by antimicrobial therapy. The risk of HUS may be increased by these treatments.

Uncooked foods increase risk for traveller's diarrhea

Chemophrophylaxis recommended only for high-risk

Traveler's diarrhea is usually little more than an inconvenience. The incidence of the disease can be greatly reduced by eating only cooked foods and peeled fruits, and drinking hot or carbonated beverages. Avoiding uncertain water, ice, salads, and raw vegetables is a wise precaution. High-priced hotel accommodations have no protective effect. Chemoprophylaxis against traveler's diarrhea is not routinely recommended. TMP-SMX or ciprofloxacin has been recommended for a short-term (<2 weeks) in people at high risk of disease because of chronic conditions such as achlorhydria, gastric resection, prolonged use of H2 blockers or antiacids, and underlying diseases such as diabetes, AIDS, or other long-term immunosuppression.

### Meningitis

Pathogenesis similar to group B streptococci

K1 polysaccharide identical to group B meningococcus

*E. coli* is one of the most common causes of neonatal meningitis, many features of which are similar to group B streptococcal disease (Chapter 16). The pathogenesis involves vaginal *E. coli* colonizing the infant via ruptured amniotic membranes or during childbirth. Failure of protective maternal immunoglobulin M (IgM) antibodies to cross the placenta, and the special susceptibility of newborns, surely play a role. Fully 75% of cases are caused by strains possessing the K1 capsular polysaccharide that contains sialic acid and is structurally identical to the group B polysaccharide of *Neisseria meningitidis*, another cause of meningitis.

### Other Opportunistic Infections

Opportunistic infection follows mechanical disruption

With the exception of urinary tract infections, extraintestinal *E. coli* infections are uncommon unless there is a significant breach in host defenses. Opportunistic infection may follow mechanical damage, such as a ruptured intestinal diverticulum or intestinal trauma, or involve a generalized impairment of immune function. Failure of local control of infection can lead to spread and eventually Gram-negative septic shock. A significant proportion of blood isolates have the K1 surface polysaccharide. The particular diseases that result depend on the sites involved and include many of the syndromes covered in Chapters 59 to 72.

# SHIGELLA

## Bacteriology

Non-lactose fermenters

*Shigella* species are closely related to *E. coli* biochemically and antigenically. Most fail to ferment lactose or to produce gas when fermenting glucose, and all are nonmotile. They cause **bacillary dysentery,** a common disease with worldwide distribution. The genus is divided into four species, or groups, on the basis of differences in O antigens and some biochemical reactions. The species (groups) are *Shigella dysenteriae* (A), *Shigella flexneri* (B), *Shigella boydii* (C), and *Shigella sonnei* (D), as shown in Appendix 20–1. All but *S. sonnei* are further subdivided into a total of more than 30 individual serotypes. *Shigella dysenteriae* type 1, also known as the **Shiga bacillus,** is the cause of classic tropical bacillary dysentery, a disease typically more severe than that produced by other *Shigella* strains.

Four species; 30 serotypes

Shiga bacillus more severe

## Shigellosis

### Epidemiology

In the United States shigellosis is largely a pediatric disease caused by *S. sonnei*, affecting those less than 10 years of age with most below the age of 5. In contrast, *S. flexneri* disease in the United States has become largely a disease of sexually active gay men. Shigellosis has been a long-standing problem in institutions plagued by crowding and poor hygienic conditions, and it is an increasing problem in day-care centers. It can be readily transmitted among family members by the fecal–oral route with secondary attack rates between 20 and 40%. This high infectivity reflects the fact that less than 200 organisms are sufficient to infect volunteers. *Shigella,* unlike *V. cholerae* and most *Salmonella* species, is acid-resistant and survives passage through the stomach to reach the intestine.

Primarily fecal-oral transmission in children

*S. somei* most common

Very low infecting dose

### Pathogenesis

The fundamental event in the pathogenesis of bacillary dysentery is invasion of the human colonic mucosa. This triggers an intense acute inflammatory response with mucosal ulceration and abscess formation. Invasion by *Shigella* is a multistep process (Fig 20–2). Initially, the invading bacteria induce their own endocytosis by epithelial cells that are not "professional" phagocytes. The precise features of the entry process are not yet known but involve accumulation of filamentous actin underneath the host cell cytoplasmic membrane at the site of bacterial entry. This penetration occurs at the level of the cellular focal adhesion plaques, which are structures in which converging filaments of intracellular actin and associated actin-binding proteins adhere to components of the extracellular matrix. The entry of *Shigella* does not occur through the apical surface of cells but rather through exposed basolateral surfaces of M cells.

Invasion a multistep process

Actin accumulation involved in entry

Enter at basolateral surface of M cells

All virulent *Shigella* carry a large 220-kb plasmid that has several genes essential for the attachment and entry process. This includes a family of **invasion plasmid antigen** (*Ipa*) genes whose products act at different stages in the pathogenic process. For example, mutants of different genes (*IpaB, IpaC, IpaD,* etc) may be adherent but unable to enter cultured animal cells or to invoke the polymerization of host cellular actin beneath the site of adherence. No information is yet available about how these gene products interact with the cell surface or the cellular cytoskeleton.

Large plasmid required for virulence

Invasion plasmid can trigger genes required for attachment and entry

The *Shigella* brought into cells are surrounded by a phagocytic vacuole, but within 15 minutes of entry, they escape and enter the cytoplasmic compartment of the host cell. Remarkably, almost immediately, short filaments of polymerized cytoplasmic actin accumulate at one extremity of a bacterium to form an actin-containing "tail" that drives the microbe forward in spurts through the cytoplasm. A bacterial ATPase is responsible for the assembly of actin at the pole of moving bacteria. Plastin, an isoform of fibrin containing two actin-binding sites, is present in the actin tail. The distribution of plastin combined with its ability to form tight actin bundles suggests that it may cross-link actin adjacent to the bacterial body so that a sphincter-like contraction of the tail is the driving force to propel the usually nonmotile *Shigella* through the cell. Thus, as the bacteria replicate intracellularly they exploit resources of the cellular cytoskeletal apparatus, in conjunction with certain bacterial factors to motor themselves through and between host cells.

Rapid escape from phagocytic vacuole

Actin "tails" propel organism through cytoplasm

Passage of *Shigella* into adjacent epithelial cells occurs through finger-like projections from the surface of an infected cell to the surface of an uninfected cell involving the cadhedrin, L-CAM. The site of the protrusion at the cell surface shows a striking cytoskeletal rearrangement and this protrusion, with the bacterium trailing its actin tail, at its tip, may elongate to as much as 20 μm. The tip of the protrusion penetrates the surface membrane

Enter adjacent cells directly by long protrusions

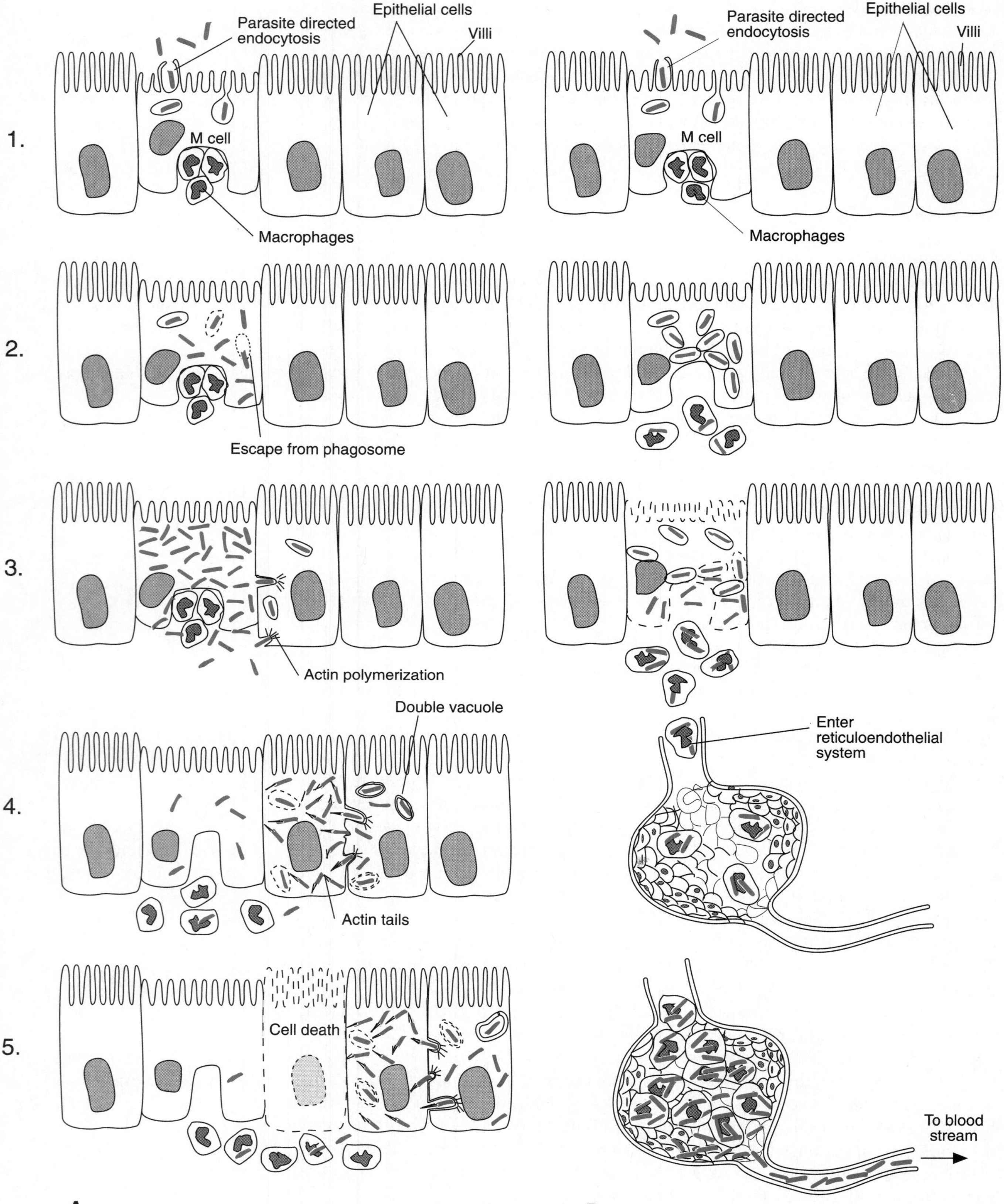


**Figure 20–2.** Invasion by *Shigella flexneri* and *Salmonella typhi.* Both invasive pathogens enter the M cell by inducing their own endocytosis. **A.** *Shigella* rapidly escapes the phagosome and uses the cell cytoskeleton to spread from cell to cell. **B.** *S. typhi* goes through the M cell to the submucosa where it enters the reticuloendothelial system. There it multiplies intracellularly, eventually seeding the blood stream.

of an adjacent cell and is then phagocytosed, thus placing the bacterium within a double membrane within the newly infected cell. The bacterium then lyses these membranes and is released into the cytoplasm, whereupon it begins to replicate and once more travel through this unusual intracellular highway system.

Must lyse double membrane in adjacent cell

The characteristics of *Shigella* entry and interaction with cellular elements are very similar to those observed with *Listeria monocytogenes* (Chapter 17), which is Gram-positive, motile, and prefers livestock over humans. Finding that such dissimilar bacteria use such similar tactics to infect their preferred host suggests that this represents a common thread to the selective pressures for a microbe to become a "successful" enteric pathogen.

Mechanisms similar to *Listeria*

There is some question about the precise host cell surface that is recognized by *Shigella* in the bowel lumen. The long-held idea that *Shigella* penetrate the apical surface of colonic cells is not borne out by the experimental observation that *Shigella* only readily enter the basolateral side of polarized cells. Current evidence suggests that *Shigella* initially transits the mucosal membrane by entering the follicle-associated M cells of the intestine, which lack the highly organized brush borders of absorptive enterocytes. There is evidence that the *Shigella,* like certain other pathogenic bacteria and viruses, adhere selectively to M cells and can transcytose through them into the underlying collection of phagocytic cells (Fig 20–3). Here, *Shigella* have another useful property, which is to cause the death of phagocytic macrophages by activating normal programmed cell death (apoptosis).

M cells act as entry and transmit sites

*Shigella* can kill phagocytes

Thus, once through the M cell the *Shigella* can presumably neutralize the first line of defense, attain the basolateral side of enterocytes, and invade them by the spectacular process just described. During natural infection, *Shigella* usually reach the lamina propria to evoke a profound inflammatory response; extension of the infection beyond the lamina is unusual in well-nourished individuals. Some *Shigella* produce Shiga toxin, which has the same mechanism and effects described above for the EHEC. Shiga toxin is not an essential determinant of the invasion process, but its presence can contribute to the severity of the disease, and as in the case of EHEC disease, infection can lead to the hemolytic uremic syndrome.

Extension beyond lamina propria unusual

Shiga toxin contributes to severity of disease

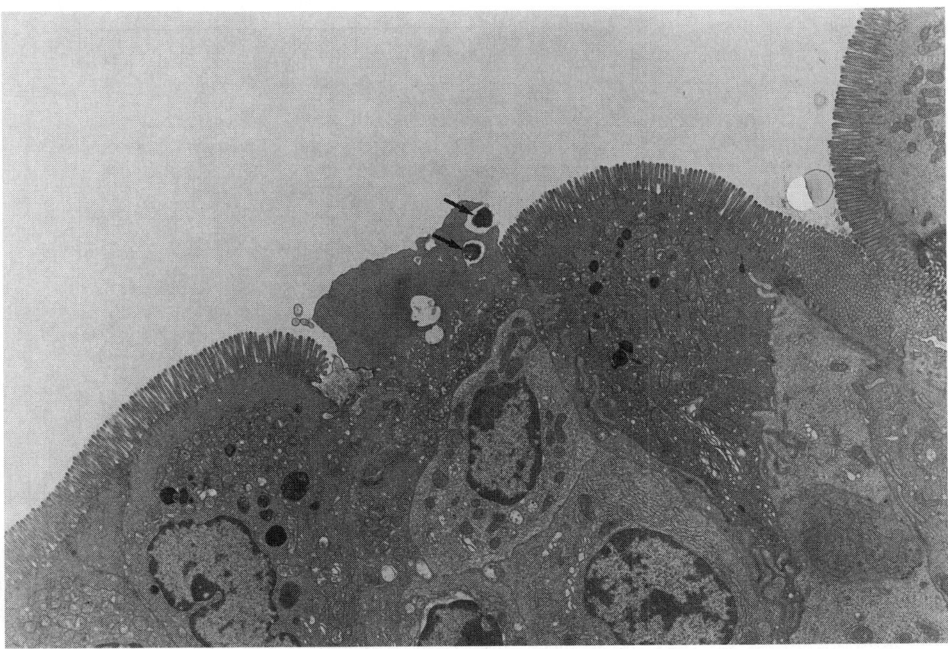

**Figure 20–3.** *Salmonella* entering an M cell. Two organisms (arrows) are seen attaching to the M cell surface. Note the contrast with the flanking enterocytes and the macrophage just below the M cell.

## Shigellosis: Clinical Aspects

### Clinical Manifestations

Watery diarrhea followed by fever, bloody mucoid stools, and cramping

*Shigella* organisms cause an acute inflammatory colitis and bloody diarrhea, which in the most characteristic state presents as a dysentery syndrome—a clinical triad consisting of cramps, painful straining to pass stools (tenesmus), and a frequent, small-volume, bloody, mucoid discharge. However, most clinical shigellosis due to *S. sonnei* in the United States is a watery diarrhea that is often indistinguishable from that of other bacterial or viral diarrheal illness. The disease usually begins with fever and systemic manifestations of malaise, anorexia, and sometimes myalgia. These nondescript symptoms are followed by the onset of watery diarrhea containing the large numbers of leukocytes detectable by light microscopy. The diarrhea may turn bloody with or without the other classical signs of dysentery. The more severe manifestations of the disease occur when *S. flexneri,* the species that predominates in the developing world, is isolated or, as in the past 20 years during epidemics of *S. dysenteriae* type 1 (Shiga) in Asia, Latin America, and Africa. Mortality in outbreaks of Shiga dysentery have been as high as 10 to 20%.

Mortality significant with *S. dysenteriae* type 1

### Treatment

Most infections self-limiting
Treatment may shorten illness and period of excretion

Several antimicrobics have proved effective in the treatment of shigellosis. Because the disease is usually self-limiting, the beneficial effect of treatment is in shortening the illness and the period of excretion of organisms; however, resistance may develop by plasmid transfer. The original discovery of in vivo plasmid transfer occurred during treatment of cases of shigellosis in which the infecting *Shigella* acquired multidrug resistance from an *E. coli* present simultaneously in the bowel. Resistance rates of 5 to 50% to ampicillin, once considered the treatment of choice, have caused a shift to trimethoprim-sulfamethoxazole in many areas. In recent years, quinolones and third-generation cephalosporins have been turned to in the face of resistance to other agents. Antispasmodic agents may make the patient worse and are contraindicated in shigellosis and other invasive diarrheas.

Ampicillin resistance common

### Prevention

Sanitation, insect control, hand washing, cooking important

Standard sanitation practices such as sewage disposal and water chlorination are important in preventing the spread of shigellosis. In certain circumstances insect control may also be important, because flies can serve as passive vectors when open sewage is present. Good individual sanitary practices, such as hand washing and proper cooking of food, are highly protective.

Live attenuated vaccines under investigation

*Shigella* infection produces relatively short-lived immunity to reinfection with homologous serogroups. Parenteral vaccines have been disappointing, and current efforts are directed towards orally administered live vaccines that could stimulate mucosal IgA. There are many candidate strains including attenuated *Shigella* mutants, *E. coli–Shigella* genetic hybrids, and *E. coli* with genes for some (but not all) the invasive (Ipa) proteins. The general idea is to find a strain that will go through enough of the multistage process described above to stimulate an immune response but stop short of full penetration and spread.

# SALMONELLA

## Bacteriology

Usually lactose negative, $H_2s$ positive

Members of the genus *Salmonella* are ubiquitous pathogens found in humans and their livestock, wild mammals, reptiles, birds, and even insects. The failure to ferment lactose and the ability to produce hydrogen sulfides from sulfur-containing amino acids are features used to identify colonies on primary isolation media. Panels of biochemical tests are used for confirmation. Antigenic analysis based on cell wall (O), capsular (K), and flagellar (H) antigens has led to the identification of over 1500 distinct antigenic variants of *Salmonella,* each of which was given a species designation. Although these are clearly not species, many of these colorful names (*S. budapest, S. seminole, S. tamale, S. oysterbeds,* etc) have been preserved, and serologic typing of salmonellae is a useful epi-

Large numbers of species based on antigenic diversity and biochemical tests

demiologic tool for investigating outbreaks of disease. However, the fact is that most human disease is caused by only about ten different serotypes of *Salmonella,* and one of these, *S. typhimurium,* has been the strain of *Salmonella* most frequently isolated worldwide.

## Salmonellosis

### Epidemiology

GASTROENTERITIS

*Salmonella* gastroenteritis is predominantly a disease of industrialized societies and improper food handling. The incidence of human *Salmonella* infection in the United States has more than doubled in the past decade to about 50,000 reported cases per year. This is felt to reflect only about 1% of the actual number of infections. As noted earlier, several serotypes, particularly *S. typhimurium* and *S. enteritidis*, are the major causes of disease. Poultry products, including eggs infected transovarially, are most often implicated as the vehicle of infection. There is a seasonal variation with peak incidence in summer and fall. Inadequate cooking practices that affect relatively large numbers of people are most commonly involved.

Disease related to improper food handling

Poultry products most common

The classic example of *Salmonella* "food poisoning" is the community picnic or bazaar, where volunteers prepare poultry, potato salad, and other potential culture media to be eaten later in the day. Because the refrigerators are filled with iced tea, beer, and soda, the food is left out in covered pans. An appropriate incubation temperature is provided by the still-warm contents and the afternoon sun, and the organisms enter logarithmic growth during the softball game. The bacteria usually produce no noticeable change in the food, and those who eat it are stricken the following day in rough proportion to their degree of consumption. This series of events also occurs frequently with other types of bacterial food poisoning (Chapter 65).

*Salmonella* + food + time lead to food poisoning

In recent years the epidemiology of salmonellosis has changed and the number of infections has increased. More and more often now one sees multistate outbreaks of salmonellosis spread through the contamination of foodstuffs during large-scale production from a single contaminated source through a massive, efficient interstate delivery system. It is also clear that in a time of rapid transport, foodstuffs from developing countries find their way to the local vegetable or meat counter. Thus, while the infection rate may be relatively low, even an attack rate of less than 0.5% in such a large number of exposures leads to many infected individuals. It is of concern to public health officials that a low incidence of disease over a massive area will be missed by most surveillance methods and by a society that increasingly forfeits infectious disease surveillance at the local level because of budgetary considerations.

Increased disease related to multistate outbreaks

Rapid transport may mark disease detection

The highest rates of infection are in children less than 5 years old, persons aged 20 to 30, and those older than 70. If one household member becomes infected, the probability that another will become infected approaches 60%. Nearly one third of all *Salmonella* epidemics occur in nursing homes, hospitals, mental health facilities, and other institutions. A recent increase in the popularity of raw milk has been associated with outbreaks of *Salmonella* (and *Campylobacter*) infection. Exotic pets such as turtles have also been the source of infection.

Readily transmitted at home

Raw milk and exotic pets are sources

TYPHOID FEVER

Typhoid fever is still an important cause of morbidity and mortality worldwide. In the United States and most other industrialized nations it is mostly seen in travelers to endemic areas such as Mexico, Latin America, Asia, and India. The decline in disease in industrialized nations largely reflects the availability of clean water supplies and improved disposal of fecal waste. The etiologic agent of typhoid is a single species, *S. typhi*, that can infect only humans under natural conditions as do the paratyphoid strains.

*S. typhi* only infects humans

### Pathogenesis of Infection

*Salmonella* is one of the best-studied bacterial species at the genetic level. A great deal is known about the regulation of *Salmonella* pathogenicity and the response of host cells to bacterial attachment and entry, but surprisingly little about the functional determinants of pathogenicity.

GASTROENTERITIS

*Salmonella* alters plasma membrane

Membrane ruffles associated with cytoskeletal changes

Enter cell by stimulating pinocytosis

The normal architecture of the brush border of intestinal cells is dramatically altered within minutes following *S. typhimurium* infection by the stimulation of membrane "ruffles" (Fig 20–4). Ruffles are specialized mammalian plasma membrane sites of filamentous actin rearrangement induced by growth factors, mitogens, or oncogene expression. Evidently, *Salmonella* have evolved an adhesin(s) on their surface that reacts with a host cell receptor to stimulate localized membrane ruffling. This ruffling is associated with cytoskeletal rearrangements at the site of bacterial–host cell contact and subsequently by a flux of intracellular free $Ca^{2+}$. The bacteria are internalized presumably by the induced pinocytosis associated with ruffles. Moreover, ruffles directly elicited by invasive *Salmonella* cells facilitate the internalization of many more nearby *Salmonella*. Thus, a single site of *Salmonella*-induced ruffling acts as a portal of entry for many adherent and adjacent bacteria by macropinocytosis. We need to learn more about the nature of the cellular receptor recognized by *Salmonella* and the bacterial adhesin mediating attachment. How *Salmonella* subverts the normal cellular machinery mediating pinocytosis for its own ends is of as much interest to mammalian cell biology as it is to understanding bacterial pathogenicity.

Because there is no effective model for *Salmonella* gastroenteritis, one can only speculate that the bacteria invade the enterocytes of the large and small bowel, transcytose through the basolateral membrane to enter the lamina propria, and induce a profound inflammatory response.

ENTERIC FEVER

*S. typhi* enter and kill M cells

Host-adapted salmonellosis, as typified by *S. typhi* in humans and *S. typhimurium* in mice, takes a more defined and specific route of infection. Both of these microorganisms bind to intestinal M cells by an unknown adhesin. The infection kills the M cell and delivers the invading bacterium into the Peyer's patch, where they invade macrophages and other cells. At least some *Salmonella* cells establish a privileged niche within macrophages. The bac-

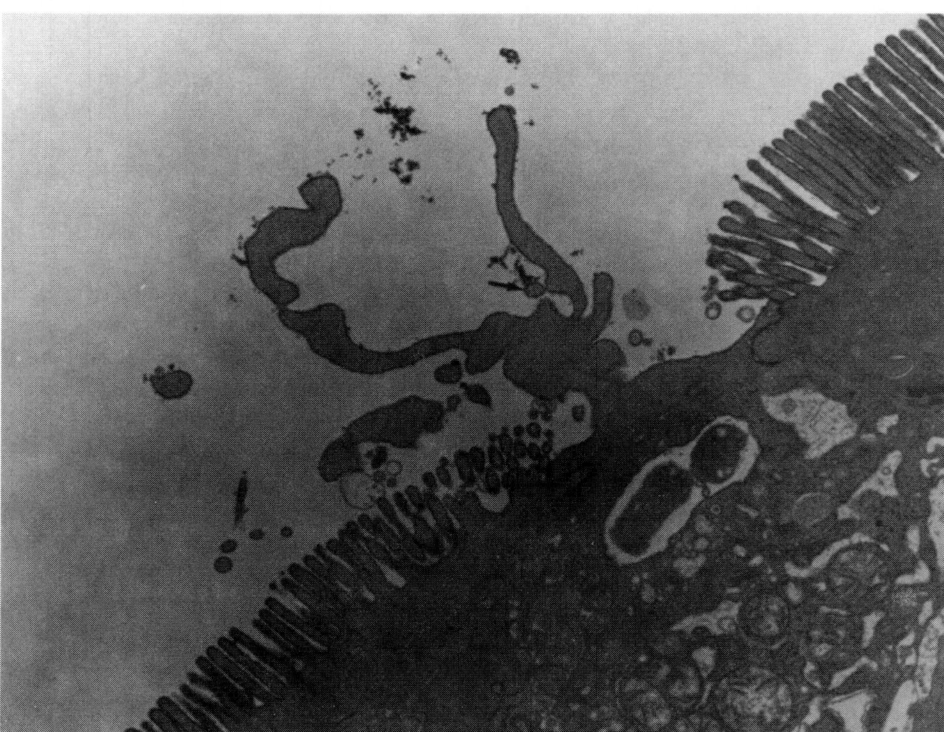

**Figure 20–4.** *Salmonella* membrane ruffles. These extensions of the plasma membrane are stimulated by the *Salmonella* (arrow) and are related to internalizing the bacteria.

teria remain within a membrane-bound vacuole that is inhibited from fusing with other host-cell organelles. The bacteria replicate at a rapid pace within a "spacious" vacuole, leading in many cases to macrophage death. The intracellular survival of *S. typhi* is associated with inhibition of the oxidative metabolic burst of host phagocytes. Typically, the bacteria spread from the intestinal Peyer's patch into the reticuloendothelial system, including the liver and spleen, eventually reaching the bloodstream. The immune response to enteric fever is both humoral and cell mediated. In nonfatal cases, humoral antibody and activated macrophages will eventually subdue the untreated infection over a period of about 3 weeks.

Enter and multiply in macrophages
Inhibit oxidative bursts

Spread to reticuloendothelial system and blood

### Genetics

A number of distinct genetic loci necessary for *Salmonella* to enter cells have been identified, the majority of which are restricted to a segment of the bacterial chromosome. Clearly, the genes governing motility and chemotaxis are important for pathogenicity. Several of the genes required for pathogenicity are environmentally regulated. Environmental cues such as oxygen tension, osmolarity, and growth state are known to have a profound influence on the capacity of *Salmonella* to enter mammalian cells. In this regard it is instructive to see that growing *Salmonella* under conditions thought to mimic the lumen of the small bowel provides the most infective cultures. Most pathogenic *Salmonella* also harbor a plasmid associated with resistance to serum killing and carrying genes important in an undefined way with the organism's capacity to replicate after entry. No structural determinants of pathogenicity have been clearly identified.

Motility and chemotaxis important

Environmental factors affect infectivity

## Salmonellosis: Clinical Aspects

It is most useful to think about the *Salmonella* on the basis of their host preference.

- ***Salmonella* serotypes highly adapted to humans.** The prototype is *S. typhi,* the typhoid bacillus, although others, such as *S. paratyphi* A, B, and C, and *S. sendai,* have no known reservoir outside of humans.
- ***Salmonella* highly adapted to specific hosts other than humans.** For example, *S. pullorum* infects avian hosts, *S. dublin* infects cattle, and *S. cholerasuis* infects swine. Some of these, such as *S. cholerasuis,* can also cause infection in humans.
- ***Salmonella* with a broad host range.** Most *Salmonella* belong to this category, and they cause most human and nonhuman infection.

### Clinical Manifestations

The clinical pattern of salmonellosis can be divided into gastroenteritis, enteric fever (typhoid-like disease), bacteremia with and without focal extraintestinal infection, and the asymptomatic carrier state. Although any *Salmonella* can probably cause any of these clinical manifestations under appropriate conditions, in practice certain serotypes are associated with particular clinical syndromes: *S. typhimurium, S. enteritidis,* and *S. newport* with gastroenteritis; *S. typhi* and the paratyphoid species with enteric fever; and *S. cholerasuis* with bacteremia and focal infection without antecedent gastrointestinal disturbance.

Enteric fever, bacteremia, gastroenteritis have limits to *Salmonella* species

#### Gastroenteritis

*Salmonella* gastroenteritis usually follows the ingestion of contaminated food or drinking water and accounts for about 15% of food-borne infection in the United States. Typically, the episode begins 24 to 48 hours after ingestion, with nausea and vomiting followed by, or concomitant with, abdominal cramps and diarrhea. Diarrhea persists as the predominant symptom for 3 to 4 days and usually resolves spontaneously within 7 days. Fever (39°C) is present in about half of the patients. The spectrum of disease ranges from a few loose stools to a severe dysentery-like syndrome.

Nausea, vomiting, diarrhea, 1–2 days after ingestion

The infecting dose is much higher than with *Shigella*; ingestion of 10,000 or more *Salmonella* bacilli are required to cause illness in 25% of healthy volunteers. Achlorhydric individuals, or those taking antiacids, can be infected with considerably smaller inocula. In most cases the disease is resolved by the host; on occasion, however, the microorganisms enter the bloodstream to cause sepsis. Individuals with impaired humoral or cell-mediated immunity, or those with a compromised reticuloendothelial system (eg, from sickle-cell or

Infecting dose higher than *Shigella*

Hodgkin's disease) are at particular risk for severe sequelae. *Salmonella* bacteremia may be the first manifestation of HIV infection.

### Treatment

Antimicrobial therapy generally not indicated

The primary therapeutic approach to *Salmonella* gastroenteritis is fluid and electrolyte replacement and the control of nausea and vomiting. Antibiotic therapy is usually not used because it has a tendency to increase the duration and frequency of the carrier state. In patients with underlying risk factors, antimicrobial therapy is applied as a prophylactic measure aimed at preventing systemic spread. No human vaccine is available.

#### Enteric Fever

Multiorgan systemic infection caused by *S. typhi* and paratyphoid strains

Enteric fever is a multiorgan-system *Salmonella* infection characterized by prolonged fever, sustained bacteremia, and profound involvement of the reticuloendothelial system, particularly the mesenteric lymph nodes, liver, and spleen. In principle, any *Salmonella* serotype can cause this syndrome, but the vast majority of enteric fever cases are caused by the typhoid bacillus and paratyphoid strains.

Two week incubation period

Fever persisting for weeks

Diarrhea not prominent

The manifestations of typhoid (Fig 20–5) have been well documented in human volunteer studies conducted during vaccine trials. A dose of $10^5$ laboratory-grown organisms ingested in milk caused disease in 30% of volunteers; 90% became ill if they swallowed $10^9$ cells. The mean incubation period following the lower dose was 13 days. The first symptom of the disease is fever associated with a headache. The fever rises in a stepwise fashion over the next 72 hours. A relatively slow pulse is characteristic and out of phase with the elevated temperature. In untreated patients the elevated temperature persists for weeks. A faint rash (rose spots) appear during the first few days on the abdomen and chest. Few in number, they are readily overlooked, especially in dark-skinned individuals. Many patients are constipated, although perhaps one third of patients will have a mild diarrhea. As the untreated disease progresses, an increasing number of patients complain of diarrhea.

Fever begins with bloodstream seeding

The evolution of the infection follows the pathogenesis (see above) in which the microorganisms traverse the M cells and Peyer's patch to become ingested by macrophages. Rather than being killed by these phagocytic cells, the bacteria proliferate, and they are carried to the lymphatic circulation to the mesenteric nodes, from which the bacteria begin to reach the bloodstream. This is the point at which the fever begins its slow, steady rise.

Obviously, chronic infection of the bloodstream is a serious disease and the effects of

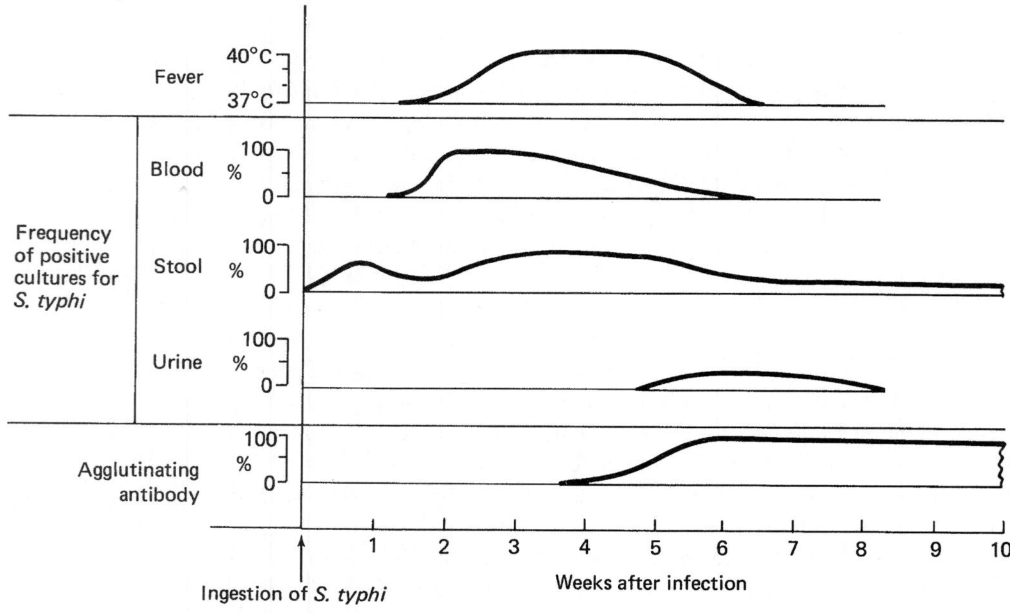


**Figure 20–5.** Natural history of enteric (typhoid) fever. The course of disease without antimicrobial therapy. Fever chart shows time course for typical patient. Culture and agglutinating antibody show timing and probability of positive results in a group of typhoid fever patients.

endotoxin can lead to myocarditis, encephalopathy, or intravascular coagulation. Moreover the persistent bacteremia can lead to infection at other sites. Of particular importance is the biliary tree with reinfection of the intestinal tract and diarrhea late in the disease. Urinary tract infection and metastatic lesions in bone joint, liver, and meninges may also occur. However, the most important complication of typhoid fever is hemorrhage from perforations through the wall of the terminal ileum at the site of necrotic Peyer's patches or in the proximal colon. These occur in patients whose disease has been progressing for 2 weeks or more.

Bacteremia may lead to infection at other sites

Intestinal perforation major complication

The organisms are probably sequestered in phagocytic cells in the liver and spleen so that blood cultures remain positive for at least 2 weeks in untreated patients, although the stool may remain positive for several months after recovery. Some patients become chronic carriers for years (hence the famous "typhoid Mary" Mallon), typically because of chronic infection of the gallbladder and the biliary tract particularly when stones are present. These individuals are important reservoirs of infection in endemic areas.

Biliary infection can lead to chronic carrier state

**Diagnosis and Treatment.** Isolation of *S. typhi* from the blood or feces confirms the diagnosis. Early in the infection, the blood is far more likely to give a positive culture result than culture from any other site. Eventually, however, positive cultures can be obtained from the stool and in some cases from urine culture. Most patients with typhoid fever develop agglutinating antibodies to the O and H antigens of *S. typhi* between the second and fourth weeks of illness, but their usefulness for diagnostic purposes is limited.

Blood culture positive early in disease

Stool culture positive later

Chloramphenicol was the first antibiotic to be used to treat typhoid in 1948, and it reduced the mortality from 15 to 25% to 1 to 1.5%. It is still a drug of choice in developing countries because it is so inexpensive, although resistance has developed to it. Ampicillin and trimethoprim-sulfonamide have been used successfully to treat infections caused by chloramphenicol-resistant strains. Newer cephalosporins (ceftriaxone) and quinolones (ciprofloxacin, norfloxacin) are also effective. With effective antimicrobial therapy, patients feel better in 24 to 48 hours, the temperature returns to normal in 3 to 5 days, and the patient is generally recovered by 10 to 14 days.

Antimicrobics are effective

Vaccines have been available since before the turn of the century. An intramuscular killed whole bacterial vaccine was widely employed by the military and in travelers, but gave poor protection against exposure to large doses of organisms. Recently, a live oral vaccine containing attenuated *S. typhi* has been licensed. It is probably as effective (or equally ineffective) as the injectable vaccine, protecting up to 70% of children in endemic areas. When all is said and done, the provision of clean water supplies and the treatment of carriers will lead to the disappearance of typhoid. The importance of carriers and sanitation was emphasized by a typhoid outbreak in 1973 among migrant workers in Florida. The source was traced to leakage of sewage into the water supply, failure of chlorination, and a chronic carrier.

Vaccines only moderately effective

General sanitation and elimination of carrier state most important

#### Bacteremia and Metastatic Infection

The acute gastroenteritis caused by many *Salmonella* serotypes can be associated with transient or persistent bacteremia. Frank sepsis may be seen in those with a compromised cell-mediated immune system. Metastatic spread by salmonellae is quite common. These organisms have a unique ability to colonize sites of preexisting structural abnormality including cardiovascular lesions, sites of malignancy, and the meninges (especially in infants). The serotype that classically caused sustained bacteremia and metastatic disease was *S. choleraesuis,* and it continues to cause the highest incidence of these events per episode of human infection. Because of improvement in the pork industry, the reservoir of this organism is decreasing and is being replaced by certain strains of *S. typhimurium* and *S. heidelberg*.

*S. choleraesuis* most common bacteremic serotype

*Salmonella* have a distinct propensity to localize on abnormal cardiovascular surfaces such as atherosclerotic plaques. Thus, endothelial and endocardial infection by *Salmonella* is predominantly a disease of the older patient. *Salmonella* infection of the bone typically involves the long bones and the spine at sites of injury or abnormality. Hence, sites of trauma, sites of sickle-cell injury, and skeletal prothesis are particularly at risk.

Tendency to localize in blood vessels and bone

Diagnosis is generally made by blood culture. In a surprising number of cases, there is no obvious prior history of an antecedent acute diarrheal episode. Antimicrobial therapy, together with surgical intervention, is usually successful.

Asymptomatic Carrier State

The chronic carrier state refers to the persistence of salmonellae in the stool or urine for periods longer than 4 months to a year. The carrier state can be residual from a known previous symptomatic episode of disease or the result of asymptomatic infection. Fully 5% of patients recovering from gastroenteritis still shed the organisms 20 weeks later. Chronic carriers who are food handlers are an important reservoir in the epidemiology of food-borne disease. Antibiotic treatment to eradicate the carrier state meets with erratic success and usually fails in the presence of co-existent biliary tract disease.

Food handlers carrying *Salmonella* are important reservoir

*Salmonella* in the AIDS Patient and other High-risk Groups

*Salmonella* infection in the AIDS patient is very common and is also often very severe. Bacteremia occurs in 70% of these patients and can cause septic shock and death. Despite adequate antimicrobial coverage, relapses are very common. Patients with lymphoproliferative disease, perhaps owing to the same T-cell defect as AIDS patients, are also highly susceptible to disseminated salmonellosis.

High frequency of bacteremia in AIDS and other T-cell deficiencies

Patients with schistosomiasis (Chapter 55) are at risk for developing a chronic, systemic *Salmonella* infection. Apparently, the bacteria infect the parasites and are protected from antimicrobial therapy and host humoral defenses. The clinical syndrome is one of chronic bacteremia that can persist for years, along with a profound hypertrophy of the reticuloendothelial system. The schistosomes must be eradicated to eliminate the *Salmonella.*

Many infect schistosomes

# YERSINIA

## Bacteriology

*Yersinia* are primarily animal pathogens, with occasional transmission to humans through direct or indirect contact. *Y. pestis* is the cause of plague, one of the greatest pandemic infectious diseases in human history. Morphologically, *Yersinia* tend to be coccobacillary and to retain staining at the ends of the cells (bipolar staining). Their general growth and metabolic characteristics are the same as those of other Enterobacteriaceae, although some strains grow more slowly or have optimal growth temperatures below 37°C. *Y. pestis* is antigenically homogenous, but *Y. pseudotuberculosis* and *Y. enterocolitica* have multiple O and H antigens (see Appendix 20–1).

Animal pathogens transmitted to humans

## Yersinia Diseases

### Pathogenesis

The enteropathogenic *Yersinia, Y. enterocolitica* and *Y. pseudotuberculosis,* invade the M cells of the Peyer's patch; *Y. pestis* enters the dermal lymphatics by the bite of an infected flea. Virulence factors produced by *Yersinia* include (1) invasin, an attachment protein; (2) an ST-like enterotoxin; (3) AIL, a complement resistance factor; and (4) the plasmid-mediated *Yersinia* outer membrane proteins or Yops, which have a variety of actions. These virulence factors are regulated in a complex fashion to support *Yersinia*'s pathogenic strategy, which is to paralyze the phagocytic activity of defending macrophages and neutrophils and to nullify the host cellular immune response.

Multiple virulence factors nullify phagocytic and cellular immune response

The determinants that promote cellular attachment and entry are encoded both on the bacterial chromosome and on an essential common 70-kb plasmid found in all pathogenic *Yersinia*. Virulence expression is controlled by two independent feedback loops, each of which responds to an environmental signal, one involving temperature and the other involving free calcium ($Ca^{2+}$). The enteropathogenic *Yersinia* entering the human host in contaminated food or drink at a temperature below 37°C produce only invasin and the ST-like enterotoxin. Invasin provides strong attachment of bacteria to host cells expressing $\beta_1$ integrins on their surface. Under some circumstances, invasin can actually mediate the entry of bacteria into Peyer's patch epithelial cells by stimulating a phagocytic response. It seems

Temperature and $Ca^{2+}$ regulate virulence factor expression

Invasin is attachment protein

likely that the intimate invasin–integrin attachment of the bacteria to host cells induces a host–cell transmembrane signaling process. Some *Y. enterocolitica* strains produce the ST-like enterotoxin, which is chromosomal. If this factor plays a role in the pathogenesis of infection, it is likely early, because like invasin, its synthesis ceases almost completely at 37°C.

ST-like enterotoxin produced by some strains

At 37°C, the invading *Yersinia* stop synthesizing invasin and ST but begin to synthesize AIL, the product of a chromosomal gene, that mediates resistance to complement-mediated killing. However, the plasmid-mediated outer membrane protein Yops produced at 37°C after cellular attachment are the hallmark of *Yersinia* pathogenicity, and form a multiprotein structure on the bacterial surface that interacts with host cells. Yops are also maximally produced at $Ca^{2+}$ concentrations that are below those found in human body fluids but are found inside cells.

AIL and Yops synthesized at 37°C

The virulence effector Yops (YopH, YopE, YopM and YpkA) share no homology with other known bacterial proteins but rather have homologous sequences in common with several eukaryotic factors. YopM shares homology with the platelet receptor of the von Willebrand factor and prevents platelet aggregation through its interaction with thrombin. YpkA possesses serine-threonine kinase activity and shares homology with corresponding eukaryotic enzymes. YopH and YopE act in concert to obstruct phagocytosis by macrophages and other professional phagocytes. YopH has tyrosine phosphatase activity and acts on host cell substrates. YopE mediates a contact-dependent cytotoxic activity that depolymerizes the actin microfilament network of the target cell.

Yops are more like eukaryotic proteins than those from other bacteria

Yops have multiple antiphagocytic and toxic actions

Recent work suggests that pathogenic *Yersinia* bind to integrins on the surface of macrophages through either invasin early in infection or through a plasmid protein YadA. The Yop complex is secreted to the bacterial surface and one of these, YopN, helps create a channel through the host cell surface through which the effector Yops are translocated into the host cell cytoplasm. The biological outcome of this extraordinary multifactorial process is the capacity of the pathogenic *Yersinia* to enter and replicate within the reticuloendothelial system and to delay the cellular immune response. The systemic symptoms seen in infected animals and humans accompanying yersiniosis can be traced largely to the effects of endotoxin.

Yops can create their own entry pores into host cells

Endotoxin creates systemic effects

*Y. pestis* is a specialized variant. This organism is very closely related to *Y. pseudotuberculosis* but it does not express either invasin or YadA. It does express yet another adhesin, called the pH 6 antigen, which probably plays a similar role. The plague bacillus also possess a unique small plasmid that encodes a fibrinolysin that may play a role in the pathogenesis of infection and that has been suggested to play an important role in the capacity of this microorganism to survive the environment of the flea. *Y. pestis* also produces a capsular protein antigen termed F1, which has antiphagocytic properties.

*Y. pestis* has its own adhesin

Capsular protein has antiphagocytic properties

## Yersinia Infections: Clinical and Epidemiologic Aspects

### Y. pestis

*Y. pestis* causes plague in both man and animals. The pathogenesis, epidemiology, and clinical features of this important disease are covered in Chapter 31.

### Y. pseudotuberculosis

In animals *Y. pseudotuberculosis* causes pseudotuberculosis, a disease characterized by lesions ranging from local necrosis to granulomatous inflammation in the lymph nodes, spleen, and liver. The organisms have been shown to survive and grow within mammalian cells. In humans the most common manifestation is an acute mesenteric lymphadenitis. The portal of entry is the gastrointestinal tract, and in most cases wild animals are a possible source of infection. The primary clinical manifestations are fever and abdominal pain, often mimicking acute appendicitis. Diagnosis is by isolation of *Y. pseudotuberculosis* from lymph nodes or from blood in the small proportion of cases that are bacteremic. The role of antimicrobial therapy in mesenteric lymphadenitis is uncertain, as the disease is usually self-limiting. The organism is usually susceptible to ampicillin, cephalosporins, aminoglycosides, tetracyclines, and chloramphenicol.

Mesenteric adenitis mimics acute appendicitis

### Y. enterocolitica

May also cause diarrhea and sepsis syndromes

*Y. enterocolitica,* a more recently described pathogen, produces a wider variety of infections than other members of the genus. The most common infection is enterocolitis, usually occurring in children and characterized by fever, diarrhea, and abdominal pain. It also causes an acute mesenteric lymphadenitis similar to that produced by *Y. pseudotuberculosis,* terminal ileitis, septicemia, and a polyarthritic syndrome associated with its diarrheal manifestations.

Wide geographic variation in isolation of *Y. enterocolitica*

Geographic variation in the frequency of *Y. enterocolitica* infections is marked. The highest rates have been reported from some Scandinavian and other European countries, with much lower rates in the United Kingdom and the United States. Low isolation rates may be partially attributable to the difficulty of growing *Y. enterocolitica* from stool specimens. Few laboratories in the United States routinely screen stools for *Yersinia* because the yield has been low and good selective media are not available.

*Y. enterocolitica* enterocolitis is usually self-limiting, and the influence of antimicrobics on its course is not clear. The organism is susceptible to the same antimicrobics as *Y. pseudotuberculosis,* with the exception of penicillins and cephalosporins, to which it is usually resistant through production of beta-lactamases.

## OTHER ENTEROBACTERIACEAE

All of the Enterobacteriaceae listed in Appendix 20–1 are capable of producing opportunistic infections of the type discussed above for *E. coli.* None can be considered proven causes of enteric disease although, no doubt, some will be in the future. This list includes only those isolated in at least moderate frequency. There are many other rare species. The most common genera are discussed briefly below.

### Klebsiella

Polysaccharide capsule with antiphagocytic properties

The most distinctive bacteriologic features of the genus *Klebsiella* are the absence of motility and the presence of a polysaccharide capsule. This gives colonies a glistening, mucoid character and forms the basis of a serotyping system. Over 70 capsular types have been defined, including some that cross-react with those of other encapsulated pathogens, such as *Streptococcus pneumoniae* and *Haemophilus influenzae.* Limited studies suggest that the capsule interferes with complement activation in a way similar to the other encapsulated pathogens. Multiple types of pili are also present on the surface and probably aid in adherance to respiratory and urinary epithelium.

Pneumonia and resistance to antimicrobics common

*K. pneumoniae,* the most common species, is able to cause classic lobar pneumonia, a characteristic of other encapsulated bacteria. Most *Klebsiella* pneumonias are indistinguishable from those produced by other members of the Enterobacteriaceae. *Klebsiellae* are now among the most resistant to antimicrobics of all the Enterobacteriaceae. This resistance may be chromosomal or plasmid mediated, and multiresistant strains are encountered that are highly resistant to all the common agents.

### Enterobacter

*Enterobacter* species generally ferment lactose promptly and produce colonies similar to those of *Klebsiella,* although not as mucoid. A differential feature is motility by peritrichous flagella, which are generally present in *Enterobacter* species but uniformly absent in *Klebsiella.*

Linked to contaminated IV fluids

*Enterobacter* species appear to be less virulent than *Klebsiella.* They are usually found in mixed infections, in which their significance must be decided on clinical and epidemiologic grounds. Several hospital outbreaks traced to contaminated parenteral fluid solutions have implicated *Enterobacter* species. In addition to ampicillin most isolates are resistant to first-generation cephalosporins, but may be susceptible to second- or third-generation cephalosporins, although mutants derepressed for beta-lactamase production occur at relatively high frequency and confer resistance to many cephalosporins.

## Serratia

May produce red pigment

*Serratia* strains ferment lactose slowly (3 to 4 days), if at all. Some produce distinctive brick-red colonies. Although less common, this genus produces the same range of opportunistic infections seen with the rest of the Enterobacteriaceae. *Serratia* strains show consistent resistance to ampicillin and cephalothin, with the frequent addition of plasmid-determined resistance to many other antimicrobics, including the aminoglycosides. Sporadic infections and nosocomial outbreaks with multiresistant strains have often been difficult to control.

β-lactam resistance common

## Citrobacter

The genus *Citrobacter,* although biochemically and serologically similar to *Salmonella,* does not cause enterocolitis or enteric fever. *Citrobacter* strains may be present in the normal intestinal flora, and cause opportunistic infections like many other Enterobacteriaceae. Despite reports of association with diarrheal disease, present evidence does not indicate that *Citrobacter* should be considered an enteric pathogen.

## Proteus, Providencia, and Morganella

Some species swarm over the surface of agar plates

*Proteus, Morganella,* and *Providencia* (see Appendix 20–1) are also opportunistic pathogens found with varying frequencies in the normal intestinal flora. *Proteus mirabilis,* the most commonly isolated member of the group, is one of the most susceptible of the Enterobacteriaceae to the penicillins; this characteristic includes moderate susceptibility to penicillin G. Other Proteeae are regularly resistant to ampicillin and the cephalosporins. *Proteus mirabilis* and *Proteus vulgaris* share the ability to swarm over the surface of media, rather than remaining confined to discrete colonies (Fig 20–6). This characteristic makes them readily recognizable in the laboratory—often with dismay, because the spreading growth covers other organisms in the culture and thus delays their isolation. *Proteus* and *Morganella* differ from other Enterobacteriaceae in the production of a very potent urease, which aids their rapid identification. It also leads to production of alkalinity and an ammoniac odor in

Some potent urease producers

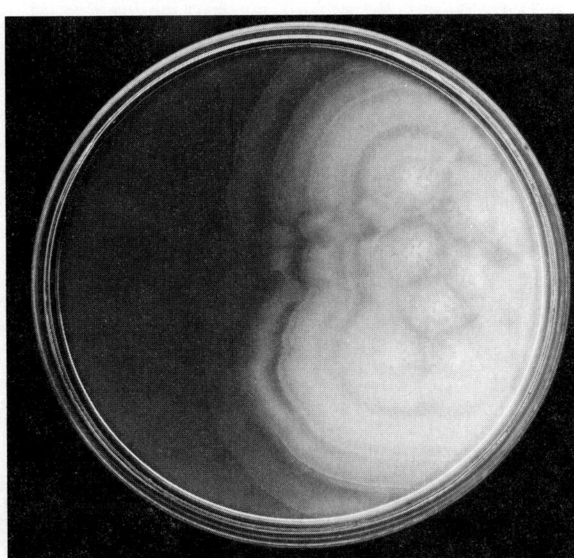

**Figure 20–6.** Swarming *Proteus.* This strain of *Proteus mirabilis* was inoculated at one spot on the blood agar plate. Note the waves of the spreading growth, which have covered the entire plate. On media containing bile salts (MacConkey agar) the swarming is inhibited and discrete colonies are formed.

urinary tract infections. *Providencia* species do not produce urease, are the least frequently isolated, and are generally the most resistant of the group to antimicrobics.

## LABORATORY DIAGNOSIS OF ENTEROBACTERIACEAE INFECTIONS

Easily isolated on routine media

Selective media required for enteric pathogens

EHEC require serotyping

For the opportunistic Enterobacteriaceae, culture on routine media, as described in Chapter 14, is the standard approach. Selective media for isolation of *Shigella* and *Salmonella* are long established as part of the routine stool culture, but *Yersinia* isolation requires additional procedures. Distinguishing diarrhea-causing *E. coli* from the many other strains in stools is a special problem. EHEC colonies can be screened using failure to ferment sorbitol and confirmed with O157 antisera. Extending serotyping to the EPEC would be helpful but impractical, particularly in the developing countries, where the strains are most prevalent.

Molecular methods can detect virulence properties directly

Most recently, better understanding of the genetic and molecular basis for virulence has led to the development of specific immunodiagnostic, DNA probe, and other molecular techniques directed at detecting toxin(s), adhesins, or invasins. Some can be used to detect specific organisms directly in clinical material. These methods are not yet commonly used in clinical laboratories because they are expensive and most of the diarrheal diseases are self-limiting. They are, however, of extraordinary value in epidemiologic work.

## TREATMENT

Susceptibility to antimicrobics to highly variable

With the exception of some enteric infections discussed above, antimicrobial therapy is crucial to the outcome of infections with members of the Enterobacteriaceae. Unfortunately, combinations of chromosomal and plasmid-determined resistance (Chapter 13) render them the most variable of all bacteria in susceptibility to antimicrobial agents. They are usually resistant to high concentrations of penicillin G, erythromycin, and clindamycin, but may be susceptible to the broader-spectrum beta-lactams, aminoglycosides, tetracycline, chloramphenicol, sulfonamides, quinolones, nitrofurantoin, and the polypeptide antibiotics. Because the probability of resistance varies among genera and in different epidemiologic settings, the susceptibility of any individual strain must be determined by in vitro tests. Typical frequencies of resistance for the more common Enterobacteriaceae appear in Appendix 13–1.

## ADDITIONAL READING

Bliska JB, Galán JE, Falkow S: Signal transduction in the mammalian cell during bacterial attachment and entry. *Cell* 1993;73:903–920.

Donnenberg M, Kaper J: Minireview: Enteropathogenic *E. coli*. *Infect Immun* 60:3953–3961;1992. A course summary of the current status of the many *E. coli* enteropathogenic mechanisms.

Johnson JR: Virulence factors in *Escherichia coli* urinary tract infection. *Clin Microbiol Rev* 1991;4:80–128. This review focus on the pathogenesis of UTI but also includes much material of general relevance to other *E. coli* infections.

Sansonetti PJ: Genetic and molecular basis of epithelial cell invasion by *Shigella* species. *Rev Infect Dis* 1991;13(suppl 4):S285–292.

APPENDIX 20–1. GENERAL CHARACTERISTICS OF SOME ENTEROBACTERIACEAE

| Organism | Serologic Type(s) (Antigens) | Bacteriologic Features | | | | | | Major Disease(s) | Found in Normal Flora |
|---|---|---|---|---|---|---|---|---|---|
| | | *Lactose* | *Indole* | *Urease* | *Hydrogen Sulfide* | *Motility* | *Other* | | |
| *Escherichia coli* | 150+ (O, K, H) | + | + | – | – | + | | Urinary tract infections; diarrhea; opportunistic | Yes |
| *Shigella dysenteriae* | 10 (O) | – | v | – | – | – | | Dysentery (type 1, severe) | No |
| *Shigella flexneri* | 6 (O) | – | – | – | – | – | | Dysentery | No |
| *Shigella boydii* | 15 (O) | – | v | – | – | – | | Dysentery | No |
| *Shigella sonnei* | 1 (O) | – | – | – | – | – | | Dysentery | No |
| *Klebsiella pneumoniae* | 72 (K) | + | – | +[a] | – | – | Encapsulated | Pneumonia; opportunistic | Yes |
| *Enterobacter* sp. | | + | – | – | – | + | | Opportunistic | Yes |
| *Serratia marcescens* | | – | – | v[a] | – | + | Red pigment | Opportunistic | Yes |
| *Salmonella* serotypes | 1500+ (O, H) | – | – | – | + | + | | Diarrhea | No |
| Salmonella choleraesuis | 1 (O, H) | – | – | – | v | + | | Bacteremia | No |
| *Salmonella typhi* | 1 (O, H, K) | – | – | – | + | + | | Enteric (typhoid) fever | No |
| *Salmonella paratyphi A.* | (O, H) | – | – | – | + | + | | Diarrhea; enteric fever | No |
| *Citrobacter* sp. | | v | – | v[a] | + | + | | Opportunistic | Yes |
| *Proteus mirabilis* | | – | – | + | + | + | Swarming[b] | Opportunistic | Yes |
| *Proteus vulgaris* | | – | + | + | + | + | Swarming[b] | Opportunistic | Yes |
| *Morganella morganii* | | – | + | + | – | + | | Opportunistic | Yes |
| *Providencia* | | – | + | v | – | + | | Opportunistic | Yes |
| *Yersinia pestis* | | – | – | – | – | – | | Plague | No |
| *Yersinia pseudotuberculosis* | 10 (O, H) | – | v | +[c] | – | +[c] | | Mesenteric lymphadenitis | No |
| *Yersinia enterocolitica* | 50+ (O, H) | – | – | +[c] | – | +[c] | | Mesenteric lymphadenitis; enteric fever; diarrhea | No |

*Abbreviations:* + = more than 90% of strains positive; – = less than 10% of strains positive; v = variable (some strains positive, others negative).

[a] Positive reactions weak or delayed compared to those of Proteeae.

[b] Growth swarms over surface of agar plates.

[c] Positive reactions seen at 25°C but not at 37°C.

**APPENDIX 20–2. EXOTOXINS PRODUCED BY ENTEROBACTERIACEAE**

| Toxin | Target | Enzymatic Activity | Primary Action | Effect | Genetic Control |
|---|---|---|---|---|---|
| *Escherichia coli* LT | G regulatory protein | ADP-ribosylation | Adenylate cyclase stimulation | Fluid loss | Plasmid |
| *Escherichia coli* ST | Glycoprotein receptor | Unknown | Guanylate cyclase stimulation | Fluid loss | Plasmid |
| *Shigella dysenteriae,* type 1 Shiga toxin | 60S ribosome | Modifies 28S ribosomal RNA | Inhibits protein synthesis | Cell death | Chromosomal |
| Shigalike toxins | 60S ribosome | Modifies 28S ribosomal RNA | Inhibits protein synthesis | Cell death | Temperate phage |

Chapter 21

# *Vibrio, Campylobacter,* and *Helicobacter*

*Kenneth J. Ryan and Stanley Falkow*

Despite the fact that this group includes some of the most common of all microbial pathogens, only *Vibrio cholerae,* the cause of classical Asiatic cholera, has been recognized as such for more than two decades. Study of cholera toxin has improved our understanding of other infectious diarrheas, and cholera itself, far from restricted to its historic locale, has resurged in the last half of the 20th century. *Campylobacter jejuni* is now established as one of the most important causes of diarrhea throughout the world. *Helicobacter pylori* causes gastritis, leading to peptic ulcer disease and possible gastric cancer.

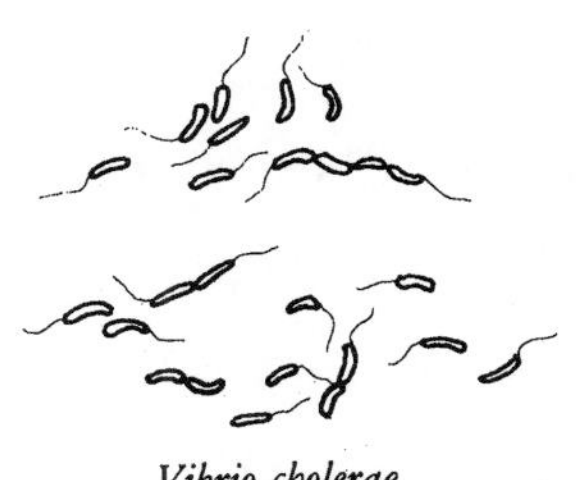

*Vibrio cholerae*

## VIBRIO

Vibrios are curved, Gram-negative rods commonly found in saltwater. Cells may be linked end to end, forming S shapes and spirals. They are highly motile with a single polar flagellum, non-spore forming, oxidase positive, and can grow under aerobic or anaerobic conditions. The cell envelope structure is similar to that of other Gram-negative bacteria. *Vibrio cholerae* is the prototype cause of a toxigenic water-loss diarrhea called **cholera.** Other species cause diarrhea, wound infections, and, rarely, systemic infection.

Rapidly motilite curved rods

Found in seawater

### ■ Vibrio cholerae

*V. cholerae* has a low tolerance for acid, but grows under alkaline (pH 8.0 to 9.5) conditions that inhibit many other Gram-negative bacteria. It is facultatively anaerobic, but grows best under aerobic conditions on routine bacteriologic media. It is distinguished from other vibrios by its biochemical reactions, O antigenic structure, and production of a potent enterotoxin. The nomenclature of the genus *Vibrio* is somewhat confusing, because many strains with essentially the same biochemical reactions may or may not produce enterotoxin and cholera. The strains associated with epidemic cholera are limited to a single serogroup, 0:1, and a biochemical variant, *V. cholerae* biotype eltor, sometimes called *Vibrio eltor.* Each may be subdivided into at least two serotypes. Noncholera vibrios have worldwide distribution and are frequently found in water, sewage, and various marine environments. They have occasionally been associated with diarrhea and enterotoxin production but not epidemic cholera.

Preference for alkaline over acid conditions

Epidemic cholera limited to serotype 0:1 strains including Eltor biotype

Isolates from marine environments worldwide

## Cholera

### Epidemiology

Usual transmission of epidemic cholera through water supply

Interepidemic maintenance may be in crustaceans

Epidemic cholera is spread primarily by contaminated water under conditions of poor sanitation. During epidemics, numerous vibrios purged from the intestines of infected individuals reach the primary water supply and are transmitted to others via drinking, food preparation, or bathing. The maintenance of the organism in nature between epidemics is more obscure. It is fragile, surviving only a few days in the environment, but may be maintained longer in marine and fresh-water crustaceans. Convalescent human carriage is usually brief, and prolonged carriage very rare.

Eltor biotype has spread in recent years

Sporadic cases in United States associated with eating crabs and shrimp caught in Southeast

South American epidemic widespread

New serotype may complicate control

The eltor biotype of *V. cholerae* has a longer survival in nature and is more likely to produce subclinical cases of cholera, both of which would aid its geographic spread and survival. This organism, first discovered in 1905 at El Tor quarantine camp for Mecca pilgrims, has been of increasing importance in the spread of epidemic cholera beyond its historic location in Africa and southern Asia to Indonesia, south and central Asia, Africa, and western Europe. This pandemic reached the United States in 1973, and continued with occasional cases related to eating inadequately cooked crabs and shrimp caught off the Gulf Coast of Louisiana and Texas. In 1991 South America was hit with devastating results due to persistence in locales with poor sanitation. For example, in Peru alone over 500,000 cases were documented in 1991 and 1992, with over 4500 deaths. Western Hemisphere cases reported from 21 countries are also of the El Tor biotype, although the Gulf Coast and South American outbreaks do not appear to be linked. The short incubation period of cholera makes imported cases less likely but possible. One case was linked to a man who ate ceviche (marinated uncooked fish) at an airport in Ecuador before departing to Florida. In early 1993 the cholera situation was further complicated by the detection of a novel vibrio serotype in Bangladesh that caused severe disease even in those who had previously suffered from El Tor disease.

### Pathogenesis

Large doses required to pass stomach acid barrier

Penetration of mucus related to mucinase and motility

Pili regulated together with toxin

To produce disease, *V. cholerae* must reach the small intestine in sufficient numbers to multiply and colonize. In healthy people, ingestion of large numbers of bacteria is required to offset the acid barrier of the stomach. *V. cholerae*'s colonization of the entire intestinal tract from the jejunum to the colon must be aided by the ability of the organism to penetrate the surface mucus covering of the intestinal mucosa and to adhere to the epithelial surface. The organism's motility, chemotaxis, and a mucinase may bring the organism to the host cell surface. The *V. cholerae* possess long filamentous pili that form bundles on the bacterial surface. These pili, called Tcp pili (for *T*oxin *C*o-regulated), are regulated similarly to cholera toxin and other virulence determinants. Mutants that are defective in Tcp pilus biosynthesis are avirulent in human volunteers. The genetic locus determining the synthesis and assembly of the Tcp pili is complex but it is clear that they belong to the family of *N*-methylphenylalanine type pili similar to those seen for the gonococcus, *Moraxella*, and other bacterial pathogens.

Cholera toxin has active (A) and multiple binding (B) units

Ganglioside receptor for B units found on surface of many cell types

A unit separates with A1 entering cytoplasm

A1 subunit ADP-ribosylates G protein regulating adenylate cyclase system

The outstanding feature of *V. cholerae* pathogenicity is the ability of virulent strains to secrete a potent enterotoxin responsible for the disease cholera. The structure and mechanism of action of cholera toxin has been studied extensively (Fig 21–1). Cholera toxin is an A-B type ADP-ribosylating toxin. Its molecule is an aggregate of multiple polypeptide chains organized into two toxic subunits (A1, A2) and five binding (B) units. The B units mediate tight binding to a GM1-ganglioside receptor, a sialic acid residue linked to a ceramide lipid, found on the surface of many types of cells. Once bound, the A1 subunit is released from the toxin molecule by reduction of the disulfide bond that binds it to the A2 subunit, and it enters the cell by translocation, where it exerts its effect on the membrane-associated adenylate cyclase system at the basolateral membrane surface. The precise mechanism whereby the toxin enters the cell at the apical surface of the epithelium and translocates to the basolateral membrane is still uncertain, but may involve trafficking of membrane vesicles through the Golgi apparatus. The target of the toxic A1 subunit is a guanine nucleotide (G) protein, Gs alpha, that regulates activation of the adenylate cyclase system. Cholera toxin catalyzes the ADP ribosylation of the G protein, rendering it unable to dissociate from the active adenylate cyclase complex. This causes persistent activation of

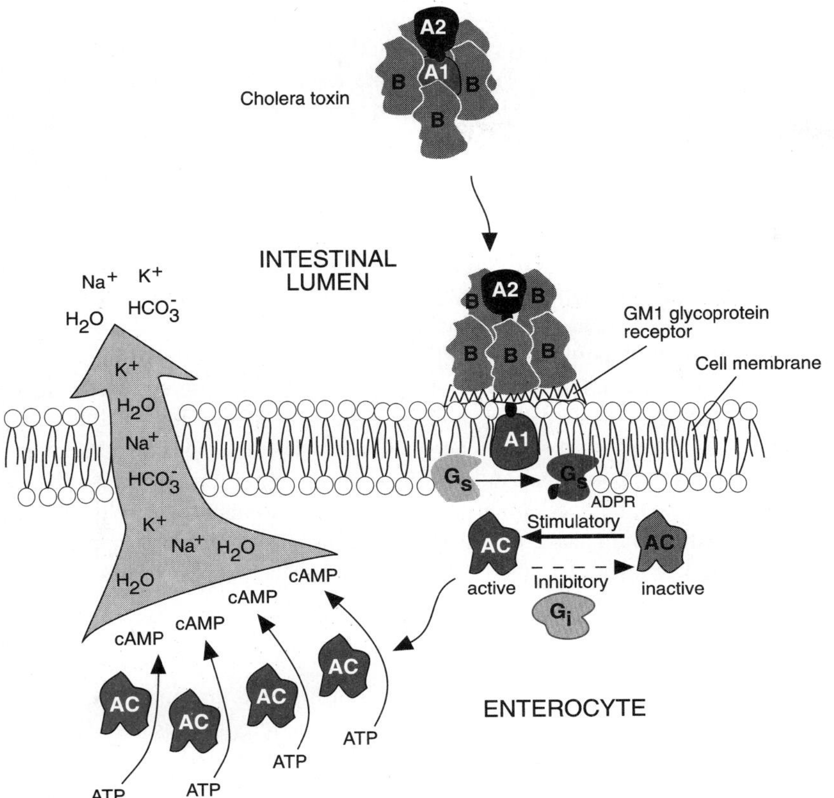


**Figure 21–1.** The action of cholera toxin. The complete toxin is shown binding to the GM1-ganglioside receptor on the cell membrane via the binding (B) subunits. The active portion ($A_1$) of the A subunit catalyzes the ADP-ribosylation of the $G_s$ (stimulatory) regulatory protein, "locking" it in the active state. Because the $G_s$ protein acts to return adenylate cyclase from its inactive to active form, the net effect is persistent activation of adenylate cyclase. The increased adenylate cyclase activity results in accumulation of cyclic adenosine 3′, 5′-monophosphate (cAMP) along the cell membrane. The cAMP causes the active secretion of sodium ($Na^+$), chloride ($Cl^-$), potassium ($K^+$), bicarbonate ($HCO_3^-$), and water out of the cell into the intestinal lumen.

intracellular adenylate cyclase, which in turn stimulates the conversion of adenosine triphosphate to cyclic adenosine 3′, 5′-monophosphate (cAMP). The net effect is excessive accumulation of cAMP at the cell membrane, which causes hypersecretion of chloride, potassium, bicarbonate, and associated water molecules out of the cell. The water and electrolyte shift from the cell to the intestinal lumen is the fundamental cause of the watery diarrhea of cholera.

Adenylate cyclase "locked" in active state

Hypersecretion of water and electrolytes from increased cAMP causes diarrhea

Mutants that are defective in cholera toxin biosynthesis are reduced in their virulence. Not only are such mutants less likely to cause the classical watery diarrhea but they also do not colonize the small bowel as well as toxigenic strains. The role of the toxin in colonization is not clear. Understanding the mechanism of action of cholera toxin has acquired additional importance with the discovery that other enterotoxins, such as the heat-labile toxin (LT) of *Escherichia coli* (Chapter 20), use the same mechanism. Interestingly, synthesis of cholera toxin is controlled by a chromosomal gene, whereas the *E. coli* LT gene is located on a plasmid.

Nontoxigenic strains do not colonize

Cholera toxin and *E. coli* LT mechanism the same

It was widely thought that an appropriate strain of *V. cholerae* deficient in toxin production would be a useful vaccine candidate. However, in volunteer studies, several such derivatives caused mild diarrhea, leading to the realization that *V. cholerae* possesses other enterotoxins. These include the *zot* toxin, which affects the tight junctions between cells, and the *ace* toxin, which also produces a secretory response in experimental animals. The *zot* and *ace* genes are closely linked to the cholera toxin genes, *ctxA* and *ctxB*, on the bacterial chromosome.

Other toxins probably have a role in disease

Transcription of the cholera toxin operon is affected by a number of environmental factors including pH, low osmolarity, and temperature. As many as 20 other *V. cholerae* genes are regulated similarly as part of a regulon that is controlled by three transcriptional activators, *ToxR, ToxS,* and *ToxT*. *ToxR* and *ToxS* comprise a two-component regulatory system in which *ToxS* "senses" environmental changes and causes *ToxR* to activate transcription of a constellation of genes including *ToxT,* which in turn activates the *Tcp* group of genes controlling pilin biosynthesis and assembly. Yet another level of regulation allows *V. cholerae* to produce a siderophore and a receptor that binds hemin and hemoglobin in response to iron concentration.

Regulatory system senses environmental changes and turns on multiple virulence genes

The fluid loss that results from the adenylate cyclase stimulation of cells depends on the balance between the amount of bacterial growth, toxin production, fluid secretion, and fluid absorption in the entire gastrointestinal tract. In general, an alkaline environment ideal for continued growth of the organism is produced, and fluid loss in the form of voluminous, watery stools results. The outpouring of fluid and electrolytes is greatest in the small intestine, where the secretory capacity is high and absorptive capacity low. The diarrheal fluid can amount to many liters per day, with approximately the same sodium content as plasma but two to five times the potassium and bicarbonate concentrations. The result is dehydration (isotonic fluid loss), hypokalemia (potassium loss), and metabolic acidosis (bicarbonate loss). The diarrheal fluid also contains mucus flecks, giving it a gross appearance called **rice-water stools.** The intestinal mucosa remains unaltered except for some hyperemia because *V. cholerae* does not invade.

Cholera toxin causes extensive fluid, potassium, and bicarbonate loss

Intestinal mucosa is structurally unaffected; no invasion

### Immunity

Nonspecific defenses such as gastric acidity, gut motility, and intestinal mucus are important in preventing colonization with *V. cholerae*. For example, in persons who lack gastric acidity (gastrectomy or achlorhydria from malnutrition), the attack rate of clinical cholera is higher. Natural infection provides long-lasting immunity, which current evidence indicates is attributable more to mucosal than to humoral immune mechanisms. The immune state has been associated with production of secretory IgA by lymphocytes in the subepithelial areas of the gastrointestinal tract, but the precise protective mechanism remains to be established.

Attach rate higher with achlorhydria

Immunity associated with sIgA

## Cholera: Clinical Aspects

### Clinical Manifestations

Typical cholera has a rapid onset, beginning with abdominal fullness and discomfort, gurgling, rushes of peristalsis, and loose stools. Vomiting may also occur. The stools quickly become watery, voluminous, almost odorless, and contain mucus flecks (rice-water stools). There is no pus or blood in the stools, and the patient is afebrile. Clinical features of cholera result from the extensive fluid loss and electrolyte imbalance, which can lead to extreme dehydration, hypotension, and death within hours if untreated.

Extreme watery diarrhea with large fluid loss

Disease manifestations from dehydration and electrolyte imbalance

### Diagnosis

The initial suspicion of cholera depends on recognition of the typical clinical features in an appropriate epidemiologic setting. A bacteriologic diagnosis is accomplished by isolation of *V. cholerae* from the stool. The organism grows on common clinical laboratory media such as blood agar and MacConkey agar, but its isolation is enhanced by the use of thiosulfate-citrate-bile salt-sucrose agar. Once isolated, the organism is readily identified by biochemical reactions. In parts of the world where cholera is not endemic, these procedures are not routinely used in clinical laboratories and must be requested specifically.

Stool culture using selective media required

### Treatment

The outcome of cholera is dependent on balancing the diarrheal fluid and ionic losses with adequate fluid and electrolyte replacement. This is accomplished by oral and/or intravenous administration of solutions of glucose with near physiologic concentrations of sodium and chloride and higher than physiologic concentrations of potassium and bicarbonate. Exact formulas are available as packets to which a given volume of water is added. Oral replacement, particularly if begun early, is sufficient for all but the most severe cases and has sub-

Oral or intravenus fluid and electrolyte replacement most important

stantially reduced mortality from the disease. Antimicrobial therapy with tetracycline shortens the duration of diarrhea and magnitude of fluid loss.

Antimicrobial therapy useful

### Prevention

Epidemic cholera, a disease of poor sanitation, does not persist where treatment and disposal of human waste is adequate. As good sanitary conditions do not exist in much of the world, secondary local measures such as boiling or chemical treatment of water during epidemics are required. The occasional cases associated with crustaceans could be prevented by adequate cooking (10 minutes) and avoidance of recontamination from containers and surfaces.

Water sanitation required

Cook shellfish at least 10 minutes

Vaccines prepared from whole cells, lipopolysaccharide, and cholera toxoid have been disappointing, providing some protection that is not long-lasting. Current interest includes live attenuated vaccine strains because of their potential to stimulate the local sIgA immune response that appears to be of primary importance in cholera. Through use of recombinant DNA technology, strains have been constructed that have the A subunit of toxin gene deleted, leaving only the binding B subunits. Strains with deleted *zot* and *ace* as well as cholera toxin genes are currently being tested as well, and preliminary results are said to be promising.

Attenuated vaccines may stimulate local sIgA

Genetically engineered vaccine deletes A subunit

## Other Vibrios

Several less common infections have been associated with *Vibrio* species other than *V. cholerae*. Because of their salt requirement and normal habitat in seawater, these species are sometimes called halophilic vibrios. Bacteriologically, they resemble *V. cholerae* in many respects, but are readily distinguished on the basis of biochemical and serologic characteristics.

Halophilic vibrios found in seawater

The most common of these species is *V. parahemolyticus*, which causes an acute illness characterized by severe cramping, abdominal pain, vomiting, and watery diarrhea. The incubation period is short, typically 24 to 48 hours after ingestion. *V. parahemolyticus* is commonly present in coastal waters throughout the world. Infection develops after ingestion of raw or incompletely cooked seafood. In the United States, most cases have been detected in common source outbreaks involving shellfish. In countries such as Japan, where raw fish is commonly eaten, *V. parahemolyticus* accounts for a significant portion of all diarrheal illnesses. The disease is usually self-limiting, and the course is not affected by antimicrobial therapy.

*V. parahemolyticus* infections from undercooked or raw seafood

Other halophilic *Vibrio* species may cause diarrhea or infections of cuts and wounds contaminated with seawater. Such infections typically involve seashore bathers or fishermen, or follow ingestion of raw shellfish. The most virulent member of this group is *V. vulnificus,* which in addition to wound infections and gastroenteritis, can produce a life-threatening bacteremia. Over a 10-year period there were 40 deaths in Florida from *V. vulnificus* infection; in 35 of these the organism was acquired by eating raw oysters. The risk of severe disease is much greater in persons with liver disease or iron-overload states (eg, thalassemia and hemochromatosis).

*V. vulnificus* causes sepsis or wound infections

Deaths linked to raw oysters, iron overload states

# CAMPYLOBACTER

Campylobacters are motile, curved, oxidase-positive, Gram-negative rods similar enough morphologically to vibrios for them to be classified together until recently. The cells have polar flagella and are often attached in pairs to give a "seagull" appearance. Campylobacters grow well only on enriched media under microaerophilic conditions (reduced oxygen tension but not strict anaerobiosis). Growth usually requires 2 to 4 days, sometimes as much as a week. In contrast to the vibrios and members of the *Enterobacteriaceae,* campylobacters are biochemically inactive. Of the *Campylobacter* species associated with human disease, *C. jejuni,* a common cause of diarrhea is the most important.

Gram morphology similar to vibrio

Require microaerophilic conditions for growth

In contrast to the marine habitat of vibrios, campylobacters are commonly found in the normal gastrointestinal and genitourinary flora of animals, including sheep, cattle, chick-

Commonly found in animals

ens, wild birds, and many others. Domestic animals such as dogs may also carry the organisms and probably play a significant role in transmission to humans.

## Campylobacter jejuni

One of the most common causes of diarrhea

Before 1973, *C. jejuni* was not recognized as a cause of human disease. It was not until selective media for its isolation were developed in the late 1970s that its importance was appreciated. This organism is now recognized as one of the most common causes of infectious diarrhea. Some other *Campylobacter* species are potential causes of diarrhea, but only *C. jejuni* will be discussed here.

## Campylobacter Enteritis

### Epidemiology

Up to 30% of all cases

It is humbling to consider how a pathogen as common as *C. jejuni* could have been missed for so many years. Studies throughout the world show isolation of *C. jejuni* from 4 to 30% of all cases of infectious diarrhea with less than 1% of healthy persons carrying the organism. The primary reservoir is in animals. Usually the source is raw or partially cooked poultry, but outbreaks have been caused by contaminated rural water supplies and unpasteurized milk often consumed as a "natural" food. Sometimes a direct association can be made as with a sick household pet.

Pets and undercooked foods common sources

### Pathogenesis and Immunity

Low infecting dose

Infection is established by oral ingestion followed by colonization of the intestinal mucosa. The infecting dose is probably low, as volunteers have been infected with as few as 500 cells. Adherence of *C. jejuni* to a number of cell types has been demonstrated, but the binding ligand has not been identified. A candidate enterotoxin and a cytotoxin have been described but their role in human disease is not yet established. *C. jejuni* is one of only a few organisms where flagella have been implicated in pathogenesis. Nonflagellated mutants are much less virulent in animal models of infection. *Campylobacter* entry into cultured animal cells has been described, but intracellular replication has not been shown to be part of the pathogenesis of infection. All in all, the virulence determinants of this microorganism remain uncertain. In its natural hosts, it resides in the caecum and is asymptomatically carried by adult animals. Acquired immunity following natural infection with *C. jejuni* has been demonstrated in volunteer studies, but the mechanisms involved are unknown.

Pathogenesis uncertain

## Campylobacterosis: Clinical Aspects

### Clinical Manifestations

Fever, abdominal pain, and diarrhea

The illness typically begins 1 to 7 days after ingestion with lower abdominal pain, which may be severe enough to mimic acute appendicitis. The abdominal pain is followed by diarrheal stools that usually contain blood and pus. Fever is commonly present. The illness is typically self-limiting after 3 to 5 days, but may last 1 to 2 weeks. The diagnosis is confirmed by isolation of the organism from the stool using a special medium made selective for *Campylobacter* by inclusion of antimicrobics that inhibit the normal facultative flora of the bowel. Plates must be incubated in a microaerophilic atmosphere that can now be conveniently generated in a sealed jar by hydration of commercial packs similar to those used for anaerobes.

Selective medium in microaerophilic atmosphere used for isolation

### Treatment

Usually self-limiting

*C. jejuni* is generally susceptible to erythromycin, tetracycline, chloramphenicol, the aminoglycosides, and the quinolones, but not to penicillins and cephalosporins. Because the disease is usually self-limiting, the effects of antimicrobics on its course remain unclear. Limited clinical experience indicates erythromycin may be effective if given early in the course of the illness.

Antimicrobics may shorten course

## C. fetus

*C. fetus* has long been recognized as a common cause of abortion in sheep and cattle and a rare cause of sepsis in humans. The most common human presentation is of intermittent fever without evidence of localized infection. Occasionally the meninges and heart valves may become infected, and thrombophlebitis is considered a typical feature although it occurs in only 10% of cases. The diagnosis is established by isolation of *C. fetus* from the blood.

A rare cause of sepsis without an obvious source

# HELICOBACTER

Barely a decade has passed since the first suggestion that chronic gastritis and peptic ulcers could be an infectious disease. Within some limits that suspicion has now been confirmed, and antimicrobial treatment regimens have provided the first lasting relief for one of the most common of all intestinal diseases. The causative agent, *Helicobacter pylori,* had long been observed in association with the gastric mucosa but dismissed as a commensal or secondary invader. It is now clear that this organism is one of a small family of microaerophilic Gram-negative bacilli uniquely adapted to take advantage of the ecologic niche of the stomach.

Long dismissed, *Helicobacter* now accepted cause of gastritis and ulcers

## Helicobacter pylori

*H. pylori* has many similarities to the campylobacters and was classified with them until recently. The cells are slender, curved rods that grow slowly (4 to 7 days) under microaerophilic conditions on the same media used for campylobacters. Their outstanding bacteriologic feature is the production of a urease so potent that its action can be demonstrated within minutes of inoculation of urea-containing test media. *H. pylori* is exclusive to humans, but other species have been found in the stomachs of many animals ranging from dogs to ferrets, where they are also associated with gastritis. It is difficult to imagine the old "stress ulcer" theories surviving the recent discovery of a cheetah with *Helicobacter* gastritis.

Many features similar to campylobacter

Potent urease is distinguishing feature

Animals have *Helicobacter* gastritis

## Helicobacter Gastritis

### Epidemiology

*H. pylori* is found in the most common form of gastritis, that occurring in the stomach antrum, formerly thought to be caused by stress, chemical irritation, bile reflux, or ischemia. Once established it shows remarkable ability to persist and cause inflammation, perhaps for life. Chronic and acute inflammation are present in both the epithelium and lamina propria often with epithelial destruction. This condition may progress no further but is a prerequisite for peptic ulceration. Helicobacters can be linked to virtually all gastric and duodenal ulcers other than those associated with use of nonsteroidal anti-inflammatory agents. Chronic gastritis is also a percussor of gastric adenocarcinoma. Epidemiologic studies have now shown gastric infection with *H. pylori* to increase the risk for this malignancy approximately six-fold.

Persistent cause of gastritis of the stomach antrum

Gastritis precedes peptic ulcer

Adenocarcinoma risk increased by *H. pylori*

### Pathogenesis

The importance of the above associations have stimulated intensive search for the molecular mechanisms involved. The role of cytotoxins, urease, mucinase, flagella, and other structures is under investigation. Urease currently occupies the dominant focus because of its ability to allow *H. pylori* to survive the extreme acid (pH 2.0) conditions of the stomach by splitting ammonia from urea, thus creating its own relatively alkaline microenvironment.

Urease aids survival in extreme acid environment of stomach

The ammonia and other urease products may also be responsible for injury by disruption of mucosal permeability via a toxic effect on the tight cell junctions of gastric epithelial cells. Injury may also be related to a cytotoxin belonging to the RTX family similar to

Urease and cytotoxin may cause injury

the *Escherichia coli* alpha-hemolysin and the *Bordetella pertussis* adenylate cyclase. This toxin may be the cause of vacuolation of gastric epithelial cells, a prominent histopathologic feature of the disease. It is still difficult to adequately exploit genetic and molecular methods because of the lack of an adequate animal model other than humans.

Organisms adhere to fucose and blood group antigens

Adhesin not yet identified

Recently, in-situ adherence assays have revealed the pattern of receptors for *H. pylori* in human tissues. Fluorescent-labeled *H. pylori* adhere selectively to epithelial cells of the gastrointestinal tract with the highest numbers in the gastric mucosa. In the gastric mucosa, adhesion was exclusive to the gastric pits and the luminal surface and with binding to fucose-containing carbohydrates. Fucose is a terminal component of the human ABO(H) and Lewis blood group antigens, which are expressed on the mucosal cells of the bowel. It is striking that Lewis and blood group O phenotypes are associated with an increased risk of ulcer disease. No specific bacterial adhesin has been identified, although electron microscopy shows binding to gastric mucosa by pilus-like structures.

## Helicobacter Gastritis: Clinical Aspects

### Clinical Manifestations and Diagnosis

Nausea, epigastric pain, leading to perforation

Culture or urease tests diagnostic

The clinical findings of both gastritis and peptic ulcer disease include nausea, anorexia, vomiting, epigastric pain, and even less specific symptoms such as belching. Many patients are asymptomatic for decades, even up to perforation of an ulcer. The diagnosis is best established by endoscopic examination with biopsy and culture of the gastric mucosa. Indirect diagnostic methods include antibody detection and a "breath test," which detects *H. pylori* urease in expired air. The advantage of direct detection of the organism is that culture is the most sensitive indicator of cure following therapy.

### Treatment and Prevention

Cures with low relapse rate using antimicrobics and bismuth salts

*H. pylori* is susceptible in vitro to a wide variety of classical antimicrobics and to bismuth salts. Cure rates approaching 95% have been achieved with a three-drug regimen combining bismuth salts and metronidazole with either tetracycline or amoxicillin. More importantly, relapse rates are low, something that was not true with the old ulcer treatment regimens. Immunization seems a distant goal for an organism that lives for decades with its host despite evidence of at least a humoral immune response.

## ADDITIONAL READING

Blake PA, Allegra DT, Snyder JD, et al: Cholera—A possible endemic focus in the United States. *N Engl J Med* 1980;302:305–309. This study was the first to detail the epidemiologic features of cholera cases along the Gulf Coast of Louisiana.

Falk P, Roth KA, Borén T, et al: An in-vitro adherence assay reveals that *Helicobacter pylori* exhibits cell lineage-specific tropism in the human gastric epithelium. *Proc Natl Acad Sci USA* 1993;90:2035–2039. This study describes an important experimental step in the direction of understanding *Helicobacter* gastritis.

Lee A, Fox J, Hazell S: Pathogenicity of *Helicobacter pylori*: A perspective. *Infect Immun* 1993;61:1601–1610. This brief review pinpoints the current status and future direction of *H. pylori* research.

Spangler BD: Structure and function of cholera toxin and the related *Escherichia coli* heat-labile enterotoxin. *Microbiol Rev* 1992;56:622–647. This review covers the pathogenic effects as well as structure of cholera toxin and its relation to other bacterial exotoxins.

Wachsmuth IK, Evins GM, Fields PI, Olsvik O, et al: The molecular epidemiology of cholera in Latin America. *J Infect Dis* 1993;167:621–626. This epidemiologic study applies the techniques of modern molecular biology to the spread of this historic disease.

Chapter 22

# *Pseudomonas* and Other Opportunistic Gram-negative Bacilli

*Kenneth J. Ryan and Stanley Falkow*

A number of opportunistic Gram-negative rods of several genera not considered in other chapters are discussed in this chapter. With the exception of *Pseudomonas aeruginosa,* they rarely cause disease, and all are frequently encountered as contaminants and superficial colonizers. The significance of their isolation from clinical material thus depends on the circumstance and site of culture and on the clinical situation of the patient.

## *PSEUDOMONAS AERUGINOSA*

### Bacteriology

*Pseudomonas aeruginosa* is an aerobic, motile, Gram-negative rod; its outstanding bacteriologic feature is the production of colorful water-soluble pigments. It is commonly found free living in moist environments, but is also a pathogen of plants, animals, and humans. As a cause of infection, it is particularly important in patients with severe burns, cystic fibrosis (CF), hematologic malignancies, and other immunocompromised states. *P. aeruginosa* also demonstrates the most consistent resistance to antimicrobics of all the medically important bacteria.

Gram-negative motile rod

#### Morphology and Structure

*P. aeruginosa* is generally slimmer and more pale staining than members of the *Enterobacteriaceae* family, but its length is comparable (0.5 × 2.5 μm). Its flagella are polar, but other morphologic differences from other Gram-negative bacteria are not sufficiently consistent to be diagnostically useful. Ultrastructural features are similar to those of other Gram-negative bacteria. The lipopolysaccharide (LPS) present in the cell wall has a core-lipid A structure with both common and variable components. The polysaccharide side chains extending from the outer membrane LPS are believed to determine serologic specificity of the variable component. A mucoid exopolysaccharide slime layer may be present and is prominent in some strains. Pili composed of repeating monomers of the pilin structural subunit extend from the cell surface.

Polar flagella, slime layer, and pili present

## Growth and Metabolism

Aerobes with simple growth requirements

*P. aeruginosa* is an aerobe sufficiently versatile in its growth and energy requirements to use simple molecules such as ammonia and carbon dioxide as sole nitrogen and carbon sources. Thus, it does not require enriched media for growth, and it can survive and multiply over a wide temperature range (20 to 42°C) in almost any environment, including those with a high salt content. The organism uses oxidative energy-producing mechanisms and has high level of cytochrome oxidase (oxidase positive). Although an aerobic atmosphere is necessary for optimal growth and metabolism, most strains will multiply slowly in an anaerobic environment if nitrate is present as an electron acceptor.

Oxidase positive

Growth on all common isolation media is luxurious, although not as rapid as that of the *Enterobacteriaceae*. Colonies are well developed after overnight incubation, usually show blue/green pigmentation, and have a delicate, fringed edge. Confluent growth often has a characteristic metallic sheen and intense "fruity" odor. Hemolysis is usually produced on blood agar. In broth, a surface pellicle is formed, reflecting the organism's preference for aerobic conditions and chemotaxis toward oxygen.

Fringed, irregular colonies with metallic sheen

## Classification

*P. aeruginosa* is one of several oxidase-positive, motile organisms to produce non-lactose-fermenting colonies on MacConkey agar. Its oxidase reaction differentiates it from the *Enterobacteriaceae*, and its production of blue, yellow, or rust-colored pigments differentiates it from most other Gram-negative bacteria. The blue pigment, **pyocyanin,** is produced only by *P. aeruginosa*; its demonstration, however, requires balance of metallic ions not found in all media that support its growth. **Pyoverdin,** a yellow pigment that fluoresces under ultraviolet light, is also produced by free-living nonpathogenic pseudomonads. Pyocyanin and pyoverdin combined produce a bright green color that diffuses throughout the medium. A rust-colored pigment, **pyorubrin,** is produced by a small proportion of strains. The combination of pyocyanin production and the ability to grow at 42°C is sufficient to distinguish *P. aeruginosa* from other pseudomonads.

No lactose fermentation

Blue pyocyanin and yellow pyoverdin combine for green color diffusing through medium imparts green color to growth

Several systems for subtyping *P. aeruginosa* have been developed. The most generally accepted includes 17 serotypes based on lipopolysaccharide O antigens. *Pseudomonas* bacteriocins (pyocins) and bacteriophages that lyse *P. aeruginosa* in up to 30 patterns have been isolated and organized into typing systems. Recently, a wide range of molecular techniques have proved useful in distinguishing strains involved in outbreaks.

Systems for subtyping include serologic, bacteriocin, and phage types

## Toxins and Extracellular Products

Most strains of *P. aeruginosa* produce extracellular products, including a toxin termed **exotoxin A,** proteolytic enzymes destructive to tissues, lecithinase, collagenase, and an elastase that could account for the destruction seen in arterial walls. Hemolysins (one of which is a phospholipase C) and a leukocidin have also been described. *P. aeruginosa* LPS endotoxin has biologic activities similar to other Gram-negative bacilli, but is roughly 10-fold less toxic than the endotoxin of *Enterobacteriaceae*.

Multiple extracellular enzymes produced

LPS less toxic than that of *Enterobacteriaceae*

**Exotoxin A** is 10,000 times more toxic to experimental animals than *Pseudomonas* endotoxin, and is found in more than 90% of clinical isolates. Mutants that lack exotoxin A have much decreased virulence for experimental animals, and antitoxin protects animals against otherwise fatal challenge with exotoxin-A-producing strains. The exotoxin A molecule possesses separate domains for cell membrane binding, translocation, and catalytic activity, all of which are distinct from diphtheria toxin. Exotoxin A enters cells via receptor-mediated endocytosis and is internalized into a low pH vesicle from which it translocates and reaches its target molecule. The toxin acts to inhibit protein synthesis by a mechanism identical to that of diphtheria toxin (Chapter 17). It catalyzes the ADP-ribosylation and thus the inactivation of elongation factor 2, leading to shutdown of protein synthesis and cell death.

Exotoxin A strongest correlate of virulence

Action same as diphtheria toxin

**Exoenzyme S** has been implicated as a virulence factor required by *P. aeruginosa* for dissemination from burn wounds and for tissue destruction in patients with chronic lung infection. In vitro it ADP-ribosylates several proteins including vimentin and a *ras* protein, but the physiologically important target protein(s) is not yet identified. *P. aeruginosa* also expresses an **elastase** that acts to inactivate a variety of biologically important proteins and processes. Its role as a virulence factor is supported by the list of substrates that it attacks,

Another ADP-ribosylating toxin

including elastin, human IgA and IgG, complement components, and some collagens. *P. aeruginosa* elastase shows homology with other proteases including those produced by *Legionella pneumophila* and *Vibrio cholerae*.

## P. aeruginosa Disease

### Epidemiology

The primary habitat of *P. aeruginosa* and other pseudomonads is environmental. They are found in water, soil, and various types of vegetation throughout the world. *P. aeruginosa* has been isolated from the throat and stool of 2 to 10% of healthy persons. Colonization rates may be higher in hospitalized patients. Infection with *P. aeruginosa,* rare in previously healthy persons, is one of the most important causes of invasive infection in compromised patients with serious underlying disease, such as leukemia, CF, and extensive burns. The organism's ability to survive and proliferate in water with minimal nutrients can lead to heavy contamination of any unsterile water, such as that in the humidifiers of respirators. Inhalation of aerosols from such sources can bypass the normal respiratory defense mechanisms and initiate pulmonary infection. Infections have resulted from the growth of *Pseudomonas* in medications, contact lens solutions, and even in some disinfectants. Sinks and faucet aerators may be heavily contaminated and serve as the environmental source for contamination of other items. It is important to recognize, however, that the simple finding of a few *P. aeruginosa* in solutions or sites not normally sterile (for example, drinking water or food) is not in itself abnormal or a cause for alarm. The risk lies in the proximity between items susceptible to contamination and patients uniquely predisposed to infection.

Primary habitat environmental

Produces invasive infections in immunocompromised hosts

Multiplication in humidifiers, solutions, and medications

### Pathogenesis and Immunity

Although *P. aeruginosa* is an opportunistic pathogen, it is one of particular virulence. The organism usually requires a significant break in first-line defenses (such as a wound) or a route past them (such as a contaminated solution or intratracheal tube) to initiate infection. Attachment to epithelial cells is the first step in infection and is likely mediated by pili that belong to the family of *N*-methylphenylalanine type pili similar to those of the gonococcus, and *V. cholerae*. Several other adhesins have been described that could be involved in the pathogenesis of respiratory infection. As yet, it is unclear which of these adhesins are operative during the infectious process. Epithelial cells from CF patients are less highly sialylated than normal epithelial cells and reportedly have increased receptors for *P. aeruginosa* attachment. These findings are experimentally consistent with a role for *Pseudomonas* pili in the initial recognition of asiloganglioside receptors on epithelial cells. Surface polysaccharides produced as a slime layer may also aid adherence to cells or the mucus blanket that covers them. A special case of the later occurs in patients with CF (see "Clinical Manifestations" later in the chapter). These strains produce large amounts of a copolymer of mannuronic and glucuronic acids referred to as alginate. This extracellular polysaccharide forms a glycocalyx that may promote adherence to respiratory epithelium and interfere with effective phagocytosis.

Need for break in first-line defenses

Pili similar to those of gonococci

Polysaccharide slime may mediate adherence

Alginate polymer forms glycocalyx

The relative roles of the cellular LPS and extracellular enzymes in virulence have been a source of some debate, but current opinion favors the latter as most important, particularly exotoxin A, exotoxin S, and elastase. The toxicity of *Pseudomonas* LPS is weak compared to that of the *Enterobacteriaceae*; it is a potent immunogen, however, and LPS-directed antibody may decrease the incidence of fatal burn infections. Exotoxin A production is associated with a fatal outcome in bacteremic patients, and antitoxin against it is associated with survival. No diphtheria-like systemic effect of exotoxin has been demonstrated, but its cytotoxic action correlates with the primarily invasive and locally destructive lesions seen in *P. aeruginosa* infections. The other exoenzymes are also associated with virulence in experimental systems and have actions destructive to cells including the cytoskeleton. Pyocyanin is able to kill cells through generation of reactive oxygen intermediates and has been shown to disrupt the function of human cilia, inhibit lymphocyte proliferation, and alter the function of phagocytes.

Extracellular enzymes of prime importance

LPS and exotoxin A are immunogenic

Pyocyanin inhibits ciliary action

The virulence of *P. aeruginosa* is therefore multifactorial and is under control of several regulatory pathways. Exotoxin A is controlled by a transcriptional activator that is subject to iron regulation. In contrast, environmental stimuli other than iron appear to be relevant for exotoxin S expression, which is regulated by its own transcriptional activator. Elastase expression requires the transcriptional activator LasR, which also enhances exotoxin A expression. Recently, it has been shown that LasR requires a diffusible inducer molecule called *Pseudomonas* autoinducer. This autoinducer provides *Pseudomonas* cells with a means of cell-to-cell communication for the regulation of virulence-associated genes. In response to cell density or other environmental and nutritional stimuli, this communication can coordinate the response of the microbe to varying conditions within the human host.

Multiple virulence factors regulated by iron and other environmental stimuli

Human immunity to *Pseudomonas* infection is not well understood, although some inferences can be drawn from animal studies and clinical observations. The importance of humoral immunity is supported by demonstration of a protective effect of various experimental vaccines and passive transfer of immunity with immune globulin. The strong propensity of *P. aeruginosa* to infect the immune-compromised host, particularly those with defective cell-mediated immunity, indicates that these responses are also important. Knowledge of the specific mechanisms involved is, however, lacking.

Humoral and cellular immune responses both important

## *P. aeruginosa* Disease: Clinical Aspects

### Clinical Manifestations

*P. aeruginosa* can produce any of the opportunistic extraintestinal infections caused by members of the *Enterobacteriaceae* family. Burn, wound, urinary tract, skin, eye, ear, and respiratory infections all occur and may progress to bacteremia. *P. aeruginosa* is also one of the most common causes of infection in environmentally contaminated wounds (for example, osteomyelitis after compound fractures).

Multiple opportunistic infections including burns and environmentally contaminated wounds

*P. aeruginosa* pneumonia is a severe infection particularly in patients with granulocytopenia. It is associated with alveolar necrosis, vascular invasion, infarcts, and bacteremia. It is also a common cause of otitis externa, including "swimmer's ear" and a rare but life-threatening "malignant" otitis externa seen in diabetics. Folliculitis of the skin may follow soaking in inadequately decontaminated hot tubs that can become heavily contaminated with the organism.

Common cause of otitis externa

The organism can cause conjunctivitis, keratitis, or endophthalmitis when introduced into the eye by trauma or contaminated medication or contact lens solution. Keratitis can progress rapidly and destroy the cornea within 24 to 48 hours. In some cases of *P. aeruginosa* bacteremia, cutaneous papules develop that progress to black, necrotic ulcers. It is called **ecthyma gangrenosum** and is the result of direct invasion and destruction of blood vessel walls by the organism.

Eye infections form contamination of contact lenses

Bacteremia leads to ecthyma gangrenosum

### *P. aeruginosa* and Cystic Fibrosis

*P. aeruginosa* is now the most common bacterial pathogen to complicate the management of patients with CF, an inherited disease of exocrine glands associated with excessive viscid mucus in the smaller respiratory passages. In a high proportion of cases the respiratory tract becomes colonized with *P. aeruginosa*, which, once established, becomes almost impossible to eradicate. This infection is a leading cause of morbidity and eventual death of these patients.

Respiratory colonization of CF patients becomes chronic

In CF patients the organisms do not invade the lung tissue, but remain in the bronchi, forming a kind of biofilm with associated microcolonies. A striking feature of this association is the presence of alginate-producing mucoid strains rarely seen in other circumstances. Several enzymes are involved in alginate biosynthesis, including a GDP mannose dehydrogenase that effectively channels carbohydrate intermediates into alginate. No less than four gene loci are involved in the transcriptional regulation of alginate biosynthesis. The environmental stimuli regulating the mucoid phenotype is unknown, although some investigators propose osmolarity and desiccation signals that may exist in the lung of CF patients. The end result is enhanced survival of *P. aeruginosa* through adherence and avoidance of phagocytosis. Some studies indicate that the alginate also interferes with the access and/or action of antimicrobics.

Environmental signals trigger multiple genes

Carbohydrates channeled to alginate

Biofilm enhances survival

### Treatment and Prevention

Of the pathogenic bacteria, *P. aeruginosa* is the organism most consistently resistant to antimicrobics. To a considerable extent this resistance is due to outer membrane porins that restrict the entry of antimicrobics to the periplasmic space. *P. aeruginosa* strains are regularly resistant to penicillin, ampicillin, cephalothin, tetracycline, chloramphenicol, sulfonamides, and the earlier aminoglycosides (streptomycin, kanamycin). Much effort has been directed toward the development of antimicrobics with anti-*Pseudomonas* activity. The aminoglycosides, gentamicin, tobramycin, and amikacin, are all active against most strains despite the presence of mutational and plasmid-mediated resistance. Carbenicillin and ticarcillin are active and can be given in high doses, but plasmid-mediated resistance and permeability mutations occur more frequently than with the aminoglycosides. A primary feature of the third-generation cephalosporins (ceftazidime), carbapenems (imipenem), or monobactams (azthreonam) is their activity against *Pseudomonas*. In general, urinary infections may be treated with a single drug; but more serious systemic *P. aeruginosa* infections are usually treated with a combination of an anti-*Pseudomonas* beta-lactam antimicrobic and an aminoglycoside, particularly in neutropenic patients. Ciprofloxacin is also used in treatment of such cases. In all instances susceptibility must be confirmed by in vitro susceptibility tests.

Multiresistance to antimicrobics by restricting permeability

Mutational and plasmid mediated resistance occurs to penicillins and aminoglycosides

Third-generation cephalosporins generally active

Vaccines incorporating somatic antigens from multiple *P. aeruginosa* serotypes have been developed and proved immunogenic in humans. The primary candidates for such preparations are patients with burn injuries, cystic fibrosis, or immunosuppression. Although some protection has been demonstrated, these preparations are still experimental.

Vaccines are experimental

## P. PSEUDOMALLEI AND P. MALLEI

*P. pseudomallei* can cause primary infections in otherwise healthy individuals. It is not found in temperate climates, but exists as a saprophyte in soil, ponds, rice paddies, and produce in Southeast Asia, the Philippines, Indonesia, and other tropical areas. Infection is acquired by direct inoculation or by inhalation of aerosols or dust containing the bacteria. The disease, **melioidosis,** is usually an acute pneumonia; however, it is sufficiently variable that subacute, chronic, and even relapsing infections may follow systemic spread. The clinical and radiologic features may resemble tuberculosis. In fulminant cases, rapid respiratory failure may ensue and metastatic abscesses develop in the skin or other sites. Tetracycline, chloramphenicol, sulfonamides, and trimethoprim-sulfamethoxazole have been effective in therapy.

Melioidosis acquired in tropical areas but relapses occur

**Glanders** is a disease of horses and some other mammals caused by *P. mallei.* Transmission to humans is extremely rare. The disease manifests as local suppurative or acute pulmonary infections.

## OTHER PSEUDOMONADS

There are a large number of other *Pseudomonas* species. They are classified into five groups based on ribosomal RNA/DNA homology together with biochemical and cultural tests. The total number of infections produced by these species is far lower than those produced by *P. aeruginosa* alone. They are most frequently seen as colonizers and contaminants. Those of medical importance are shown in Table 22–1, which does not include all the known rRNA groups or species. *P. cepacia* is an opportunistic organism that has been found to contaminate reagents, disinfectants, and medical devices in much the same manner as *P. aeruginosa.* It has also complicated the course of cystic fibrosis patients but without the mucoid colony type seen with *P. aeruginosa*. These pseudomonads cause only opportunistic infections, and the assignment of species names has little clinical importance beyond differentiation from *P. aeruginosa*. Reports vary regarding the frequency of their isolation from cases of bacteremia, arthritis, abscesses, wounds, conjunctivitis, and urinary tract infections. In general, unless isolated in pure culture from a high-quality (direct) specimen, it is difficult to attach pathogenic significance to any of the miscellaneous *Pseudomonas* species.

Ribosomal RNA homology used to classify

*P. cepacia* seen in same settings as *P. aeruginosa*

**TABLE 22–1. PSEUDOMONADS ASSOCIATED WITH HUMAN INFECTION**

| | Bacteriologic Features | | | | | |
|---|---|---|---|---|---|---|
| **Species** | ***Pyocyanin*** | ***Other Pigments*** | ***Fluo-rescence*** | ***Growth at 42°C*** | ***Amino-glycoside Resistance***[a] | **Disease** |
| *P. aeruginosa*[b] | + | + | + | + | 5–20% | Opportunistic |
| *P. fluorescens*[b] | – | + | + | – | Uncommon | Opportunistic |
| *P. putida*[b] | – | + | + | – | Uncommon | Opportunistic |
| *P. mallei*[b] | – | – | – | – | — | Glanders |
| *P. pseudomallei*[c] | – | – | – | + | 90% | Melioidosis |
| *P. cepacia*[c] | – | – | – | v | 90% | Opportunistic |
| *P. alcaligenes*[b] | – | – | – | v | Uncommon | Opportunistic |
| *P. stutzeri*[b] | – | – | – | v | Uncommon | Opportunistic |
| *P. acidovorans*[d] | – | – | – | v | Uncommon | Opportunistic |

*Abbreviations:* v, variable; +, usually positive (more than 90%); –, usually negative (less than 10%).
[a] Aminoglycoside resistance refers to gentamicin, tobramycin, amikacin, etc.
[b] rRNA group I.
[c] rRNA group II.
[d] RNA group III.

## ACINETOBACTER

Confused with Neisseria on Gram stain

Frequent in environment

The genus *Acinetobacter* comprises Gram-negative coccobacilli that occasionally appear sufficiently round on Gram smears to be confused with *Neisseria.* On primary isolation they closely resemble the *Enterobacteriaceae* in growth pattern and colonial morphology, but are distinguished by their failure to ferment carbohydrates or reduce nitrates. As with most of the organisms discussed in this chapter, the isolation of *Acinetobacter* from clinical material does not define infection, because they appear most frequently as colonizers and contaminants. Pneumonia is the most common infection, followed by urinary tract and soft tissue infections. Nosocomial respiratory infections have been traced to contaminated inhalation therapy equipment, and bacteremia to infected intravenous catheters. Treatment is complicated by frequent resistance to penicillins, cephalosporins, chloramphenicol, and occasionally aminoglycosides.

## MORAXELLA

Otitis media and respiratory infection

*Moraxella* is another genus of coccobacillary, Gram-negative rods that are usually paired end to end. Some species require enriched media, such as blood or chocolate agar. Their morphology, fastidious growth, and positive oxidase reaction can result in confusion with *Neisseria.* This is particularly true for *M. catarrhalis,* which for many years was classified with *Neisseria.* More recently it was called *Branhamella catarrhalis,* and is an occasional cause of otitis media and lower respiratory tract infection. Both infections relate to the presence of *M. catarrhalis* in the normal oropharyngeal flora.

Frequent β-lactamase producers

The organism now called *M. lacunata,* originally described as a cause of angular conjunctivitis, is an uncommon isolate from the eye and respiratory tract. With the exception of *M. catarrhalis,* which frequently produces beta lactamase, *Moraxella* species are generally susceptible to penicillin.

## AEROMONAS AND PLESIOMONAS

Colonies resemble *Enterobacteriaceae*

The genera *Aeromonas* and *Plesiomonas* have features similar to those of both the *Enterobacteriaceae* and *Pseudomonas.* They are aerobic and facultatively anaerobic, attack carbohydrates fermentatively, and demonstrate various other biochemical reactions. Their colonies and growth pattern resemble those of the *Enterobacteriaceae.* The major taxo-

**TABLE 22–2. CHARACTERISTICS OF MISCELLANEOUS GRAM-NEGATIVE BACILLI**

| | | Bacteriologic Features | | | | |
|---|---|---|---|---|---|---|
| **Organism** | **Usual Habitat** | ***Growth on MacConkey Agar*** | ***Oxidase*** | ***Motility*** | ***Other*** | **Infection** |
| *Alkaligenes* | Respiratory tract, intestinal tract | + | + | + | | Blood, urine, wounds |
| *Cardiobacterium* | Respiratory tract, intestinal tract | – | + | – | $CO_2$ required | Endocarditis |
| *Chromobacterium* | Environmental (tropical) | + | + | v | Blue to yellow pigments | Blood, abscesses |
| *Actinobacillus* | Oral | – | + | + | $CO_2$ required | Endocarditis |
| *Flavobacterium* | Environmental | – | + | – | Yellow pigment | Meningitis, nosocomial |
| *Eikenella* | Respiratory tract | – | + | – | $CO_2$ required; pits agar | Abscesses, endocarditis |
| *Xanthomonas maltophilia*[a] | Environmental | + | ± | + | — | Pneumonia, bacteremia |

*Abbreviations:* +, usually positive (more than 90%); –, usually negative (less than 10%); v, variable.
[a] Formerly *Pseudomonas maltophilia.*

nomic resemblance to *Pseudomonas* is that both *Aeromonas* and *Plesiomonas* are oxidase positive with polar flagella. Their habitat is basically environmental (water and soil), but they can occasionally be found in the human intestinal tract.

Found in soil and water

In addition to opportunistic infection, some evidence suggests an occasional role for *Aeromonas* in gastroenteritis through production of a toxin with enterotoxic and cytotoxic properties. This association is not yet strong enough to justify attempts to routinely isolate them from diarrheal stools. Resistance to penicillins and cephalosporins is common. Most strains show susceptibility to chloramphenicol and tetracycline, with variable susceptibility to aminoglycosides, including gentamicin.

Some strains produce gastroenteritis

## OTHER GRAM-NEGATIVE RODS

The terms "miscellaneous" or "nonfermenter" are used loosely by bacteriologists to describe Gram-negative rods that do not ferment carbohydrates or that fail to react in many of the tests used to characterize other bacteria. Identification is frequently delayed as additional tests are tried or the organism is sent to a reference laboratory. As the clinical significance of all these organisms is essentially the same, the clinician will usually receive a report of a "nonfermenter" or another descriptive term and a susceptibility test result. The significance of the isolate is then decided on clinical grounds. The major characteristics of some of these organisms are shown in Table 22–2. The types of infection listed represent the most common among scattered case reports, and should not be interpreted as typical for each organism.

Many isolates beyond routine identification procedures of clinical laboratories

Some Gram-negative bacilli fail to conform to any of the species currently recognized. If clinically important, such strains are sent to reference centers, such as the Centers for Disease Control (CDC) in Atlanta. Eventually, some are given designations such as "CDC group IIF," which may appear in clinical reports. Much later, a new genus and/or species name may be issued if agreement among taxonomists is sufficient.

## ADDITIONAL READING

May TB, Shinaburger D, Maharaj R, Litto J, et al: Alginate synthesis by *Pseudomonas aeruginosa:* A key pathogenic factor in chronic cystic fibrosis patients. *Clin Microbiol Rev* 1991;4:191–206. This review gives a complete account of the current clinical, pathogenesis, and genetic aspects of this unique infection.

Passador L, Cook JM, Gambello MJ, et al: Expression of *Pseudomonas aeruginosa* virulence genes requires cell-to-cell communication. *Science* 1993;260:1127–1130.

Prince A: Adhesins and receptors of *Pseudomonas aeruginosa* associated with infection of the respiratory tract. *Microbiol Pathogen* 1992;13:251–260.

Chapter 23

# *Haemophilus* and *Bordetella*

Kenneth J. Ryan and Stanley Falkow

*Haemophilus* and *Bordetella* are small, Gram-negative rods that tend to assume a coccobacillary shape. They are nonmotile, non-spore forming, with complex nutritional growth requirements for blood-containing media. Historically, these organisms were grouped together, although their biology is very different. Nevertheless, members of both genera contain species exclusively found in humans that cause respiratory infections; in addition, one species, *Haemophilus influenzae,* is responsible for a variety of systemic infections, including purulent meningitis.

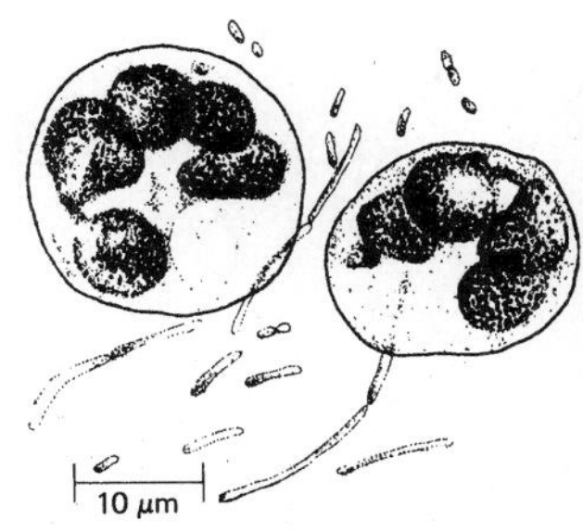

*Haemophilus influenzae in CSF*

## HAEMOPHILUS

### H. influenzae

#### Morphology and Structure

*Haemophilus* organisms are among the smallest of bacteria. The curved ends of the short (1.0 to 1.5 μm) bacilli makes many appear round, hence the term coccobacilli. The tiny cells are usually of uniform shape except in cerebrospinal fluid (CSF), where some may be elongated to several times their usual length.

The cell wall has a lipopolysaccharide–protein surface similar to that of other Gram-negative bacteria. *H. influenzae* may have a polysaccharide capsule, but other species of *Haemophilus* are not encapsulated. Capsulate *H. influenzae* are divided into six serotypes, designated a to f, based on the capsular polysaccharide antigen. The type b capsule is made up of a polymer of ribose, ribitol, and phosphate, called polyribitol phosphate (PRP). These surface polysaccharides are strongly associated with virulence, particularly *H. influenzae* type b (Hib), which is responsible for most cases of serious systemic infection. Cell-wall (somatic) antigens of capsulated and non-encapsulated *Haemophilus* have not been associated with virulence.

Six serotypes based on polysaccharide capsule

Type b capsule is polyribotol phosphate

#### Growth

In addition to the usual components of enriched culture media, *Haemophilus* (Greek "haema," blood, and "philos," loving) species require added blood products for optimal growth. This requirement is attributable to the need for hematin and/or nicotinamide adenine dinucleotide (NAD) as growth factors. These growth factors, also termed X factor (hematin) and V factor (NAD), are both present in erythrocytes. In culture media, optimal concentrations of X and, particularly, V factors are not available to *Haemophilus* from blood unless the red blood cells are lysed by gentle heat (chocolate agar) or digested and added separately as a supplement. Although erythrocytes are the only convenient source of hematin, the V factor is present in a variety of biologic materials and is produced by some

Growth requirement for hematin (X) and NAD (V)

Chocolate agar has X and Y

Satellitism around colonies of *S. aureus* based on V factor

other bacteria and yeast. These conditions are responsible for the "satellite phenomenon," in which *H. influenzae* grows on blood agar only in the vicinity of a colony of *Staphylococcus aureus* that is producing V factor.

Broth media need supplements

When their nutritional needs are met, most *Haemophilus* species grow rapidly, producing 1- to 2-mm translucent colonies after overnight incubation under aerobic or anaerobic conditions. Encapsulated strains may produce larger colonies with a glistening mucoid quality. Commonly used broth media fail to support good growth of *Haemophilus,* unless whole blood is added with the inoculum (as in blood cultures). Even then, the organisms may not become sufficiently numerous to produce turbidity unless supplements are added.

## H. influenzae Disease

### Epidemiology

Meningitis in children under 2 years

Prior to the introduction of effective vaccines, approximately 1 in every 200 children developed invasive Hib disease by the age of 5 years. Meningitis is the most common form and most often attacks those under 2 years of age. Cases of epiglottitis and pneumonia tend to peak in the 2- to 5-year age range. The rates of disease have declined dramatically since 1989 (see "Prevention" later in the chapter).

Spread unless protected by vaccine or prophylaxis

At one time *H. meningitis* was believed to be an isolated endogenous infection, but reports of outbreaks in closed populations and careful epidemiologic studies of secondary spread in families have changed this view. The risk of serious infection for unimmunized children under 4 years of age living with an index case is more than 500-fold that for nonexposed children. This risk indicates a need for prophylaxis for contacts in the susceptible age group. Rifampin is currently recommended for this purpose.

### Pathogenesis

Carrier rates in health high

Various *Haemophilus* species are common inhabitants of the upper respiratory tract. Carrier rates for *H. influenzae* as high as 80% have been found in children, and are commonly 20 to 50% in healthy adults. Most strains are non-encapsulated, but healthy carriers of encapsulated strains are common. The events that cause these organisms to initiate disease are poorly understood and differ for encapsulated and unencapsulated *Haemophilus* strains.

Invasion of Hib from nasopharynx

Limited number of Hib clones account for disease

Systemic spread is typical only for encapsulated *H. influenzae* strains, and over 90% of invasive strains are type b. Virulent Hib strains occasionally invade into the deeper tissues beyond the nasopharynx. Bacteremia then leads to spread to the central nervous system and metastatic infections at distant sites such as bones and joints. It is of interest that 182 distinct Hib clones characterized by enzyme profiles have been identified in natural populations worldwide, but only 9 account for about 80% of all invasive disease. Conversely, one *H. influenzae* clone rarely associated with invasive disease is frequently carried in the upper respiratory tract without associated symptoms. When we understand the full significance of these molecular epidemiologic findings we will have a better grasp on the true pathogenesis of *H. influenzae* invasive disease.

Localized infections primarily nonencapsulated strains

Adherence of noncapsulate strains related to pili and surface proteins

Consistent with their relative prevalence in the respiratory tract, nontypeable organisms account for more than 90% of localized *H. influenzae* disease, particularly otitis media, sinusitis, and exacerbations of chronic bronchitis. Like other Gram-negative bacteria, nontypeable *H. influenzae* have common pili capable of promoting attachment to host cells and that are probably involved in the process of colonization. However, a family of nonpilus, surface-exposed, high-molecular-weight proteins has also been identified recently in nontypeable strains but not in encapsulated strains. The high-molecular-weight proteins HMW1 and HMW2 show homology with the filamentous hemagglutinin that plays an essential role in adherence of *Bordetella pertussis* to ciliated epithelial cells (see below). Yet HMW1 and HMW2 interact with different specific host cell receptor molecules whose distribution varies from one cell type to another. It is possible that these proteins contribute to the tissue tropism demonstrated by nontypeable *H. influenzae* for the conjunctiva, middle ear, larynx, and even the genitalia.

Antiphagocytic effect of capsule

The pathogenic mechanisms involved in Hib infection remain to be fully understood. The capsule is antiphagocytic and probably the most significant determinant of virulence. There is some evidence to suggest that there is a complex regulatory cascade coordinating capsular biosynthesis and adherence factors that act cooperatively in establishing the microbe within susceptible hosts. Infection is a very common consequence of the bacteria–host cell interaction; disease is less common and seems to occur within a short period (less than 3 days) after the initial encounter. *H. influenzae* can be seen to transcytose through the cells of the epithelial layer in organ cultures of nasopharyngeal tissue. The microbial factors determining this property have not yet been identified. Endotoxin in the cell wall is toxic to ciliated respiratory cells, but endotoxemia is not a prominent feature of *Haemophilus* infection to the extent that it is with *Neisseria meningitidis. H. influenzae* produces no exotoxin, but elaborates an IgA protease that may facilitate colonization.

Capsule and adherence factors regulated together

Disease follows soon after initial encounter

Endotoxin acts on ciliated cells

### Immunity

Immunity to Hib infections has been clearly associated with the presence of anticapsular (PRP) antibodies, which are bactericidal in the presence of complement. The infant is usually protected by passively acquired maternal antibody for the first few months of life. Thereafter the presence of actively acquired antibody increases with age; it is present in the serum of most children by age 10. The peak incidence of Hib infections is 6 to 18 months of age, when serum antibody is least likely to be present. This inverse relationship between infection and serum antibody is similar to that for *N. meningitidis* (see Fig 19–2). The major difference is that immunity requires antibody directed against only a single type (Hib) rather than several serogroups. Thus, systemic *H. influenzae* infections (meningitis, epiglottitis, cellulitis) are rare in adults. When such infections develop, however, the immunologic deficit is probably the same as that with meningococci: lack of circulating antibody.

Anticapsular and bactericidal antibody is protective

Hib infections most common at ages when antibody titer is lowest

Like many polysaccharides, Hib PRP behaves as a T-cell-independent antigen. B cells mount the primary response without significant involvement of T-helper cells. Antibody responses from disease or immunization with PRP are variable and typically poor under 18 months of age. Significant secondary responses from boosters are not elicited. Conjugation of PRP to protein dramatically improves the immunogenicity by eliciting the T-cell responses typical of protein antigens while preserving the specificity for PRP.

T-cell-independent response to PRP poor under 18 months

## H. influenzae Disease: Clinical Aspects

### Clinical Manifestations

#### Hib Meningitis

Hib meningitis follows the same pattern as other causes of acute purulent bacterial meningitis (Chapter 67). Meningitis is often preceded by signs and symptoms of an upper respiratory infection, such as nasopharyngitis, sinusitis, or otitis media. Whether these represent a predisposing viral infection or early invasion by the organism is not known. Just as often, meningitis is preceded only by vague malaise, lethargy, irritability, and fever. Mortality is currently 3 to 6% despite appropriate therapy, and roughly one third of all survivors have significant neurologic sequelae.

Acute purulent meningitis may follow sinusitis or otitis media

Outset may be vague

#### Hib Acute Epiglottitis

Hib is one cause of acute epiglottitis. It is a dramatic infection in which the inflamed epiglottis and surrounding tissues obstruct the airway. The onset is sudden, with fever, sore throat, hoarseness, a barking cough, and rapid progression to severe prostration within 24 hours. The child has air hunger, inspiratory stridor, and retraction of the soft parts of the chest with each inspiration. The hallmark of the disease is an inflamed, swollen, cherry-red epiglottis that protrudes into the airway and can be visualized on lateral x-rays. As with meningitis, this infection is treated as a medical emergency with prime emphasis on antimicrobics and maintenance of an airway (tracheostomy). Manipulations, including routine examination or attempting to take a throat swab, can be fatal by triggering laryngospasm and acute obstruction.

Cherry-red swollen epiglottis and barking cough

Airway maintenance needed

#### Hib Cellulitis

A tender, reddish-blue swelling in the cheek or periorbital areas is the usual presentation of Hib cellulitis. Fever and a moderately toxic state are usually present, and the infection may follow an upper respiratory infection or otitis media. A large proportion of cases are bacteremic, and some develop infections at other sites.

ARTHRITIS

Large joints involved

Joint infection may follow another manifestation of *H. influenzae* infection or appear as the primary illness. Local signs of inflammation in single, large, weight-bearing joints with fever and irritability are the usual features. *Haemophilus* arthritis is occasionally the cause of a more subtle set of findings, in which fever occurs without clear clinical evidence of joint involvement. Bacteremia is usually present.

OTHER RESPIRATORY INFECTIONS

Displacement of normal flora into lumina

Noncapsulate strains common in otitis media, sinusitis, and bronchitis

Bronchitis linked to underlying damage

*H. influenzae* is the second most common cause of otitis media and acute and chronic sinusitis, as well as one of several common respiratory organisms that can cause and exacerbate chronic bronchitis. These infections usually result from displacement of the normal flora into normally sterile luminal structures. Thus, most of these *H. influenzae* infections are caused by non-encapsulated and thus nontypable strains found commonly in the respiratory flora. Infection usually remain localized without bacteremia. Disease may be acute or chronic, depending on the anatomic site and underlying pathology. For example, otitis media is acute and painful because of the small, closed space involved, but usually clears without sequelae after antimicrobic therapy and reopening of the eustachian tube. The association of *H. influenzae* with chronic bronchitis is more complex. There is evidence that *H. influenzae* and other bacteria play a role in inflammatory exacerbations, but a unique cause and effect relationship is difficult to prove. The underlying cause of the bronchitis is usually related to chronic damage resulting from smoking or other factors.

*Haemophilus* pneumonia may be caused by either encapsulated or non-encapsulated organisms. Encapsulated strains have been observed to produce a disease much like pneumococcal pneumonitis; however, unencapsulated strains may also produce pneumonia, particularly in patients with chronic bronchitis.

## Diagnosis

Blood cultures useful in systemic infections

The combination of clinical findings and a typical Gram smear is usually sufficient to make a presumptive diagnosis of *Haemophilus* infection. This diagnosis must then be confirmed by isolation of the organism from the site of infection or from the blood. Blood cultures are particularly useful in systemic *H. influenzae* infections, because it is often difficult to get an adequate specimen directly from the site of infection. A large proportion of these cases are bacteremic and thus the organism can be detected with blood cultures.

Demonstration of growth factor requirements

Bacteriologically, small coccobacillary Gram-negative rods that grow on chocolate agar but not blood agar strongly suggest *Haemophilus.* Confirmation and speciation depends on demonstration of the requirement for X and V factors and/or biochemical tests. Serotyping, despite the importance of antibody in pathogenesis, is usually unnecessary for clinical purposes.

Type b capsular PRP antigen present in body fluids

Hib PRP is released into body fluids and circulates during the course of infection. It may be demonstrated in CSF, blood, or urine by antigen-detection methods such as latex agglutination (Chapter 14). These procedures are not dependent on the presence of live organisms and are particularly helpful when cultures are negative because of prior antimicrobial therapy.

## Treatment

Ampicillin-resistant strains produce β-lactamase

Resistance rate highly variable

*H. influenzae* is usually susceptible in vitro to ampicillin and amoxicillin, the newer cephalosporins, chloramphenicol, tetracycline, aminoglycosides, and sulfonamides. It is less susceptible to other penicillins and to erythromycin. *Haemophilus* meningitis has been treated effectively with ampicillin, chloramphenicol, and the newer cephalosporins. Since 1974, the therapy of systemic infections has been complicated by the emergence of strains that produce a plasmid-mediated beta-lactamase identical to that found in some enterics, such as *Escherichia coli.* The frequency of resistant strains varies between 5 and 50% in different geographic areas. Although ampicillin-resistant strains that do not produce beta-lactamase have also been described, they are uncommon, as are chloramphenicol-resistant *H. influenzae*. Current practice is to start empiric therapy with a third-generation cephalosporin (eg, ceftriaxone, cefotaxime), which can be changed to ampicillin if susceptibility tests indicate that the infecting strain is susceptible.

Third-generation cephalosporin used

### Prevention

Purified PRP vaccines became available in 1985, but due to the typically poor immune response of infants to polysaccharide antigens their use was limited to children 24 months of age and older. Because immunization at this age misses the peak incidence of Hib invasive disease, a new vaccine strategy was needed that included improved stimulation of T-cell-dependent immune responses in infants. To achieve this three PRP-protein conjugate vaccines were developed using proteins derived from *Corynebacterium diphtheriae* (toxoid, CRM 197) or *Neisseria meningitidis* (outer membrane protein). The first PRP-protein conjugate vaccines were licensed in 1989 and by late 1990 were recommended for universal immunization beginning at two months of age. The impact has been dramatic (Fig 23–1). In a large surveillance study conducted by the Centers for Disease Control, the incidence of invasive Hib disease dropped 71% between 1989 and 1991. All evidence indicates this trend has continued to the point where this long-dominant pathogen of childhood is becoming a rarity where immunization is universal. An unexpected concomitant finding has been a dramatic drop in *H. influenzae* colonization rates in immunized populations. This suggests a role for PRP beyond confounding opsonophagocytosis.

Early vaccines missed peak age of disease

PRP conjugated to other bacterial proteins

Universal immunization at 2 months produced dramatic reduction in Hib disease

## Other Species of Haemophilus

Several other *Haemophilus* species exist and are defined by their requirement for X and/or V factor, $CO_2$ dependence, and other cultural characteristics (Table 23–1). The respiratory species, of which *H. parainfluenzae* is the most common, have the same biology as the non-encapsulated strains of *H. influenzae*. An organism isolated from outbreaks of conjunctivitis, formerly assigned the name *H. aegyptius,* is now considered a specific biotype of *H. influenzae*. One clonal variant of the *aegyptius* type is responsible for a systemic syndrome called Brazilian purpuric fever, which is a fulminant pediatric disease characterized by fever, shock, and often death. Preceding the dramatic systemic findings is a purulent conjunctivitis that resolves before the onset of fever. It is a rare complication of conjunctivitis leading to speculation that a particular clone of *aegyptius* affects patients with a particular immune constitution. Most of these other *Haemophilus* species have been reported to cause systemic illness, including pneumonia, meningitis, arthritis, endocarditis, and soft tissue in-

Other species similar to noncapsulated *H. influenzae*

*Aegyptius* biotypes can produce fulminant fever

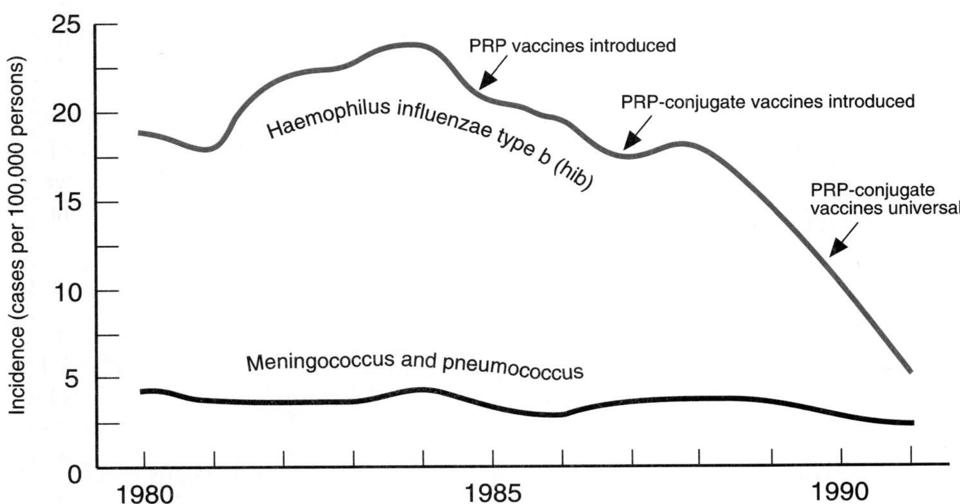


**Figure 23–1.** The decline of Hib meningitis. Recent decline in *H. influenzae* type b (Hib) meningitis and its association with the introduction of new vaccines is shown. (*Adapted from Adams WG, Deaver KA, Cochi SL, et al: Decline of childhood* Haemophilus influenzae *type b (Hib) disease in the Hib vaccine era.* JAMA *1993;269:221–226.*)

**TABLE 23–1. CHARACTERISTICS OF HAEMOPHILUS SPECIES**

| Haemophilus Species | Growth Factor Requirement | | Hemolysis | Enhanced Growth With $CO_2$ | Polysaccharide Capsular Antigen |
|---|---|---|---|---|---|
| | *X* | *V* | | | |
| *H. influenzae* (encapsulated) | + | + | – | – | Types a–f |
| *H. influenzae* (nonencapsulated) | + | + | – | – | – |
| *H. parainfluenzae* | – | + | – | – | – |
| *H. haemolyticus* | + | + | + | – | – |
| *H. aphrophilus* | – | – | – | + | – |
| *H. paraaphrophilus* | – | + | – | + | – |
| *H. ducreyi* | + | – | – | – | – |

*Abbreviations:* X, hematin; V, nicotinamide adenine dinucleotide.

fections. Such cases are rare, as are those in which non-encapsulated *H. influenzae* causes invasive disease.

### H. ducreyi

Soft chancre a genital ulcer with satellite lesions

*H. ducreyi* causes chancroid, a common venereal disease in developing countries. Although much less frequent, it has caused occasional outbreaks in North America. The typical lesion is a tender papule on the genitalia that develops into a painful ulcer with sharp margins. Satellite lesions may develop by autoinfection, and regional lymphadenitis is common. The incubation period is usually short (2 to 5 days). The lack of induration around the ulcer in chancroid has caused the primary lesion to be called "soft chancre" to distinguish it from the primary syphilitic chancre, which is typically indurated and painless. The presence of open genital sores due to *H. ducreyi* enhances the risk of transmission of HIV. This may contribute to the heterosexual spread of AIDS on the African continent, where chancroid is common.

May contribute to spread of AIDS in Africa

Culture of *H. ducreyi* is difficult, but the organism can be isolated on chocolate agar, particularly if vancomycin is added to inhibit interfering flora. The bacteria are present in small numbers and may take up to 10 days to grow. Clinical laboratories must be specifically instructed to search for the organism when the disease is suspected. Little is known about the pathogenic determinants of *H. ducreyi*. Indeed, on the basis of 16S ribosomal sequence analysis it may be that this microbe is more closely related to *Pasteurella* species than to other *Haemophilus* species. In any event, recent findings suggest that *H. ducreyi* isolates possess a capsule and have the ability to bind to and even enter certain types of epithelial cell.

Isolation is difficult

## BORDETELLA

## ■ B. pertussis

*B. pertussis* is a coccobacillus with Gram-stain morphology similar to that of *Haemophilus*. The organisms are strict aerobes and nonmotile. Infection of the human tracheobronchial epithelium produces pertussis (whooping cough), a prolonged disease marked by paroxysmal coughing.

### Structure and Growth

Small piliated Gram-negative coccobacilli

*B. pertussis* is a tiny (0.5 to 1.0 μm), Gram-negative coccobacillus with highly regular staining characteristics. The cell wall has the structure typical of Gram-negative bacteria. The surface exhibits pili and a rodlike protein called the filamentous hemagglutinin (Fha), which can bind to and agglutinate erythrocytes.

*B. pertussis* is slow growing and requires special medium for isolation. The organism is also very susceptible to environmental changes and survives only briefly outside the human respiratory tract. Aerobic incubation for 3 to 7 days is required for growth of tiny, glistening, compact colonies with the appearance of bisected pearls.

### Virulence Factors

ADHESINS

*B. pertussis* produces a number of adhesins, the most important of which is thought to be the filamentous hemagglutinin (Fha). Fha is a large 220-kd protein that may have separate domains to interact with ciliated epithelial cells and macrophages. In addition, the organism produces pili and an adhesin called pertactin that may have binding properties similar to Fha. These adhesins act in concert with a consortium of toxins that are responsible for most of the features of clinical disease.

Fha and other adhesins mediate adherence to ciliated cells

PERTUSSIS TOXIN (PT)

Pertussis toxin (PT) is the major virulence factor of *B. pertussis*. It is a classic A-B toxin produced from a single operon as an enzymatic subunit (S1) and five distinct binding subunits that are assembled into the complete toxin presumably on the bacterial surface. The binding subunits mediate attachment of the toxin to carbohydrate moieties on the host cell surface, and the enzymatic subunit is internalized and ADP-ribosylates a G-protein that affects adenylate cyclase activity. Unlike cholera toxin, which in essence keeps cyclase activity "turned on," pertussis toxin freezes the opposite side of the regulatory circuit and cripples the capacity of the host cell to inactivate cyclase activity.

PT is an A-B toxin

ADP-ribosylates G protein

The biologic effects of PT depend on the host cell type involved. These include histamine sensitization, promotion of lymphocytosis, insulin secretion, and a variety of actions involving immune effector cells. The toxin is unusual in that its binding subunits also act in concert with Fha as adhesins in binding to both ciliated cells and the CR3 receptor of macrophages. It has been speculated that the latter binding leads to an uptake pathway that does not stimulate the oxidative killing pathway within the phagocytic cells. The concerted binding of toxin and adhesive factors to the host cell results in the efficient delivery of the bacterial virulence factors to specific targeted cell types.

Multiple actions depending on the cell type

OTHER TOXINS

Another potent toxin, an invasive adenylate cyclase, enters the host cell and raises host cell cAMP levels. This extracellular enzyme is hemolytic and interferes with chemotaxis and superoxide production by polymorphonuclear leukocytes. Remarkably, it is activated by calmodulin, a eukaryotic $Ca^{2+}$-binding protein. Such activation of a bacterial enzyme by an intracellular mammalian protein is unusual, but is also seen with another bacterial adenylate cyclase, anthrax toxin (Chapter 17).

*B. pertussis* produces its own adenylate cyclase

Tracheal cytotoxin resembles a fragment of cell-wall peptidoglycan: (1,6 anhydromuramic acid-*N*-acetyl-glucosamine-tetrapeptide). This substance is released by multiplying bacterial cells and causes the death and extrusion ciliated cells in tracheal ring organ cultures. Concomitantly there is a release of the cytokine Il-1. *B. pertussis* cells also encode a dermonecrotic toxin, and like other Gram-negative rods produce LPS.

Peptidoglycan fragments injure tracheal cells

## ■ Pertussis (Whooping Cough)

### Epidemiology

*B. pertussis* is spread by airborne droplet nuclei to those in close contact with a patient in the early stages of illness. It is highly infectious. Secondary spread in families, schools, and hospitals is common although often not recognized due the mildness of symptoms in immunized persons. Sporadic epidemics occur, and there is no strong seasonal pattern to the disease. Adult cases with symptoms resembling the common cold are a significant reservoir of the organism, and have been the source of outbreaks in highly susceptible populations, such as newborns.

High infectivity, spread by airborne droplet nuclei

Atypical or subclinical disease in adults acts as reservoir

The incidence of pertussis decreased markedly in the United States after the introduction of immunization in the 1940s, but then increased through the 1980s to a 20-year peak of 1.8 cases per 100,000 population in 1990. In general, pertussis has increased when immunization rates have decreased. For example, when immunization rates in England fell below

Effectiveness of immunization repeatedly demonstrated

Fatal cases in infants

50% in 1981 pertussis cases rose dramatically; there were 47,000 cases in the first 9 months of 1982 alone. Mortality has dropped in accordance with the decreased incidence of disease, but remains highest in infants. Over 70% of fatal cases are in children under 1 year of age.

## Pathogenesis

Only infects humans

*B. pertussis* is a strict human pathogen. When introduced into the respiratory tract, the organism has a remarkable tropism for ciliated bronchial epithelium mediated by the adhesins described above. The bacteria first attach to and immobilize the cilia. This action begins a sequence in which the ciliated epithelial cells are progressively destroyed and extruded from the epithelial border (Fig 23–2) primarily by the action of the tracheal cytotoxin. Pertussis toxin is clearly responsible for many of the systemic manifestations of the disease such as lymphocytosis, but its role in local injury, cough, or the prolonged course of the illness is unclear. The adenylate cyclase probably plays an antiphagocytic role by virtue of its direct action on phagocytes. Although considerable local inflammation and exudate are produced in the bronchi, *B. pertussis* does not directly invade the cells of the respiratory tract.

Attachment to cilia progresses to death of cell

### Regulation of Pathogenicity

Single locus controls multiple unlinked virulence genes

The expression of virulence genes by *B. pertussis* is often used as a model for the coordinated control of bacterial pathogenicity. *B. pertussis* regulates the synthesis of pertussis toxin, the invasive adenylate cyclase, Fha, pili, dermonecrotic toxin, and many other genes through the pleiotropic *bvg* (*B. pertussis* virulence gene) genetic locus. This locus controls the expression of at least 20 unlinked chromosomal genes at the transcriptional level; expression is modulated by changes in specific environmental parameters, including temperature. *Bordetella* also possesses genes whose expression is silenced by *bvg*.

Regulatory genes respond to temperature and ionic changes in the environment

Transcriptional regulation is controlled by a two-gene operon consisting of BvgA and BvgS (Fig 23–3). BvgS is a member of the histidine kinase sensor class of bacterial regulatory proteins that spans the bacterial cytoplasmic membrane where it probably exists as a multimer. A periplasmic domain responds to temperature or ionic changes. At 37°C, BvgS autophosphorylates two domains and subsequently donates a phosphate group to the cytoplasmic protein BvgA, a member of the class of bacterial protein response regulators. BvgA then binds to a DNA recognition sequence located upstream of both the bvgAS operon and at least the Fha and fimbrial structural genes and promotes the transcription of these genes. Although BvgA and BvgS are also required for expression of pertussis toxin and the invasive cyclase, their direct participation has not yet been clearly defined. It is clear that *Bvg-*

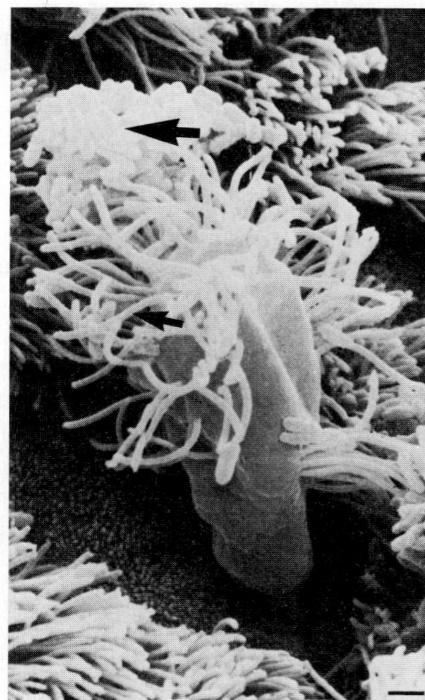

**Figure 23–2.** A tracheal organ culture 72 hr after infection with *B. pertussis*. The organisms have attached to the cilia of some cells and killed them. These balloon-like cells with attached bacteria are extruded from the epithelium. The large arrow shows the *Bordetella* and the small arrow the cilia. Note the background of uninfected ciliated cells and denuded epithelium where nonciliated cells remain. (*Reproduced with permission from Muse, K. E., Collier, A. M., and Baseman, J. B. 1977.* J. Infect Dis. *136:768–777. Figure 3, copyright 1977 by University of Chicago, publisher.*)

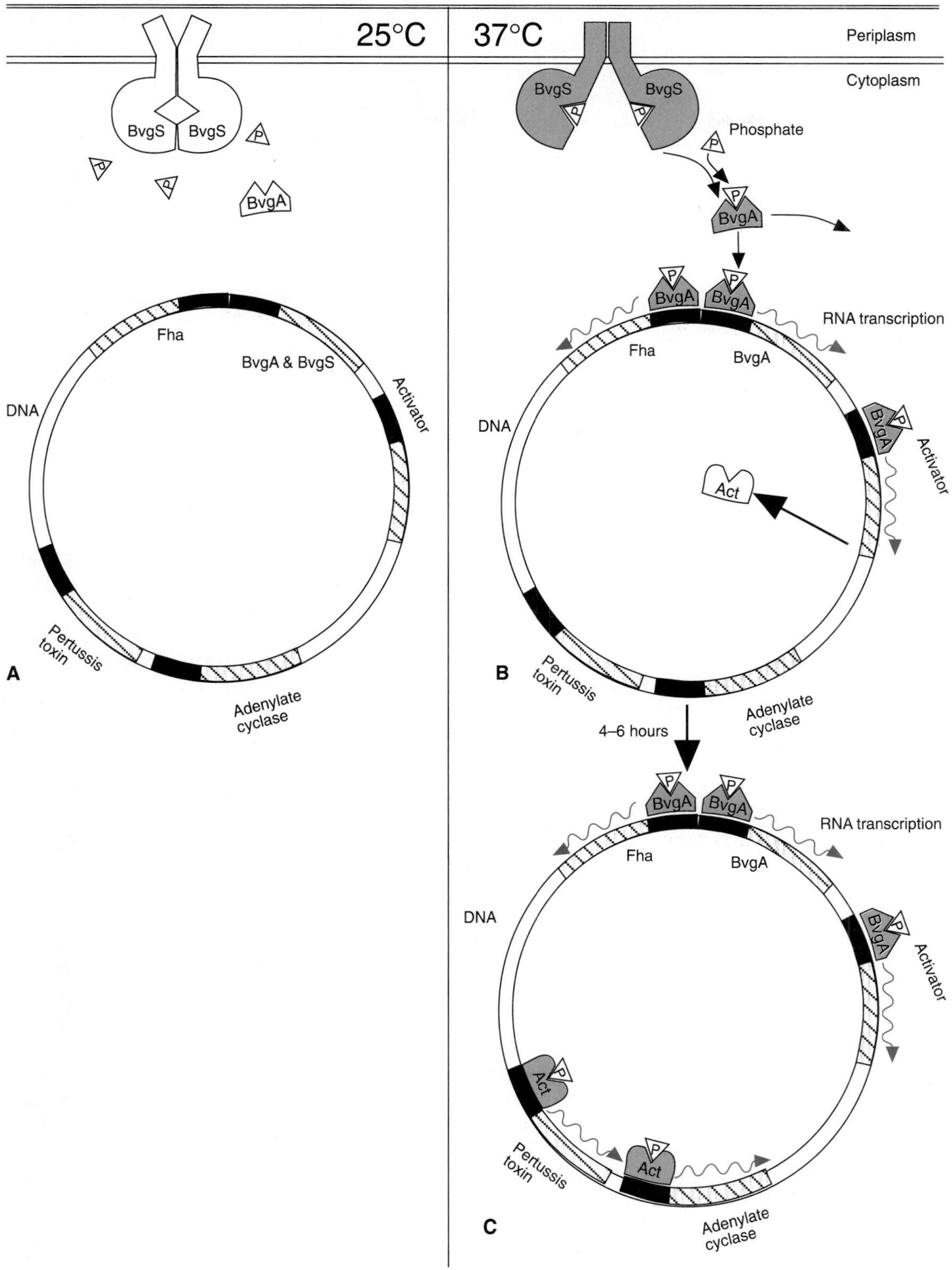


**Figure 23–3.** Regulation of *B. pertussis* virulence factors. **A.** At 25°C the membrane-associated regulatory protein BvgS is inactive as are the genes for virulence factors filamentous hemagglutinin (Fha), pertussis toxin, and adenylate cyclase. **B.** At 37°C BvgS autophosporylates and activates a cytoplasmic regulatory protein, BvgA, by phosphorylation. BvgA activates transcription of genes for production of BvgS, BvgA, Fha, and a postulated second regulator, Act. **C.** Hours later transcription of the pertussis toxin and adenylate cyclase is activated by Act. (*Adapted from Melton, AR, Weiss AA: Characterization of environmental regulators of* Bordetella pertussis. *Infect Immun 1993;61:807–815.*)

Virulence factor genes are sequentially activated

dependent gene activation is temporally regulated. The first step in shifting a culture from 25 to 37°C involves the transcriptional activation of Fha and pilin genes. The level of BvgA protein increases, and subsequently, about 6 hours later under laboratory conditions, the levels of pertussis toxin and adenylate cyclase mRNA increase proportionally.

Thus, the induction of virulence factors in *B. pertussis* is sequential with adhesin expression (Fha and pili) preceding expression of factors involved in tissue injury. The finely honed response of *B. pertussis* virulence factors to changes in temperature and ionic conditions presumably play a role in the pathogenesis of infection and help it adapt in a stepwise fashion to the diverse local conditions within the human respiratory tract.

### Immunity

Immune mechanisms not well known

Although antibodies are produced during the course of pertussis and by immunization, their role in immunity is not well understood. Naturally acquired immunity is not lifelong, although second attacks, when recognized, tend to be mild. The high susceptibility of newborns and infants before immunization may reflect a low level of antibody in adults and thus lack of passive transfer to the infant at birth.

## Pertussis: Clinical Aspects

### Clinical Manifestations

After an incubation period of 7 to 10 days, pertussis follows a prolonged course consisting of three overlapping stages: (1) catarrhal, (2) paroxysmal coughing, and (3) convalescent. In the catarrhal stage, the primary feature is a profuse and mucoid rhinorrhea that persists for 1 to 2 weeks. Nonspecific findings such as malaise, fever, sneezing, and anorexia may also be present. The disease is most communicable at this stage, as large numbers of organisms are present in the nasopharynx and the mucoid secretions.

Catarrhal phase, highly communicable

Paroxysmal coughing phase lasts for weeks

The appearance of a persistent cough marks the transition from the catarrhal to the paroxysmal coughing stage. At this time, episodes of paroxysmal coughing occur up to 50 times a day for 2 to 4 weeks. The characteristic inspiratory whoop follows a series of coughs as air is rapidly drawn through the narrowed glottis. Vomiting frequently follows the whoop. The combination of mucoid secretions, whooping cough, and vomiting produces a miserable, exhausted child barely able to breathe. Apnea may follow such episodes, particularly in infants. Marked lymphocytosis reaches its peak at this time with absolute lymphocyte counts of up to 40,000/mm$^3$.

Inspiratory whoop, coughing may lead to apnea

Absolute lymphocytosis

During the 3- to 4-week convalescent stage the frequency and severity of paroxysmal coughing and other features of the disease gradually fade. Partially immune persons and infants under 6 months of age may not show all the typical features of pertussis. Some evolution through the three stages is usually seen, but paroxysmal coughing and lymphocytosis may be absent.

Convalescent phase a gradual fading

The most common complication of pertussis is pneumonia caused by a superinfecting organism such as *Streptococcus pneumoniae*. Atelectasis is also common but may be recognized only by radiologic examination. Other complications, including convulsions, hemorrhage, and hernias, are related to the pressure effects of the paroxysmal coughing and the anoxia produced by inadequate ventilation and apneic spells.

Pulmonary complications include superinfection

### Diagnosis

A clinical diagnosis of pertussis is confirmed by isolation of *B. pertussis* from a nasopharyngeal swab. The organism is not found in the blood or at distant sites. Specimens collected early in the course of disease (during the catarrhal or early paroxysmal stage) provide the greatest chance of successful isolation. Unfortunately, the diagnosis is frequently not considered until paroxysmal coughing has been present for some time, and the number of organisms has decreased significantly. The nasopharyngeal swab is best collected by the pernasal route and plated directly onto a special charcoal blood agar medium, which has replaced the classic Bordet–Gengou agar. Low concentrations a cephalosporin are usually added to these plates to inhibit members of the normal flora and thus allow the slow-growing *B. pertussis* to be isolated. Characteristic colonies appear after 3 to 5 days of incubation and the organisms are identified serologically, because *B. pertussis* shows few specific metabolic activities.

Nasopharyngeal swab plated on charcoal blood agar

Organisms often not present by paroxysmal phase

A direct immunofluorescent technique has been successfully applied to nasopharyngeal smears for rapid diagnosis of pertussis. Smears are stable on transport to the laboratory, whereas the organisms themselves may not survive without special precautions. Positive smears should always be confirmed by culture, if possible.

Direct immunofluorescence allows rapid diagnosis

### Treatment

Once the paroxysmal coughing stage has been reached, the treatment of pertussis is primarily supportive. Antimicrobial therapy is useful at earlier stages and for limiting spread to other susceptible individuals. Of a number of antimicrobics active in vitro against *B. pertussis*, erythromycin is preferred because of its clinical effectiveness and relative lack of toxicity.

Erythromycin treatment effective catarrhal phase

### Prevention

Active immunization is the primary method of preventing pertussis. Vaccines are produced from inactivated whole cell suspensions or from partially purified preparations derived from whole cells. In the United States, the vaccine is combined with diphtheria and tetanus toxoids to produce a triple vaccine, DPT. Three doses given at monthly intervals are begun as early in life as possible (6 to 8 weeks) because of the high susceptibility and mortality in infants. Booster doses later in childhood are recommended. Recent immunization reduces the attack rate upon exposure and the severity of disease upon infection. Side effects and vaccine-related complications have been a problem with some pertussis vaccine preparations. Local inflammation and febrile reactions are common, and rarely febrile seizures have occurred.

Whole cell and partially purified vaccines available

Included in universal DPT course

Pertussis immunization has become a controversial, even emotional, issue in many countries. Small but vocal groups argue that permanent neurologic sequelae are occasionally caused by the vaccine. Critical epidemiologic analysis of all available data does not support these claims. However, the whole-cell vaccine is among the crudest preparations routinely injected into humans and is associated with significant morbidity. Purified acellular vaccines containing primarily pertussis toxin and filamentous hemagglutinin are now available, but have not yet been shown to be as effective as the whole-cell preparation. In the United States they are licensed for use only as boosters following the whole-cell vaccine. With the recent advances in understanding the relative roles played by the *B. pertussis* virulence factors, it is simply a matter of time before we will have an improved vaccine composed of purified pertussis toxoid and probably Fha or another adhesin.

Whole cell vaccine has side effects

Acellular vaccines are less effective

## ADDITIONAL READING


Adams WG, Deaver KA, Cochi SL, et al: Decline of childhood *Haemophilus influenzae* type b (Hib) disease in the Hib vaccine era. *JAMA* 1993;269:221–226. This paper and others in the same issue of *JAMA* document one of the most difficult and successful episodes in the history of immunization.

Daum RS, Granoff DM, Makela PH, et al (eds): Epidemiology, pathogenesis, and prevention of *Haemophilus influenzae* disease. *J Infect Dis* 1992;165(suppl 1):S1–S206. This supplement contains the findings of an international symposium on all aspects of *H. influenzae* disease.

Fothergill LD, Wright J: Influenzal meningitis: The relation of age incidence to the bactericidal power of blood against the causal organism. *J Immunol* 1933;24:273–284. A classic study, the first to advance the currently accepted concepts of humoral immunity in *H. influenzae* disease.

Jorgensen JH: Update on mechanisms and prevalence of antimicrobial resistance in *Haemophilus influenzae*. *Clin Infect Dis* 1992;14:1119–1123. The current status of the multiple resistance mechanisms of *H. influenzae* is reviewed.

Muse KE, Collier AM, Baseman JB: Scanning electron microscopic study of hamster tracheal organ cultures infected with *Bordetella pertussis*. *J Infect Dis* 1977;136:768–777. The unique tropism of *B. pertussis* for ciliated cells and the subsequent destruction of those cells are shown experimentally and visually.

Stephens DS, Farley MM: Pathogenic events during infection of the human nasopharynx with *Neisseria meningitidis* and *Haemophilus influenzae*. *Rev Infect Dis* 1991;13:22–33. A well-illustrated review that demonstrates steps in invasion for both pathogens.

Weiss A, Hewlette E. Virulence factors of *Bordetella pertussis*. *Ann Rev Microbiol* 1986;40:661-686. A comprehensive summary of major virulence determinants.

# Mycoplasma and Ureaplasma

W. Lawrence Drew

*Mycoplasma* and *Ureaplasma* resemble other bacteria except in their lack of a cell wall. They are ubiquitous in nature as the smallest of free-living microorganisms. Numerous *Mycoplasma* species have been isolated from animals and humans, but only three species have been associated with human disease (Table 24–1). *Mycoplasma pneumoniae* is a lower respiratory tract pathogen. *Mycoplasma hominis* and *Ureaplasma urealyticum* cause genitourinary tract infections.

## GENERAL CHARACTERISTICS

No cell walls

Cell membrane contains sterols

Not stained well by common methods

Slow growth in specialized artificial media

Hemadsorption a feature of *M. pneumoniae*

The organisms have diameters of about 0.2 to 0.3 μm, but they are highly plastic and pleomorphic and may appear as coccoid bodies, filaments, and large multinucleoid forms. They do not have a cell wall and are bounded only by a single triple-layered membrane (Fig 24–1) that, unlike other bacteria, contains sterols. The sterols are not synthesized by the organism, but are acquired as essential components from the medium or tissue in which the organism is growing. Lacking a cell wall, *Mycoplasma* and *Ureaplasma* stain poorly or not at all with the usual bacterial stains. Their double-stranded DNA genome is small, probably because of lack of genes encoding a complex cell wall. *Mycoplasma pneumoniae* is an aerobe, but most other species are facultatively anaerobic. All grow slowly in enriched liquid culture medium and on special *Mycoplasma* agar to produce minute colonies only after several days of incubation. The center of the *M. pneumonia* colony grows into the agar and appears denser, giving the appearance of an inverted "fried egg." Growth in culture is inhibited by specific antisera directed at the particular species. Colonies of *M. pneumoniae* bind red blood cells onto the surface of agar plate cultures (hemadsorption). This is due to binding by the mycoplasma to sialic acid-containing oligosaccharides present on the red cell surface.

## ■ MYCOPLASMA PNEUMONIAE

## ■ Mycoplasma pneumoniae Disease

### Epidemiology

Very low infecting dose

*M. pneumoniae* accounts for approximately 20% of all cases of pneumonia. Infection is acquired by droplet spread. Experimental challenges indicate that the human infectious dose is very low, possibly less than 100 colony-forming units.

Worldwide endemic infection with intermittent epidemics

Endemic infections with *M. pneumoniae* occur worldwide, but they are especially prominent in temperate climates. Epidemics at 4- to 6-year intervals have been noted in both civilian and military populations. The most common age for symptomatic *M. pneumoniae*

**TABLE 24–1. PATHOGENIC MYCOPLASMA AND UREAPLASMA SPECIES OF HUMANS**

| Organism | Site | Prevalence | Disease |
|---|---|---|---|
| *M. pneumoniae* | Upper and lower respiratory tract | Common | Primary atypical pneumonia |
| *M. hominis* | Genitourinary tract | Common | Postpartum fever; pelvic inflammatory disease |
| *U. urealyticum* | Genitourinary tract | Very common | Nongonococcal urethritis |

Most common in teenagers

Outbreaks occur in families and closed communities

infection is between 5 and 15 years, and the disease accounts for more than one third of all cases of pneumonia in teenagers, but is also seen in older persons. Infections in children less than 6 months old are uncommon. The disease often appears as a sporadic, endemic illness in families or closed communities because its incubation period is relatively long (2–15 days) and because prolonged shedding in nasal secretions may cause infections to be spread over time. Attack rates in susceptible individuals within families approach 60%. Asymptomatic infections occur, but most studies have suggested that more than two thirds of infected cases develop some evidence of respiratory tract illness.

## Pathogenesis

Adherence to bronchial epithelial cells by surface protein respiratory epithelium

Damage to ciliary action and epithelium

Initially, the organism attaches to the cilia and microvilli of the cells lining the bronchial epithelium. This attachment is mediated by a surface mycoplasmal cytadhesin (P1) protein which binds to complex oligosaccharides containing sialic acid found in the apical regions of bronchial epithelial cells. The oligosaccharide receptors are chemically similar to those on the surface of erythrocytes and are not found on the nonciliated goblet cells or mucus to which *M. pneumoniae* does not bind. The organisms interfere with ciliary action and initiate a process that leads to desquamation of the involved mucosa and a subsequent inflammatory reaction and exudate. The inflammatory response is at first most pronounced in the bronchial and peribronchial tissue, although the alveoli may also be involved. Lymphocytes, plasma cells, and macrophages then infiltrate and thicken the walls of the alveoli and bronchioles.

Organisms are shed in upper respiratory secretions for 2 to 8 days before the onset of symptoms, and shedding continues for as long as 14 weeks after infection.

## Immunity

Complement fixing antibody titers peak at 2–4 weeks

Cold hemagglutinins are IgM

Both local and systemic specific immune responses occur. Local IgA antibody is produced, but disappears 2 to 4 weeks after the onset of the infection. Complement-fixing serum antibody titers reach a peak 2 to 4 weeks after infection and gradually disappear over 6 to 12 months. Nonspecific immune responses to the glycolipids of the outer membrane of the organism often also develop. The most common of these responses involves the production of cold hemagglutinins, which are IgM antibodies that react with the I antigen of human red

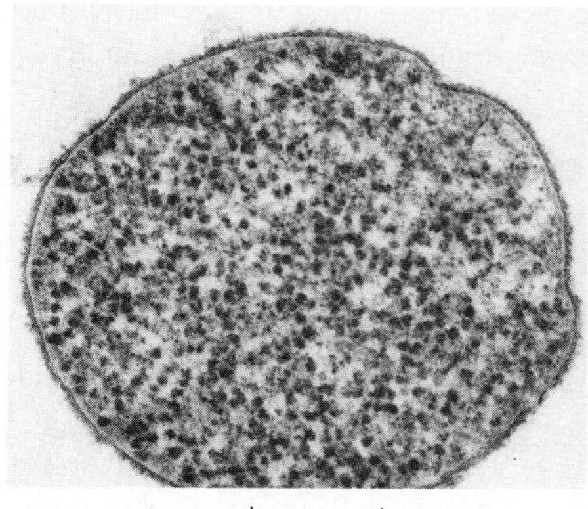


**Figure 24–1.** Electron micrograph of *Mycoplasma*. Note cytoplasmic membrane ribosomes and surface amorphous material with absence of cell wall. (*Courtesy of the late Dr. E. S. Boatman.*)

blood cells and cause agglutination at temperatures of 0 to 4°C. They are seen in about two thirds of symptomatic patients infected with *M. pneumoniae*.

Immunity is not complete, and reinfection with *M. pneumoniae* is common. Clinical disease appears to be more severe in older than in younger children, which has led to the suggestion that many of the clinical manifestations of disease are the result of cellular immune responses rather than invasion by the organism.

Immunity incomplete and reinfection common

## Mycoplasma pneumoniae Disease: Clinical Aspects

### Clinical Manifestations

A mild tracheobronchitis with fever, cough, headache, and malaise is the most common syndrome associated with acute *M. pneumoniae* infection. The pneumonia is typically less severe than bacterial pneumonia. It has been described as "walking" pneumonia, as most cases do not require hospitalization. The disease is of insidious onset, with fever, headache, and malaise for 2 to 4 days before the onset of respiratory symptoms. Pulmonary symptoms are generally limited to a non- or minimally productive cough. X-rays reveal a unilateral or patchy pneumonia, usually in a lower lobe, although multiple lobes are sometimes involved. Small pleural effusions are seen in 25% of cases.

Primary atypical (walking) pneumonia

Insidious onset leads to patchy pneumonia

Pharyngitis with fever and sore throat may also occur. Nonpurulent otitis media or myringitis occurs concomitantly in approximately 15% of patients with *M. pneumoniae* pneumonitis. The presence of nonpurulent otitis media and lower respiratory illness in a teenager suggests *M. pneumoniae* infection.

Pharyngitis and otitis media also common

### Laboratory Diagnosis

Clinical diagnosis of *M. pneumoniae* infection may be difficult because the manifestations overlap with those of other bacterial and viral infections. Gram-stained sputum usually shows some mononuclear cells, but, lacking a cell wall, *M. pneumoniae* is not seen. The absence of organisms, however, may help to suggest an etiology. The organism can be isolated from throat swabs or sputum of infected patients using special culture media and methods, but because of its slow growth, isolation usually requires incubation for a week or longer. Thus, serologic tests rather than cultures are more commonly used for specific diagnosis. A fourfold rise in serum antibody during acute infection or convalescence from the disease indicates *M. pneumoniae* infection. The most widely used serologic method is complement fixation. With the relatively long incubation period and insidious onset of the disease, many patients already have high antibody titers at the time they are first seen. In these situations a single high titer, such as a complement fixation titer greater than 1:128, indicates recent or current infection, because these antibodies are generally of short duration. There have been many efforts to develop enzyme immunoassays for IgM-specific antibody that would, it is hoped, identify patients with active infections. In research settings, these tests have been successful but they are not yet generally available.

Diagnosis usually serologic because *M. pneumoniae* grows slowly

Single high complement fixing titer may be diagnostic

Because more than two thirds of patients with symptomatic lower respiratory *M. pneumoniae* infection develop high titers of cold hemagglutinins, their demonstration can be useful in some clinical situations. It must be remembered that cold hemagglutinins are nonspecific and have been observed in adenovirus infections, infectious mononucleosis, and some other illnesses. The test is simple, however, and can be performed rapidly in any clinical laboratory.

Cold agglutinins are nonspecific but helpful

Direct detection of the organism in respiratory secretions has been attempted using immunoassay methods, DNA hybridization, and the polymerase chain reaction. These, too, are successful in research settings but have not been developed into clinically practical procedures.

### Treatment

Erythromycin and tetracycline are the agents used for treatment of *M. pneumoniae* infections. They shorten the course of infection, although eradication from the nasopharynx may take much longer. Clarithromycin appears comparable to erythromycin in limited clinical studies.

Erythromycin, tetracycline, and clarithromycin used

## MYCOPLASMA HOMINIS

Found in genitourinary tract

Association with postpartum fever

Erythromycin resistant

*Mycoplasma hominis* is a common inhabitant of the genitourinary tract. Although some strains grow on ordinary blood agar as nonhemolytic pinpoint colonies, the organism is best detected on *Mycoplasma* agar, on which it grows rapidly. *Mycoplasma hominis* and *Ureaplasma* can be differentiated by demonstrating arginine breakdown by the former and urease activity by the latter. At least seven antigenic variants of *M. hominis* have been described. To date, the major clinical condition associated with *M. hominis* infection is postabortal or postpartum fever. *Mycoplasma hominis* is isolated from the blood of about 10% of women with this condition.

The diseases appear to be self-limiting, although antibiotic therapy may decrease the duration of fever and hospitalization. Recently, serologic studies and animal experiments have indicated that pelvic inflammatory disease syndromes in women may be associated with *M. hominis* infection of the fallopian tubes. The organism is sensitive to tetracycline. In contrast to *U. urealyticum* and *M. pneumoniae, M. hominis* is resistant to erythromycin.

## UREAPLASMA UREALYTICUM

Urease production marks the species

The genus *Ureaplasma* contains a single species, *U. urealyticum*, of which some 14 serotypes have been described. *Ureaplasma* is distinguished from *Mycoplasma* by its production of urease. On special *Ureaplasma* agar media, colonies are small and circular and grow downward into the agar. In liquid media containing urea and phenol red, growth of *Ureaplasma* results in production of ammonia from the urea, with a resultant increase in pH and a change in color of the indicator.

### Epidemiology

Acquired by sexual activity

The main reservoir of human strains of *U. urealyticum* is the genital tract of sexually active men and women; it is rarely found before puberty. Colonization, which probably results primarily from sexual contact, occurs in more than 80% of individuals who have had three or more sexual partners.

### Clinical Manifestations

Association with urethritis

Because of the high colonization rate, it has been difficult to associate specific illness with *Ureaplasma*; however, recent studies suggest that approximately one half of cases of nongonococcal, nonchlamydial urethritis in men may be caused by *U. urealyticum.* In women, *Ureaplasma* has been shown to cause chorioamnionitis and postpartum fever. The organism has been isolated from 10% of women with the latter syndrome.

#### Diagnosis and Treatment

Tetracycline and spectinomycin effective

Men with nongonococcal urethritis should be treated on the assumption that *Ureaplasma* infection may be involved. Tetracycline is the treatment of choice because it is also active against *Chlamydia*, but tetracycline-resistant strains of *Ureaplasma* have been reported that have been associated with recurrences of nongonococcal urethritis in men. In such cases, spectinomycin treatment or treatment with quinolone antimicrobics is also effective. Women with postpartum fever due to *U. urealyticum* may respond to tetracycline treatment.

## ADDITIONAL READING

Broughton RA. Infections due to *Mycoplasma pneumoniae* in childhood. *Pediatr Infect Dis.* 1986;5:71–85. A review of clinical manifestations, diagnosis, and treatment of *Mycoplasma pneumoniae* infections in children.

Cassell GH, Cole BC. Mycoplasmas as agents of human disease. *N Engl J Med.* 1981;304:80–89. A review of mycoplasmas and their contribution to respiratory, extrapulmonary, and urogenital disease.

Crawshaw SC, Stocker DI, Sugrue DL, Haran MV. Evaluation of the significance of *Mycoplasma hominis* and *Ureaplasma urealyticum* in female genital tract infection—A retrospective case note study. *Int J STD AIDS.* 1990;1(3):191–194. Erythromycin was ineffective in eradicating the organisms in 62.5% of patients with *Mycoplasma hominis* infection and 70% of those with *Ureaplasma urealyticum* infection.

Embree J. *Mycoplasma hominis* in maternal and fetal infections. *Ann NY Acad Sci.* 1988;549:56–64. Reviews the evidence for *Mycoplasma* hominis as a cause of chorioamnionitis, septic abortion, postpartum fever, and neonatal infection.

Kanamoto Y, Miyakey Y, Suginaka H, Usui T. In vitro susceptibility of *Ureaplasma urealyticum* clinical isolates to new macrolides. *Chemotherapy.* 1991;37(4):256–259. Nine antimicrobial agents were studied for their antimicrobial activity against 100 strains of *Ureaplasma urealyticum.* The $MIC_{90}$ values of erythromycin, josamycin, doxycycline, minocycline, and tetracycline ranged from 0.1 to 0.78 μg/mL. Norfloxacin was least active, with a $MIC_{90}$ or 12.5 μg/mL. Of 100 strains tested, 5 were resistant (MIC ≥ 12.5 μg/mL) to tetracycline, and 2 were resistant to minocycline and doxycycline.

Marais NF, Wessels PH, Smith MS, Gericke A. *Chlamydia trachomatis*, *Mycoplasma hominis* and *Ureaplasma urealyticum* infections in women. Prevalence, risks and management at a South African infertility clinic. *J Reprod Med.* 1991;36(3):161–164. *Mycoplasma hominis* was isolated from three (7.5%) endocervical swabs. None of the endocervical swabs yielded a culture positive for *Ureaplasma urealyticum.* The prevalence of 35.9% for *Chlamydia trachomatis* was surprisingly high.

Taylor-Robinson D, McCormack WM. The genital mycoplasmas. *N Engl J Med.* 1980;302:1003–1010, 1063–1067. A comprehensive review of the laboratory diagnosis, epidemiology, and treatment of genital mycoplasmas and their role in the etiology of urethritis, prostatitis, epididymitis, vaginitis, cervicitis, pelvic inflammatory disease, and postpartum fever.

Uldum SA, Jensen JS, Sondergard-Anderson J, Lind K. Enzyme immunoassay for detection of immunoglobulin M (IgM) and IgG antibodies to *Mycoplasma pneumoniae. J Clin Microbiol.* 1992;30(5):1198–1204. An enzyme immunoassay (EIA) for detection of IgM and IgG antibodies to *Mycoplasma pneumoniae* was developed. The combined measurement of specific IgM and IgG gave a specificity of 99.7% and a sensitivity of 97.8%.

Waites KB, Crouse DT, Cassell GH. Antibiotic susceptibilities and therapeutic options for *Ureaplasma urealyticum* infections in neonates. *Pediatr Infect Dis J.* 1992;11:23–29.

Chapter 25

# *Legionella*

Kenneth J. Ryan

The widely publicized outbreak of pneumonia among attendees of the 1976 American Legion convention in Philadelphia led to the isolation of a new infectious agent, *Legionella pneumophila*. The event was unique in medical history; for months the American public had entertained theories of its cause that ranged from sabotage to viroids, only to find that a previously undescribed Gram-negative rod was responsible. It was an outstanding example of the benefits of pursuing sound epidemiologic evidence until it is explained by equally sound microbiologic findings. We now know the disease had occurred for many years: specific antibodies and organisms have been detected in material preserved from the 1950s, and a mysterious hospital outbreak in 1965 has been solved retrospectively. The primary reasons the organism escaped detection for so long are that it stains poorly or not at all with common methods and it does not grow on the usual bacteriologic media. *Legionella pneumophila* is only one of a growing list of more than 30 *Legionella* species.

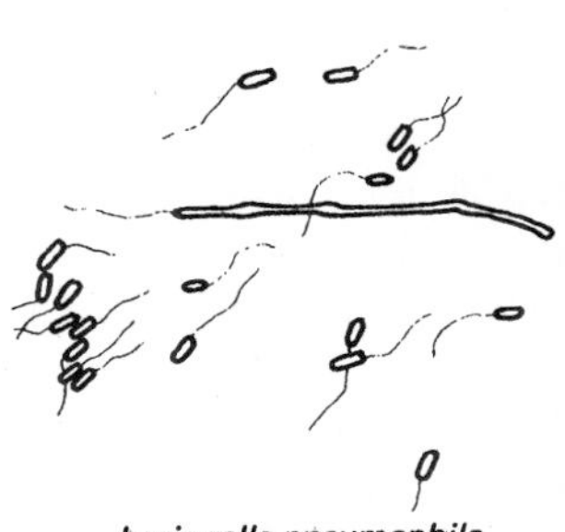

*Legionella pneumophila*

## BACTERIOLOGIC FEATURES

### Morphology

*Legionella pneumophila* is a thin, pleomorphic, Gram-negative rod 0.5 to 0.7 μm wide and 2 to 20 μm in length or longer. Elongated, filamentous forms are common. In clinical specimens, the organism stains poorly or not at all by Gram stain or the usual histologic stains; it can be demonstrated, however, by certain silver impregnation methods (Dieterle stain) and by some simple stains that omit decolorization steps. Ultrastructurally, *L. pneumophila* has features similar to those of Gram-negative bacteria with a typical outer membrane, thin peptidoglycan layer, and cytoplasmic membrane. Polar, subpolar, and lateral flagella may be present. Most species of *Legionella* are motile. Spores are not found.

Gram-negative cell wall structure but stains with difficulty

### Growth

*Legionella* species do not grow on common enriched bacteriologic media such as blood agar, but require a medium containing amino acids supplemented with L-cysteine and a source of ferric ions. The latter may be provided by hemoglobin or soluble ferric pyrophosphate. *Legionella pneumophila* grows optimally at a pH of 6.9, and it is sensitive to major variations from this pH. Growth occurs in 2 to 5 days on agar media under aerobic conditions at 35°C. Colonies have a surface resembling ground glass. Growth in fluid media is generally poor.

Growth requires iron and low pH

## Classification

Identification based antigenic structure and DNA homology
Original *L pneumophila* type 1 still most common
Many other *Legionella* species and serotypes

*Legionella* possess catalase, oxidase (weak), gelatinase, and β-lactamase activity, but do not grow or react positively in most other taxonomic tests used to classify other bacteria. Their identification and classification depend largely on antigenic features, chromatographic analysis of cellular fatty acid content, and DNA homology tests. In addition to *L. pneumophila,* 32 other species (*L. bozemanii, L. dumoffii, L. micdadei,* etc) and 52 serotypes within the *Legionella* genus have been identified. Of the 15 species that have been isolated from human infections, *L. pneumophila* still accounts for 80 to 90% and most of these are the original Philadelphia serotype 1.

The most commonly encountered *Legionella* other than *L. pneumophila* is *L. micdadei. Legionella micdadei* is distinctive in demonstrating acid-fastness in sputum and tissue, a characteristic that is lost in culture. Other species may differ in some cultural features, such as fluorescence of colonies under ultraviolet light, but DNA homology is the primary taxonomic tool in assigning new species.

# ■ LEGIONELLOSIS

## Epidemiology

Water habitat is where organism survives best

Amoebas act as reservoir

Infections associated with aerosols distributed by humidifying and cooling systems

No person-to-person transmission

In nature *Legionella* species are found in fresh water and soil and as parasites of protozoa including numerous species of amoebae. Cases can almost always be linked with water habitats where amoebas act as the environmental reservoir for virulent legionellas. The organism is known to survive as long as a year in unchlorinated tap water. Most outbreaks have occurred in or around large buildings such as hotels, factories, and hospitals. The water sources have involved cooling towers or some other part of the building's air-conditioning system. Organisms contaminating the water are aerosolized and spread either directly or through the air ducts of the system. Some hospital outbreaks have implicated respiratory devices and potable water coming from parts of the hot water system such as faucets and shower heads.

Person-to-person transmission has not been documented, and the organisms have not been isolated from healthy individuals. It is difficult to ascertain the overall incidence of *Legionella* infections, as most information has been from outbreaks. Serologic surveys indicate that outbreaks constitute only a small part of the total cases, many of which currently go undetected. Estimates based on seroconversions suggest approximately 25,000 cases in the United States each year. Both serologic and environmental studies indicate that *Legionella* has low virulence for humans.

## Pathogenesis and Pathology

Strong tropism for the lung

Necrotizing multifocal pneumonia with intracellular bacteria

Facultative intracellular pathogen that enters and multiplies in macrophages

Enters phagocyte by specialized process

*Legionella pneumophila* is striking in its propensity to attack the lung, producing a necrotizing multifocal pneumonia. Microscopically, the process involves the alveoli and terminal bronchioles, with relative sparing of the larger bronchioles and bronchi. Microabscess formation is common. The inflammatory exudate contains fibrin, polymorphonuclear leukocytes (PMNs), macrophages, and erythrocytes. A striking feature is the preponderance of bacteria within phagocytes and the lytic destruction of inflammatory cells.

*Legionella pneumophila* is a facultative intracellular pathogen. Its pathogenicity depends on its ability to survive and multiply within cells of the monocyte–macrophage series. In fact, there is little evidence that the organism multiplies outside of cells in the alveolar space. Inhaled legionellas reach the alveoli where their ability to bind C3 enhances phagocyte recognition and uptake. In PMNs they have enhanced survival, probably through inhibiting activation of the respiratory burst, but the events involving alveolar macrophages and blood-derived monocytes are of prime importance.

*Legionella pneumophila* is taken into monocytes/macrophages by a process called **coiling phagocytosis** (Fig 25–1). Once in the phagocyte, the *Legionella*-containing phagosome becomes lined with ribosomes and clusters of mitochondria. At this stage, instead of being

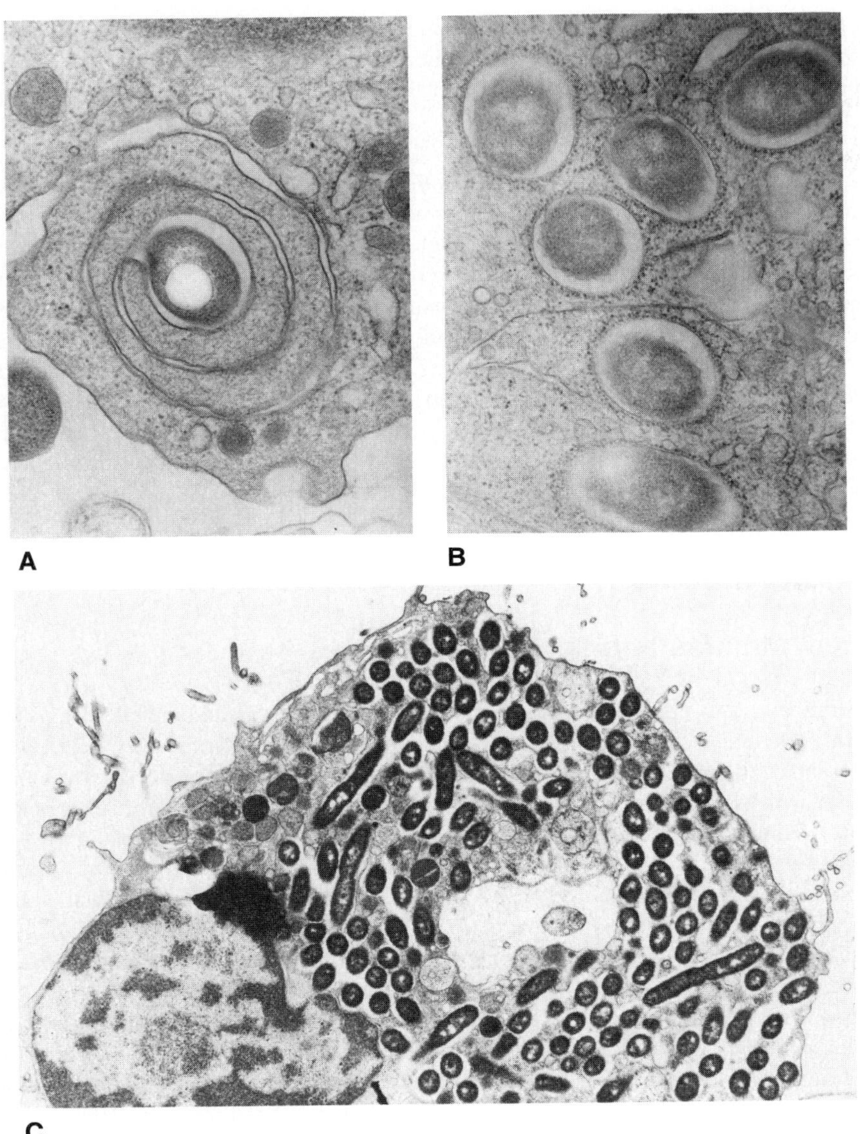


**Figure 25–1.** Multiplication of *Legionella pneumophila* in human macrophages. *Legionella pneumophila* enters the cell by coiling phagocytosis **(A)**, and the phagosome created is lined by ribosomes and mitochondria **(B)**. The bacteria multiply within the macrophages to reach very high numbers **(C)**. (*Courtesy of Dr. Marcus Horwitz.*)

killed by the bactericidal mechanisms of the macrophage, the bacteria multiply extensively, eventually lysing the cell. The factors involved in this process must be complex. One genetic study showed more than 30 new *Legionella* proteins activated and 30 others suppressed with the organism's move from the extracellular to the intracellular environment. Some of these probably relate to metabolic adaptation such as the demonstrated ability of *L. pneumophila* to use intracellular iron from transferrin inside the cell. Others relate to confounding the macrophage bactericidal systems. In this aspect *Legionellas* have been shown to prevent phagolysosomal fusion and the acidification of the phagosome.

Multiple genes involved in switch from extracellular to intracellular environment

Blocks phagolysomal fusion and acidification

Although it is not yet possible to generalize across the many species and serotypes of *Legionella*, some associations that relate to this organism's unique pathogenesis have been found. An outer membrane porin binds C3, facilitating phagocyte recognition, and another outer membrane protein called **macrophage invasion potentiator** (Mip) determines cell entry. Mip is thus associated with both invasiveness and virulence. All *Legionella* species investigated so far produce a peptide toxin that inhibits activation of the oxidative killing mechanisms of PMNs. A number of extracellular enzymes have been identified, although any contribution to virulence remains to be determined.

Toxin inhibits oxidative killing mechanisms

Intracellular events similar in amoeba

The progression of intracellular events in free-living amoebae is remarkably similar to that in human alveolar macrophages and monocytes. Legionellas may well represent a food source for the environmental protozoa rather than a threat.

### Immunity

Activated macrophages limit growth

Iron restriction may be involved

Just as intracellular multiplication is the key to *L. pneumophila* virulence, its inhibition by cell-mediated mechanisms appears to be the most important aspect of immunity. Whether *L. pneumophila* is able to interfere with development of these responses is not known, but hypoexpression of major histocompatibility complex class I and II molecules has been observed in phagosomes containing the organisms. Cytokine-activated macrophages inhibit intracellular multiplication and limit growth of *Legionella*. One possible mechanism for this effect is downregulation of systems that give *L. pneumophila* access to the iron it needs for growth. The role of antibody in immunity appears to be less. In the presence of activated cellular immune responses antibody may play an ancillary role through enhancement of phagocytosis. It is unknown whether humans who have had Legionnaires' disease have increased immunity to reinfection and disease.

## LEGIONELLOSIS: CLINICAL ASPECTS

### Clinical Manifestations

Two clinically and epidemiologically distinct syndromes are associated with *L. pneumophila*. The first, a severe pneumonia with an incubation period of 2 to 10 days, is called **Legionnaires' disease** and has mortality as high as 60%. The other, **Pontiac fever** (named for a 1968 Michigan outbreak), is a nonpneumonic febrile illness with an incubation period of 20 to 48 hours. Pontiac fever is a self-limiting illness that is not life threatening. The attack rate for Legionnaires' disease has been estimated at less than 5% of those exposed to infection, whereas more than 90% have had clinical illness in outbreaks of Pontiac fever.

Severe toxic pneumonia in 5% of those exposed

High mortality among immunocompromised

Legionnaires' disease is a severe toxic pneumonia that begins with myalgia and headache, followed by a rapidly rising fever. A dry cough may develop and later become productive, but sputum production is not a prominent feature. Chills, pleuritic chest pain, vomiting, diarrhea, confusion, and delirium may all be seen. Radiologically, patchy or interstitial infiltrates with a tendency to progress toward nodular consolidation are present unilaterally or bilaterally. Liver function tests often indicate some hepatic dysfunction. In the more serious cases the patient becomes progressively ill and toxic over the first 3 to 6 days, and the disease terminates in shock, respiratory failure, or both. The overall mortality is about 15%, but has been higher than 50% in some hospital outbreaks. It is particularly high in patients with serious underlying disease or suppression of cell-mediated immunity. Disease caused by *L. micdadei* occurs almost exclusively in immunosuppressed persons.

Non-progressive, self-limiting disease may be immune response

Pontiac fever begins similarly with fever and myalgia, and one half of all patients have a dry cough. The disease does not progress, however, and recovery usually begins after 2 to 5 days. It would be considered a mild form of Legionnaires' disease were it not for the rather uniform clinical and epidemiologic features in documented outbreaks. In the Pontiac outbreak there were 144 cases with no deaths. It is much less common than Legionnaires' disease and may represent an immune reaction to dead or low-virulence *Legionella* strains.

### Diagnosis

High-quality specimens needed

Direct immune fluorescence most rapid

The possibility of Legionnaires' disease should be considered in any patient with severe progressive pneumonia not shown to be caused by another organism. The best means of diagnosis for clinical purposes is direct microscopic examination and culture of infected tissues. For this purpose, a high-quality specimen such as that from a transtracheal aspirate, lung aspirate, or lung biopsy is usually necessary, because the organism is rarely found in sputum. Typically, the Gram smear shows no bacteria; the organisms are demonstrated by direct immunofluorescence examination using *Legionella*-specific conjugates. This method is the most rapid means of diagnosis, but it is positive in only 25 to 50% of culture-proved cases.

Cultures should be made on routine media as well as on special agar media that meet the growth requirements of *Legionella*. Currently, the best agar medium is buffered charcoal yeast extract (BCYE). It contains amino acids, vitamins, L-cysteine, iron, and charcoal to adsorb toxic fatty acids. It is buffered to an acid pH (below 7.0), which is optimal for *Legionella* growth. The isolation of characteristic Gram-negative rods on BCYE after 2 to 5 days that have failed to grow on routine media (blood agar, chocolate agar), is presumptive evidence of *Legionella*. Diagnosis is confirmed by direct immunofluorescent staining of smears prepared from the colonies. BCYE also allows isolation of most other *Legionella* species. Occasional cases with positive direct immunofluorescent smears but negative cultures are still seen. These results are probably caused by strains for which growth conditions remain unmet.

Culture on special media required for isolation

Cultures may be negative

The diagnosis of legionellosis can also be established by demonstrating a significant rise in specific serum antibody titer using an indirect immunofluorescence technique. As with most other serodiagnostic tests, this method requires paired (acute and convalescent) sera; it is used primarily for retrospective diagnosis and in epidemiologic studies. In some communities elevated titers in single serum samples have been detected in as much as 25% of the population.

Serodiagnosis by rising titer

Diagnostic procedures for legionellosis may not be available in some hospital laboratories. This is particularly true for the direct immunofluorescence test. Clinicians should advise the laboratory of the suspicion of Legionnaires' disease in advance so that these procedures can be set up or the material sent to a reference laboratory. Searching for *Legionella* from environmental sources requires the use of specialized procedures including polymerase chain reaction amplification.

### Treatment and Prevention

The best information on antimicrobial therapy is still provided by the original Philadelphia outbreak. Because the etiology was completely obscure at the time, the cases were treated with many different regimens. Patients treated with erythromycin clearly did better than those given the penicillins, cephalosporins, or aminoglycosides; subsequently, it was shown that most *Legionella* produce of β-lactamases. In vitro susceptibility tests and animal studies confirmed the activity of erythromycin and showed that tetracycline, rifampin, and the newer quinolones are also active. Although the other antimicrobics are sometimes used in combination, erythromycin remains the treatment of choice.

Erythromycin treatment of choice

The prevention of legionellosis involves avoiding or minimizing contamination of aerosol sources in cooling towers and in water supplies of buildings. This is complicated by the fact that, compared with the Enterobacteriaceae, legionellas are relatively resistant to chlorine and heat. They have been isolated from hot water tanks held at over 50°C. Methods for decontaminating water systems are still under evaluation, although some outbreaks appear to have been aborted by using disinfectants, by correcting malfunctions in air-conditioning systems, or by temporarily elevating water system temperature above 70°C.

Preventive measures involve treatment or heating of water sources

## ADDITIONAL READING

Dowling JN, Saha AK, Glew RG. Virulence factors of the family Legionellaceae. *Microbiol Rev.* 1992;56:32–60. The review provides comprehensive coverage of all aspects of virulence and molecular pathogenesis.

Fraser DW, Tsai TR, Orenstein W, et al. Legionnaires' disease: Descriptions of an epidemic of pneumonia. *N Engl J Med.* 1977;297:1189–1197.

McDade JE, Shepard CC, Fraser DW, et al. Legionnaires' disease: Isolation of a bacterium and demonstration of its role in other respiratory disease. *N Engl J Med.* 1977;297:1197–1203. This study and the report by Fraser et al describe the 1976 outbreak at the Philadelphia American Legion convention and the methods that led to the discovery of the cause of this "new" disease. It makes good reading as an example of medical discovery and the requirements of proof.

Winn WC Jr. Legionnaires' disease: Historical perspective. *Clin Microbiol Rev.* 1988;1:60–81. This review focuses on the events leading to the discovery and definition of this disease but delivers much more than indicated by the title.

Chapter 26

# Spirochetes

*James J. Plorde*

The spirochetes are helical organisms; their morphology differs from that of other bacteria in that they have a flexible, peptidoglycan cell wall around which several axial fibrils are wound. These fibrils have the structure of flagella and are referred to as **endoflagella** (Fig 26–1). The cell wall and endoflagella are completely covered by an outer bilayered membrane similar to the outer membrane of other Gram-negative bacteria. In some species, a hyaluronic acid slime layer forms around the exterior of the organism and may contribute to its virulence. Spirochetes are motile, exhibiting rotation and flexion; this motility is believed to result from movement of the endoflagellar filaments, although the mechanism is not clear. Like other bacteria, spirochetes divide by transverse fission.

Outer membrane is external to endoflagella wound around cell wall

Many spirochetes are very slim (0.15 μm or less) and can be visualized only by dark-field microscopy, electron microscopy, or special staining techniques that effectively increase their diameter to bring them within the resolving power of the light microscope. Other spirochetes (*Borrelia*) are larger and visible in stained preparations. They are Gram negative, although they are more easily detected by other staining methods.

Many are too slim to be seen by light microscopy

Some spirochetes are free living; some are members of the normal flora of humans and animals; and three genera, *Treponema*, *Leptospira*, and *Borrelia*, include the causative agents of important human and zoonotic diseases.

Parasitic spirochetes grow more slowly in vitro than most disease-causing bacteria, and some, including the causative agent of syphilis, have not been grown beyond several generations in cell culture. Some are strict anaerobes, others require low concentrations of oxygen, and still others are aerobic.

Spirochetes grow slowly or not at all in culture

## TREPONEMA

### Treponema pallidum

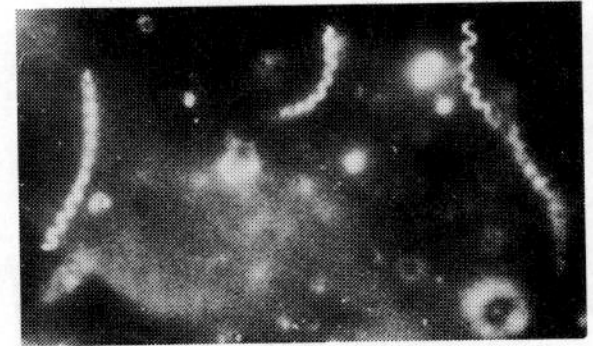

*Treponema pallidum.* **Dark-field microscopy**

*Treponema pallidum* is the causative agent of syphilis, a venereal disease first recognized in the 16th century as an acute and often fatal disease that rapidly spread through Europe as a concomitant of the extensive military campaigns of the century. Over the intervening years, a state of more balanced parasitism developed; the disease is now a more chronic illness, but it can nonetheless have devastating effects.

#### Morphology

*Treponema pallidum* is a slim (0.15-μm) spirochete 5 to 15 μm long with regular spirals of a wavelength of 1 μm and an amplitude of about 0.3 μm. It is not visible by transmitted light under the microscope, because its width is below the resolving power of the instrument and its refractive index is similar to that of the usual suspending medium. It is read-

Very thin spirals

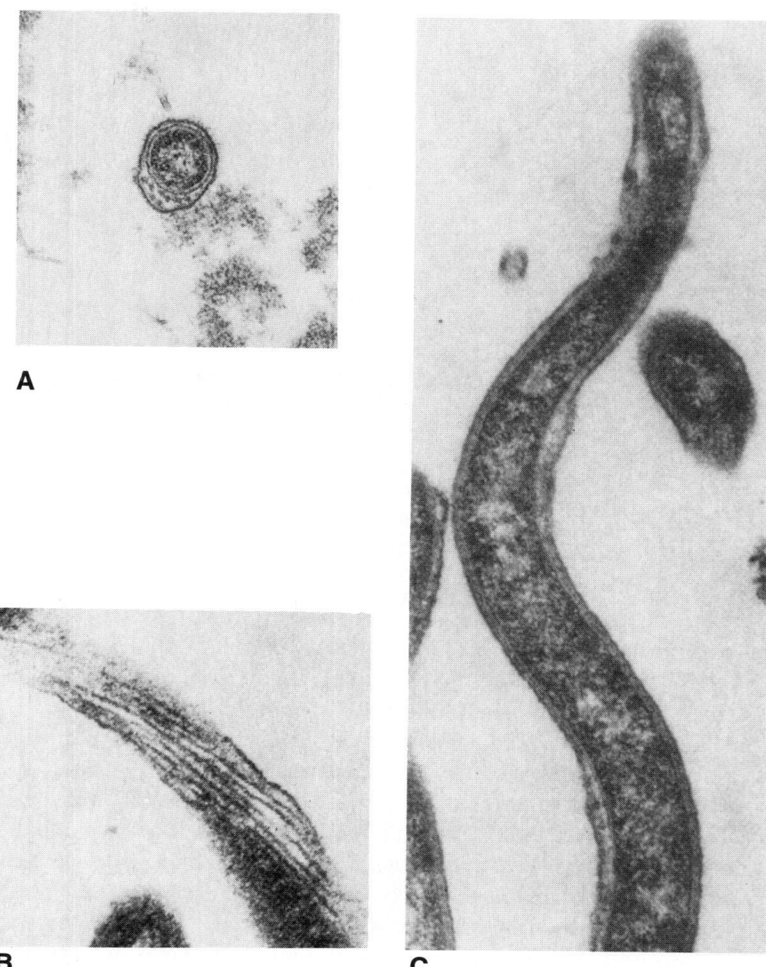


**Figure 26–1.** Spirochete of Lyme disease. Original magnification × 40,000. **A,B.** Note endoflagella. **C.** Note outer membrane. (*Reprinted with permission from Dr. Steere AC.* N Engl J Med. *1983;308:736.*)

Fails to stain by routine methods; visualized by dark-field

Characteristic flexional and rotational motility

ily seen by immunofluorescence techniques and by dark-field microscopy, which depends on reflection of light from the surface of particles (see Chapter 14). It cannot be visualized with the usual bacteriologic stains; however, its width can be effectively increased by the use of techniques that deposit silver on its surface, and silver impregnation techniques are used to demonstrate it in histologic preparations. Viable *T. pallidum* shows characteristic slow, corkscrew motility with sudden 90-degree angle flexions at its center.

## Cultivation

Brief growth in some primary cell cultures only

Little known of metabolism

Until recently, *T. pallidum* had not been shown to multiply in vitro. With the use of special tissue culture techniques and careful control of oxygen tension and pH, the organism has now been shown to multiply through several generations in primary cell culture, but has not been passed in subculture. It was previously thought that *T. pallidum* was an anaerobe, but it is now known to be capable of carrying out oxidative dissimilation of glucose and to incorporate radiolabeled amino acids in the presence of low concentrations of oxygen. The organism retains viability for considerable periods in liquid medium in the absence of oxygen. Other information about its metabolic properties is limited because of the extreme difficulty in obtaining sufficient organisms for study.

## Resistance

Rapid death in environment

*Treponema pallidum* dies rapidly on drying and is readily killed by a wide range of disinfectant agents. These properties account for its almost exclusive transmission by direct contact. It is exquisitely sensitive to penicillin and is inhibited by low concentrations of tetracyclines, erythromycin, and many other antimicrobics. No resistance to chemotherapeutically useful agents appears to have developed.

High susceptibility to disinfectants, penicillin, other antimicrobics

### Antigenic Structure

The outer membrane of the spirochete contains few proteins and is only weakly antigenic; however, during the course of a syphilitic infection, antibodies are produced that react with it and, in the presence of complement, immobilize the spirochete. These are referred to as **antitreponemal antibodies.** A number of somatic proteins have been detected and purified by recombinant DNA techniques and antibodies to them demonstrated in the sera of infected patients, but their role in immunity and diagnosis remains to be established. During infection, antibodies termed **nontreponemal antibodies** also develop that react with a phospholipid component, cardiolipin (diphosphatidyl glycerol), of normal human and animal tissues that is found in mitochondrial membranes. It remains unclear whether the antigen that stimulates production of this antibody is a product of the spirochete itself or a modified component of host cells. The difficulty in answering this question is compounded, because *T. pallidum* adsorbs lipids from the tissues in which it is multiplying.

Treponemal antibodies formed to protein antigens

Nontreponemal antibodies directed at host tissue components

## Syphilis

### Epidemiology

In most cases, *T. pallidum* infection is acquired from direct sexual contact with an individual who has an active primary or secondary syphilitic lesion. Transmission occurs in approximately one third of such contacts. Less commonly, the disease may be spread by nongenital contact with a lesion (eg, of the lip), sharing of needles by intravenous drug users, or transplacental transmission to the fetus within approximately the first 3 years of the maternal infection (see Chapters 69 and 70). Occasional cases result from accidental inoculation of infected material. Modern precautions have essentially eliminated blood transfusion as a source of the disease. With the introduction of penicillin, the number of reported cases of syphilis in the United States has dropped to approximately 100,000 per year but has been increasing since 1985.

Infection usually from sexual contact with primary or secondary lesions

Transplacental and other transmission mechanisms occur

### Pathogenesis

*Treponema pallidum* is an exclusively human pathogen under natural conditions. In the laboratory, it can produce lesions when inoculated into the skin, cornea, or testicle of the rabbit. The latter yields large numbers of *T. pallidum,* which are a source of antigen for serologic tests. Infection in rabbits is nonprogressive and does not mimic the disease in humans. Some degree of passive protection is provided by sera from recovered animals.

Exclusively human pathogen

The spirochete reaches the subepithelial tissues through inapparent breaks in the skin or possibly by passage between the epithelial cells of a mucous membrane. It multiplies locally with a generation time of about 30 hours; although the primary lesion is local, the organism also disseminates rapidly to local lymph nodes and then to other organs by way of the bloodstream.

Penetration through mucosa or breaks in skin

Spirochete disseminates to local lymph nodes and blood

Initially, there is little tissue reaction to multiplication of *T. pallidum,* which appears to produce neither endotoxins nor exotoxins, but the primary lesion develops 2 to 10 weeks after infection as an indurated swelling at the site of infection. The surface necroses to yield a hard-based ulcerated lesion, termed the **chancre,** which is teeming with spirochetes and is highly infectious. The basic pathologic lesion is an endarteritis. The small arterioles show swelling and proliferation of their endothelial cells. This reduces or obstructs local blood supply and probably accounts for the necrotic ulceration. Dense, granulomatous cuffs of lymphocytes, monocytes, and plasma cells surround the vessels. Untreated, the lesion heals within 3 to 8 weeks, frequently with considerable fibrosis. During this time, antibodies and cell-mediated immunity to spirochetal antigens develop. The primary lesion is not always apparent, especially when it involves the female genital tract.

Primary chancre highly infectious with numerous spirochetes

Basic lesion endarteritis

Primary lesion may be inapparent

For reasons that are not understood, the disease is then silent for 2 to 10 weeks, during which a disseminated secondary stage develops with varying degrees of severity. Lesions are heavily infected with *T. pallidum* and do not appear to differ antigenically from

Latent for many weeks

Secondary stage involves generalized superficial lesions with high infectivity

those causing the primary lesions. Immune complexes of antibody, spirochetal components, and complement are present in arteriolar walls and account for some of the clinical manifestations. This stage may last several weeks and may relapse. It may be mild, however, and go unnoticed by the patient. Secondary lesions are highly infectious. The factors that control the secondary stage are unclear: humoral antibody has not been shown to play a role, and high titers of both treponemal and nontreponemal antibodies are present throughout. It has been suggested that the relapsing course of early syphilis is a reflection of a finely poised balance between a developing cellular immunity and suppression of T lymphocytes.

Infection progresses to latency, tertiary disease, or spontaneous cure

Tertiary gummatous lesions have protean manifestations depending on location

Tertiary stage noninfectious

After the secondary stage, nontreponemal antibody test results of one fourth of patients revert to negative, possibly the result of spontaneous cure. In another 45%, serologic tests remain positive, but no further clinical manifestations appear. The remaining untreated cases develop tertiary manifestations several months to 30 years later. Most late syphilitic manifestations are destructive gummatous lesions, again associated with the characteristic endarteritis of syphilis. They can affect skin, bone, joints, oral and nasal cavities, parenchymatous organs, the cardiovascular system, and the meninges and nervous system. Too few spirochetes are in the lesions to be demonstrated by microscopic techniques, except in general paresis, when large numbers are found in the cerebral cortex. Late disease is not infectious to others. It appears probable that late manifestations involve delayed-type hypersensitivity responses to the spirochete or its products or an autoimmune reaction to host tissues in areas in which spirochetes persist. Once again, however, the processes are unclear.

### Immunity

Immunity is not lasting

In the early stages of syphilis, the patient rapidly becomes immune to reinfection, but immunity is short-lived if the patient is successfully treated. In the later stages, immunity to reinfection is more solid and continues after treatment. From experiments in rabbits, it appears that both antibody and cell-mediated immunity are significant, but as in humans they are not sufficiently effective to eradicate established disease in most instances. Syphilis in immunocompromised patients such as those suffering from the acquired immunodeficiency syndrome may present with unusually aggressive or atypical manifestations.

## Syphilis: Clinical Aspects

### Clinical Manifestations

#### Primary Syphilis

Chancre is indurated, painless ulcer

The primary syphilitic lesion is an ulcer with regional lymphadenopathy. Syphilis must always be considered in the differential diagnosis of a genital ulcer. The median incubation period from contact until the appearance of the primary syphilitic chancre is about 21 days; the period is proportional to the size of the infecting inoculum. The chancre (Fig 26–2) develops at the site of infection. Typically, it begins as an indurated, painless papule, usually of the penis, external genitalia, anal area, or lips, that becomes ulcerated. Bilateral, firm, nonsuppurative, painless enlargement of the inguinal lymph nodes usually develops within

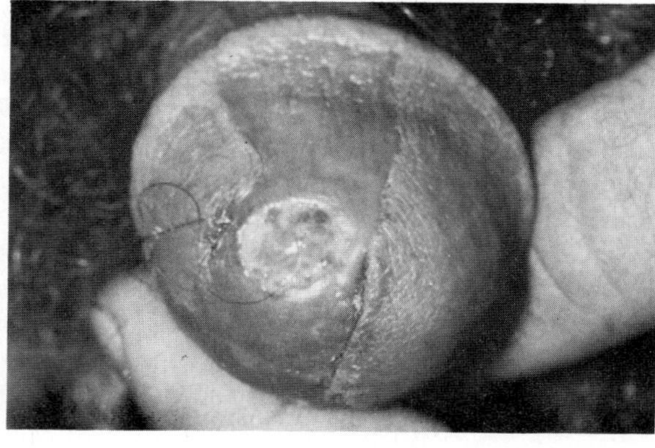

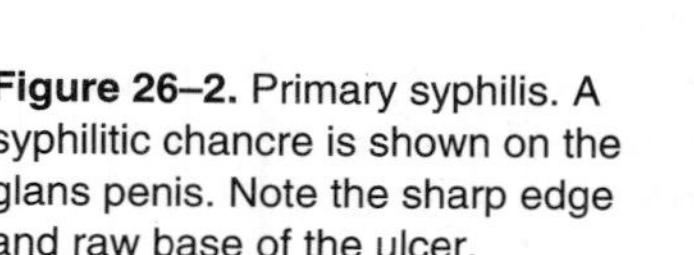

**Figure 26–2.** Primary syphilis. A syphilitic chancre is shown on the glans penis. Note the sharp edge and raw base of the ulcer.

1 week of the primary lesion and may persist for months. Primary lesions teeming with *T. pallidum* can be found by dark-field or direct fluorescence antibody microscopy. They heal spontaneously after 4 to 6 weeks.

Chancre lasts for weeks

SECONDARY SYPHILIS

Secondary syphilis may develop 2 to 10 weeks after the primary lesion has healed. It is characterized by a symmetric mucocutaneous maculopapular rash and generalized nontender lymph node enlargement with manifestations of systemic infection. Skin lesions are distributed on the trunk and extremities, often including the palms, soles, and face, and can mimic a variety of infectious and noninfectious skin eruptions. About one third of cases develop painless mucosal warty erosions called **condylomata lata.** These erosions usually develop in warm, moist sites such as the genitals and perineum. In one third of untreated cases, host immune responses appear to resolve the infection. In the remainder, the illness enters a dormant or latent state.

Maculopapular rash extending to palms and soles

Warty condylomata lata appear on genitalia

LATENT SYPHILIS

Latent syphilis is characterized by positive results of serologic tests in the absence of clinical signs or symptoms or of abnormal findings in cerebrospinal fluid. It is divided into two stages. Early latent syphilis, which occurs within 2 years of infection, is potentially transmissible because relapses associated with spirochetemia are possible. Late latent syphilis, which occurs more than 2 years after infection, is associated with immunity to relapse and resistance to reinfection: About one third of cases do not progress beyond this stage.

Serologic tests still positive

TERTIARY SYPHILIS

About one third of patients with untreated syphilis develop tertiary syphilis. The manifestations may appear as early as 5 years after infection, but characteristically occur after 15 to 20 years. Meningovascular syphilis involves vascular changes of the meninges associated with increased cells and protein in the cerebrospinal fluid and focal neurologic changes. In general paresis, there is extensive cortical degeneration of the brain, with mental changes ranging from decreased memory to hallucinations or frank psychosis. Tabes dorsalis involves demyelination of the posterior columns and dorsal roots and damage to dorsal root ganglia. The latter produces ataxia, wide-based gait, foot slap, and loss of the sensations of position, pain, and temperature. Not all patients with central nervous system involvement have symptomatic disease.

One third of untreated progress to tertiary

Cortical degeneration in generalized paresis

The most characteristic lesion of late cardiovascular syphilis is the development of an aneurysm of the ascending and transverse segments of the aortic arch as a result of gummatous changes in the middle coat of the aorta and loss of elasticity. This aneurysm can lead to aortic valve incompetence, pressure necrosis of structures adjacent to the aorta, or rupture of the aorta. The isolated gumma is a granulomatous reaction to *T. pallidum* infection. It occurs most often in skin, bones, or joints, but may involve any organ. Clinical manifestations of gumma are similar to those of other mass-producing lesions in the tissues, such as tumors.

Aortic aneurism from gummatous changes in wall

CONGENITAL SYPHILIS

The fetus is susceptible to syphilis only after the fourth month of gestation, and adequate treatment of an infected mother before that time will prevent fetal damage. Thereafter, treatment of the mother involves treatment of an already infected fetus. Because active syphilitic infection is devastating to the infant, routine serologic testing is performed in early pregnancy and should be repeated in the last trimester in women at high risk of acquiring syphilis. Untreated maternal infection may result in fetal loss or congenital syphilis, which is analogous to secondary syphilis in the adult, with involvement of the eyes, meninges, bones, and skin. Anemia, jaundice, and thrombocytopenia may also occur, and the disease in the infant must be differentiated from other congenital infections such as toxoplasmosis, rubella, and cytomegalovirus.

Fetus infected after fourth month of pregnancy

Detected by serologic testing

## Laboratory Diagnosis

*Treponema pallidum* can be detected in primary and secondary lesions by dark-field microscopy or by treatment of smears from lesions with polyclonal fluorescent antitrepone-

Dark-field positive in primary and secondary lesions

Indirect immunofluorescence test available

mal antibody preparations derived from sera of infected rabbits. The recent introduction of monoclonal antibodies specific for *T. pallidum* has improved both sensitivity and specificity of the direct immunofluorescence test. Dark-field microscopy requires considerable skill and experience and is prone to misinterpretation in the examination of oral and rectal lesions, in which other spirochetes from the normal flora may be numerous.

Nontreponemal tests use cardiolipin antigen

Most cases of syphilis are diagnosed serologically. Nontreponemal tests such as the VDRL (Venereal Disease Research Laboratory), RPR (rapid plasma reagin), and several more recently introduced procedures depend on immune flocculation of cardiolipin in the presence of lecithin and cholesterol. They become positive in the early stages of the primary lesion and, with the possible exception of some patients with advanced HIV infection, are uniformly positive during the secondary stage. They slowly wane in the later stages of the disease. In neurosyphilis, VDRL tests on cerebrospinal fluid may be positive when the serum VDRL has reverted to negative. Cardiolipin tests are nonspecific: they may become positive in a variety of autoimmune diseases or in those involving substantial tissue destruction or liver involvement, such as lupus erythematosus, viral hepatitis, infectious mononucleosis, and malaria. False-positive results can also occur occasionally in pregnancy and in patients with HIV infection. Nontreponemal tests are thus used as screening procedures for diagnosis and are confirmed by one of the treponemal tests to be described next. They are, however, of substantial value as tests of cure after treatment, because they slowly revert to negative or their titer of reactivity decreases substantially after successful therapy. In contrast, treponemal tests more commonly remain positive.

False-positive test results in other diseases

Nontreponemal tests are used for screening and as tests of response to treatment

FTA-ABS is an indirect immunofluorescent test

Treponemal tests involve direct detection of antibody to *T. pallidum*. The spirochetes used in the tests are derived from rabbit testicular lesions. Two procedures are now used most frequently, the fluorescent treponemal antibody absorption test (FTA-ABS) and, increasingly, the microhemagglutination test for *T. pallidum* antibody (MHA-TP). The FTA-ABS procedure is an indirect immunofluorescence serodiagnostic test (see Chapter 14). It involves treatment of the patient's serum with extracts of a cultivated treponeme that is not *T. pallidum*. This treatment blocks potential nonspecific cross-reacting antibodies. The treated (absorbed) serum is then applied to a slide to which *T. pallidum* has been fixed. After any specific antibody is allowed to react, nonbound constituents of serum are removed by washing, and the presence of antibody on *T. pallidum* is detected by application of a fluorescein-labeled anti-human globulin serum prepared by immunizing rabbits with human immunoglobulin. Positive results are indicated by the bright fluorescence of *T. pallidum* under the ultraviolet microscope.

MHA-TP involves adsorption of treponemal antigens to erythrocytes

The MHA-TP is simpler than the FTA-ABS and only slightly less sensitive. It is a hemagglutination test employing *T. pallidum* antigens adsorbed to erythrocytes that have been stabilized by tannic acid and formaldehyde. Appropriate blocking antigens are added to avoid nonspecific reactions.

Several treponemal tests capable of detecting specific IgM antibodies have been developed. Potentially, they could be valuable in the diagnosis of congenital syphilis in children newly born of syphilitic mothers. The diagnosis in such infants is currently confused by the presence of circulating, maternally acquired, antitreponemal IgG antibodies. Unfortunately, reliable commercial IgM tests are not yet generally available.

Treponemal tests are specific, but unaffected by treatment

Treponemal tests are considerably more specific than those using cardiolipin, but the titers of positive tests do not decrease rapidly with cure. Thus, they are valuable confirmatory tests, but they are not helpful in monitoring therapy. Until recently, it was believed that a negative treponemal test excluded the possibility of prior syphilis. It is now known that therapy-induced seroreversal occurs with regularity in symptomatic HIV-positive patients and in up to a quarter of immunocompetent patients treated for a first episode of primary infection.

## Nonvenereal Treponemal Diseases

Etiologic agents indistinguishable from *T. pallidum*

Three nonvenereal treponematoses, bejel (endemic syphilis), yaws, and pinta, occur in different geographic locations. In each case, the etiologic spirochete is indistinguishable morphologically and antigenically from *T. pallidum*, and the same difficulties have been encountered in attempting to grow them. Patients exhibit serologic responses in nontreponemal and treponemal tests similar to those of patients with syphilis, and it seems probable that each disease, and venereal syphilis itself, is caused by organisms that have diverged in evolution under particular local conditions. It has not been possible to determine which, if any, was the first human disease.

The nonvenereal treponematoses all occur in developing countries in which hygiene has been poor, little clothing is worn, and direct skin contact is common, often because of overcrowding. They frequently develop in childhood. The major manifestations of pinta and yaws involve the skin, and infection is transmitted by direct contact. In bejel, primary and secondary lesions usually involve the oral cavity, and spread may occur during suckling, by oral contact, or through fomites. All three diseases have primary and secondary stages, and tertiary manifestations may develop. Their features are summarized in Table 26–1. These infections are rarely transmitted venereally, and congenital infections do not occur. All are susceptible to penicillin. Their manifestations are well recognized by affected populations, and all have been greatly reduced in incidence by public health procedures designed to eradicate them.

Occur under poor hygienic conditions

Major clinical manifestations involve the skin or oral cavity

Penicillin treatment effective

## LEPTOSPIRA

Leptospirosis is a worldwide disease of a variety of animal species. It can be transmitted to humans, usually through water contaminated with animal urine. It is caused by *Leptospira interrogans*, the pathogenic member of the genus *Leptospira*. In the past, multiple species of pathogenic leptospires were recognized (eg, *L. icterohaemorrhagiae*, *L. canicola*, *L. pomona*, and *L. autumnalis*) based on geographic occurrence, differences in host species, and associated clinical syndromes, as well as antigenic differences. Now, however, 18 serogroups are recognized, many of which bear the names of the previously described species (eg, *L. interrogans*, serogroup *pomona*), and more than 170 serotypes are recognized within these groups. The clinical syndromes caused by the different serogroups have special features, but they show considerable overlap. The distinction between serogroups and serotypes is of epidemiologic and epizoologic importance rather than clinical significance.

Zoonotic disease transmitted through animal urine

*L. interrogans* has many serogroups and serotypes

### ■ Leptospira interrogans

#### Morphology and Cultivation

*Leptospira interrogans* is a slim (approximately 0.15-μm) spirochete 5 to 15 μm long, with a single axial filament, fine, closely wound spirals, and hooked ends. As it is not visualized with the usual bacteriologic staining procedures, detection is most easily accomplished by

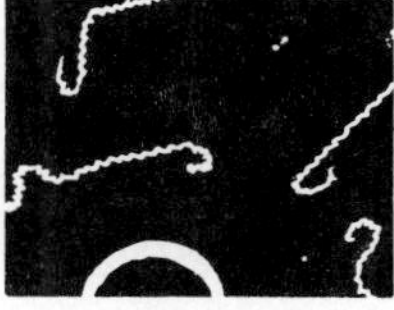

*Leptospira,* dark-field microscopy

**TABLE 26–1. NONVENEREAL TREPONEMES**

| Disease | Cause | Major Geographic Location | Primary Lesion | Secondary Lesions | Tertiary Lesions |
|---|---|---|---|---|---|
| Bejel | *T. pallidum*, subspecies *endenicum*[a] | Middle East; arid, hot areas | Oral cavity[b] | Oral mucosa | Rare; gummatous lesions of skin, periosteum, bone, and joint |
| Yaws | *T. pallidum*, subspecies *pertenue* | Humid, tropical belt | Skin, papillomatous | Systemic; resemble syphilis | Rare; gummatous lesions of skin, periosteum, bone, and joint[c] |
| Pinta | *T. carateum* | Central and South America | Skin, erythematous papule | Skin; merge into primary lesion; altered pigmentation | Areas of altered skin pigmentation and hyperkeratoses |

[a] Probably a variant of that causing venereal syphilis.
[b] Often inapparent.
[c] Neurologic manifestations usually absent.

Grows in artificial culture

dark-field or immunofluorescence microscopy. It is an aerobe and can be grown in certain special enriched semisolid media.

### Resistance

Survives in water under alkaline conditions

*Leptospira interrogans* can survive days or weeks in some waters in the environment at a pH above 7.0. Acidic conditions, such as those that may be found in urine, rapidly kill the organism. It is highly sensitive to drying and to a wide range of disinfectants. The organism is also susceptible to a number of antimicrobics, including penicillin and tetracycline.

### Antigenic Structure

As indicated previously, *L. interrogans* can be divided into multiple serogroups and serovars (serotypes), although some antigens are common to all members of the species. Seroidentification is accomplished in reference laboratories by agglutination tests using highly specific absorbed antisera against the various antigenic components.

### Animal Pathogenicity

Chronic renal infections in rodents, cattle, and household pets

The various serogroups of *L. interrogans* are pathogenic to a wide range of wild and domestic animal species, particularly rats, cattle, and dogs. These animals constitute the zoonotic reservoirs of the diseases. Infection is often subclinical, with organisms persisting in the renal tubules and being excreted in the urine for many weeks. Guinea pigs and some other small laboratory animals susceptible to intraperitoneal infection have been used to isolate the organism from clinical and environmental sources.

## Leptospirosis

Transmitted by occupational or recreational exposure to contaminated water

Infection usually results from contact with water contaminated with the urine of infected animals or, in the case of the serogroup canicola, by direct contact with canine urine. Sewer workers, miners, farm workers, veterinarians, and slaughterhouse employees are all subject to exposure, although most clinical cases in North America are now associated with recreational exposure to contaminated water (eg, children playing in irrigation ditches or other bodies of water receiving farmland drainage). Human cases of leptospirosis peak during the summer months.

Infection occurs through upper alimentary tract or skin

Bacteremic phase may spread to CNS

Disease sometimes biphasic

Weil's disease with hemorrhage, hepatitis, and renal involvement has significant mortality

The organism gains entrance to the tissues through small skin lesions or the conjunctiva or, most commonly, through ingestion and the upper alimentary tract mucosa. Most infections are subclinical and only detectable serologically, but after an incubation period of 7 to 13 days an influenza-like febrile illness with fever, chills, headache, conjunctival suffusion, and muscle pain may develop. This disease is associated with bacteremia. Leptospires are also found in the cerebrospinal fluid at this stage, but without clinical or cytologic evidence of meningitis. The fever often subsides after about a week coincident with the disappearance of the organisms from the blood, but may recur with a variety of clinical manifestations depending partly on the serogroup involved. This second phase of the disease usually lasts 3 or more weeks and may present as an aseptic meningitis resembling viral meningitis (see Chapter 67) or as a more generalized illness with muscle aches, headache, rash, pretibial erythematous lesions, biochemical evidence of hepatic and renal involvement, or all of these. In its most severe form (Weil's disease, usually caused by the *icterohaemorrhagiae* group), there is extensive vasculitis, jaundice, renal damage, and sometimes a hemorrhagic rash. The mortality in such cases is as high as 10%.

Probable immunologic component to second phase

The onset of the second phase of the disease correlates with the appearance of circulating IgM antibodies, and it appears probable that there is a major immunologic component to its pathogenesis. This is supported by absence of response to antimicrobics when given at this stage and failure usually to recover the organism from the cerebrospinal fluid in cases of leptospiral meningitis. Leptospirosis is essentially blind-ended in humans, with transmission to others being virtually unknown.

### Laboratory Diagnosis

Blood culture positive in first week, urine later

Leptospires can be isolated from the blood or cerebrospinal fluid during the first week of the disease. Thereafter, they can often be isolated from the urine if precautions are taken to initiate cultures immediately after the specimen is collected. Antibodies begin to appear within the first week of clinical disease, and the diagnosis is usually made by agglutination tests using serotypes common in particular regions as antigens. A titer of 1:100 or greater is suggestive of infection in the presence of a compatible clinical picture. A fourfold increase in titer is diagnostic.

Serodiagnosis is usual diagnestic method

### Treatment

Penicillin and tetracycline (including doxycycline) treatment appears to modify the course of the disease if given within the first 4 days of the bacteremic phase. Later treatment is ineffective.

Antimicrobic treatment only effective early

### Prevention

Vaccines are used extensively in cattle and household pets to prevent the disease, and this has reduced its occurrence in humans. Doxycycline, given once weekly, prevents leptospirosis in individuals working in high-risk environments for short periods. Other measures include rodent control, drainage of waters known to be contaminated, and care on the part of those subject to occupational exposure to avoid contamination of food or skin lesions. Clinical disease is now unusual in the United States, and fewer than 100 cases are reported annually; however, many cases are probably unreported. It is impossible to eliminate the disease because of its reservoir in rodents. The infection is much more common in developing countries in which exposure to irrigated crops is extensive.

Rodent control and limiting high-risk environments

# BORRELIA

## Borrelia recurrentis

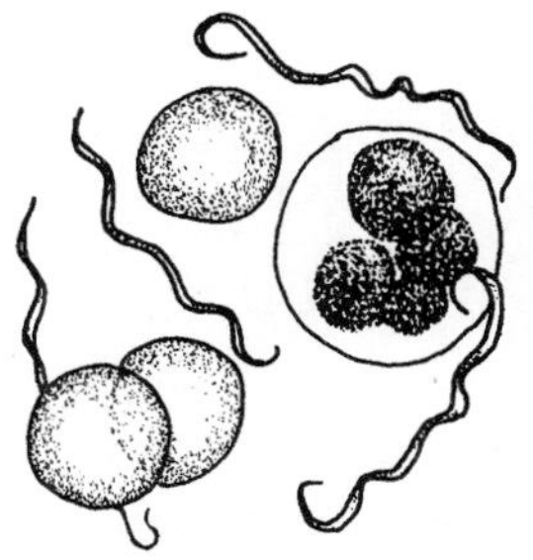

*Borrelia recurrentis* in blood smear

Relapsing fever is a disease transmitted to humans by ticks in the case of endemic relapsing fever or by body lice in the case of epidemic relapsing fever. The causative spirochetes have remarkable antigenic variability. In the past, various specific names have been given to strains associated with different species of ticks; similarities outweigh differences, however, and it has been shown experimentally that strains are not restricted to single vectors and that some tickborne strains can infect lice and vice versa. Pending definitive DNA base composition and homology studies of different strains, it is reasonable to regard them all as members of a single species, *Borrelia recurrentis,* and they are so considered here. The disease is characterized by two or more relapses associated with selection of antigenic variants.

## ■ Bacteriology

MORPHOLOGY, STAINING, AND CULTURE

*Borrelia recurrentis* is a large spirochete 10 to 30 μm long and approximately 0.3 μm wide, containing 15 to 20 axial flagella. In contrast to those of *Treponema* and *Leptospira,* spirals are irregular, with a wavelength of 2 to 4 μm. The basic organizational structure of the cell and its motility conform to that of other spirochetes, but unlike most, it is readily stained by aniline dyes. The organism is Gram negative, but it is seen most easily with Giemsa or Wright staining of smears of blood sampled during the bacteremic phase of the disease. *Borrelia recurrentis* is microaerophilic and has been successfully grown in artificial cultures containing long-chain fatty acids.

Large and easily stained

ANTIGENIC STRUCTURE AND VARIATION

The most characteristic antigenic property of *Borrelia* is its variability. Major surface protein antigens that are partly responsible for virulence and determine immunity vary dramatically at a frequency of about $10^4$ per generation, a much higher rate than is usual for expressed mutations. It is now known that genes responsible for the different proteins exist in all cells of the *Borrelia,* but are transposed intermittently from a silent storage locus to an active expression site at which they displace the previously active gene. In some cases,

High-frequency variation of major protein antigens

Silent genes for each variable antigen are transposed sequentially to an expression site

it appears that genes encoding such proteins are carried extrachromosomally on linear plasmids. The characteristic relapses of the disease are due to selection of variants with major surface protein antigens that do not react with the antibodies produced in response to the original infection or a previous relapse. Antigenic switching by *Borrelia* is, thus, an important mechanism for avoiding host defenses resembling those used by gonococci (see Chapter 19) and trypanosomes (see Chapter 54).

Antigenic switching allows *Borrelia* to avoid immune defenses; accounts for relapses

PATHOGENICITY

Tickborne strains of *B. recurrentis* infect a range of small rodents and other mammals and are pathogenic to humans. Soft-bodied ticks of the genus *Ornithodorus* can be infected from the animal reservoir; infected ticks are found in mountainous areas of North America and in other parts of the world in which the endemic disease occurs. The survival of the tick is not influenced by the infection, and the organism can be passed transovarially to subsequent generations. In louseborne relapsing fever, the human body louse is infected by ingesting *Borrelia* from a case of the disease, but the infection is not transmitted transovarially. The relapsing nature of the disease in humans is reproduced in susceptible laboratory animals.

Rodents are reservoir for tick-borne strains

Ticks transmit transovarially

## Relapsing Fever

EPIDEMIOLOGY

Endemic relapsing fever occurs in most areas of the world. It is contracted from the bite of an infected tick and is ultimately derived from the rodent reservoir. In addition to their ability to pass the infection to their progeny, ticks may remain infectious for several years when deprived of hosts. Human cases of endemic relapsing fever are usually sporadic; in the United States they often develop after exposure to ticks during recreational activities. The largest reported outbreak occurred in 62 National Park employees and tourists who slept in tick- and rodent-infested cabins on the Northern Rim of the Grand Canyon in 1973. A second outbreak involved 42 boy scouts who camped in a log cabin located in eastern Washington State.

Endemic infection is tick-borne

Epidemic relapsing fever involves human-to-human spread by the body louse. In this case there is no transovarial spread, and the life span of the infected louse is not longer than 2 months. Infection results from scratching and crushing the infected louse into its bite or other superficial wounds. The disease is associated with overcrowding, war, poverty, and social breakdown, and without treatment the mortality may approach 30%. Currently, this variety of relapsing fever appears to be limited to east and central Africa (particularly Ethiopia), China, and the Peruvian Andes. As the life span of the infected louse is brief and human carriage is not documented, it is quite possible that epidemic relapsing fever can originate from cases of endemic tickborne relapsing fever. This hypothesis remains to be proved, however, because outbreaks have occurred in areas where the endemic disease is not documented, and there are differences in some pathogenic characteristics of strains isolated from tick- or louseborne disease.

Epidemic infection is louse-borne between humans

Association of epidemics with overcrowding, poverty, and war

IMMUNITY

Immunity to the disease is largely humoral and appears to involve lysis of the organism in the presence of complement. The disease is controlled when variants from the antigenic repertoire are no longer able to avoid the immune response. For further information on this antigenic variability, the reader should consult the reference to the work of Barbour cited at the end of this chapter.

Immunity primarily humoral

## Relapsing Fever: Clinical Aspects

CLINICAL MANIFESTATIONS

After a mean incubation period of 7 days, massive spirochetemia develops with high fever, rigors, severe headache, muscle pains, and weakness. The organism produces an endotoxin-like substance, which probably accounts for some of the manifestations. The febrile period lasts about a week and terminates abruptly with the development of an adequate immune response. The disease relapses 2 to 4 days later, usually with less severity, but following the same general course. Epidemic relapsing fever is usually limited to one or two relapses, but with endemic disease three or four may occur.

Spirochetemia and endotoxin-like effects

Relapses 2–4 days later

Epidemic relapsing fever is more severe than endemic disease, possibly because of the social conditions that predispose to it. Fatalities in endemic relapsing fever are rare. Most organs of the body are invaded by *Borrelia* during the disease, and mortality is usually associated with myocarditis.

Epidemic disease more severe

LABORATORY DIAGNOSIS

Diagnosis is readily made during the febrile period by Giemsa or Wright staining of blood smears. The appearance of the spirochete among the red cells is characteristic. Cultural and animal inoculation procedures are also used for recovery of the infecting organism. Specific serodiagnostic tests are unhelpful.

Spirochetes seen in direct blood smears during fever

TREATMENT

The disease responds well to tetracycline or erythromycin therapy, and single-dose treatment with these agents can be effective. As in the case of syphilis and leptospirosis, treatment often produces a Jarisch–Herxheimer reaction, associated with sharp rises in plasma tumor necrosis factor, interleukin-6, and interleukin-8 concentrations; the reaction may occasionally be fatal.

Tetracycline or erythromycin treatment

PREVENTION

Prevention of endemic relapsing fever involves attention to deticking and insecticide treatment and rodent control around habitations, such as mountain cabins, shown to be associated with infection. Epidemic relapsing fever is controlled by delousing, particularly dusting of clothing with appropriate insecticides. Ultimately, improved hygiene will stop an outbreak and prevent further occurrences.

Louse and tick removal when around habitat

## Borrelia burgdorferi

Lyme disease is a recently defined zoonotic disease that is transmitted to humans by *Ixodes* ticks. Human cases have been reported from the United States, Europe, Australia, the former Soviet Union, China, and Japan. The disease is named for the town in Connecticut in which a cluster of cases was first recognized. It is initially characterized by a chronic migratory erythematous skin rash, fever, muscle and joint pains, and often some evidence of meningeal irritation. Later, the patient may develop meningoencephalitis, evidence of myocarditis, and a recurrent arthritis which can be severely disabling and develop over several years.

Zoonotic disease transmitted by *Ixodes* deer ticks

### ■ Bacteriology

MORPHOLOGY AND STAINING

*Borrelia burgdorferi* is a large spirochete measuring 10 to 30 μm long and 0.2 μm wide with loose and irregular spirals. Its basic cell structure and motility conform to those of other spirochetes (see Fig 26–1); it possesses 7 to 11 flagella. Like other borrelias, *B. burgdorferi* is Gram negative, but is most easily visualized with Giemsa, Wright, or acridine orange stain. In histopathologic sections, the spirochete can sometimes be visualized with silver impregnation or immunofluorescence staining procedures.

Stains with Giemsa or Wright stain

CULTURE AND STRAIN IDENTIFICATION

*Borrelia burgdorferi* is microaerophilic and can be grown, with some difficulty, in artificial culture. Although this procedure has been useful for both detection and antimicrobial susceptibility testing, its diagnostic value is limited by the organism's fastidious nature, prolonged doubling time (8–24 hours), and paucity of number in human tissues and fluids. Polyclonal antibodies prepared against purified cell components and monoclonal antibodies have indicated that there are probably several distinct strains of *B. burgdorferi*.

Microaerophil that can be grown in culture

### ■ Lyme Borreliosis

EPIZOOLOGY AND EPIDEMIOLOGY

In the United States, the disease is transmitted by *I. dammini* ticks in the eastern and central states and by *I. pacificus* in the west. Adult *Ixodes* ticks attach to, feed, and mate on deer in the late fall and winter. In the spring, fertile females, engorged from their blood meals,

*I. dammini* and *I. pacificus* are usual vectors in United States

Adults feed on deer

Larvae feed on murine reservoir of *B. burgdorferi*

Nymphs feed on vertebrate host (including humans); transmit disease if infected

Deer are essential to maintaining tick cycle

fall to the ground and deposit their eggs. During the summer, the tick larvae seek out and obtain a blood meal from the white-footed mouse, which is the main reservoir of *B. burgdorferi*. The spirochetes ingested by the larvae are maintained through the subsequent development stages of the tick. The following spring or summer, the small (1–2 mm) nymphs feed on a vertebrate host (including, again, white-footed mice) to obtain the blood required for maturation to adulthood; in the process they amplify the reservoir and may transmit the disease to humans among other mammals. The engorged, satiated nymphs fall off their host, mature into adult male and female ticks, and parasitize any available deer, thus completing a life cycle that has occupied a full 2 years. Deer are essential to the mating and survival of the tick and thus the disease does not occur in areas in which deer are absent. Transovarial transmission of *B. burgdorferi* is rare, but its occurrence contributes to maintenance and spread of the organism in nature.

Human infection usually follows bite of infected nymph

Spread throughout United States

Infection most common in summer months

Vertebrates other than deer can be infected by both the adult and nymph stages of the tick, but human Lyme disease is acquired primarily from nymphs, because they are active when humans are most likely to invade their ecosystem. Many other mammals have been shown to develop infection with *B. burgdorferi*, including raccoons, opossums, voles, cattle, and the domestic dog. Lyme disease has been spreading rapidly in the United States and has now been reported from 43 states. It is prominent in the northeastern states, Wisconsin, Minnesota, and parts of California, Nevada, and Oregon. In 1988, 5000 cases were reported, and it is probable that very many more were unreported. The reason for the extension of the habitat of infected ticks is not completely understood, but may involve carriage by birds and increasing deer populations. The increase in human cases partly reflects greater recreational use of infested areas and progression of suburbs into the habitats of the ticks and their primary hosts. The disease is usually acquired from infected nymphs between May and September and is most common in children, probably because of greater skin exposure.

#### Pathogenesis

Injury may involve endotoxin, immune mechanisms

Pathogenetic mechanisms remain to be established clearly. It is known that the outer membrane of the spirochete contains proteins and a toxic lipopolysaccharide that differs, however, from the usual Gram-negative endotoxin. The spirochetal peptidoglycan has inflammatory properties, survives considerable periods in tissues, and may contribute to arthritis when deposited in joint tissues.

In the early stages of the disease, circulating immune complexes and elevated levels of IgM are present in most patients. These disappear from the serum during the late stage of disease but are found in joint fluid. The rarity of spirochetes in affected tissues at this stage indicates that autoimmune responses probably contribute to the chronic arthritis and other late clinical manifestations.

### ■ Lyme Borreliosis: Clinical Aspects

#### Clinical Manifestations

Multiple stage disease

As with syphilis, Lyme borreliosis presents in stages. These comprise a primary lesion, a period of spirochetemia associated with fever and generalized manifestations of illness, and finally persistence of viable spirochetes in various organ systems leading to immunologically mediated damage. The disease is rarely fatal, but if untreated, it is often a source of chronic ill health.

Primary chronic migrating erythema at site of tick bite

The primary lesion occurs at the site of the tick bite, usually the thigh, groin, or axilla, 3 to 30 days after the feed. It begins as a macule or papule that expands to become an annular lesion with a raised, red border and central clearing. The lesion, known as **erythema chronicum migrans**, slowly expands. The center may become necrotic and new adjacent rings may form. Roughly half of untreated patients develop metastatic skin lesions that closely resemble the primary one. Skin biopsies show the presence of the spirochete and perivascular infiltrates of lymphocytes and histocytes. The patient frequently develops fever, muscle and joint pains, and some evidence of meningeal irritation. In the untreated patient, the skin lesions usually disappear over a period of weeks, but constitutional symptoms may persist for months.

The second stage of the disease usually begins weeks to months after the resolution of the primary lesion and generally involves the nervous system, the heart, or both. Approximately 15% of patients develop neurologic abnormalities. Typically, these present as a fluctuating meningitis accompanied by facial palsy and a peripheral neuropathy, which completely resolves within several months; facial palsy may be seen in isolation of other neurologic manifestations. Heart disease occurs in about 10% of patients, usually as an atrioventricular block. In some cases, however, an acute myocarditis develops that can lead to cardiac enlargement. Cardiac abnormalities may also fluctuate in intensity but generally resolve completely in a matter of weeks.

Some untreated patients develop fluctuating meningitis or cardiac manifestations

Arthritis marks the third stage of the disease and develops in almost two thirds of patients weeks to years after the onset of infection. Typically, it too follows a fluctuating or intermittent course, generally infecting the large joints, particularly the knees. In 10% of patients, the arthritis becomes chronic with erosion of the bone and cartilage; such individuals are often of HLA type DR4 or DR2. Synovial biopsies show vascular proliferations, perivascular infiltrates of lymphocytes and histiocytes, and fibrin deposits. The spirochetes are rarely demonstrable in the lesions by staining techniques. Occasionally, mild neurologic dysfunctions or even frank encephalitis has been reported. Another late disease manifestation most frequently seen in Europe is acrodermatitis chronica atrophicans, chronic violaceous plaques or nodules located on the extensor surfaces of the body.

Fluctuating arthritis develops months or years later

### Diagnosis

Although *B. burgdorferi* certainly exists in blood, joint fluid, and cerebrospinal fluid, cultures and direct microscopic examinations of these materials are only occasionally positive. Organisms can be cultured more frequently from the initial skin lesions, but few laboratories currently possess the techniques required. Organisms may also occasionally be demonstrated in ticks that have been allowed to feed on infected patients under controlled conditions; the procedure, however, is impractical for routine diagnosis. It is hoped that the recent development of polymerase chain reaction procedures capable of amplifying *B. burgdorferi*-specific DNA sequences in body fluids and tissues will facilitate diagnosis.

Culture possible but not usually available

Presently, the laboratory diagnosis of the disease usually rests on the demonstration of circulating antibodies to the borrelia. These often take 4 weeks to develop, but IgG antibodies are almost uniformly present in symptomatic patients thereafter. Several enzyme immunoassay tests for detecting IgM and IgG antibodies against *B. burgdorferi* are available commercially. Unfortunately, these tests are not well standardized and frequently demonstrate nonspecific reactivities, substantially decreasing their sensitivity and specificity. Western immunoblotting procedures have demonstrated improved specificity, but are, as yet, not well standardized. The recent identification of a 39-kilodalton antigen specific for *B. burgdorferi,* raises hope that its use in an enzyme immunoassay will, at last, provide an immunoserologic test of high sensitivity and specificity. Although borrelial antibodies cross-react with many other spirochetes, patients with Lyme disease do not give positive VDRL or other cardiolipin antigen tests for syphilis.

Diagnosis primarily by serology

Methods not well standardized

### Treatment

Doxycycline, amoxicillin, and erythromycin are all effective in the treatment of early Lyme disease. Approximately 15% of patients experience a febrile (Jarisch–Herxheimer-like) reaction early in the course of therapy. In the second and third stages of the disease, prolonged administration of parenteral penicillin or ceftriaxone is usually necessary; a recent controlled study suggests that the latter agent is superior. In patients with chronic arthritis, antibiotic therapy is effective in only half the affected individuals, and nonresponders may require surgical intervention.

Antimicrobics effective in primary disease, less so later

### Prevention

There is currently no vaccine available for Lyme borreliosis. In areas where the disease occurs, the most useful preventive measures are the use of clothes that reduce the likelihood of the infected nymph reaching the legs or arms, careful search for nymphs after potential exposure, and removal of the tick by its head with tweezers. Some insect repellents may provide added protection. Early diagnosis and treatment prevent the more serious compli-

Protective clothing and insect repellants

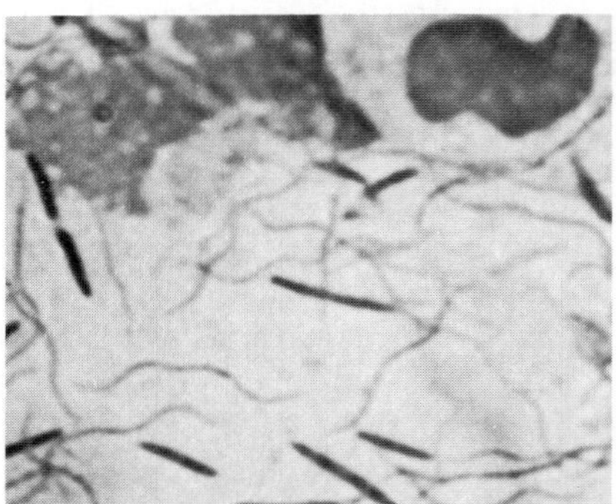

**Figure 26–3.** Fusospirochetal disease. Note the large number of fusiform organisms and spirochetes. (*Reproduced with kind permission from Leon J. Lebeau, Ph.D., Department of Pathology, University of Illinois Medical Center.*)

cations of later disease, and the public must be educated in the early manifestations of the infection. Current data do not support the administration of antimicrobics prophylactically to individuals incurring tick bites in endemic areas.

## SPIROCHETES OF THE NORMAL ORAL FLORA AND FUSOSPIROCHETAL DISEASES

Vincent's infection and ulcerative gingivitis associated with immunodeficiencies

The oral cavity, particularly the dental crevice, harbors spirochetes of the genera *Treponema* and *Borrelia* as part of its normal flora. As described in Chapter 62, spirochetes from this source, together with fusobacteria (see Chapter 18) and leptotrichia can cause an anaerobic, synergistic, necrotizing, ulcerative infection of the gums or similar ulcerations in the oral cavity or pharynx termed **Vincent's infection** or **trench mouth.** This opportunistic infection is usually seen with severe malnutrition, in leukemia, or in the immunocompromised host, particularly with deficient phagocytic defenses. It may also follow trauma or complicate herpes simplex infections. The term **trench mouth** was derived from the common occurrence of infections of this type in troops under the appalling conditions that existed in the trenches during World War I, when reasonable oral hygiene could not be maintained.

The disease is readily diagnosed by examining specially stained smears of material taken directly from the ulcerated lesion. Its appearance is illustrated in Figure 26–3 in which the characteristic fusiform and spirochetal organisms are seen. Resolution is rapid with penicillin therapy supplemented with careful oral hygiene.

## ADDITIONAL READING


Barbour AG. Antigenic variation of surface proteins of *Borrelia* species. *Rev Infect Dis.* 1988;10(suppl 2):S399–S402. A review of the molecular genetics of antigenic variation in relapsing fever borrelias by a major contributor to the field.

Burgdorfer W. The enlarging spectrum of tick-borne spirochetoses. R. R. Parker Memorial Lecture. *Rev Infect Dis.* 1986;8:932–940. An overview of *Borrelia* infections by the discoverer of *B. burgdorferi.*

Hook EW III, Marra CM. Acquired syphilis in adults. *N Engl J Med.* 1992;326:1060–1069. A recent, concise review.

Horton JM, Blaser MJ. The spectrum of relapsing fever in the Rocky Mountains. *Arch Intern Med.* 1985;145: 871–875. This article analyzes the clinical manifestations, epidemiology, and treatment of 22 cases of tickborne relapsing fever that occurred between 1944 and 1983 and describes in detail several of the later cases.

Keller TL, Halperin JJ, Whitman M. PCR detection of *Borrelia burgdorferi* DNA in cerebrospinal fluid of Lyme neuroborreliosis patients. *Neurology.* 1992;42:32–42.

Lastavica CC, Wilson ML, Berardi VP, et al. Rapid emergence of a focal epidemic of Lyme disease in coastal Massachusetts. *N Engl J Med.* 1989;320:133–137. A fascinating account of an outbreak of the disease associated with an adjacent nature reserve. An excellent source of recent references.

Musher DM, Hamill RJ, Baughn RE. Effect of human immunodeficiency virus (HIV) infection on the course of syphilis and the response to treatment. *Ann Intern Med.* 1990;113:872–881.

Penn CW. Pathogenicity and immunology of *Treponema pallidum. J Med Microbiol.* 1987;24:1–9. An account of the subject that discusses both the limitations of present knowledge and the opportunities offered by biotechnology for future advances.

Rahn DW. Lyme disease: Clinical manifestations, diagnosis and treatment. *Semin Arthritis Rheum.* 1991;20: 201–218. The most recent, comprehensive review of this disease.

Romanowski B, Sutherland R, Fick GH, Mooney B, Love EJ. Serologic response to treatment of infectious syphillis. *Ann Intern Med.* 1991;114:1005, 1009. The first careful analysis of the serologic responses to current therapy for infectious syphillis.

Stamm LV, Dallas WS, Ray PH, et al. Identification, cloning, and purification of protein antigens of *Treponema pallidum. Rev Infect Dis*. 1988;10(suppl 2):S403–S407. A description of the application of recombinant DNA technology to obtaining purified protein antigens of an organism that has not been grown. These approaches are being used by several research groups and are beginning to clarify the immunology of syphilis and to produce improved diagnostic reagents.

Steere AC. Lyme disease. *N Engl J Med.* 1989;321:586–596. A review of the subject by an author whose work led to recognition of the disease and its importance.

Chapter

27

# Mycobacteria

*James J. Plorde*

*Mycobacterium* is a genus of Gram-positive bacilli that demonstrate the staining characteristic of acid-fastness. The most important species, *Mycobacterium tuberculosis,* the cause of tuberculosis, has been one of the most devastating of all infectious agents and remains the leading cause of infectious death worldwide. *Mycobacterium tuberculosis* and other mycobacterial species are assuming increasing importance in immunocompromised patients, particularly those with AIDS.

## MYCOBACTERIUM: GENERAL CHARACTERISTICS

### Morphology and Structure

The mycobacteria are slim, rod-shaped organisms 0.2 to 0.4 × 2 to 10 μm in size. They are nonmotile and do not form spores. The unusual cell wall contains *N*-glycolylmuramic acid instead of the *N*-acetylmuramic acid present in the murein sac of most bacteria. It is also characterized by a very high concentration (60%) of lipids complexed to a variety of peptides and polysaccharides; the principal component of these complexes is mycolic acid, a long-chain fatty acid. The lipids make the cell surface hydrophobic, rendering mycobacteria resistant to staining with basic aniline dyes unless they are applied with heat or for prolonged periods. Once stained, however, mycobacteria resist decolorization with up to 3% hydrochloric acid, 95% ethanol, or both. These properties, which depend on the integrity of the cell wall, are described as acid fastness and acid–alcohol fastness, and the bacteria possessing them as acid-fast bacilli (AFB). Details are described in Chapter 14. This characteristic allows mycobacteria to be distinguished from other genera and species using the Ziehl–Neelsen stain or various modifications of this procedure, including the use of fluorochromes as the primary stain. In this case, mycobacteria, but not other genera, fluoresce when examined microscopically at the excitor wavelength of the stain.

Cell wall has high lipid content

Difficult to stain, but once stained difficult to decolorize

Acid fastness distinguishes from most other bacteria

### Growth

Mycobacteria are strictly aerobic, and the most important pathogen, *M. tuberculosis,* shows enhanced growth in 10% carbon dioxide and at a pH of about 6.5 to 6.8. Nutritional requirements vary among species and range from the ability of some nonpathogens to multiply on the washers of water faucets to the strict intracellular parasitism of *Mycobacterium leprae,* which does not grow in artificial media or cell culture.

Strict aerobes

Mycobacteria grow more slowly than most human pathogenic bacteria because of their

Many species grow slowly

hydrophobic cell surface, which causes them to clump and inhibits permeability of nutrients into the cell. Addition of the surfactant Tween 80 to cultures of *M. tuberculosis* wets the surface and leads to dispersed and more rapid growth.

## Classification

Distinguished by cultural features, biochemical reactions, and pathogenicity

The major distinguishing features among different species of mycobacteria are nutritional and temperature requirements, growth rates, pigmentation of colonies grown in light or darkness, some key biochemical tests, cellular constellation of free fatty acids, and range of pathogenicity in experimental animals. Some of the more important characteristics are summarized in Appendix 27–1. The improved means of in vitro characterization have essentially eliminated the need for animal pathogenicity tests.

## Pathogenicity

Includes human and animal pathogens

Mycobacteria include a wide range of species pathogenic for humans and animals. Some, such as *M. tuberculosis,* occur exclusively in humans under natural conditions. Others, such as *Mycobacterium intracellulare,* can infect various species, including humans, but also appear able to exist in the free-living state. Most nonpathogenic species are widely distributed in the environment.

Slowly progressive diseases

Diseases caused by mycobacteria tend to develop slowly, follow a chronic course, and elicit a granulomatous response. Infectivity of pathogenic species is quite high, but virulence for healthy humans is low; for example, disease following infection with *M. tuberculosis* is the exception rather than the rule.

Lack exotoxins or endotoxins

Mycobacteria do not produce classic exotoxins or endotoxins, and disease processes are largely a result of delayed-type hypersensitivity reactions to mycobacterial proteins. The hypersensitive state can be detected by intradermal injections of purified proteins from the mycobacteria. Cross-reaction of responses to proteins from different species is considerable.

# MYCOBACTERIUM TUBERCULOSIS

*Mycobacterium tuberculosis* is the cause of almost all cases of human tuberculosis in developed countries. In the past a significant number of tuberculous infections were caused by the animal pathogen *Mycobacterium bovis,* usually from drinking milk from infected herds; now, however, the disease has been almost eliminated by eradication programs in cattle and by pasteurization of milk.

## ■ Bacteriology

### Morphology, Staining, and Cultural Characteristics

Growth requires rich medium, $CO_2$

*Mycobacterium tuberculosis* is a slim, strongly acid–alcohol-fast rod. It frequently shows irregular beading in its staining, appearing as connected series of acid-fast granules (Fig 27–1). It grows at 37°C, but not at room temperature, and requires enriched or complex media for primary growth from clinical specimens. Growth is enhanced by 5 to 10% carbon dioxide, but is still very slow, with a mean generation time of 12 to 24 hours.

Multiple media available including rapid radiometric system

The classic Löwenstein–Jensen medium is composed of 60% homogenized egg in nutrient base with malachite green to inhibit the growth of nonmycobacterial contaminants. Colonies usually appear after 3 to 6 weeks of incubation. They become raised, warty, and adherent, with a buff pigmentation, and are difficult to emulsify because of their high lipid content. Other commonly used media are oleic acid–albumin agar (7H-11), a semisynthetic plating medium that grows *M. tuberculosis* more rapidly, and oleic acid–albumin broth (7H-12), which is used in some rapid radiometric detection systems. On 7H-11 agar, virulent strains show cording in which multiplying organisms remain attached in parallel bundles

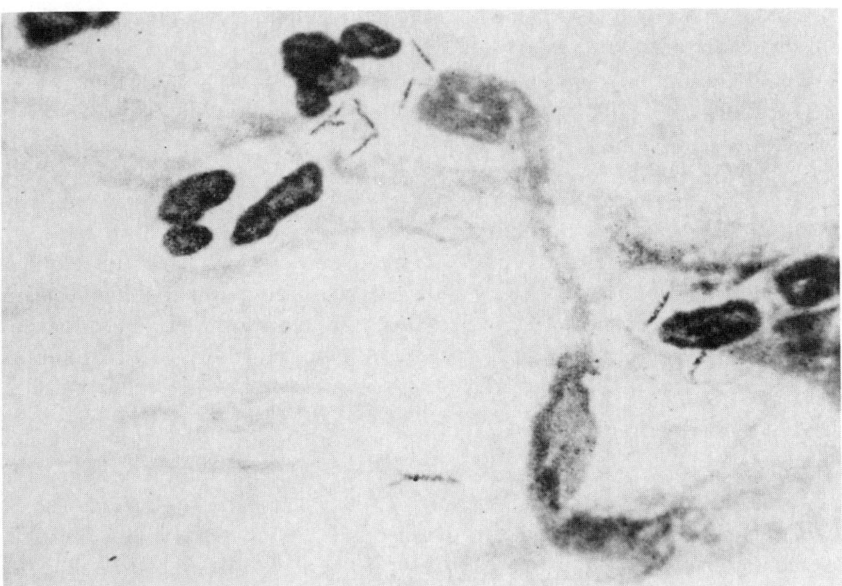

**Figure 27–1.** *Mycobacterium tuberculosis* in sputum stained by Ziehl–Neelsen technique. The mycobacteria retain the red carbol fuchsin through the decolorization step. The cells, background, and any other organisms stain with methylene blue counterstain.

and form long intertwining cords or ropes. This phenomonon is caused by a glycolipid known as **cord factor.** Although complex media are needed for primary isolation, a heavy inoculum of *M. tuberculosis* will grow well on the surface of a liquid medium containing only inorganic salts, asparagine, and glycerol.

The major phenotypic tests for identification of *M. tuberculosis* are summarized in Appendix 27–1. Of particular importance is the ability of *M. tuberculosis* to produce large quantities of niacin, which is uncommon in other mycobacteria.

## Range of Pathogenicity

*Mycobacterium tuberculosis* is highly virulent for guinea pigs, but much less so for other commonly used experimental animals; thus, much of our knowledge of the pathogenesis and immunity of tuberculosis has been derived from the guinea pig model. The minimal infecting dose for this animal is usually less than 10 cells, and after subcutaneous or intramuscular injection, a local and systemic infection develops with extensive involvement of lymph nodes, liver, and spleen. Untreated, the animal dies, usually after 6 to 12 weeks. Monkeys in captivity are also very susceptible to *M. tuberculosis* infection and can pose a serious source of infection to those working with them.

Highly virulent for guinea pigs

## Resistance

*Mycobacterium tuberculosis* is unusually resistant to drying, to most disinfectants except formaldehyde and glutaraldehyde, and to acids and alkalis. This resistance, attributable to its hydrophobic lipid surface, is exploited in preparing contaminated clinical specimens for culture. Tubercle bacilli are quite heat sensitive; they are killed in milk by pasteurization for 30 minutes at 62°C. Individual organisms in droplet nuclei are susceptible to inactivation by ultraviolet light.

Unusual resistance to drying and disinfectants but not to heat

## Antigenic Structure

*Mycobacterium tuberculosis* has a complex antigenic structure; humoral immune responses are mounted to many protein and polysaccharide antigens which do not appear to be involved in protective immunity. More than a dozen somatic and secreted antigens of *M. tuberculosis* have been cloned. If serologic tests against these antigens prove to have sufficient sensitivity and specificity, they would have significant diagnostic value, particularly in patients with extrapulmonary forms of tuberculosis. Likewise, monoclonal antibodies against

Responses occur to antigens but are not involved in immunity or used for diagnostic tests

any specific antigens would be of value in seroidentification or even serotyping. At present, however, there are no practical tests for these purposes.

Cellular immunity and cell-mediated hypersensitivity, directed against an array of protein antigens (tuberculoproteins), develop during the course of infection and contribute to both the pathology of and the immunity to the disease. Attempts to isolate a single, specific responsible antigen have so far been unsuccessful, although modern procedures for detecting, separating, and producing protein antigens or synthetic peptides are only now being exploited. Tuberculin, the most studied antigen preparation, consists of heat-stable proteins liberated into liquid culture media. A purified protein derivative (PPD) of tuberculin is now used for skin testing for hypersensitivity and is standardized in tuberculin units according to skin test activity. Hypersensitivity does not result from repeated PPD injections in those who are skin test negative; however, the degree of hypersensitivity may be somewhat increased for a few weeks in those already allergic.

Tuberculin and PPD are heat stable proteins extracted from liquid media

### Virulence Mechanisms

The basis for *M. tuberculosis* virulence is largely unknown. It produces no toxins, and both the intact cell and cellular components are remarkably innocuous to humans and experimental animals not previously sensitized to tuberculin. A number of cell wall lipids have been studied for their contribution to organism virulence. Two, Wax D and cord factor, elicit granulomatous lesions, but the amounts required are considerably in excess of those to be expected in a natural lesion. Cord factor has also been shown to be lethal to mice and inhibitory to neutrophil migration, but its direct role in human disease remains unclear. A third group of lipids, the sulfolipids, inhibit lysosome fusion to the phagocytic vacuole and suppress the production of superoxide anion, permitting mycobacteria to survive and multiply within macrophages, even those activated by the cellular immune response. This and the ability of mycobacteria to survive under the physical and chemical conditions (low pH, high lactic acid, high $CO_2$) present in developing lesions appear to be central to their virulence, but specific details are unknown. To date, not a single virulence gene has been defined and the molecular basis for invasion of, and multiplication within, host cells remain obscure. Disease manifestations result primarily from hypersensitivity to the tuberculoproteins.

Ability to multiply in macrophages and in developing lesions central to virulence

Sulfolipids inhibit lysosome-phagosome fusion

Molecular mechanisms unknown

## Tuberculosis

Tuberculosis is a disease of great antiquity that reached epidemic proportions during the major periods of urbanization in the 18th and 19th centuries. Mortality reached 200 to 700 per 100,000 population each year, accounting for 20 to 30% of all deaths in urban centers and winning tuberculosis the appellation of the "White Plague." Morbidity was many times higher. The disease has major sociologic components, flourishing with ignorance, poverty, overcrowding, and poor hygiene and during the social disruptions of war and economic depression. Under these conditions, the poor are the major victims, but all sectors of society are at risk. Chopin, Paganini, Thoreau, Keats, Elizabeth Barrett Browning, and the Brontës, to name but a few, were all lost to the disease in their intellectual prime. With knowledge of its cause and transmission, the disease was increasingly brought under control in Western countries, but mortality and morbidity remain at 19th-century levels in many developing countries despite extensive national and international control programs. Presently, it is estimated that half of the world's population is infected with *M. tuberculosis,* 30 million have active disease, an additional 8 million develop new disease annually, and 3 million die of this "captain of all the men of death" yearly. This makes tuberculosis the leading cause of death from an infectious disease. Worldwide, it is now thought responsible for 6% of all deaths and 26% of avoidable adult deaths. Particularly concerning for the future control of tuberculosis is the marked susceptibility of patients with AIDS and the growing resistance of *M. tuberculosis* to the currently available antimicrobic agents.

History and prevalence

Attack rates still high in many developing countries

Resistance to antimicrobics increasing

### Epidemiology

The great majority of tuberculous infections are first contracted by inhalation of droplet nuclei carrying the causative organism; occasionally, infection occurs through the gastrointestinal tract or skin.

Most infections by respiratory route

It has been estimated that a single cough can generate as many as 3000 infected droplet nuclei and that less than 10 bacilli may initiate a pulmonary infection in a susceptible individual. The likelihood of acquiring infection thus relates to the numbers of organisms in the sputum of an open case of the disease, the frequency and efficiency of the coughs, the closeness of contact, and the adequacy of ventilation in the contact area. Epidemiologic data indicate that large doses or prolonged exposure to smaller infecting doses is usually needed to initiate infection in humans. In some closed environments, such as a submarine or a crowded nursing home, a single open case of pulmonary tuberculosis can infect the majority of PPD-negative individuals sharing sleeping accommodations.

Repeated coughing generates infectious dose into air

Poor ventilation increases risk

The decline in mortality and occurrence of the disease in the United States over the last century is shown in Figure 27–2. By the mid-1980s, it was estimated that only 4 to 5% of American citizens, and less than 1% of American children, demonstrated positive tuberculin skin tests. The decline was not, however, uniform throughout the American populace, case rates among nonwhites and the urban poor remaining significantly higher than the national average. As the incidence of infection in the United States and other developed countries decreased, there was also a major shift in the age of tuberculosis patients. Most were over 50 and represented cases in which an old primary lesion, quiescent for decades, became reactivated. The grandfather who has developed "chronic bronchitis" is a classic source of infection to children. In 1985, the steady decline in reports of active cases and of deaths in the United States ceased, and in the ensuing 7 years active cases increased nearly 20% This is partly attributable to infections developing in immigrants from countries in which primary infections are common, partly to social and economic changes that have left a subpopulation of impoverished and often homeless individuals living under conditions reminiscent of the 19th century, partly to an increase in the numbers of intravenous drug users, and partly because of the AIDS epidemic. The last three risk factors are often found in the same individuals. It is estimated that patients with latent tuberculosis increase their risk of reactivation disease by factors of 200 to 300 with the development of a human immunodeficiency virus coinfection. The per annum reactivation rate of such individuals is estimated at 8%.

Overall decline masks increases in some subpopulations

Reactivation among older persons

Immigrants, impoverished, homeless, AIDS patients, drug abusers

Accompanying the increase in reactivation tuberculosis among high-risk American populations has been an increase in the transmission of *M. tuberculosis*. Annual tuberculin

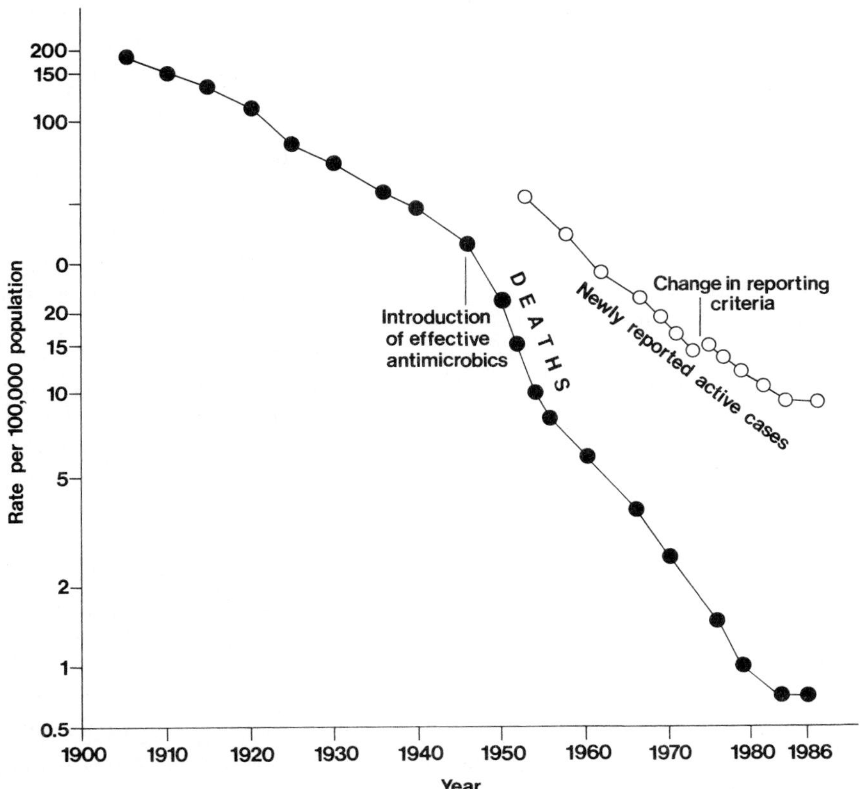


**Figure 27–2.** Morbidity and mortality of tuberculosis in the United States, 1900–1986.

Rates increasing in children

skin conversions among intravenous drug abusers have reached 6 to 7% in some areas of the United States, and the number of cases of tuberculosis among children born in the United States under the age of 5 increased by a third between 1987 and 1990. A few single-source epidemics of tuberculosis occur each year, sometimes involving schoolchildren and a teacher with unrecognized cavitary pulmonary tuberculosis or tuberculous bronchopneumonia. Often the majority of such children exposed over time become PPD positive, and some develop clinical and radiologic evidence of primary infection. Such exposure in childhood is an indication for chemoprophylaxis. Recently, similar outbreaks have been described in association with shelters for the homeless and nursing homes for the elderly and among medical personnel exposed during aerosol therapy to unusually large numbers of infected droplets from unrecognized cases of tuberculosis.

## Pathogenesis

### Primary Infection

Inhaled organisms multiply in aveolar macrophages

Primary tuberculosis is the response to initial infection in an individual not previously infected and sensitized to tuberculoprotein. The infection is usually pulmonary and develops at the periphery of the midzone of the lung. Tubercle bacilli that reach the small bronchi or alveoli with inhaled droplets are engulfed by macrophages. Those that survive continue to multiply within the macrophages and are carried to the hilar lymph nodes that drain the infected site. Multiplication of the organisms is relatively unimpeded, and the inflammatory reaction is minor and nonspecific. Dissemination of some bacilli through the lymphatic vessels and bloodstream is common at this time, and they may be deposited in many organs, including the liver, spleen, kidney, bone, brain, meninges, and apices or other parts of the lung. Symptoms and signs of infection are usually absent or manifest as a mild influenza-like disease; however, the primary site of infection and some enlarged hilar lymph nodes can often be detected radiologically. In infants and immunocompromised adults, hematogenous dissemination of organisms may occasionally produce a life-threatening meningitis.

Low reactivity to the organism allows multiplication and dissemination to lymph nodes, bloodstream

Hypersensitivity and cell-mediated immunity develop in 2–6 weeks

Mycobacterial antigens presented by infected macrophages

Cell-mediated immunity to *M. tuberculosis* and hypersensitivity to tuberculoprotein, probably manifestations of the same process, develop 2 to 6 weeks after infection, with formation of classic histologic tubercles at the sites of bacillary multiplication. This process is initiated when competent T lymphocytes recognize mycobacterium–Ia antigen complexes on the surface of *M. tuberculosis*-containing macrophages. In the presence of macrophage-produced interleukin-1, the activated lymphocytes respond to the presented antigens with the elaboration of several cytokines. Some of these proteins attract circulating monocytes. Others, including interferon $\gamma$ and possibly tumor necrosis factor $\alpha$, activate local tissue macrophages and the recruited monocytes to enhanced destruction of ingested mycobacteria, resulting in a slowing or discontinuation of intracellular bacterial growth. Nitrous oxide or other reactive nitrogen intermediates probably mediate the destruction of the mycobacteria. Another cytokine, interleukin-2, induces clonal expansion of the activated lymphocytes, thus amplifying the host's immunologic response. Still others stimulate accumulation of fibroblasts and deposition of collagen, which helps to wall off the area of infection and prevent further dissemination.

Cytokines mediate destruction, further inflammation

The tubercle includes activated macrophages and other cell types

Caseation occurs with high levels of antigen and hypersensitivity

Morphologically, the tubercle is a microscopic granuloma consisting of some multinucleated giant cells formed by the fusion of several macrophages (Langhans cells), many epithelioid cells (activated macrophages), and a surrounding collar of lymphocytes (Fig 27–3) and fibroblasts. When many bacteria are present and there is a high degree of hypersensitivity, enzymes, reactive oxygen intermediates, and reactive nitrogen intermediates are released by dying macrophages and lead to necrosis of the center of the granuloma, which is termed caseous because of its cheesy, semisolid character.

Most primary infections are controlled; lesions fibrose and sometimes calcify

Organisms remain viable for long periods

Primary infection may progress to reactivation or miliary tuberculosis

Primary infections are usually handled well by the host. Bacterial multiplication ceases. Most organisms die, and the lesions in the lung and draining lymph nodes fibrose and sometimes calcify to produce the classic Ghon complex on x-ray. Most microscopic lesions in other areas of the body also heal by fibrosis, and the organisms in them slowly die. In others, the tubercle bacilli remain viable for long periods and serve as a potential source of reactivation many months or years later if host defenses weaken. In approximately 5% of patients, the primary disease is not controlled and merges into the reactivation type of tuberculosis, or it disseminates to many organs to produce active miliary tuberculosis. The latter may result from a necrotic tubercle eroding into a small blood vessel.

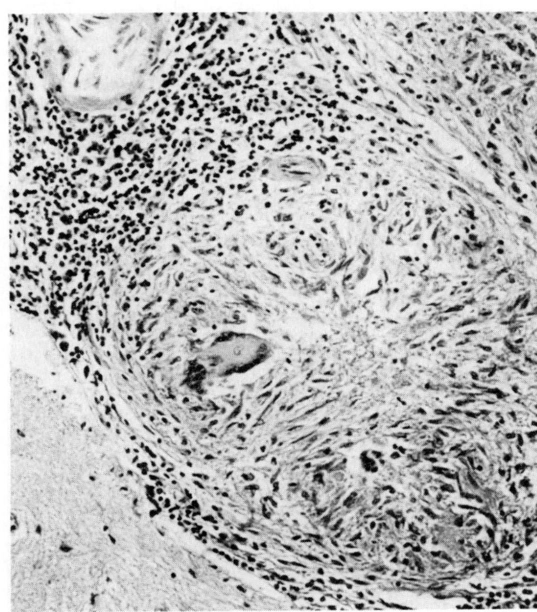

**Figure 27–3.** Microscopic tubercule of brain, showing giant cell and surrounding epithelioid cells and lymphocytes.

REACTIVATION (ADULT) TUBERCULOSIS

Approximately 10% of those recovering from a primary infection develop clinical disease sometime during their lifetime. In Western countries, reactivation of previous quiescent lesions occurs most often after the age of 50 and is more common in men. Frequently, reactivation is associated with malnutrition, alcoholism, diabetes, old age, and a dramatic change in the individual's life, such as loss of a spouse. When the disease was more common, reactivation tuberculosis was more often seen in young adults of both sexes. Recently, reactivation and progressive primary tuberculosis among younger adults have increased as a complication of AIDS.

Reactivation is most common in older men

Predisposing factors include underlying disease, life events

Reactivation usually occurs in body areas of relatively high oxygen tension and low lymphatic drainage, most often in the apex of the lung. The lesions show spreading, coalescing tubercles with numerous tubercle bacilli, and large areas of caseous necrosis. Necrosis often involves the wall of a small bronchus from which the necrotic material is discharged, resulting in a pulmonary cavity and bronchial spread. Frequently, small blood vessels are also eroded. As a result, the sputum in these patients is often blood stained and contains caseous material and numerous tubercle bacilli. Sputum droplets from such patients are the major source of infection to others. The disease is characterized by chronic fever and weight loss, probably mediated in part by macrophage-derived tumor necrosis factor (cachectin). Night sweats, productive coughing, and hemoptysis are frequent manifestations.

Lung apex has high oxygen low lymphatic drainage

Discharge of caseous material forms pulmonary cavities

Cavitary pulmonary tuberculosis most infectious form

Less commonly, reactivation tuberculosis can also occur in other organs, such as the kidneys, bones, lymph nodes, brain, meninges, bone marrow, and bowel and, again, is an important complication in some AIDS patients.

## Immunity

As discussed previously, humans generally have a rather high innate immunity to development of disease. This immunity was dramatically illustrated in the Lübeck disaster of 1926: As a result of a laboratory error, 249 infants were fed a virulent culture of *M. tuberculosis* in place of the intended bacillus Calmette–Guérin (BCG) vaccine. Although the dose was very large, 173 of the children developed only minor lesions and survived; 76 children, however, died of acute disease. Among humans, there is excellent epidemiologic and historic evidence for differences in racial immunity. Races with a long history of urbanization and exposure to the epidemics of the 18th and 19th centuries have greater resistance than rural peoples or those whose exposure to infection was recent. Native Americans and Eskimos, whose exposure was quite recent, are very susceptible and had high morbidity and mortality when the infection was introduced. Studies on attack rates in identical and nonidentical

Innate immunity high

Racial differences in immunity reflect extent of exposure of forebears twins, however, have clearly shown genetic differences in susceptibility. When one twin is clinically infected, the attack rate in an identical twin is 75%; that in a nonidentical twin is 25%.

Immunity is cell mediated, but incomplete; both CD4+ and CD8+ T lymphocytes involved

Acquired immunity is cell mediated but incomplete. Both helper–inducer (CD4+) and cytotoxic (CD8+) T lymphocytes are involved. Macrophages are activated at the site of infection by lymphokines from antigen-stimulated CD4+ T lymphocytes and limit the multiplication and spread of *M. tuberculosis*. Cytotoxic T cells release bacilli from unactivated phagocytic cells and allow them to be ingested and handled by the activated macrophages. The concomitant delayed-type hypersensitivity to tuberculoprotein plays an important part in immunity to reinfection by mobilizing immune cells and macrophages to the site of deposition of tubercle bacilli. In the past, it was believed that reinfection from external sources was extremely rare, but it is now clear that loss of hypersensitivity and cell-mediated immunity can occur over time and that reinfection can develop into clinical tuberculosis.

Delayed-type hypersensitivity enhances immunity to reinfection

Hypersensitivity can precipitate caseation and spread in established disease

The role of delayed-type hypersensitivity in immunity of established tuberculosis is more complex, because high degrees of sensitivity can precipitate caseous necrosis and lead to spread of the disease. Therapy by inoculation with large doses of tuberculin, as attempted at the turn of the century, leads to a systemic tuberculin reaction with hyperemia and even necrosis in tuberculous lesions, marked constitutional signs, and often spread of the disease.

Lesions in AIDS patients related to degree of immunosuppression

The importance of cell-mediated immunity and hypersensitivity in modulating the course of tuberculosis is, perhaps, most dramatically illustrated in patients with AIDS. Those with minimal impairment of cellular immune responses develop typical tubercles containing relatively few bacilli. Those with advanced impairment demonstrate abundant acid-fast bacilli without epithelioid cell accumulation or associated tissue necrosis.

## Diagnosis

### Tuberculin Test

PPD text measures hypersensitivity to tuberculoprotein

The tuberculin skin test measures delayed-type hypersensitivity to tuberculoprotein. Purified protein derivative (PPD), derived from culture filtrates of *M. tuberculosis*, is standardized biologically against an international reference preparation and its activity expressed in tuberculin units (TU). Most initial skin tests employ 5 TU (intermediate strength). When an unusually high degree of hypersensitivity or eye or skin tuberculosis is suspected, then 1 TU (first strength) or less is used initially to avoid the risk of an excessive reaction locally or at the site of a mycobacterial lesion.

PPD test interpreted by degree of induration

The test most commonly performed involves intradermal injection of 0.1 mL of PPD containing 5 TU. It is read 48 to 72 hours later. An area of measured induration of 10 mm or more accompanied by erythema constitutes a positive reaction, although smaller areas of induration and erythema indicate a lesser degree of sensitization to mycobacterial proteins. No induration indicates a negative reaction.

Positive PPD indicates past or current infection

A positive PPD test indicates that the individual has been infected at some time with *M. tuberculosis* or with a strongly cross-reacting mycobacterium of another species. It carries no implication about the activity of the infection, which may have been simply a primary complex contracted 20 years previously.

Anergy may develop with therapy or disease affecting cell-mediated immunity

A negative PPD test in a healthy individual indicates that he or she has not been infected with *M. tuberculosis*, is in the prehypersensitive stage of a primary infection, or has finally lost tuberculin sensitivity along with disappearance of antigen from an old primary complex. Patients with severe disseminated disease, those on steroid or immunosuppressive drugs, or those with certain other diseases such as AIDS and measles may also become anergic, lose their tuberculin hypersensitivity, and become more susceptible to the disease. Induration below the 10-mm-diameter criterion for positivity indicates low-level sensitization, which may be attributable to *M. tuberculosis* infection or to a cross-reacting mycobacterial infection.

Clinical value of skin test depends on prevalence of reactivity in population

The clinical value of the PPD test depends on the occurrence of primary infection in different age groups. Now, in much of the Western world, primary infection is sufficiently uncommon that a negative test is frequently important in excluding tuberculosis, and a positive test in infancy or childhood has significance in diagnosis and can often be used to trace a household or school source of infection. Epidemiologic surveys of tuberculin reactivity indicate trends in the incidence of infection and constitute the simplest way of monitoring the effectiveness of control measures.

Laboratory Diagnosis

If present in sufficient numbers, acid-fast bacilli can be detected microscopically in direct smears of clinical specimens or in smears of material concentrated for culture (see below). Smears are stained by the Ziehl–Neelsen procedure or one of its modifications, including the fluorescence staining method. About 65% of culture-positive sputum samples yield positive smears from concentrated specimens. These procedures are not specific for *M. tuberculosis* because other mycobacteria may have a similar morphology and may be etiologic agents of disease, members of the normal flora, or external contaminants. Their significance depends on the specimen. Acid-fast bacilli in sputum collected into a container not subject to contamination are highly significant for mycobacterial infection. A clean-voided male urine specimen, on the other hand, is often contaminated with *Mycobacterium smegmatis* from the prepuce, and the finding of acid-fast bacilli does not per se indicate infection. Bronchoscopy equipment and nasotracheal tubes or their lubricants are prone to contamination with free-living mycobacteria, and false conclusions have been drawn from smears of such preparations. The polymerase chain reaction has been reported to be useful in the direct diagnosis of tuberculosis by a number of investigators. To date, none of these techniques are practical for routine use in the clinical laboratory.

Mycobacteria detected in direct smears of clinical material

*M. smegmatis* and contaminating mycobacteria may yield "false" positives in some specimens

Cultural confirmation of a tentative diagnosis of tuberculosis is thus essential, and the organism must be isolated for identification and susceptibility testing. Specimens from protected sites, such as cerebrospinal fluid, bone marrow, pleural fluid, and ureteric urine, can be seeded directly to culture media used for *M. tuberculosis* isolation. Those samples inevitably contaminated with normal flora, such as sputum, gastric aspirations (cultured when sputum is not available, eg, in young children), or voided urine, are treated with alkali, acid, or a detergent germicide under conditions that kill the normal flora, but allow many mycobacteria to survive because of their resistance to these agents. The most commonly used treatment now employs *N*-acetylcysteine, to dissolve mucus, combined with the antibacterial effect of a weak sodium hydroxide solution. The material is concentrated by centrifugation or filtration, neutralized or washed, and inoculated onto culture media.

Material contaminated with normal flora must be treated

Mucolytic agents used in sputum

NaOH used as antibacterial

Cultures on solid media usually take 3 weeks or longer to show visible colonies. Growth may be detected radiometrically in about half the time by using liquid oleic acid–albumin broth containing $^{14}C$-labeled palmitic acid, which is metabolized by mycobacteria to liberate $^{14}CO_2$. The labeled $CO_2$ is detected in the space above the medium using an automated sampling procedure. Incorporation of a specific inhibitor of *M. tuberculosis* in a parallel vial increases the specificity of the test.

Traditional cultures take 3+ weeks; labeled substrate procedures are twice as fast

Whichever procedure is used, specific identification of an isolated mycobacterium is essential. It may be achieved with a number of cultural and biochemical tests, including those shown in Appendix 27–1, but the process usually takes several weeks. More rapid results can be obtained by high-resolution gas chromatographic analysis of fatty acids in mycobacterial colonies or by testing for homology between genetic probes of labeled mycobacterial DNA and ribosomal RNA extracted from the strain under test. Specific probes are now available commercially for detecting *M. tuberculosis* and the *M. avium–intracellulare* complex.

Traditional speciation uses cultural and biochemical tests

DNA/RNA homology useful

Susceptibility testing is important with newly diagnosed cases. When sufficient numbers of acid-fast bacilli are seen on direct smears, the treated clinical specimen can be seeded directly onto antimicrobic-containing media for susceptibility tests, thereby saving several weeks. If numbers are scanty, the initiation of tests must await primary isolation. More rapid test results can be obtained by incorporating antimicrobics into the medium used for radiometric detection of mycobacterial growth. These results show good concordance with conventional tests and are available 1 to 2 weeks earlier.

Susceptibility testing by conventional and labeled substrate procedures

## Treatment and Prophylaxis

*Mycobacterium tuberculosis* is susceptible to several effective antimicrobics (Table 27–1). Isoniazid, ethambutol, rifampin, pyrazinamide, streptomycin, and combinations of these agents constitute the primary drugs of choice for treatment of tuberculosis. All of these, except ethambutol, are bactericidal. Isoniazid and rifampin are active against both intra- and extracellular organisms, and pyrazinamide, a nicotinamide analog, acts at the acidic pH found within cells. Streptomycin does not penetrate into cells and is thus active only against extracellular organisms. The modes of action of these agents are considered in Chapter 13;

Multiple antimicrobics act intra- and extracellularly

**TABLE 27–1. ANTIMICROBICS COMMONLY USED IN TREATMENT OF TUBERCULOSIS**

| First-Line Drug | Second-Line Drug[a] |
|---|---|
| Isoniazid | *para*-Aminosalicylic acid |
| Ethambutol | Ethionamide |
| Rifampin | Cycloserine |
| Pyrazinamide | Fluoroquinolones |
| Streptomycin | Kanamycin, etc |

[a] Second-line drugs added to combinations if resistance or toxicity contraindicates first-line agent.

Resistance or toxicity may limit some agents

except for isoniazid and rifampin, their molecular targets have yet to be defined. *Mycobacterium tuberculosis* is also susceptible to other drugs that may be used to replace those of the primary group if they are inappropriate because of resistance or drug toxicity. The fluoroquinolones, such as ciprofloxacin and ofloxacin, are active against *M. tuberculosis* and penetrate well into infected cells. Their role in the treatment of tuberculosis is under evaluation.

Combined therapy used to prevent resistance

Mutational resistance to antituberculous drugs occurs at frequencies of $10^{-7}$ to $10^{-10}$, and mutants often come to predominate and produce clinical relapse when a single drug is used to treat serious tuberculosis. The resistance develops because organisms in many tuberculous lesions are sufficiently numerous to include resistant mutants, which can grow under the conditions that exist in lesions during treatment and cause clinical relapse. Adequate, continuous treatment with two or three antituberculous drugs with different modes of action greatly reduces this problem, because the chance of a doubly resistant mutant being present among the number of organisms in a lesion is very low. Primary infections with drug-resistant strains appear to be increasing, and susceptibility tests are indicated for organisms from active cases of tuberculosis.

Even "short" courses of treatment last 9 months

Resistance, HIV infection require longer time

Compliance a major problem

Treatment of established tuberculosis always involves double or triple therapy to prevent the selection of resistant mutants. Such treatment with antimicrobics to which the organism is susceptible usually renders the patient noninfectious within a week or two, which has shifted the care of the tuberculous patient from isolation hospitals and sanatoriums to the home or the general hospital. After an initial intense phase of systemic chemotherapy, treatment is usually continued with oral antimicrobics for several months. Until recently, therapy with two oral agents, isoniazid and ethambutol, was continued for a total of 18 to 24 months. Studies have now demonstrated that therapy can be shortened to 9 months when isoniazid and rifampin are used concomitantly, and to 6 months when pyrazinamide is added as a third agent. In patients whose organisms display resistance to one or more of these drugs, and in those with HIV infection, a more prolonged treatment course is used. The effectiveness of chemotherapy on most forms of tuberculosis has been dramatic and has greatly reduced the need for surgical procedures such as pulmonary lobectomy. Failure of chemotherapy is often associated with lack of adherence to the regimen by the patient, the presence of resistant organisms, or both. Unfortunately, both situations are increasingly encountered. A 1991 study by the US Centers for Disease Control indicated that nearly 15% of American *M. tuberculosis* isolates were resistant to one or more agents; 3% of new and 7% of recurrent cases were resistant to multiple agents. Rates were much higher in areas such as New York City.

Prophylactic chemotherapy, usually with isoniazid alone, is now used in situations in which known or suspected primary tuberculous infection poses the risk of clinical disease. Some indications for prophylaxis are summarized in Table 27–2. Isoniazid can be used alone

**TABLE 27–2. SOME INDICATIONS FOR ISONIAZID PROPHYLAXIS OF TUBERCULOSIS**

Radiologic evidence of active primary complex

PPD-positive close contact of infectious case

Child who is close contact of infectious case, whether or not PPD positive (retest after 12 weeks)

Known recent PPD converter (eg, laboratory worker who is regularly tested)

Patient with skin test, radiologic, or other evidence of primary infection who is immunosuppressed, is undergoing corticosteroid treatment, or has a disease (eg, AIDS) predisposing to tuberculosis

*Abbreviations:* PPD, purified protein derivative; AIDS, acquired immunodeficiency syndrome.

in prophylaxis because the load of tubercle bacilli in a subclinical primary lesion is small in relation to that in reactivation tuberculosis, and experience has shown that the development of subsequent clinical disease from isoniazid-resistant strains selected by prophylaxis can be discounted. Unfortunately, isoniazid may cause a form of hepatitis, and the risk increases progressively after age 20. Its use in older subjects involves balancing risk against potential benefit and requires monitoring with liver function tests.

Chemoprophylaxis may use single drug

### Immunoprophylaxis

At present the BCG vaccine (named for its originators, Calmette and Guérin) is the only available vaccine. It has been used for prophylaxis of tuberculosis in various countries since 1923; administration is usually intradermal. It is a live vaccine derived originally from a strain of *M. bovis* that was attenuated by repeated subculture. Since then, it has had a checkered history, with results in different controlled trials ranging from ineffectiveness to 80% protection. In most studies, however, it has substantially decreased the highly lethal miliary and meningeal forms of tuberculosis among young children. On the basis of these results, massive immunization campaigns sponsored by the World Health Organization have been organized in underdeveloped countries.

BCG vaccine is a live attenuated derivative of *M. bovis*

Effectiveness of BCG variable

Bacillus Calmette–Guérin is used only in tuberculin-negative subjects. Successful vaccination leads to a minor local lesion, self-limiting multiplication of the organism locally and in draining lymphatic vessels, and development of tuberculin hypersensitivity. The latter results in loss of the PPD test as a diagnostic and epidemiologic tool, and when infection rates are low, as they are now in most Western countries, this loss may offset the possible immunity produced. In general, tuberculosis rates in the West have declined as rapidly in countries that have not used the BCG vaccine as in those that have adopted mass vaccination with its occasional complications. Its potential value in these countries is restricted to population groups at particular risk. Its role in developing countries remains a matter of some contention. The BCG vaccination is contraindicated for individuals in whom cell-mediated immune mechanisms are compromised, such as those infected with the human immunodeficiency virus.

PPD conversion caused by BCG

BCG contraindicated for AIDS patients

## OTHER MYCOBACTERIA CAUSING TUBERCULOSIS-LIKE DISEASES

Mycobacteria causing diseases that often resemble tuberculosis are listed in Appendix 27–1. With the exception of *M. bovis*, they have become relatively more prominent as the incidence of tuberculosis has declined. All have known or suspected environmental reservoirs, and all the infections they cause appear to be acquired from these sources. Immunocompromised individuals or those with chronic pulmonary conditions or malignancies are more likely to develop disease with these organisms. There is no evidence of case-to-case transmission. The organisms grow on the same media as *M. tuberculosis*, but usually more rapidly. Colonies of some species produce yellow or orange pigment in the light (photochromogenic), and some in the light and dark (scotochromogenic). Species are distinguished by these characteristics and by biochemical reactions. Environmental mycobacteria that cause tuberculosis-like infections are usually more resistant than *M. tuberculosis* to some of the antimicrobics used in the treatment of mycobacterial diseases, and susceptibility testing is often needed as a guide to therapy.

Acquired from the environment; no case-to-case transmission

Some species are pigmented

Resistance common

### ■ Mycobacterium kansasii

*Mycobacterium kansasii* is a photochromogenic mycobacterium that usually forms yellow-pigmented colonies after about 2 weeks of incubation in the presence of light. In the United States, infection is most common in Illinois, Oklahoma, and Texas and tends to affect urban residents; it is uncommon in the Southeast. There is no evidence of case-to-case transmission, but the reservoir has yet to be identified. It causes about 3% of mycobacterial disease in the United States.

*Mycobacterium kansasii* infections resemble tuberculosis and tend to be slowly progressive without treatment. Cavitary pulmonary disease, cervical lymphadenitis, and skin

Resembles tuberculosis

infections are most common, but disseminated infections also occur. They are an important cause of disease in patients with HIV infection and CD4+ T lymphocyte counts of less than 200 cells/μL; clinical features closely resemble tuberculosis in patients with AIDS. Hypersensitivity to proteins of *M. kansasii* develops and cross-reacts almost completely with that caused by tuberculosis. Positive PPD tests may thus result from clinical or subclinical *M. kansasii* infection. Prolonged combined chemotherapy with isoniazid, rifampin, and ethambutol is usually effective.

Infection may cause PPD conversion

## Mycobacterium avium–intracellulare Complex

*Mycobacterium avium–intracellulare* complex is a group of related acid-fast organisms that grow only slightly faster than *M. tuberculosis* and can be divided into a number of serotypes. Among them are organisms that cause tuberculosis in birds (and sometimes swine), but rarely cause disease in humans. Others may produce disease in mammals, including humans, but not in birds. They are found worldwide in soil and water and in infected animals. In the United States they are most common in the Southeast, Pacific Coast, and north-central regions. They are second only to *M. tuberculosis* in significance and frequency of the diseases they cause.

*Mycobacterium avium-intracellulare* complex associated with birds and mammals

Second only to *M. tuberculosis* as cause of disease in United States

The most common infection in humans is cavitary pulmonary disease, often superimposed on chronic bronchitis and emphysema. Most of those infected are white men aged 50 or more. Cervical lymphadenitis, chronic osteomyelitis, and renal and skin infections also occur. The organisms in this group are substantially more resistant to antituberculous drugs than most other species, and treatment with the three or four agents found to be most active often requires supplementation with surgery. About 20% of cases relapse within 5 years of treatment.

Wide range of diseases; most common are pulmonary

Relative resistance to antituberculous drugs

Disseminated *M. avium–intracellulare* infections, once considered rare, are now the most common systemic bacterial infection in patients with AIDS. They usually develop when the patient's general clinical condition and CD4+ helper T lymphocyte concentrations are declining. Clinically, the patient experiences progressive weight loss and intermittent fever, chills, night sweats, and diarrhea. Histologically, granuloma formation is muted, and there are aggregates of foamy macrophages containing numerous intracellular acid-fast bacilli. The diagnosis is most readily made by blood culture, using a variety of specialized cultural techniques. Identification can be rapidly accomplished with the use of specific DNA probes. Response to chemotherapeutic agents is marginal, and the prognosis is grave.

Disseminated infection is a common complication of AIDS

Organisms isolated from blood

## Mycobacterium scrofulaceum

*Mycobacterium scrofulaceum* is an acid-fast scotochromogen that occurs in the environment under moist conditions. It forms yellow colonies in the dark or light within 2 weeks, and it shares several features with the *M. avium–intracellulare* complex.

*Mycobacterium scrofulaceum* is now one of the more common causes of granulomatous cervical lymphadenitis in young children. It derives its name from **scrofula,** an old descriptive term for tuberculous cervical lymphadenitis. The infection manifests as an indolent enlargement of one or more lymph nodes with little, if any, pain or constitutional signs. It may ulcerate or form a draining sinus to the surface. It does not cause PPD conversion. Treatment usually involves surgical excision.

Granulomatous cervical lymphadenitis in children

# MYCOBACTERIUM LEPRAE

*Mycobacterium leprae,* the cause of leprosy, is an acid-fast bacillus that has not been grown in artificial medium or tissue culture beyond, possibly, a few generations. It can, however, be grown in the footpads of normal mice, in thymectomized irradiated mice, and in the armadillo, which may also be infected naturally. The central reservoir of *M. leprae*, however, appears to be infected humans. Very rarely, cases develop in nonendemic areas without known case contacts. The infectivity of *M. leprae* is low. Most new cases have had prolonged close contact with an infected individual in the past. Transmission probably occurs

*M. leprae* fails to grow in culture

Low infectivity human reservoir is the source

most commonly by contamination of the nasal mucosa or minor skin lesions with infected nasal secretions from cases of lepromatous leprosy. Biting insects may also be involved. In vivo growth is very slow; as a consequence, the incubation period is measured in years or decades.

Slow growth in vivo contributes to incubation period measured in years

Leprosy is a chronic granulomatous disease of the peripheral nerves and nasal mucosa. It is rare in the United States and other Western countries and, for this reason, is considered only briefly. It remains a major problem on a worldwide scale, however, with an estimated 10 to 12 million cases. Immigration into Western countries from areas where the disease occurs has increased the numbers of cases seen.

Skin and nerve involvement

Two major forms of the disease are recognized, tuberculoid and lepromatous; intermediate forms occur, however, and the first form may merge into the second.

## Tuberculoid Leprosy

Tuberculoid leprosy involves the development of macules or large, flattened plaques on the face, trunk, and limbs with raised, erythematous edges and dry, pale, hairless centers. The organism may invade some peripheral sensory nerves, resulting in patchy anesthesia. Few *M. leprae* are seen in tuberculoid lesions, which are granulomatous with extensive epithelioid cell, giant cell, and lymphocytic infiltration. Patients show delayed hypersensitivity to **lepromin,** a tuberculin analog derived from leprous tissue. They mount an excellent cell-mediated immune response. The disease is indolent, with simultaneous evidence of slow progression and healing. Because of the small number of organisms present, this form of the disease is usually noncontagious.

Few *M. leprae* in granulomatous lesions

Strong delayed hypersensitivity and cell-mediated immunity

## Lepromatous Leprosy

In lepromatous multibacillary leprosy, cell-mediated immunity is deficient, and patients are anergic to lepromin. Growth of *M. leprae* is, thus, relatively unimpeded. Histologically, lesions show dense infiltration with leprosy bacilli, and large numbers may reach the bloodstream. Skin lesions are extensive, symmetric, and diffuse, particularly on the face, with thickening of the looser skin of the lips, forehead, and ears, resulting in the classic leonine appearance. Damage may be severe, with loss of nasal bones and septum, sometimes of digits, and with testicular atrophy in men. The organism spreads systemically, with involvement of the reticuloendothelial system.

Deficient cell-mediated immunity and anergy to lepromin

Many *M. leprae* in lesions

## Diagnosis

Laboratory diagnosis of lepromatous leprosy involves preparation of Ziehl–Neelsen-stained scrapings of infected tissue, particularly nasal mucosa or ear lobes. Large numbers of acid-fast bacilli are seen. Tuberculoid leprosy is diagnosed clinically and by histologic appearance of full-thickness skin biopsies.

Acid-fast smears and biopsies primary diagnostic methods

Recently, glycolipid antigens unique to *M. leprae* have been identified, purified, and tested for their usefulness in serodiagnostic tests. The specificity has been excellent, but the sensitivity for tuberculoid leprosy is still unsatisfactory. It is likely that suitable serologic tests will be available for this disease in the near future.

## Treatment and Prevention

Treatment has been revolutionized by the development of sulfones, such as dapsone, which blocks *para*-aminobenzoic acid metabolism in *M. leprae*. When combined with rifampin, dapsone usually controls or cures tuberculoid leprosy when given for 6 months. In lepromatous leprosy and multibacillary intermediate forms of the disease, a third agent (clofazimine) is added to help prevent the selection of resistant mutants, and treatment is continued at least 2 years.

Sulfones combined with rifampin primary treatment

Prevention of leprosy involves recognition and treatment of infectious patients and

Prevention requires early diagnosis and treatment of cases

early diagnosis of the disease in close contacts. Chemoprophylaxis with sulfones has been used for children in close contact with lepromatous cases. Immunization with BCG vaccine has been investigated, with varying results.

A possible diagnosis of leprosy elicits fear and distress in patients and contacts out of all proportion to its risks. Few clinicians in the United States have the experience to make such a diagnosis, and expert help should be sought from public health authorities before reaching this conclusion or indicating its possibility to the patient.

## OTHER MYCOBACTERIAL INFECTIONS

### Mycobacterium fortuitum Complex

Rapid growers cause abscesses and infections of prostheses

*Mycobacterium fortuitum* complex comprises free-living, rapidly growing, acid-fast bacilli that produce colonies within 3 days. Human infections are rare. Abscesses at injection sites in drug abusers are probably the most common lesions. Occasional secondary pulmonary infections develop. Some cases have been associated with implantation of foreign material, for example, breast prostheses and artificial heart valves. Except in the case of endocarditis, the infections usually resolve spontaneously with removal of the prosthetic device.

### Mycobacterium marinum

Cause of fish tuberculosis

*Mycobacterium marinum* causes tuberculosis in fish, is widely present in fresh and salt waters, and grows at 30°C but not at 37°C. It occurs in considerable numbers in the slime that forms on rocks or on rough walls of swimming pools, and it can cause skin lesions in humans. Classically, a swimmer who abrades his or her elbows or forearms climbing out of a pool develops a superficial granulomatous lesion that finally ulcerates. It usually heals spontaneously after a few weeks, but is sometimes chronic. The organism may be sensitive to tetracycline as well as to some antituberculous drugs.

### Mycobacterium ulcerans

Occurs in tropical areas

Severe, progressive ulcerations require surgical removal

*Mycobacterium ulcerans* is a much more serious cause of superficial infection. Cases usually occur in the tropics, most often in parts of Africa, New Guinea, and northern Australia, but have been seen elsewhere sporadically. Children are most often affected. The source and mode of transmission of the infection are unknown. Those infected develop severe ulceration involving the skin and subcutaneous tissue that is often progressive unless treated effectively. Surgical excision and grafting are usually needed. Antimicrobic treatment is often unsuccessful. Like *M. marinum*, M. ulcerans grows at 30°C but not at 37°C. (see Appendix 27–1)

## ADDITIONAL READING

Advisory Council for the Elimination of Tuberculosis. Initial therapy for tuberculosis in the era of multidrug resistance. *Morbid Mortal Wkly Rept*. 1993;42:No.RR-7,1–8. The multiple options for treatment are explained and tabulated.

Barnes PF, Bloch AB, Davidson PT, Snider DE Jr. Tuberculosis in patients with human immunodeficiency virus infection. *N Engl J Med*. 1991;324:1644–1650. A recent review of the impact of one of humankind's newest scourges on one of its oldest.

Bloom BR, Murray CJL. Tuberculosis: Commentary on a reemergent killer. *Science*. 1992;257:1055–1064. A recent, pithy, enlightening and disturbing review of this recurring menace and the paucity of tools available to deal with it.

Daniel TM. Selective primary health care: Strategies for control of disease in the developing world. II. Tuberculosis. *Rev Infect Dis*. 1982;4:1254–1265. A brief but excellent synopsis of the status of tuberculosis in the developing world and potential strategies for its control in areas with limited financial and personnel resources.

Daniel TM. Antibody and antigen detection in the immunodiagnosis of tuberculosis. Why not? What more is needed? Where do we stand today? *J Infect Dis*. 1988;158:678–680.

Dubos RJ, Dubos J. *The White Plague. Tuberculosis, Man, and Society*. Boston: Little, Brown; 1952. A scholarly and highly readable account of the history and impact of tuberculosis on Western culture.

Frieden TR, Sterling T, Pablos-Mendez A, Kilburn JO, Cauthen GM, Dooley SW. The emergence of drug-resistant tuberculosis in New York City. *N Engl J Med*. 1993;328:521–526. A frightening look at the future.

Gaylord H, Brennan PJ. Leprosy and the leprosy bacillus. Recent developments in characterization of antigens and immunology of the disease. *Annu Rev Microbiol*. 1987;41:645–675.

Hastings RC, Gillis TP, Krahenbuhl JL, et al. Leprosy. *Clin Microbiol Rev*. 1988;1:330–348. The preceding two references are recent comprehensive reviews of this biblical disease, with an emphasis on its microbiology and immunology.

Interlied CB, Kemper CA, Bermudez LEM. The *Mycobacterium avium* complex. *Clin Microbiol Rev*. 1993;6: 266–310. A comprehensive review of all aspects of this increasingly important group including its role in AIDS patients.

Slutsker L, Castro KG, Ward JW, Dooley SW Jr. Epidemiology of extrapulmonary tuberculosis among persons with AIDS in the United States. *Clin Infect Dis*. 1993;16:513–518.

Snider D Jr, Bridbord K, Hui F, eds. Research towards global control and prevention of tuberculosis with an emphasis on vaccine development. *Rev Infect Dis*. 1989;11(suppl 2):S335–S490. Proceedings of a Fogarty International Center Workshop with contributions by authorities covering the latest information on the topics considered in this chapter.

Wolinsky E. Mycobacterial disease other than tuberculosis. *Clin Infect Dis*. 1992;15:1–12. A recent highly readable and comprehensive summary of the mycobacteria that have been termed "atypical" and of the clinical diseases they produce.

**APPENDIX 27–1. MYCOBACTERIA OF MAJOR CLINICAL IMPORTANCE[a]**

| | Characteristics | | | | | | | | |
|---|---|---|---|---|---|---|---|---|---|
| **Species** | ***Reservoir*** | ***Virulence for Humans*** | ***Disease Caused*** | ***Case-to-Case Transmission*** | ***Growth Rate[b]*** | ***Optimum Growth Temperature*** | ***Pigment Production[c]*** | ***Substantial Niacin Production[d]*** | ***Virulence for Guinea Pigs[e]*** |
| *M. tuberculosis* | Human | +++ | Tuberculosis | Yes | S | 37 | – | + | + |
| *M. bovis* | Animals | +++ | Tuberculosis | Rare | S | 37 | – | – | + |
| Bacillus Calmette–Guérin | Artificial culture | ± | Local lesion | Very rare | S | 37 | – | – | – |
| *M. kansasii* | Environmental | + | Tuberculosis-like | No | S | 37 | Photochromogen | – | – |
| *M. scrofulaceum* | Environmental | + | Usually lymphadenitis | No | S | 37 | Scrotochromogen | – | – |
| *M. avium–intracellulare* | Environmental; birds | + | Tuberculosis-like | No | S | 37 | ± | – | – |
| *M. fortuitum* | Environmental | ± | Local abscess | No | F | 37 | ± | – | Local abscess |
| *M. marinum* | Water; fish | ± | Skin granuloma | No | S | 30 | Photochromogen | – | – |
| *M. ulcerans* | Probably environmental; tropical | + | Severe skin ulceration | No | S | 30 | – | – | – |
| *M. leprae* | Human | +++ | Leprosy | Yes | NG | NG | NG | NG | – |
| *M. smegmatis* | Human, external urethral area | – | None | – | F | 37 | – | – | – |

[a] Numerous nonpathogenic environmental mycobacteria exist and may contaminate human specimens.
[b] S = slow (colonies usually develop in 10 days or more); F = fast (colonies develop in 7 days or less); NG = not grown.
[c] Yellow–orange pigment. Photochromogen is pigment produced in light; scotochromogen is pigment produced in dark or light.
[d] Many other differential biochemical tests used, eg, nitrate reduction, catalase production, Tween 80 hydrolysis.
[e] Disease following subcutaneous injection of light inoculum (eg, $10^2$ cells).

Chapter 28

# *Actinomyces* and *Nocardia*

*Kenneth J. Ryan*

*Actinomyces* and *Nocardia* are Gram-positive rods characterized by filamentous, treelike branching growth, which has caused them to be confused with fungi in the past. They are opportunists that can sometimes produce indolent, slowly progressive diseases. A related genus, *Streptomyces*, is of medical importance as a producer of many antibiotics, but rarely causes infections. Important differential features of these groups and of the mycobacteria to which they are related are shown in Table 28–1.

## ACTINOMYCES

### Bacteriology

Slow-growing anaerobic members of normal flora

*Actinomyces* are normal inhabitants of some areas of the gastrointestinal tract of humans and animals from the oropharynx to the lower bowel. They grow after prolonged incubation (4–10 days) under microaerophilic or strictly anaerobic conditions. The organisms typically appear as elongated Gram-positive rods that branch at acute angles and often show irregular staining. In pus the most characteristic form is the sulfur granule. This yellow–orange granule, named for its gross resemblance to a grain of sulfur, is a small colony (usually less than 0.3 mm) of intertwined branching *Actinomyces* filaments solidified with elements of tissue exudate.

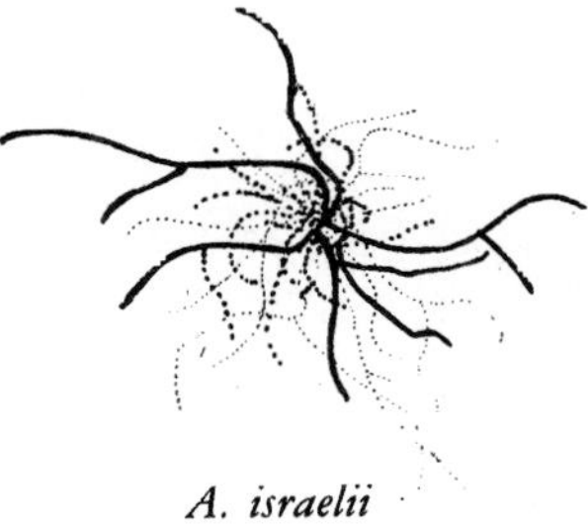
*A. israelii*

Most infections due to *A. israelii*

Species of *Actinomyces* are distinguished on the basis of biochemical reactions, cultural features, and cell wall composition. Most human actinomycosis is caused by *Actinomyces israelii,* but other species have been isolated from typical actinomycotic lesions. The related organism *Arachnia propionicus,* originally classified with the *Actinomyces,* can produce clinically similar disease. Other species of *Actinomyces* have been associated with dental and periodontal infections (see Chapter 62).

### Actinomycosis

Conditions for growth require displacement into tissues

Sinus tracts produced with pus and sulfur granules

*Actinomyces* species are highly adapted to mucosal surfaces and do not produce disease unless they transgress the epithelial barrier under conditions that produce a sufficiently low oxygen tension for their multiplication. Such conditions usually involve mechanical disruption of the mucosa with necrosis of deeper, normally sterile tissues (eg, following tooth extraction). Once initiated, growth occurs in microcolonies in the tissues and extends without regard to anatomic boundaries. The lesion is composed of inflammatory sinuses which ultimately discharge to the surface. Sulfur granules are present within the pus, but are not numerous. Free *Actinomyces* or small branching units are rarely seen, although contami-

TABLE 28–1. SOME FEATURES OF MYCOBACTERIA AND ACTINOMYCETES

| Genus | True Branching | Acid Fast | Weakly Acid Fast[a] | Aerobic Growth | Penicillin Susceptible |
|---|---|---|---|---|---|
| *Mycobacterium*[b] | – | +[c] | + | + | – |
| *Actinomyces* | + | – | – | – | + |
| *Nocardia* | + | – | +[d] | + | – |
| *Streptomyces* | + | – | Rare | + | – |

[a] Using weak decolorizer (1% $H_2SO_4$).
[b] See Chapter 27.
[c] Ziehl–Neelsen method for *M. tuberculosis.*
[d] Applies to *N. asteroides* and *N. brasiliensis* only.

Little evidence of immunity

nating Gram-negative rods are common. As the lesion enlarges, it becomes firm and indurated. Human cases provide little evidence of immunity to *Actinomyces*. Once established, infections typically become chronic and resolve only with the aid of antimicrobic therapy. Antibodies can be detected in the course of infection, but seem to reflect the antigenic stimulation of the ongoing infection rather than immunity. Infections with *Actinomyces* are endogenous, and case-to-case transmission does not appear to occur.

## Actinomycosis: Clinical Aspects

### Clinical Manifestations

Cervicofacial, thoracic, and abdominal actinomycosis most common sites

All are endogenous infections

Actinomycosis exists in several forms that differ according to the original site and circumstances of tissue invasion. Infection of the cervicofacial area, the most common site of actinomycosis, is usually related to poor dental hygiene, tooth extraction, or some other trauma to the mouth or jaw. Lesions in the submandibular region and the angle of the jaw give the face a swollen, indurated appearance.

Thoracic and abdominal actinomycoses are rare and follow aspiration or traumatic (including surgical) introduction of infected material leading to erosion through the pleura, chest, or abdominal wall. Diagnosis is usually delayed, because only vague or nonspecific symptoms are produced until a vital organ is eroded or obstructed. The firm, fibrous masses are often initially mistaken for a malignancy. Pelvic involvement as an extension from other sites also occurs occasionally. It is particularly difficult to distinguish from other inflammatory conditions or malignancies. A more localized chronic endometritis, apparently caused by *Actinomyces*, has been associated with the use of intrauterine contraceptive devices.

### Diagnosis

Paucity of *Actinomyces* in sinus drainage

Actinomycotic drainage often contaminated with other species

A clinical diagnosis of actinomycosis is based on the nature of the lesion, the slowly progressive course, and a history of trauma or of a condition predisposing to mucosal invasion by *Actinomyces*. The etiologic diagnosis can be difficult to establish with certainty: although the lesions may be extensive, the organisms in pus may be few and may remain concentrated in sulfur granule colonies deep in the indurated tissue. The diagnosis is further complicated by heavy colonization of the moist draining sinuses with other bacteria, usually Gram-negative rods. This contamination not only causes confusion regarding the etiology, but interferes with isolation of the slow-growing anaerobic *Actinomyces*. Material for direct smear and culture should include as much pus as possible to increase the chance of collecting the diagnostic sulfur granules.

Direct Gram stains of sulfur granules show branching rods

Anaerobic culture required for isolation

Sulfur granules crushed between two slides and stained show a dense, Gram-positive center with individual branching rods at the periphery. Granules should also be selected for culture, because material randomly taken from a draining sinus usually grows only superficial contaminants. Culture media and techniques are the same as those used for other anaerobes (see Chapters 14 and 18). Incubation must be prolonged, because some strains require 7 days or more to appear. Identification requires a variety of biochemical tests to differentiate *Actinomyces* from propionibacteria (anaerobic diphtheroids), which may show a tendency to form short branches in fluid culture.

Biopsies for culture and histopathology are useful, but it may be necessary to examine many sections and pieces of tissue before sulfur granule colonies of *Actinomyces* are found. The morphology of the sulfur granule in tissue is quite characteristic with routine hematoxylin and eosin (HE) or histologic Gram staining. With HE, the edge of the granule shows amorphous eosinophilic "clubs" formed from the tissue elements and containing the branching actinomycotic filaments.

Biopsy shows characteristic clubbed lesions

### Treatment

Penicillin G is the treatment of choice for actinomycosis, although a number of other antimicrobics (tetracycline, erythromycin, clindamycin) are active in vitro and have shown some clinical effectiveness. High doses of penicillin must be used and therapy prolonged for 4 to 6 weeks or longer before any response is seen. Although slow, response to therapy is often striking given the degree of fibrosis and deformity caused by the infection. Because detection of the causative organism is difficult, many patients are treated empirically as a therapeutic trial based on clinical findings alone.

Penicillin may have to be used empirically

# NOCARDIA

## Bacteriology

*Nocardia* species are Gram-positive, rod-shaped bacteria that show true branching both in culture and in clinical lesions. In contrast to *Actinomyces*, they are strict aerobes, and the species most common in human infection (*Nocardia asteroides* and *Nocardia brasiliensis*) are weakly acid fast. *Nocardia* species are commonly found in the environment, particularly in soil. They have been isolated in small numbers from the respiratory tract of healthy persons, but are not considered members of the normal human flora.

Gram-positive aerobes derived from environmental sources

The microscopic morphology is similar to that of *Actinomyces*, although *Nocardia* tend to fragment more readily and are found as shorter branched units throughout the lesion rather than concentrated in a few colonies or granules. Many strains take the Gram stain poorly, appearing "beaded" with alternating Gram-positive and Gram-negative sections of the same filament (Fig 28–1). Growth typically appears on ordinary laboratory medium (blood agar) after 2 days. Colonies initially have a dry, wrinkled, chalklike appearance, are adherent to the agar, and eventually develop white to orange pigment.

Morphology similar to *Actinomyces* but weakly acid fast

Speciation of *Nocardia* is a tedious process that involves tests for decomposition of substrates such as casein, tyrosine, and xanthine, as well as other tests not usually applied to most bacteria. Although the organism grows in a few days, these tests may require weeks

Identification may take many weeks

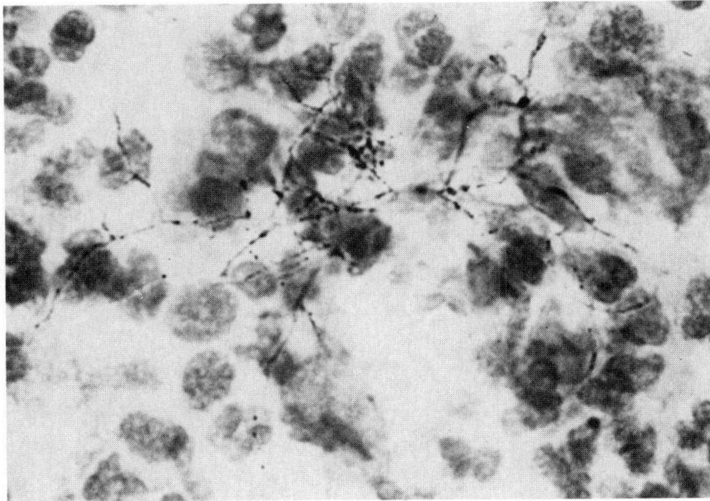

**Figure 28–1.** *Nocardia* in sputum. Note the filamentous bacteria forming treelike branches among the neutrophils. (*Reprinted with permission of Schering Corporation, Kenilworth, NJ, the copyright owner.* )

to complete. The species of medical importance are *N. asteroides, N. brasiliensis,* and *N. caviae*.

## Nocardiosis

### Pulmonary Nocardiosis

Pulmonary infection usually due to *N. asteroides*

Increased occurrence in the immunocompromised

Activated macrophages and neutrophils involved

Pulmonary nocardiosis begins with inhalation of *Nocardia* (usually *N. asteroides*) that is present in dust or soil or on contaminating mucosal surfaces. This event must be relatively common in comparison to the frequency of disease. Factors leading to disease are poorly understood, although roughly half of all patients with pulmonary nocardiosis have an underlying disease or have undergone treatment known to compromise immune defenses. These conditions include leukemia, lymphoma, chronic pulmonary disorders, and the use of immunosuppressive agents such as corticosteroids. There is evidence that effective cell-mediated immunity is important in host defense against *Nocardia* infection. Increased resistance to experimental *Nocardia* infection in animals has been mediated by cytokine-activated macrophages. Neutrophils are prominent in nocardial lesions. Although they do not kill *Nocardia*, they slow its growth while an immune response is mounted. Activated macrophages have enhanced capacity to kill *Nocardia* that they have engulfed. *Nocardia* are considered opportunists; their infectivity is low, and there is no case-to-case transmission.

Dissemination to central nervous system produces multifocal abscesses

The primary lesions in the lung show acute inflammation with suppuration and destruction of parenchyma. Multiple, confluent abscesses may occur. Unlike *Actinomyces* infections, there is little tendency toward fibrosis and localization. Dissemination to distant organs, particularly the brain, may occur. In the central nervous system, multifocal abscesses are often produced. The great majority of *Nocardia* pulmonary and brain infections are produced by *N. asteroides*.

### Skin and Subcutaneous Tissue Infections

Cutaneous infection due to *N. brasiliensis* inoculated by minor trauma

Infections can follow direct inoculation of *Nocardia*. This mechanism is usually associated with some kind of outdoor activity and with relatively minor trauma, such as a sliver or thorn prick. Infection is usually with *N. brasiliensis*, which produces a superficial pustule at the site of inoculation. If *Nocardia* gain access to the subcutaneous tissues, lesions resembling actinomycosis may be produced, complete with draining sinuses and sulfur granules. This infection may occur with *Nocardia* species or related organisms such as *Actinomadura madurae* (formerly *Nocardia madurae*), a cause of the mycetoma syndrome (see Chapter 49).

## Nocardiosis: Clinical Aspects

### Clinical Manifestations

Bronchopneumonia and cerebral abscess findings depend on localization

Pulmonary infection is usually a confluent bronchopneumonia that may be acute, chronic, or relapsing. Production of cavities and extension to the pleura are common. Symptoms are those of any bronchopneumonia, including cough, dyspnea, and fever. The clinical signs of brain abscess depend on its exact location and size; the neurologic picture can be particularly confusing when multiple lesions are present. The combination of current or recent pneumonia and focal central nervous system signs is suggestive of *Nocardia* infection. The cutaneous syndrome typically involves a pustule, fever, and tender lymphadenitis in the regional lymph nodes.

### Diagnosis

Direct Gram stain usually positive for branching, beaded rods

The diagnosis of *Nocardia* infection is much easier than that of actinomycosis, because the organisms are present in greater numbers throughout the lesions. Filaments of Gram-positive rods with primary and secondary branches can usually be found in sputum and are readily demonstrated in direct aspirates from skin or other purulent sites. Demonstration of acid-fastness, when combined with other observations, is diagnostic of *N. asteroides* or *N. brasiliensis*. The acid-fastness of *Nocardia* species differs from that of mycobacteria (see

Chapter 27) in that they are less strongly acid fast. The staining method thus employs a decolorizing agent weaker than that used for mycobacteria.

Weak acid fastness characteristic for *N. asteroides*

Culture of *Nocardia* is not difficult if the laboratory is alerted to the possibility of nocardiosis. The organisms grow on routine media used for Gram-positive bacteria (blood agar) or on those used for routine fungal cultures as long as they do not contain antibacterial agents.

Culture on routine media

### Treatment

*Nocardia* are usually highly sensitive to sulfonamides, but relatively resistant to penicillin. Combination of sulfonamides with drainage and surgery has been successful in treatment of this disease, which rarely enters spontaneous remission. Thus, nocardiosis is one of the few indications for systemic sulfonamide therapy, although a significant proportion of patients do not respond. Technical difficulties in susceptibility testing have hampered the rational selection and study of other antimicrobics, but various reports support clinical activity of ampicillin, newer β-lactams (imipenem, ceftriaxone), minocycline, aminoglycosides, cycloserine, and trimethoprim–sulfamethoxazole. Antituberculous agents and antifungal agents such as amphotericin B have no activity against *Nocardia*.

Sulfonamide therapy and drainage

Many other antimicrobics are being used

## RHODOCOCCUS

*Rhodococcus* species, aerobic actinomycetes with characteristics similar to those of *Nocardia,* have recently been recognized as opportunistic pathogens in severly immunocompromised patients, particularly those with AIDS. They are found in the soil and one species, *Rhodococcus equi*, has an epidemiologic association with horses. *Rhodococcus equi* is a facultative intracellular pathogen of macrophages with features somewhat similar to those of *Legionella* and *Listeria*. Optimal treatment is unknown although erythromycin, aminoglycosides, and some β-lactams show in vitro activity.

Intracellular pathogen from environmental sources

# Chlamydia

W. Lawrence Drew

Members of the genus *Chlamydia* are obligate intracellular bacteria containing both DNA and RNA. They have nucleoids and ribosomes and a discrete cell envelope. They multiply in host cells and are susceptible to several antibacterial antimicrobics. Three recognized species cause disease in humans, *Chlamydia psittaci*, *Chlamydia trachomatis*, and the most recently characterized species, *Chlamydia pneumoniae*. They cause infections of the respiratory tract, genital tract, and conjuctiva. One biovariant of *C. trachomatis* is the cause of trachoma, an important cause of blindness in many developing countries.

## CHLAMYDIA: GENERAL CHARACTERISTICS

*Chlamydia* species are small, generally rounded organisms that show morphologic variation during their replicative cycle. The cell envelope consists of inner and outer membranes, similar to those of Gram-negative bacteria, but differs from the latter in that there is no peptidoglycan layer between the membranes. This may account for the ineffectiveness of β-lactam agents in the treatment of *Chlamydia* infections. *Chlamydia* possess ribosomes of the eubacterial type and synthesize their own proteins. They differ from mycoplasmas in that the latter can be cultured in cell-free media and have no cell wall. The DNA genome of chlamydia is one-fourth the size of that of *Escherichia coli* and one of the smallest among prokaryotes.

Gram-negative type outer membrane but without peptidoglycan

Obligate intracellular bacteria fail to grow outside in artificial media

DNA homology between *C. psittaci*, *C. trachomatis*, and *C. pneumoniae* is less than 30%, although rRNA sequence analysis suggests they still share a common origin. The three species share a common group antigen. Their major differential features are shown in Table 29–1. With the exception of one *C. trachomatis* biovar, *C. pneumoniae* and *C. trachomatis* appear to have humans as a sole natural habitat.

*Chlamydia* species are metabolically deficient compared with free-living bacteria, because they are dependent on the host cell for energy generation and cannot synthesize adenosine triphosphate (ATP) or reoxidize reduced nicotinamide adenine dinucleotide phosphate.

Require host-derived ATP

### Replicative Cycle

The replicative cycle of *Chlamydia* is illustrated in Figure 29–1. It involves two forms of the organism, a small (0.3-μm) hardy infectious form termed the **elementary body,** and a larger (1+μm) fragile intracellular replicative form termed the **reticulate body.** The elementary body attaches to glycoprotein or glycolipid receptors found in the plasma membrane of susceptible target cells (usually columnar or transitional epithelial cells). Proteins present in elementary but not reticulate bodies are the putative chlamydial adhesins. The chlamydiae enter by endocytosis within a vacuole derived from the host cell membrane in

Elementary body infects cell by attachment to plasma membrane

**TABLE 29–1. MAJOR DIFFERENTIAL FEATURES OF CHLAMYDIA SPECIES THAT CAUSE HUMAN DISEASE**

| Feature[a] | C. psittaci | C. trachomatis | C. pneumoniae |
|---|---|---|---|
| Natural habitat | Birds | Humans | Humans |
| Diseases | Pneumonitis | Conjunctivitis, general tract infections, lymphogranuloma venereum | Upper and lower respiratory tract infections |
| Virulence in mouse | High | Variable (lymphogranuloma venereum strains only) | Less than *C. psittaci* |
| Glycogen-containing discrete inclusion bodies | No | Yes | No |
| Sensitive to sulfonamides | No | Yes | No |

[a] Information regarding serotypes is provided in Table 29–1.

Host cell metabolism used during entry

a process that uses host cell metabolism. Chlamydial elementary bodies neither expend energy nor synthesize protein. Once in the cell *Chlamydia* may evade lysosomal killing by not provoking the fusion of lysosomes with the Chlamydia-laden phagosomes.

Elementary body tranforms to reticulate body by protein modification

Multiple reticulate bodies create characteristic inclusion bodies

The metabolic changes that lead the elementary body to reorganize within 8 to 12 hours into the 10 to 100 times larger reticulate body are incompletely understood, but involve protein synthesis and modification of crosslinked outer membrane proteins to a monomeric state. Using the ATP-generating capacity of the host cell, reticulate bodies then divide by binary fission within the endocytic vacuole. The newly formed organisms finally occupy much of the infected host cell, producing a large cytoplasmic inclusion body characteristic of *Chlamydia* infections. After 24 to 72 hours, the reticulate bodies reorganize and condense to yield multiple elementary bodies with the capacity to infect other host cells when the infected cell ruptures. This process has reverse elements of initial multiplication events such as the conversion of outer membrane proteins from a monomeric state back to a crosslinked state. The proteins thought to mediate attachment to host cells are also synthesized.

Inclusion bodies contain glycogen

*Chlamydia trachomatis* reticulate bodies synthesize large amounts of glycogen, and the inclusion bodies in the cell thus stain blue with iodine. *Chlamydia psittaci* and *C. pneumoniae* inclusions do not contain glycogen.

### Antigenic Structure

Chlamydiae have common lipopolysaccharide antigens and specific cell envelope protein antigens by which they are divided into a number of serotypes. The antigenic difference between the various subtypes of *C. trachomatis* appears to reside mainly in the major outer membrane protein, which constitutes about 50% of the membrane. Each of the major disease syndromes caused by chlamydiae are associated with several different serotypes (Table 29–2). The type-specific antigens elicit protective antibody in experimental animals, but the group antigens do not. Serotyping is performed by a fluorescence antibody procedure, but is not undertaken in routine diagnostic laboratories.

# ■ CHLAMYDIA DISEASES

## Chlamydia psittaci Infections

Zoonotic respiratory disease contracted from birds

Human psittacosis (ornithosis) is a zoonosis contracted through inhalation of respiratory secretions or dust from droppings of infected birds. It was initially described in psittacines, such as parrots and parakeets, but was subsequently shown to occur in a wide range of avian species. The disease is usually latent in its natural host, but may become active, particularly with the stress of recent captivity or transport; *C. psittaci* is then excreted in large amounts.

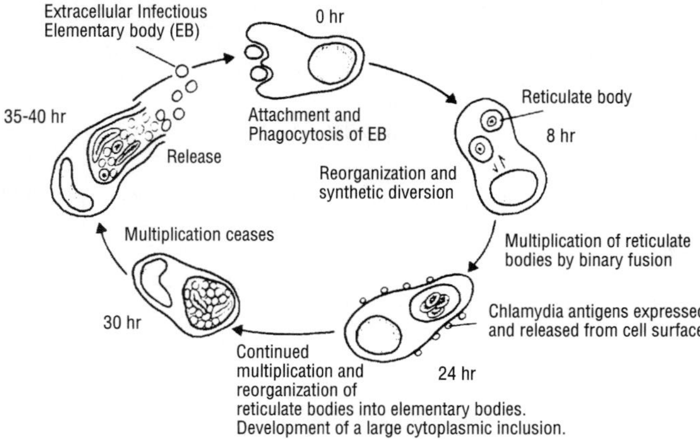


**Figure 29–1.** Reproduction cycle of *Chlamydia.*

### Epidemiology

Psittacosis in humans is seen mainly as an occupational hazard of poultry workers and bird fanciers, particularly owners of psittacine birds. Reported cases of human psittacosis in the United States decreased during the 1950s, in association with the use of antimicrobials in poultry feeds and quarantine regulations for imported psittacine birds. Currently 100 to 200 cases are reported each year. Some strains of *C. psittaci* are highly contagious and pose a hazard for laboratory workers.

Associated with poultry processing and captive psittacine birds

### Clinical Disease and Treatment

Psittacosis in humans is an acute infection of the lower respiratory tract, usually presenting with acute onset of fever, headache, malaise, muscle aches, dry hacking cough, and bilateral interstitial pneumonia. Occasionally, systemic complications such as myocarditis, encephalitis, and hepatitis may develop. The liver and spleen are often enlarged. The diagnosis of psittacosis should be suspected in any patient with acute onset of febrile lower respiratory illness with hepatosplenomegaly who gives a history of close exposure to birds. Indeed, a history of bird exposure should be especially sought in patients who appear to have a bilateral pneumonia, not caused by other agents. It must be remembered that spread can occur from both symptomatic and asymptomatic infections of birds. The specific diagnosis is usually made by demonstrating a fourfold rise in the titer of complement-fixing or indirect fluorescent antibody to chlamydial group antigen. Although *C. psittaci* can be isolated from blood or sputum early in the disease, these methods are attempted only in specialized laboratories because of the risk of laboratory infection. Treatment with tetracycline or erythromycin is effective if given early in the course of illness.

Bilateral interstitial pneumonitis

Diagnosis primarily serologic

## Chlamydia pneumoniae Infections

*C. pneumoniae* has been shown to be a cause of "walking pneumonia" in young adults worldwide. It is estimated that 10% of pneumonia and 5% of bronchitis in young adults are due to this agent. Epidemiologic evidence indicates that infection occurs throughout the year and is spread between humans by respiratory droplets. Unlike psittacosis, birds are not the reservoir. Outbreaks of community-acquired pneumonia caused by *C. pneumoniae* have been reported, as has apparent nosocomial spread. About 50% of adults have antibody and reinfections do occur. Most infections present as pharyngitis, lower respiratory tract disease, or both, and the clinical spectrum is similar to that of *Mycoplasma pneumoniae* infection. Pharyngitis or laryngitis may occur 1 to 3 weeks prior to bronchitis or pneumonia and cough may persist for weeks.

"Walking" pneumonia in young adults

Bronchitis, pharyngitis also occur

The diagnosis is established by serologic testing but this is not routinely available.

TABLE 29–2. ASSOCIATION BETWEEN CHLAMYDIAL SPECIES, SEROTYPES, AND DISEASE

| Species | Subtype | Disease |
|---|---|---|
| *C. psittaci* | Many | Psittacosis |
| *C. pneumoniae* | One | Acute respiratory infection |
| *C. trachomatis* | A, B, C | Trachoma |
| | D, E, F, H, I, J, K | Nongonococcal urethritis, cervicitis, endometritis, salpingitis, proctitis, epididymitis, inclusion conjunctivitis in newborns, infant pneumonia syndrome |
| | $L_1$, $L_2$, $L_3$ | Lymphogranuloma venereum |

Treatment with tetracycline or erythromycin for 10 to 14 days is effective in ameliorating the signs and symptoms of *C. pneumoniae* infection.

## Chlamydia trachomatis Infections

### Eye Infections

Trachoma and inclusion conjunctivitis due to different serotypes

Trachoma and inclusion conjunctivitis are distinct diseases of the eye that have some overlap in their clinical manifestations. Trachoma, a chronic conjunctivitis caused by *C. trachomatis* immunotypes A, B, Ba, and C, is usually seen in less developed countries and often leads to blindness. Inclusion conjunctivitis is an acute infection caused by immunotypes D to K, but is usually not associated with chronicity or permanent eye damage. It occurs in newborns and adults worldwide.

### Trachoma

Leading cause of blindness in some developing countries

Chronic infection leads to eyelid and corneal scarring

Trachoma, a chronic follicular conjunctivitis, afflicts several hundred million persons worldwide and has blinded millions, particularly in Africa. The disease is usually contracted in infancy or early childhood from the mother or other close contacts. First exposure results in acute conjunctivitis, which usually resolves. Persistence and reinfections and the associated inflammatory responses provide the stimulus for the major pathologic effects of the disease in untreated cases. Chronic inflammation of the eyelids and increased vascularization of the corneal conjunctiva are followed by severe corneal scarring and conjunctival deformities. Visual loss often occurs 15 to 20 years after the initial infection.

Prevention of reinfection most important control measure

Topical or systemic antimicrobic therapy effective

Control of trachoma is directed toward prevention of continued reinfection during early childhood. Improvement in general hygienic practices is the most important factor in decreasing transmission of infection within families and, of course, one of the most difficult to implement on a broad scale. Topical or systemic tetracyclines are the primary treatment, although azithromycin appears to be a promising alternative. Corrective surgery may prevent blindness and is required for severe corneal and blepharal conjunctival scarring.

### Inclusion Conjunctivitis

Neonatal conjunctivitis contracted from maternal genital infection

Inclusion conjunctivitis is seen among population groups in which the serotypes causing *C. trachomatis* genital infections are common. It is the most common form of neonatal conjunctivitis in the United States, occurring in 2 to 6% of newborn infants. The infection results from direct contact with infected cervical secretions of the mother at delivery.

High attack rate

Smears or culture from conjunctiva diagnostic

Inclusion conjunctivitis usually presents as an acute, copious, mucopurulent eye discharge 2 to 25 days after birth. Infection occurs in roughly two thirds of infants born vaginally to infected mothers, and one third of these become overtly ill. Diagnosis can be made by demonstrating characteristic cytoplasmic inclusions in smears of conjunctival scrapings (Fig 29–2) or by culture from conjunctival swabs. Systemic therapy is preferred because the nasopharynx, rectum, and vagina may also be colonized and other forms of disease may develop, such as an infant pneumonia syndrome. Erythromycin is the preferred antimicrobic for infants. Inclusion conjunctivitis is clinically similar but less common in adults, and is usually associated with concomitant genital tract disease.

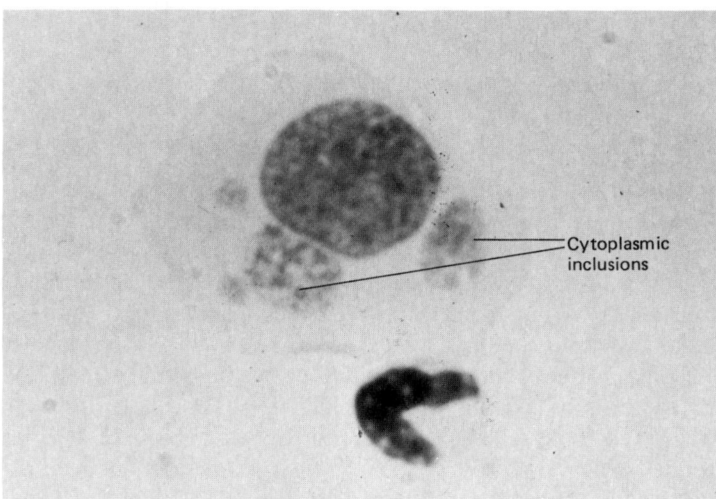


**Figure 29–2.** *Chlamydia trachomatis* cytoplasmic inclusion bodies in a conjunctival epithelial cell.

## Genital Tract Infections

The clinical spectrum of sexually transmitted infections with *C. trachomatis* is similar to that of *Neisseria gonorrhoeae*. *Chlamydia trachomatis* can cause urethritis and epididymitis in men and cervicitis, salpingitis, and urethral syndrome in women. In addition, three serotypes of *C. trachomatis* cause lymphogranuloma venereum, another sexually transmitted disease (see Table 29–2).

Clinical spectrum resembles that of *N. gonorrhoeae*

The highest prevalence of *C. trachomatis* infections is among sexually active teenagers, where the rates exceed 5% for males and 10% for females. Approximately one third to one half of male sexual contacts of women with *C. trachomatis* cervicitis develop urethritis after an incubation period of 2 to 6 weeks. The proportion of men with mild to absent symptoms is higher than in gonorrhea.

Frequent in teenagers

Urethritis in men often asymptomatic

Infections of the uterine cervix may produce vaginal discharge but are usually asymptomatic. Ascending infection in the form of salpingitis and pelvic inflammatory disease (PID) progresses in a portion of infected women estimated between 5 and 30%. The scarring produced by chronic or repeated infection is an important cause of sterility and ectopic pregnancy.

Salpingitis and pelvic inflammatory disease lead to ectopic pregnancy, sterility

More than half of all infants born to mothers excreting *C. trachomatis* during labor show evidence of infection during the first year of life. Most develop inclusion conjunctivitis (see earlier discussion), but 5 to 10% develop an infant pneumonia syndrome. *Chlamydia trachomatis* accounts for about one third to one half of all cases of interstitial pneumonia in infants. The illness usually develops between 6 weeks and 6 months of age and has a gradual onset. The child is usually afebrile, but develops difficulty in feeding, a characteristic staccato (pertussis-like) cough, and shortness of breath. The disease is rarely fatal, but may be associated with decreased pulmonary function later in life.

Infant pneumonia syndrome has delayed, gradual onset

Decreased pulmonary function a later consequence

Lymphogranuloma venereum (LGV) is a sexually transmitted infection caused by *C. trachomatis* strains of the $L_1$, $L_2$, or $L_3$ serovar. It occurs principally in South America and Africa although small outbreaks have recently occurred in North America. The clinical course is characterized by transient genital lesions followed by multilocular suppurative involvement of the inguinal lymph nodes. The primary genital lesion is usually a small painless ulcer or papule, which heals in a few days and may go unnoticed. The most common presenting complaint is inguinal adenopathy. Nodes are initially discrete, but as the disease progresses they become matted and suppurative (bubos). The skin over the node may be thinned, and multiple draining fistulas develop. Systemic symptoms such as fever, chills, headaches, arthralgia, and myalgia are common. Late complications include urethral or rectal strictures and perirectal abscesses and fistulas. In homosexual men, LGV strains can cause a hemorrhagic ulcerative proctitis. The most satisfactory method for diagnosis is isolation of an LGV strain of *C. trachomatis* from aspirated bubos or tissue biopsies. In 80 to 90% of patients, the LGV complement fixation test is positive (titer of more than 1:64)

Serotypes causing lymphogranuloma venereum distinct

Papule and inguinal adenopathy

Abscesses, strictures, and fistulas with chronic infection

shortly after the appearance of the bubo. Lymph nodes may need to be aspirated to prevent rupture.

Further consideration of genital tract infections with *C. trachomatis* is given in Chapter 70.

## Laboratory Diagnosis

Epithelial cells required for detection

All direct *C. trachomatis* diagnostic tests require the collection of epithelial cells from the site of infection. Inflammatory cells are not useful and should be cleaned away as much as possible. For genital infections, cervical specimens are preferred in females and urethral scrapings or in males. Eye infections require conjunctival scrapings.

Isolation of *Chlamydia* requires special treatment of cell lines

*Chlamydia* detected in cells by immunofluorescence

Isolation of *C. trachomatis* is the most sensitive and specific method of diagnosis. It is achieved in cell culture using idoxuridine- or cycloheximide-treated McCoy cells. Treatment of the cells with antimetabolites inhibits host cell replication and allows chlamydiae to use available cell nutrients for growth. After inoculation with samples and incubation for 3 to 7 days, the cells are stained with fluorescein-labeled monoclonal antibodies to detect intracytoplasmic chlamydiae (Fig 29–3). Staining with iodine also demonstrates the glycogen-containing inclusions but is less sensitive than immunofluorescence.

Many noncultural methods available

Noncultural methods less sensitive

A large number of procedures are now available for noncultural direct detection of *C. trachomatis* in clinical specimens. These include direct fluorescent antibody (DFA) methods using monoclonal antibodies directed against outer membrane proteins of elementary bodies in epithelial cells, enzyme immunoassays that detect chlamydial lipopolysaccharide, and nucleic acid hybridization methods that use a DNA probe to detect *C. trachomatis* ribosomal RNA sequences. These tests are faster, less expensive, and more available than culture; however, they are also less sensitive and less specific. Of the products evaluated, results vary widely but the best performers have a sensitivity of approximately 70% and a specificity of 97 to 99% compared with culture. Although noncultural tests can play an important role in controlling this disease, the results must be interpreted in light of the expected prevalence in the population tested as well as the social and medicolegal implications. In many instances confirmation by culture is required.

Value serodiagnosis limited by preexisting antibody

Serodiagnostic methods have little use in diagnosis of chlamydial genital infection because of the difficulty of distinguishing current from previous infection. Detection of IgM antibodies against *C. trachomatis* is helpful in cases of infant pneumonitis. Chlamydial serology is also useful in the diagnosis of lymphogranuloma venereum where a single high titer (>1:32) or a fourfold rise supports a presumptive diagnosis.

## Treatment

Effective antimicrobics include erythromycin, azithromycin

Strains of *C. trachomatis* are sensitive to many antimicrobics, of which those most commonly used are the tetracyclines, particularly doxycycline, and erythromycin. Azithromycin may be the antimicrobic of the future and may even be effective as a single oral dose. Erythromycin is used for pregnant women and infants because of the tooth staining that may result from tetracycline therapy and less experience with the newer agents. Ofloxacin is an alternative regimen for adults. Sulfonamides are inferior to the other agents.

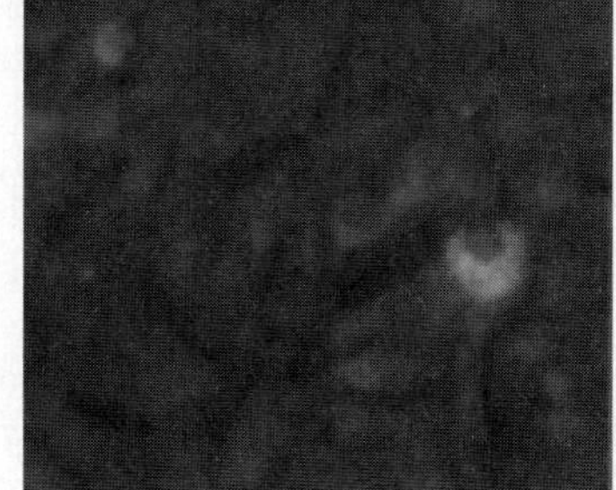

**Figure 29–3.** *Chlamydia trachomatis* cytoplasmic inclusions in tissue culture stained with fluorescein-labeled monoclonal antibodies. (*Courtesy of Syva Company, Palo Alto, California.*)

### Prevention

Routine eye prophylaxis for infants using silver nitrate or antibiotic ointments has limited effectiveness for *Chlamydia* as 15 to 25% of exposed infants still develop inclusion conjunctivitis. The primary approach to prevention of all forms of *C. trachomatis* infection comprises detection and treatment of acute and occult cases. No vaccine is available or under development.

Newborn eye prophylaxis has high failure rate

## ADDITIONAL READING

Addiss DG, Vaughan ML, Golubjatnikov R, et al. *Chlamydia trachomatis* infection in women attending urban Midwestern family planning and community health clinics: Risk factors, selective screening, and evaluation of non-culture techniques. *Sex Transm Dis.* 1990;17:138–146. Prevalence and risk factors for endocervical *Chlamydia trachomatis* infection in an urban Midwestern population were evaluated. Ninety-three (12.4%) patients had cultures positive for *C. trachomatis.*

Cates W Jr, Wasserheit JN. Genital chlamydial infections: Epidemiology and reproductive sequelae. *Am J Obstet Gynecol.* 1991;164:1771–1781. The clinical, diagnostic, and therapeutic reasons behind our failure to control chlamydial infections are examined.

Centers for Disease Control and Prevention. Recommendations for the prevention and management of *Chlamydia trachomatis*, 1993. *MMWR Morb Mortal Wkly Rep.* 1993;42(RR-12):1–39. The best source of current recommendations on diagnostic tests and treatment.

Moncada J, Schachter J, Bolan G, et al. Confirmatory assay increases specificity of the chlamydiazyme test for *Chlamydia trachomatis* infection of the cervix. *J Clin Microbiol.* 1990;28:1770–1773. This evaluation of one of the noncultural diagnostic tests illustrates the data needed for interpretation.

Reeve R, ed. *Chlamydial Infections.* Berlin/New York: Springer-Verlag; 1989. A summary of up-to-date information by leaders in the field, with particular emphasis on *Chlamydia trachomatis.*

Taylor HR, Fitch CP, Murillo-Lopez F, Rapoza P. The diagnosis and treatment of chlamydial conjunctivitis. *Int Ophthalmol.* 1988;12:95–99. The possibility of chlamydial infection must be borne in mind in neonatal conjunctivitis, in acute conjunctivitis in sexually active adults, and in chronic follicular conjunctivitis, and accurate diagnosis is based on laboratory tests.

Taylor-Robinson D, Thomas BJ. Laboratory techniques for the diagnosis of chlamydial infections. *Genitourin Med.* 1991;67:256–266. Comprehensive, thorough review of culture-, immunoassay- and DNA-based methods for detecting *Chlamydia.*

# *Rickettsia, Coxiella, Ehrlichia,* and *Rochalimaea*

W. Lawrence Drew

Bacteria of the family Rickettsiaceae, generally referred to as the rickettsiae, now include three medically important genera: *Rickettsia, Coxiella,* and the newly defined human pathogen, *Ehrlichia*. All are Gram-negative bacilli, and all are strict intracellular pathogens. Where the epidemiology is known the reservoir is animals and transmission is often by an insect vector. The diseases are typically fevers, often with a rash. The classic rickettsial disease is epidemic typhus, and the most common infections are the various spotted fevers found throughout the world.

Obligate intracellular parasites

Spotted fever and typhus groups of *Rickettsia*

Rochalimaeae are Gram-negative bacilli formerly associated with the rickettsiae, but are not strict intracellular pathogens.

## THE RICKETTSIAE: GROUP CHARACTERISTICS

### Morphology and Structure

Rickettsiae are small coccobacilli which often show a transverse septum between two bacilli, reflecting division by binary fission. They commonly measure no more than 0.3 to 0.5 μm. Although the Gram reaction is negative, they take the usual bacterial stains poorly and are better demonstrated by the Giemsa stain, particularly in infected cells. The ultrastructural morphology, which is similar to that of other Gram-negative bacteria, includes a Gram-negative type of cell envelope, ribosomes, and a nuclear body. Chemically, the cell wall contains lipopolysaccharide and at least two large proteins in the outer membrane, as well as peptidoglycan. The outer membrane proteins extend to the cell surface where they are the most abundant protein present.

Small, Gram-negative coccobacilli stained best by Giemsa

Abundant outer membrane proteins at surface

### Growth and Metabolism

*Rickettsia* grow freely in the cytoplasm of eukaryotic cells to which they are highly adapted, in contrast to *Ehrlichia* and *Coxiella,* which replicate in cytoplasmic vacuoles. They can only be grown in living host cells such as cell cultures and embryonated eggs. Infection of the host cell begins by induction of an endocytic process, which is analogous to phagocytosis, but requires expenditure of energy by the rickettsiae. Penetration of infected cells appears to be facilitated by production of a rickettsial phospholipase. Their estimated generation time is much longer than that of bacteria such as *Escherichia coli*, but more rapid than that of *Mycobacterium tuberculosis*. The organisms then escape the phagosome or endocytic vacuole to enter the cytoplasm, possibly aided by elaboration of the phospholipase. Recent studies indicate that intracellular and intercellular spread involves directional actin

Grow in cytoplasm following induced endocytosis

Growth slow compared to most bacteria

Spread involves actin polymerization

polymerization and use of the host cell cytoskeleton in a manner similar to *Listeria* (see Chapter 17) and *Shigella* (see Chapter 20). Intracytoplasmic growth eventually produces lysis of the cell.

Exogenous cofactors and ATP required

The obligate intracellular parasitism of rickettsiae has several interesting features. Failure to survive outside the cell is apparently related to requirements for nucleotide cofactors (coenzyme A, nicotinamide adenine dinucleotide) and adenosine triphosphate (ATP). In the rickettsia-infected cytoplasm, host cell ATP is exchanged for rickettsial adenosine diphosphate (ADP) by an exchange transport system similar to that found in mitochondria.

Rapidly loses infectivity outside host cell

Outside the host cell, rickettsiae not only cease metabolic activity, but leak protein, nucleic acids, and essential small molecules. This instability leads to rapid loss of infectivity, because the penetration of another cell requires energy. In summary, rickettsiae have the metabolic capabilities of other bacteria, but must borrow some essential elements from host cells for adequate growth and, thus, do not survive well in the environment.

## RICKETTSIAL DISEASE: GENERAL CHARACTERISTICS

### Epidemiology and Pathogenesis

Infect vascular endothelium with vasculitis and thrombosis

Most rickettsiae have animal reservoirs and are spread by insect vectors, which are prominent components of their life cycles. Most rickettsial infections of humans result in clinical illness. Rickettsiae infect the vascular endothelium, usually after the bite of an infected arthropod vector. The primary pathologic lesion is a vasculitis in which rickettsiae multiply in the endothelial cells lining the small blood vessels. Focal areas of endothelial proliferation and perivascular infiltration leading to thrombosis and leakage of red blood cells into the surrounding tissues account for the rash and petechial lesions; however, vascular lesions occur throughout the body, producing the systemic manifestations of the disease. They are obviously most apparent in skin, but most serious in the adrenal glands.

Multiple vascular lesions throughout body

Clinically, the infection manifests as fever and headache with widespread focal lesions, the most prominent of which is a rash. An endotoxin-like shock has been demonstrated in animals on injection of whole rickettsial cells, but the nature and role of any toxin in human disease are unknown.

### Diagnosis

In vitro cultivation is hazardous

Culture of rickettsiae is both difficult and hazardous. Their isolation in fertile eggs or cell cultures is generally attempted only in reference centers with special facilities and personnel experienced in handling the organisms. For this reason serologic tests are the primary means of specific diagnosis. In the early 1900s, the observation that serum from patients with typhus caused agglutination of certain strains of *Proteus* was developed into a serologic testing scheme called the **Weil–Felix test.** Although widely used in the past, this test lacks sensitivity and specificity and has now been replaced with a new generation of serologic tests using specific rickettsial antigens. A number of test systems have been developed, of which the indirect fluorescent antibody (IFA) method is generally the most sensitive and specific. This test is usually available only in reference laboratories.

Weil–Felix test replaced by specific serologic tests

## RICKETTSIAL DISEASE: SPECIFIC FORMS

### Spotted Fever Group

Many tick-borne rickettsioses occur in different parts of world

The most important rickettsial disease in North America is Rocky Mountain spotted fever caused by *Rickettsia rickettsii.* A number of other spotted fever rickettsioses are found in various parts of the world (Table 30–1); the name often reveals the locale (eg, Mediterranean spotted fever, and Marseille fever). They are caused by *Rickettsia conorii,* a species serologically related to, but distinct from, *R. rickettsii*. Rocky mountain spotted fever is used here to typify the spotted fevers; another less severe illness that occurs in North America, is rickettsialpox.

**TABLE 30–1. EXAMPLES OF PATHOGENIC RICKETTSIAE**

| Disease | Organism | Most Common Geographic Distribution | Zoonotic Cycle | |
|---|---|---|---|---|
| | | | *Vector* | *Reservoir* |
| Spotted fever group | | | | |
| Rocky Mountain spotted fever | *Rickettsia rickettsii* | North and South America | Tick | Rodents Dogs |
| Rickettsialpox | *Rickettsia akari* | United States, Former Soviet Union, Korea, Africa | Mite | Mouse |
| Mediterranean spotted fevers | *Rickettsia conorii* | Southern Mediterranean, Israel, Africa | Tick | Rodents, Dogs |
| Typhus group | | | | |
| Epidemic | *Rickettsia prowazekii* | Africa, Asia, South America | Body louse | Humans[a] |
| Brill's | *Rickettsia prowazekii* | Worldwide[b] | None[c] | Humans |
| Murine | *Rickettsia typhi* | Worldwide (pockets) | Flea | Rodents |
| Scrub | *Rickettsia tsutsugamushi* | South Pacific, Asia | Mite | Rodents |
| Trench fever | *Rochalimaea quintana*[d] | Europe, Africa, Asia | Body louse | Humans |
| Q fever | *Coxiella burnetii* | Worldwide | None[e] | Sheep, cattle, goats |
| Cat scratch fever | *Rochalimaea henselae*[d] | Worldwide | None | Cats, dogs |
| Human ehrlichiosis | *Ehrlichia chaffeensis* | Worldwide | Ticks | |

[a] An apparently identical organism has been isolated from flying squirrels in the United States.
[b] Related to immigration.
[c] Relapsing form of epidemic typhus.
[d] Related to *Rickettsia*, but has been grown in artificial culture.
[e] Transmission by inhalation of infected aerosols.

## Rocky Mountain Spotted Fever

Rocky Mountain spotted fever is an acute febrile illness which occurs in association with residential and recreational exposure to wooded areas where infected ticks exist. The disease has a significant mortality (25%) if untreated.

### EPIDEMIOLOGY

*Rickettsia rickettsii* is primarily a parasite of ticks. In the western United States, the wood tick (*Dermacentor andersoni*) is the primary vector. In the East the dog tick (*Dermacentor variabilis*) and in the Southwest the Lone Star tick (*Amblyomma americanum*) are the natural carriers and vectors of the disease. As *R. rickettsii* does not kill its arthropod host, the organism is passed through unending generations of ticks by transovarial spread. Adult females require a blood meal to lay eggs, and thus may transmit the disease. Infected adult ticks have been shown to survive as long as 4 years without feeding.

Ticks naturally infected with *R. rickettsii*

Transovarial spread and survival without feeding perpetuate tick infection

*Rickettsia rickettsii* is found in both North America and South America. The highest attack rates in the United States are in the central and mid-Atlantic states (Fig 30–1). The US incidence increased in the 1970s and early 1980s to more than 0.5 case per 100,000 population but has since decreased to less than half that figure. More than two thirds of cases are in children less than 15 years of age. The illness is generally seen between April and September because of increased exposure to ticks. A history of tick bite can be elicited in approximately 70% of cases.

Most cases in children

### CLINICAL MANIFESTATIONS

The incubation period between the tick bite and the onset of illness is usually 2 to 6 days, but may be as long as 2 weeks. Fever, headache, rash, toxicity, mental confusion, and myal-

Incubation period 2–6 days after tick bite

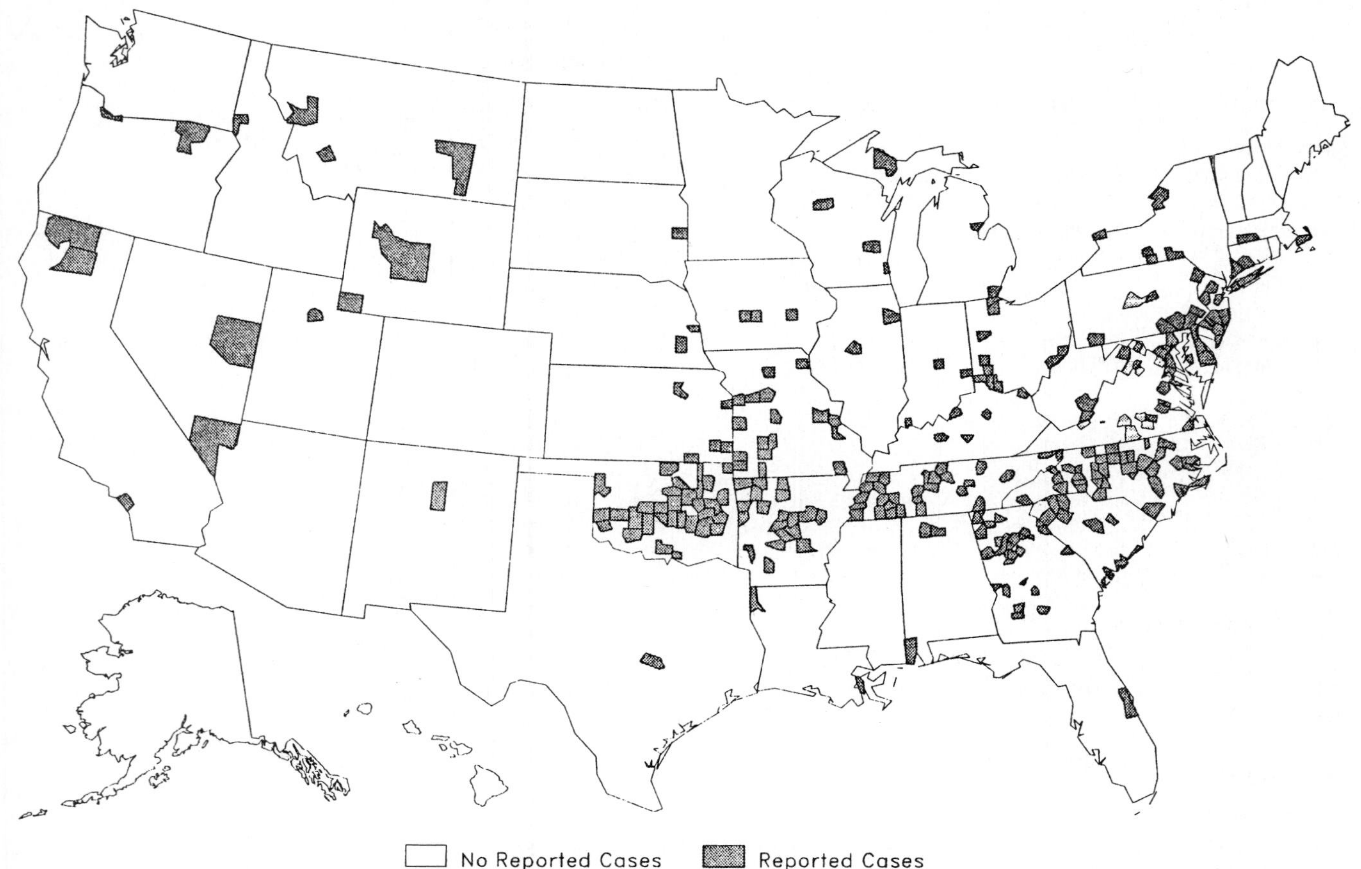


**Figure 30–1.** Rocky Mountain spotted fever. Distribution of counties in the United States reporting cases in 1992. (*Reprinted with permission from Centers for Disease Control and Prevention. Summary of Notifiable Diseases, United States 1992.* MMWR Morb Mortal Wkly Rep. *1993;41(55).*)

Rash spreads from extremities to trunk

gia are the major clinical features. The rash is the most characteristic feature of the illness. It usually develops on the second or third day of illness as small erythematous macules that rapidly become petechial. The lesions appear initially on the wrists and ankles and then spread up the extremities to the trunk in a few hours. A diagnostic feature of Rocky Mountain spotted fever is the frequent appearance of the rash on the palms and soles, a finding not usually seen in maculopapular eruptions associated with viral infections. Muscle tenderness, especially in the gastrocnemius, is characteristic and may be extreme. If untreated, or in occasional cases despite therapy, complications such as disseminated intravascular coagulation, thrombocytopenia, encephalitis, vascular collapse, and renal and heart failure may ensue.

### Diagnosis

Rising titers against rickettsial antigens confirms diagnosis

Therapy based on clinical manifestations

Because serologic tests are the primary diagnostic tests, it is difficult to establish the diagnosis of Rocky Mountain spotted fever early in the course of illness. Indirect fluorescent antibodies may appear by the sixth or seventh day of illness, however, and a fourfold rise in antibody titer between acute serum and convalescent serum establishes the diagnosis. Specific therapy must usually be started solely on the basis of clinical signs, symptoms, and epidemiologic considerations.

### Therapy

Treatment during first week most effective

Appropriate antibiotic therapy is highly effective if given during the first week of illness. If delayed into the second week or when pathologic processes such as diffuse intravascular coagulation are present, therapy becomes progressively less effective. The antibiotics of choice are tetracycline and chloramphenicol. Seriously ill patients and children less than 8 years of age are usually given chloramphenicol. Sulfonamides may enhance the disease process and are thus contraindicated. Before specific therapy became available, the mortality of Rocky Mountain spotted fever was approximately 25%. Treatment has reduced this figure to 5 to 7%. Death results primarily in patients in whom diagnosis and therapy are delayed into the second week of illness.

Tetracycline or chloramphenicol effective

PREVENTION

The major means of preventing Rocky Mountain spotted fever is avoidance or reduction of tick contact. Frequent deticking in tick-infested areas is important, because ticks generally must feed for 4 to 6 hours before they can transmit the disease. Tick surveys in the Carolinas have shown infection in about 5% of samples. Killed vaccines prepared from infected ticks, or rickettsias grown in embryonated eggs and cell cultures have been developed. None is licensed for clinical use at present.

Frequent deticking primary prevention

### Rickettsialpox

Rickettsialpox was first recognized in New York City in 1946. It is a benign rickettsial illness caused by *Rickettsia akari* and transmitted by a rodent mite. Distinguishing features of the disease include an eschar at the site of the bite and a vesicular rash. The house mouse and other semidomestic rodents are the primary reservoir. Humans acquire infection when the mite seeks an alternative host.

Benign disease transmitted by rodent mites

Rickettsialpox is a biphasic illness. The first phase is the local lesion at the bite, which starts as a papulovesicle and develops into a black eschar over 3 to 5 days. Fever and constitutional symptoms appear as the organism disseminates. The second phase of the disease is a diffuse rash similar to that of Rocky Mountain spotted fever distributed randomly in the body, which, like the local lesion, becomes papulovesicular and develops into eschars. Rickettsialpox is self-limiting after 1 week, and no deaths have been reported. Tetracycline therapy shortens the course to 1 to 2 days.

Local eschar followed by fever and rash

Tetracycline therapy

## Typhus Group

### Primary Louse-Borne Typhus Fever

Primary louse-borne typhus fever is caused by *Rickettsia prowazekii* transmitted to humans by the body louse. Historically, it has appeared during times of misery (war, famine) that create conditions favorable to human body lice (crowding, infrequent bathing). Although endemic typhus foci are thought to persist in parts of Africa and Latin America, the number of cases reported has declined in recent decades. Most come from a single country, Ethiopia, which has had more than its share of social upheaval. Epidemic typhus has not been seen in the United States for more than half a century. *Rickettsia prowazekii* has been recovered from flying squirrels and their ectoparasites in the southeastern United States, and a few human cases of sylvatic typhus have occurred in these areas.

Severe louse-borne disease due to *R. prowazekii*

Endemic foci in Africa

The chain of epidemic typhus infection starts with *R. prowazekii* circulating in a patient's blood during an acute febrile infection. The human body louse becomes infected during one of its frequent blood meals, and after 5 to 10 days of incubation, large numbers of rickettsiae appear in its feces. As the louse defecates while it feeds, the organisms can be rubbed into the louse bite wounds when the host scratches the site. Dried louse feces are also infectious through the mucous membranes of the eye or respiratory tract. The louse dies of its infection in 1 to 3 weeks, and the rickettsiae are not transmitted transovarially.

Infection involves louse feeding, defecation

Fever, headache, and rash begin 1 to 2 weeks after the bite. A maculopapular rash appears first on the trunk and then spreads centripetally to the extremities, a pattern opposite to that of Rocky Mountain spotted fever. Headache, malaise, and myalgia are prominent components of the illness. Complications include myocarditis and central nervous system dysfunction. In untreated disease, the fatality rate increases with age from 10% to as high as 60%. As with the spotted fever group, therapy with tetracycline or chloramphenicol is effective. Louse control is the best means of prevention and is particularly important in controlling epidemics. No effective vaccine is available.

Fever, headache, and rash with high mortality rate

Louse control primary prevention

### Recrudescent Typhus

Less severe relapse of typhus after many years

Recrudescent typhus (Brill's disease) is a relapse of louse-borne typhus appearing 10 to 40 years after the primary attack. Factors triggering the relapse are unknown, but may involve fading immunity to rickettsiae that have remained dormant in reticuloendothelial cells. Recrudescent typhus is usually milder than the primary infection and is less often fatal, presumably because of partial immunity.

### Murine Typhus

Transmitted by fleas from rat reservoir of *T. typhi*

Murine typhus is caused by *Rickettsia typhi* and transmitted to humans by the rat flea (*Xenopsylla cheopis*). Human illness is incidental to the natural transmission of the disease among urban rodents, which serve as the reservoir. Only 30 to 60 cases of murine typhus are reported in the United States each year. Half of these typically occur along the Gulf Coast of Texas.

Resembles typhus, but less severe

*R. typhi* shares antigens with *R. prowazekii*

The pathogenesis is similar to that of louse-borne typhus but the history includes exposure to rat, rat fleas, or both. The flea defecates when it takes a blood meal, and the infected feces gain access through the bite wound. After an incubation period of 1 to 2 weeks, illness begins with headache, myalgia, and fever. The rash is maculopapular, not petechial; it starts on the trunk and then spreads to the extremities in a manner similar to typhus. Because of antigens shared by *R. typhi* and *R. prowazekii*, serologic tests may not separate the two diseases. In the untreated patient, fever may last 12 to 14 days. With tetracycline or chloramphenicol therapy, the course is reduced to 2 to 3 days. Mortality and complications are rare, even if the disease is untreated.

### Scrub Typhus

*R. tsutsugamushi* transmitted from chiggers

Scrub typhus is found in the southwest Pacific, Southeast Asia, and Japan. The causative organism is *Rickettsia tsutsugamushi*. Mites that infest rodents are the reservoir and vectors, transmitting the rickettsiae to their own progeny via infected ova. Humans pick up the mites as they pass by low trees or brush. The mite larvae (chiggers) deposit rickettsiae as they feed.

Local eschar followed by fever, headache, rash, and lymphadenopathy

Serologic diagnosis by IFA

The typical initial lesion, a necrotic eschar at the site of the bite on the extremities, develops in only 50 to 80% of cases. Fever increases slowly over the first week, sometimes reaching 40.5°C. Headache, rash, and generalized lymphadenopathy follow later. The maculopapular rash, which appears after about 5 days, is more evanescent than that seen with louse-borne or murine typhus. Hepatosplenomegaly and conjunctivitis may also appear. Specific diagnosis requires demonstration of a serologic response using the IFA test. The prognosis is good with chloramphenicol or tetracycline therapy.

## ■ *COXIELLA*

*C. burnetii* multiplies in phagolysosome

Resistant to drying

*Coxiella burnetii,* the cause of Q fever, has morphological features similar to those of other rickettsiae, but differs in DNA composition and a number of other features. Phase variation of surface polysaccharide in response to environmental conditions has been observed and linked to virulence. The organism is taken into host cells by a phagocytic process that does not involve expenditure of energy by the parasite. It multiplies in the phagolysosome primarily because it is adapted to growth at low pH and resists lysosomal enzymes. *Coxiella burnetii* is much more resistant to drying and other environmental conditions than rickettsiae, which substantially accounts for its ability to produce infection by the respiratory route.

Transmitted by inhalation

Livestock placental tissue high risk

Occupational exposure in slaughterhouses, research facilities

Q fever is primarily a zoonosis transmitted from animals to humans by inhalation rather than by arthropod bite. Its distribution is worldwide among a wide range of mammals, of which cattle, sheep, and goats are most associated with transmission to humans. *Coxiella burnetii* grows particularly well in placental tissue, attaining huge numbers (>$10^{10}$ per gram), which at the time of birth contaminate the ground and may survive there for years. At 40°C, viability is retained for one or more years in dried fomites. The disease occurs among those exposed to infected animals or their products, particularly workers involved with slaughtering. Another high-risk environment is animal research facilities that have not provided adequate protection for personnel. Infection in all of these circumstances is believed to result from inhalation, which may be at some distance from the site of generation of the infectious aerosols. Infection can also occur from ingestion of animal products such as unpasteurized milk.

*Coxiella burnetii* has an affinity for the reticuloendothelial system, but little is known of the pathology, as fatal cases are rare. As in livestock, most human infections are inapparent. When clinically evident, Q fever usually begins 9 to 20 days after inhalation, with abrupt onset of fever, chills, and headache. A mild, dry, hacking cough and patchy interstitial pneumonia may or may not be present. There is no rash. Hepatosplenomegaly and abnormal liver function tests are common. Complications such as myocarditis, pericarditis, and encephalitis are rare. Chronic infection is also rare, but particularly important when it takes the form of endocarditis. There is evidence that the strains associated with endocarditis constitute an antigenic subgroup of *C. burnetii.*

Systemic infection without rash

Lung involvement, hepatosplenomegaly, and endocarditis occur

The diagnosis is usually made by demonstrating high or rising titers of antibody to Q fever antigen by complement fixation, IFA, or enzyme immunoassay procedures. Although most infections resolve spontaneously, tetracycline therapy is felt to shorten the duration of fever and reduce the risk of chronic infection. Vaccines have been shown to stimulate antibodies and some studies have suggested a protective effect for heavily exposed workers.

Diagnosis is serologic

## EHRLICHIA

The *Ehrlichia* genus includes a number of species of white blood cell-associated rickettsiae. They were first reported to cause human disease in the 1950s, but since 1986 more than 250 cases have been reported in the United States. They are tick borne, and human ehrlichiosis is clinically similar to Rocky Mountain spotted fever less the rash. Serologic findings and analysis of PCR-amplified DNA fragments suggest that human disease is due to a new species, *Ehrlichia chaffeensis,* but there have been few isolations of any *Ehrlichia* from humans. On rare occasions the diagnosis may be suggested by observation of characteristic ehrlichial intracytoplasmic inclusions within leukocytes (Fig 30–2), but it is most often confirmed serologically. These tests require the assistance of specialized laboratories.

Tick borne and WBC associated

Intracytoplasmic inclusions

## ROCHALIMAEA

*Rochalimaea* species differ from other rickettsiae in that they can be cultured on artificial media. Recent evidence indicates they are related to the genus *Bartonella,* which also grows in artificial media. *Rochalimaea quintana* is the best known species of this genus as the cause of trench fever, which has a worldwide distribution. The name derives from its prominence in the trenches of World War I. This disease has a reservoir in humans and its vector is the body louse. Most cases are mild or subclinical. When symptomatic, the patient has sudden onset of chills, headache, relapsing fever, and a maculopapular rash on the trunk and abdomen. Illness can last for 14 to 30 days and the disease is suggested by a history of louse contact. The diagnosis can be made by culturing the organism on special agar medium or by demonstrating seroconversion.

Grow on artificial media

Trench fever louse borne

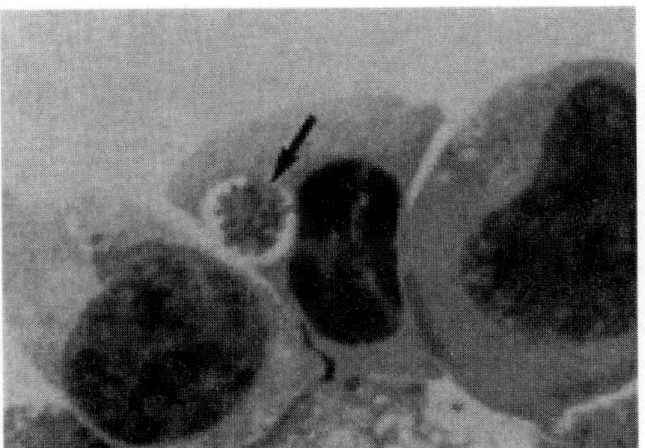

**Figure 30–2.** Mononuclear cell in the cerebrospinal fluid containing *Ehrlichia* intracytoplasmic inclusions (arrow). (*Reprinted with permission from Dunn BE, Monson TP, Dumler JS, et al. Identification of* Ehrlichia chaffeensis *morulae in cerebrospinal fluid mononuclear cells.* J Clin Microbiol. *1992;30:2207–2210.*)

Cat scratch fever a febrile lymphadenopathy

Link to *R. henselae* is serologic

Vascular infection of AIDS patients

Another species, *Rochalimaea henselae*, has recently been associated with a number of diseases, the most common of which is cat scratch disease. Cat scratch disease is a febrile lymphadenitis with systemic symptomatology; approximately 24,000 cases occur in the United States each year. The disease is thought to result from cat scratches or, less often, dog contact. Symptoms may include skin or eye rashes or even temporary blindness. *Rochalimaea henselae* has been isolated directly from cats, although the latter do not appear ill, and a serologic response to *R. henselae* antigens has been demonstrated by IFA tests in typical patients. For severe disease, rifampin may be the most useful treatment.

Bacillary angiomatosis, a proliferative disease of small blood vessels of the skin and viscera, seen in AIDS patients and other immunocompromised hosts, has been associated with *Rochalimaea* by molecular methods. The polymerase chain reaction (PCR) (see Chapter 14) was used to amplify ribosomal RNA gene fragments directly from tissue samples. Sequence analysis of DNA transcribed from these fragments pointed to the *Rochalimaea* genus. Subsequently, both *R. henselae* and *R. quintana* have been isolated from AIDS patients with bacillary angiomatosis. Other conditions seen primarily in AIDS patients, such as peliosis hepatis, have also been associated with *R. henselae*.

## ADDITIONAL READING

Dolan MJ, Wong MT, Regnery RL, et al. Syndrome of *Rochalimaea henselae* adenitis suggesting cat scratch disease. *Ann Intern Med.* 1993;118:331–336. Describes the clinical syndrome of cat scratch disease caused by *Rochalimaea henselae*, including methods for isolation of the organism from tissue and identification.

English Lt CK, Wear DJ, Margileth AM, et al. Cat-scratch disease isolation and culture of the bacterial agent. *JAMA*. 1988;259:1347–1352. A Gram-negative bacterium or its cell wall-defective variants were isolated from lymph nodes of 10 patients with cat scratch disease. Three of seven with recent cat scratch disease had fourfold or greater rises in antibody titer against the cultured bacteria; the remaining four patients had maximum titers of 1:32 to 1:128.

McDade JE, Newhouse VF. Natural history of *Rickettsia rickettsii*. *Annu Rev Microbiol.* 1986;40:287–309. A review of the basic biology, distribution, and transmission of *Rickettsia rickettsii*.

Perkocha LA, Geahan SM, Yen TSB, et al. Clinical and pathological features of bacillary peliosis hepatis in association with human immunodeficiency virus infection. *N Engl J Med.* 1990;323:1581–1585. The bacilli, which could not be cultured, were morphologically identified to those found in the skin lesions of cutaneous bacillary angiomatosis. HIV-associated bacillary peliosis hepatis is an unusual, treatable opportunistic infection, probably caused by the same organism that causes cutaneous bacillary angiomatosis.

Reimer LG. Q fever. *Clin Microbiol Rev*. 1993;6:193–198. A concise review of *Coxiella burnetii* and the epidemiology, pathogenesis, and clinical aspects of Q fever.

Tappero JW, Koehler JE, Berger TG, et al. Bacillary angiomatosis and bacillary splenitis in immunocompetent adults. *Ann Intern Med.* 1993;118:363–365. Describes five patients with cutaneous bacillary angiomatosis or bacillary splenitis without evidence of HIV infection who were determined to be immunocompetent after immunologic evaluation. In three patients with both cat and cat flea exposures, infection by *Rochalimaea henselae* was confirmed by amplification and sequencing of 16 S rDNA from an infected tissue specimen.

Chapter 31

# Some Bacteria Causing Zoonotic Diseases

*Kenneth J. Ryan*

Many bacterial, rickettsial, and viral diseases are classified as zoonoses, because they are acquired by humans either directly or indirectly from animals. This chapter considers bacteria causing four zoonotic infections that are not discussed in other chapters. All four, *Brucella, Yersinia pestis, Francisella tularensis,* and *Pasteurella multocida,* are Gram-negative bacilli that are primarily animal pathogens. The diseases they cause, brucellosis, plague, tularemia, and pasteurellosis, are now rare in humans and develop only after unique animal contact. The full range of zoonoses considered in this and other chapters is shown in Appendix 31–1.

## BRUCELLA

Brucellosis (sometimes known as undulant fever or Malta fever) is a genitourinary infection of sheep, cattle, pigs, and other animals. Humans become infected directly by occupational contact with these animals (farmers, slaughterhouse workers, veterinarians) or indirectly by consumption of contaminated animal products such as milk. In humans, the reticuloendothelial system is the primary target of infection, producing a prolonged febrile systemic illness.

### Bacteriology

Gram-negative coccobacilli may require $CO_2$ for growth

*Brucella* species are small, coccobacillary, Gram-negative rods that resemble *Haemophilus* and *Bordetella* morphologically. They are nonmotile, non-acid fast, and non-spore forming. Growth requires an aerobic environment and enriched media such as blood agar. One species, *Brucella abortus,* requires enrichment of the atmosphere to 5 to 10% carbon dioxide. Colonies are visible on solid media only after 2 to 3 days of incubation, and broth cultures may require more time depending on the size of the inoculum.

Species and biovars differentiated by cultural tests

DNA homology studies indicate that only a single *Brucella* species, *Brucella melitensis,* is justified, but the names *Brucella abortus* and *Brucella suis* (now considered biovars) have considerable medical significance and will continue to be used here. All produce catalase, oxidase, and urease, but do not ferment carbohydrates. They are differentiated by carbon dioxide requirements for growth, hydrogen sulfide production, and the ability of particular concentrations of the dyes thionin and basic fuchsin to inhibit their growth (Table 31–1).

TABLE 31–1. CHARACTERISTIC FEATURES OF BRUCELLA

| Characteristic | B. melitensis | B. abortis[a] | B. suis[a] |
|---|---|---|---|
| Carbon dioxide requirement | – | + | – |
| Hydrogen sulfide production | – | + | ± |
| Growth in presence of | | | |
| Thionin[b] | + | – | + |
| Basic fuchsin[b] | + | + | – |

[a] Considered biovars of *B. melitensis.*
[b] Concentration of 1:50,000 in nutrient medium.

Smooth to rough variation seen in culture relate to protein-lipopolysaccharide antigens

*Brucella* isolates demonstrate smooth colony forms on primary isolation which are associated with the presence of a small capsule and virulence. Rough colonies have an uneven surface and tend to replace the S form on repeated subculture. They are composed of mutants that have lost their capsules and most of their virulence. Smooth types have lipopolysaccharide antigens with two distinct epitopes designated A (*abortus*) and M (*melitensis*). They are present in different amounts in all three species.

## Brucellosis

### Epidemiology

Abortion in cattle, goats, and hogs

Brucellosis is an important cause of abortion, sterility, and decreased milk production in cattle, goats, and hogs. It is spread among animals by direct contact with infected tissues and ingestion of contaminated feed and causes chronic infection of the mammary glands, uterus, placenta, seminal vesicles, and epididymis. Although the associations are not absolute, each species is linked to a different animal: *B. abortus* tends to infect cattle; *B. melitensis,* goats; and *B. suis,* hogs.

Infection occupational and through unpasteurized dairy products

Unpasteurized "health" foods a recent risk

Humans acquire the infection by occupational exposure or consumption of unpasteurized dairy products. The organisms may gain access through cuts in the skin, contact with mucous membranes, inhalation, or ingestion. In the United States, the number of cases has dropped steadily from a maximum of more than 6000 per year in the 1940s to the current level of 100 to 150 per year. Of these cases, 50 to 60% are in abattoir employees, government meat inspectors, veterinarians, and others who handle livestock or meat products. Consumption of unpasteurized dairy products, which accounts for 8 to 10% of infections, is the leading source in persons who have no connection with the meat processing or livestock industries. Some recent cases of this type have been associated with "health" foods. In the United States, the distribution of human cases of brucellosis includes virtually every state, but is concentrated in those with large livestock industries or proximity to Mexico (California, Texas). An outbreak of *B. melitensis* in Texas was traced to unpasteurized goat cheese brought in from Mexico.

### Pathogenesis and Immunity

Multiplication in macrophages

Immunity T-cell mediated

Erythritol in animal placentas stimulates growth

After penetration of the skin or mucous membranes, the organisms are carried within polymorphonuclear leukocytes through the lymph to the systemic circulation by way of the regional lymph nodes and the thoracic duct. Virulent *Brucella* can enter and multiply in macrophages in the liver sinusoids, spleen, bone marrow, and other components of the reticuloendothelial system. Smooth (virulent) *Brucella* strains possess a currently unknown virulence factor that allows some intracellular growth despite local macrophage activation by cytokines. Thus, intracellular events in the monocyte determine the outcome of a *Brucella* infection, and control is dependent on active T-cell response. Antibodies to *Brucella* antigens can be detected in the sera of patients by a variety of methods, but there is no evidence that they alter the natural history of disease or confer immunity. Exotoxins, capsules, or antiphagocytic components are apparently not involved in virulence. In cows, sheep, pigs, and goats, erythritol, a four-carbon alcohol present in chorionic tissue, markedly stimulates growth of *Brucella*. This stimulation probably accounts for the tendency of the organism to locate in these sites. The human placenta does not contain erythritol.

If not controlled locally, infection progresses with the formation of small granulomas in the reticuloendothelial sites of bacterial multiplication and with release of bacteria back into the systemic circulation. These recurrent bacteremic episodes are largely responsible for the recurrent chills and fever of the clinical illness. The intracellular events resemble that of *Salmonella typhi*, and its disease, typhoid fever (see Chapter 20).

Recurrent bacteremia from reticuloendothelial sites

## Brucellosis: Clinical Aspects

### Clinical Manifestations

Brucellosis starts with malaise, chills, and fever 7 to 21 days after infection. Drenching sweats in the late afternoon or evening are common, as are temperatures in the range 39.4 to 40°C. The pattern of periodic nocturnal fever (undulant fever) typically continues for weeks, months, or even 1 to 2 years, and the patient becomes chronically ill with associated body aches, headache, and anorexia. Weight loss of up to 20 kg may occur during prolonged illness. Despite these dramatic effects, physical findings and localizing signs are few. Less than 25% of patients show detectable enlargement of the reticuloendothelial organs, the primary site of infection. Of such findings, splenomegaly is most common, followed by lymphadenopathy and hepatomegaly. Occasionally, localized infection develops in the lung, bone, brain, heart, or genitourinary system. These cases usually lack the pronounced systemic symptoms of the typical illness.

Night sweats and periodic nocturnal fever

Chronic illness, weight loss, and splenomegaly

### Diagnosis

Definitive diagnosis requires isolation of *Brucella* from the blood or from biopsy specimens of the liver, bone marrow, or lymph nodes. Supplementation with carbon dioxide is needed for growth of *B. abortus*. The slow growth of some strains requires prolonged incubation of culture medium to achieve isolation. Blood cultures, in particular, may require 2 to 4 weeks for growth, although most are positive in 2 to 5 days.

Diagnosis by blood culture

The diagnosis is often made serologically, but is subject to the same interpretive constraints as are all serologic tests. Antibodies that agglutinate suspensions of heat-killed organisms typically reach titers of 1:640 or more in acute disease. Lower titers may reflect previous disease or cross-reacting antibodies. Titers return to the normal range within a year of successful therapy.

Agglutinins ≥ 1:640

### Treatment and Prevention

Tetracycline is the primary antimicrobic for the treatment of brucellosis. In seriously ill patients, streptomycin, gentamicin, or rifampin may be added. The therapeutic response is not rapid; 2 to 7 days may pass before patients become afebrile. Up to 10% of cases have relapses in the first 3 months after therapy. Prevention is primarily by measures to minimize occupational exposure and by the pasteurization of dairy products. Control of brucellosis in animals involves a combination of immunization with an attenuated strain of *B. abortus* and eradication of infected stock. No human vaccine is in use.

Tetracycline effective

Pasteurization primary prevention

# *YERSINIA PESTIS*

Plague is an infection of rodents and small mammals caused by *Y. pestis*. It is transmitted to humans by the bite of infected fleas. The disease has two major cycles, urban and sylvatic, and two major clinical forms, bubonic and pneumonic. The combined pathogenic and epidemiologic potential of *Y. pestis* makes it one of the most potent and feared pathogens known.

## Bacteriology

*Yersinia pestis* is a nonmotile, non-spore-forming, Gram-negative bacillus with a tendency toward pleomorphism and bipolar staining. It is a member of the Enterobacteriaceae and is discussed in Chapter 20 with other members of the genus *Yersinia*.

# Plague

## Epidemiology

Black Death continued into 20th century

The term **plague** is often used generically to describe any explosive pandemic disease with high mortality. Medically it refers only to infection caused by *Y. pestis,* and this application was justly earned, because *Y. pestis* was the cause of the most virulent epidemic plague of recorded human history, the Black Death of the Middle Ages. In the 14th century, the estimated population of Europe was 105 million; between 1346 and 1350, 25 million died of plague. Pandemics continued through the end of the 19th century and the early 20th century despite elaborate quarantine measures developed in response to the obvious communicability of the disease. Yersin isolated the etiologic agent in China in 1894 and named it after his mentor, Pasteur (*Pasteurella pestis*). The name was later changed to honor Yersin (*Y. pestis*).

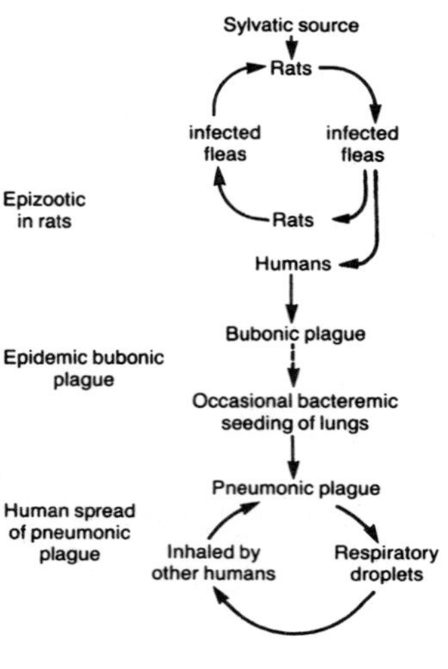


Urban plague

The plagues of the Middle Ages are examples of the urban cycle involving rats and humans. The first step probably involves infection of rats from a sylvatic rodent source. Under poor hygienic conditions and when food sources elsewhere are scarce, rat populations in cities increase, which facilitates rat-to-rat transmission of *Y. pestis* by the rat flea (*Xenopsylla cheopis*). These conditions also bring the primary rat reservoir into closer contact with humans. When the number of nonimmune rats is sufficient, epizootic plague develops among them with bacteremia and high mortality. Fleas feeding on the rat become infected, and the bacteria multiply in the intestinal tract of the flea to numbers that eventually block the proventriculus. As the infected rat dies, its hungry fleas seek a new host, which is usually another rat, but may be a human. The infected flea regurgitates *Y. pestis* from the proventriculus into the new bite wound. The probability of transmission to humans is thus greatest when both rat population and rat mortality are high. The bite of the flea is the first event in the development of a case of bubonic plague, which, even if serious enough to kill the patient, is not normally contagious to other humans. Some patients with bubonic plague, however, develop a secondary pneumonia by bacteremic spread to the lungs. They can then transmit pneumonic plague directly to others by droplet spread. It is not hard to understand how rapid spread proceeds in conjunction with crowded unsanitary conditions and continued flea-to-human transmission. An urban plague epidemic is vividly described in Albert Camus' novel *The Plague*.

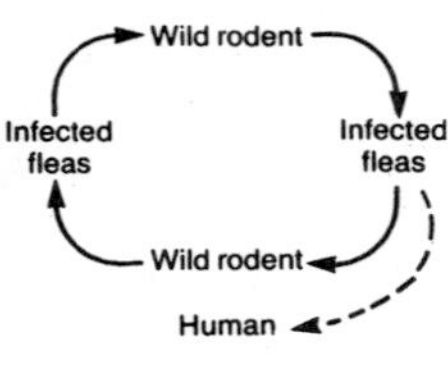


Sylvatic plague

Although urban plague epidemics have been essentially eliminated by rat control and other public health measures, a sylvatic transmission cycle persists in many parts of the world, including North America. This cycle involves nonurban mammals such as prairie dogs, deer mice, rabbits, and wood rats. Transmission between them is accomplished by fleas. Coyotes or wolves may be infected by the same fleas or by ingestion of infected rodents. By their nature, the reservoir animals rarely come in contact with humans; when they do, however, the infected fleas they carry can transmit *Y. pestis*. The most common circumstance is a child exploring the outdoors who comes across a dead or dying prairie dog and pokes, carries, or touches it long enough to be bitten by the fleas leaving the animal. The result is a sporadic case of bubonic plague, which occasionally becomes pneumonic.

Most US cases in western states

Sylvatic plague exists in most continents, is common in Southeast Asia, but is not found in Western Europe or Australia. In the United States, the primary enzootic areas are the semiarid plains of the western states. Infected animals and fleas have been detected from the Mexican border to the eastern half of Washington State.

Human disease linked to events in reservoir

The geographic focus of human plague in the United States is in the "four corners" area where Arizona, New Mexico, Colorado, and Utah meet, but cases have occurred in California, West Texas, Idaho, and Montana. Up to 15 cases are reported most years, although this number rose to 30 to 40 in the mid-1980s. These variations are strongly related to changes in the size of the sylvanic reservoir. A fatal case of pneumonic plague reported in 1992 was linked to an infected domestic cat the patient had removed from the crawlspace under a house in the endemic area.

## Pathogenesis and Immunity

*Y. pestis* multiplies in flea foregut

*Yersinia pestis* multiplies in the infected flea and blocks the foregut. The flea then regurgitates organisms into the next bite wound it produces. The organisms reach the regional lymph nodes of the newly infected individual through the lymphatic vessels. As the conditions change from the temperature (about 20–25°C) and ionic environment of the flea to that of the new host, *Y. pestis* produces the array of virulence factors discussed in Chapter 20. In the regional nodes, *Y. pestis* multiplies rapidly and produces a hemorrhagic suppurative necrosis that results in a painful swelling known as a **bubo.** The components of the organism responsible for the necrosis and extreme systemic toxicity remain unclear, although both endotoxin and exotoxins are produced. Further spread leads to bacteremia and seeding of the lungs, liver, spleen, and occasionally the meninges. Pulmonary spread produces a fatal necrotizing hemorrhagic pneumonia known as pneumonic plague. Progression of plague pneumonia is rapid and so extensive that a terminal cyanosis is typical.

Virulence factors triggered by temperature and ionic shift

Bubo often progresses to bacteremia

Terminal cyanosis is the Black Death

Recovery from bubonic plague appears to confer lasting immunity, but for obvious reasons the mechanisms have not been extensively studied by modern immunologic methods. Animal studies suggest that antibody against the F1 capsular protein antigen is protective by enhancing phagocytosis, but cell-mediated mechanisms are required for intracellular killing. Because *Y. pestis* is a facultative intracellular parasite, the latter mechanisms must be at least as important as antibody in determining plague immunity.

## Plague: Clinical Aspects

### Clinical Manifestations

The incubation period for bubonic plague is 2 to 7 days after the flea bite. Onset is marked by fever and the painful bubo, usually in the groin (**bubo** is from the Greek **boubon** for "groin") or, less often, in the axilla. Without treatment, 50 to 75% of patients progress to bacteremia and die in Gram-negative septic shock within hours or days of development of the bubo. About 5% of victims develop pneumonic plague with mucoid, then bloody sputum. Primary pneumonic plague has a shorter incubation period (2–3 days) and begins with only fever, malaise, and a feeling of tightness in the chest. Cough, production of sputum, dyspnea, and cyanosis develop later in the course. Death on the second or third day of illness is common, and there are no survivors without specific therapy. The course of plague is identical whether it is acquired from urban or sylvatic sources.

Bubonic plague mortality 50–75% in untreated cases

Pneumonic plague fatal if untreated

### Diagnosis

Gram smears of aspirates from the bubo typically reveal bipolar-staining Gram-negative bacilli. An immunofluorescence technique is available in reference laboratories for immediate precise identification. *Yersinia pestis* is readily isolated on the media used for other members of the Enterobacteriaceae (blood agar, MacConkey agar), although growth may require more than 24 hours of incubation. The appropriate specimens are bubo aspirate, blood, and sputum. Laboratories must be notified of the suspicion of plague to avoid delay in the bacteriologic diagnosis and to guard against laboratory infection.

Direct Gram, immunofluorescent staining, and culture

### Treatment and Prevention

Streptomycin is the treatment of choice for both bubonic and pneumonic plague, because its effectiveness has been proven. Tetracycline, chloramphenicol, and sulfonamides are alternatives. Timely treatment reduces the mortality of bubonic plague to 10 to 15%. Of the 31 human cases of plague reported in the United States in 1984, 6 (19%) died.

Streptomycin primary treatment

Urban plague has been prevented by rat control and general public health measures such as use of insecticides. Sylvatic plague is virtually impossible to eliminate because of the size and dispersion of the multiple rodent reservoirs. Disease can be prevented by avoidance of sick or dead rodents and rabbits. Eradication of fleas on domestic pets, which have been known to transport infected fleas from wild rodents to humans, is recommended in endemic areas. The continued presence of fully virulent plague in its sylvatic cycle poses a risk of extension to the urban cycle and epidemic disease in the event of major disaster or social breakdown.

Avoidance of sick or dead wild rodents

Chemoprophylaxis with tetracycline is recommended for those who have had close

Tetracycline chemoprophylaxis appropriate for exposed

contact with a case of pneumonic plague. It is also used for the household contacts of a case of bubonic plague, because they may have had the same flea contact. A formalin-killed plague vaccine is used only for those in high-risk occupations.

## FRANCISELLA

Tularemia is a disease of wild mammals caused by *F. tularensis*. Humans become infected by contact with infected animals either directly or through the bite of a vector (tick or deer fly). The illness is characterized by high fever and severe constitutional symptoms. Many features of the clinical infection and its epidemiology are similar to those of plague.

### Bacteriology

Gram-negative coccobacilli

Special requirement for –SH compounds

*Francisella tularensis* is a small, facultative, coccobacillary, Gram-negative organism with much the same morphology as *Brucella*. It is one of the few bacterial species of medical importance that does not grow on the usual enriched media. This characteristic is due to a special requirement for sulfhydryl compounds, and growth occurs best on a cysteine–glucose blood agar medium incubated aerobically. On primary isolation, 2 to 10 days of incubation is required for appearance of the tiny transparent colonies. The species is antigenically homogeneous and not closely related to any other genus.

### Tularemia

#### Epidemiology

Usually acquired from infected rabbit carcass or ticks

Transovarial transmission in ticks

Humans most often acquire *F. tularensis* by contact with an infected rabbit or tick. Many other wild mammals can also be infected, including squirrels, muskrats, beavers, and deer. A common history is that of skinning wild rabbits on a hunting trip. The bite or scratch of a domestic dog or cat, probably after the animal ingested or mouthed an infected rodent or rabbit, has been implicated occasionally. Infected animals may not show signs of infection, because the organism is well adapted to its natural host. Ticks and deer flies are the usual vectors in animals. The tick may also serve as a reservoir of the organism by transovarial transmission to its offspring.

Distribution throughout Northern Hemisphere

Tularemia is distributed throughout the Northern Hemisphere, although there are wide variations in specific regions. The highly virulent tick/rabbit-associated strains are common only in North America. It is not found in the British Isles. Surveillance for human cases in the southwestern and central United States between 1981 and 1987 revealed rates between 5 and 36 cases per million population.

#### Pathogenesis and Immunity

Low infecting dose

If directly injected or inhaled, the infecting dose of *F. tularensis* is very low (less than 100 organisms). Infection can follow virtually any kind of contact with the skin or mucous membranes, and the organism probably gains access to the tissues through unnoticed breaks in the epithelium.

Survival in monocytes with focal necrosis and granulomas

Relatively little is known of the events that occur during the 2- to 5-day incubation period. The organism infects the reticuloendothelial organs, often forming granulomas, and the disease may sometimes follow a chronic relapsing course. These properties suggest multiplication within macrophages a known feature of *F. tularensis* in experimental systems. A lesion often develops at the site of infection, which becomes ulcerated. Early bacteremic spread probably occurs, although it is rarely detected. Other areas of multiplication are characterized by necrosis or granuloma production, and a mixture of abscesses and caseating granulomas may be seen in the same organ.

Cell-mediated immunity important

Naturally acquired infection appears to confer long-lasting immunity. Agglutinating antibody titers remain elevated for many years, but cellular immunity probably plays the major role in resistance to reinfection.

## Tularemia: Clinical Aspects

### Clinical Manifestations

After an incubation period of 2 to 5 days, tularemia may follow a number of courses, depending on the site of inoculation and extent of spread. All begin with the acute onset of fever, chills, and malaise. In the ulceroglandular form, a local papule at the inoculation site becomes necrotic and ulcerative. Regional lymph nodes become swollen and painful. The oculoglandular form, which follows conjunctival inoculation, is similar except that the local lesion is a painful purulent conjunctivitis. Ingestion of large numbers of *F. tularensis* (more than $10^8$) leads to typhoidal tularemia, with abdominal manifestations and a prolonged febrile course similar to that of typhoid fever. Inhalation of the organisms can result in pneumonic tularemia or a more generalized infection similar to the typhoidal form. Like plague pneumonia, tularemic pneumonia may also develop through seeding of the lungs by bacteremic spread of one of the other forms. Any form of tularemia may progress to a systemic infection with lesions in multiple organs. Without treatment, mortality ranges from 5 to 30%, depending on the type of infection. Ulceroglandular tularemia, the most common form, generally carries the lowest risk of a fatal outcome. In the US surveillance study mentioned earlier, the mortality was 2%.

Ulceroglandular, oculoglandular, typhoidal, and pneumonic forms exist

Lowest mortality with ulceroglandular

### Diagnosis

Because tularemia is uncommon and *F. tularensis* has unique growth requirements, the diagnosis is easily overlooked. Although some strains grow on chocolate agar, laboratories must be alerted to the suspicion of tularemia so that specialized media can be prepared and precautions taken against the considerable risk of laboratory infection. An immunofluorescent reagent is available in reference laboratories for use directly on smears from clinical material.

Special media needed for culture

Because of the difficulty and risk of cultural techniques, many cases are diagnosed by serologic tests. Agglutinating antibodies are usually present in titers of 1:40 by the second week of illness, rising to 1:320 or greater after 3 to 4 weeks. Unless previous exposure is known, single high antibody titers are considered diagnostic.

Serodiagnosis most common approach

### Treatment and Prevention

Streptomycin is the drug of choice in all forms of tularemia, although recent experience indicates that gentamicin may be just as effective. Tetracycline and chloramphenicol have also been effective, but relapses are more common than with streptomycin. Prevention is mainly by the use of rubber gloves and eye protection when handling potentially infected wild mammals. Prompt removal of ticks is also important. A vaccine exists, but is used only in laboratory workers and others who cannot avoid contact with infected animals.

Aminoglycosides effective

## PASTEURELLA MULTOCIDA

*Pasteurella multocida* is one of many species of *Pasteurella* included in the normal respiratory flora of some animals. It is a small, coccobacillary, Gram-negative organism that grows readily on blood agar but not on MacConkey agar. In addition, it is oxidase positive and ferments a variety of carbohydrates. Unlike most Gram-negative rods, *P. multocida* is susceptible to penicillin. Humans are usually infected by the bite or scratch of a domestic dog or cat. Infection develops at the site of the lesion, often within 24 hours. The typical infection is a diffuse cellulitis with a well-defined erythematous border. The diagnosis is made by culture of an aspirate of pus expressed from the lesion. Frequently, too few organisms are present to be seen on a direct Gram smear. *Pasteurella multocida* is by far the most common cause of an infected dog or cat bite. For unknown reasons, *P. multocida* is occasionally isolated from the sputum of patients with bronchiectasis. Infections are treated with penicillin.

Penicillin-sensitive, Gram-negative rods

Most common cause of infected animal bites or scratches

## ADDITIONAL READING

Crook LD, Tempest B. Plague. A clinical review of 27 cases. *Arch Intern Med.* 1992;152:1253–1256. A nice review of clinical aspects of plague cases seen between 1965 and 1989 at the Gallup, New Mexico, Indian Medical Center. Analysis of treatment outcomes is included.

McNeill WH. *Plagues and Peoples*. New York: Anchor Press/Doubleday; 1976. An account of the impact of infectious diseases, including zoonoses, on the course of human history.

Smith LD, Ficht TA. Pathogenesis of *Brucella*. *CRC Crit Rev Microbiol*. 1990;17:209–230. A review of known pathogenic mechanisms from both the human and veterinary standpoints.

Taylor JP, Istre GR, McChesney TC, Satalowich FT, Parker RL, McFarland LM. Epidemiologic characteristics of human tularemia in the southwest-central states, 1981–1987. *Am J Epidemiol*. 1991;133:1032–1038. This study indicates tularemia is more common in the United States than most experts thought.

## APPENDIX 31–1. SOME IMPORTANT BACTERIAL AND RICKETTSIAL ZOONOTIC INFECTIONS

| Disease | Etiologic Agent | Usual Reservoir | Usual Mode of Transmission to Humans | Transmission Between Humans | Mode of Transmission Between Humans | Special Characteristics |
|---|---|---|---|---|---|---|
| Anthrax | *Bacillus anthracis* | Cattle, sheep, goats | Infected animals or products | No[a] | | Resistant spores |
| Bovine tuberculosis | *Mycobacterium bovis* | Cattle | Milk | No[a] | | |
| Brucellosis | *Brucella* sp | Cattle, swine, goats | Milk, infected carcasses | No[a] | | |
| *Campylobacter* infection | *C. jejuni* | Wild mammals, cattle, sheep, pets | Contaminated food and water | Yes | Fecal–oral | |
| Leptospirosis | *Leptospira* sp | Cattle, rodents | Water contaminated with urine | No[a] | | |
| Lyme disease | *Borrelia bergdorferi* | Deer, rodents | Ticks; transplacentally | No[a] | | Spreading relapsing disease |
| Pasteurellosis | *Pasteurella multocida* | Animal oral cavities | Bites, scratches | No[a] | | |
| Plague | *Yersinia pestis* | Rodents | Fleas | Yes | Droplet (pneumonic) spread | Great epidemic potential |
| Other *Yersinia* infections | *Y. enterocolitica, Y. pseudotuberculosis* | Wild mammals, pigs, cattle, pets | Fecal–oral | Yes | Fecal–oral | |
| Relapsing fever | *Borrelia* species | Rodents, ticks | Ticks | Yes | Body louse[b] | Epidemic potential |
| Salmonellosis | *Salmonella* serotypes | Poultry, livestock | Contaminated food | Yes | Fecal contamination of food | |
| Rickettsial spotted fevers | *R. rickettsii* (eg) | Rodents, ticks, mites | Ticks, mites | No[a] | | |
| Murine typhus | *Rickettsia typhi* | Rodents | Fleas | No[a] | | |
| Q fever | *Coxiella burnetii* | Cattle, sheep, goats | Contaminated dust and aerosols | No[a] | | |

[a] What never? No never. What *never*? Well, hardly ever! (W. S. Gilbert, "H.M.S. Pinafore").

[b] The relationship between tickborne relapsing fever and epidemic relapsing fever by the body louse remains uncertain.

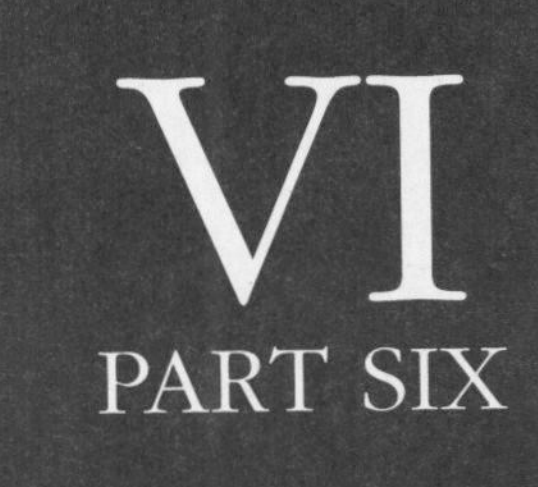


# Pathogenic Viruses

Chapter 32

# Influenza, Respiratory Syncytial Virus, Adenovirus, and Other Respiratory Viruses

C. George Ray

Respiratory disease accounts for an estimated 75 to 80% of all acute morbidity in the US population. Most of these illnesses (approximately 80%) are viral. If episodes not requiring medical attention, are included, the overall average is three to four illnesses per year per person, although incidence varies inversely with age (the frequency is greater among young children). Seasonality is also a feature; incidence is lowest in the summer months and highest in the winter.

The viruses that are major causes of acute respiratory disease (ARD) include influenza viruses, parainfluenza viruses, rhinoviruses, adenoviruses, respiratory syncytial virus, and respiratory coronaviruses. Reoviruses are of questionable importance, but are also considered. Others, such as enteroviruses and measles virus, can also cause respiratory symptoms, but are discussed in other chapters.

Respiratory viruses represented by diverse agents

In addition to the ability to cause a variety of ARD syndromes, this somewhat heterogeneous group of viruses share a relatively short incubation period (1–4 days) and mode of spread from person to person. Transmission is direct, by infective droplet nuclei, or indirect, by hand transfer of contaminated secretions to nasal or conjunctival epithelium. All of these agents are associated with an increased risk of bacterial superinfection of the damaged tissue of the respiratory tract, and all have a worldwide distribution.

Short incubation period

Transmission by droplet nuclei or direct contact

## INFLUENZA VIRUSES

### Influenza Virus Group Characteristics

Influenza viruses are members of the orthomyxovirus group, which are enveloped, pleomorphic, single-stranded RNA viruses. They are classified into three major serotypes, A, B, and C, based on different ribonucleoprotein antigens. Influenza A is the most extensively studied of the three, and much of the following discussion is based on knowledge of this type. It usually causes more severe disease and more extensive epidemics than the other types and has a greater tendency to undergo significant antigenic changes. Influenza B is

Orthomyxoviruses divided into types A, B, and C

Type A has greatest virulence and epidemic spread

somewhat more antigenically stable and usually occurs in more localized outbreaks; influenza C appears to be a relatively minor cause of disease.

Enveloped RNA virus with segmented genome

Virus-specified hemagglutinin and neuramidase spikes

Influenza A and B viruses consist of a nucleocapsid containing eight segments of negative-sense, single-stranded RNA, which is enveloped in a glycolipid membrane derived from the host cell plasma membrane. The inner side of the envelope contains a layer of virus-specified protein. Two virus-specified glycoproteins, hemagglutinin and neuraminidase, are embedded in the outer surface of the envelope and appear as "spikes" over the surface of the virion (Fig 32–1). Influenza C differs considerably from the others in that it possesses only seven RNA segments and has no neuraminidase, although it does possess other receptor-destroying capability (see below). In addition, the hemagglutinin of influenza C binds to a cell receptor different from that for types A and B.

Hemagglutinin acts in viral attachment

The virus-specified glycoproteins are antigenic and have special functional importance to the virus. Hemagglutinin is so named because of its ability to agglutinate red blood cells from certain species (eg, chickens, guinea pigs) in vitro. Its major biological function is to serve as a point of attachment to *N*-acetylneuraminic (sialic) acid-containing glycoprotein or glycolipid receptor sites on human respiratory cell surfaces, which is a critical first step in initiating infection of the cell.

Neuraminidase has role in envelope fusion and viral release

Neuraminidase is an antigenic hydrolytic enzyme that acts on the hemagglutinin receptors by splitting off their terminal neuraminic (sialic) acid. The result is destruction of receptor activity. Neuraminidase is thought to serve several functions. It may inactivate a free mucoprotein receptor substance in respiratory secretions that could otherwise bind to viral hemagglutinin and prevent access of the virus to the cell surface. It may be important in fusion of the viral envelope with the host cell membrane as a prerequisite to viral entry. It also aids in the release of newly formed virus particles from infected cells, thus making them available to infect other cells. Type-specific antibodies to neuraminidase appear to inhibit the spread of virus in the infected host and to limit the amount of virus released from host cells.

Nucleocapsid and virus assembly are at different cell sites

Nucleocapsid assembly takes place in the cell nucleus, but final virus assembly takes place at the plasma membrane. The ribonucleoproteins are enveloped by the plasma membrane, which by then contains hemagglutinin and neuraminidase. Virus "buds" are formed, and intact virions are released from the cell surface (see Chapter 6, Fig 6–11).

Viral isolation in eggs or cell cultures

Influenza A viruses were initially isolated in 1933 by intranasal inoculation of ferrets, which developed febrile respiratory illnesses. The viruses will replicate in the amniotic sac of embryonated hen's eggs, where their presence can be detected by the hemagglutination test. Most strains can also be readily isolated in cell culture systems, such as primary monkey kidney cells. Some cause cytopathic effects in culture.

Hemadsorption and hemagglutination inhibition used to detect presence of virus

Antihemagglutinin antibodies detectable in serum

The most efficient method of detection is demonstration of hemadsorption by adherence of erythrocytes to infected cells expressing hemagglutinin or by agglutination of erythrocytes by virus already released into the extracellular fluid. The virus can then be identified specifically by neutralization or inhibition of these properties by addition of antibody directed specifically at the hemagglutinin. This method is called **hemadsorption inhibition** or **hemagglutination inhibition,** depending on whether the test is performed on infected cells or extracellular virus, respectively. Also, because the hemagglutinin is antigenic, hemagglutination inhibition tests can be used to detect antibodies in infected sub-

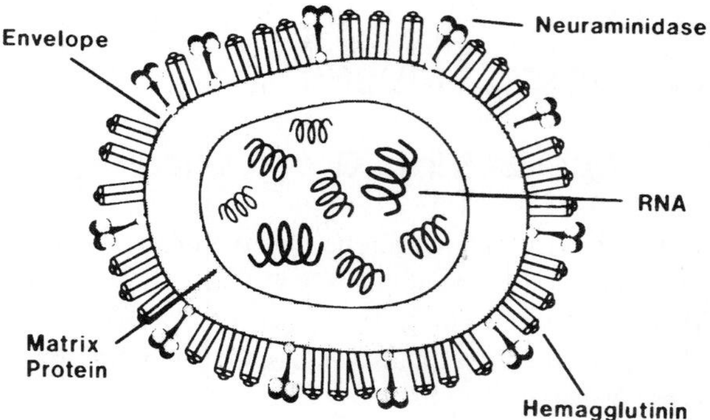


**Figure 32–1.** Diagrammatic view of influenza A or B virus, containing eight distinctive segments of single-stranded RNA.

jects. It has been shown that antibody directed against specific hemagglutinin is highly effective in neutralizing the infectivity of the virus.

## Influenza A

Influenza A is considered in detail because of its great clinical and epidemiologic importance.

The influenza A virion contains at least eight segments of single-stranded RNA with defined genetic responsibilities. These functions include coding for virus-specified proteins and antigens. A unique aspect of influenza A viruses is their ability to develop a wide variety of subtypes through the processes of mutation and recombination. These processes result in antigenic changes called **drifts** and **shifts,** which are discussed shortly.

Influenza A genome in multiple segments

Mutability of virus produces antigenic changes

A number of subtypes of hemagglutinin and neuraminidase antigens are known to exist among influenza A viruses. Of these, three hemagglutinins ($H_1$, $H_2$, and $H_3$) and two neuraminidases ($N_1$ and $N_2$) appear to be of greatest importance in human infections. These subtypes are designated according to the H and N antigens on their surface, for example, $H_1N_1$, $H_3N_2$. Within each subtype there may also be more subtle, but sometimes important, antigenic differences (drifts). These differences are designated according to the major representative virus to which they are most closely related antigenically, using the place of initial isolation, number of the isolate, and year of detection. For example, two $H_3N_2$ strains of influenza A viruses that differ antigenically only slightly are called A/Texas/1/77($H_3N_2$) and A/Bangkok/1/79($H_3N_2$).

Subtypes based on H and N antigens

Subtle changes called antigenic drift

Antigenic drifts within major subtypes can involve either the H or N antigen, as well as the genes encoding nonstructural proteins, and can result from as little as a single mutation in the viral RNA. The mutant may come to predominate under the selective immunologic pressures in the host population. Such drifts are frequent among influenza A viruses, occurring at least every few years and sometimes even during the course of a single epidemic. Drifts can also develop in influenza B viruses, but at a considerably lower frequency.

Antigenic drift every few years with type A

In contrast to the frequently occurring mutations that cause antigenic drift among influenza A strains, major antigenic changes in H, N, or both subtypes can occur suddenly and unpredictably. These are referred to as antigenic shifts. They almost certainly result from recombinational events that can be readily reproduced in the laboratory. Simultaneously infecting a cell with two different influenza A subtypes yields progeny that contain antigens derived from either of the original viruses. For example, a cell infected simultaneously with influenza A($H_3N_2$) and influenza A ($H_1N_1$) may produce a mixture of influenza viruses of the subtypes $H_3N_2$, $H_1N_1$, $H_1N_2$, and $H_3N_1$. Alternative possibilities for the emergence of "new" epidemic strains are that earlier antigenic subtypes become latent in human host tissues and reactivate later to spread to nonimmune contacts, or that they circulate into animal or avian reservoirs only to readapt and spread in human hosts when a sufficient proportion of the population has little or no immunity to the "new" subtypes.

Major antigenic shifts due to recombination

New subtype may emerge or become latent

Major antigenic shifts, which have occurred approximately every 8 to 10 years in this century, have often resulted in serious epidemics or pandemics among populations with little or no preexisting antibody to the new subtypes. Examples include the appearance of an $H_1N_1$ subtype in 1947, followed by an abrupt shift to an $H_2N_2$ strain in 1957, which caused the pandemic of Asian flu. A subsequent major shift in 1968 to an $H_3N_2$ subtype (the Hong Kong flu) led to another, but somewhat less severe epidemic. The Russian flu, which appeared in late 1977, was caused by an $H_1N_1$ subtype very similar to that which dominated between 1947 and 1957 (Table 32–1).

Major antigenic shifts correlate with epidemics

The concepts of antigenic shift and drift in human influenza A virus infections can be roughly summarized as follows. Periodic shifts in the major antigenic components appear, usually resulting in major epidemics in populations with little or no immunologic experience with the subtype. As the population of susceptible individuals is exhausted (ie, subtype-specific immunity is acquired by increasing numbers of people), the subtype continues to circulate for a time, undergoing mutations with subtle antigenic drifts from season to season. This allows some degree of virus transmission to continue. Infectivity persists because subtype-specific immunity is not entirely protective against drifting strains; for example, an individual may have antibodies reasonably protective against influenza A/Texas/77($H_3N_2$), yet be susceptible in succeeding years to reinfection by influenza A/Bangkok/79($H_3N_2$).

Minor antigenic drifts allow maintainence in population

**TABLE 32–1. MAJOR ANTIGENIC SHIFTS ASSOCIATED WITH INFLUENZA A PANDEMICS, 1947–1987**

| Year | Subtype | Prototype Strain |
|---|---|---|
| 1947 | $H_1N_1$ | A/FM$_1$/47 |
| 1957 | $H_2N_2$ | A/Singapore/57 |
| 1968 | $H_3N_2$ | A/Hong Kong/68 |
| 1977 | $H_1N_1$ | A/USSR/77 |
| 1987 | $H_3N_2$ | No pandemic occurred; various strains circulating worldwide |

Eventually, however, the overall immunity of the population becomes sufficient to minimize the epidemic potential of the major subtype and its drifting strains. Unfortunately, the battle is never entirely won, as the scene is set for the sudden and usually unpredictable appearance of an entirely new subtype that may not have circulated among humans for 20 years or more.

Anamnestic responses continue to first infecting subtype's antigens (original antigenic sin)

Another concept helpful in understanding the behavior of influenza A virus in humans is the doctrine of original antigenic sin, which states that the immune response to all subsequent influenza A infection is dominated by a persistence of antibody to the first virus with which a person has contact through constant anamnestic response. This doctrine describes primarily the antibody response to the hemagglutinin antigen, but there is evidence that it also applies to neuraminidase antigen responses. To clarify the concept, the antibody response to the hemagglutinins is illustrated in the following example. An infant or young child never infected by any influenza A virus is immunologically "virgin" in this respect. The first infection may be with an $H_1N_1$ subtype, and the patient develops an antibody response to the $H_1$ antigen. Years later, the patient becomes infected with an $H_2N_2$ subtype and develops antibodies to the $H_2$ antigen; in addition, even though the H antigen is different in the second episode, there is an anamnestic antibody response to the initial ($H_1$) antigen. Throughout life, anamnestic "recall" remains enhanced with regard to the first subtype encountered and, to a lesser extent, to subsequent subtypes, regardless of which influenza A virus later infects the patient. This phenomenon supports the presence of one or more shared (conserved) epitopes among all strains.

Age-specific attack rates relate to historical exposure

This immunologic recall response probably accounts for the variability in age-specific attack rates when newer subtypes are introduced into a population. For example, the appearance of the Russian flu ($H_1N_1$) in 1977–1978 was noteworthy in that a similar subtype had been prevalent during 1947–1956, but then disappeared. Individuals born after 1956 would not have experienced prior infection with the subtype, and the prediction that the highest attack rates would be among those less than 35 years of age was correct.

Individual variation is significant

Unfortunately, none of these generalizations can be applied with great confidence to the individual patient. People vary in their immune responses to viruses, and other host factors, such as the aging process, can modify susceptibility to infection. Therefore, even though a specific influenza A subtype might be expected to affect primarily younger individuals, it is still considered prudent to attempt to protect high-risk groups such as the elderly, who might acquire severe, potentially life-threatening infections.

## Infections Caused by Influenza Viruses

### Epidemiology

Human, animal, and avian strains are similar

Humans are the major hosts of the influenza viruses, and severe respiratory disease is the primary manifestation of infection. Influenza A viruses closely related to those prevalent in humans, however, circulate among many mammalian and avian species. Some of these may undergo antigenic mutation or genetic recombination and emerge as new human epidemic strains.

Characteristic influenza outbreaks have been described since the early 16th century and outbreaks of varying severity have occurred nearly every year. Severe pandemics occurred in 1743, 1889–1890, 1918–1919 (the Spanish flu), and 1957 (the Asian flu). These episodes were associated with particularly high mortality; for example, the Spanish flu was thought to have caused at least 20 million deaths. Usually, the elderly and persons of any age group with cardiac or pulmonary disease have the highest death rate.

Pandemic influenza may have high mortality

Direct droplet spread is the most common mode of transmission. Influenza infections in temperate climates tend to occur most frequently during midwinter months. Major outbreaks of influenza A usually occur at 2- to 3-year intervals; influenza B epidemics appear irregularly, usually every 4 to 5 years. The typical epidemic develops over a period of 3 to 6 weeks and may involve 10% of the population. Illness rates may exceed 30% among school-aged children, residents of closed institutions, and industrial groups. One major indicator of influenza virus activity is an abrupt rise in school or industrial absenteeism. In severe influenza A epidemics, the number of deaths reported in a given area of the country often exceeds the number expected for that period. This significant increase, referred to as **excess mortality,** is another indicator of severe, widespread illness. Influenza B rarely causes such severe epidemics.

Seasonality favors winter months

Epidemic intervals usually a few years

Excess mortality or increased absenteeism an indicator of epidemic

## Pathogenesis

Influenza viruses have a predilection for the respiratory tract, and viremia is rarely detected. They multiply in ciliated respiratory epithelial cells, leading to functional and structural ciliary abnormalities. This is accompanied by a switch-off of protein and nucleic acid synthesis in the affected cells, the release of lysosomal hydrolytic enzymes, and desquamation of both ciliated and mucus-producing epithelial cells. There is, thus, substantial interference with the mechanical clearance mechanism of the respiratory tract. The process of cell death results in the cleavage of complement components, leading to localized inflammation. Early in infection, the primary chemotactic stimulus is directed toward mononuclear leukocytes, which constitute the major cellular inflammatory component. The respiratory epithelium may not be restored to normal for 2 to 10 weeks after the initial insult.

Virus multiplies in respiratory epithelium

Synthetic blocks cause cilial damage and cell desquamation

Clearance mechanisms compromised

The virus particles are also toxic to tissues. This toxicity can be demonstrated by inoculating high concentrations of inactivated virions into mice, which produces acute inflammatory changes in the absence of viral penetration or replication within cells.

Viral toxicity causes inflammation

Other host cell functions are also severely impaired, particularly during the acute phase of infection. They include chemotactic, phagocytic, and intracellular killing functions of polymorphonuclear leukocytes and perhaps of alveolar macrophage activity.

Phagocytic host defenses compromised

The net result of these effects is that, on entry into the respiratory tract, the viruses cause cell damage, especially in the respiratory epithelium, which elicits an acute inflammatory response and impairs mechanical and cellular host responses. This damage renders the host highly susceptible to invasive bacterial superinfection. In vitro studies also suggest that bacterial pathogens such as staphylococci can more readily adhere to the surfaces of influenza virus-infected cells. Recovery from infection begins with interferon production, which limits further virus replication, and with rapid generation of natural killer cells. Shortly thereafter, class I major histocompatibility complex (MHC)-restricted cytotoxic T cells appear in large numbers to participate in the lysis of virus-infected cells and, thus, in initial control of the infection. This is followed by the appearance of local and humoral antibody along with an evolving, more durable cellular immunity. Finally, there is repair of tissue damage.

Damage creates susceptibility to bacterial invasion

Interferon and cytotoxic T cell response associated with recovery

## Immunity

Although cell-mediated immune responses are undoubtedly important in influenza virus infections, humoral immunity has been investigated more extensively. Typically, the patient responds to infection within a few days by the production of antibodies directed toward the group ribonucleoprotein antigen, the hemagglutinin, and the neuraminidase. Peak antibody titer levels are usually reached within 2 weeks of onset, then gradually wane over the following months to varying low levels. Antibody to the ribonucleoprotein appears to confer little or no protection against reinfection. Antihemagglutinin antibody is considered the most protective, as it has the ability to neutralize virus on reexposure; such immunity is relative, however, and quantitative differences in responsiveness exist between individuals. Furthermore, antigenic shifts and drifts often allow the virus to subvert the antibody re-

Antihemaggultinin antibody has protective effect

Antineuraminidase may limit viral spread

sponse on subsequent exposures. Antibody to neuraminidase antigen is not as protective as antihemagglutinin antibody, but may play a role in limiting virus spread within the host.

## Influenza Infections: Clinical Aspects

### Clinical Manifestations and Outcome

As stated previously, influenza A and B viruses tend to cause the most severe illnesses, whereas influenza C seems to occur infrequently and generally causes milder disease. The typical acute influenzal syndrome is described here.

Short incubation period followed by acute disease with dry cough

The incubation period is brief, lasting an average of 2 days. Onset is usually abrupt, with symptoms developing over a few hours. These include fever, myalgia, headache, and occasionally shaking chills. Within 6 to 12 hr, the illness reaches its maximum severity and a dry, nonproductive cough develops. The acute findings persist, sometimes with worsening cough, for 2 to 5 days, followed by gradual improvement. By a week after onset, the patient feels significantly better. Fatigue, nonspecific weakness, and cough, however, can remain frustrating lingering problems for an additional 2 to 3 weeks or longer.

Progressive respiratory infection and pneumonia may be lethal

Reye's syndrome may follow

Occasional patients develop a progressive infection that involves the tracheobronchial tree and lungs to a greater extent. In these situations pneumonia, which can be lethal, is the result. Other unusual acute manifestations of influenza include central nervous system dysfunction, myositis, and myocarditis. In infants and children, a serious complication known as Reye's syndrome may develop 2 to 12 days after onset of the infection; it is characterized by severe fatty infiltration of the liver and cerebral edema. This syndrome is associated not only with influenza viruses, but with a wide variety of systemic viral illnesses; the risk is enhanced by exposure to salicylates, such as aspirin.

Sudden worsening suggests bacterial superinfection

The most common and important complication of influenza virus infection is bacterial superinfection. Such infections usually involve the lung, but bacteremia with secondary seeding of distant sites can also occur. The superinfection, which can develop at any time in the acute or convalescent phase of the disease, is often heralded by an abrupt worsening of the patient's condition after initial stabilization. The bacteria most commonly involved include *Streptococcus pneumoniae, Haemophilus influenzae,* and *Staphylococcus aureus.*

In summary, there are essentially three ways in which influenza may cause death:

- **Underlying disease with decompensation.** People with limited cardiovascular or pulmonary reserves can be further compromised by any respiratory infection. Thus, the elderly and those of any age with underlying chronic cardiac or pulmonary disease are at particular risk.
- **Superinfection.** Superinfection can lead to bacterial pneumonia and occasionally disseminated bacterial infection.
- **Direct rapid progression.** Less commonly, direct rapid progression of the viral infection can lead to severe viral pneumonia with asphyxia.

### Laboratory Diagnosis

Virus isolation or direct immunofluorescence detect virus

During the acute phase of illness, influenza viruses can be readily isolated from respiratory tract specimens, such as nasopharyngeal and throat swabs. Most strains grow in primary monkey kidney cell cultures or in the amniotic cavity of embryonated hen's eggs, and they can be detected by hemadsorption or hemagglutination. Rapid diagnosis of infection is possible by direct immunofluorescence or immunoenzymatic detection of viral antigen in epithelial cells or secretions from the respiratory tract.

Serodiagnosis useful epidemiologically

Serologic diagnosis is of considerable help epidemiologically and is usually made by demonstrating a fourfold or greater increase in complement-fixing or hemagglutination inhibition antibody titers in acute and convalescent specimens collected 10 to 14 days apart.

### Prevention

Whole virus and "split" vaccines protective but variable and of short duration

The best available method of control is by use of killed viral vaccine prepared from those strains related most closely to the antigenic subtypes currently causing infections. These inactivated vaccines may contain whole virions or "split" subunits composed primarily of hemagglutinin antigens. They are commonly used, in two doses given 1 month apart, to immunize children who may not have been immunized previously; otherwise, single annual doses are recommended just prior to influenza season. Vaccine efficacy is variable, and annual revaccination is necessary to ensure maximal protection. Used in this way, the virus vaccines may be 70 to 85% effective.

It is recommended that vaccination be directed primarily toward the elderly, individuals of all ages who are at high risk (eg, those with chronic lung or heart disease), and their close contacts, including medical personnel and household members.

Vaccination indicated for high risk

Amantadine hydrochloride, a symmetric amine, has been shown to be effective in short-term (several weeks) oral prophylaxis of influenza A infections. It appears to act by blocking the ion channel of the viral M2 protein, resulting in interference with its key role in early virus uncoating and also later virion assembly. Amantadine can produce side effects, however, and is recommended only for high-risk patients until vaccine-induced immunity can be achieved. A typical example of its use would be during an epidemic in which an elderly, potentially susceptible patient may become exposed to infection within a defined period. Oral amantadine prophylaxis may be initiated concurrently with administration of a vaccine containing the most current antigens and continued for 2 weeks. The immunogenic effect of the vaccine should ensure continued protection. It must be emphasized that amantadine has been proven effective for influenza A virus infections only; it is useless in the management and prevention of infections caused by other influenza types or by any other respiratory virus. A newer related drug, rimantadine, seems to be as efficacious as amantadine and may cause fewer adverse effects. Unfortunately, virus resistance to both drugs can readily develop in vitro or in vivo. A single amino acid substitution in the transmembrane portion of the M2 protein is all that is necessary for this to occur.

Amantadine prophylaxis effective short-term for influenza A only

Blocks virus uncoating and assembly

Resistance from single amino acid substitution in target protein

### Treatment

The two basic approaches to management of influenzal disease are symptomatic care and anticipation of potential complications, particularly bacterial superinfection. Once the diagnosis has been made, rest, adequate fluid intake, conservative use of analgesics for myalgia and headache, and antitussives for severe cough are commonly prescribed. It must be emphasized that even nonprescription drugs must be used with caution. This applies particularly to those drugs containing salicylates given to children because the risk of Reye's syndrome must be considered.

Supportive therapy indicated

Bacterial superinfection is often suggested by a rapid worsening of clinical symptoms after the patient has initially stabilized. Antibiotic prophylaxis has not been shown to enhance or diminish the likelihood of superinfection, but can increase the risk of acquisition of more resistant bacterial flora in the respiratory tract and make the superinfection more difficult to treat. Ideally, the physician should instruct the patient regarding the natural history of the influenza virus infection and be prepared to respond to bacterial complications, if they occur, with a specific diagnosis and therapy.

Prophylaxis may prevent bacterial superinfection

When influenza A infection is proved or strongly suspected, 4 to 5 days of amantadine hydrochloride or rimantadine therapy may also be considered. Such treatment has been shown to benefit some patients to a modest degree, as measured by reduction of number of days of confinement to bed, of fever, and of functional respiratory impairment. These effects, however, have been observed only when the drug is administered early in the illness (within 12–24 hours of onset).

Amantadine therapy must be early

## PARAINFLUENZA VIRUSES

There are four serotypes of parainfluenza viruses: parainfluenza 1, 2, 3, and 4. These enveloped viruses belong to the paramyxovirus group, contain nonsegmented, negative-sense, single-stranded RNA; and, like the influenza viruses, possess a neuraminidase and hemagglutinin. Their mode of spread and pathogenesis is similar to that of the influenza viruses. They differ from the influenza viruses in that RNA synthesis occurs in the cytoplasm rather than the nucleus; in addition, the antigenic makeup of the individual parainfluenza serotypes is relatively stable, and significant antigenic shift or drift does not occur. Each serotype is considered separately.

Paramyxoviruses with four serotypes

Structure like influenza viruses, but with unsegmented genome

Antigenically stable

## Parainfluenza 1

Associated with croup and tracheobronchitis

Parainfluenza 1 is the major cause of acute croup (laryngotracheitis) in infants and young children, but also causes less severe diseases such as mild upper respiratory illness (URI), pharyngitis, and tracheobronchitis in all age groups. Outbreaks of infection tend to occur most frequently during the fall months.

## Parainfluenza 2

Parainfluenza 2 is of slightly less significance than parainfluenza 1 or 3. It has been associated with croup, primarily in children, with mild URI, and occasionally with acute lower respiratory disease. As with parainfluenza 1, outbreaks usually occur during the fall months.

## Parainfluenza 3

Severe lower respiratory disease in infants

Parainfluenza 3 is a major cause of severe lower respiratory disease in infants and young children. It often causes bronchitis, pneumonia, and croup in children less than 1 year old. In older children and adults, it may cause URI or tracheobronchitis. Infections are common and can occur in any season; it is estimated that nearly one half of all children have been exposed to this virus by 1 year of age.

## Parainfluenza 4

Parainfluenza 4 is the least common of the group and is generally associated with mild upper respiratory illness only.

## Summary

The parainfluenza viruses are important because of the serious diseases they can cause in infants and young children. Parainfluenza 1 and 3 are particularly common in this regard. Overall, the group is thought to be responsible for 15 to 20% of all nonbacterial respiratory diseases requiring hospitalization in infancy and childhood. The onset of illness may be abrupt, as in acute spasmodic croup, but usually begins as a mild URI with variable progression over 1 to 3 days to involvement of the middle or lower respiratory tract. Duration of acute illness can vary from 4 to 21 days but is usually 7 to 10 days.

Transient immunity

Immunity to reinfection is transient; although repeated infections can occur in older children and adults, they are usually milder than the illnesses of infancy and early childhood.

Laboratory diagnosis by isolation or direct immunofluorescence

Specific diagnosis is based on virus isolation, usually in monkey kidney cell cultures, or on serology using hemagglutination inhibition, complement fixation, or neutralization assays on paired sera to detect a rising antibody titer. Direct immunofluorescence can also be used for rapid detection of antigen in respiratory epithelial cells.

There is currently no method of control or specific therapy for these infections.

# RESPIRATORY SYNCYTIAL VIRUS

## ■ Virology

Pneumovirus causing syncytium formation in cell cultures

Respiratory syncytial virus (RSV) is now classified as a pneumovirus within the paramyxovirus family. Its name is derived from its ability to produce cell fusion in tissue culture (syncytium formation). Unlike influenza or parainfluenza viruses, it possesses no hemagglutinin or neuraminidase. The RNA genome is nonsegmented, negative sense, and single stranded and codes for at least 10 different proteins. Among these are two matrix (M) proteins in the viral envelope. One forms the inner lining of the viral envelope; the function of the other is uncertain.

Enveloped RNA virus with unsegmented genome

The antigens on the surface of the viral envelope include the G glycoprotein, which probably serves as an attachment site to host cell receptors, and the fusion (F) glycoprotein, which induces fusion of the viral envelope with the host cell surface. F glycoprotein is also responsible for fusion of infected cells in cell cultures, leading to the appearance of multinucleated giant cells (syncytium formation). Antibodies directed at the F glycoprotein are more efficient than anti-G glycoprotein antibodies in neutralizing the virus in vitro.

Two glycoproteins mediate attachment and syncytium formation

At least two antigenic subgroups (A and B) of RSV are known to exist. The epidemiologic and biological significance of these variants is not yet certain.

Respiratory syncytial virus is the single most important etiologic agent in respiratory diseases of infancy, and it is the major cause of bronchiolitis and pneumonia among infants under 1 year of age.

Most important in infants

## Respiratory Syncytial Virus Disease

### Epidemiology

Community outbreaks of RSV infection occur annually and can commence at any time from late fall to early spring. The usual outbreak lasts 8 to 12 weeks and can involve nearly one half of all families with children. In the family setting, it appears that older siblings often introduce the virus into the home, and secondary infection rates can be almost 50%. The usual duration of virus shedding is 5 to 7 days; young infants, however, may shed virus for 9 to 20 days or longer.

High attack rate, introduced by older siblings

Spread of RSV in the hospital setting is also a major problem. Control is difficult, but includes careful attention to hand washing between contacts with patients, isolation, and exclusion of personnel and visitors who have any form of respiratory illness. Masks are not effective in controlling nosocomial spread.

Nosocomial infection spread by direct contact

### Pathogenesis

The virus is spread to the upper respiratory tract by contact with infective secretions. Infection appears to be confined primarily to the respiratory epithelium, with progressive involvement of the middle and lower airways. Viremia occurs rarely. The direct effect of virus on respiratory tract epithelial cells is similar to that previously described for influenza viruses, and cytotoxic T cells appear to play a similar role in early control of the acute infection.

Confined to respiratory epithelium

The apparent enhanced severity of disease, particularly in very young infants, is not yet clearly understood, but may have an immunologic basis. Factors that have been proposed to play a role include (1) qualitative or quantitative deficits in humoral or secretory antibody responses to critical virus-specified proteins; (2) excessive damage from inflammatory cytokines or direct cell-mediated cytotoxicity; (3) formation of antigen–antibody complexes within the respiratory tract resulting in complement activation; and (4) IgE-mediated histamine release.

Possible immunological basis for enhanced disease in infants

The usual mortality among infants hospitalized with RSV infections is 0.5 to 1%; however, this rises to 15% or greater in children receiving cancer chemotherapy, infants with congenital heart disease, and those with severe immunodeficiency. Infants with underlying chronic lung disease are also considered to be at high risk for a lethal outcome.

### Pathology

The major findings are in the bronchi, bronchioles, and alveoli. These findings include necrosis of epithelial cells, interstitial mononuclear cell inflammatory infiltrates, which sometimes also involve the alveoli and alveolar ducts, and plugging of smaller airways with material containing mucus, necrotic cells, and fibrin (Fig 32–2). Multinucleated syncytial cells with intracytoplasmic inclusions are occasionally seen in the affected tracheobronchial epithelium.

Bronchiolar and alveolar necrosis and inflammation

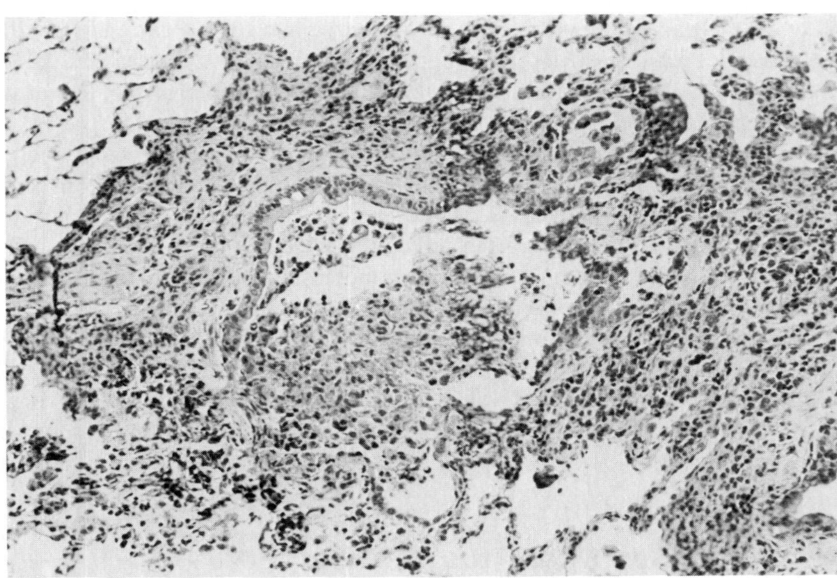

**Figure 32–2.** Photomicrograph illustrating the bronchiolar and surrounding interstitial inflammation in respiratory syncytial virus infection. (Original magnification ×100.)

### Immunity

Immunity to reinfection brief

Infection results in IgG and IgA humoral and secretory antibody responses. Immunity to reinfection is quite tenuous, however, as demonstrated by patients who have recovered from a primary acute episode and have become reinfected with disease of similar severity in the same or succeeding year. Illness severity appears to diminish with increasing age and successive reinfection.

## Respiratory Syncytial Virus Disease: Clinical Aspects

### Clinical Manifestations and Outcome

Infant bronchiolitis and pneumonitis lasting up to 2 weeks

The usual incubation period is 1 to 4 days, followed by the onset of rhinitis; severity of illness progresses to a peak within 1 to 3 days. In infants, this peak usually takes the form of bronchiolitis and pneumonitis, with cough, wheezing, and respiratory distress. Clinical findings include hyperexpansion of the lungs, hypoxemia (low oxygenation of blood), and hypercapnia (carbon dioxide retention). Interstitial infiltrates, often with areas of pulmonary collapse, may be seen on chest radiography (Fig 32–3). Fever is variable. The duration of acute illness is often 10 to 14 days. The fatality rate among hospitalized infected infants is estimated to be 0.5 to 1%. Causes of death include respiratory failure, right-sided heart failure (cor pulmonale), and bacterial superinfection. Death has sometimes resulted from unnecessary procedures in patients in whom RSV infection was not considered. Bronchoscopy, lung biopsy, or overly aggressive therapy with corticosteroids and bronchodilators for presumed asthma can all pose a danger to such patients.

Children, adults have milder illness

Older infants, children, and adults are also readily infected. The clinical illnesses in these groups are usually milder and include croup, tracheobronchitis, and URI. Respiratory syncytial virus can also cause acute flareups of chronic bronchitis and trigger acute wheezing episodes in asthmatic children.

### Laboratory Diagnosis

Virus isolation, direct immunofluorescent or immunoassay detect RSV

Rapid diagnosis of RSV infection can be made by immunofluorescence or immunoenzyme detection of viral antigen. The virus can also be isolated from the respiratory tract by prompt inoculation of specimens into cell cultures without prior freezing. Syncytial cytopathic effects develop over 2 to 7 days. The cell cultures of choice are heteroploid cell lines. Sero-

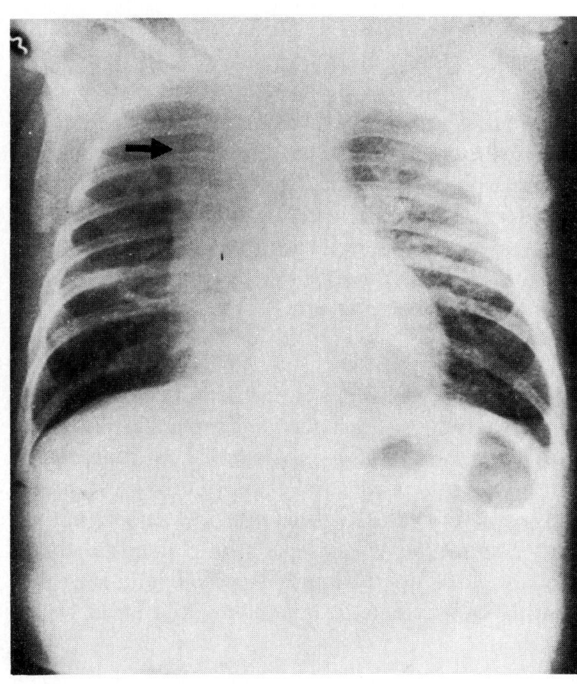

**Figure 32–3.** Chest radiograph of an infant with a severe case of respiratory syncytial virus pneumonia and bronchiolitis. Bilateral interstitial infiltrates, hyperexpansion of the lung, and right upper lobe atelectasis (arrow) are all present.

diagnosis may also be employed, but requires acute and convalescent sera and is less sensitive than antigen detection methods or culture.

### Prevention and Treatment

No vaccine is available; however, recent studies suggest that ribavirin aerosol treatment might be effective in some circumstances. Attenuated live virus vaccines and immune globulin containing high antibody titers to RSV are also under active investigation.

Ribavirin and supportive treatment indicated

Treatment is directed primarily at the underlying pathophysiology and includes adequate oxygenation, ventilatory support when necessary, and close observation for complications such as bacterial superinfection and right-sided heart failure.

## ADENOVIRUSES

## ■ Virology

Of the almost 100 different serotypes of adenoviruses, 47 are known to affect humans. These viruses are naked and icosahedral and possess double-stranded DNA. Replication and assembly occur in the nucleus, and virions are released by cell destruction. All adenoviruses share a common group-specific, complement-fixing antigen associated with the hexon component of the viral capsid. Adenoviruses are characterized by their ubiquity and persistence in host tissues for periods ranging from a few days to several years. Their ability to produce infection without disease is illustrated by the frequent recovery of virus from tonsils or adenoids removed from healthy children (the group name is derived from its discovery in 1953 as a latent agent in many adenoid tissue specimens) and by prolonged intermittent shedding of virus from the pharynx and intestinal tract after initial infection.

Multiple serotypes of naked, double-stranded DNA viruses

Potential for prolonged infection without disease

Type 1 and 2 adenoviruses are highly endemic; type 5 is the next most common. Most primary infections with these viruses occur early in life. The spread of the virus can be either respiratory or by fecal–oral contamination.

Spread by respiratory or fecal–oral route

Overall, only about 45% of adenovirus infections result in disease. Their most significant contribution to acute illness is in children, particularly those under 2 years of age (approximately 10% of acute febrile illness). They are also major causes of acute respiratory disease in military recruits, usually by types 4 and 7.

Disease in children and military recruits

## Adenovirus Disease

### Epidemiology

Swimming pool and medication-associated conjunctivitis

Infections caused by serotypes 1, 2, and 5 are generally most frequent during the first few years of life. All serotypes can occur during any season of the year, but are encountered most frequently during late winter or early spring. Sharp outbreaks of disease caused by serotypes 3 and 7 have been traced to inadequately chlorinated swimming pools. Conjunctivitis is the illness most commonly associated with these episodes. Other outbreaks of conjunctivitis have been traced to physicians' offices and appear to have been spread by contaminated ophthalmic medications or diagnostic equipment.

### Pathogenesis

Infects by droplet or oral routes

The adenoviruses usually enter the host by inhalation of droplet nuclei or by the oral route. Direct inoculation onto nasal or conjunctival mucosa by hands, contaminated towels, or ophthalmic medications may also occur. The virus replicates in epithelial cells, producing cell necrosis and inflammation. Viremia sometimes occurs and can result in spread to distant sites, such as the kidney, bladder, liver, lymphoid tissue (including mesenteric nodes), and, occasionally, the central nervous system. In the acute phase of infection, the distant sites may also show inflammation; for example, abdominal pain is occasionally seen with severe illnesses and is believed to result from mesenteric lymphadenitis caused by the viruses.

Epithelial cell replication may be followed by viremic spread and remote disease

After the acute phase of illness, the viruses may remain in tissues, particularly lymphoid structures such as tonsils, adenoids, and intestinal Peyer's patches, and become reactivated and shed without producing illness for 6 to 18 months thereafter. This reactivation is enhanced by stressful events (stress reactivation), such as infection by other agents. Integration of adenoviral DNA into the host cell genome has been shown to occur; this latent state can persist for years in tonsillar tissue and peripheral blood lymphocytes.

Latency by integration of adenoviral DNA

A potentially important pathogenic feature of the virion is the presence of pentons, which are located at each of the 12 corners of the icosahedron. They are fiberlike projections with knoblike terminal structures and appear to be responsible for a toxic effect on cells, which manifests as clumping and detachment in vitro. In addition, adenoviruses have developed other novel strategies to survive in the host, yet produce deleterious effects. These include encoding a 19K protein in its early E3 genomic region that binds class I MHC antigens in the endoplasmic reticulum, thus restricting their expression on the surface of infected cells and interfering with recognition and attack by cytotoxic T cells. This ability to evade immunosurveillance may be vital to establishment of latency. Another early protein, E1A, has been associated with increased susceptibility of epithelial cells to destruction by tumor necrosis factor and other cytokines. Other adenoviral proteins have been described that have a variety of effects on cell function and susceptibility to cytolysis. Their relative significance and interactions remain topics of great interest.

Penton projections toxic to cells

Proteins restrict cytotoxic T cells and enhance cytokine susceptibility

### Pathology

Like that of the viruses described previously, the primary pathology is epithelial cell necrosis with a predominantly mononuclear inflammatory response. In some instances, smudgy intranuclear inclusions may be seen in infected cells (Fig 32–4).

### Immunity

Immunity type-specific

Immunity after infection is serotype specific and usually long lasting. In addition to type-specific immunity, group-specific complement-fixing antibodies appear in response to infection. These antibodies are useful indicators of infection, but do not specify the infecting serotype.

## Adenovirus Disease: Clinical Aspects

### Clinical Manifestations and Outcome

Multiple upper respiratory syndromes and conjunctivitis

The diversity of major syndromes and commonly associated serotypes are summarized in Table 32–2. The acute respiratory syndromes vary in both clinical manifestations and severity. Symptoms include fever, rhinitis, pharyngitis, cough, and conjunctivitis. Adenoviruses

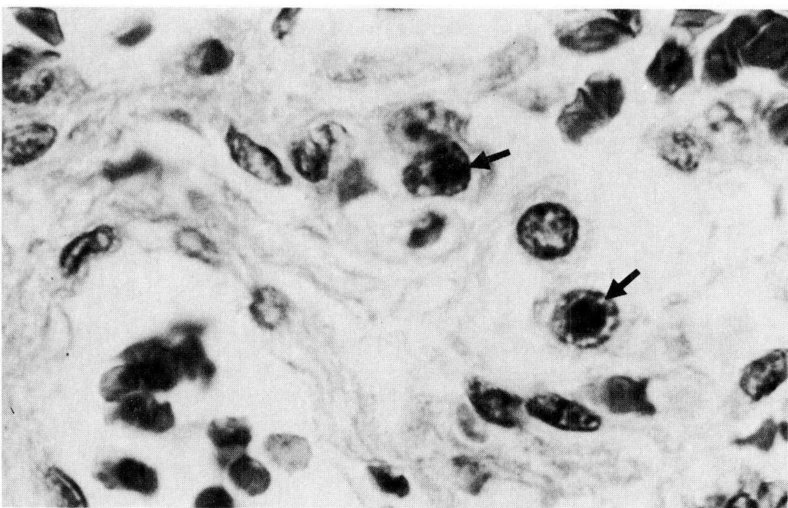

**Figure 32–4.** Lung tissue from a fatal case of adenovirus type 7 pneumonia. Large, smudgy intranuclear inclusions in alveolar epithelial cells (arrows), which are sometimes seen in adenovirus infections, are present. (Original magnification ×100.)

are also common causes of nonstreptococcal exudative pharyngitis, particularly among children less than 3 years of age. Acute, and occasionally chronic, conjunctivitis and keratoconjunctivitis have been associated with several serotypes. More severe disease, such as laryngitis, croup, bronchiolitis, and severe pneumonia, may also occur. Occasionally, the illness may be prolonged for several weeks and can clinically resemble pertussis. A syndrome of pharyngitis and conjunctivitis (pharyngoconjunctival fever) is classically associated with adenovirus infection. Adenoviruses can also cause acute hemorrhagic cystitis, in which hematuria and dysuria are prominent findings. More recently, some serotypes that are difficult to cultivate in the laboratory have been recognized as significant causes of gastroenteritis (see Chapter 38).

Significant cause of pharyngitis

More severe disease includes hemorrhagic cystitis

### Laboratory Diagnosis

Many serotypes can be readily isolated in heteroploid cell cultures. There is little difficulty in relating the virus detected to the illness in question when the isolate has been obtained from a site other than the upper respiratory or gastrointestinal tract (eg, lung biopsy, conjunctival swabs, urine); because of the known tendency for intermittent asymptomatic shedding into the oropharynx and feces, however, isolates from these sites must be interpreted more cautiously. If their significance is questionable, serologic testing of acute and convalescent sera may be necessary to confirm the relationship between the virus and the illness in question.

Viral isolation may not mean disease

### Prevention and Treatment

In the past, killed virus vaccines produced from serotypes 3, 4, and 7 were found effective in reducing illness in military recruits. The vaccine was discontinued, however, when it was found that types 3 and 7 were capable of inducing tumors in newborn hamsters. More recently, a live virus vaccine containing serotypes 4 and 7, enclosed in enteric-coated capsules and administered orally, has been used in military recruit groups. The viruses are released into the small intestine, where they produce an asymptomatic, nontransmissible infection. This vaccine has been found effective, but is neither available nor recommended for civilian groups. There is no specific therapy for infection.

Live vaccine used in military

## RHINOVIRUSES

The rhinovirus group comprises 100 accepted serotypes and many more that are not yet classified. They are picornaviruses, small (20–30 nm), naked particles containing single-stranded, positive-sense RNA, and are distinguished from enteroviruses by their acid labil-

Multiple serotypes of small, naked RNA viruses

TABLE 32–2. CLINICAL SYNDROMES ASSOCIATED WITH ADENOVIRUS INFECTION

| Syndrome | Common Serotypes Found[a] |
|---|---|
| Childhood febrile illness; pharyngoconjunctival fever | 1, 2, **3,** 5, 7, **7a** |
| Pneumonia and other acute respiratory illnesses | 1, 2, **3,** 5, 7, **7a, 7b** (4 in military recruits) |
| Pertussis-like illness | 1, 2, **3,** 5, **19,** 21 |
| Conjunctivitis | 2, 5, 7, 8, **19,** 21 |
| Keratoconjunctivitis | **3,** 8, 9, **19** |
| Acute hemorrhagic cystitis | 11 |
| Acute gastroenteritis | 40, 41 |

[a] Serotypes in boldface are those commonly associated with outbreaks.

Optimum growth temperature 33°C

Bind to ICAM intercellular adhesion molecule

ity and an optimum temperature of 33°C for in vitro replication. This temperature approximates that of the nasopharynx in the human host and may be a factor in the localization of pathologic findings at that site. These viruses are most consistently isolated in cultures of human diploid fibroblasts. The receptor for most rhinoviruses (and some coxsackieviruses) is glycoprotein intercellular adhesion molecule 1 (ICAM-1), a member of the immunoglobulin supergene family. ICAM-1 is best known for its role in immunologic cell adhesion; its ligand is lymphocyte function-associated antigen 1 (LFA-1).

## Clinical Manifestations and Epidemiology

Common cold viruses

Minimal cell injury

Rhinoviruses are known as the common cold viruses. They represent the major causes of mild URI syndromes in all age groups, especially older children and adults. Lower respiratory tract disease caused by rhinoviruses is uncommon. The usual incubation period is 2 to 3 days, and acute symptoms usually last 3 to 7 days. Interestingly, mucosal cell damage is minimal during the illness. Data suggest that activation and an increase in kinins, particularly bradykinin, may have a major role in the pathogenesis of increased secretions, vasodilation, and sore throat. Rhinovirus infections may be seen at any time of the year. Epidemic peaks tend to occur in the early fall or spring months.

## Prevention and Treatment

Multiple serotypes make vaccine different

May be able to block ICAM attachment

Currently there are no methods of prevention with vaccines and no specific therapy. Prospects for the development of an appropriate vaccine appear dim. The multiplicity of serotypes and their tendency to be type specific in the production of antibodies would seem to demand the development of a multivalent vaccine, which would be extremely difficult to accomplish. Recent studies, however, have suggested that a monoclonal antibody directed at the virus receptor or the use of a recombinant soluble receptor (ICAM-1) might block attachment of rhinoviruses. It remains to be seen whether these observations can be translated into effective preventive or therapeutic applications. At present, the attitude toward these viruses is best summed up by Sir Christopher Andrewes, who suggested that we should perhaps accept these infections as "one of the stimulating risks of being mortal."

# CORONAVIRUSES

Enveloped RNA viruses

Coronaviruses contain a single-stranded, positive-sense RNA genome. This is surrounded by an envelope that includes a lipid bilayer derived from intracellular rough endoplasmic reticulum and Golgi membranes of infected cells. Petal- or club-shaped spikes (peplomers) measuring approximately 13 nm project from the surface of the envelope, giving the appearance of a crown of thorns or a solar corona. The peplomers play an important role in inducing neutralizing and cellular immune responses. Like the rhinoviruses, coronaviruses are considered primary causes of the common cold. Based on serologic studies, it is estimated that they may cause as many as 5 to 10% of common colds in adults and a similar proportion of lower respiratory illnesses in children.

Disease similar to rhinoviruses

The number of serotypes is unknown. Two strains (229E and OC43) have been studied to some extent; it is clear that they can cause outbreaks similar to those of the rhinoviruses and that reinfection with the same serotype can occur. The cellular receptor for strain 229E is aminopeptidase N, a cell surface metalloprotease. No receptor for strain OC43 has yet been characterized.

## REOVIRUSES

The reoviruses (respiratory enteric orphans) are naked virions that contain segmented, double-stranded RNA and replicate in the cytoplasm of infected cells. They are ubiquitous and have been found in humans, simians, rodents, cattle, and a variety of other hosts. They have been studied in great detail as experimental models, revealing much basic knowledge about viral genetics and pathogenesis at the molecular level. Three serotypes are known to infect humans; however, their role and importance in human disease remain uncertain. Sporadic cases of febrile URI, exanthems, pneumonia, hepatitis, encephalitis, and gastroenteritis have all been reported to be associated with these viruses. Asymptomatic shedding of reoviruses also occurs, which makes it difficult to prove association with disease.

Uncertain association with human disease

Reoviruses can be isolated in cell cultures, particularly primary monkey kidney or human kidney monolayers.

## ADDITIONAL READING

### Influenza Viruses

Abramson JS, Mills EL. Depression of neutrophil function induced by viruses and its role in secondary microbial infections. *Rev Infect Dis.* 1988;10:326–341. This article reviews the functional neutrophil defects induced by influenza viruses, as well as what is known with respect to other viral agents.

Webster RG, Laver WG, Air GM, et al. Molecular mechanisms of variation in influenza viruses. *Nature.* 1982;296:115–121. An excellent review of "drifts," "shifts," and virulence.

### Respiratory Syncytial Virus

Henderson FW, Collier AM, Clyde WA, et al. Respiratory-syncytial-virus infections, reinfections, and immunity in young children. *N Engl J Med.* 1979;300:530–534. Examination of the effect of prior exposure on subsequent infection with the same virus suggests that illness on second infection may be no less severe than that with the first; however, the next reinfection may be modified.

Ray CG, Holberg CJ, Minnich LL, et al. Acute lower respiratory illnesses during the first three years of life: Potential roles for various etiologic agents. *Pediatr Infect Dis J.* 1993;12:10–14. The variety of viruses implicated in lower respiratory illnesses during early life and the relative importance of each agent are described.

### Rhinoviruses

Collono RJ, Callahan PL, Long WJ. Isolation of a monoclonal antibody that blocks attachment of the major group of human rhinoviruses. *J Virol.* 1986;57:7–12. The possibility of a novel immunologic approach to prevention, and even treatment, of picornavirus infections is raised.

Gwaltney JM Jr, Moskalski PB, Hendly JO, et al. Hand-to-hand transmission of rhinovirus colds. *Ann Intern Med.* 1978;88:463–467. An interesting study of the efficiency of spread of rhinoviruses by various routes.

## Reoviruses

Sharpe AH, Fields BN. Pathogenesis of viral infections: Basic concepts derived from the reovirus model. *N Engl J Med*. 1985;312:486–497. A clearly presented review of the molecular basis of reovirus pathogenesis, drawing interesting comparisons with other viruses.

Marlin SD, Staunton DE, Springer TA, et al. A soluble form of intercellular adhesion molecule-1 inhibits rhinovirus infection. *Nature*. 1990;344:70–72. The experimental approach to defining the nature of a receptor and potential therapeutic applications is well illustrated in this article.

Wold WSM, Gooding LR. Region E3 of adenovirus: A cassette of genes involved in host immunosurveillance and virus–cell interactions. *Virology*. 1991;184:1–8. This excellent review illustrates just how clever a "common" virus can be and how much more remains to be revealed.

Chapter 33

# Mumps Virus, Measles, Rubella, and Other Childhood Exanthems

*C. George Ray*

The major viruses to be described in this chapter (mumps, measles, rubella, and the human parvovirus B19) represent totally different virus families; however, they share several common epidemiologic characteristics: (1) distribution is worldwide, with a high incidence of infection in nonimmune individuals; (2) humans appear to be the sole reservoir of infection; and (3) person-to-person spread is primarily by the respiratory (aerosol) route.

The other disease discussed in this chapter, roseola infantum, is a common illness in early life.

## MUMPS

### Mumps Virus

Mumps virus is a paramyxovirus, and only one antigenic type is known. Like fellow members of its genus, it contains single-stranded, negative-sense RNA surrounded by an envelope. There are two glycoproteins on the surface of the envelope; one mediates neuraminidase and hemagglutinating activity, and the other is responsible for lipid membrane fusion to the host cell.

Enveloped single-stranded RNA virus with hemagglutinating and neuraminidase activity

### Mumps Infection

#### Epidemiology

The highest frequency of mumps infection is observed in the 5- to 15-year age group. Infection is rarely seen in the first year of life. Although about 85% of susceptible household contacts acquire infection, approximately 30 to 40% of these contacts do not develop clinical disease. The disease is communicable from approximately 7 days before until 9 days after onset of illness; however, virus has been recovered in urine for up to 14 days following onset. The highest incidence of infection is usually during the late winter and spring months, but it can occur during any season.

High infectivity both before and after onset of illness

### Pathogenesis

Viremic phase follows local replication

After initial entry into the respiratory tract, the virus replicates locally. Replication is followed by viremic dissemination to target tissues such as the salivary glands and central nervous system. It is also possible that before development of immune responses, a secondary phase of viremia may result from virus replication in target tissues, for example, initial parotid involvement with later spread to other organs. Viruria is common, probably as a result of direct spread from the blood into the urine, as well as active viral replication in the kidney. Virtually all infections are associated with transient, subclinical impairment of renal function.

Viruria and renal impairment common

### Immunity

As in most viral infections, the early antibody response is predominantly with IgM, which is replaced gradually over several weeks by specific IgG antibody. The latter persists for a lifetime, but can often be detected only by specific neutralization assays. Immunity is associated with the presence of neutralizing antibody. The role of cellular immune responses is not clear, but they may contribute both to the pathogenesis of the acute disease and to recovery from infection. It is known that acute infection can cause a transient diminution of delayed-type hypersensitivity to previously recognized antigens, such as tuberculin protein. After primary infection, immunity to reinfection is virtually always permanent.

Neutralizing antibody is protective

### Pathology

The tissue response is that of cell necrosis and inflammation with predominantly mononuclear cell infiltration. In the salivary glands swelling and desquamation of necrotic epithelial lining cells, accompanied by interstitial inflammation and edema, may be seen within dilated ducts.

## Mumps: Clinical Aspects

### Clinical Manifestations and Outcome

Incubation period 2–3 weeks

Parotitis unilateral or bilateral

After an incubation period of 12 to 29 days (average, 16 to 18 days), the typical case is characterized by fever and swelling with tenderness of the salivary glands, especially the parotid glands. Swelling may be unilateral or bilateral and persists for 7 to 10 days. Several complications can occur, usually within 1 to 3 weeks of onset of illness. All appear to be a direct result of virus spread to other sites and illustrate the extensive tissue tropism of mumps. Complications, which can occur without parotitis, include infection of the following:

1. Meninges: Approximately 10% of all infected patients develop meningitis. It is usually mild, but can be confused with bacterial meningitis. In about one third of these cases, associated or preceding evidence of parotitis is absent.
2. Brain: Encephalitis is occasionally severe.
3. Spinal cord and peripheral nerves: Transverse myelitis and polyneuritis are rare.
4. Pancreas: Pancreatitis is suggested by abdominal pain and vomiting.
5. Testes: Orchitis is estimated to occur in 10 to 20% of infected men. Although there is concern regarding subsequent sterility, it appears that such an outcome is quite rare.
6. Ovaries: Oophoritis is an unusual, usually benign inflammation of the ovarian glands.
7. Other rare and transient complications, including myocarditis, nephritis, arthritis, thyroiditis, thrombocytopenic purpura, mastitis, and pneumonia: The complications are acute and usually resolve without sequelae within 2 to 3 weeks; occasional permanent effects have been noted, however, particularly in cases of severe central nervous system infection, where sensorineural hearing loss and other impairment can occur.

### Laboratory Diagnosis

Cell culture from saliva, throat, CSF

Mumps virus can be readily isolated early in the illness from the saliva, pharynx, and other affected sites, such as the cerebrospinal fluid. The urine is also an excellent source for virus isolation. Mumps virus grows well in primary monolayer cell culture derived from monkey kidney, producing syncytial giant cells and viral hemagglutinin, and can be isolated in other cell systems as well as in the allantoic cavity of embryonated hen's eggs. Rapid diagnosis can be made by direct detection of viral antigen in pharyngeal cells or urine sediment by direct immunofluorescence.

Viral antigen detected by immunofluorescene

The best serologic tests are enzyme immunoassay (EIA) and indirect immunofluorescence to detect IgM- and IgG-specific antibody responses. Alternatively, the complement fixation test can be used, in which two virion antigens are employed: the S (soluble) nucleocapsid antigen and the V (viral) antigen, which is a component of the viral envelope. Antibody to the S antigen rises as quickly as 3 days after onset of symptoms, then usually disappears in 6 to 8 months. Antibody to the V antigen rises more slowly; it peaks 2 to 4 weeks after onset, then remains detectable for years afterward. Other serologic tests are also available, such as hemagglutination inhibition and neutralization. Of these, the neutralization test is the most sensitive for detection of immunity to infection.

EIA detects IgM and IgG responses

### Treatment

Immune serum globulin and mumps hyperimmune globulin are no longer recommended for the prevention or treatment of mumps. No specific therapy is available.

### Prevention

Since 1968, a live, attenuated vaccine has been available that is safe and highly effective. It is produced by serial propagation of virus in chick embryo cell cultures. A single dose causes seroconversion in more than 95% of recipients. Duration of immunity, although not yet established, appears to be greater than 10 years and may be lifelong. This vaccine is currently recommended for infants after the first year of life and for adults (particularly men) who may be susceptible and at high risk of exposure.

Live vaccine given in first year of life

# MEASLES

## ■ Measles Virus

The measles virus is classified in the paramyxovirus family, genus *Morbillivirus*. It contains linear, negative-sense, single-stranded RNA, which encodes at least six virion structural proteins. Of these, three are in the envelope, comprising a matrix (M) protein that plays a key role in viral assembly and two types of glycoprotein projections (peplomers). One of the projections is a hemagglutinin (H), which mediates adsorption to cell surfaces; the other (F) mediates cell fusion, hemolysis, and viral entry into the cell. No neuraminidase activity is present. Only a single serotype restricted to human infection is recognized. Two antigenically similar viruses, rinderpest of cattle and canine distemper virus, have not been shown to cause human infection.

Enveloped single-stranded RNA virus with hemagglutinating and fusion glycoproteins

## ■ Measles Infection

### Epidemiology

The highest attack rates have been in childhood, usually sparing infants less than 6 months of age because of passively acquired antibody; however, a shift in age-specific attack rates to greater involvement of adolescents and young adults was observed in the United States in the 1980s. This shift is believed to be attributable to the influence of immunization: younger children may be better immunized to limit spread of the virus, whereas older age groups may have missed effective immunization or earlier infection by the wild virus. A marked decline in measles in the early 1990s may reflect decreased transmission as increased immunization coverage takes effect. In the first half of 1993 only 167 cases were reported by US health departments compared to 13,787 during the same months of 1990, a 99% decrease.

Although childhood disease, infection in young adults important in transmission

Dramatic (99%) decrease recently

Epidemics tend to occur during the winter and spring in 1- to 3-year cycles and increasingly are limited to one dose vaccine failures or groups who do not accept immunizations. The infection rate among exposed susceptible subjects in a classroom or household

Epidemics in unimmunized groups

setting is estimated at 85%, and more than 95% of those infected become ill. The period of communicability is estimated to be 3 to 5 days before appearance of the rash to 4 days afterward.

### Pathogenesis

Respiratory cell multiplication disrupts cytoskeleton

Viremic dissemination to multiple sites

After implantation in the upper respiratory tract, viral replication proceeds in the respiratory mucosal epithelium. The effect within individual respiratory cells is profound. Even though measles does not directly restrict host cell metabolism, susceptible cells are damaged or destroyed by virtue of the intense viral replicative activity and the promotion of cell fusion with formation of syncytia. This results in disruption of the cellular cytoskeleton, chromosomal disorganization, and the appearance of inclusion bodies within the nucleus and cytoplasm. Replication is followed by viremic and lymphatic dissemination throughout the host to distant sites, including lymphoid tissues, bone marrow, abdominal viscera, and skin. Virus can be demonstrated in the blood during the first week after illness onset, and viruria persists for up to 4 days after the appearance of rash. During the viremic phase, measles virus infects T and B lymphocytes, circulating monocytes, and polymorphonuclear leukocytes without producing cytolysis. The effect on B lymphocytes has been shown to suppress immunoglobulin synthesis; in addition, generation of natural killer cell activity appears to be impaired. There is also evidence that the capability of polymorphonuclear leukocytes to generate oxygen radicals is diminished, perhaps directly by the virus or by activated suppressor T cells. This may further explain the enhanced susceptibility to bacterial superinfections. In addition, virion components can be detected in biopsy specimens of Koplik's spots and vascular endothelial cells in the areas of skin rash.

Infection of T and B lymphocytes may produce susceptibility to other infections

### Immunity

CMI may be part of the disease manifestations

Lifelong immunity associated with neutralizing antibody

Although cell-mediated immune responses to other antigens may be acutely depressed during measles infection, there is evidence that measles virus-specific cell-mediated immunity developing early in infection plays a role in mediating some of the features of disease, such as the rash, and is necessary to promote recovery from the illness. Antibodies to the virus appear in the first few days of illness, peak in 2 to 3 weeks, and then persist at low levels. Immunity to reinfection is lifelong and is associated with the presence of neutralizing antibody. In patients with defects in cell-mediated immunity, including those with severe protein-calorie malnutrition, the infection is prolonged, tissue involvement is more severe, and complications such as progressive viral pneumonia are common.

### Pathology

Vasculitis, giant cells, and inclusions are seen

In addition to necrosis and inflammatory changes in the respiratory tract epithelium, several other features of measles virus infection are noteworthy. The skin lesions show vasculitis characterized by vascular dilation, edema, and perivascular mononuclear cell infiltrates. The lymphoid tissues show hyperplastic changes, and large multinucleated reticuloendothelial giant cells are often observed (Warthin–Finkeldey cells). Some of the giant cells contain intracytoplasmic and intranuclear inclusions. Similarly involved giant epithelial cells can be found in a variety of mucosal sites, the respiratory tract, skin, and urinary sediment.

Lesions in encephalitis by cytotoxic T cell activity

The major findings in measles encephalitis include areas of edema, scattered petechial hemorrhages, perivascular mononuclear cell infiltrates, and necrosis of neurons. In most cases, perivenous demyelination in the central nervous system is also observed. The pathogenesis is thought to be related to infiltration by cytotoxic (CD8+) T cells, which react with myelin-forming or virus-infected brain cells.

## ■ Measles: Clinical Aspects

### Clinical Manifestations and Outcome

Incubation period 7–18 days

Common synonyms for measles include rubeola, 5-day measles, and hard measles. The incubation period ranges from 7 to 18 days. A typical illness usually begins 9 to 11 days after exposure, with cough, coryza, conjunctivitis, and fever. One to three days after onset, pinpoint gray–white spots surrounded by erythema (grains-of-salt appearance) appear on mucous membranes. This sign, called **Koplik's spots,** is usually most noticeable over the buccal mucosa opposite the molar teeth and persists for 1 to 2 days. Within a day of the appearance of Koplik's spots, the typical measles rash begins, first on the head, then on the trunk and extremities. The rash is maculopapular and semiconfluent; it persists for 3 to 5 days before fading. Fever and severe systemic symptoms gradually diminish as the rash progresses to the extremities. Lymphadenopathy is also common, with particularly noticeable involvement of the cervical nodes.

Koplik's spots on mucous membranes

Rash goes head to trunk and extremities

The disease can be very severe, especially in immunocompromised or malnourished patients. Death may result from overwhelming viral infection of the host, with extensive involvement of the respiratory tract and other viscera, or from other related causes. In some developing countries, mortality rates of 15 to 25% have been recorded.

## Complications

Bacterial superinfection, the most common complication, occurs in 5 to 15% of all cases. Such infections include acute otitis media, mastoiditis, sinusitis, pneumonia, and sepsis. Clinical signs of encephalitis develop in 1 of 500 to 1000 cases. This usually occurs 3 to 14 days after onset of illness and can be extremely severe. The mortality in measles encephalitis is approximately 15%, and permanent neurologic damage among survivors is estimated at 25%. Acute thrombocytopenic purpura may also develop during the acute phase of illness, leading to bleeding episodes. Abdominal pain and acute appendicitis can occur secondary to inflammation and swelling of lymphoid tissue.

Bacterial superinfection common

Thrombocytopenic purpura and bleeding in acute phase

Both wild and attenuated (vaccine) measles viruses have been shown to depress delayed hypersensitivity and cell-mediated immunity significantly for as long as several weeks. Exacerbation of chronic granulomatous infections such as tuberculosis can result. Measles has also been implicated in a rare, smoldering, usually fatal encephalitis known as subacute sclerosing panencephalitis, which is discussed later in this section.

Cell-mediated immunity depressed during vaccine infection

## Laboratory Diagnosis

The typical measles infection can usually be diagnosed on the basis of clinical findings. When the disease is atypical, laboratory confirmation may be necessary. Virus isolation from the oropharynx or urine is usually most productive in the first 5 days of illness. Measles grows on a variety of cell cultures, producing multinucleated giant cells similar to those observed in infected host tissues. If rapid diagnosis is desired, measles antigen may be identified in urinary sediment or pharyngeal cells by direct fluorescent antibody methods. Serologic diagnosis using complement fixation, hemagglutination inhibition, or indirect fluorescent antibody methods is also commonly used and requires acute and convalescent serum samples.

Virus isolation only required in atypical cases

Rapid diagnosis possible by immunofluorescence

## Treatment

No specific therapy is available other than supportive measures and close observation for the development of complications such as bacterial superinfection.

## Prevention

Live, attenuated measles vaccine is available and highly immunogenic. To ensure effective immunization, the vaccine should be administered to infants after the first year of life (preferred routine immunization is at 13–15 months of age). In children less than 1 year old, vaccine efficacy is occasionally impaired, probably because of the persistence of maternal antibody and the relatively lower immunologic responsiveness to some antigens early in life. Immunity induced by the vaccine may be lifelong. Reactions to vaccination, usually in the form of fever and occasional rash, are rarely severe. There is no clear evidence that the vaccine causes encephalitis. Because the vaccine consists of live virus, it should not be administered to immunocompromised patients and it is not recommended for pregnant women. Exceptions to these guidelines include susceptible HIV-infected persons.

Live, attenuated vaccine highly immunogenic

Vaccination contraindicated in pregnancy, immunocompromised

Exposed susceptible patients who are immunologically compromised (including small infants) may be given immune serum globulin intramuscularly. This treatment can modify or prevent disease if given within 6 days of exposure, but protection is transient.

Passive protection appropriate for immunocompromised

Killed measles virus vaccines, commonly used between 1963 and 1967, are no longer available. It has been shown that formalin-inactivated vaccine virus does not induce pro-

Killed vaccines can produce illness by sensitization

tective immunity and could additionally cause other difficulties: (1) It can sensitize some individuals, who will then develop severe local inflammatory reactions on subsequent inoculation with live vaccine; and (2) the sensitization may result in severe atypical illness (atypical measles syndrome) when the patient is exposed to the wild virus later in life. This syndrome is characterized by abrupt onset of high fever, often with abdominal pain and pneumonia, and the appearance of a rash, predominantly over the extremities. The rash may be papular, vesicular, or hemorrhagic. The pathogenesis may be related to selective formalin inactivation of F-glycoprotein antigenicity. The lack of antibodies to F may allow cell-to-cell spread of wild virus by cell fusion, facilitating production of antigens that could generate adverse cytotoxic T-cell responses or immune complexes.

### Subacute Sclerosing Panencephalitis

Progressive neurologic disease of children

Subacute sclerosing panencephalitis is a progressive neurologic disease of children, which usually begins 2 to 10 years after a measles infection. It is characterized by insidious onset of personality change, poor school performance, progressive intellectual deterioration, development of myoclonic jerks (periodic muscle spasms), and motor dysfunctions such as spasticity, tremors, loss of coordination, and ocular abnormalities, including cortical blindness. Neurologic and intellectual deterioration generally progress over 6 to 12 months, with the child eventually becoming bedridden and stuporous. Dysfunctions of the autonomic nervous system, such as difficulty with temperature regulation, may develop. Progressive inanition, superinfection, and metabolic imbalances eventually lead to death.

Inclusions in neuronal cells

Most of the pathologic features of the disease are localized to the central nervous system and retina. Both the gray and the white matter of the brain are involved, the most noteworthy feature being the presence of intranuclear and intracytoplasmic inclusions in oligodendroglial and neuronal cells.

Chronic measles virus infection

Incomplete measles virus present in brain tissue

The disease is a result of chronic measles virus infection of the central nervous system. Evidence for this conclusion includes (1) elevated measles antibody titers in the cerebrospinal fluid (CSF), (2) intranuclear and intracytoplasmic inclusions characteristic of a paramyxovirus in brain cells, (3) demonstration of measles-specific antigen by immunofluorescence testing in brain cells, and (4) isolation of measles virus from brain tissue and lymph nodes by cocultivation rescue techniques. Patients with subacute sclerosing panencephalitis have been shown to fail to respond immunologically to the M (matrix) protein of the measles virus, which plays a key role in virus assembly, probably in nucleocapsid alignment beneath the cytoplasmic membrane before budding. Further studies have shown that patients have a variety of patterns of missing measles virus structural proteins in brain tissue. Thus, any of several defects in viral gene expression may prevent normal viral assembly, allowing persistence of defective virus at an intracellular site with failure of immune eradication.

Rarely, a similar progressive, degenerative neurologic disorder may be related to persistent rubella virus infection of the central nervous system. This condition is seen most often in adolescents who have had congenital rubella syndrome. Rubella virus has been isolated from brain tissue in these patients, again using cocultivation techniques.

Reduced incidence after introduction of measles vaccine

The incidence of subacute sclerosing panencephalitis is approximately one per 100,000 measles cases. The disease appears to be twice as frequent in males as in females. Its occurrence in the United States has decreased markedly over the past 20 years with the widespread use of live measles vaccine.

At present, there is no accepted effective therapy for subacute sclerosing panencephalitis.

## RUBELLA

Rubella was considered a mild, benign exanthem of childhood until 1941, when the Australian ophthalmologist Sir Norman Gregg described the profound defects that could be induced in the fetus as a result of maternal infection. Since 1962, when the virus was first isolated, knowledge regarding its extreme medical importance and biological characteristics has increased rapidly.

## Rubella Virus

Rubella virus is classified as a member of the togavirus family. It is enveloped and contains single-stranded, positive-sense RNA. There is only one serotype, and no extrahuman reservoirs are known to exist. The virus can agglutinate some types of red blood cells, such as those obtained from 1-day-old chicks and trypsin-treated human type O cells.

Enveloped, single-stranded RNA togavirus

## Rubella Infection

### Epidemiology

Infections are usually observed during the winter and spring months. In contrast to measles, which has a high clinical attack rate among exposed susceptible individuals, only 30 to 60% of rubella-infected susceptible persons develop clinically apparent disease. Although rubella is highly contagious, an estimated 15% of young adults escape natural infection during childhood. A major focus of concern is the susceptible woman of childbearing age, who carries a risk of exposure during pregnancy. Disease in patients with primary acquired infections is contagious from 7 days before to 7 days after the onset of rash; congenitally infected infants may spread the virus to others for 6 months or longer after birth.

Low virulence, high infectivity

Childbearing woman the major concern

### Pathogenesis and Immunity

In acquired infection, the virus enters the host through the upper respiratory tract, replicates, and then spreads by the bloodstream to distant sites, including lymphoid tissues, skin, and organs. Viremia in these infections has been detected for as long as 8 days before to 2 days after onset of the rash, and virus shedding from the oropharynx can be detected up to 8 days after onset (Fig 33–1). Cellular immune responses and circulating virus–antibody immune complexes are thought to play a role in mediating the inflammatory responses to infection, such as rash and arthritis. After infection the serum antibody titer rises, with a peak within 2 to 3 weeks of onset. Natural infection also results in the production of specific secretory IgA antibodies in the respiratory tract. Immunity to disease is nearly always lifelong; however, reexposure can lead to transient respiratory tract infection, with an anamnestic rise in IgG and secretory IgA antibodies, but without resultant viremia or illness.

Upper respiratory infection with viremic spread

Cell-mediated immunity mediates arthritis, rash

Congenital infection occurs as a result of maternal viremia, placental infection, and transplacental spread to the fetus. Once fetal infection occurs, it persists chronically. Such persistence is probably related to an inability to eliminate the virus by immune or interferon-mediated mechanisms. There is too little inflammatory change in the fetal tissues to explain

Transmission to fetus by viremia

Fetal infection becomes chronic

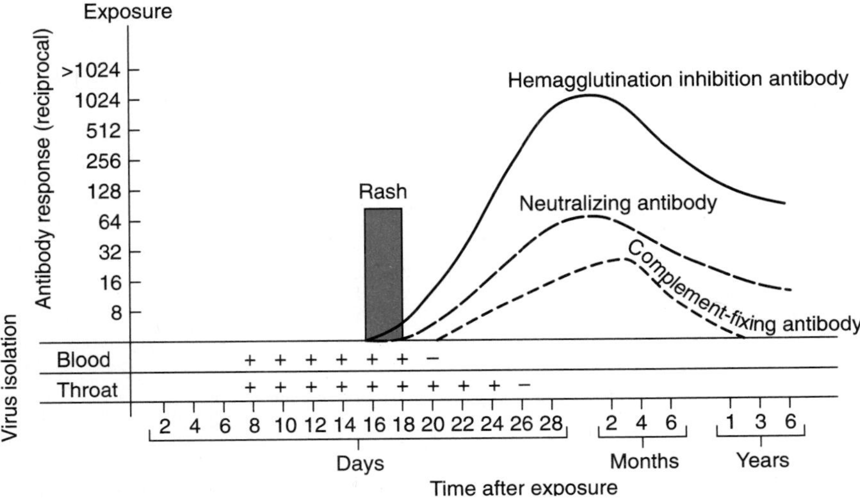


**Figure 33–1.** Antibody response and viral isolation in a typical case of acquired rubella.

the pathogenesis of the congenital defects. Possibilities include placental and fetal vasculitis with compromise of fetal oxygenation, chronic viral infection of cells leading to impaired mitosis, cellular necrosis, and induction of chromosomal breakage. Any or all of these factors may operate at a critical stage of organogenesis to induce permanent defects. Viral persistence with circulating virus–antibody immune complexes may evoke inflammatory changes postnatally and produce continuing tissue damage.

Infection and virus shedding continues long after birth

After birth, affected infants continue to excrete the virus in the throat, urine, and intestinal tract (Fig 33–2). Virus may be isolated from virtually all tissues in the first few weeks of life. Shedding of virus in the throat and urine, which persists for at least 6 months in most cases, has been known to continue for 30 months. Virus has also been isolated from lens tissue removed 3 to 4 years later. These observations underscore the fact that such infants are an important reservoir in perpetuating virus transmission.

The prolonged virus shedding is somewhat puzzling, as it does not represent a typical example of immunologic tolerance. The affected infants are usually able to produce circulating IgM and IgG antibodies to the virus (see Fig 33–2), although antibodies may decrease to undetectable levels after 3 to 4 years. Many infants show evidence of depressed rubella virus-specific cell-mediated immunity during the first year of life.

### Pathology

Because postnatally acquired disease is usually mild, little is known about its pathology. Mononuclear cell inflammatory changes can be observed in tissues, and viral antigen can be detected in the same sites (eg, skin and synovial fluid).

Fetal disease includes multiple malformations

Congenital infections are characterized primarily by the various malformations. Necrosis of tissues such as myocardium and vascular endothelium may also be seen, and quantitative studies suggest a decrease in cell quantity in affected organs. In severe cases, normal calcium deposition in the metaphyses of long bones is delayed, which creates a "celery stalk" appearance on a radiograph.

## Rubella: Clinical Aspects

### Clinical Manifestations and Outcome

Mild illness with lymphadenopathy and macular rash

Rubella is commonly known as German measles or 3-day measles. The incubation period for acquired infection is 14 to 21 days (average, 16 days). Illness is generally very mild, consisting primarily of low-grade fever, upper respiratory symptoms, and lymphadenopathy, which is most prominent in the posterior cervical and postauricular areas. A macular

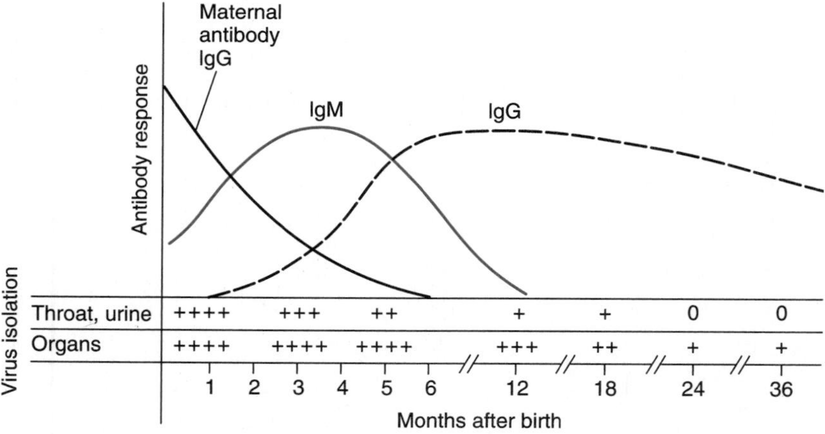


**Figure 33–2.** Persistence of rubella virus and antibody in congenitally infected infants.

rash often follows within a day of onset and lasts 1 to 3 days. This rash is usually most prominent over the head, neck, and trunk, and may be quite faint. Petechial lesions may also be seen over the soft palate during the acute phase. The most common complication is arthralgia or overt arthritis, which may affect joints of the fingers, wrists, elbows, knees, and ankles. The joint problems, which occur most frequently in women, rarely last longer than a few days to 3 weeks. Other, rarer complications include thrombocytopenic purpura and encephalitis.

Arthralgia, arthritis most common in women

Because of the rather nonspecific nature of the illness, a diagnosis of rubella cannot be made on clinical grounds alone. More than 30 other viral agents, which are discussed later in this chapter, can produce a similar illness. Confirmation of the diagnosis requires laboratory studies.

The major significance of rubella is not the acute illness, but the risk of fetal damage in pregnant women, particularly when they contract either symptomatic or subclinical primary infection during the first trimester. The risk of fetal malformation and chronic fetal infection, which is estimated to be as high as 80% if infection occurs in the first 2 weeks of gestation, decreases to 6 to 10% by the 14th week. The overall risk during the first trimester is estimated at 20 to 30%. Clinical manifestations of congenital rubella syndrome vary, but may include any combination of the following major findings: cardiac defects, commonly patent ductus arteriosus and pulmonary valvular stenosis; eye defects such as cataracts, chorioretinitis, glaucoma, coloboma, cloudy cornea, and microphthalmia; nerve deafness; enlargement of liver and spleen; thrombocytopenia; intrauterine growth retardation. Other findings include central nervous system defects such as microcephaly, mental retardation, and encephalitis; anemia; transient immunodeficiency; interstitial pneumonia, sometimes chronic; and intravascular coagulation, hepatitis, rash, and other congenital malformations. Late complications of congenital rubella syndrome have also been described, including an apparent increased risk of diabetes mellitus, chronic thyroiditis, and occasionally the development of a progressive subacute panencephalitis in the second decade of life.

High risk for fetal damage with infection in first trimester

Lesions of congenital rubella include multiple body systems

Some congenitally infected infants may appear entirely normal at birth, and sequelae such as hearing or learning deficits may not become apparent until months later. The spectrum of defects thus varies from subtle to severe.

## Laboratory Diagnosis

The virus may be isolated from respiratory secretions in the acute phase (and from urine, tissues, and feces in congenitally infected infants) by inoculation into a variety of cell cultures. The cell cultures required are not usually employed routinely in the laboratory, however, and isolation can be expensive, tedious, and time consuming, requiring as long as 2 weeks for the development of interfering or cytopathic effects.

Culture rarely used in routine diagnosis

Serologic diagnosis is usually employed in acquired infections; paired acute and convalescent samples collected 10 to 21 days apart are used. The hemagglutination inhibition test is used most often, but indirect fluorescent antibody, enzyme immunoassay, and other tests are available.

Hemagglutination inhibition test most common for serodiagnosis

Determination of IgM-specific antibody is sometimes useful to ascertain whether an infection occurred in the past several months; it has also been used in the diagnosis of congenital infections. Unfortunately, there are certain pitfalls in interpreting this test. Some individuals (less than 5%) with acquired infections may have persistent elevations of IgM-specific antibodies for 200 days or more afterward, and some congenitally infected infants do not produce detectable IgM-specific antibodies.

IgM tests can help detect acute and congenital infection

Serologic testing is also used to determine potential susceptibility or immunity to infection. The presence of antibodies at or above the technical threshold level (eg, 1:8 or 1:10 with the hemagglutination inhibition test) indicates a very high probability of immunity (titers of 1:16 or greater are particularly reassuring), whereas titers below the threshold (reported as undetectable) suggest lack of immunity. Testing is often done to determine whether individuals such as female adolescents are susceptible. Susceptible individuals require closer surveillance and consideration for immunization when such a procedure can be performed safely. It is particularly important to determine the immune status of women who are pregnant or contemplating pregnancy, in case exposure should occur subsequently. If the woman has serologic proof of prior immunity, the risk to the fetus if she is accidentally

Serologic tests to detect susceptibility particularly in young women

Results useful if there is exposure

exposed is nil; if not, and exposure occurs during pregnancy, careful serologic monitoring is necessary.

### Treatment

Other than supportive measures, there is no specific therapy for either the acquired or the congenital infection.

### Prevention

Live, attenuated rubella vaccine indicated for children, hospital workers

Since 1969, live, attenuated rubella vaccines have been available for routine immunization. The current vaccine virus, grown in human diploid fibroblast cell cultures (RA 27/3), has been shown to be highly effective: it causes seroconversion in approximately 95% of recipients. Interestingly, significant seroconversion is often associated with excretion of the vaccine virus in the pharynx; however, its transmission to others has never been documented. Routine immunization is now recommended for infants after the first year of life and for other individuals with no history of immunization and lack of immunity by serologic testing. Target groups include female adolescents and hospital personnel in a high-risk setting. Complications of the vaccine, although similar to those of the acquired, wild virus disease, are far less frequent and usually milder. They include occasional rash, fever, and joint complaints; the latter are more common in women. The vaccine is contraindicated in many immunocompromised patients and in pregnancy. To date, more than 200 instances of accidental vaccination of susceptible pregnant women have been reported, with no clinically apparent adverse effects on the fetus; however, it is strongly recommended that immunization be avoided in this setting and that nonpregnant women avoid conception for at least 3 months after receiving the vaccine.

Vaccine not known to produce defects in fetus

Artificial immunity may be lifelong

Vaccine-induced immunity may be lifelong. Further follow-up is necessary, however, before any conclusions can be made. Studies to date indicate that the duration of protection is at least 16 years. Immune serum globulin has not been shown of significant value in post-exposure prophylaxis, and it is not routinely recommended.

## PARVOVIRUS B19 INFECTIONS

Small naked, single-stranded DNA viruses

Parvoviruses are very small (18–26 nm), naked virions containing a linear single-stranded DNA molecule that encodes as few as three proteins. Diseases caused by parvoviruses have been recognized among nonhuman hosts for a number of years. Notable among these are canine parvovirus and feline panleukopenia virus, which produce particularly severe infections among puppies and kittens, respectively. These do not appear to cross species barriers. The human parvovirus, B19, has been well described, but our understanding is far from complete.

Replicates in erythroid precursor nuclei

Parvovirus B19 can be grown in primary cultures of human bone marrow cells, fetal liver cells, hematopoietic progenitor cells generated from peripheral blood, and a megakaryocytic leukemia cell line. The primary site of replication appears to be the nucleus of an immature cell in the erythrocyte lineage. Such infected cells then cease to proliferate, resulting in an impairment of normal erythrocyte development. The clinical consequences of this effect are generally trivial, unless the patient is already compromised by a chronic hemolytic process, such as sickle cell disease or thalassemia, in which maximal erythropoiesis is continually needed to counterbalance increased destruction of circulating erythrocytes. Primary infection by parvovirus B19 in such patients often produces an acute, severe, sometimes fatal anemia manifested as a rapid fall in red blood cell counts and hemoglobin. This may present initially with no clinical symptoms other than fever, and is commonly referred to as **transient aplastic crisis.** Immunocompromised patients, such as individuals with AIDS, sometimes have difficulty clearing the virus and develop persistent anemia with reticulocytopenia. Parvovirus B19 has also been occasionally implicated as a cause of persistent bone marrow failure and an acute hemophagocytic syndrome.

Aplastic crisis may persist in AIDS patients

A more common disease that is clearly attributable to parvovirus B19 is erythema infectiosum (also referred to as fifth disease or academy rash). After an incubation period of 4 to 12 days, a mild illness appears, characterized by fever, malaise, headache, myalgia, and itching in varying degrees. A confluent, indurated rash appears on the face, giving a

Erythema infectiosum usually mild "slapped cheek" rash

"slapped-cheek" appearance. The rash spreads in a day or two to other areas, particularly exposed surfaces such as the arms and legs, where it is usually macular and reticular (lace-like). During the acute phase, generalized lymphadenopathy or splenomegaly may be seen, along with a mild leukopenia and anemia. The illness lasts 1 to 2 weeks, but rash may recur for periods of 2 to 4 weeks thereafter, exacerbated by heat, sunlight, exercise, or emotional stress. Arthralgia sometimes persists or recurs for weeks to months, particularly in adolescent or adult females. Overt arthritis has also been reported in some. Serious complications are extremely rare; however, like rubella, active transplacental transmission of parvovirus B19 can occur during primary infections in pregnancy, sometimes resulting in stillbirth of fetuses that are profoundly anemic. The progress can be so severe that hypoxic damage to the heart, liver, and other tissues leads to extensive edema (hydrops fetalis). The frequency of such adverse outcomes is as yet undetermined.

Occasional severe fetal infection

Epidemiologic evidence suggests that spread of the virus is primarily by the respiratory route, and high transmission rates occur in households. Outbreaks tend to be small and localized, particularly during the spring months, with the highest rates among children and young adults. Seroepidemiologic studies have demonstrated evidence of past infection in 30 to 60% of adults. Laboratory confirmation of infection is presently difficult to obtain. Viremia, which usually lasts 7 to 12 days, may be detected by specific DNA probe, polymerase chain reaction, or immunoprecipitation methods. Alternatively, the presence of IgM-specific antibody late in the acute phase or during convalescence strongly supports the diagnosis. It is important to be aware that erythema infectiosum is extremely variable in its clinical manifestations, and even the "classic" presentation can be mimicked by other agents, such as rubella and echoviruses. Before a firm diagnosis is made on clinical grounds, especially during outbreaks, it is wise to exclude the possibility of atypical rubella infection.

Detection requires specialized methods or serology

## ROSEOLA INFANTUM (EXANTHEM SUBITUM)

Roseola infantum is a common disease of infants and children 6 months to 4 years of age. Its alternative name, exanthem subitum, means "sudden rash." There may be more than one cause: the most common is now thought to be human herpesvirus type 6 (see Chapter 37). The illness is characterized by abrupt onset of high fever, sometimes accompanied by brief, generalized convulsions and leukopenia. After 3 to 5 days, the fever diminishes rapidly, followed in a few hours by a faint, transient, macular rash.

Associated with human herpesvirus Type 6

Several other agents, including adenoviruses, coxsackieviruses, and echoviruses, have occasionally been noted to cause this syndrome.

## OTHER CAUSES OF RUBELLA-LIKE RASHES

In addition to erythema infectiosum, diseases caused by numerous other agents can mimic rubella clinically. These agents include at least 17 echoviruses, 9 coxsackieviruses, several adenoviral serotypes, arboviruses such as dengue, Epstein–Barr virus, scarlet fever, and toxic drug eruptions, among others. Because of the wide variety of diagnostic possibilities, it is not possible to diagnose or rule out rubella confidently on clinical grounds alone. Therefore, a specific diagnosis requires specific laboratory studies. Because rubella is an infection with such significant impact on the fetus, serologic study to rule out this possibility is mandatory if the diagnosis is suspected during early pregnancy.

## ADDITIONAL READING

### Mumps

Beard CM, Benson RC, Kelalis PP, et al. The incidence and outcome of mumps orchitis in Rochester, Minnesota, 1935–1974. *Mayo Clin Proc*. 1977;52:3–7. Long-term follow-up and incidence and sequelae of mumps orchitis are discussed.

## Measles

Baczko K, Leibert UG, Billeter M, et al. Expression of defective measles virus genes in brain tissues of patients with subacute sclerosing panencephalitis. *J Virol.* 1986;59:472–478. A molecular study that helps clarify our current concepts of measles virus persistence.

Griffin DE, Ward BJ, Juaregui E, et al. Immune activation during measles: $\beta_2$-Microglobulin in plasma and cerebrospinal fluid in complicated and uncomplicated disease. *J Infect Dis.* 1992;166:1170–1173. This and a series of prior publications cited by the authors provide excellent insight into the immunopathologic mechanisms induced by measles virus.

## Rubella

Miller E, Cradock-Watson JE, Pollock TM. Consequences of confirmed maternal rubella at successive stages of pregnancy. *Lancet.* 1982;2:781–784. A precise analysis of the risks of infection at various times during gestation.

Polk BF, White JA, DeGirolami PC, Modlin JF. An outbreak of rubella among hospital personnel. *N Engl J Med.* 1980;303:541–545. The contagiousness of the virus and its impact in high-risk settings are illustrated.

## Parvovirus B19

Munshi NC, Zhou S, Woody MJ, et al. Successful replication of parvovirus B19 in the human megakaryocytic cell line MB-02. *J Virol.* 1993;67:562–566. An approach to development of an in vitro system for use in diagnosis and molecular pathogenesis is provided.

Chapter 34

# Poxviruses

C. George Ray

The poxvirus family includes viruses that infect birds, mammals, and even insects. They are large, brick-shaped or ovoid, double-stranded DNA-carrying virions (Fig 34–1) measuring approximately 100 × 200 × 300 nm; their structure is complex, and replication occurs in the cytoplasm of infected cells. They possess an envelope, which is not acquired by budding and not essential for infectivity. The agents most important in human disease are variola, vaccinia, molluscum contagiosum, orf, cowpox, and pseudocowpox.

## VARIOLA

Smallpox has had a significant role in world history with respect to both the serious epidemics recorded since antiquity and the sometimes dangerous measures taken to prevent infection.

### Variola Virus

Two types are known: variola major and variola minor (alastrim). Although the viruses are indistinguishable antigenically, their fatality rates differ considerably (less than 1% for variola minor, 3–35% for variola major). They are also difficult to distinguish in the laboratory; variola major, however, has slightly greater virulence in embryonated hen's eggs. It is remarkable that although these viruses are exceedingly infectious, they have been eradicated worldwide. Thus, any discussion of smallpox is now of more historic than practical interest.

Variola major and minor difficult to distinguish

### Smallpox

The first major step toward modern prevention and subsequent eradication of smallpox can be credited to Edward Jenner, who noted that milkmaids who develop mild cowpox lesions on their hands appeared immune to smallpox. He published evidence in 1798 indicating that purposeful inoculation of individuals with cowpox material could protect them against subsequent infection by smallpox. The concept of vaccination gradually evolved, with the modern use of live vaccinia virus, a poxvirus of uncertain origin, to produce specific immunity.

Jenner vaccinated with cowpox

In 1967, the World Health Organization launched an ambitious program aimed at eradication of smallpox. This goal was considered realistic for two major reasons: (1) no extrahuman reservoir of the virus was known to exist, and (2) asymptomatic carriage

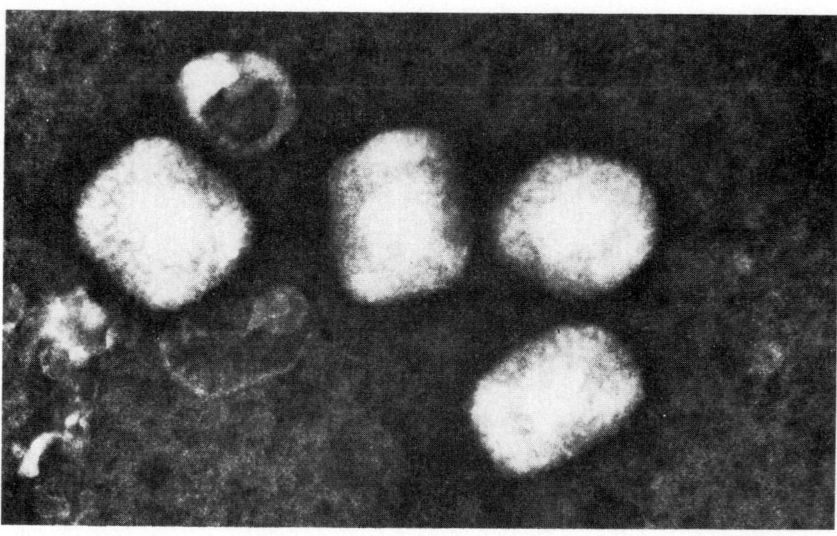

**Figure 34–1.** Electron microscopic appearance of a poxvirus (vaccinia). (Negative stain; original magnification × 60,000.) (*Courtesy of Dr. Claire M. Payne.*)

apparently did not occur. The basic approach included intensive surveillance for clinical cases of smallpox, prompt quarantine of such patients and their contacts, and vaccination of contacts to prevent further spread. A tremendous amount of effort was involved, but the results were astonishing: the last recorded case of naturally acquired smallpox occurred in Somalia in 1977. Global eradication of smallpox was confirmed in 1979 and accepted by the World Health Organization (WHO) in May 1980. Vaccination is therefore no longer deemed necessary, except for a very few laboratory workers who may handle the virus in WHO-restricted laboratories.

Multiple features of smallpox made it a candidate for eradication campaign

Surveillance continues, including studies of poxviruses of animals (eg, buffalopox, monkeypox) that are antigenically somewhat similar to smallpox. Some virologists remain legitimately concerned that an animal poxvirus could mutate to become highly virulent to humans, although the probability of such an occurrence seems very low.

## Smallpox: Clinical Aspects

### Clinical Manifestations and Outcome

Single stage rash and sometimes fatal outcome

Modifying effects of previous vaccination modified disease

Respiratory and fomite spread

The incubation period of smallpox was usually 12 to 14 days, although in occasional fulminating cases it could be as short as 4 to 5 days. The typical onset was abrupt, with fever, chills, and myalgia, followed by a rash 3 to 4 days later. The rash evolved to firm papulovesicles that became pustular over 10 to 12 days, then slowly healed. In contrast to varicella, only a single crop of lesions (all in the same stage of evolution) developed; these lesions were most prominent over the head and extremities (Fig 34–2). Some cases of variola major were fulminant, with a hemorrhagic rash ("sledgehammer" smallpox). Death could result from the overwhelming primary viral infection or from bacterial superinfection. Previous vaccination, usually more than 3 years before the onset of infection, could shorten the evolution of illness or modify it to a degree that sometimes made diagnosis difficult. The disease was highly contagious, and the virus could survive well in the extracellular environment. Acquisition of infection by respiratory spread or by exposure to dried crusts from skin lesions, contaminated articles, and fomites has been well documented.

### Laboratory Diagnosis

Variola produces lesions (pocks) on the chorioallantoic membranes of embryonated hen's eggs; it also infects a variety of cell cultures in vitro. Cytology of lesions shows cytoplas-

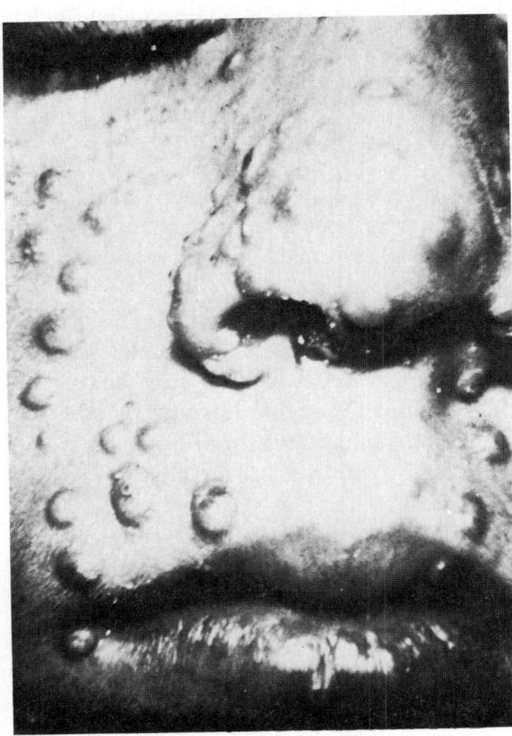

**Figure 34–2.** Closeup of facial lesions of smallpox during the first week of the illness.

mic inclusions, but neither intranuclear inclusions nor giant cells. Direct electron microscopy has also been used for rapid diagnosis.

## VACCINIA

Vaccinia virus is serologically related to smallpox, although its exact origin is unknown. Some virologists believe it is a recombinant virus derived from smallpox and cowpox; others suggest it originated from a poxvirus of horses. The virus is usually propagated by dermal inoculation of calves, and the resultant vesicle fluid ("lymph") is lyophilized and used as a live virus vaccine in humans. The vaccine is inoculated into the epidermis and produces a localized lesion, which indicates successful immunization. The lesion becomes vesicular, then pustular, followed by crusting and healing over 10 to 14 days. The local reaction is sometimes severe and accompanied by systemic symptoms such as fever, rash, and lymphadenopathy. Vaccinia-produced immunity to smallpox wanes rapidly after 3 years, becoming virtually absent after 20 years.

Unknown origin

Vaccination produces strong local reactions

Immunity wanes after 3 years

In addition to the local reactions, several other potentially serious and lethal complications can occur with vaccinia infection. These include encephalitis, progressive vaccinia (vaccinia gangrenosum, usually seen in immunocompromised patients), disseminated vaccinia, autoinoculation into the eye or mucous membranes, allergic reactions, and bacterial superinfection.

Severe reactions seen in immunocompromised

There has been a resurgence of scientific interest in vaccinia as a possible vector for active immunization against other diseases, such as hepatitis B, herpes simplex, and even human immunodeficiency virus. It has been shown that gene sequences coding for specific immunogenic proteins of other viruses can be inserted into the vaccinia virus genome, with subsequent expression as the virus replicates. For example, a recombinant vaccinia strain carrying the gene sequence for hepatitis B surface antigen (HbsAg) can infect cells, lead to production of HbsAg, and stimulate an antibody response to it. Theoretically, gene sequences coding for a variety of antigens could be packaged in a single viable vaccinia virus, thus allowing simultaneous active immunization against multiple agents. Recently, it has been shown that use of an avian poxvirus, such as canarypox, may be an even safer, yet ef-

Vaccinia of interest as mechanism for delivering the proteins of other viruses

fective vector for use in humans. Whether such approaches become routinely applicable to clinical medicine remains to be seen.

## MOLLUSCUM CONTAGIOSUM

Molluscum contagiosum is a benign, cutaneous poxvirus disease of humans, spread by direct contact with infected cells. It is usually acquired by inoculation into minute skin abrasions; events that commonly lead to transmission include roughhousing in shower rooms and swimming pools, sharing of towels, and sexual contact.

After an incubation period of 2 to 8 weeks, nodular, pale, firm (pearl-like) lesions usually 2 to 10 mm in diameter develop in the epidermis. These lesions are painless and umbilicated in appearance. A cheesy material may be expressed from the pore at the center of each lesion. Local trauma may cause spread of lesions in the involved skin area. The lesions are not associated with systemic symptoms, and they disappear in 2 to 12 months without treatment. Specific treatment, if desired, is usually by curettage or careful removal of the central core by expression with forceps.

The pathologic findings, which are limited to the epidermis, include hyperplasia, ballooning degeneration, and acanthosis. The diagnosis, made on clinical grounds, can be confirmed by demonstration of large, eosinophilic cytoplasmic inclusions (molluscum bodies) in the affected superficial epithelial cells.

## ORF

**Orf** is an old Saxon term for a human infection caused by a parapoxvirus of sheep and goats. Synonyms for the infection in animals include contagious pustular dermatitis, ecthyma contagiosum, pustular ecthyma, and "scabby mouth." Humans usually acquire the infection by close contact with infected animals and accidental inoculation through cuts or abrasions on the hand or wrist. The typical skin lesion is solitary; it begins as a vesicle and then evolves into a nodular mass that later develops central necrosis. Regional lymphadenopathy sometimes develops; dissemination is rare. The average duration of the lesion is 35 days, followed by complete resolution. The diagnosis is usually made on the basis of clinical appearance and occupational history. Serologic confirmation or electron microscopy of the lesion can be done, but is rarely necessary.

## MILKER'S NODULES AND COWPOX

Milker's nodules (pseudocowpox) is a cutaneous poxvirus disease of cattle, distinct from cowpox, that can cause local skin infections similar to orf in exposed humans. Healing of the skin lesions may take 4 to 8 weeks. There is no cross-immunity to cowpox.

Cowpox is now very rare in the United States. It produces a vesicular eruption on the udders of cows and similar, usually localized, vesicular lesions in humans who are accidently exposed.

## ADDITIONAL READING

Cadoz M, Strady A, Meignier B, et al. Immunization with canarypox virus expressing rabies glycoprotein. *Lancet*. 1992;339:1429–1432. A nonhuman poxvirus that undergoes only abortive replication in mammalian cells is exploited as a potentially safe vector for immunization. The editorial on pages 1448–1449 is also worthwhile reading.

Moss B. Vaccinia virus: A tool for research and vaccine development. *Science*. 1991;252:1662–1667. A concise summary of the broader applications of this virus.

Smith GL, Mackett M, Moss B. Infectious vaccinia virus recombinants that express hepatitis B virus surface antigen. *Nature*. 1983;302:490–495. This paper details the potential novel use of vaccinia virus recombinants as immunogens against totally unrelated infectious agents.

White PJ, Shackelford PG. Edward Jenner, M.D. and the scourge that was. *Am J Dis Child*. 1983;137:864–869. An informative review of the history of smallpox and its eradication.

Chapter 35

# Enteroviruses

*C. George Ray*

Enteroviruses constitute a major subgroup of small RNA viruses (picornaviruses) that readily infect the intestinal tract. They include the polioviruses, coxsackieviruses, echoviruses, and more recently discovered agents that are simply designated enteroviruses. The number of serotypes that can infect humans has grown to a total of 68, and more are likely to be found in the future.

Enteroviruses cause paralytic disease, mild acute aseptic meningitis syndromes, pleurodynia, exanthems, pericarditis, nonspecific febrile illness, and occasional fulminant encephalomyocarditis of the newborn. As more has been learned, it is apparent that the spectrum of disease is even broader. Some infections can result in chronic, active disease processes.

These viruses, which have many characteristics in common, are first considered as a group. Some of the special features of important serotypes will be discussed in more detail later in this chapter.

## ENTEROVIRUSES

The enteroviruses of humans and animals are ubiquitous and have been found worldwide. Their name is derived from their ability to infect intestinal tract epithelial and lymphoid tissues and to be shed into the feces.

### Enteroviruses: Group Characteristics

#### Morphologic and Biological Features

As a group, the enteroviruses are extremely small (22–30 nm in diameter), naked virions with icosahedral symmetry. They possess single-stranded, positive-sense RNA and four major polypeptides. Following replication and assembly in the cellular cytoplasm, new virus is released by cell destruction.

**Small, single-stranded RNA viruses**

Enteroviruses are distinguished from rhinoviruses, which are also members of the picornavirus family, by their resistance to acid (pH 3.0), capability to replicate efficiently at 37°C, and higher buoyant density. Another feature is cationic stability; in the presence of molar magnesium chloride, the viruses become more resistant to thermal inactivation. They are also resistant to many common disinfectants such as 70% alcohol, substituted phenolics, ether, and various detergents that readily inactivate most enveloped viruses. Chemical agents, such as 0.3% formaldehyde or free residual chlorine at 0.3 to 0.5 ppm, are effective; however, if sufficient extraneous organic debris is present, the virus can be protected and survive long periods.

**Resistant to acid, detergents, and many disinfectants**

**Formaldehyde and hypochlorite are active against enteroviruses**

Antigenic mutations and drifts occur

Some of the enterovirus serotypes share common antigens, but there are no significant serologic relationships between the major classes listed in Table 35–1. Genetic variation within specific strains occurs, and mutants that exhibit antigenic drift and altered tropism for specific cell types are now recognized. There may also be a single, highly conserved epitope that is shared by all serotypes.

Antibody to surface proteins neutralize

Polioviruses, which have been most extensively studied as enterovirus prototypes, are known to have epitopes on three surface structural proteins (VP1, VP2, and VP3) that induce type-specific neutralizing antibodies. This appears to be generally the case for all enteroviruses; definitive identification of isolates usually requires neutralization tests.

### Growth in the Laboratory

Grow in primate cell cultures

Coxsackie A and B viruses have different effects on newborn mice

Most of these agents can be isolated in primate (human or simian) cell cultures and show characteristic cytopathic effects; some strains, however, particularly several coxsackievirus A serotypes, are grown with difficulty in cell cultures, and inoculation of newborn mice may be necessary for detection of virus. The newborn mouse, in fact, is one basis for originally classifying group A and B coxsackieviruses. After inoculation of mice at 24 hours of age or less and observation for 2 to 12 days, A coxsackieviruses cause primarily a widespread, inflammatory, necrotic effect on skeletal muscle, leading to flaccid paralysis and death; similar inoculation of B coxsackieviruses causes encephalitis, resulting in spasticity and occasionally convulsions. Other organs are variably affected, and histopathologic examination is sometimes helpful in distinguishing the two. Echoviruses and polioviruses rarely have an adverse effect on mice, unless special adaptation procedures are first employed. The higher-numbered enteroviruses (types 68–72), which have overlapping, variable growth and host characteristics, have been classified separately. Hepatitis A virus has been classified as enterovirus 72 or as a heparnavirus.

## ■ Enterovirus Disease

### Host Range

Animals not involved in human disease

Humans are the major natural host for the polioviruses, coxsackieviruses, and echoviruses. There are enteroviruses of other animals with limited host ranges that do not appear to extend to humans. Conversely, viruses thought to be identical or related to human enteroviruses have been isolated from dogs and cats. Whether these agents cause disease in such animals is debatable, and there is no evidence of spread from animals to humans.

### Epidemiology

Proportion of asymptomatic infections varies with strain

The enteroviruses have a worldwide distribution, and asymptomatic infection is common. The proportion of infected individuals who develop illness varies from 2 to 100%, depending on the serotype or strain involved and the age of the patient. Secondary infections in households are common and range as high as 40 to 70%, depending on factors such as family size, crowding, and sanitary conditions.

Dominant epidemic strains come and go

In some years, certain serotypes emerge as dominant epidemic strains; they then may wane, only to reappear in epidemic fashion years later. For example, echovirus 16 was a major cause of outbreaks in the eastern United States in 1951 and 1974. Coxsackievirus B1

**TABLE 35–1. HUMAN ENTEROVIRUSES**

| Class | Number of Serotypes |
|---|---|
| Poliovirus | 3 |
| Coxsackievirus | |
| Group A | 23 |
| Group B | 6 |
| Echovirus | 31 |
| Enterovirus | 5[a] |

[a] More recently discovered enteroviruses, which have overlapping biological characteristics, are identified numerically (types 68–72).

was common in 1963; echovirus 9 in 1962, 1965, 1968, and 1969; and echovirus 30 in 1968 and 1969. The emergence of dominant serotypes is quite unpredictable from year to year.

All enteroviruses show a seasonal predilection; epidemics are usually observed during the summer and fall months. In subtropical and tropical climates, the duration of greatest transmission sometimes extends into the winter months.

Strong prevalence for summer and fall

Direct or indirect fecal–oral transmission is considered the most common mode of spread. After infection, the virus persists in the oropharynx for 1 to 4 weeks, and it can be shed in the feces for 1 to 18 weeks. Thus, sewage-contaminated water, fecally contaminated foods, or passive transmission by insect vectors (flies, cockroaches) may occasionally be the source of infection. More commonly, however, spread is directly from person to person. This mode of transmission is suggested by the high infection rates seen among young children, whose hygienic practices tend to be less than optimal, and in crowded households. Approximately two thirds of all isolates are from children 9 years of age or younger.

Person-to-person fecal–oral transmission correlates with predominance in children

Incubation periods vary, but relatively short intervals (2–10 days) are frequent. Often, illness is seen concurrently in more than one family member, and the clinical features vary within the household.

Incubation periods typically short

## Pathogenesis and Pathology

Initial binding of an enterovirus to the cell surface is commonly between an attachment protein in a "canyon" configuration on the virion surface and cell receptors belonging to the immunoglobulin gene superfamily. Recently, a different receptor, belonging to the integrin group of adhesion molecules, has been identified for at least one echovirus serotype. After primary replication in the epithelial cells and lymphoid tissues in the upper respiratory and gastrointestinal tracts, viremic spread to other sites can occur. Potential target organs vary according to the virus strain and its tropism, but may include the central nervous system, heart, vascular endothelium, liver, pancreas, lungs, gonads, skeletal muscles, synovial tissues, skin, and mucous membranes. Histopathologic findings include cell necrosis and mononuclear cell inflammatory infiltrates; in the central nervous system, the inflammatory cells are localized most prominently in perivascular sites. The initial tissue damage is thought to result from the lytic cycle of virus replication; secondary spread to other sites may ensue. Viremia is usually undetectable by the time symptoms appear, and termination of virus replication appears to correlate with the appearance of circulating neutralizing antibody, interferon, and mononuclear cell infiltration of infected tissue. The early antibody response is with immunoglobulin M (IgM), which usually wanes 6 to 12 weeks after onset to be replaced progressively by IgG-specific antibodies. The important role of antibodies in termination of infection, demonstrated in mouse models of group B coxsackievirus infections, is supported by the observation of persistent echovirus and poliovirus replication in patients with antibody deficiency diseases.

Initial attachment binds viral surface protein to cell surface receptors

Host receptor may relate to immunoglobulin or integrin families

Initial replication in epithelial and lymphoid cells followed by viremic spread

Injury by cell lysis localized in perivascular sites

Antibody response terminates replication

Although initial acute tissue damage may be caused by the lytic effects of the virus on the cell, the secondary sequelae may be immunologically mediated. Enterovirus-caused poliomyelitis, disseminated disease of the newborn, aseptic meningitis, encephalitis, and acute respiratory illnesses, thought to represent primary lytic infections, can usually be identified through routine methods of virus isolation and determination of specific antibody titer changes. On the other hand, syndromes such as myopericarditis, nephritis, and myositis have been associated with enteroviruses primarily because of serologic and epidemiologic evidence. In many of these cases, viral isolation is the exception rather than the rule. The pathogenesis of these latter infections is not clear; however, observations suggest that the acute infectious phase of the virus may be mild or subclinical and often subsides by the time clinical illness becomes evident. Illness may represent a host immunologic response to tissue injury by the virus or to viral or virus-induced antigens that persist in the affected tissues. In experimental group B coxsackievirus myocarditis, mononuclear inflammatory cells (monocytes, natural killer lymphocytes) seem to play a greater role than antibody in termination of infection, and the persistence of inflammation after disappearance of detectable virus or viral antigen appears to be mediated by cytotoxic T lymphocytes. Experimental findings have led to another hypothesis regarding pathogenic mechanisms that is called **molecular mimicry.** This is best conceptualized as a form of virus-induced autoimmune response. It is known that small peptide sequences on viral epitopes can sometimes be shared by host tissues. Thus, an immune response produced by the virus may also generate anti-

In addition to lytic effects of virus there are probable immunopathologic manifestations

Disease may follow the acute infection

Coxsackie B myocarditis may involve virus-induced cross reacting antibody

bodies or cytotoxic cross-reactive effector lymphocytes that recognize shared determinants located on host cells. For example, a monoclonal antibody directed against a neutralizing site of a group B coxsackievirus has also been shown to react strongly with normal myocardial cells.

### Immunity

Immunity is serotype specific

Infection by a specific serotype in an immunologically normal host is followed by a humoral antibody response, which can often be detected by neutralization methods for many years thereafter (Fig 35–1). There is relative immunity to reinfection by the same serotype; however, reinfection has been reported, usually resulting in subclinical infection or mild illness.

### Laboratory Diagnosis

Viral isolation from pharynx or closed space significant

In acute enterovirus-caused syndromes, diagnosis is most readily established by virus isolation from throat swabs, stool or rectal swabs, body fluids, and occasionally tissues. Viremia is usually undetectable by the time symptoms appear. When there is central nervous system involvement, cerebrospinal fluid cultures taken during the acute phase of the disease may be positive in 10 to 85% of cases (except in poliovirus infections, in which virus recovery from this site is rare), depending on the stage of illness and the viral serotype involved. Direct isolation of virus from affected tissues or body fluids in enclosed spaces (eg, pleural, joint, pericardial, or cerebrospinal fluid) usually confirms the diagnosis. Isolation of an enterovirus from the throat is highly suggestive of an etiologic association, as the virus is usually detectable at this site for only 2 days to 2 weeks after infection; isolation of virus from fecal specimens only must be interpreted more cautiously, as asymptomatic shedding from the bowel may persist for as long as 4 months (see Fig 35–1). It has also been shown that the polymerase chain reaction can be used to amplify conserved enteroviral RNA sequences in tissues and body fluids, thus greatly enhancing detection. Further evaluation is underway to determine the feasibility of this approach.

Prolonged shedding in stool

Serodiagnosis usually impractical

The diagnosis may be further supported by fourfold or greater neutralizing antibody titer changes between paired acute and convalescent serum samples. This method is often expensive and cumbersome, however, requiring careful selection of serotypes for use in antigens. Serodiagnosis is generally reserved for critical situations in which the etiology is questioned, such as isolation of a virus only from a peripheral source such as the feces, or in illnesses such as myopericarditis, in which the yield on routine culture is low and the number of serotypes that might be expected to be involved is limited. Quantitative inter-

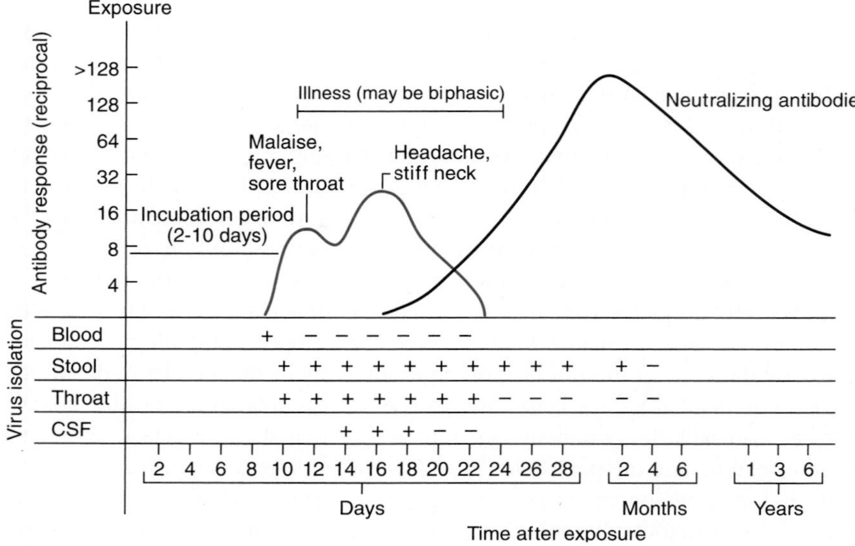


**Figure 35–1.** Antibody response and viral isolation in a typical case of enteroviral infection. CSF, cerebrospinal fluid.

pretations of antibody titers on single serum samples are rarely helpful, because of the wide range of titers to different serotypes that can be found among healthy individuals. In acute poliovirus infections, antibody titer determinations on acute and convalescent sera can aid in diagnosis.

### Prevention

Vaccines for the prevention of poliovirus infections are discussed later in this chapter. Although proper disposal of feces and careful personal hygiene are recommended, the usual quarantine or isolation measures are relatively ineffective in controlling the spread of enteroviruses in the family or community.

Difficult to prevent spread

### Treatment

None of the currently available antiviral agents has been shown effective in treatment or prophylaxis of enterovirus infections. Treatment is entirely symptomatic and supportive.

## Enteroviruses: Specific Groups

### Polioviruses

#### ■ Poliovirus: Epidemiology and Pathogenesis

Worldwide, the most important enteroviruses are the three poliovirus serotypes (types 1–3). They first emerged as important causes of disease in developed temperate zone countries during the latter part of the 19th century, and they have become increasingly important elsewhere as living conditions improve in developing countries. This somewhat paradoxical situation is related to the fact that the risk of paralytic disease resulting from infection increases with age. Improvement of sanitary conditions tends to impede spread of the viruses; thus, individuals may become infected not in early infancy but later in life, when paralysis is more likely to occur.

Risk of paralysis from infection increases with age

The particular tropism of polioviruses for the central nervous system (CNS), which they usually reach by passage across the blood–CNS barrier, is perhaps favored by reflex dilatation of capillaries supplying the affected motor centers of the anterior horn of the brain stem or spinal cord. An alternate pathway is via the axons or perineural sheaths of peripheral nerves. Motor neurons are particularly vulnerable to infection and variable degrees of neuronal destruction. The histopathologic findings in the brain stem and spinal cord include necrosis of neuronal cells and perivascular "cuffing" by infiltration with mononuclear cells, primarily lymphocytes (Fig 35–2).

CNS tropism by blood or peripheral nerves

Motor neuron cells destroyed

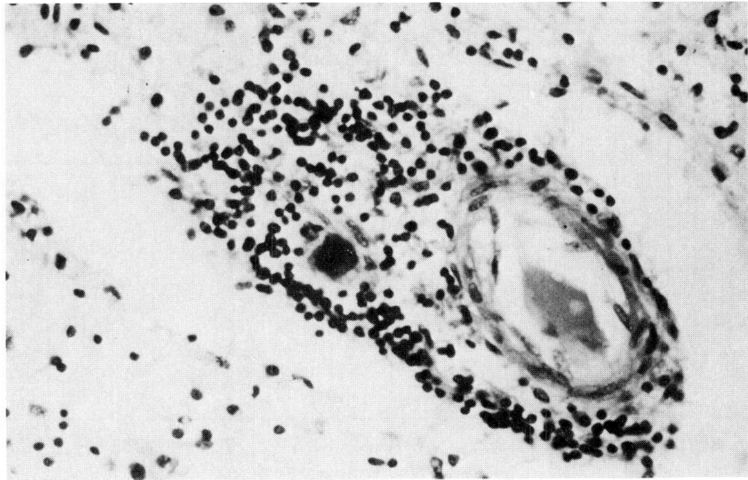

**Figure 35–2.** Section of spinal cord from a fatal case of poliomyelitis, demonstrating perivenous mononuclear cell inflammatory reaction. (*Courtesy of Dr. Peter C. Johnson.*)

## ■ Polio: Clinical Aspects

Subclinical and abortive poliomyelitis common

Aseptic meningitis recovers rapidly

Paralytic poliomyelitis manifests flaccid paralysis without sensory loss

Recovery of function up to 6 months

**Clinical Manifestations and Outcome.** Most infections (perhaps 90%) are either completely subclinical or so mild that they do not come to attention. When disease does result, the incubation period ranges from 4 to 35 days, but is usually between 7 and 14 days. Three types of disease can be observed: Abortive poliomyelitis is a nonspecific febrile illness of 2- to 3-day duration with no signs of CNS localization. Aseptic meningitis (nonparalytic poliomyelitis) is characterized by signs of meningeal irritation (stiff neck, pain, and stiffness in the back) in addition to the signs of abortive poliomyelitis. Recovery is rapid and complete, usually within a few days. The third manifestation, paralytic poliomyelitis, is the major possible outcome of infection and is often preceded by a period of minor illness, sometimes with 2 or 3 symptom-free days intervening. There are signs of meningeal irritation, but the hallmark of paralytic poliomyelitis is asymmetric flaccid paralysis, with no significant sensory loss. The extent of involvement varies greatly from case to case; in its most serious forms, however, all four limbs may be completely paralyzed or the brain stem may be attacked, with paralysis of the cranial nerves and muscles of respiration (bulbar polio). The maximum extent of involvement is evident within a few days of first paralysis. Thereafter, as temporarily damaged neurons regain their function, recovery begins and may continue for as long as 6 months; paralysis persisting after this time is permanent.

Inactivated (Salk) vaccine used in many countries

Live (Sabin) vaccine is given orally (OPV)

**Prevention.** Two types of poliovirus vaccines are currently licensed in the United States: inactivated polio vaccine and live oral attenuated virus vaccine. Each contains the three serotypes of poliomyelitis virus.

Inactivated polio vaccine (IPV, also known as killed polio vaccine or Salk vaccine) was introduced in 1955; its use was associated with a dramatic decline in paralytic cases (Fig 35–3). It remains the only vaccine used in some countries, notably Sweden and The Netherlands, and its efficacy has been generally excellent. Vaccination is by subcutaneous injection. Primary vaccination with three doses of the present enhanced-potency IPV (two doses 6–8 weeks apart and the third 8–12 months later) produces antibody responses in more than 98% of recipients. The current product is considered quite safe, with no significant deleterious side effects.

Oral polio vaccine (OPV), also known as trivalent oral polio vaccine (TOPV) or Sabin vaccine, is composed of live, attenuated viruses that have undergone serial passage in cell

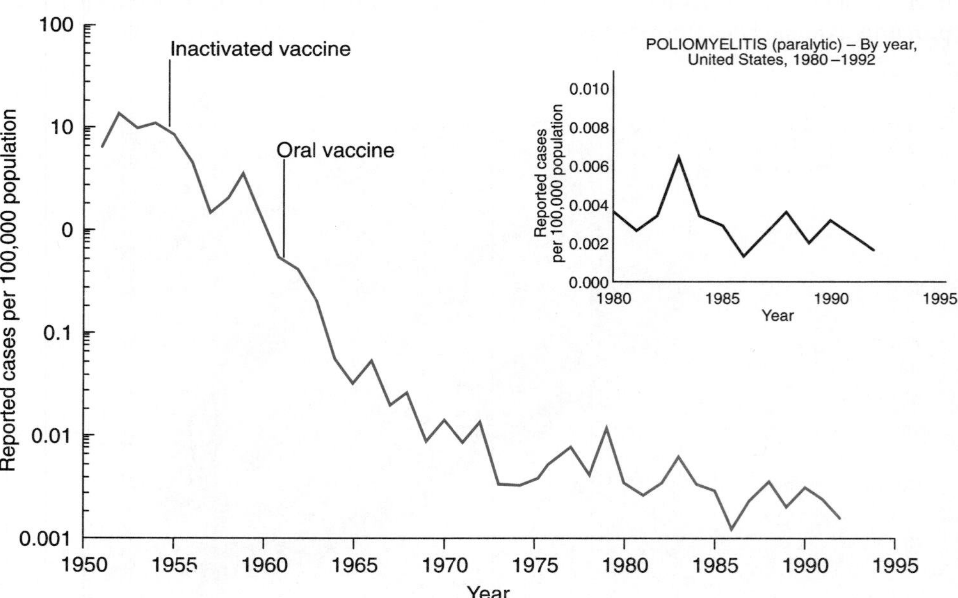


**Figure 35–3.** Reported paralytic poliomyelitis attack rates in the United States, 1951–1992. (*From the Centers for Disease Control, Summary of Notifiable Diseases United States, 1992,* Morbid Mortal Wkly Rep. *1993;41(5):46.*)

cultures from humans and subhuman primates. It was first licensed in the United States in 1963. The vaccine is given orally as a primary series of three doses (the first two doses usually 6–8 weeks apart and the third 8–12 months later) and produces antibodies to all three serotypes in more than 95% of recipients; these antibodies persist for several years. As with IPV, recall boosters are recommended to maintain adequate antibody levels. Like wild poliovirus, OPV viruses infect and replicate in the oropharynx and intestinal tract and can be spread to other persons.

Vaccine virus replicates and can spread

One disadvantage of OPV is the remote risk of vaccine-associated paralytic disease in some recipients or their household contacts, including immunocompromised persons. There is speculation that some instances of vaccine-associated paralytic disease may be related to reversion of attenuated virus to more virulent characteristics in vivo after serial passage from person to person. The incidence of vaccine-associated paralytic poliomyelitis is estimated at approximately 1 per 2.6 million doses distributed.

Vaccine-associated poliomyelitis a remote risk with OPV

Although there are no currently recognized areas of wild poliovirus prevalence in the United States, it must be kept in mind that importation of these strains can readily occur from endemic areas in developing nations. Once introduced into a community, the virus can spread rapidly among susceptible individuals. Thus, continuing immunization programs are of utmost importance in preventing spread of this disease.

## COXSACKIEVIRUSES AND ECHOVIRUSES

The coxsackieviruses and echoviruses are widespread throughout the world. Their epidemiology and pathogenesis are much the same as those of the polioviruses. Unlike polioviruses, they have a greater tendency to affect the meninges and occasionally the cerebrum, but rarely affect anterior horn cells.

Do not affect motor neurons

The consequences of infection with these agents are highly variable and related only in part to virus subgroup and serotype. Up to 60% of infections are subclinical. The main interest in these agents stems from their ability to cause more serious illness, which becomes most evident during epidemics of infection with a particular agent.

Most infections subclinical

Inapparent infection is common. Illness manifestations vary from mild to lethal. Table 35–2 lists the major syndromes and serotypes commonly associated with each. Considerable overlap occurs, however, and one should not be surprised if an enteroviral serotype found in connection with a specific syndrome differs from that most often encountered.

Wide range of clinical manifestations

Aseptic meningitis is the most frequently recognized clinical illness associated with enterovirus infections. This syndrome can be mild and self-limiting, lasting 5 to 14 days; however, it is sometimes accompanied by encephalitis, which can lead to permanent neurologic sequelae.

Asepetic meningitis most common syndrome

Acute inflammation of the heart muscle (myocarditis), its covering membranes (peri-

**TABLE 35–2. CLINICAL SYNDROMES AND COMMONLY ASSOCIATED ENTEROVIRUS SEROTYPES[a]**

| Syndrome | Coxsackievirus | | Echovirus and Enterovirus (E) |
|---|---|---|---|
| | *Group A* | *Group B* | |
| Aseptic meningitis, encephalitis | 2, 4, 7, **9**, 10 | 1, **2, 3, 4, 5** | **4, 6, 9, 11, 16, 30,** E70, E71 |
| Muscle weakness and paralysis (poliomyelitis-like disease) | **7, 9** | 2, 3, 4, 5 | 2, 4, 6, 9, 11, 30, E71 |
| Cerebellar ataxia | 2, 4, **9** | 3, 4 | 4, 6, 9 |
| Exanthems and enanthems | **4, 5, 6, 9, 10, 16** | 2, 3, 4, 5 | **2, 4, 5, 6, 9, 11, 16, 18, 25** |
| Pericarditis, myocarditis | 4, 16 | **2, 3, 4, 5** | 1, 6, 8, 9, 19 |
| Epidemic myalgia (pleurodynia), orchitis | 9 | 1, **2, 3, 4, 5** | 1, 6, 9 |
| Respiratory | 9, 16, **21,** 24 | 1, 3, 4, 5 | **4, 9, 11,** 20, 25 |
| Conjunctivitis | **24** | 1, 5 | **7, E70** |
| Generalized disease (infants) | — | 1, **2, 3, 4, 5** | 3, 6, 9, 11, 14, 17, 19 |

[a] Serotypes most commonly associated with syndrome are in boldface.

Myocarditis often associated with Coxsackle B viruses

carditis), or both can be caused by a variety of viral agents; Group B coxsackieviruses are the most commonly implicated enteroviruses. Such infections are usually self-limiting, but may be fatal in the acute phase (arrhythmia or heart failure) or progress to chronic dilated myocardiopathy.

Exanthems can mimic other diseases

The exanthems are often not associated with CNS inflammation. They can resemble rubella, roseola infantum, or adenoviral macular or maculopapular exanthems, but may also appear as vesicular or hemangioma-like lesions. One interesting syndrome is hand-foot-and-mouth disease, which usually affects children and is characterized by a vesicular eruption over the extremities and the oral cavity. Coxsackie virus A16 is most commonly implicated, but others, such as enterovirus 71, can cause a similar illness. Herpangina is an enanthematous (mucous membrane-affecting) febrile disease in which small vesicles or white papules (lymphonodules) surrounded by a red halo are seen over the posterior palate, pharynx, and tonsillar areas. This mild, self-limiting (1 to 2 week) illness has usually been associated with infection by several different group A Coxsackievirus serotypes.

Herpangina infection of palate and tonsils

Epidemic myalgia

Epidemic myalgia (pleurodynia or Bornholm disease) is characterized by fever and sudden onset of intense upper abdominal or thoracic pain. The pain may be aggravated by movement, such as breathing or coughing, and can persist as long as 14 days. Group B coxsackieviruses are often implicated.

Generalized disease of the newborn is a disseminated, often lethal enteroviral infection characterized by pathologic changes in the heart, brain, liver, and other organs.

It is apparent from Table 35–2 that the spectrum of disease produced by these viruses is enormous and that many other illnesses may also result from infections by this subgroup. Epidemics of acute hemorrhagic keratoconjunctivitis associated with enterovirus 70 and localized outbreaks of disease resembling paralytic poliomyelitis caused by enterovirus 71 infection have been described. In addition, there is evidence that certain enteroviruses, particularly group B coxsackievirus serotypes, may sometimes participate in the pathogenesis of insulin-dependent diabetes mellitus, acute arthritis, polymyositis, and idiopathic acute nephritis. Further investigations are required to establish whether or not such associations are significant.

## ADDITIONAL READING


Diamond DC, Kohara M, Abe S, et al. Antigenic variation and resistance to neutralization in poliovirus type 1. *Science*. 1985;229:1090–1093. This article illustrates how a single point mutation can cause significant changes in an enteroviral phenotype.

Ray CG, Fulginiti VA. Coxsackievirus and echovirus infections. In: Hoeprich PD, Jordan MC, eds. *Infectious Diseases*. 4th ed. Philadelphia: JB Lippincott; 1989:1142–1149, 1360–1369. Reviews of the clinical and epidemiologic features of enteroviral infections.

Wright PF, Kim-Farley RJ, deQuandros CA, et al. Strategies for the global eradication of poliomyelitis by the year 2000. *N Engl J Med*. 1991;325:1774–1779. The World Health Organization has made a commitment to the eradication of poliomyelitis in this decade. The authors outline how this could be done and what further research is needed to facilitate it.

Chapter 36

# Hepatitis Viruses

W. Lawrence Drew

Hepatitis means inflammation of the liver, and as a disease entity, it has been recognized since the days of Hippocrates. The causes of hepatitis are varied and include viruses, bacteria, and protozoa, as well as drugs and toxins (eg, isoniazid, carbon tetrachloride, and ethanol). The clinical symptoms and course of acute viral hepatitis can be similar, regardless of etiology, and determination of a specific cause depends primarily on the use of laboratory tests. Hepatitis may be caused by at least five different viruses whose major characteristics are summarized in Table 36–1. *Non-A, non-B hepatitis* is a term previously used to identify cases of hepatitis not due to hepatitis A or B. With the discovery of the hepatitis viruses C and E, virtually all the viral etiologies of non-A, non-B disease can be specifically identified. Other viruses, such as Epstein–Barr virus, cytomegalovirus, varicella–zoster virus, and yellow fever viruses, can also cause inflammation of the liver, but hepatitis is not the primary disease caused by them.

Hepatitis has multiple causes

## HEPATITIS A

### Hepatitis A Virus

Hepatitis A virus is the cause of what was formerly termed infectious hepatitis or short-incubation hepatitis. It was first detected in the early 1970s in stools of patients incubating the disease. Subsequently, the virus has been successfully cultivated in primary marmoset liver cell cultures and in fetal rhesus monkey kidney cell cultures.

Hepatitis A virus is an unenveloped, single-stranded RNA virus with cubic symmetry and a diameter of 27 nm (Fig 36–1). It is not inactivated by ether and is stable at –20°C and low pH. These properties are similar to those of enteroviruses, and hepatitis A virus has now been classified as enterovirus type 72. There is only one serotype of hepatitis A virus which is distinct from other picornaviruses.

Unenveloped, single-stranded, small RNA virus; grows in specialzed cell cultures

Humans appear to be the major natural hosts of hepatitis A virus. Several other primates (including chimpanzees and marmosets) are susceptible to experimental infection, and natural infections of these animals may occur.

Humans are natural hosts

### Hepatitis A Disease

#### Epidemiology

The major mode of spread of hepatitis A is fecal–oral. Inoculation of infectious material intramuscularly can produce disease; transmission through blood transfusion, although possible, is not an important means of spread. Most cases of hepatitis A are not linked to a

Fecal–oral spread

**TABLE 36–1. COMPARISON OF A, B, D (DELTA), C, AND E HEPATITIS**

| Feature | A | B | D | C | E |
|---|---|---|---|---|---|
| Virus type | Single-stranded RNA | Double-stranded DNA | Single-stranded RNA | RNA, similar to flavivirus | RNA, similar to calicivirus |
| % of viral hepatitis | 50 | 41 | <1 | 5 | <1 |
| Incubation period (days) | 15–45 (mean, 25) | 7–160 (mean, 60–90) | 28–45 | 15–160 (mean, 50) | ? |
| Onset | Usually sudden | Usually slow | Variable | Insidious | ? |
| Age preference | Children, young adults | All ages | All ages | All ages | Young adult |
| Transmission | | | | | |
| Fecal–oral | +++ | ± | ± | – | +++ |
| Sexual | + | ++ | ++ | + | +? |
| Transfusion | – | ++ | +++ | +++ | – |
| Severity | Usually mild | Moderate | Often severe | Mild | Variable |
| Chronicity (%) | None | 10 | 50–70 | >50% | None |
| Carrier state | None | Yes | Yes | Yes | ? |
| Immune serum globulin protective[a] | Yes | Yes | Yes[b] | Uncertain | ? |

*Abbreviation:* Plus signs indicate relative frequencies.
[a] Hyperimmune globulin more protective.
[b] Prevention of hepatitis B prevents hepatitis D.

Associated with crowding and poor hygiene

No chronic carriers

single contaminated source, but occur sporadically. The disease is common under conditions of crowding, and it occurs at high frequency in mental hospitals, schools for the retarded, and day-care centers. As a chronic carrier state has not been observed with hepatitis A, perpetuation of the virus in nature presumably depends on sporadic subclinical infections and person-to-person transmission. Outbreaks of hepatitis A have been linked to the ingestion of undercooked seafood, usually shellfish from waters contaminated with human feces. Common-source outbreaks related to wholesale distribution of other foods, including vegetables, have also been reported.

Attack rates vary for different populations

High incidence in developing countries

The disease is widespread but seroepidemiologic studies have shown marked variation in infection rates among various population groups. For example, rates are higher among those of lower socioeconomic status and among male homosexuals. Less than one half of the general population of the United States now has serologic evidence of prior hepatitis A virus infection, however, and rates have been decreasing since 1970, apparently because of better sanitation and less crowding. In contrast, in many underdeveloped countries, more than 90% of the adult population shows evidence of previous hepatitis A infection; in most cases, however, the evidence is of asymptomatic infection during childhood. The risk

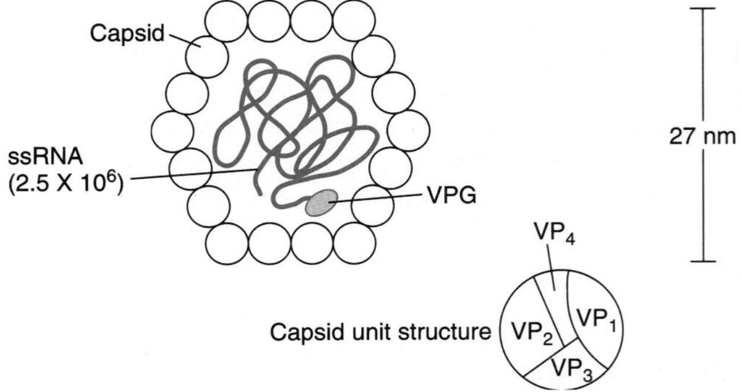


**Figure 36–1.** Diagram of the proposed structure of the hepatitis A virus. The protein capsid is made up of four viral polypeptides ($VP_1$ to $VP_4$). Inside the capsid is a single-stranded (ss) molecule of RNA (molecular weight $2.5 \times 10^6$), which has a genomic viral protein (VPG) on the 5′ end. (*Reprinted with permission of Dr. J. A. Hoofnagle and of Abbott Laboratories, Diagnostic Division, North Chicago, Illinois.*)

of overt disease is much higher in nonimmune infected adults than in children; travelers from developed countries who enter endemic areas are particularly susceptible.

Risk of disease greatest in nonimmune adults

### Pathogenesis

The virus is believed to replicate initially in the enteric mucosa. It can be demonstrated in feces by electron microscopy for 10 to 14 days before onset of disease. In most patients with symptoms of the disease, complete virus is no longer found in fecal specimens; viral antigen, however, has been demonstrated in feces for up to 14 days thereafter. Multiplication in the intestines is followed by a period of viremia with spread to the liver. The response to replication in the liver consists of lymphoid cell infiltration, necrosis of liver parenchymal cells, and proliferation of Kupffer cells. The extent of necrosis often coincides with the severity of disease. A variable degree of biliary stasis may be present.

Virus replicates in intestinal mucosa during incubation period

Viremic spread to liver parynchymal cells with necrosis

### Immunity

Antibody to hepatitis A virus can be detected during early illness when the virus is still found in feces, and most patients with symptoms or signs of acute hepatitis A already have detectable antibody in serum. Early antibody responses are predominantly IgM, which can be detected by radioimmunoassay for several weeks or months. During convalescence, antibody of the IgG class predominates. Detectable levels of IgG antibody to hepatitis A virus persist indefinitely in serum, and patients with anti-hepatitis A virus antibodies are immune to reinfection. Although virus-specific IgA has been demonstrated in stool, secretory immunity has not been shown to be important for hepatitis A.

IgM antibody response develops before symptoms

Later IgG response gives long-term immunity

## Hepatitis A Disease: Clinical Aspects

### Clinical Manifestations

In hepatitis A virus infection an incubation period of 14 to 40 days (mean, 25 days) is usually followed by the onset of fever, anorexia (poor appetite), nausea, pain in the right upper abdominal quadrant, and, within several days, jaundice. Dark urine and clay-colored stools may be noticed by the patient 1 to 5 days before the onset of clinical jaundice. The liver is enlarged and tender, and serum transaminase, aminotransferase, and bilirubin levels are elevated as a result of hepatic inflammation and damage.

Mean incubation period of 25 days

Fever, pain, jaundice, and elevation of bilirubin and hepatic enzymes

Many persons who have serologic evidence of acute hepatitis A infection are asymptomatic or only mildly ill, without jaundice (anicteric hepatitis A). The infection-to-disease ratio is dependent on age; it may be as high as 20:1 in children and approximately 7:1 in older adults. The vast majority of cases of hepatitis A are self-limiting. Chronic hepatitis such as that seen with hepatitis B is very rare. In rare cases, fulminant fatal hepatitis associated with extensive liver necrosis may occur.

Most infections are subclinical

Does not lead to chronic viral hepatitis

### Laboratory Diagnosis

The best method for documentation of acute hepatitis A virus infection is the demonstration of high titers of virus-specific IgM antibody in serum drawn during the acute phase of illness. Because IgG antibody persists indefinitely, its demonstration in a single serum sample is not indicative of recent infection; a rise in titer between acute and convalescent sera must be documented. Immune electron microscopic identification of the viral antigen in fecal specimens and isolation of the virus in cell cultures remain research tools.

Serodiagnosis requires IgM demonstration

### Prevention

#### Passive Immunization

Passive (ie, antibody) prophylaxis for hepatitis A has been available for many years. Immune serum globulin (ISG), manufactured from pools of plasma from large segments of the general population, is protective if given before or during the incubation period of the disease. It has been shown to be about 80 to 90% effective in preventing clinically apparent type A hepatitis. In some cases, infection occurs, but disease is ameliorated; that is, the patient develops anicteric, usually asymptomatic, hepatitis A. At present, ISG should be administered to household contacts of hepatitis A patients and those known to have eaten

Passive immunization with ISG is protective

ISG indicated for some travel

uncooked foods prepared or handled by an infected individual. Once clinical symptoms have appeared, the host is already producing antibody, and administration of ISG is not indicated. Persons from areas of low endemicity traveling to areas with high infection rates should receive ISG before departure and at 3- to 4-month intervals as long as potential heavy exposure continues.

ACTIVE IMMUNIZATION

Killed vaccine most promising

For hepatitis A, live attenuated vaccines have been evaluated but have demonstrated poor immunogenicity and have not been effective when given orally. Formalin-killed vaccines are more promising. They induce antibody titers similar to those of wild-virus infection and they have demonstrated efficacy in children. They will be expensive compared with the hepatitis B vaccines but may be approved in the United States soon.

### Treatment

There is no specific treatment for patients with acute episodes of hepatitis A infection. Supportive measures include adequate nutrition and rest.

# HEPATITIS B

## Hepatitis B Virus

### Structure

Enveloped, double-stranded DNA virus

Hepatitis B virus is an enveloped DNA virus belonging to the family Hepadnaviridae. It is unrelated to any other human virus; however, related hepatotropic agents have been identified in woodchucks, ground squirrels, and kangaroos. A schematic of the hepatitis B virus is illustrated in Fig 36–2. The complete virion is a 42-nm, spherical particle that consists of an envelope around a 27-nm core. The core comprises a nucleocapsid that contains the DNA genome.

Core comprises DNA genome, DNA polymerase, core and e antigens

The viral genome consists of partially double-stranded DNA with a short, single-stranded piece. It comprises 3200 nucleotides, making it the smallest DNA virus known. Closely associated with the viral DNA is a DNA polymerase. Other components of the core are a hepatitis B core antigen (HBcAg) and the hepatitis B e antigen (HBeAg), which is a low-molecular-weight glycoprotein. The major genes of hepatitis B virus and their products are shown in Table 36–2.

Envelope contains HBsAg

The envelope of the virus contains the hepatitis B surface antigen (HBsAg), which is

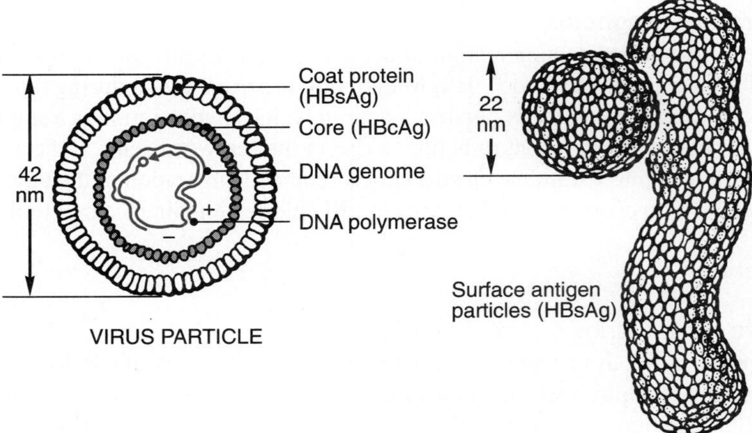


**Figure 36–2.** Schematic diagram of hepatitis B virion. The 42-nm particle is the "Dane particle" or the hepatitis B virus. The 22-nm particles are the filamentous and circular forms of hepatitis B surface antigen or protein coat.

**TABLE 36–2. MAJOR GENES OF THE HEPATITIS B VIRUS AND THEIR PRODUCTS**

| Gene | Product (Molecular Weight) | Function of Product |
|---|---|---|
| S | 25,000 and 30,000 | Major envelope protein, HBsAg |
| C | 17,000–22,000 | Internal core proteins HBcAg and HBeAg |
| P | 65,000 | Virus-associated DNA polymerase |
| X | 17,000–28,000 | 5′ protein linking to negative strand of viral DNA |

composed of one major and two other proteins. Antigenically there exist a group-specific determinant, termed *a*, and a number of subtypes that are important in epidemiologic typing, but not in immunity, because there is antigenic cross-reactivity and cross-protection between subtypes. Aggregates of HBsAg are often found in great abundance in serum during infection. They may assume spherical or filamentous shapes with a mean diameter of 22 nm and may contain portions of the nucleocapsid (see Fig 36–2). Hepatitis B DNA can also be detected in serum and is an indication that infectious virions are present there. In infected liver tissue, evidence of HBcAg, HBeAg, and hepatitis B DNA is found in the nuclei of infected hepatocytes, whereas HBsAg is found in cytoplasm.

Aggregates of HBsAg present in serum

Despite extensive attempts, hepatitis B virus has not been propagated in the laboratory. Humans appear to be the major host; as with hepatitis A, however, infection of subhuman primates has been accomplished experimentally.

Virus not yet propagated in tissue culture

### Replication Cycle

The replication of hepatitis B virus involves a reverse transcription step and, as such, is unique among DNA viruses. The double-stranded DNA is organized as two strands. One, a short strand, is associated with the viral DNA polymerase and is of positive polarity. The complete or long strand is complementary and thus of negative polarity. In viral replication, full-length "positive" viral RNA transcripts are inserted into maturing core particles late in the replicative cycle. These mRNA strands form a template for a reverse transcription step in which negatively stranded DNA is synthesized. The RNA template strands are then degraded by ribonuclease activity. A positive-stranded DNA is then initiated, although this is not completed prior to virus maturation and release and thus results in the variable-length short positive DNA strands found in the virions.

DNA organized as short-positive strand and complete negative strand

Replication involves a reverse transcription step

One positive DNA strand is not completed before viral release

## Hepatitis B Disease

### Epidemiology

Hepatitis B infection is found worldwide, with prevalence rates varying markedly between countries. Chronic carriers constitute the main reservoir of infection: in some tropical countries as many as 5 to 15% of all persons carry the virus although most are asymptomatic.

HBsAg-positive carriers main reservoir

In the United States, it is estimated that 0.1 to 0.5% of the population are chronic carriers of hepatitis B. Approximately 50% of infections in the United States are sexually transmitted and the occurrence of HBsAg is higher in certain populations, such as male homosexuals, patients on hemodialysis or immunosuppressive therapy, patients with Down syndrome, and drug addicts using injection methods. Routine screening of blood donors for HBsAg has markedly decreased the incidence of posttransfusion hepatitis B; 90% of cases developing after transfusion are now caused by hepatitis C or delta hepatitis viruses. Multiple-pool blood products cause occasional cases, and inadequately sterilized, blood-contaminated needles are still significant vehicles of transmission. Exposure to hepatitis viruses from direct contact with blood or other bodily fluids, probably through small lesions, has resulted in sporadic outbreaks of acute viral hepatitis B in medical personnel. Attack rates are also high in spouses and sexual partners of affected patients.

Half of US infections sexually transmitted

Some population groups have much higher carrier rates

Screening blood donors reduces post-transfusion risk

Most hepatitis B infections of infants do not appear to be transplacentally transmitted to the fetus in utero, but are acquired during the birth process by the swallowing of infected blood or fluids or through abrasions. The rate of virus acquisition is high in infants born to mothers who are suffering from acute hepatitis B infection or carrying HBsAg and HBeAg.

Transmitted to infant during childbirth

Infection at birth associated with development of chronic carriage

Most infants do not develop clinical disease; infection in the neonatal period is associated with failure to produce antibody to HBsAg, however, and thus with chronic carriage and epidemiologic perpetuation by transmission in the family setting.

Associated with hepatic carcinoma

Hepatocellular carcinoma has been strongly associated with persistent carriage of hepatitis B virus by serologic tests and detection of viral nucleic acid sequences integrated in tumor cell genomes. In many parts of Africa and Asia, primary liver cancer accounts for 20 to 30% of all types of malignancies, but for only 1 to 2% in North and South America and Europe. The estimated risk of developing the malignancy for persons with chronic hepatitis B is increased between 10- and more than 300-fold in different populations. The mechanism of the association is unclear. Integration of hepatitis B viral DNA in hepatocellular cancer tissue occurs at variable sites for both viral and cellular DNA, but no activation of oncogenes has yet been identified. Chromosomal deletions have been shown in one hepatocellular cell line that is infected with hepatitis B virus.

## Pathogenesis and Pathology

HBsAg found in most body fluids and secretions

Transmission by contact with infected blood or secretions

Only small amount of blood required

In the past, hepatitis B was best known as a form of posttransfusion hepatitis or as hepatitis associated with the use of illicit parenteral drugs (serum hepatitis). Over the past few years, however, it has become clear that the major mode of acquisition is through close contact with infected secretions or blood of acute cases of disease or of chronic carriers of the virus. Hepatitis B surface antigen has been found in most body fluids, including saliva, semen, and cervical secretions. Transmission by person-to-person contact has been documented, as has vertical mother-to-child transmission, usually at the time of birth. Under experimental conditions, as little as 0.0001 mL of infectious blood has produced infection. Transmission is therefore possible by vehicles such as inadequately sterilized hypodermic needles or instruments used in tattooing and ear piercing.

Rash and arthritis early in disease from immune complexes

Anti-HBsAg protective

Depressed cell-mediated immunity associated with chronic infection

The factors determining the different clinical manifestations of acute hepatitis B are largely unknown; however, some appear to involve the immunologic responses of the host. The serum sickness-like rash and arthritis that may precede the development of symptoms and jaundice appear related to circulating immune complexes that activate the complement system. Antibody to the HBsAg is protective and associated with resolution of the disease. Cellular immunity also may be important in the host response, because patients with depressed T-lymphocyte function have a high frequency of chronic infection with the hepatitis B virus. Antibody to the HBcAg, which appears during infection, is present in chronic carriers with persistent hepatitis B virion production. It does not appear to be protective.

Hepatocyte necrosis and postnecrotic cirrhosis

The morphologic lesions of acute hepatitis B resemble those of hepatitis A and non-A, non-B hepatitis. In chronic active hepatitis B, the continued presence of inflammatory foci of infection results in necrosis of hepatocytes, collapse of the reticular framework of the liver, and progressive fibrosis. The increasing fibrosis can result in the syndrome of postnecrotic hepatic cirrhosis.

Integrated viral genome may activate oncogenes

Hepatocellular carcinoma potentially preventable by immunization

Integrated hepatitis B viral DNA can be found in nearly all hepatocellular carcinomas. The virus has not been shown to possess a transforming gene, but may well activate a cellular oncogene. It is also possible that the virus does not play such a direct molecular role in oncogenicity, because the natural history of chronic hepatitis B infection involves cycles of damage or death of liver cells interspersed with periods of intense regenerative hyperplasia. This significantly increases the opportunity for spontaneous mutational changes that may activate cellular oncogenes. Whatever the mechanism, the association between chronic viral infection and hepatocellular carcinoma is clear, and liver cancer is a major cause of disease and death in countries in which chronic hepatitis B infection is common. The proven success of combined active and passive immunization in aborting hepatitis B infection in infancy or childhood makes hepatocellular carcinoma of the liver a potentially preventable disease.

## Antigenemia and Immunity

Serum HBsAg associated with acute disease and chronic carriage

Anti-HBs associated with elimination of infection and immunity

The nomenclature of hepatitis B antigens and antibodies is shown in Table 36–3. During the acute episode of disease, when there is active viral replication, large amounts of HBsAg and hepatitis B virus DNA can be detected in the serum, as can fully developed virions and high levels of DNA polymerase and HBeAg. Although HBcAg is also present, antibody against it invariably occurs and prevents its detection. With resolution of acute hepatitis B, HBsAg and HBeAg disappear from serum with the development of antibodies (anti-HBs

**TABLE 36–3. NOMENCLATURE FOR HEPATITIS B VIRUS ANTIGENS AND ANTIBODIES**

| Abbreviation | Description |
|---|---|
| HBV | Hepatitis B virus; 42-nm double-stranded DNA virus; Dane particle |
| HBsAg | Hepatitis B surface antigen; found on surface of virus; formed in excess and seen in serum as 22-nm spherical and tubular particles; four subdeterminants (*adw, ayw, adr,* and *ayr*) identified |
| HBcAg | Core antigen (nucleocapsid core); found in nucleus of infected hepatocytes by immunofluorescence |
| HBeAg | Glycoprotein; associated with the core antigen; used epidemiologically as marker of serious potential infectivity; seen only when HBsAg is also present |
| Anti-HBs | Antibody to HBsAg; correlated with protection against and/or resolution of disease; used as marker of past infection or vaccination |
| Anti-HBc | Antibody to HBcAg; seen in acute infection and chronic carriers; anti-HBc IgM used as indicator of acute infection; anti-HBc IgG used as marker of past or chronic infection; apparently not important in disease resolution |
| Anti-HBe | Antibody to HBeAg |

and anti-HBe) against them. The development of anti-HBs is associated with elimination of infection and protection against reinfection. Anti-HBc is detected early in the course of disease and persists in serum for years. It is an excellent epidemiologic marker of infection, but is not protective. A schematic diagram of these responses is shown in Figure 36–3.

In patients with chronic hepatitis B, evidence of viral persistence can be found in serum. HBsAg can be detected throughout the active disease process and anti-HBs does not develop, which probably accounts for the chronicity of the disease. Anti-HBc is, however, detected. Two types of chronic hepatitis can be distinguished. In one, HBsAg is detected, but not HBeAg; these patients usually show minimal evidence of liver dysfunction. In the other, both antigens are found; the process is more active, with continued hepatic damage that may result in cirrhosis. The occurrence of serum antigen and antibody is shown in Fig 36–4.

Presence of both HBeAg and HBsAG in chronic carriage suggests continued hepatic damage

## Hepatitis B Disease: Clinical Aspects

### Clinical Manifestations

The clinical picture of hepatitis B is highly variable. The incubation period may be as brief as 7 days or as long as 160 days (mean, approximately 10 weeks). Acute hepatitis B is usually manifested by the gradual onset of fatigue, loss of appetite, nausea, pain, and fullness in the right upper abdominal quadrant. Early in the course of disease, pain and swelling of the joints and occasionally frank arthritis may occur. Some patients develop a rash. With increasing involvement of the liver, there is increasing cholestasis and, hence, clay-colored

Incubation period up to 160 days (mean, 10 weeks)

Gradual onset abdominal and joint pain

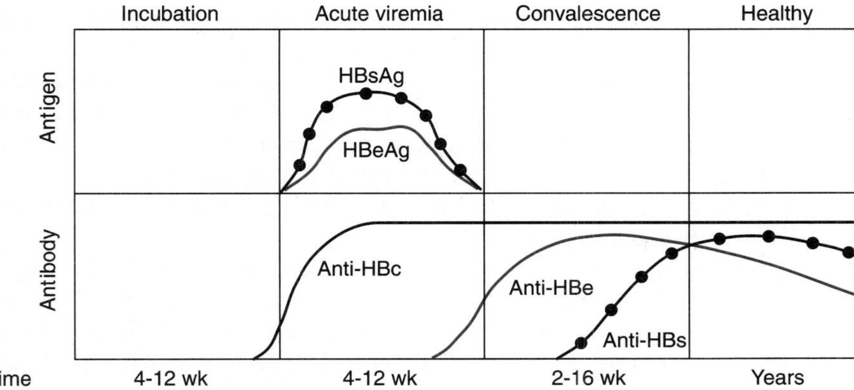


**Figure 36–3.** Sequence of appearance of viral antigens and antibodies in acute self-limiting cases of hepatitis B. HBsAg, hepatitis B surface antigen; HBeAg, hepatitis B e antigen; anti-HBc, antibody to hepatitis B core antigen; anti-HBe, antibody to HBeAg; anti-HBs, antibody to HBsAg.

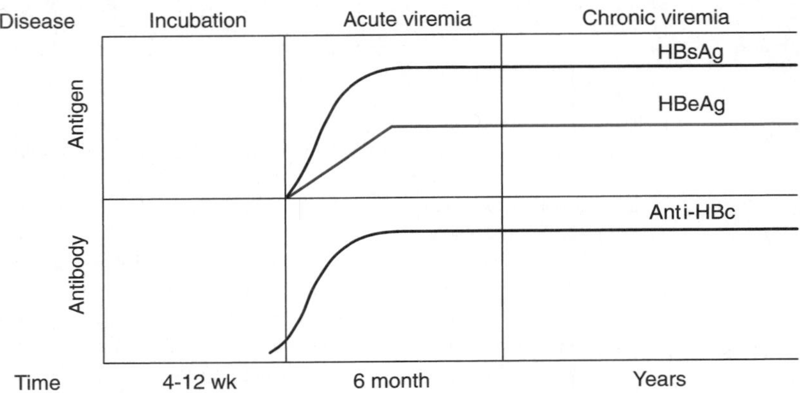


**Figure 36–4.** Sequence of appearance of viral antigens and antibodies in chronic active hepatitis B. HBsAg, hepatitis B surface antigen; HBeAg, hepatitis B e antigen; anti-HBc, antibody to hepatitis B core antigen. Antibodies to HBsAg and HBeAg not detected.

stools, darkening of the urine, and jaundice. Symptoms may persist for several months before finally resolving.

More severe than hepatitis A but anicteric cases common

In general, the symptoms associated with hepatitis B are more severe and more prolonged than those of hepatitis A; however, anicteric disease and asymptomatic infection occur. The infection-to-disease ratio, which varies according to age and method of acquisition, has been estimated to be approximately 6:1 or 7:1. One important difference between hepatitis A and hepatitis B is the development of chronic hepatitis. This occurs in approximately 10% of all patients with hepatitis B infection, but the risk is much higher for newborns and the immunocompromised. Chronic infection is associated with ongoing replication of virus in the liver and usually with the presence of HBsAg in serum. Fulminant hepatitis, leading to extensive liver necrosis and death, develops in less than 1% of cases.

Chronic hepatitis risk greatest in newborns, immunocompromised

## Laboratory Diagnosis

Acute infection diagnosed by demonstrating serum anti-HBc IgM

The laboratory diagnosis of acute hepatitis B is best made by demonstrating the IgM antibody to hepatitis B core antigen in serum. Almost all patients who develop jaundice will be anti HBc IgM positive at the time of clinical presentation. In patients with self-limiting anicteric disease, HBsAg detection in serum may also occur. Past infection with hepatitis B is best determined by detecting anti-HBc, anti-HBs, or both. Chronic infection with hepatitis B is best detected by persistence of HBsAg in blood for more than 6 to 12 months.

## Prevention

Passive immunization with HBIG protects exposed subjects

Both active prophylaxis and passive prophylaxis of hepatitis B infection can be accomplished. Most preparations of ISG contain only moderate levels of anti-HBs; however, hepatitis B immune globulin (HBIG) with significant protective activity is now available. HBIG is prepared from sera of subjects who have high titers of antibody to HBsAg, but are free of the antigen itself. Administration of HBIG soon after exposure to the virus greatly reduces acquisition of symptomatic disease. Inactivated hepatitis B vaccines have been available for several years. The first was developed by purification and inactivation of HBsAg from the blood of chronic carriers but this is no longer in use. The current vaccine is a recombinant product derived from HBAg grown in yeast. Excellent protection has been shown in studies on homosexual men and medical personnel. These groups and others, such as laboratory workers, who come into contact with blood or other potentially infected materials should receive hepatitis B vaccine.

Active immunization with recombinant HBsAg vaccine recommended for healthcare workers

A combination of active and passive immunization is the most effective approach to prevent neonatal transmission and, thus, the development of chronic carriage in the neonate. Most hospitals recommend routine screening of pregnant women for the presence of HBsAg. Infants born to those who are positive should receive HBIG in the delivery room followed by three doses of hepatitis B vaccine beginning 24 hours after birth.

Combined active and passive immunization protects exposed infants

A similar combination of passive and active immunization is used for unimmunized persons who have been exposed by needle-stick or similar injuries. The procedure varies depending on the hepatitis B status of the case linked to the injury.

### Treatment

There is no specific treatment for typical acute hepatitis B. A high-calorie diet is desirable. Corticosteroid therapy has no value in uncomplicated typical acute viral hepatitis, and recent studies suggest that it may increase the severity of chronic hepatitis caused by hepatitis B virus. Interferon alpha as a therapy is useful in a minority of patients with chronic hepatitis B infection, especially those who already demonstrate an acute immune response with low serum viral DNA levels.

Interferon may be useful

## DELTA HEPATITIS

### Hepatitis D Virus

Delta hepatitis is caused by the hepatitis D virus. This small single-stranded RNA virus requires the presence of hepatitis B surface antigens for its transmission but not its replication. Delta hepatitis is thus found only in persons with acute or chronic hepatitis B infection. Strategies directed at preventing hepatitis B are also effective in preventing delta hepatitis.

Small, single-stranded RNA virus that requires coinfection with hepatitis B virus

The method of transcription of hepatitis D viral RNA is not clear. Associated with the RNA are proteins of 27 and 29 kilodaltons that constitute the delta antigen. This protein–RNA complex is surrounded by hepatitis B surface antigen (Fig 36–5). Thus, although the delta virus produces its own antigens, it co-opts the hepatitis B surface antigen in assembling its coat. Methods are available to detect both delta antigen and IgM and IgG antibodies directed against it. These are the means by which delta infection is diagnosed.

Protein–RNA complex surrounded with HBsAg coat

### Hepatitis D Disease

Delta hepatitis is most prevalent in groups at high risk of hepatitis B. Drug addicts are those at greatest risk in the United States, and localized epidemics have occurred in this group. Because blood is not yet routinely screened for the delta agent, blood products and dialysis transmission are possible sources for those who have prior hepatitis B. Nonparenteral and vertical transmission can also occur.

Epidemics in intravenous drug abusers

### Hepatitis D Disease: Clinical Aspects

#### Clinical Manifestations

Two major types of delta infection have been noted: simultaneous delta and hepatitis B infection or delta superinfection in those with chronic hepatitis B. Simultaneous infection with both delta and hepatitis B results in clinical hepatitis that is indistinguishable from acute hepatitis A or B; however, fulminant hepatitis is much more common than with hepatitis B virus alone. The delta agent causes its greatest morbidity by increasing the severity and accelerating the pace of chronic hepatitis B infection.

Greater disease severity than with hepatitis B alone

Persons with chronic hepatitis B who acquire infection with hepatitis D suffer relapses of jaundice and have a high likelihood of developing chronic cirrhosis. Epidemics of delta

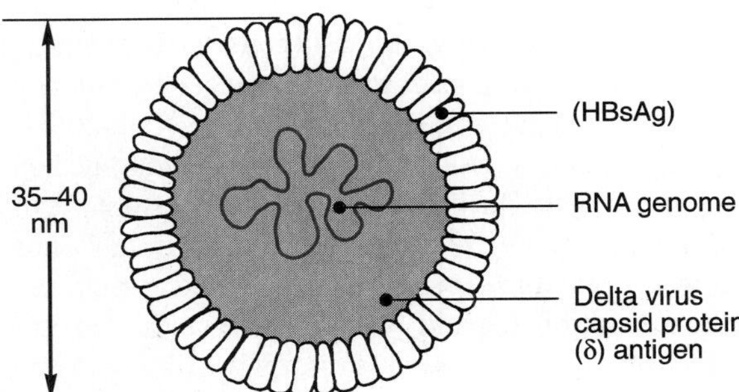


**Figure 36–5.** Schematic of delta hepatitis virus. Note outer layer derived from hepatitis B surface antigen.

infection have occurred in populations with a high incidence of chronic hepatitis B and have resulted in rapidly progressive liver disease, causing death in up to 20% of infected persons.

### Diagnosis

Diagnosis is made most commonly by demonstrating IgM or IgG antibodies, or both, to the delta antigen in serum. IgM antibodies appear within 3 weeks of infection and persist for several weeks. IgG antibodies persist for years.

### Prevention

Because the capsid of delta hepatitis is HBsAg, measures aimed at limiting the transmission of hepatitis B prevent the transmission of delta hepatitis.

# HEPATITIS C

## Hepatitis C Virus

Disease usually mild, but may cause chronic liver damage

Virus detected without isolation

Recently, it has been shown that most community-acquired and 70 to 75% of transfusion-associated hepatitis previously called non-A, non-B (NANB) are due to an RNA virus termed *hepatitis C virus.* This agent has not yet been isolated in cell culture; however, evidence for its existence and role in the etiology of transfusion-associated hepatitis was acquired by preparing numerous complementary DNA clones from the presumed RNA virus in infectious serum. Peptides encoded in these clones were then tested for reaction with antibody from cases of NANB hepatitis and one was found to be highly specific. The data derived on the nature of the viral genome suggest that it is most closely related to flaviviruses. This technical tour-de-force has provided a serologic test for screening donated blood.

Hepatitis C is usually insidious in onset, mild, and anicteric, but results in chronic liver disease in many patients. As most transmitters of the disease are asymptomatic, a chronic carrier state is presumed.

## Hepatitis C Disease

Transmitted by transfusion, possibly other means

The transmission of hepatitis C by blood is well documented: indeed, it caused the great majority of posttransfusion NANB hepatitis. The transmission of this virus in nontransfusion, community-acquired cases is less clear-cut. It may be sexually transmitted but to a much lesser degree than hepatitis B. Vertical transmission and occult needle sharing may account for some cases.

## Hepatitis C Disease: Clinical Aspects

### Prevention

It is not clear whether prophylactic immune serum globulin protects against hepatitis C. Also, it is questionable whether a vaccine will be effective as patients may be reinfected by wild-type virus.

### Diagnosis

Diagnosis by antibody detection

Antibody delayed and absent in some

Antigens of hepatitis C are not detectable in blood so diagnostic tests consist of attempts to demonstrate antibody. Unfortunately, the antibody responses in acute disease remain negative for 1 to 3 weeks after clinical onset and may never become positive in up to 20% of patients with acute, resolving disease. These antibody assays can be helpful in chronic hepatitis, especially when multiple antigens are sought. The first test developed to assist the diagnosis of hepatitis C measured antibody to the C-100 antigen of the virus. It is now acknowledged that this antibody is an inaccurate marker for the disease, and current second-generation tests measure antibodies to multiple hepatitis C antigens by either enzyme immunoassay or immunoblot testing. Even with these newer assays, IgG antibody to hepatitis C may not develop for up to 4 months, making the serodiagnosis of acute hepatitis C difficult.

### Treatment

Interferon alpha is approved for the treatment of chronic hepatitis C but it often provides only a transient benefit.

## HEPATITIS E

Hepatitis E is the cause of another form of hepatitis but this virus is spread by the fecal–oral route and therefore resembles hepatitis A. Hepatitis E virus is an RNA virus that appears similar to caliciviruses. The viral particles in stool are spherical, 27 to 34 nm in size, and unenveloped and exhibit spikes on their surface. Like hepatitis A, this virus causes only acute disease and may fulminate, especially in pregnant women. Most cases have been identified in India and in other countries with poor sanitation. Rarely have cases been identified in the United States, and these have been in visitors or immigrants from endemic areas. The diagnosis may be confirmed by demonstrating the presence of specific IgM antibody. It is not known if immune serum globulin provides protection and no treatment is available.

Transmission similar to hepatitis A

Found in areas with poor sanitation

## ADDITIONAL READING

Advisory Committee on Immunization Practices. Protection against viral hepatitis: Recommendation of the Immunization Practices Advisory Committee (ACIIP). *Morb Mort Wkly Rep.* 1990;39:1–26. A good review of the hepatitis viruses and prophylaxis.

Alter HJ. Descarts before the horse: I Clone, therefore I am: The hepatitis C virus in current perspective. *Ann Int Med.* 1991; 115:644–649. Reviews the discovery, epidemiology, and diagnosis of hepatitis C.

Davis GL, Balart LA, Schiff ER et al. Treatment of chronic hepatitis C with recombinant interferon alpha: A multicenter randomized controlled trial. *N Engl J Med.* 1989;321:1501–1506. A demonstration of successful antiviral therapy for patients with chronic non-A, non-B hepatitis, although relapse is common.

Franchis R, Meucci G, Vecchi M, et al. The natural history of asymptomatic hepatitis B. *Ann Int Med.* 1993;118:191–194. A follow-up of HBsAg positive blood donors.

Johnson Y, Lau N, Wright TL. Molecular virology and pathogenesis of hepatitis B. *Lancet.* 1993;342:1335–1339. This short review covers details of molecular structure and replication of the virus.

Tremolade F, Casarin C, Alberti A, et al. Long-term follow-up of non-A, non-B (type C) post-transfusion hepatitis. *J Hepatol.* 1992;16:273–281. 135 patients were followed for a mean of 8.5 years to determine the incidence of resolution, chronic hepatitis, cirrhosis, and hepatocellular cancers.

Werzberger A, et al. A controlled trial of a formalin-inactivated hepatitis A vaccine in healthy children. *N Engl J Med.* 1992;327:453–457. The inactivated purified hepatitis A vaccine is well tolerated, and a single dose is highly protective against clinically apparent hepatitis A.

Chapter 37

# Herpesviruses

*W. Lawrence Drew*

The group Herpesvirus, of the family Herpesviridae, comprises large, enveloped, double-stranded DNA viruses found in both animals and humans. They are ubiquitous and produce infections ranging from painful skin ulcers to chickenpox to encephalitis. The major members of the group to infect humans are two herpes simplex viruses (HSVs), cytomegalovirus (CMV), varicella–zoster virus (VZV), Epstein–Barr virus (EBV), and the recently discovered human herpesvirus types 6 and 7. Occasionally, the simian herpesvirus, herpes B virus, has caused human disease.

Large-enveloped, double-stranded DNA viruses

## GROUP CHARACTERISTICS

All herpesviruses are morphologically similar. The nucleic acid core is about 30 to 45 nm in diameter, surrounded by an icosahedral capsid. The capsid is covered by a lipoprotein envelope derived from the nuclear membrane of the infected host cell. The envelope contains multiple embedded glycoproteins that protrude beyond it as spikelike structures. Despite the morphologic similarity between these agents, substantial differences in the molecular composition of the genome are reflected in their structural glycoproteins and polypeptides. Immunologic tests are the primary means for differentiation among herpesviruses despite some cross-reactions (eg, between HSV and VZV).

Morphology similar among herpesviruses

Differentiation immunologic

Growth conditions for the individual agents vary significantly. Herpes simplex virus has the widest range; it replicates in numerous animal and human host cells, although it affects only humans in nature. Varicella–zoster virus infects only primates and is best grown in cells of human origin, although some laboratory-adapted strains can grow in primate cell lines. Human CMV replicates well only in human fibroblast cell lines. Epstein–Barr virus does not replicate in most commonly used cell culture systems, but can be grown in continuous human or primate lymphoblastoid cell cultures. Human herpesvirus type 6 grows in lymphocyte cell cultures.

Characteristically, all of these agents produce an initial overt infection followed by a period of latent infection in which the genome of the virus is present in the cell, but infectious virus is not recovered (Table 37–1). Reactivation of virus may then result in recurrent infection. Complex host–virus interactions determine the expression of disease. With all of these agents, immunocompromised patients, especially those with altered cellular immunity, have more frequent and severe episodes, including clinically severe disease from reactivation of virus.

Viral latency and disease reactivation typical for all agents

TABLE 37–1. MAJOR CLINICAL SYNDROMES OF HERPESVIRUSES IN HUMANS

| Virus | Major Clinical Syndrome | Site of Latent Infection | Diagnostic Test |
|---|---|---|---|
| Herpes simplex virus Type 1 | Gingivostomatitis in children and young adults; recurrent oral–labial infection (cold sores); infection of the cornea (keratitis); herpes encephalitis | Trigeminal nerve root ganglion and autonomic ganglia of superior cervical and vagus nerves | Culture, lesion<br>IFA, lesion |
| Type 2 | Genital herpes; neonatal herpes | Sacral nerve root ganglia | Culture, lesion<br>IFA, lesion |
| Varicella–zoster | Chickenpox (primary infection); shingles (zoster) | Thoracic cervical or lumbar nerve root ganglia | Culture, lesion<br>IFA, lesion |
| Cytomegalovirus | Asymptomatic infection; heterophile-negative mononucleosis; fever hepatitis syndrome in neonates and transplant patients; interstitial pneumonia in immunocompromised patients | Leukocytes (neutrophils and lymphocytes) | Culture, blood<br>Culture, lung lavage<br>IFA, lung |
| Epstein–Barr virus | Heterophile-positive mononucleosis | B lymphocytes | Serology |
| Human herpesvirus type 6 | Roseola (Exanthem subitum) | B and T lymphocytes | Serology |

*Abbreviation:* IFA, immunofluorescent antibody staining.

## HERPES SIMPLEX VIRUS

HSV-1 and HSV-2 distinct epidemiologically, antigenically, and by DNA homology

The term *herpes* (from the Greek *herpein*, "to creep") and the clinical description of cold sores date back to Hippocrates. Two distinct epidemiologic and antigenic types of HSV exist (HSV-1 and HSV-2). The DNA genomes of both are linear, double-stranded molecules with molecular weights of approximately $10^8$. Their nucleic acids demonstrate approximately 50% base sequence homology, which is considerably greater than that shown between these viruses and other herpesviruses. HSV-1 and HSV-2 share antigens in almost all their surface glycoproteins and other structural polypeptides. Numerous strains of both HSV-1 and HSV-2 exist. In fact, by restriction endonuclease analysis of the viral genome, most strains of HSV-1 or HSV-2 are found to differ somewhat, except in epidemiologically related cases such as mother–infant and sexual partner transfer.

Individual strains differ by restriction endonuclease techniques

## Herpes Simplex Virus Disease

### Epidemiology

No animal reservoirs

Herpes simplex viruses have worldwide distribution. There are no known animal vectors, and humans appear to be the only natural reservoir. Direct contact with infected secretions is the principal mode of spread. Seroepidemiologic studies indicate that the prevalence of HSV antibody varies according to the age and socioeconomic status of the population studied. In most underdeveloped countries, 90% of the population have HSV-1 antibody by the age of 30. In the United States, HSV-1 antibody is currently found in approximately 50 to 60% of middle-class populations; among lower socioeconomic groups, however, the percentage approaches 90%.

HSV-1 more common with lower socioeconomic status

Infection with HSV-2 linked to sexual activity

Detection of HSV-2 antibody before puberty is unusual. The virus is associated with previous sexual activity, and direct sexual transmission is the major mode of spread. Approximately 15 to 30% of sexually active adults in Western industrialized countries have HSV-2 antibody. The virus can also be isolated from the cervix and urethra of approximately 5 to 12% of adults attending sexually transmitted disease clinics; many of these patients are asymptomatic or have small, unnoticed lesions on penile or vulvar skin. Genital herpes is not a reportable disease in the United States, but it is estimated that 500,000 new cases occur per year.

## Pathogenesis

### Acute Infection

Herpes simplex virus produces both acute and latent infections, in which the virus–cell interactions and the manifestations of infection differ. In acute infections, the initial stages entail envelope glycoprotein-mediated attachment of the virus to the host cell membrane and entry into the cytoplasm. Viral DNA released in the cytoplasm is transported to nuclear pores and the viral DNA is released into the nucleus. New viral DNA synthesis and transcription of mRNA occur in the nucleus in a sequence controlled by viral regulatory proteins; mRNA then migrates to the cytoplasm. After translation of virus-specified protein in the cytoplasm, these proteins migrate back to the nucleus, where they encapsulate the viral DNA. The virus "buds" through the nuclear membrane; this process adds the envelope material to the virus particles, which are then transported through the cytoplasm and out of the cell in a manner similar to other proteins.

HSV DNA replication and viral assembly occur in the nucleus

Viral proteins synthesized in cytoplasm migrate back to nucleus

The molecular events involving synthesis of virus-specific gene products are coordinated and regulated. Three classes of mRNA coding for three groups of virus polypeptides have been identified. The initial products, designated the alpha polypeptides, are synthesized 2 to 4 hours after infection. The exact function of these alpha polypeptides, five of which have been identified, is unknown; however, some authorities believe that they may be related to the development of latent infection. The beta polypeptides include virus-specified thymidine kinase and DNA polymerase. These virus-specified enzymes differ from host cell enzymes and are therefore important targets of antiviral chemotherapy, as currently available antiviral drugs inhibit their activity. The synthesis of beta polypeptides shuts off the synthesis of alpha polypeptides and induces the synthesis of a third group of polypeptides. The gamma polypeptides, synthesized 12 to 15 hours after infection, largely represent the structural components of the viral particle.

Alpha-polypeptides produced initially

Later beta-polypeptides include virus-specified thymidine kinase

Gamma-polypeptides are structural components of virus

Pathologic changes during acute infections consist of development of multinucleated giant cells, ballooning degeneration of epithelial cells, focal necrosis, eosinophilic intranuclear inclusion bodies (Fig 37–1), and an inflammatory response characterized by an initial polymorphonuclear neutrophil infiltrate and a subsequent mononuclear cell infiltrate. The virus can spread intra- or interneuronally or through supporting cellular networks of an axon or nerve, resulting in latent infection of sensory and autonomic nerve ganglia. Spread of virus can occur by cell-to-cell transfer and can therefore be unaffected by circulating immune globulin.

Infection produces inflammation and giant cells

Virus can infect and spread in axons and ganglia

### Latent Infection

In humans, latent infection by HSV-1 has been demonstrated by cocultivation techniques in trigeminal, superior cervical, and vagal nerve ganglia, and occasionally in the S2–3 dorsal sensory nerve root ganglia. Latent HSV-2 infection has been demonstrated in the sacral

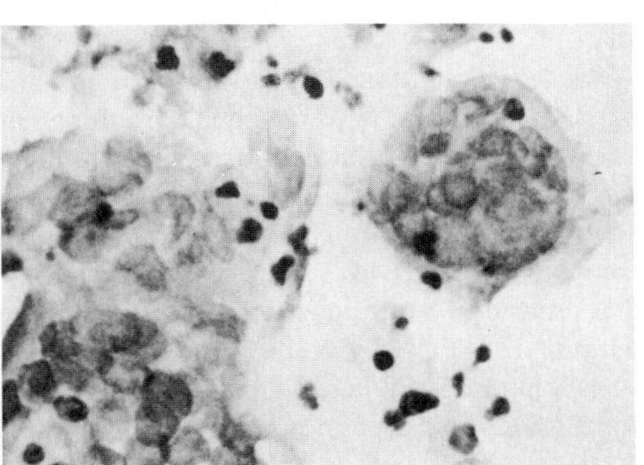

**Figure 37–1.** Multinucleated giant cells from herpes simplex virus lesion.

(S2–3) region. Latent infection of nervous tissue by HSV does not result in the death of the cell; however, the exact mechanism of viral genome interaction with the cell is incompletely understood. It has been shown that the HSV genome exists in a circular form in latently infected neuronal cells. It appears that transcription of only a small portion of the viral genome occurs. As latent infection does not appear to be associated with detectable amounts of beta or gamma polypeptides, antiviral drugs directed at the viral DNA polymerase or thymidine kinase enzymes do not eradicate the virus in its latent state.

Latency not associated with detectable beta- or gamma-polypeptides or whole virions

Reactivation of virus from latently infected ganglionic cells with subsequent release of infectious virions appears to account for most recurrences of both genital and oral–labial infections. The mechanisms by which latent infection is maintained and reactivated are unknown. Two theories have been advanced to explain how latent virus reaches peripheral sites. According to the *ganglionic theory,* metabolic changes in latently infected cells "switch on" the viral replicative cycle; the virus then travels down the peripheral nerves to the skin, where it replicates in epidermal cells and produces the lesions. An alternative explanation, the *skin trigger theory,* suggests chronic multiplication of virus in the ganglion with intermittent shedding of the virus through the nerve axon to the skin. Local alterations in host immune status then initiate replication in skin. Precipitating factors that initiate reactivation of herpes simplex are largely unknown; exposure to ultraviolet light appears to be important in some patients with recurrent oral–labial herpes. Experimentally, mucocutaneous herpes may be caused by exogenous reinfection with different strains of the same subtype; but this is uncommon in nature.

Two theories proposed to explain reactivation and release from infected ganglionic cells

### Immunity

Host factors have a major effect on clinical manifestations of HSV infection. Many episodes of HSV infection are either asymptomatic or mildly symptomatic. Initial symptomatic clinical episodes of the disease are more severe than recurrent episodes, probably because of the presence of anti-HSV antibodies and immune lymphocytes in persons with recurrent infections. Prior infection with HSV-1 shortens the duration of symptoms and lessens the severity of first infections with HSV-2.

Both cellular and humoral immune responses are important in immunity to herpes. Neutralizing antibodies directed against HSV envelope glycoproteins appear to be the most important, particularly those that mediate antibody-dependent cellular cytotoxicity (ADCC, see Chapter 8) reactions. ADCC may be important in limiting early spread of HSV. By the second week of infection cytotoxic T lymphocytes can be detected that are able to destroy HSV-infected cells prior to completion of the replication cycle. Recurrences of HSV are clinically of shorter duration and more localized than primary infections. In immunosuppressed patients, especially those with depressed cell-mediated immunity, reactivation of HSV may be associated with prolonged viral excretion and persistence of lesions. Viremia and dissemination through visceral organs have been shown to occur occasionally, even in the presence of detectable neutralizing antibody to HSV.

Evidence for cell-mediated immunity

ADCC important in limiting early spread

Cytotoxic T cells destroy infected cells

## Herpes Simplex Virus Disease: Clinical Aspects

### Clinical Manifestations

Herpes Simplex Virus Type 1

Infection with HSV-1 is usually "above the waist." It consists characteristically of grouped or single vesicular lesions that become pustular and coalesce to form single or multiple ulcers. On dry surfaces, these ulcers scab before healing; on mucosal surfaces, they reepithelialize directly. Herpes simplex virus can be isolated from almost all lesions until the crusting stage, but the titer of virus decreases as the lesions progress. Infections generally involve embryonic ectoderm (skin, mouth, vagina, conjunctiva, nervous system). The major clinical manifestations of HSV-1 disease include mucocutaneous superficial infection of the pharynx, skin, and eye and infection of the brain.

Vesicular lesions become pustular and then ulcerate

Primary infection with HSV-1 is often asymptomatic. When symptomatic, it appears most frequently as gingivostomatitis, usually in 3- to 5-year-old children. There can be fever,

Primary infections often asymptomatic

irritability, and vesicular or ulcerative lesions involving the buccal mucosa, tongue, gums, and pharynx. The lesions are quite painful, and the illness usually lasts 5 to 12 days. After this initial infection, HSV may become latent within sensory nerve root ganglia of the trigeminal nerve.

May become latent after primary gingivostomatitis

Lesions usually recur over the anterior buccal mucosa, lips, or perioral area of the face and, because reactivation is usually from a single latent source, are typically unilateral. Usually these lesions involve an area of the lip and the immediate adjacent skin; these lesions are referred to as mucocutaneous and are commonly called cold sores or fever blisters. Their recurrence may be signaled by premonitory tingling or burning in the area. Local symptoms are similar but milder than those with primary infections because of the development of partial immunity. Systemic complaints are unusual, and the episode generally lasts approximately 7 days. It should be noted that HSV may be reactivated and excreted into the saliva with no apparent mucosal lesions present. Herpes simplex virus has been isolated from saliva in 5 to 8% of children and 1 to 2% of adults who were asymptomatic at the time.

Recurrent cold sores ususally unilateral

Virus in saliva with asymptomatic reactivation

Herpes simplex virus sometimes infects the finger or nail area. This infection, termed *herpetic whitlow,* usually results from the inoculation of infected secretions through a small cut in the skin. Painful vesicular lesions of the finger develop and pustulate.

Herpes simplex virus infection of the eye is one of the most common causes of corneal damage and blindness in industrialized nations. Infections usually involve the conjunctiva and cornea, and characteristic dendritic ulcerations are produced. With recurrence of disease, there may be deeper involvement with corneal scarring. Occasionally there may be extension into deeper structures of the eye, especially if topical steroids are used.

Herpetic corneal and conjunctival infection cause of blindness

Encephalitis may rarely result from HSV-1 infection. Herpes encephalitis accounts for up to 10% of all cases of viral encephalitis in the United States. Most cases occur in adults with high levels of anti-HSV-1 antibody, suggesting reactivation of latent virus in the trigeminal nerve root ganglion and extension of productive (lytic) infection into the temporoparietal area of the brain. Primary HSV infection with neurotropic spread of the virus from peripheral sites up the olfactory bulb into the brain may also result in parenchymal brain infection.

Herpes encephalitis may be reactivation

Classically, the disease affects one temporal lobe, leading to focal neurologic signs and cerebral edema. If untreated, mortality is 70%. Clinically, the disease can resemble brain abscess, tumor, or intracerebral hemorrhage. The virus is easily isolated from brain tissue, and diagnostic brain biopsy remains the most definitive method of diagnosis. Intravenous acyclovir effectively reduces the mortality of the disease. Rapid diagnosis is very important and there are encouraging results suggesting that HSV can be detected in cerebrospinal fluid by the polymerase chain reaction (PCR), although the virus is rarely, if ever, cultured from this site. If PCR of cerebrospinal fluid proves to be sensitive and specific, the need for brain biopsy would be eliminated.

Encephalitis typically localized to temporal lobe

Rapid diagnosis allows antiviral therapy

### Herpes Simplex Virus Type 2

Genital herpes is an important sexually transmitted disease. Both HSV-1 and HSV-2 can cause genital disease and the symptoms and signs of acute infection are similar for both viruses. Seventy percent of first episodes of genital HSV infection in the United States are caused by HSV-2, and genital HSV-2 disease is also more likely to recur than genital HSV-1 infection.

HSV-2 associated with genital herpes

**Primary Genital Herpes Infection.** The mean incubation period from sexual contact to onset of lesions is 5 days. Lesions begin as small erythematous papules that soon form vesicles and then pustules (Fig 37–2). Within 3 to 5 days the vesiculopustular lesions break to form painful coalesced ulcers that subsequently dry; some form crusts and heal without scarring. With primary disease the genital lesions are usually multiple (mean, 20), bilateral, and extensive. The urethra and cervix are also infected frequently, with discrete or coalesced ulcers on the exocervix. Bilateral tenderness of the inguinal lymph nodes and slight enlargement are usually present and may persist for months. About one third of patients show systemic symptoms such as fever, malaise, and myalgia, and 1 to 10% develop aseptic meningitis with neck rigidity and severe headache. First episodes of disease usually abate after 20 to 30 days of illness.

Multiple painful vesicopustular lesions

Systemic symptoms and adenopathy common

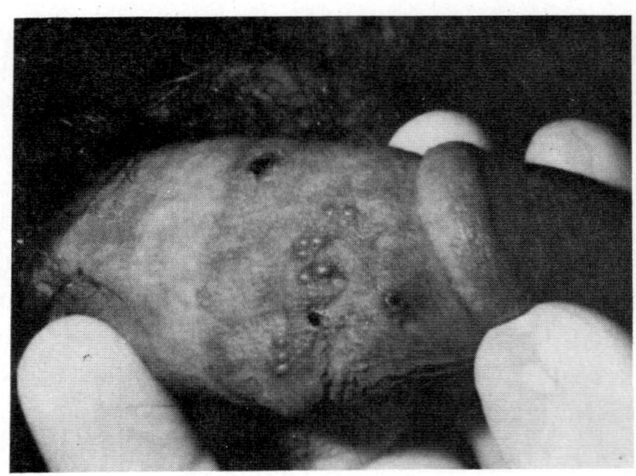

**Figure 37–2.** Multiple grouped vesicles of genital herpes.

**Recurrent Genital Infection.** In contrast to primary infection, recurrent genital herpes is a disease of shorter duration, usually localized in the genital region, without systemic symptoms. One of the characteristic symptoms is prodromal paresthesia in the perineum, genitalia, or buttocks 12 to 24 hours before the appearance of lesions. Recurrent genital herpes usually presents with grouped vesicular lesions in the external genital region. Local symptoms such as pain and itching are mild and last 4 to 5 days. The mean duration of viral shedding is 4 days, and lesions usually last 10 to 14 days.

Prodromal parasthesias and shorter duration

At least 80% of patients with primary genital HSV-2 infection develop recurrent episodes of genital herpes within 12 months. Genital HSV-1 infection appears to recur less frequently. In patients whose lesions recur, the median number of recurrences is four or five per year. They are not evenly spaced, and some patients experience a succession of monthly attacks followed by a period of quiescence. Most recurrences result from reactivation of virus from S3–S4 dorsal root ganglia. Rarely, recurrent infections may be due to reinfections with different strains of HSV-2.

Genital HSV-1 less common

**Neonatal Herpes.** Neonatal herpes usually results from transmission of disease during delivery by contact with infected genital secretions from the mother. In utero infection, although possible, is uncommon. The prevalence rate of neonatal herpes varies greatly among populations, but is estimated at approximately 1 per 2500 live births in the United States. This estimate is based on the observation that about 0.5 to 1.0% of women excreting HSV from the cervix at the onset of labor and about 6% of babies born through infected birth canals develop neonatal HSV. Because a normal immune response is absent in the neonate, neonatal HSV infection is an extremely severe disease with an overall mortality of approximately 60%, and neurologic sequelae are high in those who survive. Manifestations vary; some infants show disseminated vesicular lesions with a widespread internal organ involvement and necrosis of the liver and adrenal glands. The mortality of such disseminated disease is more than 90%. Some infants have involvement of the central nervous system only, with listlessness and seizures.

Transmitted from mother at birth or in utero

High mortality if disseminated

### Laboratory Diagnosis

Herpes simplex viruses are best demonstrated by isolation in fibroblast or a variety of other cell lines inoculated with infected secretions or lesions. The cytopathic effects of HSV can usually be demonstrated 24 to 96 hours after inoculation. Isolates of HSV-1 and HSV-2 can be differentiated by staining virus-infected cells with type-specific monoclonal antibodies to the two types or by analyzing restriction enzyme digests of purified viral DNA (see Chapter 14). Restriction endonuclease digests can also be used to define epidemiologic relationships, that is, strains acquired between sexual partners or through mother–infant transmission. A smear prepared from the base of the lesions and stained by either the Giemsa or Papanicolaou method may show intranuclear inclusions or multinucleated giant cells typical of herpes (Tzanck test), but is less sensitive than viral culture. Enzyme immunoassays have been developed for direct detection of herpes antigen in lesions. Although early versions of these noncultural tests lacked sensitivity, more recent procedures have correlations with culture that approach 90%. Serology should not be used to diagnose active HSV in-

Grow rapidly in many cell culture systems

HSV-1 and -2 distinguished by type-specific monoclonal antibodies

Direct detection EIAs have improving sensitivity

fection, for example, genital or encephalitis; frequently there is no change in antibody titer when reactivation occurs.

### Prevention

No specific form of prevention is available. Avoiding contact with individuals with lesions reduces the risk of spread; however, virus may still be shed asymptomatically from the saliva, urethra, and cervix. Because of the high morbidity and mortality of neonatal infection, special attention must be paid to prevention of spread from infected mothers. In many cases abdominal delivery (caesarean section) may be used to minimize contact of the infant with infected maternal genital secretions. Caesarean section may not be effective if rupture of the membranes precedes delivery.

Caesarean section may be done to prevent neonatal infection

### Treatment

Several antiviral drugs directed at inhibiting virus-specified enzymes have been developed. The most effective and commonly used is the nucleoside analog acyclovir (see Chapter 13), which is converted by viral enzymes to a monophosphate and then by cellular enzymes to the triphosphate form, which is a potent inhibitor of the viral DNA polymerase. Acyclovir decreases the duration of primary infection and recurrent mucocutaneous HSV infections but does not eliminate viral shedding. If taken daily it can also suppress recurrences of genital and oral–labial HSV. In its intravenous form it is effective in reducing mortality of HSV encephalitis and neonatal herpes. Acyclovir-resistant HSV has been recovered from immunocompromised (especially AIDS) patients with persistent lesions. Foscarnet is active against acyclovir-resistant HSV and is an alternative to acyclovir. No antiviral agents have been developed that decrease the risk of subsequent reactivation of disease.

Acyclovir can decrease duration of acute and recurrent disease

## VARICELLA–ZOSTER VIRUS

Varicella–zoster virus (VZV), the cause of both varicella (chickenpox) and herpes zoster, has the same general structure as herpes simplex but its own set of envelope glycoproteins and other structures. Cellular features of infected cells such as ballooning degeneration, formation of giant cells, and nuclear eosinophilic inclusion bodies are similar to those of HSV. VZV is more difficult to isolate in cell culture than HSV and grows best in diploid fibroblast cells. Compared with HSV, it has a narrower host range and a slower replicative cycle. The virus has a marked tendency to remain attached to the membrane of the host cell with less release of virions into fluids.

Slower growth and narrower range of infected cell types

## Varicella–Zoster Virus Disease

### Epidemiology

Varicella–zoster virus infection is ubiquitous. Nearly all persons contract chickenpox before adulthood, and 90% of cases occur before the age of 10. The virus is highly contagious, with attack rates among susceptible contacts of 75%. Varicella occurs most frequently during the winter and spring months. The incubation period is 11 to 21 days. The major mode of transmission is respiratory, although direct contact with vesicular or pustular lesions may result in disease. Infectivity is greatest 24 to 48 hours before the onset of rash and lasts 3 to 4 days into the rash. Virus is rarely isolated from crusted lesions.

Chickenpox acquired by respiratory route and before adulthood

Infectivity greatest before rash

### Pathogenesis

The relationship between zoster and varicella was first described by Von Bokay in 1892, when he observed several instances of varicella in households after the introduction of a case of zoster. On the basis of these epidemiologic observations, he proposed that zoster and varicella were different clinical manifestations of a single agent. The cultivation of VZV in vitro by Weller in 1954 confirmed Von Bokay's hypothesis: the viruses isolated from chickenpox and from varicella–zoster were identical. Latency of varicella–zoster occurs in

Varicella virus latent in ganglion cells and reactivation produces zoster

ganglia, and VZV genome has been demonstrated by in situ hybridization methods in dorsal root ganglia of adults many years after varicella infection.

### Immunity

Circulating antibody prevents reinfection; cell-mediated immunity controls reactivation

Both humoral immunity and cell-mediated immunity are important factors in determining the frequency of reactivation and severity of varicella–zoster. Circulating antibody prevents reinfection, and cell-mediated immunity appears to control reactivation. In patients with depressed cell-mediated immune responses, especially those with bone marrow transplants, Hodgkin's disease, AIDS, and lymphoproliferative disorders, reactivation can occur and VZV infections are more frequent and more severe.

## ■ Varicella–Zoster Disease: Clinical Aspects

### Clinical Manifestations

Chickenpox and herpes zoster (shingles)

Varicella–zoster virus produces a primary infection in normal children characterized by a generalized vesicular rash termed *chickenpox*. After clinical infection resolves, the virus may persist for decades in the absence of clinical manifestation. Reactivation of latent virus results in a unilateral vesicular eruption, generally in a dermatomal distribution, that is clinically diagnosed as herpes zoster or "shingles."

Chickenpox lesions widespread and pruritic

Chickenpox lesions generally appear on the back of the head and ears, then spread centrifugally to the face, neck, trunk, and extremities. Involvement of mucous membranes is common, and fever may occur early in the course of disease. Lesions appear in different stages of evolution; this characteristic was one of the major features used to differentiate varicella from smallpox, in which lesions were concentrated on the extremities and appeared at the same stage of disease. Varicella lesions are pruritic (itchy), and the number of vesicles may vary from 10 to several hundred.

Severe disease in immunocompromised patients

Immunocompromised children may develop progressive varicella, which is associated with prolonged viremia, visceral dissemination, and the development of pneumonia, encephalitis, hepatitis, and nephritis. Progressive varicella has an estimated mortality of approximately 20%.

Reactivation to zoster most common in elderly

Zoster lesions follow sensory nerve distribution

Reactivation of VZV is associated with the disease herpes zoster. Although zoster is seen in patients of all ages, it increases in frequency with advancing age. Clinically, pain in a sensory nerve route distribution may herald the onset of the eruption, which occurs several days to a week or two later. The vesicular eruption is usually unilateral, involving one to three dermatomes (Fig 37–3). New lesions may appear over the first 5 to 7 days. Multiple attacks of VZV infection are uncommon; if recurrent attacks of a vesicular eruption occur in one area of the body, HSV infection should be considered.

Postherpetic neuralgia after zoster

The complications of VZV infection are varied and depend on age and host immune factors. Postherpetic neuralgia is a common complication of herpes zoster in elderly adults.

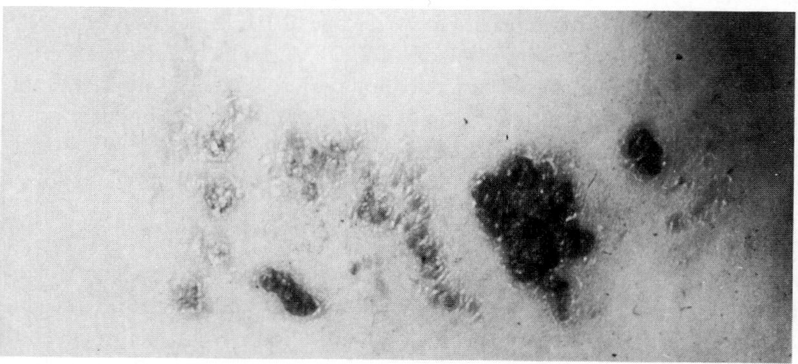

**Figure 37–3.** Herpes zoster lesion of the thorax. Note dermatomal distribution and presence of vesicles, pustules, and ulcerated and crusted lesions.

It involves persistence of severe pain in the dermatome after resolution of the lesions of zoster and appears to result from damage to the involved nerve root. Immunosuppressed patients may develop localized zoster followed by disseminated virus with visceral infection, which resembles progressive varicella. Bacterial superinfection is also possible.

Disseminated zoster and visceral spread in the immunocompromised

### Laboratory Diagnosis

Varicella or herpes zoster lesions can be readily diagnosed clinically although they may occasionally be difficult to distinguish from those caused by HSV. For confirmation, scrapings of lesions in which to look for multinucleated giant cells may be useful. The virus can be isolated from aspirated vesicular fluid inoculated onto human diploid fibroblasts; however, the virus is difficult to grow from zoster ("shingles") lesions older than 5 days and cytopathic effects are usually not seen for 5 to 9 days. For rapid viral diagnosis, varicella–zoster antigen may be demonstrated in cells from lesions by immunofluorescent antibody staining.

Diagnosis usually clinical

Rapid confirmation by immunofluorescent staining

### Prevention

High-titer immune globulin administered within 96 hours of exposure is useful in preventing infection or ameliorating disease in patients at risk for primary infection (ie, varicella) and serious complications. Immunosuppressed children who are household or play contacts of patients with primary varicella are candidates for this immunoprophylaxis. Once infection has occurred, high-titer immune globulin has not proved useful in ameliorating disease or preventing dissemination. Immune globulin is not indicated for the treatment or prevention of reactivation (ie, zoster or "shingles"). In nonimmunosuppressed children varicella is a relatively mild disease, and passive immunization is not indicated. Varicella is a highly contagious disease, and rigid isolation precautions must be instituted in all hospitalized cases.

Passive immunization for immunocompromised

Need for isolation of cases in hospital

A live vaccine developed by a group of Japanese workers appears to be effective in both immunosuppressed and immunocompetent persons. Given the relative benignity of varicella in immunocompetent children, it is not clear that VZV vaccine should be given to healthy infants, especially if immunity wanes and thus places the patient at risk of varicella as an adult, but the vaccine is being used routinely for infants in Japan and several European countries. In immunocompromised children who are susceptible to varicella, chickenpox can be extremely serious, even fatal. In these children, the live vaccine appears to be protective and indicated to prevent severe disease.

Live vaccine under evaluation

### Treatment

Acyclovir has been shown to reduce fever and skin lesions in patients with varicella and some authorities feel its use is indicated in healthy children and adults. In immunosuppressed patients, controlled trials of acyclovir have shown efficacy in reducing dissemination and its use is definitely indicated. In addition, controlled trials of acyclovir have demonstrated effectiveness in the treatment of herpes zoster in immunocompromised patients. Acyclovir may be used to treat herpes zoster in immunocompetent adults, but it appears to have only a modest impact on the development of postherpetic neuralgia, the most important complication of zoster.

Acyclovir chemotherapy in immunocompromised patients

## ■ CYTOMEGALOVIRUS

Human cytomegalovirus (CMV) possesses the largest genome of the herpesviruses. In addition to the nuclear inclusions characteristic of HSV and varicella–zoster, CMV produces perinuclear cytoplasmic inclusions and enlargement of the cell (cytomegaly). Strains of CMV demonstrate considerable genomic and phenotypic heterogeneity. Antigenic variations have been observed, but are not of clinical importance. As with HSV, restriction endonuclease analysis of viral DNA has been useful for distinguishing strains epidemiologically.

Nuclear and perinuclear cytopolasmic inclusions and cell enlargement

## Cytomegalovirus Disease

### Epidemiology

High infection rates in early childhood and early adulthood

Present in saliva, urine, semen, and cervical secretions

Cytomegalovirus is ubiquitous, and in the developed countries approximately 50% of adults have antibody to it. Age-specific prevalence rates show that approximately 10 to 15% of children are infected by CMV during the first 5 years of life, after which the rate of new infections levels off. The rate subsequently increases during young adulthood, probably through sexual transmission of disease. The virus has been isolated from saliva, cervical secretions, semen, urine, and white blood cells; it may be isolated from patients with circulating neutralizing antibody. Latent infection, which may reside in leukocytes and their precursors, accounts for transfusion-associated disease. More than one third of infants born to CMV-negative mothers who received blood from donors with CMV antibody may subsequently develop infection. Although most infections from transfusions of CMV-contaminated blood may be asymptomatic, persistent fever, hepatitis, pneumonitis, or all three may occur. Granulocyte transfusions may also lead to transmission of CMV. Excretion of virus is prolonged after congenital and perinatal infections, probably because of immunologic tolerance. High titers of virus have been isolated for more than 5 years after birth. Transmission of infection in day-care centers has been shown to occur from asymptomatic excretors to other children and seronegative parents. Immunocompromised adults, as well as sexually promiscuous homosexual men, also excrete virus for prolonged periods.

Viral latency in leukocytes: transmission by transfusions

Prolonged excretion and infectivity with congenital or perinatal infections

### Pathogenesis and Immunity

CMV DNA in normal monocytes

Cytomegalovirus infects epithelial cells and leukocytes. In epithelial cells it produces intranuclear inclusions and eccentrically placed intracytoplasmic inclusions surrounded by a clear halo, resulting in an "owl's eye" appearance. In vitro, CMV DNA can be demonstrated in monocytes showing no cytopathology, indicating a restricted growth potential in these cells.

Disease in immunocompetent individuals related only to primary infection

Both humoral and cellular immune responses are important in CMV infections. In immunocompetent persons, almost all clinical disease is related to primary infection, but subclinical reactivation with viral excretion in cervical excretions or semen can occur despite high circulating levels of antibody. During primary infections, CMV infection of monocytes results in dysfunction of these phagocytes. In immunocompromised patients this increases predisposition to fungal and bacterial superinfection.

## Cytomegalovirus Disease: Clinical Aspects

### Clinical Manifestations

Teratogenicity when primary CMV infection occurs during pregnancy

Worldwide, 1% of infants excrete CMV in urine or nasopharynx at delivery as a result of infection in utero. On physical examination, 90% of these infants appear normal; however, long-term follow-up has indicated that 20% go on to develop sensory nerve hearing loss, psychomotor mental retardation, or both. The infants with symptomatic illness (about 0.1% of all births) may have a variety of congenital defects or other disorders (hepatosplenomegaly, jaundice, anemia, thrombocytopenia, low birth weight, microcephaly, and chorioretinitis). Almost all babies with clinically evident congenital CMV infection are born of mothers who experience primary CMV infection during the pregnancy. Congenital infection frequently also results from reactivation in the mother with spread to the fetus, but such infection rarely, if ever, leads to congenital abnormalities.

Perinatal infection asymptomatic or relatively benign

In contrast to the devastating findings with some congenital infections, neonatal infection acquired during or shortly after birth appears to be associated with no adverse outcome. Most population-based studies have indicated that 10 to 15% of all mothers are excreting CMV from the cervix at delivery. Approximately one third to one half of all infants born to these mothers acquire infection. Almost all of these perinatally infected infants have no discernible illness unless the baby is premature or immunocompromised. CMV can also be efficiently transmitted from mother to child by breast milk, but these postpartum infections are also usually benign.

Most childhood CMV infections are asymptomatic

As with intrapartum acquisition of infection most CMV infections during childhood and adulthood are totally asymptomatic. In young adults, CMV may cause a mononucleosis-like syndrome. In immunosuppressed patients, latent CMV may be reactivated, possibly resulting in diffuse involvement of the lung and severe hypoxia (CMV pneumonia). In patients receiving bone marrow transplants, interstitial pneumonia caused by CMV is the leading cause of death (90% mortality). In AIDS patients CMV often disseminates to visceral organs, causing chorioretinitis, gastroenteritis, neurologic disorders, and disease in other organs.

CMV pneumonia, visceral, and eye infections in immunosuppressed and AIDS patients

### Laboratory Diagnosis

Laboratory diagnosis of CMV infection depends on (1) detecting CMV cytopathology antigen or DNA in infected tissues, (2) isolating the virus from tissue or secretions, or (3) demonstrating seroconversion. Cytomegalovirus can be grown readily in serially propagated diploid fibroblast cell lines. Demonstration of cytopathic effect generally requires 3 to 14 days, depending on the concentration of virus in the specimen. The presence of large inclusion-bearing cells in urine sediment may be detected in widespread CMV infection. This technique is insensitive, however, and provides positive results only when large quantities of virus are present in the urine.

Culture, antigen detection and, serodiagnosis useful

Because of the high prevalence of asymptomatic carriers and the known tendency of CMV to persist weeks or months in infected individuals, it is frequently difficult to associate a specific disease entity with the isolation of the virus from a peripheral site. Thus, the isolation of CMV from urine of immunosuppressed patients with interstitial pneumonia does not constitute evidence of CMV as the etiology of that illness. CMV pneumonia or gastrointestinal disease is best diagnosed by demonstrating CMV inclusions in biopsy tissue.

Difficulty in establishing relationship of viral isolation to disease

CMV inclusion cells in urine insensitive

### Prevention and Therapy

The use of blood from CMV seronegative donors or blood that is treated to remove white cells decreases transfusion-associated CMV. Similarly, the disease can be avoided in seronegative transplant recipients by using organs from CMV seronegative donors. Hyperimmune human anti-CMV globulin has been used to ameliorate CMV disease associated with renal transplants. There are experimental data suggesting that the use of condoms would decrease sexual transmission of CMV. A live attenuated CMV vaccine has been evaluated but not generally accepted for use in prospective transplant recipients.

Use of CMV seronegative donors decreases risk

Ganciclovir, a nucleoside analog of acyclovir, has been shown to inhibit CMV replication and reduce the severity of some CMV syndromes, such as retinitis and possibly gastrointestinal disease. When given with hyperimmune globulin, ganciclovir reduces the very high mortality of CMV pneumonia in bone marrow transplant patients. Foscarnet is a second approved drug for therapy of CMV disease and is equally efficacious. Its toxic effects are primarily renal with electrolyte disturbances, whereas ganciclovir is most apt to inhibit bone marrow function. Ganciclovir inhibits CMV DNA polymerase as does foscarnet, but they act on different sites and cross resistance is rare.

Ganciclovir given with hyperimmune globulin

## ■ EPSTEIN–BARR VIRUS

Epstein–Barr virus is the etiologic agent of infectious mononucleosis and African Burkitt's lymphoma. Although morphologically similar to the other herpesviruses, EBV is unique in that it can be cultured easily only in lymphoblastoid cell lines derived from B lymphocytes of humans and higher primates. The virus generally does not produce cytopathic effects or the characteristic intranuclear inclusions of other herpesvirus infections. After infection with EBV, lymphoblastoid cells containing viral genome can be cultivated continuously in vitro; they are thus transformed, or immortalized. Recent studies suggest that most of the viral DNA in transformed cells remains in circular, nonintegrated form as an episome. Viral antigen expression has been studied by immunofluorescent staining of transformed cell lines under various conditions. One group of proteins called EBV nuclear antigens (EBNAs) appear in the nucleus prior to virus-directed protein synthesis. Viral capsid antigen (VCA) can be detected in cell lines that produce mature virions. Other cell lines, called nonproducers, contain no mature virions, but express certain virus-associated antigens called early antigens (EAs).

Etiologic agent of infectious mononucleosis and Burkitt's lymphoma

Cultivated only in lymphoblastoid cell lines

EBNA, VCA, EA represent stages of viral replication

Epstein–Barr virus has been shown to replicate in vitro and in vivo in epithelial cells

Replication in epithelial cells of mouth and cervix

of both the mouth and cervix. This helps explain the observation that EBV can be cultured from saliva of some asymptomatic patients. Excretion may persist weeks to months. At present there appears to be much fewer genomic strain variations among EBV isolates than other herpesviruses.

## Epstein–Barr Virus Disease

### Epidemiology

Low contagiousness requires spread by repeated contact

Transfusion associated

Infection with EBV is acquired by contact with infected secretions such as saliva. The virus can be cultured from throat washings from 10 to 20% of normal healthy adults and from 50% of renal transplant recipients. It is of low contagiousness, and most cases of infectious mononucleosis are contracted after repeated contact between susceptible persons and those asymptomatically shedding the virus. Secondary attack rates of infectious mononucleosis are low (less than 10%), because most family or household contacts already have antibody to the agent. Infectious mononucleosis has also been transmitted by blood transfusion, and infections have developed after open heart surgery. Most transfusion-associated mononucleosis syndromes, however, are attributable to CMV.

Association with Burkitt's lymphoma and nasopharyngeal carcinoma

Epstein–Barr virus has been implicated in several malignancies including African Burkitt's lymphoma, anaplastic nasopharyngeal carcinoma (a common neoplasm in southeast China), and certain B-cell lymphomas. Epstein–Barr virus DNA is found in cells of nearly all Burkitt's lymphomas and nasopharyngeal carcinomas and in half of the cases of B-cell lymphomas that occur in immunosuppressed and AIDS patients. The precise etiologic relationship between EBV and these tumors still remains unclear. One theory is that polyclonal stimulation and proliferation of B cells increase the chance of a chromosomal translocation occurring with selective proliferation of the aberrant B-cell clone.

### Pathogenesis

Productive infection of B lymphocytes

Infected B lymphocytes produce antibody and surface antigens

Although EBV initially infects epithelial cells, the hallmark of EBV disease is productive infection of B lymphocytes. The virus enters B lymphocytes by means of envelope glycoprotein binding to surface complement (C3d) receptor; 18 to 24 hours later EBV nuclear antigens are detectable within the nucleus of infected cells. Expression of the viral genome, which encodes at least two viral proteins, is associated with immortalization and proliferation of the cell. The EBV-infected B lymphocytes are polyclonally activated to produce immunoglobulin and express a lymphocyte-determined membrane antigen that is the target of host cellular immune responses to virus-infected B lymphocytes. Only a minority of virus-infected cells transcribe all the viral proteins; these cells are, thus, lytically infected and succumb. During the acute phase of infectious mononucleosis, up to 20% of circulating B lymphocytes demonstrate EBV antigens. After infection subsides, EBV can be isolated from only about 1% of such cells.

Tumors may involve cofactors

The Epstein–Barr virus has been associated with two types of tumors, African Burkitt's lymphoma and nasopharyngeal carcinoma. The factors that render the EBV infections oncogenic in these two cases are obscure. The distribution of EBV infections in Africa has suggested an infectious cofactor, such as human immunodeficiency virus or malaria infections, which may cause immunosuppression and predispose to EBV-related malignancy. Parts of the EBV genome are found in Burkitt's lymphoma cells.

EBV DNA integrated or as plasmid

In vitro, EBV transforms B lymphocytes into lymphoblast-like cells that are able to multiply indefinitely. The DNA genome of the virus is present in the nucleus of transformed cells either integrated into the genome or more often as an extrachromosomal plasmid in multiple copies. Only partial transcription of viral proteins occurs (about 10 of the 60 to 70 genes). Two of these have been shown to be transforming genes, but the precise mechanisms by which transformation occurs are unclear.

Translocations may lead to clonal activation

In the in vivo situation, EBV-associated lymphomas have been shown to be of both monoclonal and polyclonal origin. Chromosomal translocations in B cells are characteristic of Burkitt's lymphoma and involve specific breaks in chromosomes at sites of genes encoding immunoglobulins. These translocations lead to expression of oncogenes that may contribute to clonal activation and ultimately to malignancy. Some breakdown in immune surveillance also appears to play a role in the development of malignancy because immunosuppressed patients are more prone to develop B-cell lymphomas.

The two classes of cancer associated with EBV are most common in restricted geographic areas, which offers the possibility of prevention by immunization with virus-specific antigen(s). This approach is under exploration at present. A subunit vaccine has proved effective in preventing the development of tumors in tamarin monkeys, which are highly susceptible to the oncogenic effects of the virus under experimental conditions.

### Immunity

Virus-induced infectious mononucleosis results in the synthesis of circulating antibodies against viral antigens, as well as against unrelated antigens found in sheep, horse, and some beef red blood cells. These heterophile antibodies, a heterogeneous group of predominantly IgM antibodies long known to correlate with episodes of infectious mononucleosis, are commonly used as diagnostic tests for the disease. They do not cross-react with antibodies specific for EBV, but there is no good correlation between the heterophile antibody titer and the severity of illness. Some other immunologic functions are also affected by EBV infection. Cutaneous anergy and decreased cellular immune responses to mitogens and antigens are seen early in the course of mononucleosis.

Antiviral and heterophile antibodies produced

Decreased cellular immune responses

The lymphocytosis associated with infectious mononucleosis is caused by an increase in the number of circulating T cells. It has been hypothesized that the atypical lymphocytes are activated cells developed in response to the virus-infected B lymphocytes. With recovery from illness, the atypical lymphocytosis gradually resolves and cell-mediated immune functions return to preinfection levels, although memory T cells maintain the capacity to limit proliferation of infected B cells.

Atypical lymphocytes in infectious mononucleosis are T cells

## Epstein–Barr Virus Disease: Clinical Aspects

### Infectious Mononucleosis

Infection is widespread. Antibodies to EBV occur in all population groups studied and are usually found in 90 to 95% of adults. Most early infections are asymptomatic; clinically apparent EBV infection occurs most frequently in populations in which primary EBV exposure has been delayed until the second decade of life. The disease is thus seen most often in young adults; it consists of a constellation of clinical findings, including fever, lymphadenopathy (especially in the cervical area), sore throat, and fatigue and malaise, which may last from days to several weeks.

Widespread asymptomatic infection: disease most common in young adults

Infectious mononucleosis syndrome includes fever, fatigue

### Laboratory Diagnosis

Laboratory analysis of EBV-induced infectious mononucleosis is usually documented by the demonstration of atypical lymphocytes, heterophile antibodies, or positive EBV-specific serologic findings. Hematologic examination reveals a markedly raised lymphocyte and monocyte count with more than 10% atypical lymphocytes, called Downey cells (Fig 37–4). Atypical lymphocytes, although not specific for EBV, are present with the onset of symp-

Tests for heterophile or specific antiviral antibodies used

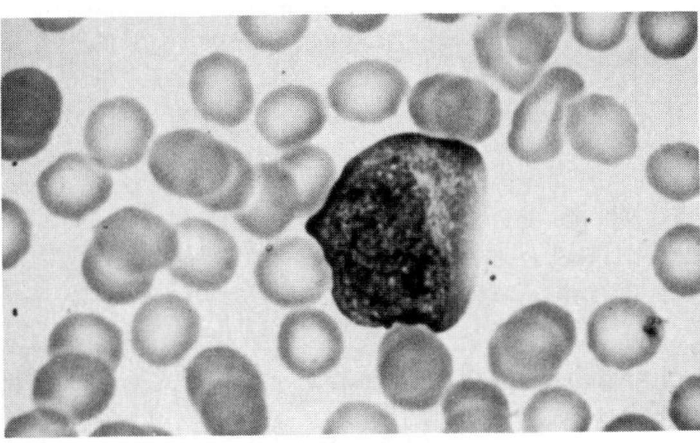

**Figure 37–4.** Atypical lymphocyte (Downey cell) in blood smear from a patient with infectious mononucleosis. Note indented cell membrane.

toms and disappear with resolution of disease. Alterations in liver function tests may also occur, and enlargement of the liver and spleen is a frequent finding.

Heterophile antibodies non-specific but appear early

Although not specific for EBV, tests for heterophile antibodies are used most commonly for diagnosis of infectious mononucleosis. In commercial kits animal erythrocytes are used in simple slide agglutination methods which incorporate absorptions to remove cross-reacting antibodies that may develop in other situations, such as serum sickness. The infectious mononucleosis heterophile antibody is absorbed by sheep erythrocytes but not by a guinea pig kidney homogenate. Heterophile antibodies can usually be demonstrated by the end of the first week of illness, but may occasionally be delayed until the third or fourth week. They may persist many months.

EBV VCA antibody typical for acute disease

Approximately 5 to 15% of EBV-induced cases of infectious mononucleosis in adults and a much greater proportion in young children and infants fail to induce detectable levels of heterophile antibodies. In these cases the EVB-specific serologic tests summarized in Table 37–2 may be used to establish the diagnosis. The most commonly used test is for antibodies to VCA which rise quickly in disease and persists for life. The presence of IgM antibody to VCA is theoretically diagnostic of acute, primary EBV infection, but low levels may occur during reactivation of EBV and cross-reactivation with antigens of other herpesviruses occur. Antibodies to EBNAs rise later in disease (after about 1 month) and also persist in low titers for life. Thus, a high titer to VCA and no titer to EBNAs are indicative of recent EBV infection, whereas antibody titers to both antigens are indicative of past infection. Isolation of EBV from clinical specimens is not practical because it requires fresh human B cells or fetal lymphocytes obtained from cord blood.

## Treatment and Prevention

Treatment supportive

Treatment of infectious mononucleosis is largely supportive. More than 95% of patients recover uneventfully. In a small percentage of patients, splenic rupture may occur; thus, restriction of contact sports or heavy lifting during the acute illness is recommended. The DNA polymerase enzyme of EBV has been shown to be sensitive to acyclovir, and acy-

**TABLE 37–2. EPSTEIN–BARR VIRUS-SPECIFIC ANTIBODIES**

| Antibody Specificity | Time of Appearance in Infectious Mononucleosis | Duration | Comments |
|---|---|---|---|
| Viral capsid antigen | | | |
| IgM | Early in illness | 1–2 months | Indicator of primary infection |
| IgG | Early in illness | Lifelong | Standard EBV titer reported by most commercial and state labs; major utility is as a marker for prior infection in epidemiologic studies; if present in the absence of EBNA antibody, indicates current infection |
| EBNA IgG | 3–6 weeks after onset | Lifelong | Late appearance of anti-EBNA IgG antibodies in IM makes absence or seroconversion a useful marker for primary infection; persists for life |
| Early antigen | | | |
| EA diffuse protein | Peaks 3–4 weeks after onset | 3–6 months | Present in IM patients; IgA antibodies useful for prediction of NPC in high-risk populations |
| EA restricted | Several weeks after onset | Months to years | Present in higher titer in African Burkitt's lymphoma; may be useful as indicator of reactivation of EBV |

*Abbreviations:* EA, early antigen; EBV, Epstein–Barr virus; IM, infectious mononucleosis; NPC, nasopharyngeal carcinoma; EBNA, EBV nuclear antigen.

clovir can decrease the amount of replication of EBV in tissue culture and in vivo. Despite this antiviral activity, systemic acyclovir makes little impact on the clinical illness. No vaccine is available.

## ■ HUMAN HERPESVIRUS TYPE 6

In 1986 a new human herpesvirus, now called human herpesvirus type 6 (HHV-6), was identified in cultures of peripheral blood mononuclear cells from patients with lympoproliferative diseases. The virus, which is genetically distinct but morphologically similar to other herpesviruses, replicates in lymphoid tissue and is cytopathic for T lymphocytes in cell culture. It appears to be the etiologic agent of exanthema subitum (roseola infantum, see Chapter 33), but its relationship to other human infections is presently unclear.

Associated with roseola infantum

Initially it was thought that HHV-6 would grow only in freshly isolated B lymphocytes and the virus was referred to as the human B-lymphotropic virus. Now it is clear that the virus is preferentially tropic for T lymphocytes. HHV-6 establishes a latent infection in T cells but may be activated to a productive lytic infection by mitogenic stimulation. Resting lymphocytes and lymphocytes from normal immune individuals are resistant to HHV-6 infection. In vivo, HHV-6 replication is controlled by cell-mediated immune factors. It appears to be capable of reactivating in immunosuppressed patients, but its clinical significance in this situation is unknown.

Latent infection of T cells

Serologic studies indicate that almost all children are infected by age 5. This makes HHV-6 the most communicable of all human herpesviruses. Most likely, it is spread by close personal contact or by the respiratory route.

## ■ HUMAN HERPESVIRUS TYPE 7

Isolation of human herpesvirus type 7 (HHV-7) was first reported in 1990. The virus was isolated from activated CD4$^+$ T lymphocytes of a healthy individual. HHV-7 is distinct from all other known human herpesviruses but is most closely related to HHV-6. Seroepidemologic studies indicate that this virus infects most children by the age of 2 years, and 97% of adults are seropositive. As of 1993 the clinical correlates of HHV-7 were not yet clear. Culture of this virus is performed only in specialized virology laboratories and is not available on a routine basis. The diagnosis of acute infection can be made by the demonstration of seroconversion.

## ADDITIONAL READING


Corey LC, Spear PG. Infections with herpes simplex viruses. *N Engl J Med.* 1986;314:686–691, 749–757. A two-part series reviewing the biology and pathogenesis of herpes simplex virus infections.

Drew L. Cytomegalovirus infection in patients with AIDS. *Clin Infect Dis.* 1992;14:608–615.

Gershon AA, et al. Varicella vaccine: The American experience. *J Infect Dis.* 1992;166(suppl 1):S63–S68. Live attenuated varicella vaccine is safe and effective in preventing chickenpox. The best immune responses occur in healthy children. Leukemic children have a 50% incidence of mild-to-moderate adverse effects but have a high degree of protection once immune reactions to varicella–zoster virus have developed.

Ho M. *Cytomegalovirus, Biology and Infection.* New York: Plenum; 1991. A valuable monograph on cytomegalovirus.

Mertz GJ, et al. Risk factors for the sexual transmission of genital herpes. *Ann Intern Med.* 1992;116:197–202. Despite clear recognition of genital herpes in source partners, there was substantial risk for transmission; in 70% of patients, transmission appeared to result from sexual contact during periods of asymptomatic viral shedding.

Niza F, et al. Isolation of a new herpesvirus from human CD4$^+$ T cells. *Proc Natl Acad Sci USA.* 1990;87:748–752. A new human herpesvirus has been isolated from CD4$^+$ T cells purified from peripheral blood mononuclear cells of a healthy individual, following incubation of the cells under conditions promoting T-cell activation.

Oren I, Sobel JD. Human herpesvirus type 6: Review. *Clin Infect Dis.* 1992;14:741–746. Human herpesvirus type 6 (HHV-6), a newly recognized human herpesvirus, is morphologically similar to other herpesviruses but is distinguishable from all of them by restriction digest analysis of DNA. Infection in infancy develops as levels of maternal antibody wane, thus resulting in either subclinical infection or an acute febrile illness termed *exanthema subitum* (roseola infantum).

Van der Horst C, et al. Lack of effect of peroral acyclovir for the treatment of acute infectious mononucleosis. *J Infect Dis*. 1991;164:788–792. One hundred twenty patients received 600 mg of acyclovir or placebo five times daily for 10 days. Analysis of mean values and time to resolution of fever, lymphadenopathy, weight change, hepatomegaly, splenomegaly, liver function tests, atypical lymphocytes, hours of bed rest, sense of well-being, and return to normal activities revealed no significant differences. There was a trend toward suppression of Epstein–Barr virus excretion in the oropharynx in acyclovir recipients. No toxicity was detected in patients treated with acyclovir.

Chapter 38

# Viruses of Diarrhea

C. George Ray

Acute diarrheal disease is an illness, usually of rapid evolution (within several hours), that lasts less than 3 weeks. A variety of infectious agents can be responsible; overall, bacteria and protozoa have been implicated as etiologic agents in approximately 20 to 25% of cases. In many of the remaining cases, viruses have been considered as the cause. Unfortunately, investigations have been hampered because most of these viruses cannot be readily cultivated in the laboratory.

Most cultivated with difficulty or not at all

Until the 1970s, proof of viral causation of acute diarrhea was usually based on exclusion of known bacterial or protozoan pathogens and supported by feeding cell-free filtrates of diarrheal stools to volunteers in an attempt to reproduce the disease. As might be expected, the results of such experiments were variable, and the methods were impractical for routine laboratory diagnosis.

One aspect of such infections that proved of great help was the frequent association with abundant excretion of virus particles during the acute phase of illness. Virion numbers in excess of $10^8$ per gram of diarrheal stool are relatively common, allowing ready visualization with an electron microscope. Direct electron microscopy and immunoelectron microscopy have been frequently employed to detect and identify the presumed causative viruses; the latter method can also be used to detect humoral antibody responses to infection.

Many viral particles in stool

Visualization by electron microscopy

Visualization of a specific virus in the stools of symptomatic patients is not sufficient to establish the role of the virus in causing disease. Other criteria to be fulfilled include the following: (1) establish that the virus is detected in ill patients significantly more frequently than in asymptomatic, appropriately matched controls and that virus shedding temporally correlates with symptoms; (2) demonstrate significant humoral or secretory antibody responses, or both, in patients shedding the virus; (3) reproduce the disease by experimental inoculation of nonimmune human or animal hosts (usually the most difficult criterion to fulfill); (4) exclude other known causes of diarrhea, such as bacteria, bacterial toxins, and protozoa. Using these criteria, four groups of viruses have been clearly established as important causes of gastrointestinal disease: rotaviruses, Norwalk or Norwalk-like viruses, astroviruses, and some adenovirus serotypes. Other viruses have also been implicated, but all of the preceding criteria have not been fulfilled, however, they are currently regarded only as "candidate" causes of gastrointestinal disease.

Multiple criteria for establishing etiologic relationship

Rotaviruses, Norwalk viruses, astroviruses, adenoviruses, and other "candidate" viruses

The currently established and candidate viruses are listed in Table 38–1 and all have several features in common, including a tendency toward brief incubation periods, fecal–oral spread by direct or indirect routes, and production of vomiting, which generally precedes or accompanies the diarrhea. The last feature has influenced physicians to use the term **acute viral gastroenteritis** to describe the syndrome associated with these agents.

TABLE 38–1. BIOLOGIC AND EPIDEMIOLOGIC CHARACTERISTICS OF VIRUSES CAUSING DIARRHEA

| Special Features | Rotavirus | Norwalk and Norwalk-like Viruses | Astrovirus | Adenovirus | Coronavirus-like |
|---|---|---|---|---|---|
| Biological | | | | | |
| Nucleic acid | Double-stranded RNA | Single-stranded RNA | ?Single-stranded RNA | Double-stranded DNA | Unknown |
| Diameter, shape | 65–70 nm, naked, double-shelled capsid | 27–38 nm, naked, round | 28–38 nm, naked, star-shaped | 70–90 nm, naked, icosahedral | 80–300 nm, enveloped, pleomorphic |
| Replication in cell culture | Usually incomplete | None | None | None or incomplete | None |
| Number of serotypes | 4 important to humans | More than 4 | 5, perhaps more | Unknown | Unknown |
| Pathogenic | | | | | |
| Site of infection | Duodenum, jejunum | Jejunum | ?Small intestine | ?Small intestine | ?Small intestine |
| Mechanism of immunity | Local intestinal IgA | Unknown | Unknown | Unknown | Unknown |
| Epidemiologic | | | | | |
| Epidemicity | Epidemic or sporadic | Family and community outbreaks | Sporadic | Sporadic | Sporadic |
| Seasonality | Usually winter | None known | None known | None known | None known |
| Ages primarily affected | Infants, children <2 y old | Older children and adults | Infants, children | Infants, children | Neonates, immuno-compromised children and adults |
| Method of transmission | Fecal–oral | Fecal–oral; contaminated water and shellfish | ?Fecal–oral | Fecal–oral | ?Fecal–oral; ?perinatal |
| Incubation period (days) | 1–3 | 0.5–2 | ?1–2 | 8–10 | ?1–2 |
| Major diagnostic tests | EIA, LA, EM[a] | EM, IEM | EM | EIA, EM | EM |

[a] EM, electron microscopy; IEM, immunoelectron microscopy; LA, latex agglutination; EIA, enzyme immunoassay.

# ROTAVIRUSES

The human intestinal rotaviruses were first found in 1973 by electron microscopic examination of duodenal biopsy specimens from infants with diarrhea. Since then, they have been found worldwide and are believed to account for 40 to 60% of cases of acute gastroenteritis occurring during the cooler months in infants and children less than 2 years of age. These viruses have been detected in intestinal contents and in tissues from the upper gastrointestinal tract.

Most common cause of winter gastroenteritis in children <2 years old

## Rotaviruses: Group Characteristics

The rotaviruses belong to the family Reoviridae. They are naked, spherical particles 65 to 75 nm in diameter (smaller forms have also been described) with a genome containing 11 segments of double-stranded RNA and a double-shelled outer capsid. Their name is derived from the Latin **rota** ("wheel") because of the outer capsid, which resembles a wheel attached by short spokes to the inner capsid and core (Fig 38–1). Three serogroups have been associated with disease in humans (groups A, B, and C). Four group A serotypes (1, 2, 3, and 4), based on type-specific antigens on the outer capsid, are of major epidemiologic importance. Rotaviruses can replicate in the cytoplasm of infected cell cultures in the labora-

Double-stranded RNA viruses

Antigenic types based on capsid structure

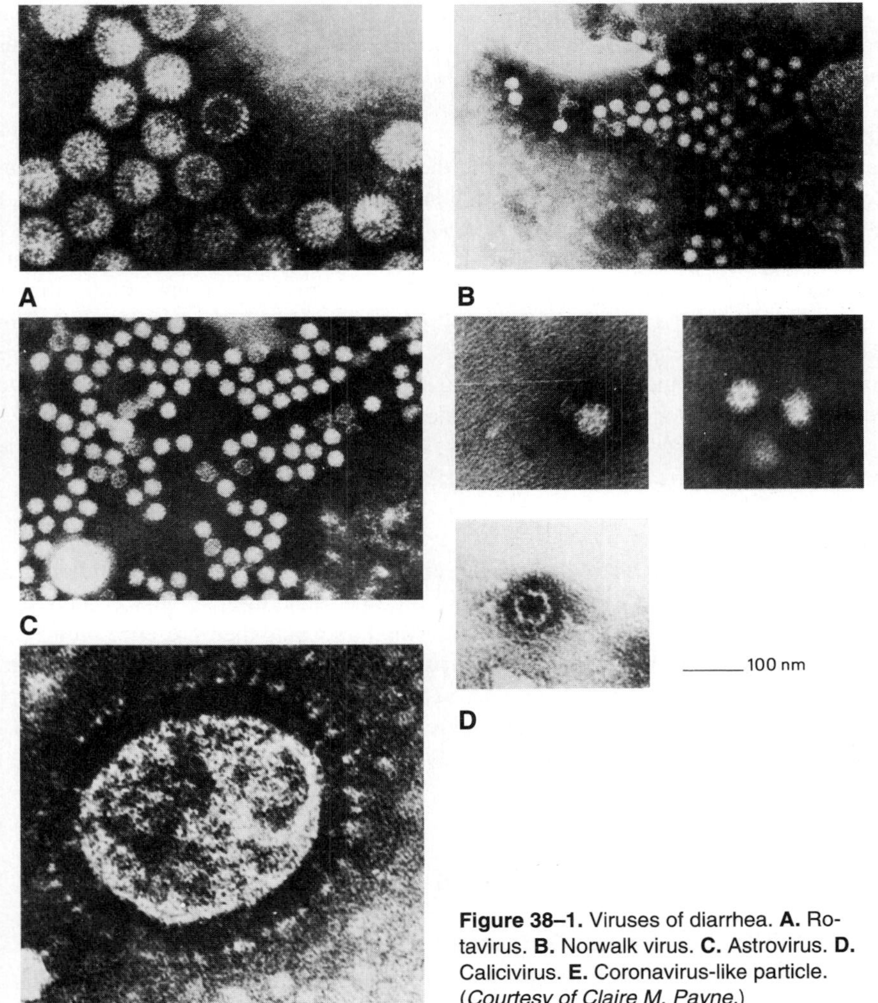


**Figure 38–1.** Viruses of diarrhea. **A.** Rotavirus. **B.** Norwalk virus. **C.** Astrovirus. **D.** Calicivirus. **E.** Coronavirus-like particle. (*Courtesy of Claire M. Payne.*)

tory, but are difficult to propagate because the replicative cycle is usually incomplete, and mature, infectious virions are often not produced. Successful propagation of human strains in vitro has, however, been achieved in some instances.

Animal rotaviruses produce diarrhea but interspecies spread not demonstrated in nature

Rotaviruses of animal origin are also highly prevalent and produce acute gastrointestinal disease in a variety of species. The very young, such as calves, suckling mice, piglets, and foals, are particularly susceptible. The animal rotaviruses can often replicate in cell cultures, and infection across species lines has been accomplished experimentally; there is, however, no evidence that such interspecies spread occurs in nature (eg, animal rotaviruses are not known to affect humans and vice versa).

## Human Rotavirus Infections

### Epidemiology

Primarily children in colder months

Outbreaks of rotavirus infection are common, particularly during the cooler months, among infants and children 1 to 24 months of age. Older children and adults can also be affected, but attack rates are usually much lower. Outbreaks among elderly, institutionalized patients have also been recognized.

Infection common in infants without disease

Although newborn infants can be readily infected with the virus, such infections often result in little or no clinical illness. This finding is illustrated by reported infection rates of 32 to 49% in some neonatal nurseries, but mild illness in only 8 to 28% of the infants. It is unclear whether this transient resistance to disease is a result of host maturation factors or transplacentally conferred immunity.

Most older children and adults immune from exposure

Seroepidemiologic studies have been useful in demonstrating the ubiquity of these viruses and, perhaps, help to explain the age-specific attack rates. By the age of 4 years, more than 90% of individuals have humoral antibodies, suggesting a high rate of virus infection early in life.

### Pathogenesis and Pathology

Destroy villus cells of jejunum and duodenum

Decreased absorptive surface

Rotaviruses appear to localize primarily in the duodenum and proximal jejunum, causing destruction of villous epithelial cells with blunting (shortening) of villi and variable, usually mild, infiltrates of mononuclear and a few polymorphonuclear inflammatory cells within the villi. The gastric and colonic mucosa are unaffected; however, for unknown reasons, gastric emptying time is markedly delayed. The primary pathophysiologic effects are a decrease in absorptive surface in the small intestine and decreased production of brush border enzymes, such as the disaccharidases. The net result is a transient malabsorptive state, with defective handling of fats and sugars. It may take as long as 3 to 8 weeks to restore the normal histologic and functional integrity of the damaged mucosa.

Viral excretion usually lasts 2 to 12 days but can be greatly prolonged, with persistent symptoms, in malnourished or immunodeficient patients.

### Immunity

Type-specific humoral and secretory IgA antibodies protective

IgA and mucin glycoproteins confer protective role of breast-feeding

Patients with rotavirus infection respond with production of type-specific humoral antibodies that appear to last for years, perhaps a lifetime. In addition, type-specific secretory IgA (sIgA) antibodies are produced in the intestinal tract, and their presence seems to correlate best with immunity to reinfection. Breastfeeding also seems to play a protective role against rotavirus disease in young infants. Secretory IgA antibodies to rotaviruses appear in colostrum and continue to be secreted in breast milk for several months postpartum. Human breast milk mucin glycoproteins have also been shown to bind to rotaviruses, inhibiting their replication in vitro and in vivo.

## Rotavirus Infections: Clinical Aspects

### Clinical Manifestations and Outcome

Short incubation period, vomiting, and watery diarrhea

After an incubation period of 1 to 3 days, there is usually an abrupt onset of vomiting, followed within hours by frequent, copious, watery, brown stools. In severe cases, the stools may become clear; the Japanese refer to the disease as **hakuri,** the "white stool diarrhea."

Fever, usually low grade, is often present. Vomiting may persist for 1 to 3 days, and diarrhea for 5 to 8 days.

The major complications result from severe dehydration, occasionally associated with hypernatremia. This complication can lead to death, particularly in very small or malnourished infants.

Dehydration major problem

### Laboratory Diagnosis

Diagnosis of acute rotavirus infection is usually by detection of virus particles in the stools during the acute phase of illness. Detection can be accomplished by direct examination of the specimen by electron microscopy or by immunologic detection of antigen with latex agglutination or enzyme immunoassay (EIA) methods (see Chapter 14).

Electron microscopic or EIA detection of virus

### Treatment and Prevention

There is no specific treatment. Vigorous replacement of fluids and electrolytes, is required in severe cases, and can be life-saving.

The rotaviruses are highly infectious and can spread quickly in family and institutional settings. Control consists of rigorous hygienic measures, including careful hand washing and adequate disposal of enteric excretions. Live, attenuated vaccines have been developed and are being tested in humans. The findings to date suggest that such an approach to control or amelioration of the natural infection may be safe and feasible. In addition, live recombinant viruses containing genomic combinations of human and animal strains are being developed for clinical testing as vaccines.

Live, attenuated, or recombinant vaccines feasible

## NORWALK VIRUSES

Although the Norwalk viruses were the first to be clearly associated with outbreaks of gastroenteritis, considerably less is known about their biology than about that of the rotaviruses. They were first associated with an outbreak in Norwalk, Ohio, in 1968, and their role was confirmed by production of disease in volunteers fed fecal filtrates. The original virus was thus called the Norwalk agent, and similar viruses have been given names such as Hawaii agent, Montgomery County agent, Ditchling agent, and so on.

## ■ Norwalk Viruses: Group Characteristics

The viruses are small, naked, round RNA-containing particles 27 to 38 nm in diameter; their appearance is similar to that of the DNA-containing parvoviruses and hepatitis A virus (see Fig 38–1). They are tentatively classified as members of the Caliciviridae family. The viruses appear to be extremely hardy; their infectivity persists after exposure to acid, ether, and heat (60°C for 30 minutes). They have not been grown in cell culture.

Small, round unenveloped RNA containing viruses

At least four different serotypes have been demonstrated by immunoelectron microscopy with convalescent sera from affected patients. Knowledge of the antigenic characteristics and biology of these viruses has been seriously hampered by the current inability to grow them in the laboratory and by their lack of known pathogenicity for animals. In addition to the recognized Norwalk viruses, other small round viruses (SRVs) and caliciviruses have been described in association with gastroenteritis. Recent molecular studies suggest these may also be related to Norwalk agents, and they are now often referred to as "Norwalk-like" viruses; however, some investigators still prefer to consider the classically appearing caliciviruses separately.

Several serotypes but not yet grown

Other small, round viruses are similar

## ■ Norwalk and Norwalk-like Virus Infections

### Epidemiology

Sharp family and community outbreaks are common and can occur in any season. Unlike rotaviruses, Norwalk and Norwalk-like viruses are much more common causes of gastrointestinal illness in older children and adults. This difference in age-specific predilection

Sharp outbreaks include older children and adults

Fecal–oral transmission

is perhaps reflected in serosurveys, which have shown that the prevalence of antibodies rises slowly, reaching approximately 50% by the fifth decade of life, a striking contrast to the frequent acquisition of antibodies to rotaviruses early in life. Transmission is primarily fecal–oral; outbreaks have also been associated with consumption of contaminated water, uncooked shellfish, and other foods.

### Pathogenesis and Pathology

Both the pathogenesis and the pathology are similar to those described for rotaviruses. The mucosal changes usually revert to normal within 2 weeks of onset of illness. Virus shedding in the feces generally lasts no more than 3 to 4 days.

### Immunity

Reinfection can occur with same serotypes

Patients and experimentally infected volunteers respond to infection with the production of humoral antibodies, which persist indefinitely; their role in protection from reinfection, however, appears minimal. Reinfection and illness with the same serotype occur, and the role of local antibody has not been well defined. It is possible that nonimmune or genetic factors are essential for protection.

## Norwalk Infections: Clinical Aspects

### Clinical Manifestations and Outcome

Clinical picture similar to that of rotavirus infection

The incubation period is 10 to 51 hours, followed by abrupt onset of vomiting and diarrhea, a syndrome clinically indistinguishable from that caused by rotaviruses. Respiratory symptoms rarely coexist, and the duration of illness is relatively brief (usually 1–2 days).

### Laboratory Diagnosis

Diagnostic tests similar to rotavirus

These viruses can be detected by electron microscopy or immunoelectron microscopy in stools during the acute phase of illness. In addition, EIA methods have been developed for detection of antigen as well as for measurement of humoral antibody responses to infection.

### Prevention and Treatment

As with rotavirus infection, there is no specific treatment other than fluid and electrolyte replacement. Prevention requires good hygienic measures.

## ADENOVIRUSES AND CANDIDATE VIRUSES

Some adenoviruses, most of which are exceedingly difficult to cultivate in vitro (in contrast to those associated with respiratory diseases), are now recognized as significant intestinal pathogens. They may account for an estimated 5 to 15% of all viral gastroenteritis in young children. These include serotypes 40, 41, and perhaps 38.

Other viruses associated with gastrointestinal diseases include astroviruses, coronavirus-like agents, and some group A coxsackieviruses (the latter primarily cause gastrointestinal symptoms in severely immunocompromised patients). Characteristics of the major ones are listed in Table 38–1. This list may grow in the future; however, much remains to be learned about their biology and epidemiologic behavior.

## ADDITIONAL READING

Blacklow NR, Greenberg HB. Viral gastroenteritis. *N Engl J Med* 1991;325:252–264. A thorough review of the biology and epidemiology of the proven and candidate agents.

Hedberg CW, Osterholm MT. Outbreaks of food-borne and water-borne viral gastroenteritis. *Clin Microbiol Rev.* 1993;6:199–210. A review emphasizing epidemiologic aspects.

Kapikian AZ. Viral gastroenteritis. *JAMA.* 1993;269:627–630. This prominent researcher in the field presents a concise, well-referenced overview of the relative importance of these various agents and current progress in prevention.

Morse DL, Guzewich JJ, Hanrahan JP, et al. Widespread outbreaks of clam and oyster-associated gastroenteritis: Role of Norwalk virus. *N Engl J Med.* 1986;314:678–681. This report illustrates the potential magnitude of Norwalk agent-caused outbreaks. The accompanying editorial on pages 707–708 will provide the reader with further reason to avoid eating raw or slightly steamed shellfish.

Chapter 39

# Arthropod-Borne and Other Zoonotic Viruses

C. George Ray

The zoonotic viruses comprise more than 400 agents, one or more of which occur in most parts of the world. Members of the group have their ultimate reservoirs in lower vertebrates or insects. They are from diverse taxonomic families of RNA viruses including, primarily the togaviruses, bunyaviruses, reoviruses, arenaviruses, and filoviruses. Their major morphologic and genetic features were summarized in Table 5–1 of Chapter 5. Certain DNA viruses (poxviruses) are also transmissible from animals to humans. These are considered in Chapter 34.

The zoonotic viruses discussed here are divided into two groups. The arboviruses are transmitted to humans by infected bloodsucking insects such as mosquitoes, ticks, and *Phlebotomus* flies (sandflies). The other zoonotic RNA viruses are generally believed to be transmitted by inhalation of infected animal excretions, by the conjunctival route, or occasionally by direct contact with infected animals. Rabies virus, which is commonly transmitted by animal bites, is discussed separately in Chapter 40.

## GENERAL VIROLOGY

In most cases, the zoonotic viruses were first named after the place of initial isolation (eg, St Louis encephalitis) or after the disease produced (eg, yellow fever). More recent studies have assigned the majority to families and genera on the basis of properties indicated in Table 5–1. The major characteristics of these families are summarized below.

Generally named after place of isolation

### Togaviruses and Flaviviruses

Togaviruses and flaviviruses are enveloped virions containing single-stranded, positive-sense RNA measuring 40 to 70 nm in external diameter. The envelope contains a hemagglutinin and lipoproteins. The lipid of the envelope is an essential component, and lipid solvents such as ether and detergents can readily inactivate the viruses. They mature by budding from cellular membranes. Replication can occur in cells of infected arthropods and vertebrate hosts.

Envelope RNA viruses containing hemagglutinin and lipoproteins

The *Alphavirus* and *Flavivirus* genera within these families include most arthropod-borne viruses. Each genus possesses its own unique primary structure of the RNA genome. Viruses within these genera are frequently serologically related to one another, but not to others. Representatives are listed in Table 39–1.

TABLE 39–1. SELECTED ARBOVIRUSES OF MAJOR IMPORTANCE TO HUMANS

| Genus and Member | Major Geographic Distribution | Primary Arthropod Vector | Usual Disease Expression |
|---|---|---|---|
| **Togaviruses** | | | |
| *Alphavirus* | | | |
| Western equine encephalitis | North America | Mosquito | Encephalitis |
| Eastern equine encephalitis | North America | Mosquito | Encephalitis |
| Venezuelan equine encephalitis | Central and South America | Mosquito | Encephalitis |
| Chikungunya | Africa and Asia | Mosquito | Febrile illness |
| **Flaviviruses** | | | |
| *Flavivirus* | | | |
| St. Louis encephalitis | North America | Mosquito | Encephalitis |
| Dengue | All tropical zones | Mosquito | Febrile illness or hemorrhagic fever |
| Yellow fever | Africa, South America, and Caribbean | Mosquito | Hemorrhagic fever |
| West Nile fever | Africa | Mosquito | Febrile illness |
| Murray Valley encephalitis | Australia | Mosquito | Encephalitis |
| Russian spring–summer encephalitis | Eastern Soviet Union and Central Europe | Tick | Encephalitis |
| Powassan | Canada | Tick | Encephalitis |
| Japanese B encephalitis | Japan, Korea, and Philippines | Mosquito | Encephalitis |
| **Bunyaviruses** | | | |
| *Bunyavirus* | | | |
| California | North America | Mosquito | Encephalitis |
| Bunyamwera | Africa | Mosquito | Febrile illness |
| Rift Valley fever | Africa | Mosquito | Febrile illness |
| Sandfly fever | Mediterranean | *Phlebotomus* | Febrile illness |
| **Reoviruses** | | | |
| *Orbivirus* | | | |
| Colorado tick fever | North America | Tick | Febrile illness |

## Bunyaviruses

Spherical, enveloped RNA includes hantavirus

Bunyaviruses are spherical, enveloped, and single-stranded negative-sense RNA viruses approximately 90 to 100 nm in external diameter. They mature by budding into smooth-surfaced vesicles in or near the Golgi region of the infected cell. California virus and hantavirus are the major disease-causing bunyaviruses in North America.

## Reoviruses

Unenveloped RNA prominent in North America

Reoviruses are spherical, unenveloped, double-stranded RNA viruses that measure about 80 nm in diameter with a segmented genome. The most important North American arbovirus of this family is that causing Colorado tick fever which is a member of the genus *Orbivirus*.

## Arenaviruses

Spherical, enveloped RNA

The arenaviruses are enveloped, spherical or pleomorphic viruses containing single-stranded, negative-sense RNA in several segments and measuring 50 to 300 nm in diameter. They mature by budding from host cell cytoplasmic membranes and contain host cell ribosomes in their interior. These ribosomes confer a granular appearance to the viruses, hence their name (from the Latin **arenosus** for "sandy"). The most significant arenavirus infections in humans are the hemorrhagic fevers including Lassa fever. The virus of lymphatic choriomeningitis is occasionally transmitted to humans from infected mice.

Contain host cell ribosomes

## Filoviruses

Filoviruses are enveloped, single-stranded, negative-sense RNA viruses. They are filamentous and highly pleomorphic, averaging 80 nm in diameter and 300 to 14,000 nm in length as they bud from the cell membrane. They are the cause of Marburg and Ebola fevers, two highly fatal hemorrhagic fevers.

Enveloped filamentous RNA viruses causing hemorrhagic fevers

# ARBOVIRUSES

## ■ Arbovirus Disease

### Natural History and Epidemiology

Arboviruses of major importance in human disease are listed in Table 39–1 with summaries of their geographic distribution, the arthropod vectors that transmit them, and the usual disease syndromes that can result from infection.

With the exception of urban dengue and urban yellow fever in which the virus may simply be transmitted between humans and mosquitoes, other arboviral disease involve non-human vertebrates. These are usually small mammals, birds, or, in the case of jungle yellow fever, monkeys. Infection is transmitted within the host species by arthropods (eg, mosquitoes or ticks) that become infected. In some cases the infection can be maintained from generation to generation in the arthropod by transovarial transmission. Infection in the arthropod usually does not appear to harm the insect; however, a period of virus multiplication (termed **extrinsic incubation period**) is required to enhance the capacity to transmit infection to vertebrates by bite. The consequences of infection transmitted from the arthropod to susceptible vertebrate hosts are variable; some develop illness of varying severity with viremia, whereas others may have long-term viremia without clinical disease. Vertebrate hosts are then a source of further spread of the virus by amplification in which noninfected arthropods feeding on viremic hosts acquire the virus, thereby increasing the risk of transmission.

Reservoirs in non-human vertebrates

Sometimes maintained by vertical transmission in vector

Multiplication in vector required

Transient viremia is a feature of many of these diseases in hosts other than their reservoir and is often insufficient to sustain transmission of the viruses; those affected, including humans and higher vertebrates (eg, horses and cattle), are often referred to as blind-end hosts. In contrast, if viremia is sustained for longer periods (eg, weeks to months in a variety of togavirus, flavivirus, and bunyavirus infections in lower vertebrates), the vertebrate host becomes highly important as a reservoir for continuing transmission. Viremia may last a week or more in human dengue and yellow fever infections, and humans may then serve as a reservoir in urban disease.

Sustained viremia required for vertebrate host to be significant reservoir

Obviously, the usual arthropod vectors are rarely present during all seasons. The question then arises as to how the arboviruses survive between the time the vector disappears and the time it reappears in subsequent years. Several mechanisms can operate to sustain the virus between transmission periods (often referred to as **overwintering**): (1) sustained viremia in lower vertebrates such as small mammals, birds, and snakes, from which newly mature arthropods can be infected when taking a blood meal; (2) hibernation of infected adult arthropods that survive from one season to the next; and (3) transovarial transmission, whereby the infected female arthropod can transmit virus to its progeny.

Season-to-season survival has multiple mechanisms

The three basic cycles of arbovirus transmission are urban, sylvatic, and arthropod-sustained.

#### Urban

As the term suggests, the urban cycle is favored by the presence of relatively large numbers of humans living in close proximity to arthropod (usually mosquito) species capable of virus transmission. The cycle is:

Urban cycle exists with dengue, yellow fever

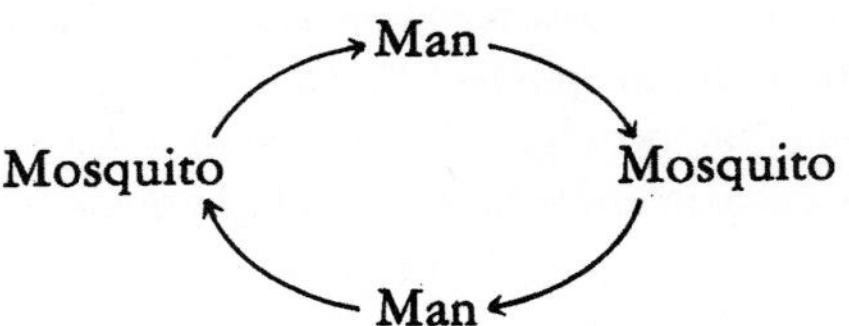


Examples of this cycle include urban dengue, urban yellow fever, and the occasional urban outbreaks of St Louis encephalitis.

SYLVATIC

In the sylvatic cycle a single nonhuman vertebrate reservoir may be involved:

Sylvanic cycle with many viruses

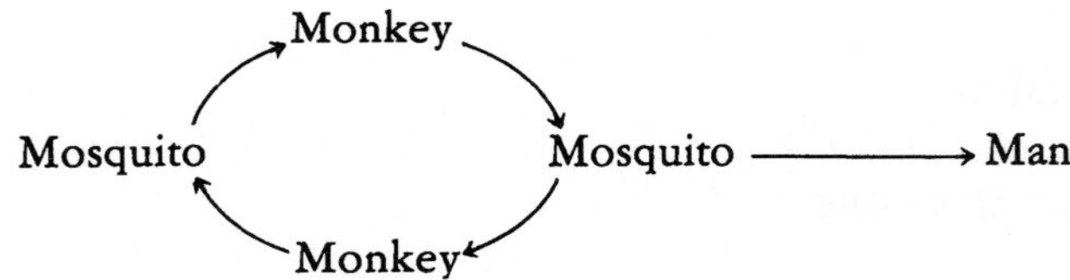


Humans are tangential hosts

In this situation the human, who becomes a tangential host through accidental intrusion into a zoonotic transmission cycle, is not important in maintaining the infection cycle. An example of this cycle is jungle yellow fever.

In other sylvatic cycles, multiple vertebrate reservoirs may be involved:

Sylvanic cycles with multiple reservoirs

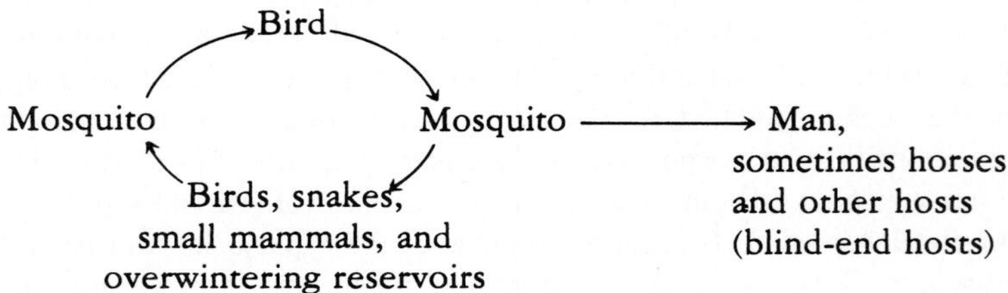


Examples include western equine encephalitis, eastern equine encephalitis, and California viruses. In some situations, such as St Louis encephalitis and yellow fever, the urban and sylvatic cycles may operate concurrently.

ARTHROPOD-SUSTAINED

Arthropods, especially ticks, may sustain the reservoir by transovarial transmission of virus to their progeny, with amplification of the cycle by spread to and from small mammals:

Arthropod sustained linked to tick transovarial transmission

Small mammals ⟺ Tick → Tick → Tick → { Man, Cattle, Goats (Blind-end hosts) } → Man (via milk, an aberrant pathway)

Tick-borne encephalitis in Russia is transmitted by this cycle. In temperate climates such as the United States, arboviruses are major causes of disease during the summer and early fall months, the season of greatest activity of arthropod vectors (usually mosquitoes or ticks). When climatic conditions and ecologic circumstances (eg, swamps and ponds) are optimal for arthropod breeding and egg hatching, arbovirus amplification may begin.

Weather, swamps, ponds, alter the conditions

An example of amplification is provided by western equine encephalitis. When the mosquito vectors become abundant, the level of transmission among the basic reservoir hosts (birds and small mammals) increases, and the mosquitoes also turn to other susceptible species such as the domestic fowl. These hosts experience a rapidly developing asymptomatic viremia which permits still more arthropods to become infected on biting. At this point, spread to blind-end hosts such as humans or horses and the development of clinical disease become likely. This occurrence depends on the accessibility of the host to the in-

Mosquito increases create risk for blind-end human infection

fected mosquito and on mosquito feeding preferences which, for unknown reasons, vary from one season to another.

## Pathogenesis and Pathology

There are three major manifestations of arbovirus diseases in humans associated with different tropisms of various viruses for human organs, although overlap can occur. In some, the central nervous system is primarily affected, leading to aseptic meningitis or meningoencephalitis. A second syndrome involves many major organ systems, with particular damage to the liver as in yellow fever. The third is manifested by hemorrhagic fever in which damage is particularly severe to the small blood vessels, with skin petechiae and intestinal and other hemorrhages.

CNS, visceral, and hemorrhagic fever the major syndromes

Infection of the human by a biting, infected arthropod is followed by viremia, which is apparently amplified by extensive virus replication in the reticuloendothelial system and vascular endothelium. After replication the virus becomes localized in various target organs, depending on its tropism, and illness results. The viruses produce cell necrosis with resultant inflammation which leads to fever in nearly all infections. If the major viral tropism is for the central nervous system (CNS), virus reaching this site by crossing the blood–brain barrier or along neural pathways can cause meningeal inflammation (aseptic meningitis) or neuronal dysfunction (encephalitis). The CNS pathology consists of meningeal and perivascular mononuclear cell infiltrates, degeneration of neurons with neuronophagia, and occasionally destruction of the supporting structure of neurons.

After bite, viremia and viral tissue tropism define disease

In CNS, aseptic meningitis, encephalitis from cell injury

In some infections, especially yellow fever, the liver is the primary target organ. Pathologic findings include hyaline necrosis of hepatocytes which produces cytoplasmic eosinophilic masses called **Councilman bodies.** Degenerative changes in the renal tubules and myocardium may also be seen, as may microscopic hemorrhages throughout the brain. Hemorrhage is a major feature of yellow fever, largely because of the lack of liver-produced clotting factors as a result of liver necrosis.

Liver often the target with necrosis of hepatocytes

Hemorrhagic fevers other than those related to primary hepatic destruction have a somewhat different pathogenesis which has been studied most extensively in dengue infections. In uncomplicated dengue fever, which is associated with a rash and influenza-like symptoms, there are changes in the small dermal blood vessels. These alterations include endothelial cell swelling and perivascular edema with mononuclear cell infiltration. More severe infection (dengue hemorrhagic fever [DHF] often complicated by shock) is characterized by perivascular edema and widespread effusions into serous cavitities such as the pleura and hemorrhages from the upper respiratory and intestinal tracts. The spleen and lymph nodes show hyperplasia of lymphoid and plasma cell elements and there is focal necrosis in the liver. The pathophysiology seems related to increased vascular permeability and disseminated intravascular coagulation (DIC), which is further complicated by liver and bone marrow dysfunction (eg, decreased platelet production, decreased production of liver-dependent clotting factors). The major vascular abnormalities may be provoked by circulating virus–antibody complexes (immune complexes) which mediate activation of complement and subsequent release of vasoactive amines. The precise reason for this phenomenon is not clear; it may be related to intrinsic virulence of the virus strains involved and to host susceptibility factors.

Dengue hemorrhagic fevers involve perivascular and endothelial injury

May progress to shock

Lymphoid hyperplasia seen

Virus–antibody complexes may trigger complement activation

Two hypotheses are based on the existence of four distinct but antigenically related serotypes of dengue virus, any of which can generate group-specific cross-reacting antibodies that are not necessarily protective against other serotypes. One possibility is that preexisting group-specific antibody at a critical concentration serves as "enhancing" rather than neutralizing antibody. In the presence of enhancing antibody, virus–antibody complexes are more efficiently adsorbed to and engulfed by monocytes and macrophages. Subsequent replication leads to extensive spread throughout the host. Alternatively, or in concert with this, activation of previously sensitized T cells by viral antigen present on the surfaces of macrophages may result in release of cytokines which mediate the development of shock and hemorrhage.

Cross reacting antibodies may enhance immune reactions more than neutralization of virus

## Immunity

The usual humoral responses (hemagglutination inhibition, complement fixation, neutralization, precipitation) in relation to onset of illness are illustrated in Figure 39–1. One exception to this general pattern is Colorado tick fever, in which increases in complement

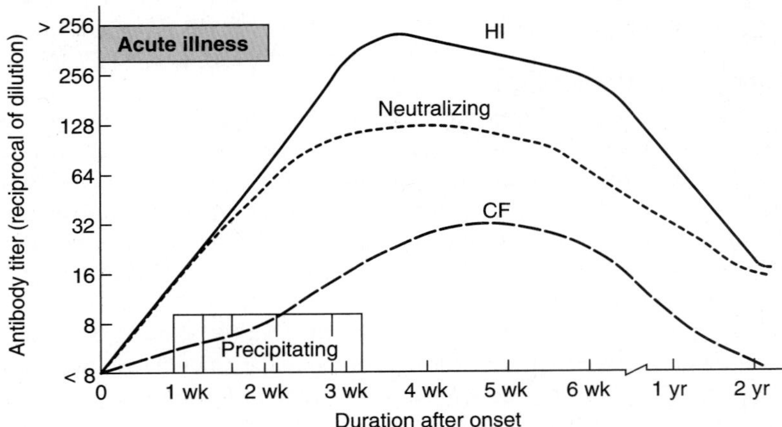


**Figure 39–1.** Typical patterns of antibody response after arbovirus infection. HI, hemagglutination inhibition antibodies; CF, complement fixation antibodies; precipitating, precipitating antibodies detected by immunodiffusion (sometimes used in diagnosis of California virus encephalitis).

Neutralizing antibodies protective and last for years

Immunity serotype specific

fixation antibody titer may be delayed by 3 to 6 weeks. The rise in antibody titer generally correlates with recovery from infection. Neutralizing antibodies, which are the most serotype specific, generally persist many years after infection. Hemagglutination inhibition and complement fixation antibodies to togaviruses and bunyaviruses are group specific; that is, they do not always clearly distinguish between members of a specific genus, such as the flaviviruses. Hemagglutination inhibition antibodies may persist several years after infection, whereas complement fixation antibodies are relatively short-lived; the presence of the latter suggests relatively recent infection (within 1–2 years). The presence of IgM-specific antibodies indicates that primary infection likely occurred within the previous 2 months. Immunity to reinfection is serotype specific and appears to be permanent.

## Arbovirus Disease: Specific Arboviruses

### Western Equine Encephalitis

Western US in horses

Encephalitis more likely in young infants

The agent that causes western equine encephalitis is prevalent in the western United States in the central valley of California, eastern Washington (Yakima valley), Colorado, and Texas. It has also been responsible for outbreaks in midwestern states (Minnesota, Wisconsin, Illinois, Missouri, and Kansas) and as far east as New Jersey. Horses and humans represent blind-end hosts; both are susceptible to infection and illness, commonly manifested as encephalitis. Although human infection in endemic areas is commonplace, overall only 1 of 1000 infections causes clinical symptoms. In young infants (under 1 year of age), however, 1 of every 25 infections may produce severe illness. The attack rates are therefore far higher in young infants than in other groups. The disease spectrum may range from mild, nonspecific febrile illness to aseptic meningitis or severe, overwhelming encephalitis. Mortality is estimated at 5% for cases of encephalitis. It is a very serious disease in infants less than 1 year of age; as many as 60% of survivors have permanent neurologic impairment.

### Eastern Equine Encephalitis

New England to South America

Vector feeds on horses and birds

The eastern equine encephalitis virus is largely confined to the Atlantic Seaboard states from New England down the coast of Central America and South America. The mosquito vector (principally *Culiseta melanura*) generally restricts its feeding to horses and birds, although occasional outbreaks among humans have occurred. The virus can cause severe encephalitis in horses and also in wild pheasants. The attack rate in humans is highest in infants and children; the mortality in this group is estimated at 20% or greater, and the incidence of severe sequelae among survivors is high.

### St Louis Encephalitis

The St Louis encephalitis virus is a major cause of arbovirus encephalitis in the United States. Its geographic distribution and major mosquito vector (*Culex tarsalis*) are similar to those of western equine encephalitis, but has been much more prevalent in eastern states and in Texas, Mississippi, and Florida. It infects but causes no disease in horses. The disease spectrum in humans is similar to that of western equine encephalitis, but the major morbidity and mortality, as well as the highest attack rates, are among adults more than 40 years of age. Infants and young children are relatively spared.

Distribution and disease similar to western equine encephalitis

More disease in adults

### California Virus

Although California virus was first isolated in that state, its major distribution in the United States has been in the Midwest; outbreaks due to the LaCrosse subtype are particularly prevalent in Wisconsin, Ohio, Minnesota, and Indiana. In Wisconsin and Minnesota, California virus is considered the most important cause of encephalitis. Studies elsewhere in North America and throughout the world, however, indicate that California virus or closely related agents are present nearly everywhere. The primary mosquito vector (*Aedes triseriatus*) is commonly encountered in suburban or rural environments. Unlike western equine, eastern equine, and St Louis encephalitis viruses, the highest attack rates are seen in those aged 5 to 18 years. Infection is often characterized by abrupt onset of encephalitis, frequently with seizures.

Virus widespread

Vector common in suburban, rural areas

Highest attack rate in those aged 5 to 18 years

### Yellow Fever

Geographically, yellow fever is distributed throughout the Caribbean, Central America, the Amazon valley in South America, and a broad central zone in Africa from the Atlantic Coast to the Sudan and Ethiopia. It continues to be a potential threat to the southeastern United States because of an urban vector (*Aedes aegypti*) in that area.

Vector persists in US

The clinical disease is characterized by abrupt onset of fever, chills, headache, and hemorrhage; it may progress to severe vomiting (sometimes with gastric hemorrhage), bradycardia, jaundice, and shock. If the patient recovers from the acute episode, there are no long-term sequelae.

### Dengue

There are four related serotypes of dengue, any of which may exist concurrently in a given endemic area. These agents are widespread throughout the world, particularly in the Middle East, Africa, the Far East, and the Caribbean Islands, and they have invaded the United States in the past. The vector (*Aedes aegypti*) is the same as the domestic vector of yellow fever. The known transmission cycle is human–mosquito–human, although a sylvatic cycle involving monkeys may also exist.

Widespread in tropical areas

Vector same as yellow fever

The characteristic clinical illness usually results in fever, an erythematous rash, and severe pain in the back, head, muscles, and joints. Especially in the Far East (Philippines, Thailand, and India), the disease has periodically assumed a severe form characterized by shock, pleural effusion, and hemorrhage often followed by death.

Severe pain in back, muscles, and joints

### Japanese B Encephalitis

The flavivirus species that causes Japanese B encephalitis is prevalent on the eastern coast of Asia, on its offshore islands (Japan, Taiwan, and Indonesia), and in India. Its transmission cycle resembles that of the St Louis encephalitis and western equine encephalitis viruses. A high proportion of human infections are subclinical, especially in children; when encephalitis does develop it is severe and often fatal.

Similar to St. Louis and western equine encephalitis

### Powassan Virus

Powassan virus is the only known tick-borne *Flavivirus* species of North America. First isolated in Ontario from a fatal human case of encephalitis, it has been found in infected ticks in Ontario, British Columbia, and Colorado. Its significance to humans is not yet established, as only a few patients with encephalitis proved to be caused by this agent have been described. Serologic evidence, however, suggests that the virus is prevalent in many areas of North America.

Tick-borne but uncertain human importance

### Colorado Tick Fever

The tick-borne *Orbivirus* species that causes Colorado tick fever has been found throughout the western United States, including Washington, Oregon, Colorado, and Idaho, and also Long Island. It is frequently found in *Dermacentor andersoni*, which are also vectors

Tick-borne throughout western US

Most infections asymptomatic

for *Rickettsia rickettsii*. The typical illness, which occurs 3 to 6 days after the tick bite, is characterized by a sudden onset with headache, muscle pains, fever, and occasionally encephalitis. Leukopenia is a consistent feature of infection. It is estimated that no more than one clinical illness occurs for every 100 infections with this agent.

## Laboratory Diagnosis

Mouse inoculation most common method

Blood best source but must be early in disease

The arboviruses may be isolated in various culture systems; for most agents, however, isolation is by intracerebral inoculation of newborn mice, which often results in encephalitis and death. The viruses may be found in the blood (viremia) from a few days before onset of symptoms through the first 1 to 2 days of illness; attempts at isolation from the blood are generally useful only when viremia is prolonged, as in dengue, Colorado tick fever, and some of the hemorrhagic fevers. Virus is not present in the stool and is rarely found in the throat; viral recovery from cerebrospinal fluid is also unusual. Virus can be isolated readily from affected tissue during the acute phase of illness, but this approach is seldom practical in diagnosis. Specific diagnosis is usually accomplished by serologic techniques using acute and convalescent sera.

Multiple serologic methods used

Various tests have been used including hemagglutination inhibition, complement fixation, virus neutralization methods, and enzyme immunoassay. Early rapid presumptive diagnosis can sometimes be made by the detection of IgM-specific antibodies that often appear within a few days of onset (except in Colorado tick fever where they may be delayed by 1 to 2 weeks), and persist 1 to 2 months.

## Treatment and Prevention

Treatment only supportive

Other than supportive care, there is no specific treatment for arboviral infections. Prevention is primarily avoidance of contact with potentially infected arthropods, a task that can be extremely difficult even with the use of adequate screening and insect repellents. In some settings, vector control can be accomplished by elimination of arthropod breeding sites (stagnant pools and the like) and sometimes by attempts to eradicate the arthropods with careful use of insecticides. Such measures have been highly effective in the control of urban yellow fever, in which elimination of urban breeding sites and other measures to eradicate the principal mosquito vector species (*Aedes aegypti*) have been used. Viruses maintained in complex sylvatic cycles are infinitely more difficult to control without risking major environmental disruption and inestimable expense.

Protection from bites and vector control primary prevention

Vaccines are available for immunization of horses against western, eastern, and Venezuelan equine encephalitis virus infections, but the latter has also been used for some laboratory personnel who work with the virus. The only other arbovirus vaccine in general use for humans is a live attenuated yellow fever virus vaccine (17-D strain), which is used to protect rural populations exposed to the sylvatic cycle and international travelers to endemic areas. In fact, many countries in tropical Africa, Asia, and South America require proof of yellow fever vaccination before allowing travelers to enter. A single subcutaneous dose results in the appearance of antibodies that persist at least 16 to 19 years, which correlates well with protective immunity. If booster doses are desired, they need not be given more than once every 10 years to maintain protection.

Yellow fever vaccine available

# OTHER RNA VIRUSES OF ZOONOTIC ORIGIN

## Arenaviruses

Sustained in small rodent reservoirs

A common feature of the arenaviruses is their zoonotic reservoir, particularly small rodents, in which they may be sustained for long periods. Primary infection of mature rodents often results in disease and death, whereas intrauterine or perinatal infection (vertical transmission) usually leads to chronic lifelong viremia with persistent shedding of virus into the feces, urine, and respiratory secretions. Although chronically infected rodents are somewhat tolerant to the virus (ie, infection is persistent without causing illness), they produce antibodies, and evidence of deleterious effects can be found in older hosts, usually in the form of immune complex glomerulonephritis. The viruses are perpetuated by vertical transmission from infected mothers to their offspring. When environmental contact becomes close, spread from the rodent reservoir to humans (and, in some instances, subhuman primates) can occur via aerosols; through exposure to infective urine, feces, or tissues; or directly by rodent bites. This is in contrast to the arthropod spread of arboviruses.

Vertical transmission in rodents

Spread to humans by aerosols, close contact

### Arenaviruses Associated With Hemorrhagic Fevers

The agents of arenavirus hemorrhagic fevers are transmitted from infected rodents to humans in the manner described above, although person-to-person spread by contact with secretions and body fluids also occurs readily. The viruses in this group include the South American hemorrhagic fever agents (Junin virus, the cause of Argentinean hemorrhagic fever, and Machupo virus, the cause of Bolivian hemorrhagic fever) and Lassa virus, the cause of Lassa fever in West Africa.

Person-to-person spread occurs by contact with body fluids

These viruses have pathogenic and pathologic features similar to those described for the arboviruses that cause hemorrhagic fevers; however, the mechanism involved in the coagulation abnormalities is not understood. All are characterized by fever, usually accompanied by hemorrhagic manifestations, shock, neurologic disturbances, and bradycardia. Lassa fever also frequently causes hepatitis, myocarditis, exudative pharyngitis, and acute deafness. The last deficit may persist after recovery. Mortality is estimated to be 10 to 50% for Lassa fever and 5 to 30% for the others. All are considered highly dangerous in terms of infectivity. Importation of cases to nonepidemic areas has occurred, with significant risk of spread to medical and laboratory personnel.

Fever, shock, and hemorrhage

Hepatitis, myocarditis with Lassa fever

High mortality and risk of further transmission

The diagnosis is suggested primarily by the recent travel history of the patient and the clinical syndromes. Although virus isolation and serologic diagnosis can be done, these procedures should not be attempted in a hospital diagnostic laboratory. Any patient suspected of having such an infection should be immediately isolated and public health authorities notified. Because of the high risk of spread of infection from body fluids and excreta, even routine laboratory studies are best deferred until the diagnosis and proper disposition of specimens can be resolved. Viremia can persist 1 month, and virus shedding in the urine may continue more than 2 months after the onset of illness.

Suggested by clinical findings and travel history

Diagnosis only in reference centers

Viremia may be prolonged

Treatment is primarily supportive; however, intravenous ribavirin, if begun within 6 days of illness onset, has been shown to be helpful in Lassa fever.

### Lymphocytic Choriomeningitis Virus

Infection with lymphocytic choriomeningitis virus is particularly common in hamsters and mice. In the United States, most human illnesses have been traced to contact with rodent breeding colonies in research or pet supply centers and to pet hamsters in the home. The illness usually consists of fever, headache, and myalgia although meningitis or meningoencephalitis also occurs occasionally. Such CNS infections may persist as long as 3 months. There is also evidence that transplacental infection can occur in humans, resulting in fetal death or hydrocephalus. The diagnosis is suggested by a history of rodent contact. The virus may be isolated in the early stages of disease by intracerebral inoculation of blood or cerebrospinal fluid into weanling mice, young guinea pigs, or cell culture. Serologic testing of acute and convalescent sera is usually performed by indirect immunofluorescence. No person-to-person transmission of infection has been documented.

Mice and hamsters in pet stores

Meningitis may persist for months

Transplacental infection in humans

## Filoviruses: Marburg and Ebola Viruses

The association of the Marburg virus with serious disease did not become apparent until 1967, when 26 cases of hemorrhagic fever occurred among persons in Germany and Yugoslavia who were handling a group of African monkeys imported from central Uganda. The agent was later identified as Marburg virus and was apparently transmitted by the infected monkeys. In 1975 the virus was associated with a similar disease in three travelers in South Africa, and in 1980 in Kenya.

Initial cases transmitted from monkeys

In 1976, severe outbreaks of hemorrhagic fever occurred in northern Zaire and south-

Viruses differ antigenically

ern Sudan. The illnesses were similar to those described for Marburg virus but were later shown to be caused by an antigenically different agent known as Ebola virus, named after a small river in Zaire. More recently, another filovirus serologically related to Ebola virus was isolated from monkeys during an epizootic of simian hemorrhagic fever at a US quarantine facility. The reservoir was determined to be monkeys imported from the Philippines.

Reservoir may be rodents

Mortality high in symptomatic infection

Ebola virus produces disease in humans and subhuman primates; onset is within 4 to 6 days of inoculation. The reservoir, although uncertain, is thought to be in small mammals, perhaps rodents. Serosurveys of humans residing in the areas where outbreaks have occurred suggest that human infections may be relatively common; as much as 7% of the survey group had antibodies, indicating past infection. In symptomatic infections, the mortality for both Marburg and Ebola viruses is extremely high (30–80%).

Diagnosis and precautions similar to arenavirus hemorrhagic fevers

As with the arenavirus-associated hemorrhagic fevers, the diagnosis of infection by these agents is suggested by a similar syndrome and recent travel history. Person-to-person transmission similar to that described for Lassa fever occurs in Ebola virus infections and may be possible with Marburg virus. Diagnosis can be confirmed in a reference center by isolation of virus in Vero cells (a continuous line derived from African green monkey kidney), mice, and guinea pigs, as well as by serologic methods employing indirect immunofluorescence or EIA. As with the arenavirus-associated hemorrhagic fevers, however, utmost care in isolation precautions and prompt notification of public health authorities are mandatory for suspected cases before any diagnostic attempts are made. There is no specific therapy for the infections.

## Hantaviruses

### Hantavirus Hemorrhagic Fever

Causes of hemorrhagic fever during Korean war

Korean hemorrhagic fever (KHF) is endemic to Korea and surrounding areas in the Far East. It is an important cause of hemorrhagic fever, often complicated by varying degrees of acute renal failure. In the 1950s thousands of military personnel developed the disease during the Korean War. The first reported isolation of KHF was in 1978, when the antigen was detected in the lung tissues of wild rodents (*Apodemus* species) by indirect immunofluorescence using convalescent sera from affected patients. No illness was apparent in the rodents, suggesting a reservoir mechanism and mode of transmission similar to those described for the arenaviruses. Additional work using the Hantaan virus (a prototype strain serially propagated in a continuous cell line from a human pulmonary carcinoma) indicated that the agent is a member of the family Bunyaviridae, and the generic designation of *Hantavirus* was given.

Detected in lung of wild rodents

Other virus similar to KHF throughout northern Eurasia

Evidence has accumulated indicating that other agents with close antigenic similarities to KHF virus are responsible for hemorrhagic–renal syndromes occurring throughout northern Eurasia, including Russia, Eastern Europe, Finland, and Scandinavia. These syndromes have been given a variety of names, including nephropathia epidemica (NE). Methods similar to those used to detect KHF have detected NE antigen in the lungs of small rodents (bank voles) in Finland.

### Other *Hantavirus* Infections

Hantavirus among rodents in US

Southwestern US outbreak related to deer, mice

Human infection by inhalation of aerosolized excreta

No human-to-human transmission

It has been known for some time that rodents in the United States may be infected with a hantavirus, but no associated human disease was recognized. In early 1993 an outbreak of fulminant respiratory disease with high mortality (67% reported to date) occurred in the Southwestern United States. This was shown to be due to a hantavirus and was associated with an increased population of infected deer mice in and around human habitations. Of the more than 30 documented infections reported in 1993, 23 patients resided in rural areas of a region bordered by the states of Arizona, New Mexico, and Colorado; however, other cases have been reported from Nevada, Texas, Louisiana, California, and North Dakota. The virus is believed to be transmitted to humans most often by inhalation of infected rodent excreta, by the conjunctival route, or by direct contact with skin breaks. Human-to-human spread has not been encountered. Public health measures to inform inhabitants of routes of spread and to reduce the rodent population appear to have controlled the outbreak. Treatment has involved aggressive respiratory support, and intravenous ribavirin appears to have been of benefit in Asian hantavirus infections; however, there are no data as yet regarding its efficacy against the U.S. strains.

Ribavirin may be useful

## Vesicular Stomatitis Virus

A rhabdovirus, vesicular stomatitis virus, that causes outbreaks of disease in cattle, pigs, and horses can be transmitted between animals by arthropods. Human infection is acquired by contact with infected animals but is unusual; it consists of a self-limited febrile illness and occasional herpeslike eruptions over the lips and mucosa.

## ADDITIONAL READING

Halstead SB. Pathogenesis of dengue: Challenges to molecular biology. *Science*. 1988;239:476–481. An excellent review of antibody-dependent enhancement in the pathogenesis of viral infection.

Homes GP, McCormick JB, Trock SC, et al. Lassa fever in the United States. Investigation of a case and new guidelines for management. *N Engl J Med.* 1990;323:1120–1123. This article is an excellent guide for appropriately suspecting and responding to importations of "exotic," potentially highly contagious viral disease.

Hughes JM, Peters CJ, Cohen ML, Mahy BWJ. Hantavirus pulmonary syndrome: An emerging infectious disease. *Science*. 1993;262:850–851. An update on the hantavirus investigations as of mid-1993.

Jahrling PB, Peters CJ. Lymphocytic choriomeningitis virus. A neglected pathogen of man. *Arch Pathol Lab Med.* 1992;116:486–488. The history, unique biology, and clinical features of this virus are well summarized.

McCormick JB, King IJ, Webb PA, et al. Lassa fever. Effective therapy with ribavirin. *N Engl J Med.* 1986; 314:20–26. This article demonstrates approaches and difficulties encountered in evaluating a new drug for a serious disease.

Nichol ST, Spiropoulou CF, Morzunov S, et al. Genetic identification of a hantavirus associated with an outbreak of acute respiratory illness. *Science*. 1993;262:914–917. This is a good example of how to use basic studies to characterize viruses and their habitat distribution.

# Rabies

*W. Lawrence Drew*

Rabies is an acute fatal viral illness of the central nervous system. It can affect all mammals and is transmitted between them by infected secretions, most often by bite. It was first recognized more than 3000 years ago and has been the most feared of infectious diseases. It is said that Aristotle recognized that rabies could be spread by a rabid dog.

## RABIES VIRUS

The rabies virus is a bullet-shaped, enveloped, single-stranded RNA virus of the rhabdovirus group (Fig 40–1). Other pathogens in this group include the vesicular stomatitis virus (see Chapter 39). Rabies virus is large, with a diameter of about 180 × 70 nm. Knoblike glycoprotein excrescences, which elicit neutralizing and hemagglutination-inhibiting antibodies, cover the surface of the virion.

Single-stranded RNA virus

The virus, which can be grown in tissue culture, produces encephalitis when injected intracerebrally into laboratory rodents. In the past, a single antigenically homogeneous virus was believed responsible for all rabies; however, differences in cell culture growth characteristics of isolates from different animal sources, some differences in virulence for experimental animals, and antigenic differences in surface glycoproteins have indicated strain heterogeneity among rabies virus isolates. These studies may help to explain some of the biological differences noted, as well as the occasional case of "vaccine failure."

Strains from different sources may vary antigenically

## RABIES VIRUS INFECTION

### Epidemiology and Epizoology

Rabies exists in two epizoologic forms: the urban form is associated with unimmunized dogs or cats; the sylvatic form occurs in wild skunks, foxes, wolves, raccoons, mongooses, and bats. Human infection, or the much more common infection of cattle, is incidental, is blind-ended, and does not contribute to maintenance or transmission of the disease. In the United States, more than 75% of reported cases of rabies in animals occur among wildlife. Human exposures may be from wild animals or from unimmunized dogs or cats. Domestic animal bites are much more important in developing countries because of lack of enforcement of animal immunization. Infection in domestic animals usually represents a spillover from infection in wildlife reservoirs. Human infection tends to occur where animal rabies is common and where there is a large population of unimmunized domestic animals. Worldwide, the occurrence of human rabies is estimated to be about 15,000 cases per year, with

Urban and sylvatic animal rabies

Infections of cattle and humans are blind ended

Human cases are derived from unimmunized dogs or cats

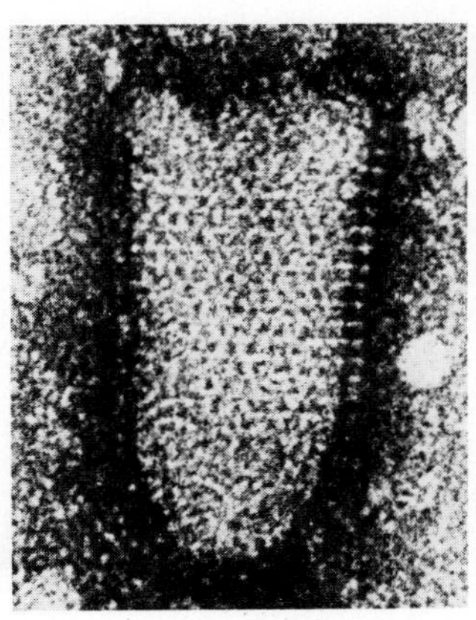

**Figure 40–1.** Rabies virus. (*Reprinted with permission from Dr. K. Hummuler, from Hummuler K, Koprowski M, Wiktor TJ.* J Virol. *1967;1:152–170.*)

the highest attack rates in Southeast Asia, the Philippines, and the Indian subcontinent. In the United States, fewer than five cases of human rabies are reported yearly.

## Pathogenesis

Infection usually injection from animal bite

Initial replication in muscle followed by spread from nerves to brain

Centrifugal spread in autonomic nerves to salivary gland, other organs

Incubation period varies depending in dose and distance to CNS

The essential first event in human or animal rabies infection is the introduction of virus through the epidermis, usually as a result of an animal bite. Inhalation of heavily contaminated material, such as bat droppings, can also cause infection. Rabies virus first replicates in striated muscle tissue at the site of inoculation. It then enters the peripheral nervous system at the neuromuscular junctions and spreads up the nerves to the central nervous system, where it replicates exclusively within the gray matter. It then passes centrifugally along autonomic nerves to reach other tissues, including the salivary glands, adrenal medulla, kidneys, and lungs. Passage into the salivary glands in animals facilitates further transmission of the disease by infected saliva. The incubation period ranges from 10 days to a year, depending on the amount of virus introduced, the amount of tissue involved, the host immune mechanisms, and the distance the virus must travel from the site of inoculation to the central nervous system. Thus, the incubation period is generally shorter with face wounds than with leg wounds. Immunization early in the incubation period frequently aborts the infection.

## Pathology

Negri body characteristic brain lesion

The neuropathology of rabies resembles that of other viral diseases of the central nervous system, with infiltration of lymphocytes and plasma cells into central nervous system tissue and nerve cell destruction. The pathognomonic lesion is the Negri body (Fig 40–2), an eosinophilic cytoplasmic inclusion distributed throughout the brain, particularly in the hippocampus, cerebral cortex, cerebellum, and dorsal spinal ganglia. As Negri bodies are not seen in at least 20% of rabies victims, their absence does not rule out the diagnosis.

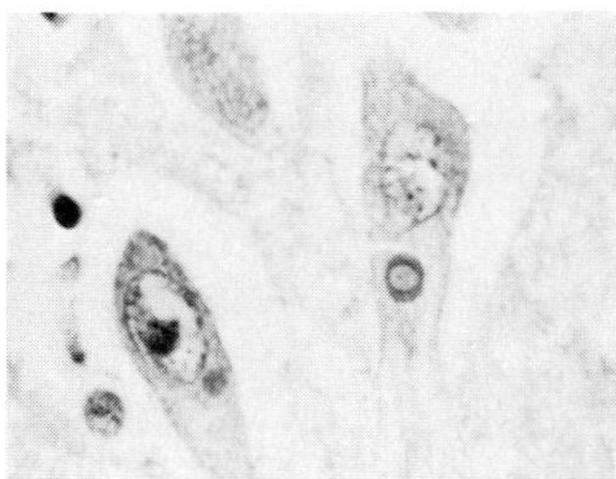

**Figure 40–2.** Negri body in cytoplasm of neuron. (*Courtesy of Dr. Daniel P. Perl.*)

# RABIES VIRUS INFECTION: CLINICAL ASPECTS

## Clinical Manifestations

Rabies in humans usually results from a bite by a rabid animal or contamination of a wound by its saliva. It presents as an acute, fulminant, fatal encephalitis; human survivors have been reported only occasionally. The disease begins as a nonspecific illness marked by fever, headache, malaise, nausea, and vomiting. Abnormal sensations at or around the site of viral inoculation occur frequently and probably reflect local nerve involvement. The onset of encephalitis is marked by periods of excess motor activity and agitation. Hallucinations, combativeness, muscle spasms, signs of meningeal irritation, seizures, and focal paralysis occur. Periods of mental dysfunction are interspersed with completely lucid periods; as the disease progresses, however, the patient lapses into coma. Autonomic nervous system involvement often results in increased salivation. Brain stem and cranial nerve dysfunction is characteristic, with double vision, facial palsies, and difficulty in swallowing. The combination of excess salivation and difficulty in swallowing produces the traditional picture of "foaming at the mouth." Hydrophobia, the painful, violent involuntary contractions of the diaphragm and accessory respiratory, pharyngeal, and laryngeal muscles initiated by swallowing liquids, is seen in about 50% of cases. Involvement of the respiratory center produces respiratory paralysis, the major cause of death. The median survival after onset of symptoms is 4 days, with a maximum of 20 days unless artificial supportive measures are instituted. Recovery is rare and has only been seen in partially immunized individuals.

Transmitted to humans from rabid animals

Encephalitic manifestations; survival very rare

Hydrophobia from dysphagia

Brief course with development of respiratory paralysis

Occasionally rabies may appear as an ascending paralysis resembling Guillain–Barré syndrome.

## Laboratory Diagnosis

Laboratory diagnosis of rabies in animals or deceased patients is accomplished by indirect or direct demonstration of virus in brain tissue. Viral antigen can be demonstrated rapidly by immunofluorescence procedures. Intracerebral inoculation of infected brain tissue or secretions into suckling mice results in death in 3 to 10 days. Histologic examination of their brain tissue shows Negri bodies; both Negri bodies and rhabdovirus particles may be demonstrated by electron microscopy. Specific antibodies to rabies virus can be detected in serum, but generally only late in the disease.

Immunofluorescent examination of infected tissue

Intracerebral inoculation of suckling mice with demonstration of Negri bodies

In many areas of the world, the dog is the most important vector of the rabies virus to humans. Other important sources of disease are the wolf in eastern Europe, the mongoose in Africa, the fox in western Europe, and the bat in Latin America and the United States.

Bats and wild animals important

## Treatment

Prevention is the mainstay of controlling human rabies. Intensive supportive care has resulted in two or three long-term survivals; despite the best modern medical care, however, the mortality still exceeds 90%. In addition, because of the infrequency of the disease, many cases die without definitive diagnosis. Human hyperimmune antirabies globulin interferon and vaccine do not alter the disease once symptoms have developed.

## Prevention

In the late 1800s Pasteur, noting the long incubation period of rabies, suggested that a vaccine to induce an immune response before the development of disease might be useful in prevention. He apparently successfully vaccinated Joseph Meister, a boy severely bitten and exposed to rabies, with multiple injections of a crude vaccine made from dried spinal cord

Pasteur's vaccine from dried spinal cord

of rabies-infected rabbits. This treatment emerged as one of the best known and most noteworthy accomplishments in the annals of medicine.

Currently, the prevention of rabies is divided into preexposure and postexposure prophylaxis. Preexposure prophylaxis is recommended for individuals at high risk of contact with rabies virus, such as veterinarians, spelunkers, laboratory workers, and animal handlers. The vaccine currently used in the United States for preexposure prophylaxis employs an attenuated rabies virus grown in human diploid cell culture and inactivated with β-propiolactone. Preexposure prophylaxis consists of two subcutaneous injections of vaccine given 1 month apart, followed by a booster dose several months later.

Preexposure prophylaxis used for individuals at special risk

Postexposure prophylaxis requires careful evaluation and judgment. Every year more than one million Americans are bitten by animals, and in each instance a decision must be made whether to initiate postexposure rabies prophylaxis. In this decision the physician must consider (1) whether the individual came into physical contact with saliva or another substance likely to contain rabies virus; (2) whether there was significant wounding or abrasion; (3) whether rabies is known or suspected in the animal species and area associated with the exposure; (4) whether the bite was provoked or unprovoked (i.e., the circumstances surrounding the exposure); and (5) whether the animal is available for laboratory examination. Any wild animal or ill, unvaccinated, or stray domestic animal involved in a possible rabies exposure, such as an unprovoked bite, should be captured and killed. The head should be sent immediately to an appropriate laboratory, usually at the state health department, for search for rabies antigen by immunofluorescence. If examination of the brain by this technique is negative for rabies virus, it can be assumed that the saliva contains no virus and that the exposed person requires no treatment. If the test is positive, the patient should be given postexposure prophylaxis. It should be noted that rodents and rabbits are not important vectors of rabies virus.

Postexposure prophylaxis decision weighs many factors influencing decision to immunize after possible exposure

Postexposure prophylaxis is based on immediate, thorough washing of the wound with soap and water; passive immunization with hyperimmune globulin, of which at least half the dose should be instilled around the wound site; and active immunization with antirabies vaccine. With human diploid vaccine, five doses given on days 1, 3, 7, 14, and 28 are recommended.

Postexposure combines concurrent active and passive immunization

Physicians should always seek the advice of the local health department when the question of rabies prophylaxis arises.

## ADDITIONAL READING

Baer GM, Bridbord K, Hui FW, et al (eds). Research towards rabies prevention. *Rev Infect Dis.* 1988;10(suppl 4):S573–S815. A symposium dealing with a worldwide perspective. It includes consideration of control of rabies in wildlife.

Recommendation of the Immunization Practices Advisory Committee. Rabies prevention—United States. *Morb Mortal Wkly Rep.* 1991;40(RR-3):1–19. Authoritative guide to rabies prophylaxis in humans.

Wunner WH, Larson JK, Dietzchold B, et al. The molecular biology of rabies viruses. *Rev Infect Dis.* 1988;10(suppl 4):S771–S784. Overview of the molecular biology of rabies viruses and the current state of knowledge of immunobiologic characteristics of different rabies virus components.

Chapter 41

# Retroviruses, Human Immunodeficiency Virus, and Acquired Immunodeficiency Syndrome

*James J. Champoux and W. Lawrence Drew*

The retroviruses are enveloped, single-stranded RNA viruses. They encode reverse transcriptase (an RNA-dependent DNA polymerase) that copies the genome into double-stranded DNA that becomes integrated into the host cell genome. Representatives of two major groups are considered in this chapter: the oncoviruses (*onco-*, "related to a tumor") and the lentiviruses (*lenti-*, "slow"). Like most enveloped viruses, all retroviruses are highly susceptible to factors that affect surface tension and are thus not transmissible through air, dust, or fomites under normal conditions, but require intimate contact with the infecting source.

Enveloped RNA viruses encode reverse transcriptase

Rapidly inactivated outside the body

Oncoviruses of this group have long been associated with a variety of cancers in animals, including leukemias, lymphomas, and sarcomas, but until recent years had not been found to infect humans. The first human retrovirus, human T-lymphotropic virus type 1 (HTLV-1), was discovered in the late 1970s. It was shown to cause adult T-cell leukemia, a rare malignancy found only in Japan, Africa, and the Caribbean, although serologic evidence shows that the virus also occurs in the United States and has raised the possibility of an association with some chronic neurologic conditions. A relative of HTLV-I, HTLV-II, has been associated with some cases of human leukemias, including hairy cell leukemia, but its precise role in these diseases remains unclear.

Oncoviruses cause tumors in many animals

HTLV-I and -II associated with human leukemias

The most important disease resulting from human retrovirus infection, the acquired immunodeficiency syndrome (AIDS), is caused by one of two lentiviruses termed *human immunodeficiency viruses* (HIV-1 and HIV-2). This devastating disease, for which there is no present cure, has spurred unprecedented research efforts to determine the nature and pathogenic mechanisms of HIV and other retroviruses in the hope of finding effective drugs and vaccines. Most of our present knowledge of HIV is derived from studies on HIV-1, which is the major cause of AIDS worldwide.

HIV-1 and -2 are lentiviruses that cause AIDS

Oncoviruses do not kill the cell they infect, but instead usually continue to produce new virus indefinitely. This property, combined with the fact that they can transduce growth-promoting genes called *oncogenes* into the recipient cell, accounts in part for their ability

Oncoviruses usually not cytolytic; transduce or activate oncogenes

Lentiviruses become cytopathic after long latency

to cause malignancies (see below). With lentivirus infections, the cell–virus relationship is quite different. Lentiviruses can persist for years in a latent state without causing much cell killing, only to become highly cytolytic when the infected cells are subjected to certain stimuli. The prototype lentivirus is the visna virus, which causes a slow degenerative neurologic disease in sheep. Like visna, HIV-1 can persist for long periods without serious effects, but eventually is induced to replicate to high levels resulting in cell death. Although HIV-1 can infect a variety of human cell types, its most drastic effects appear to result from destruction of the CD4+ subclass of T lymphocytes, which play a central role in the capacity of the host to mount effective and protective immunologic responses to a wide range of infections.

HIV attacks and destroys CD4+ T lymphocytes

## RETROVIRUSES

### Structure

Virion contains two single-stranded RNA molecules

Envelope acquired during budding contains two viral glycoproteins

Viral genome encodes structural and replicative proteins

All retroviruses are remarkably similar in their basic composition. The structure of HIV-1 is depicted in Fig 41–1. The virion is about 100 nm in diameter. It contains two copies of a single-stranded RNA genome and is thus diploid. The RNA genome is coated with the nucleocapsid protein (NC), and the RNA–protein complexes are enclosed in a capsid (CA) composed of multiple subunits. Like all enveloped viruses, the membrane is acquired during budding from the host cell, but the surface (SU) and transmembrane (TM) glycoproteins found in the envelope are virally encoded. Between the capsid and the envelope is a matrix (MA) protein. In addition to the structural proteins shown in Fig 41–1, the virion contains three virus-specific proteins that are essential for viral replication: reverse transcriptase, (RT), protease (PR), and an integrase (IN). The relationships between viral genes (*gag*, *pol*, and *env*) and the proteins they encode are presented in Table 41–1.

### Life Cycle

Figure 41–2 depicts the life cycle of a typical retrovirus and serves to illustrate the many unique aspects of retroviral replication that could be potential targets of therapeutic intervention.

#### Viral Entry

HIV-1 surface glycoprotein gp120 attaches to CD4 cell receptor

Transmembrane gp41 protein mediates fusion of viral and cell membranes

Can infect cells without CD4 molecule

The virions adsorb to cellular membrane receptors and enter the cell probably by direct fusion with the plasma membrane. For HIV-1, the virion attachment protein is the SU glycoprotein gp120, and the cell receptor is the CD4 molecule that occurs primarily on the plasma membrane of CD4+ T lymphocytes, cells of the monocyte–macrophage series, and some other target cells. The HIV-1 transmembrane (TM) protein gp41 is responsible for fusion of viral and cell membranes, a process that apparently is important for entry of the virus into the host cell.

HIV-1 can also infect cells such as fibroblasts and certain brain cells that lack the CD4 surface molecule, apparently because the fusion-inducing activity of the TM protein is sufficient in these cases to promote entry. Fusion activity may also play an important role in

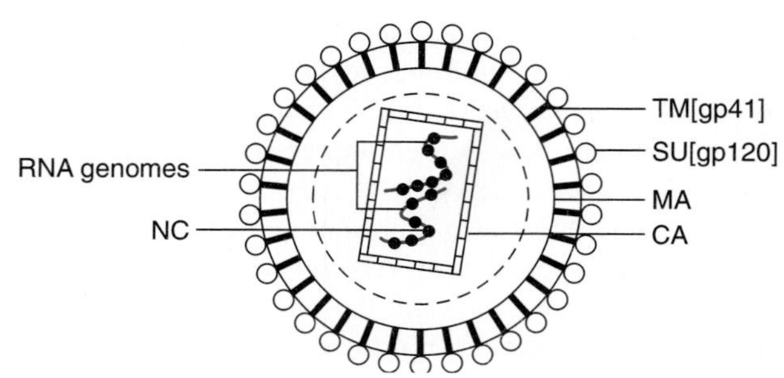


**Figure 41–1.** Structure of HIV particle. The two RNA molecules enclosed within the capsid (CA) are coated with the nucleocapsid protein (NC). The matrix protein (MA) lies just inside the membrane envelope. The envelope contains two membrane glycoproteins, gp41 and gp120, also called transmembrane protein (TM) and surface protein (SU), respectively.

TABLE 41–1. RETROVIRAL PROTEINS

| Gene[a] | Protein Products | Function |
|---|---|---|
| *gag* | Matrix (MA) | Structural |
| | Capsid (CA) | Structural |
| | Nucleocapsid (NC) | Structural |
| | Protease[b] (PR) | Protein processing |
| *pol* | Protease[b] (PR) | Protein processing |
| | Reverse transcriptase (RT) | DNA synthesis |
| | Integrase (IN) | Integration |
| *env* | Surface glycoprotein (SU) | Adsorption |
| | Transmembrane protein (TM) | Anchor for surface glycoprotein |

[a] Each gene encodes a polyprotein that is subsequently processed by proteolysis to yield the individual proteins.
[b] The protease is encoded in either the *gag* gene or the *pol* gene, depending on the virus.

amplification of the effects of the virus infection, because infected cells expressing viral glycoproteins in their membranes readily fuse with uninfected CD4+ T lymphocytes to form large syncytia. This process appears to provide a means for cell-to-cell transmission of the virus that bypasses the usual extracellular phase and also damages the membrane of uninfected cells and affects their viability.

Fusion provided direct cell-to-cell transmission

### Viral RNA Replication

Among the RNA viruses, retroviral replication is unique. Soon after entry of the viral core into the cytoplasm of the infected cell, the RNA is copied into double-stranded DNA by reverse transcriptase, the virion-associated DNA polymerase. The overall process is referred to as *reverse transcription* and results in a linear DNA molecule that enters the nucleus and integrates more or less at random into a host cell chromosome. Once the viral genetic information has been converted to DNA and integrated, it essentially becomes part of the cellular genome. The viral genes, called the *provirus,* are therefore replicated and faithfully inherited as long as the infected cell continues to divide.

Reverse transcriptase copies RNA to double-stranded DNA

DNA integrates into host chromosome and replicates with the cell as a provirus

Special sequences contained within the RNA are duplicated during the reverse transcription process so that the integrated provirus contains identical long terminal repeats (LTRs) at its ends. The LTR sequences contain the appropriate promoter, enhancer, and other signals required for transcription of the viral genes by the host RNA polymerase II. Transcription produces both a full-length RNA genome and one or more spliced mRNAs. The predominant spliced mRNA is translated to produce the envelope glycoproteins, but in HIV-1 a series of spliced mRNAs are produced that also encode a variety of viral regulatory proteins. Unlike most retroviruses, HIV-1 apparently exerts considerable control over whether primary transcripts are allocated to full-length RNA or are spliced to produce mRNAs (see below). With the exception of these regulatory proteins, all retroviral proteins are initially translated as polyproteins that are subsequently processed by proteolysis into the individual protein molecules. The enzyme responsible for most of these protein cleavages is the virus-specific protease (PR) that is encoded in either the *gag* gene or the *pol* gene of the virus (see Table 41–1).

Provirus includes its own promoter and signals that control transcription by host RNA polymerase

Genomic RNA and spliced mRNAs are both produced: the latter encode surface glycoproteins and regulatory proteins

HIV-1 can control extent of genomic or spliced mRNA production

A simplified view of retroviral RNA replication is presented in Fig 41–3. In addition to a DNA polymerase activity, the reverse transcriptase possesses an RNase H activity that is responsible for degrading the RNA portion of the DNA–RNA hybrid (+RNA/–DNA) produced in the first phase of reverse transcription. The immediate product of reverse transcription is a linear double-stranded DNA molecule that is flanked by the LTR sequences. The viral integrase (IN) catalyzes the reaction required for the integration of the linear DNA into host DNA. The integration process is highly specific with respect to the viral DNA and 2 base pairs are generally lost from each end of the DNA. The choice of a target site for integration into the cellular DNA appears, however, to be nearly random. A short sequence of base pairs in the target DNA (4 to 6 depending on the virus) is duplicated during the integration process and the sequences immediately flank the integrated provirus. The replication process is completed by transcription of the proviral DNA by the host RNA polymerase II.

RNase H activity degrades original RNA genome

Integrase catalyzed integration is random in host DNA

Integrated DNA is transcribed by host RNA polymerase

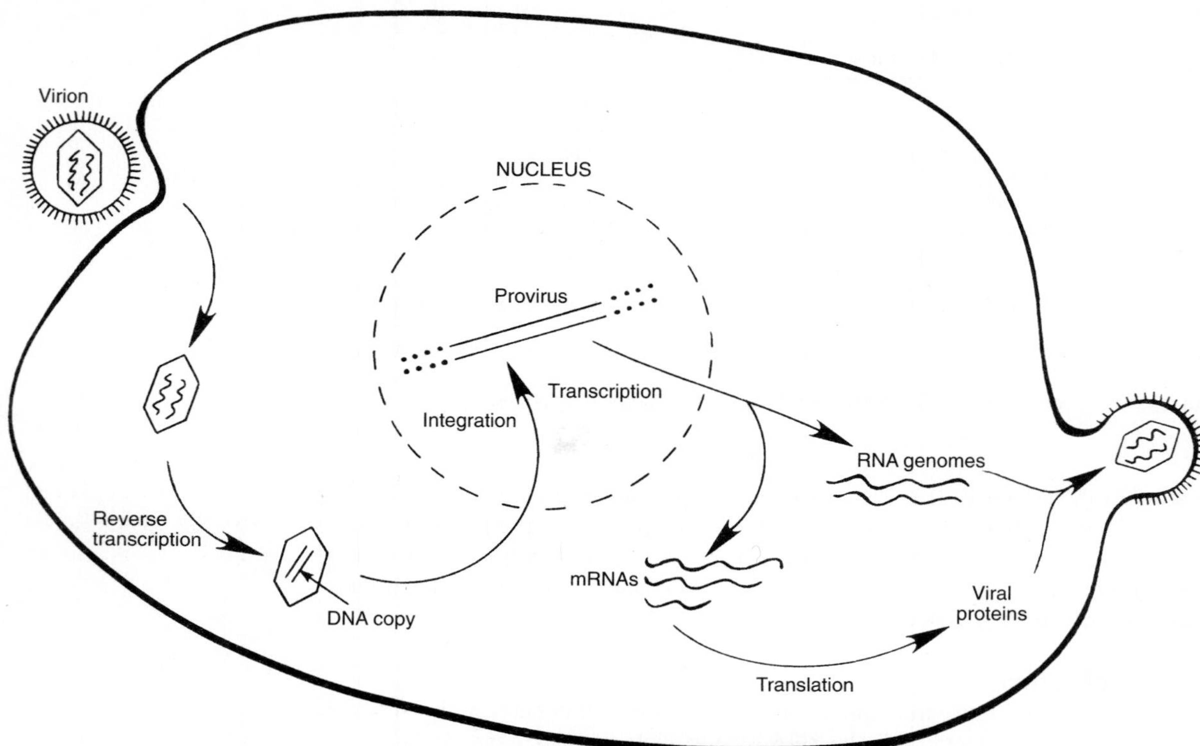


**Figure 41–2.** Retroviral life cycle.

It should be noted that the scheme represented in Fig 41–3 also describes the replication cycle for hepatitis B virus (see Chapter 36). Instead of packaging the RNA form of the genome as occurs with retroviruses, hepatitis B virus packages the double-stranded DNA that is the immediate product of reverse transcription.

### Variation in HIV-1

HIV reverse transcriptase error prone

Isolates from the same patient can differ in multiple properties

Of all the known retroviruses, HIV-1 possesses the most error-prone reverse transcriptase. This property accounts for the many nucleotide differences observed between different isolates (even from the same infected individual) and for the variability of the gp120 antigen. It may explain in part the failure of the immune system to control the infection and the increases in viral virulence that appear to occur during the course of the infection.

## Retroviral Genes

Genome organized into *gag*, *pol*, and env *genes*

The organization of the genome of different types of retroviruses is shown in Fig 41–4 (see also Table 41–1). The order of the genes for a typical retrovirus is *gag–pol–env*. The *gag* (group-specific antigen) gene encodes the structural proteins of the virus and, in some cases, the protease. The *pol* (polymerase) gene encodes the reverse transcriptase, the integrase, and sometimes the protease. The *env* (envelope) gene encodes the two membrane glycoproteins found in the viral envelope. Not surprisingly, the surface protein (gp120 in HIV-!) is responsible for the host range of the virus and its antigenicity. As indicated previously, the HIV-1 *env* gene is found to exhibit extensive variation from one isolate to another, resulting in considerable polymorphism of gp120.

Some retroviruses carry host genes rendering them oncogenic

The genomes of acute transforming oncoviruses have a variety of structures, but one feature is common to nearly all of them: some viral genes are replaced by genes derived from their hosts that render them oncogenic (see below). In every case, the signals required for reverse transcription and transcription of the provirus, which are located near the ends of the RNA, are retained in the infecting virus. In the example shown in Fig 41–4, the *pol* gene and parts of both the viral *gag* and *env* genes are deleted, but other configurations are

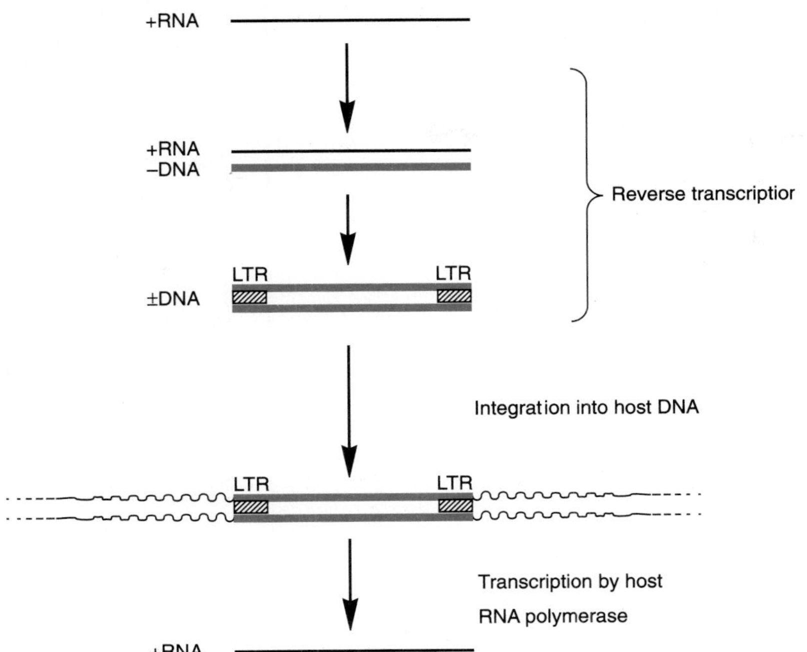


**Figure 41–3.** Retroviral RNA replication. LTR, long terminal repeat.

possible. Such oncoviruses are defective and replicate only in the presence of a helper virus that can supply the missing functions.

Defective transforming oncogenic viruses require helper virus

A comparison of the genetic makeup of HIV-1 with that of a typical retrovirus (see Fig 41–4) reveals a larger number of genes and a much more complex organization. HIV-1 contains, in addition to the usual ensemble of genes, an array of other genes (*tat, rev, nef, vif, vpr,* and *vpu*). Expression of these genes requires mRNA splicing, and all apparently encode proteins that serve regulatory roles important in determining the long period of latency exhibited by the virus (see below). HTLV-1 encodes a similar array of regulatory proteins. The names of the genes that have been best characterized and the proteins and functions they determine are listed in Table 41–2.

HIV-1 has multiple regulatory genes regulating latency

## Transformation by Retroviruses

Oncogenic retroviruses appear to transform cells to an oncogenic state by three distinct mechanisms (see Chapter 7).

First, the acute transforming viruses (see Fig 41–4) have acquired a cellular gene (called an *oncogene*) that when expressed in the infected cell results in loss of normal growth control. On infection, the oncogene is expressed from the viral LTR promoter, resulting in a rapid and acute onset of malignant disease. Persistent transformation by oncogene transduction is possible only for those retroviruses that are not cytocidal. More than 25 different oncogenes have been identified in a variety of animal retroviruses, but no human retroviruses are known that transform by this mechanism.

Noncytocidal viruses carrying cellular oncogenes can produce persistent transformation

The second mechanism is called *insertional mutagenesis.* Integration of a retrovirus in the vicinity of particular cellular genes can cause inappropriate expression of the gene, resulting in uncontrolled cell growth. These cellular genes are called *protooncogenes,* and insertional activation by the virus is apparently due to the close proximity of the integrated viral promoter or enhancer to the gene. Cancers that are caused by this mechanism have very long latent periods, because integration is random and only rarely occurs near a cellular protooncogene. No human cancers are known to be caused by this mechanism.

Integration adjacent to cellular protooncogenes can activate them

The causative agent of adult T-cell leukemia, HTLV-1, exemplifies the third mechanism. In this case, the integrated provirus in the leukemic cells from any one patient is found at a unique location on a particular chromosome. Thus, the tumors are probably monoclonal.

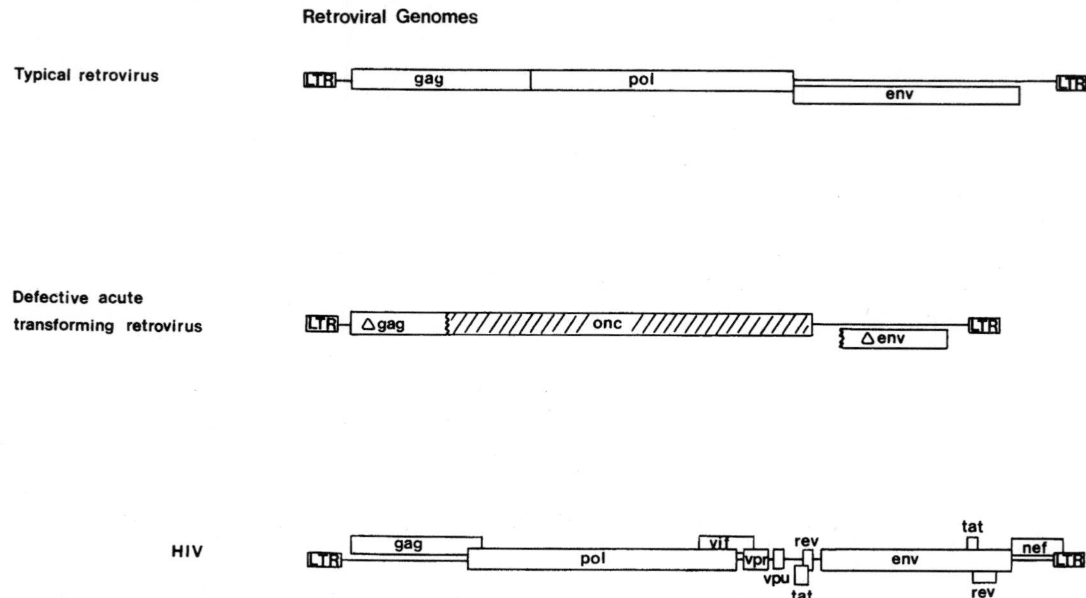


**Figure 41–4.** Maps of the integrated forms of various retroviral genomes are drawn with the genes and long terminal repeats (LTRs) shown as boxes. The vertical displacements of the boxes above and below the lines depict the relative reading frames of the coding segments.

HTLV-1 transforms by production of TAX, which activates cellular transforming genes

The cancer is not the result of insertional mutagenesis, however, because the chromosomal location of the provirus is never the same in any two patients. Instead, transformation results from the continual expression of the viral *tax* gene (the HTLV-1 homolog of the HIV-1 *tat* gene, see Table 41–2). Apparently, the TAX protein not only can activate viral transcription in the same manner as TAT (see below), but can also activate the expression of one or more cellular genes (possibly protooncogenes) resulting in malignant transformation.

## Human Immunodeficiency Virus Latency

Prolonged HIV-1 latency may include periods without protein expression

A unique feature of HIV-1 and other members of the lentivirus subfamily is the ability to produce a complex array of regulatory proteins that appear to be responsible for latent periods that can extend for months or years. In some cases, virus-specific DNA has even been detected in individuals who show no immunologic response, suggesting that the viral genome can exist for prolonged periods in a quiescent state without expressing viral proteins.

HIV-1 regulation is at three levels

Although much remains to be determined about the regulatory circuits that modulate HIV-1 gene expression, the following features of the process have been established. Regulation appears to occur at three levels: mRNA production, transport of unspliced versus spliced mRNAs from the nucleus to the cytoplasm, and maturation of viral proteins during budding. It may also occur at the level of mRNA translation. The HIV-1 regulatory proteins and their functions are listed in Table 41–2. In the absence of the viral regulatory proteins, two features of the expression of the HIV-1 proviral DNA are significant. First, the viral promoter in the LTR is intrinsically weak. Second, transport of the full-length, unspliced mRNA to the cytoplasm is so inefficient that only spliced mRNAs are translated. Extensive splicing precludes production of the virion structural proteins and the enzymes required for virus production. Thus, shortly after integration, viral gene expression is restricted to the viral envelope glycoproteins and the regulatory proteins. One of these regulatory proteins is the NEF protein, which is apparently responsible for maintaining the latent state. NEF acts on a DNA sequence (NRE) in the viral LTR near the promoter to further suppress the transcription of the integrated proviral DNA.

The HIV viral promoter is weak

Transport of unspliced HIV genome to the cytoplasm is inefficient

Integrated virus initially expresses only surface and regulatory products from spliced mRNAs

**TABLE 41–2. HUMAN IMMUNODEFICIENCY VIRUS AND HUMAN T-LYMPHOTROPIC VIRUS REGULATORY PROTEINS**

| Gene | Protein | Function |
|---|---|---|
| HIV-*tat* | TAT | Increases rate of viral transcription |
| HTLV-*tax* | TAX | Same as for TAT |
| HIV-*rev* | REV | Increases transport of unspliced mRNAs |
| HTLV-*rex* | REX | Same as for REV |
| HIV-*nef* | NEF | Negative regulator of transcription |
| HIV-*vif* | VIF | Facilitates virus maturation during budding |

Two of the regulatory proteins, TAT and REV, play a positive role in promoting viral gene expression. The TAT protein increases the rate of viral mRNA synthesis, and REV promotes the transport of full-length mRNA to the cytoplasm before it can be spliced. The combined action of these two regulatory proteins is to promote the production of virus particles. Therefore, TAT acts to counter the activity of NEF, whereas REV promotes the production of virion structural proteins at the expense of its own production and that of other regulatory proteins. The VIF protein promotes virus production at the level of maturation.

Regulatory protein NEF maintains the latent state and counters effects of TAT and REV

Superimposed on this complex regulatory network is the fact that the viral promoter contains elements that are sensitive to specific cellular transcription factors. This observation may help explain why virus production in CD4+ T lymphocytes is greatly increased when the cells are activated. Clearly the outcome of an HIV-1 infection is determined by a complex interplay between a very large number of different factors.

Viral production is enhanced when CD4+ T lymphocytes are activated

## ACQUIRED IMMUNODEFICIENCY SYNDROME

There must now be few literate people in the world who are unaware of the AIDS pandemic and of its basic features. HIV-1 and HIV-2 disable the immune system and thus predispose to a wide range of opportunistic infections and some tumors. The viruses can also cause damage to brain cells, and the dementia that ensues is one of the most serious effects of the disease. It has become increasingly difficult to define AIDS, as the spectrum of opportunistic infections and secondary neoplasms indicating AIDS has widened. As of 1993, the Centers for Disease Control and Prevention define as AIDS patients all those who are HIV antibody positive and have CD4+ T-lymphocyte counts below 200/mm$^3$ or less than 14% of total T lymphocytes. Table 41–3 tabulates the current definition using indicator diseases in patients either who have not been tested for antibody to HIV or who have tested positive for such antibody. The purpose of this section is to give a broader overview of AIDS and associated syndromes and to consider the epidemiology, diagnosis, and treatment of HIV infection and the possibilities for control in the future.

**TABLE 41–3. 1993 REVISED CLASSIFICATION SYSTEM FOR HIV INFECTION AND EXPANDED AIDS SURVEILLANCE CASE DEFINITION FOR ADOLESCENTS AND ADULTS**

| | Clinical categories | | |
|---|---|---|---|
| CD4+ T-cell categories | (A) Asymptomatic, acute (primary) HIV or PGL[a] | (B) Symptomatic, not (A) or (C) conditions | (C) AIDS-indicator conditions[b] |
| (1) ≥ 500/μL | A1 | B1 | C1 |
| (2) 200—499/μL | A2 | B2 | C2 |
| (3) ≤ 200/μL AIDS-indicator T-cell count | A3 | B3 | C3 |

[a] PGL persistent generalized lymphadenopathy. Clinical Category A includes acute (primary) HIV infection.

[b] Kaposi's sarcoma, opportunistic infection, see text.

*Adapted from Centers for Disease Control. Morbid Mortal Weekly Rept. 1993; 41: RR-17, p. 2, table 1.*

## Historical Background

AIDS first recognized in 1981

The AIDS syndrome was first recognized in the United States in 1981, when it became apparent that an unusual number of rare skin cancers (Kaposi's sarcoma) and opportunistic infections were occurring among male homosexuals. These patients were found to have a marked reduction in CD4+ T lymphocytes and were subject to a wide range of opportunistic infections normally controlled by an intact immune system. The disease was found to progress relentlessly to a fatal outcome and was first identified in male homosexuals, hemophiliacs who were receiving blood-derived coagulation factors, and intravenous drug abusers.

Skin cancers and opportunistic infection associated with reduction in T4 lymphocytes

As a result of the work of groups lead by Montagnier in France and Gallo in the United States a retrovirus (lentivirus) now known as HIV-1 was isolated, and serologic methods were developed that showed it to be responsible for the disease. Within an amazingly short time, the mode of replication of the virus, its genome, and most of the products that it encodes were characterized. It was also recognized that the extraordinary complexity and variability of the virus together with its affinity for the master cell of the immune system would make AIDS unusually difficult to control.

HIV-1 isolated and characterized as complex retrovirus

Growth of the virus in cell culture and identification of its antigens allowed development of effective test procedures for detecting HIV infection. These almost eliminated the risk of transmission by blood transfusion and allowed assessment of the modes of transmission of the disease and the extent of infection nationally and worldwide. It became apparent that heterosexual transmission could occur and that the infection could be transmitted from mother to infant either by intrauterine spread or during the birth process. It was also found that the disease had its greatest prevalence in parts of Africa where the spread was predominantly heterosexual.

New serologic tests restricted transmission by transfusion

Vertical and heterosexual transmission recognized

Retrospective serologic studies with material saved from patients with immunodeficiencies indicate that the disease was already occurring in Africa in the 1950s and in the United States in the 1970s. In 1985, a related but distinct virus, HIV-2, was also found to be endemic in parts of West Africa and to cause AIDS. To date, this virus has been relatively restricted geographically although infections with it have occurred in the western hemisphere. Simian immunodeficiency viruses have also been discovered that cause a disease in monkeys analogous to AIDS. These agents are genomically more closely related to HIV-2 than to HIV-1 and provide some insight into the biologic heritage of their human counterparts.

HIV-2, a second virus of AIDS, is still geographically restricted

## Epidemiology of HIV Infection

### Transmission

The HIV virus is transmitted between humans in three ways: sexually, perinatally, and by exposure to contaminated blood or body fluids. The virus has been demonstrated in particularly high titers in semen and cervical secretions, and the majority of cases result from sexual contact. Infection is facilitated by breaks in epithelial surfaces, which provide direct access to the underlying tissues or bloodstream. The relative fragility of the rectal mucosa probably contributed to the predominance of the disease among male homosexuals. Heterosexual transmission accounts for an increasing proportion of new cases and is frequent in the developing world. Transmission appears to be more efficient from men to women, but the reverse is clearly documented. The risk of perinatal transmission from an infected mother to her child is unknown but has been estimated at 30%.

Sex, blood, and birth primary risks

Heterosexual transmission of increasing importance

Until serologic tests for the infection became available in 1985, more than 10,000 cases were probably acquired in the United States through blood transfusion, and about 80% of hemophiliacs treated with coagulation factors derived from pooled blood sources became infected. Testing of donors and the use of recombinant or specially treated coagulation factors have now virtually eliminated these sources of infection. Transmission of infection by blood is now largely associated with sharing of needles and syringes by injecting drug users and this has been an increasing source of the disease. In some areas of the world the seroprevalence of HIV positivity among injecting drug users has been as high as 70%.

Blood transfusion continues among IV drug abusers

Transmission of infection to health care workers after accidental sticks with potentially contaminated needles is very rare (considerably less than 1% of occurrences), presumably because the amount of infectious virus in the blood of infected cases is small and larger volumes or repeated exposures are needed for a significant chance of infection. Nevertheless, cases have occurred from both clinical and laboratory exposure, and the universal precautions described in Chapter 72 are directed primarily at further reducing this risk.

Risk of transmission from accidental needle sticks is very low

Transmission does not occur through day-to-day nonsexual contact with infected individuals or through insect vectors. This is because of the fragility of the virus and the need for direct mucosal or blood contact. It is of interest that the virus has been detected in saliva, tears, urine, and breast milk. With the possible exception of breast milk, these sources have not been shown to be infectious.

No transmission by day-to-day nonsexual contact or by insects

### Occurrence

In the United States the highest prevalence rates of HIV infections are in homosexual and bisexual males, intravenous drug abusers, prostitutes, and sexual partners of HIV-infected persons. In some areas of the United States, 40 to 60% of homosexual males attending sexually transmitted disease clinics were found to be infected. Rates in prostitutes vary from 0 to 40%, depending partly on the degree of associated drug abuse. Prevalence rates in the heterosexual population, in general, are currently less than 1%, but have been increasing. In the United States in 1985 only 7% of AIDS cases were in women; by 1991 the percentage had risen to 13%. Approximately 2000 newborns per year are infected by HIV perinatally.

Most common in male homosexuals, bisexuals, drug abusers, prostitutes, and sex partners of HIV infected

Prevalence increasing in women

In contrast to the situation in the Western world, heterosexual transmission is the primary route of transmission in Africa, where there is an approximately equal distribution of infection and disease between the sexes. This may be due to a high frequency in affected areas of ulcerative genital lesions caused by other sexually transmitted diseases. These lesions facilitate passage of virus into the tissues of others during heterosexual intercourse.

Heterosexual transmission primary in Africa

Facilitated by genital ulcerative lesions from other infections

Acquired immunodeficiency syndrome has been reported in more than 150 countries, and it has been estimated that by the year 2000, 30 to 50 million people will be infected with HIV worldwide. In the United States, more than 300,000 cases had been reported by October of 1993, and it is believed that well over a million people are infected. HIV-2 infection is found primarily in West Africa and is spread by heterosexual transmission. Infection by this virus has, however, been reported in Europe in homosexual men, injecting drug users, transfusion recipients, and hemophiliac men. As of July 1992, 32 cases of HIV-2 infection had been identified in the United States, most of whom were immigrants from West Africa.

Millions of HIV-1 infected people worldwide

Imported HIV-2 cases seen in US

The epidemiology of HIV infection is changing in the United States as the pandemic evolves and as the modes of transmission become more generally understood. The homosexual communities that were first afflicted have modified their behavior and adopted prophylactic procedures that are tending to prevent new infections. On the other hand, the numbers and proportions of heterosexually transmitted, drug abuse-related, and neonatal cases are increasing, particularly among the poor and disadvantaged racial minorities. On a worldwide scale, the disease continues to spread rapidly in Africa and South America. In some areas of Africa, up to one tenth of the population is infected. The impact on the future development of these countries will be severe and the health care systems throughout the world will be hard pressed to meet the challenge of AIDS in the 1990s.

Increasing proportion of infections in heterosexuals, drug abusers, and newborns

Increasing devastation of developing world

## Pathogenesis of HIV-1 Infection

The pathogenesis of HIV-1 infection is incompletely understood and very complex, but the following factors are likely to be important in the disease-causing process.

### Infection

The initial target of HIV-1 is CD4 molecules, particularly on the surface of CD4+ helper T lymphocytes, monocytes, and macrophages. The virus can also infect other human tissues expressing CD4, and a wide range of CD4–cells including enterocytes, renal epithelium, and brain astrocytes. The mechanism for infection of non-CD4-bearing cells is unknown, but may involve other receptors or fusion with cells already infected with HIV. Other

HIV primarily infects cells bearing CD4

Other receptors and fusion may be important

viruses, particularly the herpesviruses, may act as cofactors for HIV infection, possibly by inducing surface receptors on cells they infect.

### Latency

Latency may be determined by proviral mutational changes

The long asymptomatic period following HIV infection (clinical latency) is surely related to the aspects of cellular latency described above, but other factors may be involved. For example, there is evidence that clinical latency can continue despite active virus replication in the host. Several factors can terminate the long latent period of HIV-1. Mutations occur during viral replication that appear to enhance induction of virulent virus forms of increased cytopathic capacity and altered cell tropisms. In the same patient, the mutated forms of HIV-1 isolated from later stages of disease infect a broader range of cell types and grow more rapidly than those isolated in the asymptomatic period. If this is the case, the more virulent mutants are unlikely to be the transmitted form of the virus, because the natural history of the disease does not appear to have changed. A second factor may be a requirement for activation of infected T cells to permit virus production and cell death, and this may involve a variety of mitogenic and antigenic stimuli occurring after infection.

Cytopathic capacity and cell tropisms change as the virus mutates

Production correlates with T cell activation

### Disease Progression

Macrophages may be significant in infection and spread by cell fusion

The virus replicates in macrophages, which may well be the first cells infected, as few activated CD4+ T lymphocytes are normally circulating in the blood. The virus replicates slowly in macrophages but these cells could serve as a reservoir for continued expansion of the infection to other cell types by cell-to-cell fusion, which allows the virus to spread without being exposed to neutralizing antibody. In addition to CD4+ T lymphocytes, the most prominent cell types infected are glial cells and astrocytes in the brain and the bowel mucosa. Infected macrophages may participate in breakdown of the blood–brain barrier, allowing enhanced exposure of the central nervous system (CNS). Although CNS and intestinal disturbances are a prominent part of full-blown AIDS, it is not clear whether they are a direct result of infection of these cells or mediated by cytokines from macrophages and T lymphocytes.

Brain and bowel cells can be infected

### HIV-Induced Immunodeficiency

Primary defect is virual or immunological destruction of CD4+ lymphocytes or their functional impairment

The primary immune defect in AIDS results from the reduction in the numbers and effectiveness of CD4+ helper-inducer T lymphocytes, both in absolute numbers and relative to CD8+ suppressor T lymphocytes. This is due to direct killing of CD4+ T lymphocytes by the virus, but may also involve other effects on immune function. These include secondary killing of uninfected (bystander) cells during cell fusion, autoimmune processes that lead to the elimination of CD4+ T lymphocytes by opsonophagocytosis, and antibody-dependent cell-mediated cytotoxicity (ADCC) directed at gp120 expressed on the CD4+ cell surface. There are also functional defects in CD4+ T lymphocytes affecting lymphokine production and leading to inhibition of some macrophage functions including low levels of interleukin-1 and interferon alpha.

AIDS involves generalized failure of cell-mediated immune response and of specific antibody responses

Effects on CD4+ T lymphocytes thus lead to a generalized failure of cell-mediated immune responses, but there is also an effect on antibody production due to polyclonal activation of B cells, possibly associated with other viral infections of these cells. This overwhelms the capacity of infected individuals to respond to specific antigens. The end result of these processes is a disturbance of immune balance that can give rise to malignancies as well as the susceptibility of AIDS patients to a range of viral, fungal, and bacterial infections to which they ultimately succumb.

## ACQUIRED IMMUNODEFICIENCY SYNDROME: CLINICAL ASPECTS

### Clinical Manifestations

Initial infection is often asymptomatic, but may be mononucleosis-like

Infection with HIV results in a wide spectrum of disease varying from silent infection to the presence of multiple opportunistic infections and cerebral damage. The initial infection with HIV is usually asymptomatic, although in some cases a mononucleosis-like illness develops 2 to 4 weeks after infection and lasts about 2 to 6 weeks. This illness manifests as fever, malaise, lymphadenopathy, hepatosplenomegaly, arthralgias, and rash. Sometimes there is also a mild aseptic meningitis. Whether or not these early manifestations of infection occur, the virus persists and integrates into the genome of some host cells, and the individual is thus infected for life.

Virus integrates into genome

The initial infection is followed by an asymptomatic period that, in most cases, continues for years before the disease becomes clinically apparent. During this time virus can be isolated from blood, semen, and the cervix. Approximately 50% of infected individuals develop significant disease within 10 years of infection, and the number continues to increase thereafter (Fig 41–5). It is expected that nearly all HIV-infected individuals will eventually develop some clinical aspects of this infection.

Virus may be isolated during latent period

Disease can manifest in one of three ways:

1. Persistent generalized lymphadenopathy syndrome (PGL), characterized by enlarged lymph nodes at multiple sites persisting longer than 3 months.
2. AIDS-related complex (ARC), or the presence of two or more signs and symptoms such as fever, fatigue, diarrhea, weight loss, and night sweats, together with laboratory findings indicating immune dysfunction.
3. Full-blown AIDS, which involves the occurrence of opportunistic infections, malignancies (eg, Kaposi's sarcoma), progressive wasting, and/or encephalopathy.

One commonly used clinical classification for HIV infections is that developed by the Centers for Disease Control (CDC) (see Table 41–3).

As the disease progresses, the number of CD4+ T lymphocytes declines, there is increasing immunodeficiency, and opportunistic infections become more frequent, severe, and difficult to treat. One of the best markers of the severity of AIDS is the absolute number of CD4+ T lymphocytes. Those individuals with overt AIDS almost always have fewer than 400 CD4+ T lymphocytes per microliter of blood (normal = 800–1200 cells/μL).

Severity of disease increases with declining CD4+ T lymphocyte numbers

Patients with full-blown AIDS experience a wide spectrum of infections depending on the severity of their immune defect and on the opportunistic organisms in their normal flora or with which they come in contact (Table 41–4). Some clinical manifestations of AIDS may thus vary by locale. For example, disseminated histoplasmosis is a common complication in the Midwest of the United States, as disseminated toxoplasmosis is in France. These infections are uncommon in areas where the diseases are not endemic. The diversity and anatomic sites of infection vary between patients, and any one patient may have several infections. The most common infection is pneumocystosis, and approximately 50% of patients develop *Pneumocystis carinii* pneumonia. In the past, about a quarter of all AIDS

Fully developed AIDS is associated with severe opportunistic infections

50% develop *P. carinii* pneumonia

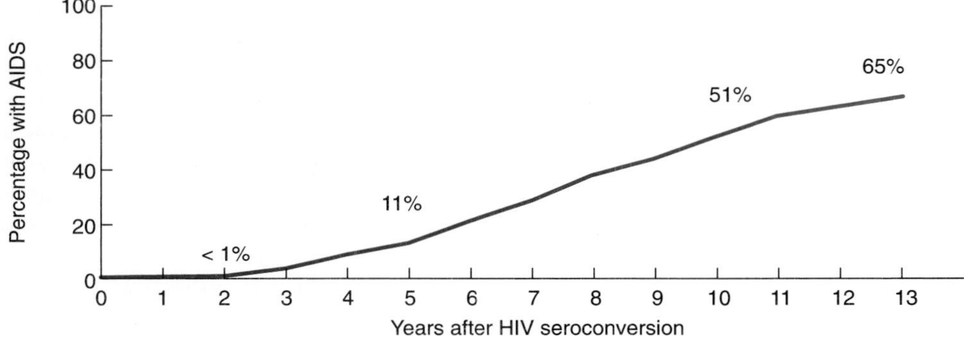


**Figure 41–5.** Progression time to AIDS. Data taken from 562 patients followed by the San Francisco City Clinic cohort. (*Reprinted with permission from Lifson AR, Hessol NA, Rutherford GW. Progression and clinical outcome of infection due to human immunodeficiency virus.* Clin Infect Dis. *1992;14:966–972.*)

**TABLE 41–4. COMMON OPPORTUNISTIC INFECTIONS IN PATIENTS WITH AIDS**

**Protozoan**
Pneumocystosis (*P. carinii* classification uncertain)
Toxoplasmosis
*Isospora belli* infection
Cryptosporidiosis

**Fungal**
Cryptococcosis
Candidiasis
Histoplasmosis (disseminated)

**Mycobacterial**
Disseminated tuberculosis (especially extrapulmonary)
*Mycobacterium avium–intracellulare* complex infections

**Viral**
Persistent mucocutaneous herpes simplex
Pulmonary cytomegalovirus, retinitis, gastrointestinal, or disseminated infection
Varicella–zoster, persistent or disseminated
Progressive multifocal leukoencephalopathy

Kaposi's sarcoma declining in US

patients developed Kaposi's sarcoma, but the number of cases has been falling in the United States despite increasing numbers of cases of AIDS. One explanation is that Kaposi's sarcoma is due to a transmitted agent different from HIV and that the spread of this organism has diminished as high-risk sexual behavior has decreased especially among gay men. Mycobacteria of the *avium–intracellulare* complex are very common agents of infection, and AIDS patients are also highly susceptible to *Mycobacterium tuberculosis* infection. Oral thrush and esophagitis due to *Candida albicans* and meningitis due to *Cryptococcus* are commonly encountered fungal infections. Persistent progressive mucocutaneous herpes simplex and herpes–zoster infections are common. Disseminated cytomegalovirus infection is often seen and presents with fever and visceral (eg, adrenal) organ involvement. Cytomegalovirus chorioretinitis is one of the most common opportunistic infections and may result in unilateral or bilateral blindness.

Mycobacterial, fungal, and viral infections are common

Specific opportunistic infections are associated with differing levels of CD4+ T-lymphocyte counts. For example, fungal and tuberculous pneumonia may occur with CD4+ T-lymphocyte counts of 200 to 500 cells/mm$^3$, whereas cytomegalovirus and *Mycobacterium avium–intracellulare* disease are seen almost exclusively in those whose counts are below 50 cells/mm$^3$.

Neurologic manifestations and lymphomas appear in later stages

As the duration of survival of AIDS patients has extended, an increasing number are developing neurologic manifestations of the disease and lymphoid neoplasms, especially non-Hodgkin's lymphomas. HIV is a neurotropic virus and can be isolated from the cerebrospinal fluid of 50 to 70% of patients with CDC class III or IV infection. Central nervous system involvement may be asymptomatic, but many patients develop a subacute neurologic illness that produces clinical symptoms varying from mild cognitive dysfunction to severe dementia. Loss of complex cognitive function is usually the first sign of illness. Progression to severe memory loss, depression, seizures, and coma may ensue. There is cerebral atrophy involving primarily cortical white matter which can be demonstrated by computed tomography or magnetic resonance imaging. Histologically, focal vacuolation of the affected brain tissue with perivascular infiltration of macrophages is noted. Multinucleated giant cells with syncytium formation surround the perivascular infiltrates. Neurologic symptoms do not usually occur until CD4+ T-lymphocyte counts are below 200 cells/mm$^3$.

Encephalopathy may progress to dementia, coma

Wasting disease in Africa

In children, a lymphocytic interstitial lung disease often occurs, possibly as a result of direct HIV infection of the lung. The disease spectrum in Africa is similar in many respects to that in the Western world, but many more patients present with severe intractable wasting and diarrhea called *slim disease*. Tuberculosis is also more commonly encountered in AIDS patients in Africa, reflecting the higher incidence of the disease in the population in general.

The 2-year mortality of AIDS, once the disease has been fully established, was initially 75%, with nearly all cases eventually dying of opportunistic infections or neoplasms.

Recent advances in therapy have slowed progression of the disease, but have not thus far prevented its relentless progress. In the United States AIDS has now overtaken unintentional injuries as the leading cause of death in men aged 25 to 44. The dramatic increase in AIDS deaths since 1982 is shown in Fig 41–6.

Therapy has slowed progress but not ultimate fatal outcome

## Diagnosis of Human Immunodeficiency Virus Infection

The diagnosis of AIDS is most commonly made by demonstrating antibody to the virus or its components. Initial screening tests are made using whole viral lysates as the target antigens in enzyme immunosoassay (EIA) tests (see Chapter 14). These have a high level of sensitivity, but because false positives occur, all positive EIA tests must be confirmed. The confirmatory test is a Western blot analysis which detects antibodies to specific viral proteins. In this procedure, viral proteins are separated by electrophoresis, transferred to nitrocellulose paper, and incubated with antisera; antibody bound to the individual proteins is detected by enzyme-labeled anti-human globulin sera (see Fig 41–7). Sera from infected patients have antibodies that react with the envelope glycoproteins or core proteins, or both. Tests made with HIV-1 detect antibody in 60 to 90% of patients infected by HIV-2.

Detection of HIV-1 antibody by EIA primary screening test

Western blot confirms by detecting antibody against specific HIV envelope and core proteins

60–90% crossreaction with HIV-2

The combination of EIA and Western blot tests gives a high degree of specificity to test results, but antibody is not detectable by these procedures in the first 2 to 4 weeks after infection. During this period the individual can still transmit the infection to others by sexual contact or blood donation. Closing this detection gap is particularly important for protection of blood products for transfusion. Although the virus can be grown during this time in mixed lymphocytic cell culture, the methods are impractical and may not be positive for up to a month. More promising approaches include direct detection of HIV core p24 antigenemia and exploitation of the polymerase chain reaction (PCR). Commercial PCR methods using primers to amplify part of the viral genome have been developed and are undergoing standardization. In addition to blood screening, these methods will be useful in detecting the very rare individuals who remain seronegative for up to 20 months. They may also be useful in determining if infants born to seropositive mothers are infected or simply demonstrating transplacental antibody.

Antibodies may not be detectable for several weeks after infection

Culture methods impractical for screening

Direct detection of core p24 by PCR under development

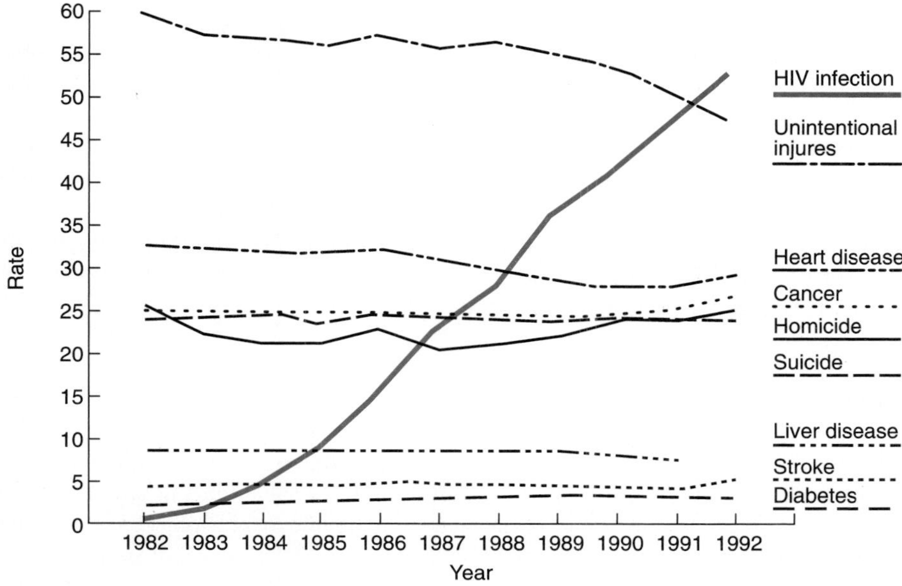


**Figure 41–6.** Death rates per 100,000 population among men aged 25 to 44 by year—United States, 1982–1992. (*Reprinted with permission from Update: Mortality attributable to HIV infection among persons aged 25–44 years—United States, 1991 and 1992.* Morb Mortal Wkly Rep. *1993;42:871.*)

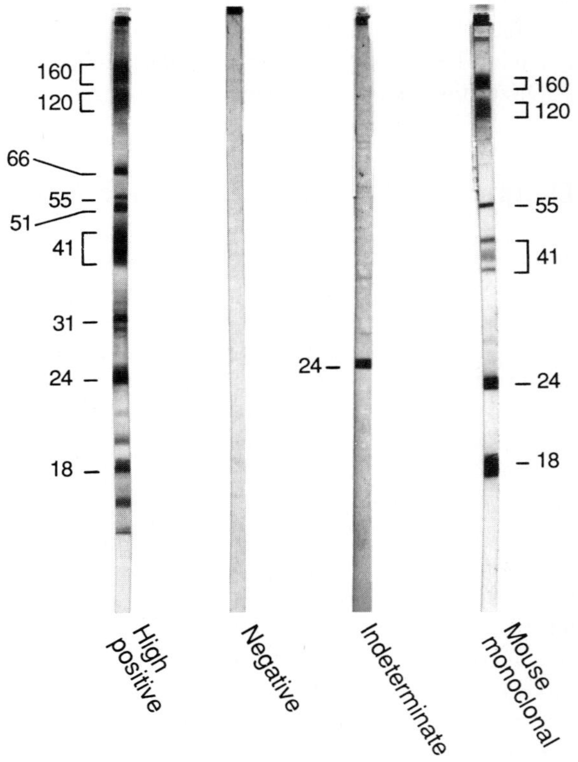

**Figure 41–7.** Western blot detection of HIV-1 antibodies. Note that the "high positive" serum exhibits antibodies to the HIV-1 envelope glycoproteins of 160, 120 and 41 kilodaltons (kD), to the GAG (core) proteins of 24 and 18 kD, and to other HIV proteins (55 and 51 kD). The "indeterminate" serum exhibits antibody to only the GAG (core) 24-kD protein. The mouse monoclonal blot is a positive control and contains antibodies to key HIV antigens. A positive sample should exhibit antibodies to both envelope and GAG proteins or to both envelope proteins (41 and 120/160 kD).

## Treatment

Zidovudine slows or controls progression but does not cure

At present, zidovudine (AZT, see Chapter 13) is the initial drug of choice for treating HIV infection. This drug delays the spread of progression of the disease, but is ineffective against integrated virus and is, thus, not curative. Moreover, the virus has been demonstrated to develop resistance in some cases during the course of therapy. It has significant toxicity for bone marrow cells, and its use is complicated by anemia, especially when higher doses (>500 mg per day) are used. Two other antiretroviral drugs, dideoxyinosine and dideoxycytidine, have been approved for use. These are also reverse transcriptase inhibitors. Drugs that inhibit HIV replication at other sites, for example, protease and transactivation, are under study for use as single agents or in combination with reverse transcriptase inhibitors. Treatment directed toward controlling or preventing opportunistic infections is an additional important part of AIDS therapy.

Reverse transcriptase inhibitors now in use

Prophylactic trimethoprim-sulfamethoxazole pentamidine aerosols can prevent PCP

One serious and often lethal opportunistic infection that has been particularly difficult to control is *Pneumocystis carinii* pneumonia (PCP). Trimethoprim–sulfamethoxazole therapy has proven to be the most economical and effective prophylaxis for PCP, but approximately 20% of patients exhibit major allergic reactions to this drug. In patients unable to take trimethoprim–sulfamethoxazole prophylaxis, aerosol pentamidine may be given monthly to reduce the frequency of disease.

## Prevention

Changes in behavior direct the spread of AIDS

The spread of AIDS has been facilitated by changing sexual mores, increased drug abuse, and, in some parts of the world, disruption of family and tribal units as a consequence of industrialization and urbanization. These factors are obviously not subject to early change. Immediate prevention has to be based on education about the means of transmission and easy access to condoms and safe needles for those large numbers of people who continue to place themselves at risk. The epidemiologic and laboratory methods used to control foci of other major epidemic diseases pose particular problems in AIDS control at present. Quite apart from questions of potential discrimination against infected individuals and the calami-

Immediate prevention is dependent on education to reduce risk

tous effects of false-positive serologic test results on the individual, the sheer magnitude and cost of case finding and contact tracing at present limit this approach.

Much research is underway to develop vaccines against the virus, but the marked mutability of HIV greatly complicates this approach, although conserved epitopes of the surface glycopeptides provide possible targets. Furthermore, passage of virus between fused cells and in syncytia protects it from antibody neutralization in established disease. Finally, the cells most adversely affected by HIV are those that contribute to cell-mediated immunity. Nevertheless, the possibility that immunization with a vaccine may block the earliest process of infection is being explored.

Vaccine approach particularly difficult

Blocking earliest stages of infection best hope

Another possible approach to the control of HIV infection involves chemoprophylaxis beginning during the clinically silent phase of the disease, using agents that specifically block viral replication. Unfortunately, agents with these properties may well control but not cure the disease.

Chemoprophylaxis not known to prevent disease

## ADDITIONAL READING

Centers for Disease Control. Revised classification systems for HIV infection and expanded surveillance case definitions for AIDS among adolescents and adults. *Morb Mortal Wkly Rep*. 1993;41(RR-17). The most recent attempt to define AIDS.

Farizo KM, Buehler JW, Chamberland ME, et al. Spectrum of disease in persons with human immunodeficiency virus infection in the United States. *JAMA*. 1992;267:1798–1805.

Levy JA. Pathogenesis of human immunodeficiency virus infection. *Microbiol Rev*. 1993;57:183–289. Detailed review of the mechanisms involved in the initiation and all stages of HIV infection.

Lifson AR, Hessol NA, Rutherford GW. Progression and clinical outcome of infection due to human immunodeficiency virus. *Clin Infect Dis*. 1992;14:966–972. Summary of the clinical events due to HIV in a cohort of homosexual men followed since the 1970s.

# Papovaviruses

W. Lawrence Drew

The papovaviruses of medical interest include the polyomaviruses and papillomaviruses.

## PAPILLOMAVIRUSES

Papillomaviruses are small, unenveloped, double-stranded DNA viruses exhibiting cubic symmetry. About 55 nm in diameter, they cause epidermal papillomas and warts in a wide range of higher vertebrates. Different members of the group are generally species specific. For example, bovine and human papillomaviruses infect only the hosts reflected in their names. In some cases, tumors caused by these agents can become malignant.

Unenveloped DNA viruses

The genomes of many of the papillomaviruses have now been cloned from infected lesions into bacterial plasmids and compared by restriction endonuclease and DNA homology procedures (see Chapters 4 and 14). These studies have shown a wide genomic diversity among papillomaviruses that infect different species and also among those that infect humans and have led to the allocation of numbers for the different genotypes.

Human genotypes differ from animal papillomaviruses

More than 50 genotypes of human papillomaviruses (HPVs) have been identified in human papillomas and warts. Some of the genotypes are serologically (phenotypically) different, and groups of genotypes are associated with specific lesions. Viral components can be detected in infected cells by labeled specific antibody or by in situ hybridization with cloned viral DNA. Human papillomaviruses have been identified in plantar warts, in flat and papillomatous warts of other skin areas, in juvenile laryngeal papillomas, and in a variety of genital hyperplastic epithelial lesions, including cervical, vulvar, and penile warts and papillomas.

Viral components detectable in infected cells by in situ hybridization

Lesions caused by HPVs include warts and papillomas

### Papillomavirus Infection

#### Epidemiology

Twelve HPV genotypes have been identified in genital lesions of humans, and there are many apparently silent infections with these viruses. The incidence of HPV infections has almost certainly been increasing, and they now constitute perhaps the most common sexually transmitted disease. From 20 to 60% of adult women in the United States are infected with one or another of the genotypes. Human papillomavirus types 6 and 11 are associated most commonly with benign genital warts in males and females and with some cellular dysplasias of the cervical epithelium, but these lesions rarely become malignant. They can be perinatally transmitted and cause infantile laryngeal papillomas. Types 16, 18, and 31 may also cause warty lesions of the vulva, cervix, and penis, and infections with these viral types more often progress to malignancy. Viral genomes of these types are found in a large pro-

Twelve genotypes found in human genital lesions; silent infections are common

HPV types 6 and 11 associated with benign genital warts

Types 16, 18, and 31 infections may progress to malignancy

HPV associated with cervical carcinoma

portion of markedly dysplastic uterine cervical cells, in carcinomas in situ, and in cells of frankly malignant lesions. Human papillomavirus infection is now considered to be associated with the majority of carcinomas of the cervix. Papillomavirus infection of the anus is a clinical problem in homosexual men, especially those with AIDS. This infection may be related to anal neoplasia as well.

### Pathogenesis

Shope rabbit papillomas can become malignant; cofactors hasten the progress

Papillomaviruses have not been grown in cell culture

Papillomaviruses were the first DNA viruses linked to malignant changes. In the mid-1930s Shope demonstrated that benign rabbit papillomas were due to filterable agents and could advance to become malignant squamous cell carcinomas. External cofactors, such as coal tar, could hasten this process. Work on the biology and mechanism by which these agents foster malignant transformation has, however, been impeded by the inability to cultivate papillomaviruses in vitro. Molecular probes to detect viral products in vivo indicate that replication and assembly of these viruses take place only in the differentiating layers of squamous epithelia, a situation that has not been reproduced in vitro.

The first evidence that HPVs could be associated with human malignant disease came from observations on epidermodysplasia verruciformis. This disease has a genetic basis that results in unusual susceptibility to HPV types 5 and 8, which produce multiple flat warts. About a third of affected patients develop squamous cell carcinoma from the lesions. The HPV genomic material is detectable in the nuclei of both benign and malignant tumors.

Both integrated and extrachromosomal viral genomes occur

Viral genome carries transforming genes

The mechanism of oncogenicity of HPV is less clear, and much of what follows has been extrapolated from studies on a bovine papillomavirus that can be grown in mouse cell lines. Cells infected with this virus are transformed and produce tumors when injected into nude (T lymphocyte-deficient) mice. The viral genome exists as multiple copies of a circular episome within the nucleus of transformed cells, but is not integrated into the cellular genome. This appears also to be the case with benign human lesions. In malignant tumors, part of the viral genome is found integrated into the cellular genome, but integration is not site specific. Both the integrated viral genome and the extrachromosomal form carry their own transforming genes. Host cells normally produce a protein that inhibits expression of papillomavirus transforming genes, but this can be inactivated by products of the virus and possibly by other infecting viruses, thus allowing malignant transformation to occur.

## Papillomavirus Infection: Clinical Aspects

### Diagnosis

Cytologic changes in cervix or vagina

EIAs detect antigen

Papillomavirus infection leads to perinuclear cytoplasmic vacuolization and nuclear enlargement, "koilocytosis," in epithelial cells of the cervix or vagina. These changes can be seen in a routine Papanicolaou smear. More sensitive is the use of immunoassays to detect viral antigen and in situ hybridization or polymerase chain reaction to detect specific viral DNA in cervical swabs or tissue (Fig 42–1). HPV does not grow in routine tissue culture and antibody tests are rarely used.

### Treatment

Infected epithelium removed

Current treatment of HPV is undergoing modification, but at present is designed mainly to destroy or remove the affected epithelium. Recurrences are common because of survival of virus in the basal layers of the epithelium. Systemic and local interferon therapy has shown some promise as a treatment, although lesions tend to recur after cessation of therapy.

# POLYOMAVIRUSES

Polyomaviruses usually cause no disease in natural hosts; transform cells in culture

The polyomaviruses include the JC virus (JCV) and BK virus (BKV) of humans and simian virus 40 (SV40). Polyomaviruses, like papillomaviruses, are members of the papovavirus family. They are also double-stranded, naked capsid DNA viruses and are widely distributed among various animal species, usually without causing apparent disease. They are, however, able to transform cells of a variety of heterologous cell lines in culture. JCV is the etiologic agent of progressive multifocal leukoencephalopathy, a fatal demyelinating dis-

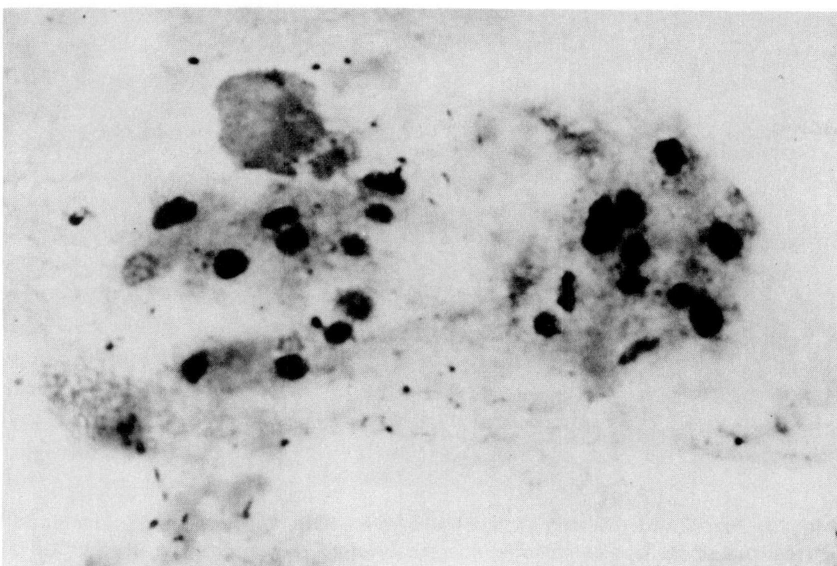

**Figure 42–1.** Human papillomavirus (HPV) type 16 DNA demonstrated in a cervical smear by in situ hybridization. The dark circles represent detection of HPV DNA sequences by the DNA probe.

ease of the central nervous system. Approximately 70% of adults show serologic evidence of JCV infection with no known clinical manifestations, but it remains latent and may reactivate in immunocompromised patients. BKV also infects a large proportion of the population. This infection is primarily latent, but can reactivate to produce cystitis in immunocopromised patients.

Serologic evidence for JCV and BKV infection common

Polyomaviruses can produce malignant tumors in certain experimental animals, but, interestingly, do not do so in their natural hosts. For example, SV40 can produce lymphocytic leukemia and a variety of reticuloendothelial cell sarcomas in baby hamsters, but is not oncogenic in its natural monkey host. Fortunately, even though it can transform some human cells in vitro, it fails to produce disease in humans, a fact that became apparent on follow-up of recipients of early batches of poliomyelitis vaccine that were contaminated with live SV40.

May produce tumors in experimental animals, but not in their natural hosts

The reason polyomaviruses fail to produce tumors in their natural hosts is uncertain, but may be because they are usually cytocidal under these conditions. From a biological point of view, the polyomaviruses are particularly useful models of oncogenicity because they can be readily studied in vitro and interact with cells in different ways. In some, they produce lytic infections and cell death with production of complete virions. In others, they integrate randomly into the cell genome and cause transformation by the expression of one or more of the viral genes. No human tumor has been shown to be caused by polyomaviruses.

Valuable experimental models of oncogenicity

No human tumors

## Progressive Multifocal Leukoencephalopathy

Progressive multifocal leukoencephalopathy (PML) is a rare, subacute, degenerative disease of the brain found primarily in adults with other chronic diseases, especially AIDS and reticuloendothelial malignancies, or those receiving immunosuppressive agents. The disease is characterized by the development of impaired memory, confusion, and disorientation, followed by a multiplicity of neurologic symptoms and signs that include hemiparesis, visual disturbances, incoordination, seizures, and visual abnormalities. PML is progressive, with death usually occurring 3 to 6 months after onset of symptoms. The incidence of PML has increased concomitantly with the AIDS epidemic.

Progressive demyelinating disease seen in AIDS patients

Cerebrospinal fluid (CSF) findings are often normal, although some patients show a slight increase in lymphocytes, and protein levels may be elevated. Pathologically, foci of demyelination are found, surrounded by giant, bizarre astrocytes containing intranuclear inclusions. The demyelination is due to viral damage to oligodendroglial cells, which syn-

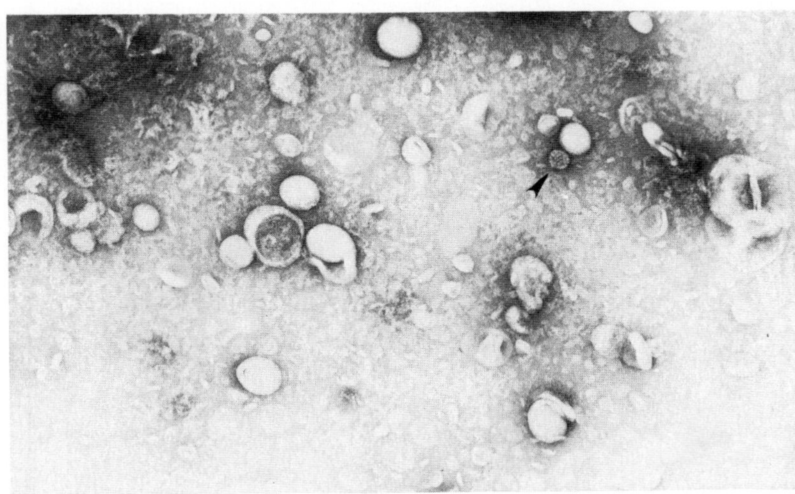

**Figure 42–2.** JC virus (arrow) among debris of cells from a brain biopsy of a case of progressive multifocal leukoencephalopathy. (*Reprinted with permission from Palmer E, Martin ML.* An Atlas of Mammalian Viruses. *Boca Raton, FL: CRC Press; 1982. Copyright 1982 by CRC Press, Inc.*)

JCV particles seen in brain

Latent infection suggested

thesize and maintain myelin. Abundant JCV particles can be seen in the brain by electron microscopy (Fig 42–2) and may be concentrated within the nuclei of oligodendrocytes. JCV DNA sequences have been demonstrated by the polymerase chain reaction in the brain of patients without PML or demyelinating lesions, suggesting that the virus may be latent in the brain prior to immunosuppression. There is no specific treatment for PML, although reducing the immunosuppression, if possible, may have some clinical benefit.

## Urinary Tract Infection

BKV may produce hemorrhagic cystitis

Infection of the urinary tract with JCV and BKV can be demonstrated frequently in immunocompromised patients but usually without symptoms or evidence of renal injury. BKV has been associated with a hemorrhagic cystitis, particularly in bone marrow transplant patients.

## Diagnosis of Infection With BK and JC Viruses

Culture impractical

Antigen demonstrated in tissue

Urine from patients excreting these polyomaviruses may contain cells similar to those from patients excreting cytomegalovirus. The nucleus of cytomegalovirus-infected cells is smaller with a larger halo effect, that is, a clear zone around the inclusion but within the nuclear membrane. The brain oligodendrocytes exhibit similar changes in patients with PML. BKV can be isolated by routine culture in diploid fibroblast or Vero monkey kidney cells, but JCV requires human fetal glial cells, which are not readily available. Viral antigens can be demonstrated in tissue by a variety of immunoassays. Recently JCV DNA has been demonstrated in brain and spinal fluid of PML patients by polymerase chain reaction.

## ADDITIONAL READING

Arthur RR, Shah KV, Charache P, Saral R. BK and JC virus infection in recipients of bone marrow transplants. *J Infect Dis.* 1988;158:563–569. Clinical significance of human polyomavirus infection in immunocompromised patients.

Bauer HM, Ting V, Greer CE, et al. Genital human papillomavirus infection in female university students as determined by a PCR-based method. *JAMA.* 1991;265:472–477. Good report on the epidemiology of human papillomavirus and current means of diagnosis.

Berger JR, Kaszwitz B, Post MJD, Dickson G, et al. Progressive multifocal leukoencephalopathy associated with human immunodeficiency virus infection. *Ann Intern Med.* 1987;107:78–87. Comprehensive review of current knowledge about progressive multifocal leukoencephalopathy in AIDS patients.

*Ciba Foundation Symposium 120*: *The Papillomaviruses*. New York: Wiley; 1986:1–246. Excellent monograph on the molecular biology and epidemiology of human papillomaviruses.

Meyer MP, Markiw CA, Matuscak RR, et al. Detection of human papillomavirus DNA in genital lesions by using a modified commercially available in situ hybridization assay. *J Clin Microsc*. 1991;29:1308–1311. The prevalences of human papillomavirus DNA for cervical intraepithelial neoplasia I, II, and III lesions by the in situ hybridization test were 42, 54, and 55%, respectively. The combined prevalence of human papillomavirus type 16/18 and 31/33/35 DNAs increased with the severity of the lesion.

Palefsky JM, Gonzales J, Greenblatt RM, et al. Anal intraepithelial neoplasia and anal papillomavirus infection among homosexual males with group IV HIV disease. *JAMA*. 1990;263:2911–2916.

The prevalence of anal human papillomavirus infection and anal intraepithelial neoplasia among immunosuppressed male homosexuals is high.

Telenti A, Marshall WF, Aksamit AJ, et al. Detection of JC virus by polymerase chain reaction in cerebrospinal fluid from two patients with progressive multifocal leukoencephalopathy. *Eur J Clin Infect Dis*. 1992;11: 253–254. Detection of JC virus in spinal fluid by polymerase chain reaction may be the first noninvasive technique available for the diagnostic confirmation of progressive multifocal leukoencephalopathy.

# Persistent Viral Infections of the Central Nervous System

*W. Lawrence Drew*

Evidence has accumulated during the past 30 years that a variety of progressive neurologic diseases in both animals and humans are caused by viral or other filterable agents that share some of the properties of viruses (Table 43–1). These illnesses have been termed *slow viral diseases* because of the protracted period between infection and the prolonged course of the illness, but a better term is *persistent viral infection*.

Progressive neurologic diseases

It is of interest that most persistent viral infections involve well-differentiated cells, such as lymphocytes and neuronal cells. They can be classified as (1) diseases associated with "conventional" viral agents that possess nucleic acid genomes and protein capsids, induce immune responses, and can be grown in cell culture systems and (2) diseases associated with "unconventional" viruses that are small, filterable infectious agents transmissible to certain experimental animals, but that do not appear to be associated with immune or inflammatory responses by the host and have not been cultivated in cell culture.

Involve conventional viruses and unconventional agents; do not produce immune or inflammatory responses

Viral persistence can result from integration of viral nucleic acid into the host genome, mutations that interfere with or severely limit viral replication or antigenicity, failure of host immune systems to recognize virus or infected cells, or perhaps encoding of the causative "virus" itself in the normal host cell genome.

Viral persistence has multiple possible mechanisms

## DISEASES ASSOCIATED WITH CONVENTIONAL AGENTS

The following are the major persistent infections caused by conventional viral agents. They are summarized in Table 43–1.

### Subacute Sclerosing Panencephalitis

Subacute sclerosing panencephalitis is considered in Chapter 33. It is a rare chronic measles virus infection of children that produces progressive neurologic disease characterized by an insidious onset of personality change, progressive intellectual deterioration, and both motor and autonomic nervous system dysfunctions.

Chronic measles infection of children

TABLE 43–1. PERSISTENT VIRUS INFECTIONS

| Disease | Agent |
|---|---|
| **Conventional Viruses** | |
| Subacute sclerosing panencephalitis | Measles virus |
| Progressive panencephalitis after congenital rubella | Rubella virus |
| Progressive multifocal leukoencephalopathy | Papovavirus (JC virus) |
| AIDS dementia complex | Human immunodeficiency virus |
| Persistent enterovirus infection of the immunodeficient | Picornaviruses |
| **Unconventional Viruses**[a] | |
| Kuru | |
| Creutzfeldt–Jakob disease | |
| Scrapie (sheep and goats) | |
| Transmissible mink encephalopathy | |

[a] Subacute spongiform encephalopathies.

## Progressive Postrubella Panencephalitis

Even more rarely, a degenerative neurologic disorder similar to measles (subacute sclerosing panencephalitis) may be related to persistent rubella virus infection of the central nervous system. This condition is seen most often in adolescents who have had congenital rubella syndrome. Rubella virus has been isolated from brain tissue in these patients using cocultivation techniques.

## Progressive Multifocal Leukoencephalopathy

Progressive neurologic disease of immunocompromised adults

Progressive multifocal leukoencephalopathy (PML) is a subacute, degenerative disease of the brain found primarily in adults with other chronic diseases, especially AIDS and reticuloendothelial malignancies, and those receiving immunosuppressive agents. PML is considered in Chapter 42.

## Persistent Enterovirus Infection

Associated with immunodeficiency

Temporary improvement with hyperimmune globulin

Persons with congenital or severe acquired immunodeficiency, especially those with agammaglobulinemia, may develop a chronic central nervous system infection due to an echovirus or other enterovirus. Headache, confusion, lethargy, seizures, and cerebrospinal fluid pleocytosis are the common manifestations. The virus can be isolated from the cerebrospinal fluid. Clinical improvement may be achieved by the administration of human hyperimmune globulin to the infecting virus type. Relapse, however, occurs if therapy is discontinued, indicating persistence of virus despite the therapy.

## AIDS Dementia Complex

Late stages of AIDS

Human immunodeficiency virus causes a persistent infection of the central nervous system in as many as half of those with symptomatic Centers for Disease Control class B or C infection. The clinical course may vary from a mild subacute illness to severe progressive dementia (see Chapter 41).

# DISEASES CAUSED BY UNCONVENTIONAL VIRAL AGENTS: SUBACUTE SPONGIFORM ENCEPHALOPATHIES

Kuru and Creutzfeldt–Jakob disease in humans

A group of progressive degenerative diseases of the central nervous system have been shown to be caused by infectious agents with unusual physical and chemical properties. Two of the illnesses, kuru and Creutzfeldt–Jakob disease, occur in humans; two others, scrapie in sheep and goats and progressive encephalopathy in mink, occur in animals. Although the pathogenesis of these four illnesses is not well understood, they have similar features. There are varying degrees of neuronal loss, spongiform neurologic changes, and astrocyte proliferation. The incubation periods are months to years. The diseases have a protracted and inevitably fatal course.

The nature of these unconventional agents is still obscure. They are small and filterable to diameters of 5 nm or less, multiply to high titers in the reticuloendothelial system and brain, produce characteristic infections, and can remain viable even in formalinized brain tissue for many years. They are resistant to ionizing radiation, boiling, and many common disinfectants. Recognizable virions have not been found in tissues, and the agents have not been grown in cell culture. Treatment of infectious material with proteases and nucleases does not decrease infectivity. The characteristics of the agents are summarized in Table 43–2.

Infectious agents resist inactivation

Purified proteinaceous extracts of brain tissue in very high dilutions have been shown to transmit disease to experimental animals. Brain extracts from scrapie-infected animals contain a glycoprotein called PrP that is not found in the brains of normal animals. PrP has been termed a prion (proteinaceous infectious particle), and considerable evidence has been produced that it is responsible for transmission and infection. Repeated attempts to find associated nucleic acids have been generally unrewarding. PrP is encoded in a host gene, and specific prion mRNA has been found in both normal and infected tissue. Why the mRNA is translated in the disease and how prion production is apparently initiated by an external source of infectious PrP remain unanswered. During scrapie infection, prion protein may aggregate into birefringent rods and form filamentous structures termed scrapie-associated fibrils (Fig 43–1), which are found in membranes of scrapie-infected brain tissues.

Prion protein associated with infectivity

Nucleic acids absent

Prion protein encoded in host cell genome

## Kuru

Kuru was a subacute, progressive neurologic disease of the Fore people of the Eastern Highlands of New Guinea. In the local Fore dialect, *kuru* means "to tremble with fear or to be afraid." The disease was brought to the attention of the Western world by Gadjusek and Zigas in the mid-1950s. Although the illness was localized and decreasing in incidence, its study has thrown light on the transmissibility and infectious nature of similar transmissible encephalopathies. Epidemiologic studies indicated that kuru usually afflicted adult women, or children of either sex. The disease was rarely observed outside of the Fore region, and outsiders in the region did not contract the disease. The symptoms and signs were ataxia, hyperreflexia, and spasticity, which led to progressive starvation and death. Mental alertness was unaffected until the late stages of illness. Pathologic examination revealed changes only in the central nervous system, with diffuse neuronal degeneration and spongiform changes of the cerebral cortex and basal ganglia. No inflammatory response was noted. Inoculation of infectious brain tissue into primates produced a disease that caused similar neurologic symptoms and pathologic manifestations after an incubation period of approximately 40 months. Epidemiologic studies indicated that transmission of the disease in humans was associated with ritual cannibalism, practiced mainly by women and young

Women and children of the Fore people of New Guinea

Transmissible to primates

Associated with cannibalism

**TABLE 43–2. BIOLOGIC AND PHYSICAL PROPERTIES OF UNCONVENTIONAL VIRUSES**

Chronic progressive pathology without remission or recovery
No pathologic evidence of an inflammatory response
Filterable to estimated diameter of ≤5 nm
No virion-like structures visible by electron microscopy
Replication to high titers in susceptible tissue
Transmissible to experimental animals
No alteration in pathogenesis by immunosuppression or immunopotentiation
No interferon production or interference by other viruses
Unusual resistance to ultraviolet radiation
Resistance to inactivation by alcohol, 10% formalin, β-propiolactone, boiling water, proteases, and nucleases
Can be inactivated by 5% sodium hypochlorite, 1 *N* sodium hydroxide, and autoclaving; partially inactivated by acetone and ether

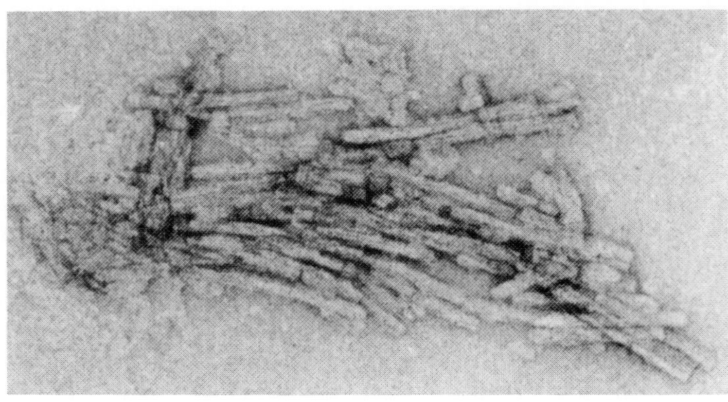

**Figure 43–1.** Amyloid-like fibrils (scrapie-associated fibrils) observed in brain extract of a patient with Creutzfeldt–Jakob disease. (*Reprinted with permission from Bockman JM, Kingsbury DT, McKinley MP, et al. Creutzfeldt–Jakob disease prion proteins in human brains.* N Engl J Med. *1985;312:73–82.*)

children and occasionally by men. This ritual involved the handling and ingestion of organs of deceased relatives. Inoculation through lesions in the skin and mucous membranes was shown to be the most likely mode of transmission, with clinical disease developing 4 to 20 years after exposure. Since the elimination of cannibalism from the Fore culture, kuru has disappeared.

## Creutzfeld–Jacob Disease

Progressive disease of the elderly

Creutzfeldt–Jakob disease is a progressive, fatal illness of the central nervous system that is seen most frequently in the sixth and seventh decades of life. The initial clinical manifestations are a change in cerebral function, usually diagnosed initially as a psychiatric disorder. Forgetfulness and disorientation progress to overt dementia, with the development of changes in gait, increased tone in the limbs, involuntary movement, and seizures. These manifestations resemble those of kuru. The disorder runs a course of 12 months to 4 to 5 years, eventually leading to death.

Very low incidence of disease; natural mode of acquisition unknown

Transmitted by tissue transplants

Creutzfeldt–Jakob disease is sporadic and found worldwide, with an incidence of disease of one case per million per year. The mode of acquisition is unknown, but a higher incidence of the disease among Israelis of Libyan origin who eat sheep eyeballs has led to speculation that the disease may be transmitted by the ingestion of scrapie-infected tissue. Infection has been transmitted by corneal transplants, by contact with infected electrodes used in a neurosurgical procedure, and by pituitary-derived human growth hormone. In these cases, the incubation period of the disease was approximately 15 to 20 months. Other evidence suggests that a longer latency may follow natural infection.

Pathologic features identical to Kuru, transmission to animals

The pathology of Creutzfeldt–Jakob disease is identical to that of kuru. It has been transmitted to chimpanzees, mice, and guinea pigs by inoculation of infected brain tissue, leukocytes, and certain organs. High levels of infectious agent have been found, especially in the brain, where they may reach $10^{-7}$ infectious doses per gram of brain. Nonpercutaneous transmission of disease has not been observed, and there is no evidence of transmission by direct contact or airborne spread.

Scrapielike structures seen in brain

Brains from patients with Creutzfeldt–Jakob disease have the birefringent rods and fibrillar structures noted in scrapie (Fig 43–1). Identification of PrP and antibodies directed against it may be a useful diagnostic adjunct to neuropathologic examination of brain tissue.

Nosocomial infections preventable by proper sterilization

There is no effective therapy of Creutzfeldt–Jakob disease, and all cases have been fatal. The small risk of nosocomial infection is related only to direct contact with brain tissue. Stereotactic neurosurgical equipment, especially that used in patients with undiagnosed dementia, should not be reused. In addition, organs from patients with undiagnosed neurologic disease should not be used for transplants. Growth hormone from human tissue has now been replaced by a recombinant genetically engineered product. The agent of

Creutzfeldt–Jakob disease has not been transmitted to animals by inoculation of body secretions, and no increased risk of disease has been noted in family members or medical personnel caring for patients. Disinfection of potentially infectious material can be accomplished by treatment for 1 hour with 0.5% sodium hypochlorite solution or by autoclaving at 121°C for 1 hour.

## ADDITIONAL READING


Adams DH. Does the infective agent of scrapie replicate without nucleic acid? An assessment. *Med Hypoth.* 1991;35:253–264. The dogma of a unique status for the scrapie agent falling outside the virologic spectrum is critically examined in the light of the circumstances that gave rise to it. It is concluded that such an extreme view cannot be justified.

Bockman JM, Kingsbury DT, McKinley MP, et al. Creutzfeldt–Jakob disease prion proteins in human brains. *N Engl J Med.* 1985;312:73–82.

Gajdusek DC. Unconventional viruses causing subacute spongiform encephalopathies. In: Fields BN, ed. *Virology.* New York: Raven Press; 1985:1519–1557. Superb review of this field by the discoverer of the epidemiology of kuru and the nature of its agent.

Lantos PL. From slow virus to prion: A review of transmissible spongiform encephalopathies. *Histopathology.* 1992;20:1–11. Spongiform encephalopathies include seven neurodegenerative diseases, three of which occur in humans (Creutzfeldt–Jakob disease, Gerstmann–Straussler–Scheinker disease, and kuru). They are all transmissible to a variety of species, and human-to-human propagation of the diseases in the form of iatrogenic transmission has been well documented. The infectious agent is highly unusual and the pathogenesis of infection remains controversial.

Prusiner SB. Prions and neurodegenerative diseases. *N Engl J Med.* 1987;317:1571–1581. Excellent consideration of this fascinating topic.

Prusiner SB. Transgenetic investigations of prion diseases of humans and animals. *Bio Sci.* 1993;339(1288):239–254. Infectious prion particles are composed largely, if not entirely, of an abnormal isoform of the prion protein (PrPSc), which is encoded by a chromosomal gene. A posttranslational process, as yet unidentified, converts the cellular prion protein (PrPC) into PrPSc.

Southern P, Oldstone MBA. Medical consequences of persistent viral infection. *N Engl J Med.* 1986;314:359–367. Excellent review of the pathogenesis and virus–host interactions of persistent viral infections.

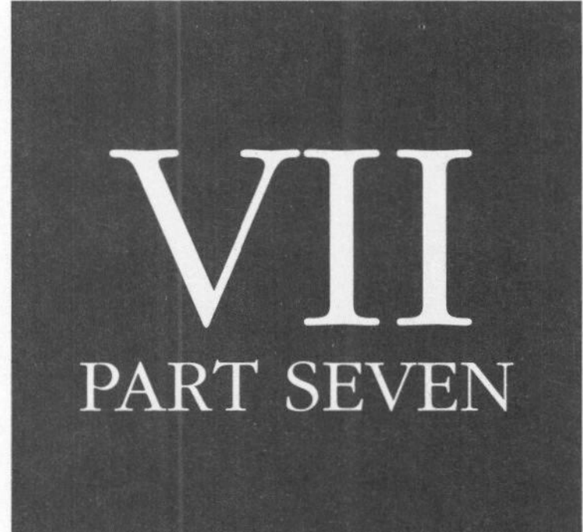


# Pathogenic Fungi

# Characteristics of Fungi

*Kenneth J. Ryan*

Fungi are a distinct class of microorganisms, most of which are free-living in nature where they function as decomposers in the energy cycle. Of the more than 200,000 known species fewer than 100 have been reported to produce disease in humans. These diseases, the mycoses, have some unique clinical and microbiologic features.

Fungi are eukaryotes with a higher level of biological complexity than bacteria. They may be unicellular or may differentiate to multicellular organization at a level of complexity between those of protozoa and plants. The mycoses vary greatly in their manifestations, but tend to be subacute to chronic with indolent, relapsing features. Acute disease such as that produced by many viruses and bacteria is uncommon in fungal infections.

## THE NATURE OF FUNGI

The fungal cell has typical eukaryotic features, including a nucleus with chromosomes, a nuclear membrane, and cytoplasmic organelles, such as mitochondria and an endoplasmic reticulum. Fungi are usually in the haploid state, although diploid nuclei are formed through nuclear fusion in the process of sexual reproduction. The cell structure includes a rigid cell wall and a cytoplasmic membrane in which ergosterol predominates; in contrast, cholesterol is the dominant sterol in mammalian membranes.

Eukaryotic cell structure

Rigid cell wall; ergosterol in cell membrane

The chemical and antigenic structure of the cell wall is markedly different from that of bacterial cells in that it does not contain peptidoglycan, glycerol or ribitol teichoic acids, or lipopolysaccharide. In their place are the polysaccharides **mannan, glucan,** and **chitin** in close association with each other and with structural proteins. Mannoproteins are mannose-based polymers (mannan) found on the surface and in the structural matrix of the cell wall where they are linked to protein. They are major determinants of serologic specificity because of variations in the composition and linkages of the polymer side chains. Glucans are glucosyl polymers, some of which form fibrils that increase the strength of the fungal cell wall, often in close association with chitin. Chitin is composed of long, unbranched chains of poly-*N*-acetylglucosamine. It is inert, insoluble, and rigid and provides structural support in a manner analogous to the chitin in crab shells or cellulose in plants. It is a major component of the cell wall of filamentous fungi. In yeasts, chitin appears to be of most importance in forming cross-septa and the channels through which nuclei pass from mother to daughter cells during cell division.

Cell wall mannan linked to structural proteins

Chitin and glucans add rigidity to cell wall

Fungal metabolism is heterotrophic, requiring exogenous organic energy sources. Metabolic diversity is great, but most fungi grow with only an organic carbon source and ammonium or nitrate ions as a nitrogen source. In nature, nutrients for free-living fungi are derived from decaying organic matter. A major difference between fungi and plants is that

Heterotrophic metabolism using available organic matter

Lack of photosynthetic mechanisms

fungi lack photosynthetic energy-producing mechanisms. Most are strict aerobes, although some can grow under anaerobic conditions. None are strict anaerobes.

Asexual and sexual reproductive elements are termed conidia and spores respectively

Fungi may reproduce by either asexual or sexual processes. Reproductive elements produced asexually are termed **conidia.** Those produced sexually are termed **spores.** Asexual reproduction involves mitotic division of the haploid nucleus and is associated with production by budding sporelike conidia or separation of hyphal elements. In sexual reproduction, the haploid nuclei of donor and recipient cells fuse to form a diploid nucleus, which then divides by classic meiosis. Some of the four resulting haploid nuclei may be genetic recombinants, and all may undergo further division by mitosis. Highly complex specialized structures may be involved. Detailed study of this process in fungal species such as *Neurospora crassa* has been important in gaining an understanding of basic cellular genetic mechanisms.

## FUNGAL GROWTH AND MORPHOLOGY

Vary greatly in size and complexity

Some show multicellular differentiation

The size of fungi varies immensely. A single cell without transverse septa may range from bacterial size (2–4 μm) to a macroscopically visible structure. The morphologic forms of growth vary from colonies superficially resembling those of bacteria to some of the most complex, multicellular, colorful, and beautiful structures seen in nature. Mushrooms are an example and can be regarded as complex colonies of fungi showing structural differentiation.

**Mycology,** the science devoted to the study of fungi, has many terms to describe the morphologic components that make up these structures. Fortunately, the terms and concepts that must be mastered can be limited by considering only the fungi of medical importance and accepting some simplification.

Yeasts multiply by budding off blastoconidia

Initial growth from a single cell may follow either of two courses, yeast or mold (Fig 44–1). The first and simplest is the formation of a bud, which extends out from a round or oblong parent, constricts, and forms a new cell. These buds are called **blastoconidia** (see Figure 44–1) and fungi that reproduce in this manner are called **yeasts.** On plates, yeasts form colonies that resemble those of bacteria. In broth, yeasts produce diffuse turbidity or grow as sediments in unshaken cultures.

Molds produce septate or nonseptate hyphae

Vegetative mycelium acts as a root

Aerial mycelium bears reproductive structures

Pseudohyphae are less rigid

Fungi may also grow through the development of **hyphae** (singular, hypha), which are tubelike extensions of the cell with thick, parallel walls. As the hyphae extend, they form an intertwined mass called a **mycelium.** Most fungi form hyphal **septa** (singular, septum), which are cross-walls perpendicular to the cell walls that divide the hypha into subunits (Fig 44–2). Some species are nonseptate; they form hyphae and mycelia as a single, continuous cell. In both septate and nonseptate hyphae, multiple nuclei are present, with free flow of cytoplasm along the hyphae or through pores in any septum. A portion of the mycelium (vegetative mycelium) usually grows into the medium or organic substrate (eg, soil) and functions, like the roots of plants, as a collector of nutrients and moisture. The more visible surface growth assumes a fluffy character as the mycelium becomes aerial. The hyphal walls are rigid enough to support this extensive, intertwining network, commonly called a **mold.** The aerial hyphae bear the reproductive structures of this class of fungi. Some fungi form structures called **pseudohyphae** (Fig 44–3), which differ from true hyphae in having recurring budlike constrictions and less rigid cell walls.

Morphology of reproductive conidia and spores used for identification

The reproductive conidia and spores of the molds and the structures that bear them assume a great variety of sizes, shapes, and relationships to the parent hyphae, and the morphology of these structures is the primary basis of identification of medically important molds. The mycelial structure plays some role in identification, depending on whether the hyphae are septate or nonseptate, but differences are not sufficiently distinctive to identify or even suggest a fungal species.

Conidia and thin stalks have multiple names

Exogenously formed asexual conidia may arise directly from the hyphae or on a special stalklike structure, the **conidiophore.** Occasionally, terms such as **macroconidia** and **microconidia** are used to indicate the size and complexity of these conidia. Conidia that develop within the hyphae are called either **chlamydoconidia** or **arthroconidia.** Chlamydoconidia become larger than the hypha itself; they are round, thick-walled structures that may be borne on the terminal end of the hypha or along its course. Arthroconidia conform more to the shape and size of the hyphal units, forming a series of delicately attached

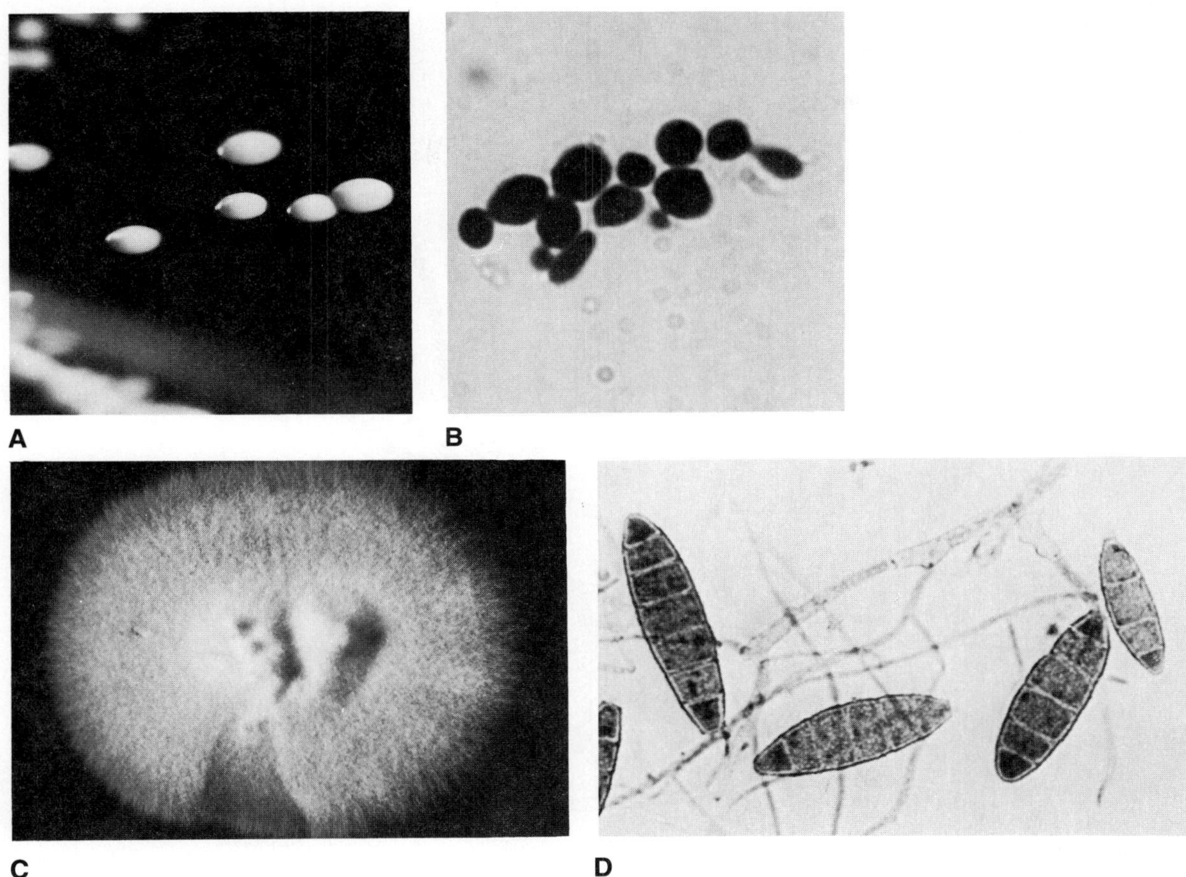


**Figure 44–1.** Yeast and mold forms of fungal growth. **A.** Yeasts form colonies similar to those of bacteria. **B.** Microscopically, they are large oval cells with occasional buds (blastoconidia). **C.** Molds form fuzzy, often pigmented colonies. **D.** Microscopically, molds are a complex of hyphae and associated conidia. (*Parts* C *and* D *reprinted with permission from Dr. E. S. Beneke and the Upjohn Company: Scope Publications, Human Mycoses.*)

conidia that break off and disseminate when disturbed. The most common sexual spore is termed an **ascospore.** Four or eight ascospores may be found in a saclike structure, the **ascus.** The structures are illustrated in Figures 44–2 and 44–3.

Ascospore the most common sexual spore

In general, fungi grow either as yeasts or as molds; mold forms show the greatest diversity. Some species can grow in either a yeast or a mold phase, depending on environmental conditions. These species are known as **dimorphic fungi.** Several human pathogens demonstrate dimorphism: they grow in the yeast form in infected tissue, but in the mold form in their environmental reservoir and in culture at ambient temperatures. For most, it is possible to manipulate the cultural conditions to demonstrate both yeast and mold phases in vitro. Yeast phase growth requires conditions similar to those of the parasitic in vivo environment, such as 35 to 37°C incubation and enriched medium. Mold growth requires minimal nutrients and ambient temperatures. The asexual spores produced in the mold phase may be infectious and serve to disseminate the fungus.

Dimorphic fungi can grow as yeasts or molds

## CLASSIFICATION

Although asexual conidia are more readily observed, the taxonomy of fungi depends on the nature of sexual spores and septation of hyphae as its differential characteristics. On this basis, four classes—Zygomycetes, Ascomycetes, Basidiomycetes, and Deuteromycetes—are defined as shown in Table 44–1. Some medically important species appear in the Zygomycetes and Ascomycetes, but none in the Basidiomycetes. Most pathogenic species, because they lack a sexual reproductive cycle, have been allocated to the class Deuteromycetes. The mycologist's dislike for this lack of symmetry is indicated by the term

Taxonomy based on sexual spores and septation

Deuteromycetes do not have sexual spores

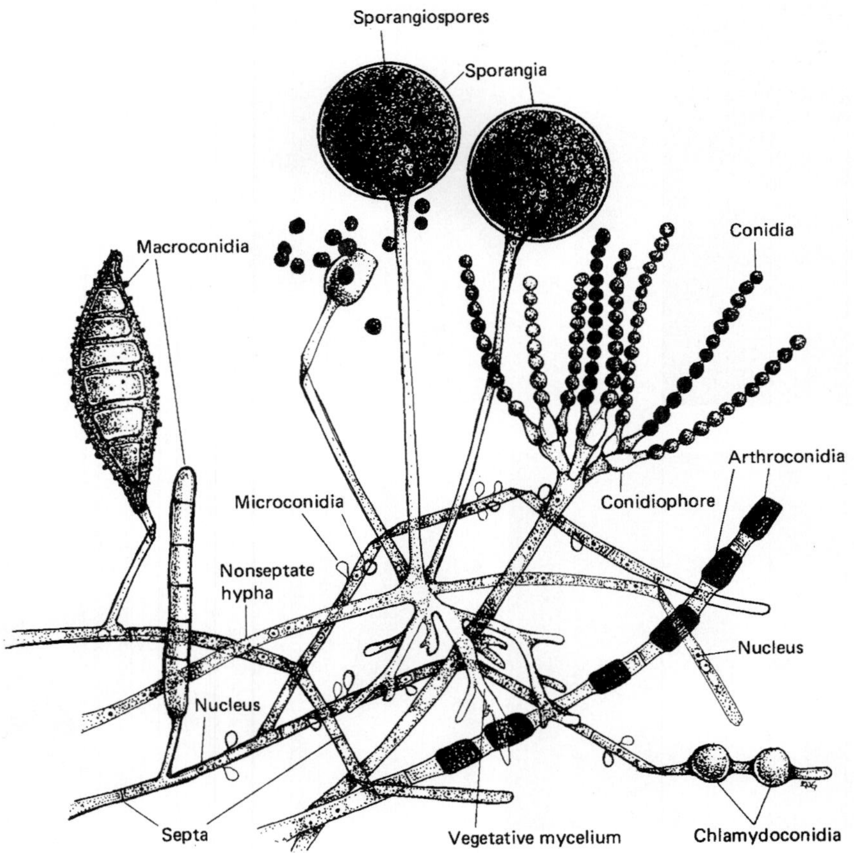


**Figure 44–2.** Mold forms. The tubelike hyphae constitute their basic structure. Examples of spores and conidia and of the structures that bear them are shown. They develop from the hyphal wall.

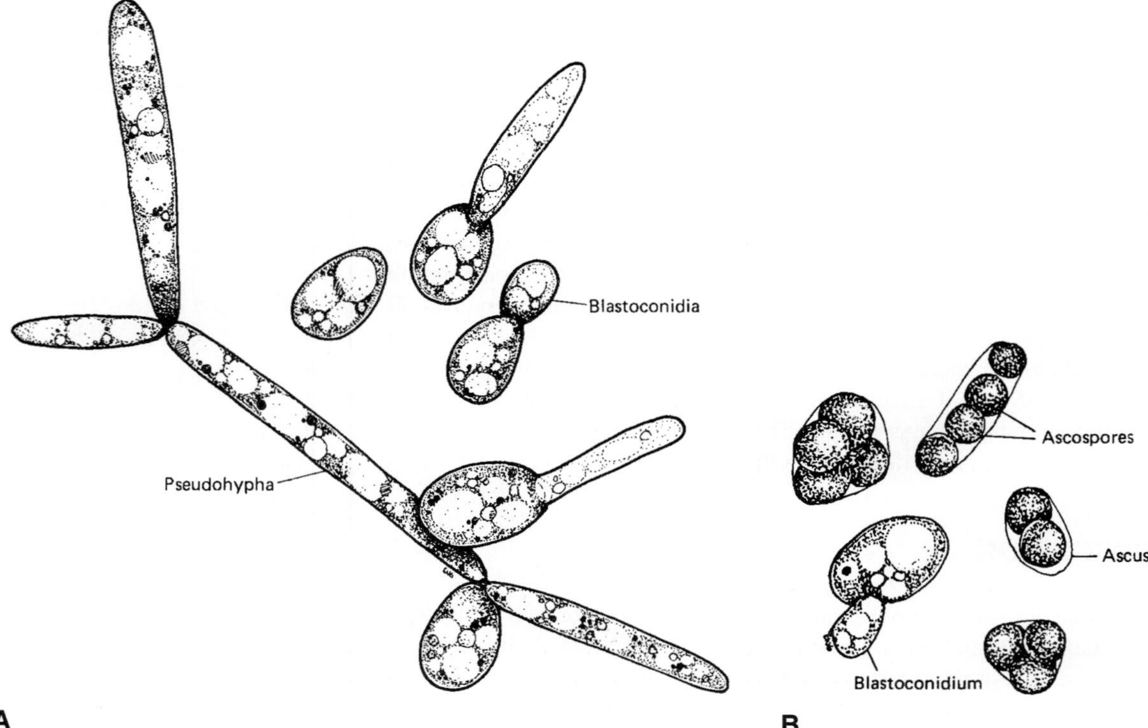


**Figure 44–3.** Yeast forms. **A.** Yeast reproduction is limited to the development of blastoconidia or longer extensions, pseudohyphae. **B.** Sexual reproduction leads to the formation of ascospores.

TABLE 44–1. TAXONOMIC CLASSES OF FUNGI

| Class | Hyphae | Reproductive Elements: Sexual | Reproductive Elements: Asexual | Biology |
|---|---|---|---|---|
| Zygomycetes | Nonseptate | Various types | Sporangioconidia | Saprophytes; rare pathogens[a] |
| Ascomycetes | Septate | Ascospores | Conidia | Saprophytes; rare pathogens |
| Basidiomycetes | Septate | Basidiospores | Conidia | Mushrooms, smuts; nonpathogenic |
| Deuteromycetes (fungi imperfecti) | Septate | None | Conidia | Common pathogens; saprophytes |

[a] Pathogenicity for humans. Many fungi are plant pathogens.

**fungi imperfecti,** which is synonymous with Deuteromycetes. It suggests that the sexual spores have been lost during evolution or are so rarely produced that they have not been detected. Indeed, some fungi originally classified in the Deuteromycetes have been transferred to the Ascomycetes on isolation of a sexual (perfect) form. These discoveries do not necessarily simplify classification; for instance, when the sexual stage of *Trichophyton mentagrophytes* was demonstrated, it was found to be identical to that of an already named ascomycete (*Arthroderma benhamiae*). This type of finding and the morphologic similarity of the asexual forms suggest a close relationship between the classes Ascomycetes and Deuteromycetes.

Sexual forms of Deuteromycetes are occasionally discovered

The grouping of medically important fungi used in the following chapters is based on the types of tissues they parasitize and the diseases they produce, rather than on the principles of basic mycologic taxonomy. The superficial fungi, such as the dermatophytes, cause indolent lesions of the skin and its appendages, commonly known as ringworm and athlete's foot. The subcutaneous pathogens characteristically cause infection through the skin, followed by subcutaneous spread, lymphatic spread, or both. The opportunistic fungi are those found in the environment or in the normal flora that occasionally produce disease, usually in the compromised host. The systemic pathogens are the most virulent fungi and may cause serious progressive systemic disease in previously healthy persons. They are not members of the normal human flora. Although their major potential is to produce deep-seated visceral infections and systemic spread (systemic mycoses), they may also produce superficial infections as part of their disease spectrum or as the initiating event. The superficial mycoses do not spread to deeper tissues. As with all clinical classifications, overlaps and exceptions occur. In the end, the organism defines the disease, and it must be isolated or otherwise demonstrated.

Discussion organized by biological behavior in humans

## EPIDEMIOLOGY

Most fungal infections arise from contact with an environmental reservoir or from the patient's own fungal flora. Some superficial mycoses can be transmitted from person to person by very close contact, such as sharing a comb with an individual who has scalp ringworm; others can be acquired from ringworm infections of animals. Other fungal infections are not communicable between humans or animals, and infected patients need not be isolated.

Infection from environment or endogenous

Only dermatophyte infections are communicable

## LABORATORY DIAGNOSIS OF FUNGAL INFECTIONS

Because of their large size, fungi often demonstrate distinctive morphologic features on direct microscopic examination of infected pus, fluids, or tissues. The simplest method is to mix the specimen with a 10% solution of potassium hydroxide (KOH preparation) and place it under a coverslip. The strong alkali digests or clears the tissue elements (epithelial cells, leukocytes, debris), but not the rigid cell walls of both yeasts and molds. After digestion of

KOH digests tissue but not fungal wall

Gram reaction of yeasts

the material, the fungi can be observed under the light microscope with or without staining (see Fig 46–1B). Some yeasts stain with common stains such as the Gram stain, to which they are usually positive. Direct examinations can be aided by the use of calciflor white, a dye that binds to polysaccharides in cellulose and chitin. Under ultraviolet light calciflor white fluoresces, enhancing detection of fungi in fluids or tissue sections.

Calciflor white enhances detection

Visible in histologic preparations

Histopathologic examination of tissue biopsy specimens is widely used and shows the relationship of the organism to tissue elements and responses (blood vessels, phagocytes, granulomatous reactions). Most fungi can be seen in sections stained with the hematoxylin and eosin (H&E) method routinely used in histology laboratories (Fig 44–4). Specialized staining procedures such as the silver impregnation methods are frequently used because they stain almost all fungi strongly but only a few tissue components. The pathologist should be alerted to the suspicion of fungal infection when tissues are submitted, because special stains and searches for fungi are not made routinely.

Periodic acid-Schiff and methenamine silver stains enhance detection

Growth in culture simple but slow

Fungi can be grown by methods similar to those used to isolate bacteria. Growth occurs readily on enriched bacteriologic media commonly used in clinical laboratories (eg, blood agar and chocolate agar). Many fungal cultures, however, require days to weeks of incubation for initial growth; bacteria present in the specimen grow more rapidly and may interfere with isolation of a slow-growing fungus. Therefore, the culture procedures of diagnostic mycology are designed to favor the growth of fungi over bacteria and to allow incubation to continue for a sufficient time to isolate slow-growing strains.

Selective media allow isolation in the presence of other flora

The most commonly used medium for cultivating fungi is Sabouraud's agar, which contains only glucose and peptones as nutrients. Its pH is 5.6, which is optimal for growth of dermatophytes and satisfactory for growth of other fungi. Most bacteria associated with humans fail to grow or grow poorly on Sabouraud's agar.

Sabouraud's agar optimal for fungi, poor for bacteria

Blood agar or another enriched bacteriologic agar medium is used when pure cultures would be expected. It is made selective for fungi by the addition of antibacterial antibiotics such as chloramphenicol and gentamicin. Cycloheximide, an antimicrobic that inhibits some saprophytic fungi, is sometimes added to Sabouraud's agar to prevent overgrowth of contaminating molds from the environment, particularly for skin cultures. Media containing these selective agents cannot be relied on exclusively because they can interfere with growth of some pathogenic fungi or because the "contaminant" may be producing an opportunistic infection. For example, cycloheximide inhibits *Cryptococcus neoformans*, and chloramphenicol may inhibit the yeast forms of some dimorphic fungi. Selective media are not needed for growing fungi from sterile sites such as cerebrospinal fluid or tissue biopsy specimens. In contrast to most parasitic bacteria, many fungi grow best at 25 to 30°C, and temperatures in this range are used for primary isolation. Paired cultures incubated at 35 to 37°C may be used to demonstrate dimorphism.

Selective media make use of antimicrobics

Incubate at 30°C for primary isolation

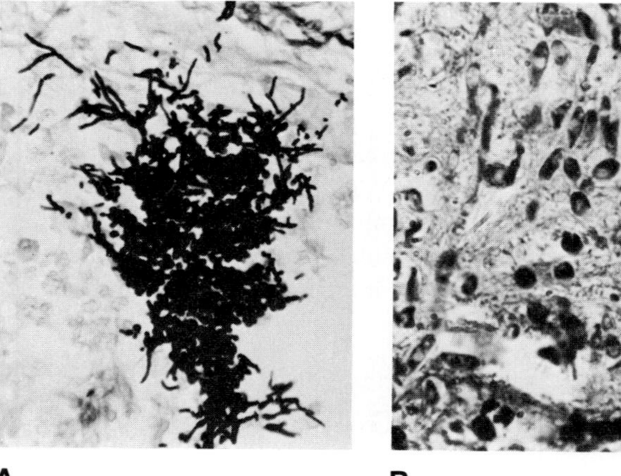


**Figure 44–4.** Direct examinations for fungi. **A.** Fungi such as *Candida albicans* are large enough to be demonstrated microscopically at low magnification. **B.** In histologic sections the invasive pseudomycelia (arrow) may be seen. (*Part* A *reproduced with permission from Dr. E. S. Beneke and the Upjohn Company: Scope Publications, Human Mycoses.*)

Once a fungus is isolated, identification procedures depend on whether it is a yeast or mold. Yeasts are identified by biochemical tests analogous to those used for bacteria, including some that are identical (eg, urease production). The ability to form pseudohyphae is also taxonomically useful among the yeasts.

Yeast identification like bacteria

Molds are most often identified by the morphology of their asexual conidia and conidiophores. Other features such as the size, texture, and color of the colonies help to characterize molds, but without demonstrating conidiation they are not sufficient for identification. The ease and speed with which various fungi produce conidia vary greatly. Minimal nutrition, moisture, good aeration, and ambient temperature favor development of conidia.

Mold identification based on morphology

Microscopic fungal morphology is usually demonstrated by methods that allow in situ microscopic observation of the fragile asexual conidia and their shape and arrangement. Morphology may also be examined in fragments of growth teased free of a mold and examined moist in preparations containing a dye called lactophenol cotton blue. The dye stains the mycelia and spores. Conidium production may not occur for days or weeks after the initial growth of the mold. It is somewhat like waiting for flowers to bloom, and it can be frustrating when the result has immediate clinical application.

Lactophenol cotton blue preparations made from mycelial growth

It is desirable, but not always possible, to demonstrate both the yeast and mold phases with dimorphic fungi. In some cases, this result can be achieved with parallel cultures at 22° and 37°C. The tissue form of *Coccidioides immitis* is not readily produced in vitro.

Dimorphism demonstration useful

An alternate approach has been developed for identification of some of the dimorphic systemic fungi, based on soluble antigens prepared from mycelial growth (exoantigens) and called the exoantigen test. When these exoantigens react with specific antibody in an immunodiffusion procedure, precipitin lines are formed between the unknown antigen and its homologous antibody. Results are usually available much more rapidly than are results of cultural tests.

Exoantigen test uses extract of fungal mycelia

Serum antibodies directed against a variety of fungal antigens can be detected in patients infected with those agents. Except for some of the systemic pathogens, the sensitivity, specificity, or both, of these tests have not been sufficient to recommend them for use in diagnosis or therapeutic monitoring of fungal infections. The tests of value are discussed in sections on specific agents.

Serologic tests useful only for systemic fungi

## ADDITIONAL READING

A number of good texts on medical mycology are available. All give more in-depth coverage of the mycologic, epidemiologic, and clinical aspects of mycoses than this book. Two are listed below.

Kwon-Chung KJ, Bennett JE. *Medical Mycology.* 3rd ed. Philadelphia: Lea & Febiger; 1992. Coverage of mycologic and pathologic features are particularly good.

Rippon JW. *Medical Mycology: The Pathogenic Fungi and Pathogenic Actinomycetes.* 3rd ed. Philadelphia: WB Saunders; 1988. Detailed, comprehensive coverage, including historic aspects, is given.

# Pathogenesis, Immunity, and Chemotherapy of Fungal Infections

*Kenneth J. Ryan*

We all have regular contact with fungi. They are so widely distributed in our environment that thousands of fungal spores are inhaled or ingested every day. Other species are so well adapted to humans that they are common members of the normal flora. Despite this ubiquity, clinically apparent systemic fungal infections are quite uncommon, even among persons living within the geographic habitat of the more pathogenic species. Progressive systemic fungal infections, however, pose some of the most difficult diagnostic and therapeutic problems in infectious disease, particularly among immunocompromised patients to whom they are a major threat. The purpose of this chapter is to give an overview of the pathogenesis and immunology of fungal infections and of the activity of antifungal agents. Details relating to specific fungi are given in Chapters 46 to 49.

## PATHOGENESIS

Compared with bacterial, viral, and parasitic disease, less is known about the pathogenic mechanisms and virulence factors involved in fungal infections. Analogies with bacterial diseases come the closest because of the apparent importance of adherence to mucosal surfaces, invasiveness, extracellular products, and interaction with phagocytes. In general, the principles discussed in Chapter 10 apply to fungal infections. Most fungi are opportunists, producing serious disease only in individuals with impaired host defense systems. Only a few fungi are able to cause disease in previously healthy persons.

Most fungi are opportunists

### Adherence

A number of fungal species, particularly the yeasts, are able to colonize the mucosal surfaces of the gastrointestinal and female genital tract. It has been shown experimentally that the ability to adhere to buccal or vaginal epithelial cells is associated with colonization and virulence. Within the genus *Candida* (see Chapter 47), the species that adhere best to epithelial cells are those most frequently isolated from clinical infections. Adherence usually requires a surface adhesin on the microbe and a receptor on the epithelial cell. In the case of *Candida albicans*, mannoprotein components extending from the cell wall have been im-

Adherence mediated by fungal adhesins and host cell receptors

Mannoprotein is the adhesin of *C. albicans* and fibronectin, the receptor

plicated as the adhesin and fibronectin and other components of the extracellular matrix as the receptor(s). Specific binding mediators have not been identified for other fungi.

## Invasion

Traumatic injection and inhalation access routes for environmental fungi

Passing an initial surface barrier, whether skin, mucous membrane, or respiratory epithelium, is an important step for most successful pathogens. Some fungi are introduced through mechanical breaks. For example, *Sporothrix schenckii* infection (see Chapter 49) typically follows a thorn prick or some other obvious trauma.

Conidia may pass air defenses

Most fungi that initially infect the lung grow as molds in the soil, and fungal spores or conidia are distributed into the air and carried in the airstream past the upper airway defenses. For example, arthroconidia of *Coccidioides immitis* can remain suspended in air for a considerable time, are small enough ($2 \times 3$–$6\ \mu m$) to reach the alveoli, and there initiate pulmonary coccidioidomycosis.

Invasion across mucosal barriers may involve enzymes

Invasion directly across mucosal barriers by the yeast *C. albicans* is associated with the formation of hyphae and pseudohyphae, but the specific mechanisms that allow them to penetrate and spread are not known. Extracellular enzymes (proteases, elastases, etc) have also been associated with virulent and invasive species of *Candida* and with some of the dimorphic systemic fungi. Although it is tempting to attribute some aspect of invasion or spread to these enzymes, their role, if any, remains to be proven.

## Phagocyte Interactions

Most fungi readily killed by neutrophils

Tissue phases of dimorphic fungi resist phagocytic killing

There is considerable evidence that normal persons have a high level of natural resistance to most fungal infections. This is particularly true of opportunistic molds. An important component of this resistance is the ability of healthy neutrophils to kill hyphae of most fungi if they reach the tissues. A small number of species, all of which are dimorphic (see Chapters 48 and 49), are able to produce mild to severe disease in otherwise healthy individuals. In vitro studies have shown these fungi to be more resistant to killing by neutrophils than the opportunists. *Candida albicans* is able to bind complement components in a way that interferes with phagocytosis.

*H. capsulatum* multiplies within macrophages

*Coccidioides immitis*, one of the best-studied species, has been shown to contain a component in the wall of its conidial (infective) phase that is antiphagocytic. As the hyphae convert to the spherule (tissue) phase, they also become resistant to phagocytic killing because of their size and surface characteristics. The tissue yeast form of *Histoplasma capsulatum* is resistant to phagocytic killing after ingestion and, in fact, multiplies within macrophages. These mechanisms of avoiding phagocytic killing appear to allow many dimorphic fungi to multiply sufficiently to produce an infection that can only be controlled by the immune response.

## Tissue Injury

No classic exotoxins known to be produced in vivo

Injury primarily due to inflammatory and immunological responses

None of the extracellular products of opportunistic fungi or dimorphic pathogens have been shown to injure the host directly during infection in a manner analogous to bacterial toxins. The presence of necrosis and infarction in the tissues of patients with invasion of fungi such as *Aspergillus* suggests a toxic effect, but direct evidence is lacking. A number of fungi do produce exotoxins, called **mycotoxins,** in the environment but not in vivo. The structural components of the cell do not cause effects similar to those of the endotoxin of Gram-negative bacteria, although mannan is known to circulate widely in the body. The injury caused by fungal infections seems to be due primarily to the inflammatory and immune responses that are stimulated by the prolonged presence of the fungus.

## IMMUNITY

A recurrent theme with fungal infections is the importance of an intact immune response in preventing infection and progression of disease. Most fungi are incapable of producing even a mild infection in an immunocompetent individual.

A small number of species (see Chapters 46, 48, and 49) are able to cause clinically apparent infection that usually resolves once there is time for activation of normal immune responses. In most instances in which it has been investigated, the action of neutrophils and T lymphocyte-mediated immune responses has been found to be of primary importance in this resolution. Progressive, debilitating, or life-threatening disease with these agents is commonly associated with depressed or absent cell-mediated immune responses, and the course of any fungal disease is worse in immunocompromised than previously healthy persons.

T-cell-mediated responses of primary importance

Progressive fungal diseases occur in immunocompromised patients

## Humoral Immunity

Antibodies can be detected at some time during the course of almost all fungal infections, but for most there is little evidence that they contribute to immunity. *Cryptococcus neoformans* (see Chapter 48) is the best example of a fungus against which antibody is probably important in controlling infection. Experimentally, opsonizing antibody enhances killing of *C. neoformans* by phagocytes, and recovery from clinical illness is associated with rising titers of antibody against the capsule of the organism. The capsule of *C. neoformans* is unique among the pathogenic fungi and has antiphagocytic properties similar to those of encapsulated bacterial pathogens (*Streptococcus pneumoniae*, *Haemophilus influenzae*, etc) against which humoral immunity is the primary defense mechanism. Antibody also plays a role in control of *C. albicans* infections by enhancing fungus–phagocyte interactions, and this is probably true for other yeasts. In some other fungal infections, the lack of protective effect of antibody is striking. In coccidioidomycosis, for example, high titers of *C. immitis*-specific antibodies are associated with dissemination and a worsening clinical course.

Opsonizing antibody effective in some yeast infections

## Cellular Immunity

Considerable clinical and experimental evidence points toward the importance of cellular immunity in fungal infections. Most patients with severe systemic disease have neutropenia, defects in neutrophil function, or depressed T lymphocyte-mediated immune reactions. These can result from factors such as steroid treatment, leukemia, Hodgkin's disease, and AIDS. In other cases, an immunologic deficit can usually be demonstrated by absence of delayed-type hypersensitivity responses or by direct in vitro assays of T-cell responsiveness to the fungus in question. In the latter case, it is possible that hyporesponsiveness is due at least in part to activation of suppressor cells or continued circulation of fungal antigen.

Systemic disease associated with deficiencies in neutrophils and T-cell-mediated immunity

Although not all fungi have been studied to the same degree, a unified picture is emerging from clinical and experimental animal studies. When hyphae or yeast cells of the fungus reach deep tissue sites, they either are killed by neutrophils or resist destruction by one of the antiphagocytic mechanisms described earlier. When the dimorphic fungi convert to yeast or spherule phases in the tissue, their growth may be slowed by macrophages, but they are not killed. The turning point comes when the macrophages are activated by cytokine mediators produced by T lymphocytes that have interacted with the fungal antigen. Where they have been identified, these mediators are interleukin 2 or interferon gamma, which can directly activate macrophages. The activated macrophages are then able to restrict the growth of the fungus, and the infection is controlled. Defects that disturb this cycle lead to progressive disease. To the extent that they are known, the specifics of these reactions are discussed in the following chapters.

Fungi that escape neutroplils grow slowly in macrophages

Growth restricted when macrophages activated by original stimulus

Immune defects lead to progressive disease

# CHEMOTHERAPY

Compared with antibacterial agents, relatively few antimicrobics are available for treatment of fungal infections. Many substances with antifungal activity have proved either to be unstable, to be toxic to humans, or to have undesirable pharmacologic characteristics, such as poor diffusion into tissues. Of the agents in current clinical use, none approach the degree of selective toxicity of the β-lactams used for antibacterial therapy, but the newer azole com-

Antifungals generally show less selective toxicity than antibacterials

pounds have significantly higher therapeutic activity and lower toxicity than earlier antifungal agents.

Fortunately, most fungal infections are self-limiting and require no chemotherapy. Superficial mycoses are often treated, but topical therapy can be used, thus limiting toxicity to the host. The remaining small group of deep mycoses that are uncontrolled by the host's immune system require the prolonged use of relatively toxic antifungals. This, combined with the fact that most of the patients have underlying immunosuppression, makes them the most difficult of all infectious diseases to treat successfully.

Most act on fungal nucleic acid synthesis or cytoplasmic membrane

The characteristics of currently used antifungal agents are discussed next and summarized in Table 45–1. Their primary targets are the nucleic acid synthesis mechanisms and the ergosterol-rich fungal cytoplasmic membrane of fungi. No clinically useful antifungal acts on the cell wall in a manner analogous to the penicillins, although inhibitors of both glucan and chitin synthesis have been discovered and are under evaluation.

## Antifungal Antibiotics

### Polyenes

Bind to ergosterol in fungal cell membranes; cause membrane disruption

The polyenes are produced by *Streptomyces* and have essentially the same modes of action and antifungal spectra. They are lipophilic and bind to sterols, particularly to ergosterol, which predominates in the fungal cytoplasmic membrane, but also to cholesterol, which predominates in mammalian membranes. Following insertion, the polyene molecules form cylindrical channels that penetrate the membrane, leading to leakage of essential small molecules with eventual cell growth inhibition and death.

Ampherotericin B most effective agent in treatment of systemic mycoses

The only polyenes in clinical use in the United States are nystatin, which is limited to topical use, and amphotericin B, which has been the most reliable antifungal for systemic use for many years. At physiologic pH amphotericin B is insoluble in water and must be administered intravenously as a colloidal suspension. Amphotericin B is not absorbed from the gastrointestinal tract.

Almost all fungi are susceptible to amphotericin B, and the development of resistance

**TABLE 45–1. CHARACTERISTICS OF ANTIFUNGAL AGENTS**

| | | Route of Administration[a] | | | |
|---|---|---|---|---|---|
| **Antifungal** | **Action** | ***Topical*** | ***Oral*** | ***Parenteral*** | **Spectrum** |
| Amphotericin B | Membrane disruption | – | – | + | All fungi |
| Nystatin | Membrane disruption | + | – | – | All fungi |
| Griseofulvin | Microtubule function | – | + | – | Dermatophytes |
| Flucytosine | Nucleic acid synthesis | – | + | – | *Candida*, *Torulopsis*, *Cryptococcus*, other yeasts |
| Potassium iodide | ? | – | + | – | *Sporothrix schenckii* |
| Clotrimazole | Ergosterol synthesis | + | – | – | Most fungi[b] |
| Ketoconazole | Ergosterol synthesis | – | + | – | Most fungi[b] |
| Fluconazole | Ergosterol synthesis | – | + | + | Most fungi[b] |
| Itraconazole | Ergosterol synthesis | – | + | – | Most fungi |
| Tolnaftate | ? | + | – | – | Dermatophytes |

[a] Indicates predominant current usage.
[b] Generally not active against *Aspergillus*.

is too rare to be a consideration in its use. The major limitation to amphotericin B therapy is the toxicity of the agent, because its affinity for fungal and mammalian membranes is relatively close. Infusion is commonly followed by chills, fever, headache, and dyspnea, but the most serious toxic effect is renal dysfunction and is seen in virtually every patient receiving a therapeutic course. Experienced clinicians learn to titrate the dosage for each patient to minimize the nephrotoxic effects. For obvious reasons, use of amphotericin B is limited to progressive, life-threatening fungal infections. In these cases, despite its toxicity, it often remains the antifungal agent of choice. Preparations that complex amphotericin B with phospholipids to form liposomes are under investigation as a way to limit toxicity.

Toxicity results from some affinity for host cell membranes

Nephrotoxicity most serious limitation on dosage

### Griseofulvin

Griseofulvin is a product of a species of the mold *Penicillium*. It is active only against the agents of superficial mycoses. Griseofulvin is actively taken up by susceptible fungi and acts on the microtubules and associated proteins that make up the mitotic spindle. It interferes with cell division and possibly other cell functions associated with microtubules. It is absorbed from the gastrointestinal tract after oral administration and concentrates in the keratinized layers of the skin. Clinical effectiveness has been demonstrated for all causes of dermatophyte infection, but the response is slow. Difficult cases may require 6 months of therapy to effect a cure.

Acts on microtubules and nuclear division

Concentrates in keratinized skin layers

## Synthetic Antifungals

### Potassium Iodide

Potassium iodide is the oldest known oral chemotherapeutic agent for a fungal infection. It is effective only for cutaneous sporotrichosis. Its activity is somewhat paradoxical, because the mold form of the etiologic agent, *Sporothrix schenckii*, can grow on medium containing 10% potassium iodide. The pathogenic yeast form of this dimorphic fungus appears to be susceptible to molecular iodine.

Used only for cutaneous sporotrichosis

### Flucytosine

Flucytosine, which was originally developed as an anticancer drug, is an antimetabolite analog of cytosine. In the cell, flucytosine is converted to 5-fluorouracil and related compounds, which can be incorporated into RNA or serve as inhibitors of thymidylate synthetase, an enzyme essential for DNA synthesis.

Product of flucytosine incorporated in RNA; disrupts protein synthesis

Flucytosine is well absorbed after oral administration. It is active against most clinically important yeasts, including *Candida albicans* and *Cryptococcus neoformans*, but has little activity against molds or dimorphic fungi. A significant limitation is the development of resistance that can occur by single-step mutation during therapy. A permease is required for entry of flucytosine into the cell. Resistance has been shown to result from mutation in the permease or any of the intracellular targets of flucytosine.

Active against yeasts but single-step mutations to resistance

Potential resistance limits flucytosine use to mild yeast infections or treatment in combination with amphotericin B for life-threatening systemic infections. Use in combination reduces the chance for expression of flucytosine resistance and allows a lower dose of amphotericin B to be used. In some instances, the combination is synergistic. The primary toxic effect of flucytosine is a reversible bone marrow suppression that can lead to neutropenia and thrombocytopenia. This effect is dose related and can be controlled by drug monitoring.

Used in combined therapy to prevent resistance

Reversible bone marrow suppression

### Azoles

The azoles are a large family of synthetic organic compounds, each containing a five-membered imidazole ring. This family includes members with antibacterial, antifungal, and antiparasitic properties. The important antifungal azoles are clotrimazole, fluconazole, ketoconazole, and itraconazole. Others are under development or evaluation. Their activity is based on inhibition of the cytochrome enzymes found in virtually all living cells. The most important component of their antifungal action is interference with the demethylase responsible for conversion of lanosterol to ergosterol, the major component of the fungal cytoplasmic membrane. This leads to formation of a defective cell membrane with altered permeability characteristics. The effect is primarily fungistatic rather than fungicidal.

Interfere with ergosterol incorporation in cytoplasmic membrane

Fungistatic activity

Ketoconazole was the first azole to be useful in systemic infections, but is now being supplanted by either fluconazole or itraconazole for most systemic mycoses, including aspergillosis and candidiasis, for which ketoconazole was not effective. Clotrimazole and miconazole are now used primarily in topical preparations.

Orally absorbed and less toxic than amphotericin B

Ketoconazole and itraconazole are given orally, and fluconazole, either orally or intravenously. Although nausea, vomiting, and elevation of hepatic enzymes complicate the treatment of some patients, the azoles are much less toxic than amphotericin B. Endocrinologic defects can be a problem because of inhibition of conversion of lanosterol to cholesterol, a precursor of several hormones. Central nervous system penetration of ketoconazole is poor, which limits its effectiveness in systemic coccidioidomycosis and cryptococcosis, but fluconazole has been more effective. Currently, fluconazole and itraconazole are the primary alternates to amphotericin B for treatment of systemic fungal infections. Azoles are also effective for superficial and subcutaneous mycoses in which the initial therapy either fails or is not tolerated by the patient.

CNS penetration a problem

### Tolnaftate

Tolnaftate is a derivative of naphthiomate. It has activity against dermatophytes (see Chapter 46), but not against yeasts. It has been effective in topical treatment of dermatophytoses and is available in over-the-counter preparations.

### Allylamines

The allylamines are a group of synthetic compounds that contain a naphthalene ring and act by inhibition of ergosterol synthesis. They include an oral agent, terbinafine, and a topical agent, naftifine. Both are used in the treatment of dermatophyte infections.

## Selection of Antifungals

Decisions on antifungal therapy balance dangers of disease against toxicity of treatment

Susceptibility testing less helpful than with bacteria

As with all chemotherapy, the selection of antifungal agents for treatment of superficial, subcutaneous, and systemic mycoses involves balancing probable efficacy against toxicity. The factors to be considered are (1) the threat of morbidity or mortality posed by the specific infection, (2) the immune status of the patient, (3) the toxicity of the antifungal, and (4) the probable activity of the antifungal agent against the fungus. Because of technical difficulties in vitro susceptibility testing has proved less helpful in individual cases of fungal infection than has been the case with bacterial infections (see Chapter 13). Molds are particularly difficult to test. Antifungal susceptibility tests done in reference laboratories can be helpful in difficult cases, but clinicians generally rely on knowledge of the etiologic agent and of the expected spectrum of each agent (see Table 45–1).

Amphotericin B followed by fluconazole or itraconazole common for serious systemic infections

In the case of superficial mycoses, the risks of appropriate therapy are small, and a number of topical agents may be tried. At the other extreme, an immunocompromised patient will most likely be treated aggressively with systemic agents for proven or even suspected systemic fungal infection. For life-threatening infections amphotericin B, despite its toxicity, is still the treatment of choice for almost all systemic fungal infections, but the newer azoles are often added. The most common regimen is an initial course of amphotericin B followed by one of the azoles.

## ADDITIONAL READING

Anaissie EL. Focus on fungal infections: An update on diagnosis and treatment. *Clin Infect Dis*. 1992;14(suppl 1):S1–S181. The proceedings of an international conference contain updates on pathogenesis and treatment.

# Superficial Fungal Pathogens

*Kenneth J. Ryan*

Dermatophytoses are superficial infections of the skin and its appendages, commonly known as ringworm, athlete's foot, and jock itch. They are caused by species of the genera *Microsporum, Trichophyton,* and *Epidermophyton,* which are collectively known as dermatophytes. These fungi are highly adapted to the nonliving, keratinized tissues of nails, hair, and the stratum corneum of the skin. The source of infection may be humans, animals, or the soil.

## ■ DERMATOPHYTES

## ■ Mycology

Dermatophytes are molds that have been classified among the Deuteromycetes (fungi imperfecti). The three genera of medical importance are *Epidermophyton, Microsporum,* and *Trichophyton,* based primarily on the morphology of their microconidia. The sexual forms have been discovered for many of the *Microsporum* and *Trichophyton* species and are assigned to a single ascomycete genus, *Arthroderma*. Dermatophytes are still called by their previous names in the medical literature for reasons of familiarity and because identification procedures continue to be based on the characteristics of asexual conidia. Many species cause dermatophyte infections; the most common of these are shown in Table 46–1. They require a few days to a week or more to initiate growth. Most grow best at 25°C on Sabouraud's agar, which is usually used for culture. The hyphae are septate, and the conidia may be borne directly on the hyphae or on conidiophores. Small microconidia may or may not be formed; however, the larger and more distinctive macroconidia (Figure 46–1C) are usually the basis for identification.

Identification of molds based on characteristics of conidia

Best growth at 25°C

Form septate hyphae, macroconidia, microconidia

## ■ Dermatophyte Disease

### Epidemiology

There are both ecologic and geographic differences in the occurrence of the various dermatophyte species. Some are primarily adapted to the skin of humans, and others to animals. Many wild and domestic animals, including dogs and cats, are infected with certain dermatophyte species and represent a large reservoir for infection of humans. Other pathogenic dermatophytes are found primarily in the soil. There are large differences between

Human, animal, or soil reservoirs

**TABLE 46–1. AGENTS OF SUPERFICIAL MYCOSES**

| Fungus | Infection Site | Fungal Growth: *In Lesion* | Fungal Growth: *In Culture (25°C)* |
|---|---|---|---|
| Dermatophytes | | | |
| *Microsporum canis* | Hair,[a] skin | Mycelia | Mold |
| *Microsporum audouini* | Hair[a] | Mycelia | Mold |
| *Microsporum gypseum* | Hair, skin | *Mycelia* | Mold |
| *Trichophyton tonsurans* | Hair, skin, nails | *Mycelia* | Mold |
| *Trichophyton rubrum* | Hair, skin, nails | Mycelia | Mold |
| *Trichophyton mentagrophytes* | Hair, skin | Mycelia | Mold |
| *Trichophyton violaceum* | Hair, skin, nails | Mycelia | Mold |
| *Epidermophyton floccosum* | Skin | Mycelia | Mold |
| Other mycoses | | | |
| *Pityrosporum orbiculare* | Skin (pink to brown)[b] | Yeast (mycelia)[c] | Yeast |
| *Cladosporium werneckii* | Skin (brown–black)[b] | Mycelia | Yeast (mold) |
| *Trichosporon cutaneum* | Hair (white)[b] | Mycelia | Mold |
| *Piedraia hortae* | Hair (black)[b] | Mycelia | Mold |

[a] Specimens fluoresce under ultraviolet light.
[b] Color of clinical lesions.
[c] Denotes less frequent findings.

temperate and tropical climates in the frequency of cases and isolations from nonhuman sources of the different species. Many of these differences are changing with shifts in population.

Human-to-human transmission requires close contact

Human-to-human transmission usually requires very close contact with an infected subject or infected materials, because dermatophytes are of low infectivity and virulence. Transmission usually takes place within families or in situations involving contact with detached skin or hair, such as barber shops and locker rooms. No special precautions beyond hand washing need be taken by the medical attendant after contact with an infected patient.

## Pathogenesis

Initial infection through minor skin breaks

Balance between fungal growth and skin desquamation determines outcome

Dermatophytoses begin when minor traumatic lesions come in contact with the fungi. Once the stratum corneum is penetrated the organism can proliferate, but does not invade deeper structures. The course of the infection is then dependent on the anatomic location, the dynamics of skin growth and desquamation, the speed and extent of the inflammatory response, and the infecting species. For example, if the organisms grow very slowly in the stratum corneum, and turnover by desquamation of this layer is not retarded, the infection will probably be short-lived and cause minimal signs and symptoms. Inflammation tends to increase skin growth and desquamation rates and helps to limit infection, whereas immunosuppressive agents such as corticosteroids decrease shedding of the keratinized layers and tend to prolong infection. Most infections are self-limiting, but those in which fungal growth rates and desquamation are balanced and in which the inflammatory response is poor tend to become chronic. The lateral spread of infection and its associated inflammation produce the characteristic sharp advancing margins that were once believed to be the burrows of worms. This characteristic is the origin of the common name **ringworm** and the Latin term **tinea** (worm) that is often applied to the clinical forms of the disease (Fig 46–1A).

Hair and nails involved primarily or by spread

Infection may spread from skin to other keratinized structures, such as hair and nails, or may invade them primarily. The hair shaft is penetrated by hyphae, which extend as arthroconidia either exclusively within the shaft (endothrix) or both within and outside the shaft (ectothrix). The end result is damage to the hair shaft structure, which often breaks off. Loss of hair at the root and plugging of the hair follicle with fungal elements may result. Invasion of the nail bed causes a hyperkeratotic reaction, which dislodges or distorts the nail.

## Immunity

The great majority of dermatophyte infections pass through an inflammatory stage to spontaneous healing. Little is known about the factors that mediate the host response in these

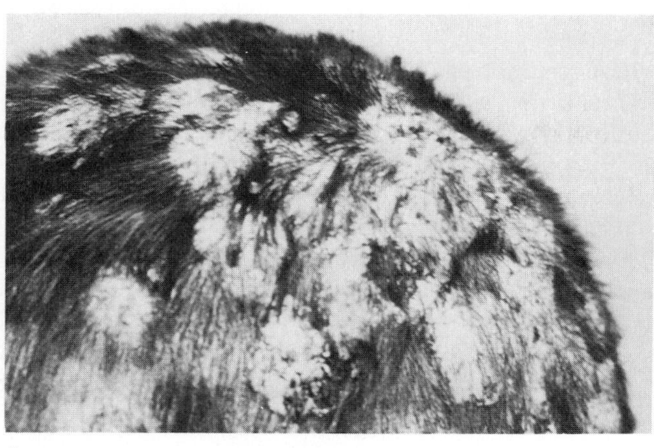

A

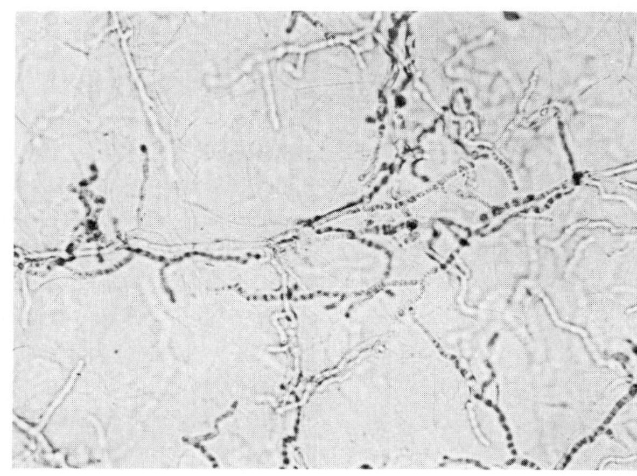

B

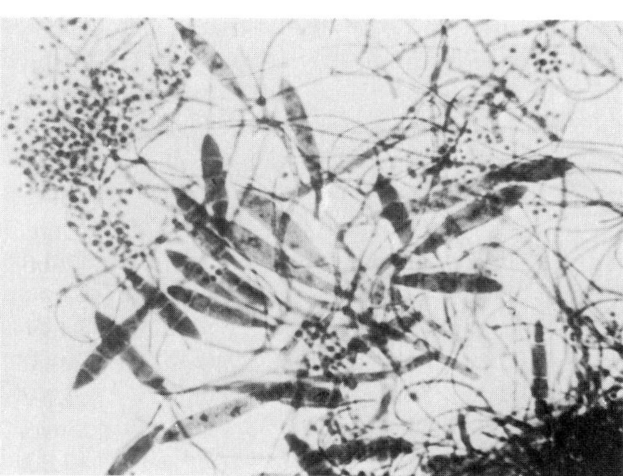

C

**Figure 46–1.** Dermatophyte infection of scalp (ringworm). **A.** Scalp lesions. Note the annular margination. **B.** Scrapings taken from the edge of the scalp lesion in KOH. Only the hyphal elements are visible. **C.** Culture. Hyphae, macroconidia, and microconidia are present. The macroconidia are characteristic of *Trichophyton*. (*Reprinted with permission from Dr. E. S. Beneke and the Upjohn Company: Scope Publications, Human Mycoses.*)

self-limiting infections or whether they confer immunity to subsequent exposures. Antibodies may be formed during infection, but they play no known role in immunity. Most clinical and experimental evidence points to the importance of cell-mediated immunity as with other fungal infections. The timing of the inflammatory response to infection correlates with appearance of delayed hypersensitivity responses. Enhanced desquamation with the inflammatory response helps remove infected skin.

Little known of immunity

Delayed hypersensitivity responses occur

Occasionally, dermatophyte infections become chronic and widespread. This progression has been related to both host and organism factors. Approximately half of these patients have underlying diseases affecting their immune responses or are receiving treatments that compromise T lymphocyte function. These chronic infections are particularly associated with *Trichophyton rubrum*, to which both normal and immunocompromised persons appear to be hyporesponsive. Although a number of mechanisms have been proposed, how this organism is able to grow without stimulating much inflammation is unexplained.

Widespread infection correlated with T lymphocyte defects

## Dermatophyte Disease: Clinical Aspects

### Clinical Manifestations

Dermatophyte infections range from inapparent colonization to chronic progressive eruptions that last months or years, causing considerable discomfort and disfiguration. Dermatologists often give each infection its own "disease" name, for example, tinea capitis (scalp), tinea pedis (feet, athlete's foot), tinea manuum (hands), tinea cruris (groin), tinea barbae (beard, hair), and tinea unguium (nail beds). Skin infections not included in this anatomic list are called tinea corporis (body). There are some general clinical, etiologic, and epidemiologic differences between these syndromes, but there is also considerable overlap.

Variations depend on skin site

Much overlap between tinea "diseases"

The primary differences between etiologic agents that infect different sites are shown in Table 46–1.

Hair infection leads to itching, hair loss

Infection of hair begins with an erythematous papule around the hair shaft, which progresses to scaling of the scalp, discoloration, and eventually fracture of the shaft. Spread to adjacent hair follicles progresses in a ringlike fashion, leaving behind broken, discolored hairs and sometimes black dots filled with fungal debris. The degree of inflammatory response markedly affects the clinical appearance and, in some cases, can cause constitutional symptoms. In most cases symptoms beyond itching are minimal.

Skin infection favors moist areas, skin folds

Skin lesions begin in a similar pattern and enlarge to form sharply delineated erythematous borders with skin of nearly normal appearance in the center. Multiple lesions can fuse to form unusual geometric patterns on the skin. Lesions may appear in any location, but are particularly common in moist, sweaty skin folds. Obesity and the wearing of tight apparel increase susceptibility to infection in the groin and beneath the breasts. Another form of infection, which involves scaling and splitting of the skin between the toes, is commonly known as athlete's foot. Moisture and maceration of the skin provide the mode of entry.

Nail bed infections can be disfiguring

Nail bed infections first cause discoloration of the subungual tissue, then hyperkeratosis and apparent discoloration of the nail plate by the underlying infection. Direct infection of the nail plate is uncommon. Progression of hyperkeratosis and associated inflammation cause disfigurement of the nail but few symptoms until the nail plate is so dislodged or distorted that it exposes or compresses adjacent soft tissue.

### Diagnosis

Direct KOH mounts of skin scrapings and infected hairs demonstrate hyphae

The goal of diagnostic procedures is to distinguish dermatophytoses from other skin diseases, such as mimicking infections caused by bacteria and other fungi, and from noninfectious inflammatory skin disorders, such as psoriasis and contact dermatitis. The most important step is microscopic examination of material taken from lesions to detect the fungus. KOH or calciflor white preparations of scales scraped from the advancing edge of a dermatophyte lesion demonstrate septate hyphae (Fig 46–1B). Examination of infected hairs reveals hyphae and arthroconidia penetrating the hair shaft. Broken hairs give the best yield. Some species of dermatophyte fluoresce, and selection of hairs for examination can be aided by the use of an ultraviolet lamp (Wood's lamp).

Culture used when KOH preparations negative

Management little influenced by species identity

The same material used for direct examination can be cultured for isolation of the offending dermatophyte. Mild infections with typical clinical findings and positive KOH preparations are often not cultured, because clinical management is not influenced significantly by the identity of the etiologic species. Clinically typical infections with negative KOH preparations require culture. The major reason for false-negative KOH results, however, is failure to collect the scrapings or hairs properly.

### Treatment and Prevention

Topical tolnaftate, naftifine, or azoles useful

Systemic treatment in more refractory cases

Many local skin infections resolve spontaneously without chemotherapy. Those that do not may be treated with topical tolnaftate, naftifine, or azoles. Nail bed and more extensive skin infections require systemic therapy with griseofulvin or ketoconazole, often combined with topical therapy. Therapy must be continued over weeks to months, and relapses are common. Keratolytic agents may be useful for reducing the size of hyperkeratotic lesions.

Dermatophyte infections can usually be prevented simply by observing general hygienic measures. No specific preventive measures such as vaccines exist.

## OTHER SUPERFICIAL MYCOSES

Tinea versicolor and tinea nigra occur primarily in tropics

Tinea (pityriasis) versicolor occurs primarily in the tropics; it is characterized by discrete areas of hypopigmentation associated with induration and scaling. Lesions are found on the trunk and arms; some assume pigments ranging from pink to yellow-brown, hence the term **versicolor.** The cause, *Pityrosporum orbiculare,* can be seen in skin scrapings as clusters of budding yeast cells mixed with hyphae. It grows primarily in the yeast form in culture.

Tinea nigra, another tropical infection, is characterized by brown to black macular lesions, usually on the hands or feet. There is little inflammation or scaling. The cause, *Cla-*

*dosporium werneckii,* is a black-pigmented fungus found in soil and other environmental sites. Scrapings of the lesion show brown–black-pigmented septate hyphae. In culture initial growth is in the yeast form, with slow development of hyphal elements.

Piedra is an infection of the hair characterized by black or white nodules attached to the hair shaft. White piedra (caused by *Trichosporon cutaneum*) infects the shaft in hyphal forms, which fragment with occasional buds. Black piedra (caused by *Piedraia hortae*) shows branched hyphae and ascopores in sections of the hair.

Piedra and infection of hair with black or white nodules

## ADDITIONAL READING

Wilson JW, Plunkett OA. The Fungus Diseases of Man. Berkeley: University of California Press; 1965. This general mycology text can still be found on the shelves of most medical libraries. Its outstanding characteristic is the photographic presentation of dermatophytoses and other cutaneous manifestations of fungal disease.

Chapter 47

# *Candida, Aspergillus,* and Other Opportunistic Fungi

*Kenneth J. Ryan*

The fungi considered in this chapter are usually found as members of the normal flora or as saprophytes in the environment. With breakdown of host defenses they can produce disease ranging from superficial skin or mucous membrane infections to systemic involvement of multiple organs. The most common opportunistic infections are caused by the yeast *Candida albicans,* a normal inhabitant of the gastrointestinal and genital floras, and a mold, *Aspergillus,* commonly found in the environment. The diseases caused by *Candida, Aspergillus,* and other opportunistic fungi are summarized in Table 47–1.

## CANDIDA: General Characteristics

*Candida* species grow as typical 4- to 6-μm, budding, round or oval yeast cells (see Fig 44–1) under most conditions and at most temperatures. Under certain conditions, including those found in infection, they can form hyphae. Some species form chlamydoconidia. Many *Candida* species have been defined; those most commonly associated with disease in humans are listed in Table 47–2. Species identification is based on a combination of biochemical and morphologic characteristics, such as carbohydrate assimilation and fermentation and the ability to produce hyphae and chlamydoconidia. Particular attention is given to the differentiation of *Candida albicans* from other species, because it is the most frequent cause of disease. It is also by far the best understood as to structure, metabolic activity, and pathogenesis.

Yeasts, hyphae, and pseudohyphae may develop

*C. albicans* most common cause of disease

Most *Candida* species, including *C. albicans,* grow rapidly on Sabouraud's agar and on enriched bacteriologic media. Smooth, white, 2- to 4-mm colonies resembling those of staphylococci are produced on blood agar after overnight incubation. Fluid cultures typically show a deposit at the bottom, but diffuse growth may occur if the broth is well aerated. *Candida albicans* forms sproutlike hyphae directly from yeast cells that are incubated in serum at 37°C. These structures are called germ tubes (Fig 47–1) and are produced within 2 to 3 hours. The organism also forms terminal thick-walled chlamydoconidia under certain conditions (see Fig 47–1).

Germ tube development and chlamydoconidia distinguish *C. albicans*

TABLE 47–1. AGENTS OF OPPORTUNISTIC MYCOSES

| Organism | Infection | Growth | | |
|---|---|---|---|---|
| | | **Tissue** | **Culture at 25 °C** | **Culture at 37 °C** |
| *Candida* | Skin, mucous membranes, urinary, disseminated | Yeast (pseudomycelia)[a] | Yeast (mycelia)[a] | Yeast |
| *Aspergillus* | Lung, disseminated | Mycelia (septate) | Mold | Mold |
| Zygomycetes[b] | Rhinocerebral, lung | Mycelia (nonseptate) | Mold | Mold |

[a] Less common feature.
[b] *Absidia, Mucor,* and *Rhizopus.*

TABLE 47–2. MEDICALLY IMPORTANT CANDIDA AND TORULOPSIS SPECIES

| Species | Germ Tubes[a] | Pseudohyphae | Chlamydoconidia |
|---|---|---|---|
| *C. albicans* | + | + | + |
| *C. krusei* | – | + | – |
| *C. parapsilosis* | – | + | – |
| *C. tropicalis* | – | + | –[b] |
| *C. guilliermondii* | – | + | – |
| *T. glabrata* | – | – | – |

[a] Rapid production (4 hours or less).
[b] Occasional strains produce chlamydoconidia morphologically different from those of *C. albicans*.

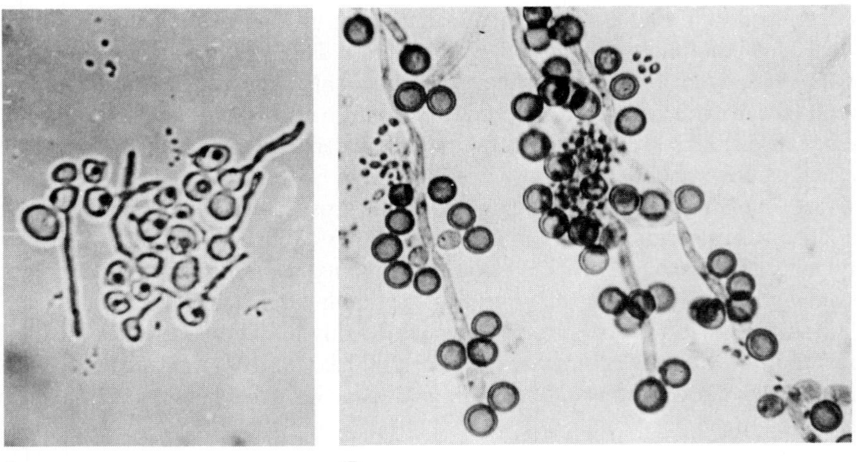


**Figure 47–1.** *Candida albicans.* **A.** When incubated at 37°C, *C. albicans* rapidly forms elongated hyphae called germ tubes. **B.** On specialized media, *C. albicans* forms thick-walled chlamydoconidia, which differentiate it from other *Candida* species. (*Reprinted with permission from Dr. E. S. Beneke and the Upjohn Company: Scope Publications, Human Mycoses.*)

# CANDIDA ALBICANS

## Mycology

The *C. albicans* cell wall is made up of a mixture of the polysaccharides mannan, glucan, and chitin alone or in complexes with protein. Ultrastructure studies have shown a fibrillar outer layer believed to be mannan and mannoprotein. The exact composition of the cell wall and surface components is known to vary under different growth and morphologic conditions.

Cell wall includes mannan, glucan, and chitin complexed with protein

*Candida albicans* grows in either of two basic morphologic forms. The yeast form with budding by blastoconidia is seen under most culture conditions. The hyphal form begins with what appear to be elongated blastoconidia extending out many times the diameter of the original cell, eventually becoming hyphae. *Candida albicans* may form hyphae or pseudohyphae. As the term **pseudohyphae** reflects morphologic rather than functional differences, the term **hyphae** is used here to encompass both forms. The biological behavior of hyphae and that of pseudohyphae appear to be the same. Many chemical, enzymatic, and functional differences have been shown between the blastoconidial and hyphal forms of *C. albicans,* some of which can be correlated with pathogenicity.

Grows by blastoconidia or hyphae

Pseudohyphae equivalent to hyphae

Features of hyphae correlate with virulence

## Candidiasis

### Epidemiology

Most *C. albicans* infections are caused by endogenous flora, except in cases of direct mucosal contact with lesions in others (eg, through sexual intercourse). Nosocomial *C. albicans* infections are also derived more frequently from the patient's own flora than from cross-infection; they are often associated with the invasive procedures mentioned previously.

Primarily endogenous infections

### Pathogenesis

*Candida albicans* is normally present in small numbers in the oral cavity, lower gastrointestinal tract, and female genital tract. This colonization is aided by the ability of *C. albicans* to adhere to mucosal cells, a feature that distinguishes it from most other *Candida* species. The pathogenic potential of *C. albicans* is strongly associated with a shift from the yeast to the hyphal form. This is based on the appearance of virulence factors associated with adherence and invasion in the hyphal phase and the clinical observation that hyphae are present in invasive lesions (see Fig 44–4). This formation of invasive hyphae is not seen with the other less virulent *Candida* species. It should, however, be noted that *Candida tropicalis* is also a virulent species although it does not form hyphae.

Adheres well to mucosal cells

Shift from yeast to hyphae form associated with virulence

*Candida albicans* hyphae have the capacity to bind to a number of molecular structures found in human tissues. These include components of the extracellular matrix (ECM) such as fibronectin, collagen, laminin, and complement C3 conversion products. This binding is mediated by mannoprotein components of the outer fibrillar surface of the organism, but it is not clear whether single or multiple adhesins are responsible. As the proteins that make up the host ECM are known to share specific structural sequences, it is possible that one *Candida* molecule could mediate adherence to multiple components of host tissues as shown in Figure 47–2.

Binds multiple components of the extracellular matrix

Surface mannoprotein acts as adhesin

Hyphae are also able to elaborate an extracellular proteinase which digests epithelial cells (see Fig 47–3). This proteinase probably facilitates invasion and may also play a role in adherence. A number of environmental factors are known to trigger conversion to the hyphal form and invasion, but how they relate to human infection is still unclear.

Hyphae produce extracellular proteinase

Factors that allow *C. albicans* to increase its relative proportion of the flora (antibacterial therapy), that compromise the general immune capacity of the host (leukopenia or corticosteroid therapy), or that interfere with T lymphocyte function (eg, AIDS) are often associated with local and invasive infection. The disruptions of the mucosa associated with chronic disease and their treatments (indwelling devices, cancer chemotherapy) may enhance the invasion process by exposing *Candida* binding sites in the ECM. Diabetes mellitus also predisposes to *C. albicans* infection, possibly because of the known greater production of the surface adherence proteins in the presence of high glucose concentrations.

Immunosuppression predisposes

Mechanical disruptions may provide access to ECM

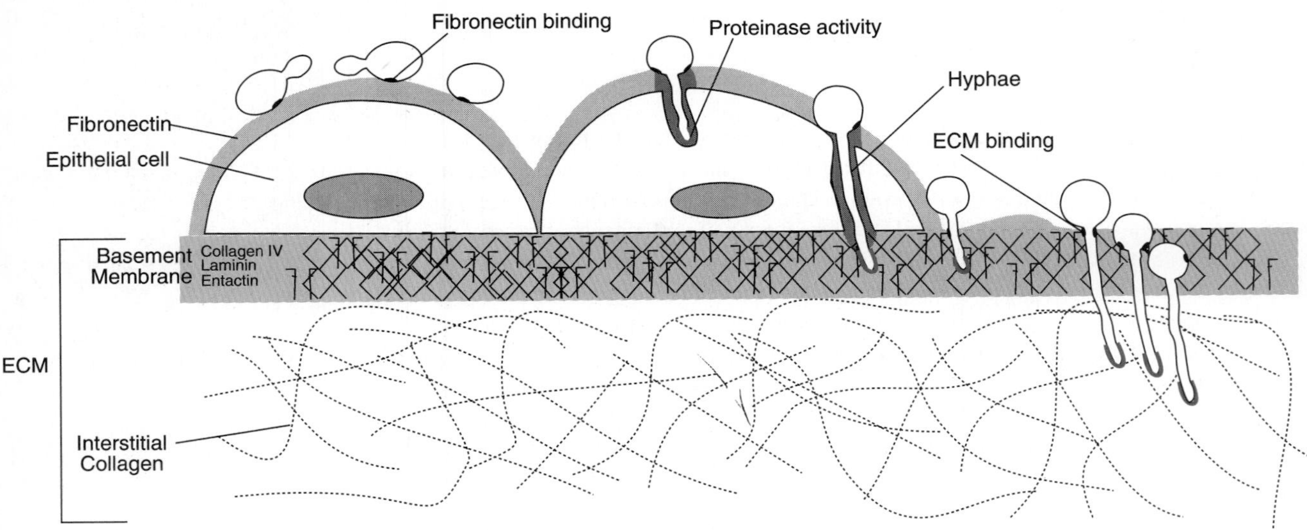


**Figure 47–2.** Pathogenesis of *Candida albicans* infections. Proposed mechanisms of *C. albicans* attachment and invasion are shown. Surface glucomannan receptor(s) on the yeast may bind to fibronectin covering the epithelial cell or to elements of the extracellular matrix (ECM) when the epithelial surface is lost or the *Candida* have invaded beyond it. Invasion is associated with formation of hyphae and production of proteinases, which may digest tissue elements.

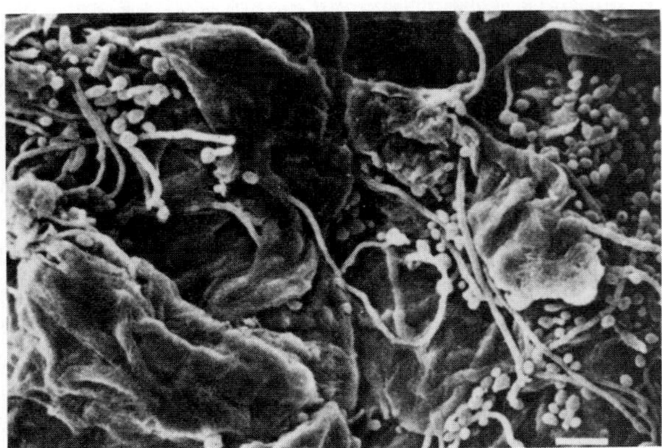

A

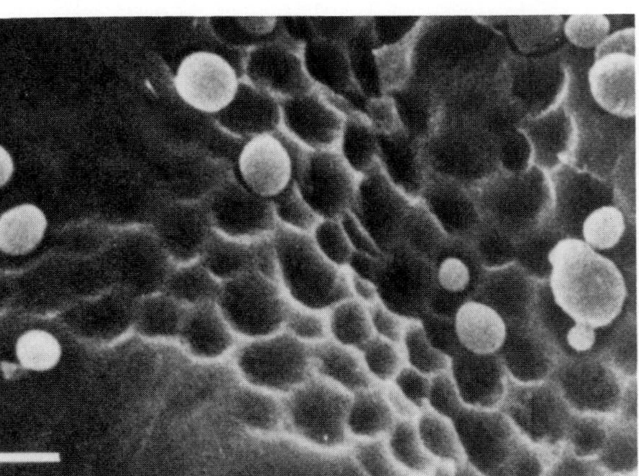

B

**Figure 47–3.** Invasiveness of *Candida albicans*. Two features of invasiveness are seen in these scanning electron micrographs taken from experiments with murine corneocytes. **A.** Both blastoconidia and mycelial elements are present. The mycelial elements spread over the surface and invade the cell cuticle. **B.** A *C. albicans* strain that produces a protease is seen producing cavity-like depressions in the cell surface. This action could play a role in invasion of the cell. (*Reprinted with permission of Thomas L. Ray and Candia D. Payne. Infect Immun. 1988;56: 1945–1947, Figures 4,6B. Copyright American Society for Microbiology.*)

### Immunity

Both humoral immunity and cell-mediated immunity are important in defense against *Candida* infections. Neutrophils are an important first-line defense. *Candida albicans* yeast forms are readily phagocytosed and killed when opsonized by antibody and complement. In the absence of antibody, the process is less efficient. Hyphal forms may be too large to be ingested by neutrophils, but neutrophils can still kill the fungi by attaching to the hyphae and discharging metabolites generated by the oxidative metabolic burst. A deficit in neutrophils or neutrophilic function is the most common correlate of serious *C. albicans* infection.

Opsonized yeast forms are phagocytosed and killed
Neutrophil products may kill extracellular hyphal forms

The *C. albicans* protein surface receptors discussed above bind the iC3b component of complement in a manner similar to that of the receptors on human neutrophils: iC3b bound to the candidal surface by these receptors is thus oriented in a fashion that makes it unavailable for opsonization. Enhanced production of these receptors under various conditions, for example, elevated glucose concentration, is associated with resistance to phagocytosis by neutrophils.

*C. albicans* receptors bind complement in an antiopsonic manner

The association of chronic mucocutaneous candidiasis (see later) with a number of T lymphocyte immunodeficiencies emphasizes the importance of this arm of the immune system in *Candida* infections. The increased frequency of vaginal candidiasis in AIDS patients suggests that even superficial infections involve T lymphocyte mediated immune responses. In animal studies *Candida* cell wall mannan has been shown to play an immunoregulatory function by downregulating cell-mediated immune responses. As with other fungi, incubation of macrophages with cytokines such as interferon gamma and tumor necrosis factor enhances their ability to kill *C. albicans*.

Compromised cell-mediated immunity associated with progressive infection
*Candida* mannan may downregulate CMI responses

## Candidiasis: Clinical Aspects

### Clinical Manifestations

Superficial invasion of the mucous membranes by *C. albicans* produces a white, cheesy plaque that is loosely adherent to the mucosal surface. The lesion is usually painless, unless the plaque is torn away and the raw, weeping, invaded surface is exposed. Oral lesions, called thrush, occur on the tongue, palate, and other mucosal surfaces as single or multiple, ragged white patches. A similar infection in the vagina, vaginal candidiasis, produces a thick, curdlike discharge and itching of the vulva. Although most women have at least one episode of vaginal candidiasis in a lifetime, approximately 5% suffer recurrent infections. This may be linked to deficient cell-mediated immune responses as in chronic mucocutaneous candidiasis.

Superficial infections include thrush, vaginal candidiasis

*Candida albicans* skin infections occur in crural folds and other areas in which wet, macerated skin surfaces are opposed. For example, one type of diaper rash is caused by *C. albicans*. Other infections of the skin folds and appendages occur in association with recurrent immersion in water (eg, dishwashers). The initial lesions are erythematous papules or confluent areas associated with tenderness, erythema, and fissures of the skin. Infection usually remains confined to the chronically irritated area, but may spread beyond it, particularly in infants.

Skin infections primarily in moist areas

In rare persons with specific defects in T cell-mediated immune defense against *Candida,* a chronic, relapsing form of candidiasis called chronic mucocutaneous candidiasis develops. Infections of the skin, hair, and mucocutaneous junctions fail to resolve with adequate therapy and management. There is considerable disfigurement and discomfort, particularly when the disease is accompanied by a granulomatous inflammatory response. Although lesions may become extensive, they usually do not disseminate. To some degree this disease may represent a clinical example of immunologic tolerance. Cutaneous anergy to *C. albicans* antigens is commonly seen in these patients and is often reversed during antifungal chemotherapy, suggesting that it is due to chronic antigen excess.

Chronic mucocutaneous candidiasis associated with specific T cell defects

Inflammatory patches similar to those in thrush may develop in the esophagus with or without associated oral candidiasis. Painful swallowing and substernal chest pain are the most common symptoms. Extensive ulcerations, deformity, and occasionally perforation of the esophagus may ensue. In immunocompromised patients similar lesions may also develop in the stomach, together with deep ulcerative lesions of the small and large intestine.

Esophagitis, intestinal candidiasis similar to thrush

Urinary tract candidiasis associated with immune compromise, diabetes

Infection of the urinary tract via the hematogenous or ascending routes may produce cystitis, pyelonephritis, abscesses, or expanding fungus ball lesions in the renal pelvis. *Candida* infections of visceral organs with or without further dissemination to multiple organs have a particularly strong association with diabetes mellitis, immunologic compromise, or some other violation of normal defense mechanisms. The organs most commonly involved are the kidneys, brain, heart, and eye. The clinical findings in disseminated infections are generally not sufficiently characteristic to suggest *C. albicans* rather than bacterial pathogens, which more commonly produce infection of deep organs.

Expanding lesion of retina or vitreous

*Candida* endophthalmitis has the characteristic funduscopic appearance of a white cotton ball expanding on the retina or floating free in the vitreous humor. Endophthalmitis and infections of other eye structures can lead to blindness.

### Laboratory Diagnosis

KOH and Gram smears of superficial lesions show yeast and hyphae

Superficial *C. albicans* infections provide ready access to diagnostic material. Exudate or epithelial scrapings examined by KOH preparations or Gram smear demonstrate abundant budding yeast cells; if associated hyphae are present, the infection is almost certainly caused by *C. albicans*.

Systemic candidiasis requires direct specimens

Deep organ involvement is much more difficult to prove without direct sampling. Cultures from specimens such as sputum run the risk of contamination from the normal flora or a superficial mucous membrane lesion. A direct aspirate, biopsy, or bronchoalveolar lavage (BAL) is often required to establish the diagnosis.

Aeration of blood cultures enhances yield

*Candida albicans* is readily isolated from the blood in media used for bacteriologic culture, but specialized procedures such as aeration enhance the yield. Even positive blood cultures may not diagnose deep organ involvement as they may represent colonization of the intravenous catheters often used in patients prone to systemic candidiasis. *Candida* endocarditis represents a special diagnostic problem, because the yeasts seeding the blood from the valve may be filtered out in the capillary beds and thus prevented from reaching the venous circulation where blood culture samples are routinely collected. Arterial blood cultures may be required in this situation.

Endocarditis may require arterial cultures

Culture and identification use standard tests

Isolation of *Candida* species is not difficult as the organisms grow rapidly as yeasts on blood or Sabouraud's agar. The primary identification procedure involves presumptive differentiation of *C. albicans* from other *Candida* species with the germ tube test. Germ tube-negative strains may be further identified biochemically or reported as "yeast not *C. albicans*," depending on their apparent clinical significance.

Serodiagnostic procedures and detection of *C. albicans* products not yet useful

Although many serologic tests have been developed for detection of *C. albicans* antibodies, none of the methods developed to date has the sensitivity or specificity needed for clinical diagnosis. Immunologic techniques for detection of circulating *Candida* cell components such as mannan show promise, but none are yet ready for clinical use.

### Treatment

Local treatment for superficial lesions

Recovery without treatment of underlying disease common

Amphotericin B, flucytosine, and azole therapy for progressive disease

*Candida albicans* is usually susceptible to amphotericin B, nystatin, flucytosine, and the azoles. Superficial infections are generally treated with topical nystatin or azole preparations. Measures to decrease moisture and chronic trauma are important adjuncts in treating *Candida* skin infections. Deeper *C. albicans* infections may resolve spontaneously with elimination or control of predisposing conditions. Removal of an infected catheter, control of diabetes, or a rise in peripheral leukocyte counts is often associated with recovery without antifungal therapy. Persistent relapsing or disseminated candidiasis is treated with amphotericin B, flucytosine, fluconazole, or combinations of amphotericin B with other drugs. Ketoconazole has been effective treatment for chronic mucocutaneous candidiasis but is being replaced with fluconazole.

## OTHER OPPORTUNISTIC YEASTS

Species of *Candida* other than *C. albicans* (Table 47–2) produce infections in circumstances similar to those described previously, but less frequently. When contamination of an indwelling device is the portal of entry, the probability of infection by these other species increases. The adherence and invasive properties of *C. albicans* are also seen with *Candida tropicalis*. Both experimental and clinical evidence indicate that *C. tropicalis* has virulence at least equal to that of *C. albicans*. *Candida tropicalis* produces an extracellular proteinase similar to that of *C. albicans* which may enhance its invasiveness.

*C. tropicalis* demonstrates virulence

Another common organism is *Torulopsis glabrata*. This species is a small (2- to 4-μm) yeast with characteristics similar to those of *Candida*. It is a member of the normal gastrointestinal and genital flora. The most common infections are in the urinary tract, but occasionally other deep tissue involvement and fungemia occur. The organisms are small enough to be confused with *Histoplasma capsulatum* in histologic preparations. Therapy is similar to that for *C. albicans* infections, although *T. glabrata* is more likely to be resistant to flucytosine.

*T. glabrata* is small for a yeast

## ASPERGILLUS

### Mycology

Aspergillus species are rapidly growing molds with septate hyphae and characteristic asexual conidia (Fig 47–4A). Fluffy colonies appear in 1 to 2 days and, by 5 days, may cover an entire plate with pigmented growth. Species are defined on the basis of differences in the

Mold differentiation on basis of conidiophores and conidia

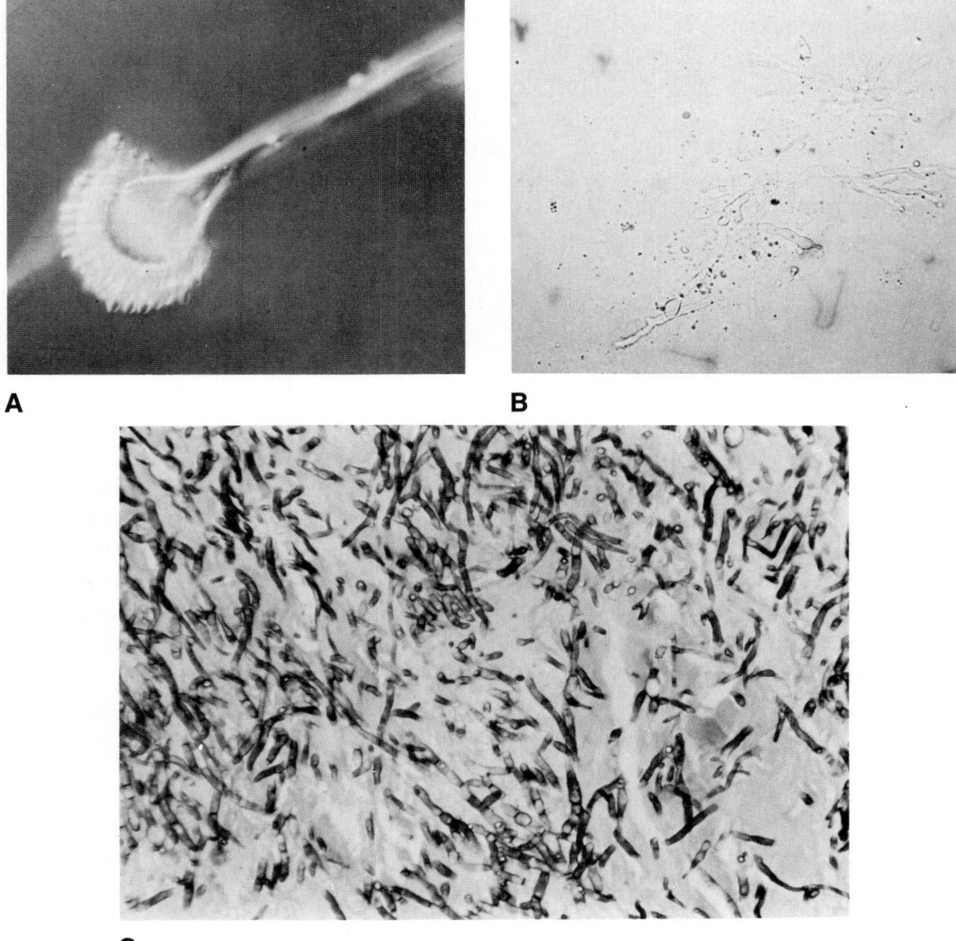


**Figure 47–4.** *Aspergillus.* **A.** This asexual conidium-forming structure is characteristic of *Aspergillus* species. The conidia are borne at the end of the fingerlike extensions at the end of the conidiophore. These structures are rarely produced in vivo. **B.** This tissue aspirate mixed with KOH shows branching, septate hyphae. **C.** Histologic sections also show branching, septate hyphae, but because the conidia shown in **A** are not seen the findings are not diagnostic of *Aspergillus.* (*Reprinted with permission from Dr. E. S. Beneke and the Upjohn Company: Scope Publications, Human Mycoses.*)

structure of the conidiophore and the arrangement of the conidia. The most important in human infections are *Aspergillus fumigatus* and *Aspergillus flavus,* but others, such as *Aspergillus niger,* can be involved.

## Aspergillosis

### Epidemiology

Environmental organisms spread by disruption

*Aspergillus* species are widely distributed in nature and found throughout the world. They seem to adapt to a wide range of environmental conditions, and the heat-resistant conidia provide a good mechanism for dispersal. Hospital air and air ducts have received attention as sources of nosocomial *Aspergillus* isolates. Occasionally, building remodeling or other kinds of major environmental disruption have been associated with increased frequency of *Aspergillus* contamination, colonization, or infection.

### Pathogenesis and Immunity

Conidia have some antiphagocytic properties

*Aspergillus* conidia must be inhaled frequently, but disease is rare in those without compromised defenses. Factors that aid the fungus in the initial stages are not known, but the ability of the conidia to bind fibrinogen and complement components has been demonstrated. *Aspergillus fumigatus* possesses an extracellular inhibitor of the alternate complement pathway that interferes with opsonophagocytosis. Production of extracellular elastase and proteinase has been associated with the more virulent species, but the pathogenic role of these enzymes remains to be demonstrated. As with *Candida,* neutrophilic killing of hyphae is a crucial step in defense against this common mold.

## Aspergillosis: Clinical Aspects

### Clinical Manifestations

Allergic responses to aspergilli often transient

*Aspergillus* can cause clinical allergies or occasional invasive infection. In both cases, the lung is the organ primarily involved. Allergic aspergillosis, which can be a mechanism of exacerbation in patients with asthma, is characterized by transient pulmonary infiltrates, eosinophilia, and a rise in *Aspergillus*-specific IgG. These conditions follow direct inhalation of fungal elements or, more commonly, colonization of the respiratory tract. Areas of the bronchopulmonary tree with poor drainage because of underlying disease or anatomic abnormalities may serve as a site for growth of organisms and continuous seeding with antigen.

Invasive pulmonary aspergillosis may erode blood vessels

Invasive aspergillosis occurs in the settings of preexisting pulmonary disease (bronchiectasis, chronic bronchitis, asthma, tuberculosis) or immunosuppression. Colonization with *Aspergillus* can lead to invasion into the tissue by branching septate hyphae. Mycelial masses can grow to such an extent that they form a radiologically visible fungus ball within a cavity. Lung tissue invasion may penetrate blood vessels, causing hemoptysis or erosion into other structures with development of fistulas. Invasive disease outside the lung is rare unless the patient is immunocompromised.

Acute pneumonia in immunocompromised host has grave prognosis

An acute pneumonia may occur in severely immunocompromised patients, particularly those with depressed neutrophil counts. Multifocal pulmonary infiltrates expanding to consolidation are present with high fever. In contrast to immunocompetent hosts, the prognosis is grave and dissemination to other organs common.

### Diagnosis

Difficult to distinguish infection from contamination

Direct aspirate or biopsy with histology and culture required

*Aspergillus* is relatively easy to isolate and identify. Its rapidly spreading mold growth and all too frequent contamination of cultures cause it to be regarded by microbiologists as a kind of weed. The diagnostic problem is distinguishing contamination and colonization with *Aspergillus* from invasive disease. The diagnosis cannot be made for certain without the use of lung aspiration, biopsy, or bronchoalveolar lavage. With material directly from the lesion, the presence of large, branching, septate hyphae (Figs 47–4B and C) and a positive culture are diagnostic. Occasionally, the complete fruiting bodies are produced in vivo, creating a striking and diagnostic histologic picture. Serologic methods have been developed to demonstrate *Aspergillus* antibodies. Although these tests may be helpful in suggesting allergic aspergillosis, they have little value in invasive disease because anti-*Aspergillus* antibody is common in healthy persons.

Serodiagnostic procedures not useful for invasive aspergillosis

### Treatment

Amphotericin B has long been the only effective treatment for invasive or disseminated aspergillosis, but clinical experience with itraconazole suggests it may be an alternative. It is not clear whether flucytosine is effective either alone or in combination with amphotericin B. In cases with pulmonary structural abnormalities and fungus balls, chemotherapy has little effect. Surgical intervention is sometimes needed.

## ZYGOMYCETES AND ZYGOMYCOSIS

**Zygomycosis** (mucormycosis) is the term applied to infection with any of a group of zygomycetes, the most common of which are *Absidia*, *Rhizopus*, and *Mucor*. These fungi are ubiquitous saprophytes in soil and are commonly found on bread and many other foodstuffs. They occasionally cause disease in persons with diabetes mellitus and in immunosuppressed patients receiving corticosteroid therapy. Diabetic acidosis has a particularly strong association with zygomycosis.

Zygomycetes are soil saprophtes

Infection in immunocompromised hosts, particularly diabetics

Pulmonary or rhinocerebral disease is acquired by inhalation of conidia. The pulmonary form has clinical findings similar to those of other fungal pneumonias; the rhinocerebral form, however, produces a dramatic clinical syndrome in which agents of zygomycosis show striking invasive capacity. They penetrate the mucosa of the nose, paranasal sinuses, or palate, often resulting in ulcerative lesions. Once beyond the mucosa, they progress through tissue, nerves, blood vessels, fascial planes, and often the vital structures at the base of the brain. The clinical syndrome begins with headache and may progress through orbital cellulitis and hemorrhage to cranial nerve palsy, vascular thrombosis, coma, and death in less than 2 weeks.

Pulmonary disease similar to other fungi

Rhinocerebral infections may penetrate to brain

The pathologic cerebral and pulmonary findings are distinctive: the zygomycetes involved all show large, nonseptate hyphae in tissue, although conidia are not seen. As with *Aspergillus*, tissue biopsies are necessary to demonstrate the invasive hyphae, unless they can be seen on scrapings from palatal or nasal ulcers. For reasons that are obscure, cultures are sometimes negative, even those from tissue containing characteristic hyphae. Therapy involves control of underlying disease, amphotericin B, and occasionally surgery.

Very large nonseptate hyphae seen in tissues

## ADDITIONAL READING


Calderone RA, Braun PC. Adherence and receptor relationships of *Candida albicans*. *Microbiol Rev*. 1991;55:1–20.

Hostetter MK. Adhesins and ligands involved in the interaction of *Candida spp*. with epithelial and endothelial surfaces. *Clin Microbiol Rev*. 1994;7:29–42.

Klotz SA. Fungal adherence to the vascular compartment: A critical step in the pathogenesis of disseminated candidiasis. *Clin Infect Dis*. 1992;14:340–347. These reviews present the most current ideas on the steps involved in the pathogenesis of this common fungal pathogen.

# Systemic Fungal Pathogens

*Kenneth J. Ryan*

The fungi discussed in this chapter cause a variety of infections, each ranging in severity from subclinical to progressive, debilitating disease. Most species are dimorphic, growing in the infectious mold form in the environment but switching to a yeast form in tissues to produce infection. They differ from the opportunistic fungi in their ability to cause disease in previously healthy persons, but the most serious disease still occurs in the immunocompromised. With the exception of *Cryptococcus neoformans* each of these species is restricted to a geographic niche corresponding to the environmental habitat of the mold form of the species. None are transmitted from human to human.

## CRYPTOCOCCUS

### Cryptococcus neoformans

*Cryptococcus neoformans* (cryptococcus) is a yeast 4 to 6 μm in diameter that produces a characteristic capsule (Fig 48–1) extending the overall diameter to 25 μm or more. This capsule is unique among pathogenic fungi and is a complex polysaccharide polymer, the major component of which is glucuronoxylomannan. There are some structural differences between serogroups based on acetylation and substitution of carbohydrates. *Cryptococcus neoformans* gives a positive test for urease, in contrast to *Candida* and most other yeasts. It grows in 2 to 5 days at 35 to 37°C on a variety of media, including blood agar, chocolate agar, and Sabouraud's agar, to produce mucoid, bacteria-like colonies. A sexual state can be demonstrated for *C. neoformans* by mating under defined conditions but has not been associated directly with disease.

Yeast with large polysaccharide capsule

Growth and urease production similar to bacteria

### Cryptococcosis

#### Epidemiology

*Cryptococcus neoformans* is found throughout the world, particularly in soil contaminated with pigeon or other bird droppings, where concentrations can exceed $10^6$ per gram. The birds themselves are not ill. Cases appear sporadically, with no particular occupational predisposition. Surprisingly, no increased risk of disease has been found in pigeon fanciers or in those who work with the organism in the laboratory. Case-to-case transmission has not been documented.

Reservoir in birds and soil

No occupational association or communicability

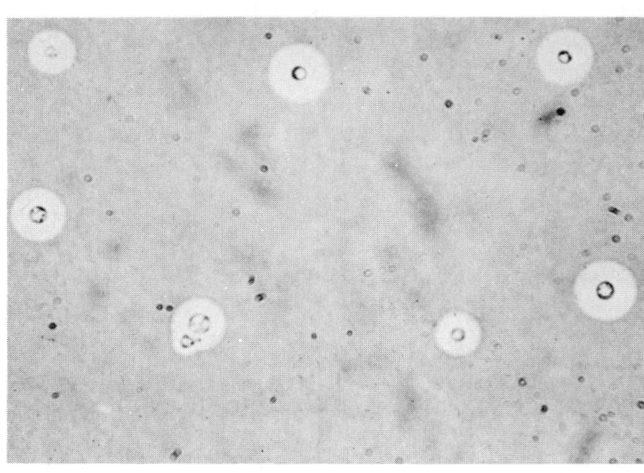

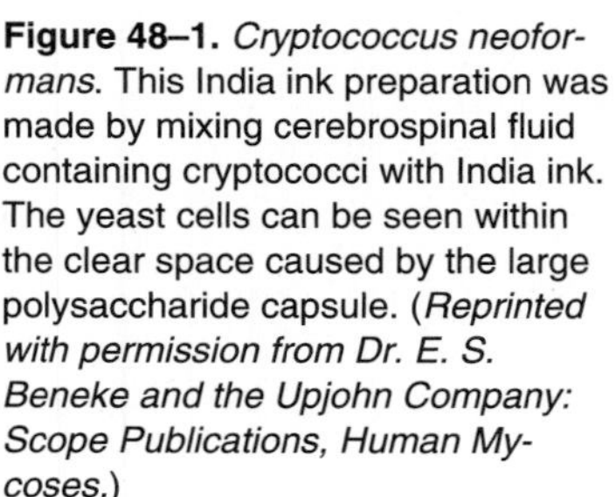

**Figure 48–1.** *Cryptococcus neoformans.* This India ink preparation was made by mixing cerebrospinal fluid containing cryptococci with India ink. The yeast cells can be seen within the clear space caused by the large polysaccharide capsule. (*Reprinted with permission from Dr. E. S. Beneke and the Upjohn Company: Scope Publications, Human Mycoses.*)

### Pathogenesis and Immunity

Pulmonary infection by inhalation

Most infections are unrecognized

Leading fungal infection of AIDS patients

Cryptococcal infection is presumed to begin with inhalation of yeast or conidia from an environmental source, followed by pulmonary infection or disease. In most instances symptoms and signs must be minimal, because cryptococcal pulmonary infections are rarely diagnosed although exposure is common. Occasionally the infection progresses in the lungs or spreads to the central nervous system. Roughly half of all such patients have received chemotherapy or have underlying disorders that compromise immunity. Cryptococcal disease is among the most common infectious complications of AIDS.

Capsule interferes with alternate pathway opsonization

T-cell responses crucial to outcome

Tissue reaction may be minimal

Initial interactions with phagocytes such as alveolar macrophages are crucial in the outcome of cryptococcal infection. Polymorphonuclear leukocytes (PMNs) and macrophages are able to phagocytose and kill cryptococci, but encapsulated cells are more resistant. The capsule seems to block opsonophagocytosis via the classic pathway and slows deposition of complement components via the alternate pathway. Nonencapsulated variants are opsonized by the classic pathway and are avirulent. Specific antibody enhances phagocytosis and killing. The circumstances are analogous to the encapsulated bacterial pathogens such as group B streptococci and pneumococci (see Chapter 16). Circulating capsular polysaccharide is also associated with immunomodulating effects such as tolerance and anergy. Animal studies indicate that T lymphocyte-mediated immune responses are crucial to the outcome of cryptococcal infection. This is supported by clinical experience particularly in AIDS patients, in whom induction of suppressor T cells may further aggravate an already compromised cellular response. Tissue reaction to *C. neoformans* may vary from little or none to purulent or granulomatous. Many cases of pulmonary, cutaneous, and even meningeal cryptococcal infection show a remarkable paucity of inflammatory cells. The propensity for cryptococci to spread to the central nervous system is unexplained but could be related to the organism's known metabolic affinity for catecholamines.

Antibody associated with clinical recovery

Cellular response to cryptococcal antigens may be depressed

Anticryptococcal antibodies are formed in the course of infection, and their appearance is associated with control of infection. The presence and extent of antigenemia with capsular antigen also has prognostic significance. A declining antigen level and rising antibody titer are favorable signs. Cryptococcosis in immunocompromised patients occurs primarily in those with defects in T lymphocyte function, particularly AIDS, or in those treated with immunosuppressive agents (eg, steroids). There is also evidence that patients with cryptococcosis who have no known immune defects often have subnormal cellular immune functions as measured by lymphocyte blastogenesis or absent or reduced delayed hypersensitivity responses to cryptococcal and other antigens. Clinical recovery in such cases is associated with return of cellular immune functions.

## ■ Cryptococcosis: Clinical Aspects

### Clinical Manifestations

CENTRAL NERVOUS SYSTEM

Meningitis is the most commonly recognized form of cryptococcal disease; it usually has a slow, insidious onset with relatively nonspecific findings until late in its course. Intermittent headache, irritability, dizziness, and difficulty with complex cerebral functions appear over weeks or months with no consistent pattern. Behavioral changes have been mistaken for psychoses. Fever is usually, but not invariably, present. Seizures, cranial nerve signs, and papilledema may appear later in the clinical course, as may dementia and decreased levels of consciousness. A more rapid course may be seen in AIDS patients, 5 to 15% of whom become infected with *C. neoformans*.

Meningitis follows chronic course

Course more rapid with AIDS

#### Other Infections

Cryptococcal pneumonia is often asymptomatic or mild. Sputum production is minimal, and no findings are sufficiently specific to suggest the etiology. Skin and bone are the sites most frequently involved in disseminated disease; skin lesions are sometimes the presenting sign and are often remarkable for their lack of inflammation. The diagnosis is sometimes made when lesions are biopsied as suspected neoplasms.

Cryptococcal pneumonia usually asymptomatic

### Diagnosis

In all attempts to demonstrate *C. neoformans* it is important to remember that the number of organisms present may be quite small. The typical cerebrospinal fluid (CSF) findings in cryptococcal meningitis are increased pressure, CSF pleocytosis (usually 100 cells or more) with predominance of lymphocytes, and depression of CSF glucose levels. In some cases, one or all of these findings may be absent, yet cryptococci are isolated on culture. Cryptococcal capsules are often demonstrable in CSF by mixing centrifuged sediment with India ink and examining the mixture under the microscope (see Fig 48–1). Some experience is necessary to avoid confusion of lymphocytes with cryptococci. Although this examination is positive in roughly 50% of cases, only a few cryptococci may be present in any single preparation. *Cryptococcus neoformans* stains poorly or not at all with routine histologic stains; thus, it is easily missed unless special fungal stains are used.

Number of organisms typically small

Direct India ink preparation diagnostic in 50% of cases

In the culture of *C. neoformans* from CSF, the more material cultured the better the chance of isolation as the number of organisms may be small. In cases with negative cultures, the polysaccharide capsular antigen may be detected in the CSF or serum by latex agglutination or enzyme immunoassay methods.

Antigen detection methods useful when culture negative

### Treatment

Amphotericin B (with or without flucytosine) or fluconazole is the usual treatment for systemic cryptococcal disease. Flucytosine use alone is limited by development of resistance during therapy. Although three fourths of cases of meningitis respond to treatment, a significant portion suffer relapses after antifungal therapy is stopped; many become chronic and require repeated courses of therapy. One half of those cured have some kind of residual neurologic damage.

Amphotericin plus flucytosine; fluconazole usual antifungals

## HISTOPLASMA

## ■ Histoplasma capsulatum

*Histoplasma capsulatum* is a dimorphic fungus that grows in the yeast phase in tissue (Fig 48–2) and in cultures incubated at 37°C. The mold phase grows in cultures incubated at 22 to 25°C and as a saprophyte in soil. The yeast forms are small for fungi (2 to 4 μm) and reproduce by budding (blastoconidia). The mycelia are septate and produce microconidia and macroconidia. The diagnostic structure is termed the **tuberculate macroconidium** because of its thick wall and radial, fingerlike projections (see Fig 48–2). Growth is obtained on blood agar, chocolate agar, and Sabouraud's agar, but may take many weeks. As with *C. neoformans,* a sexual stage has now been discovered (*Ajelomyces capsulatum*), but the asexual name continues to be used in the medical literature. The designation *H. capsulatum* is actually a misnomer, because no capsules are formed: the unstained areas seen around the yeasts in tissue sections (see Fig 48–2) are artifacts of the staining and fixation procedures.

Small dimorphic fungus producing tuberculate macroconidia

Growth may take weeks

### Dimorphism

The morphologic and physiologic events associated with conversion from the mold to the yeast phase of *H. capsulatum* have been extensively studied. They are understandably com-

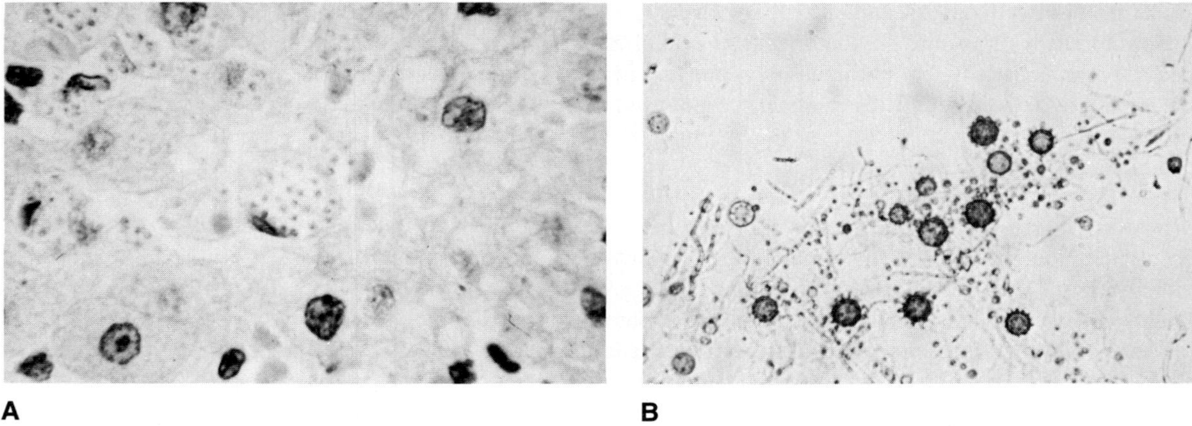

**Figure 48–2.** *Histoplasma capsulatum.* **A.** Multiple organisms are present within macrophages in the liver. **B.** The mold is shown with characteristic tuberculate macroconidia. (*Reprinted with permission from Dr. E. S. Beneke and the Upjohn Company: Scope Publications, Human Mycoses.*)

Shift from mold to yeast begins with heat shock response

Metabolic shift toward sulfhydryl compounds

Dimorphism is reversible and linked to virulence

plex given the dramatic change of milieu encountered by the fungus when its mold conidia float from their soil habitat to the pulmonary alveoli. Conversion to the yeast phase is then triggered by the host temperature (37°C) and possibly by other aspects of the new environment. In vitro studies show that the earliest events in this shift from the mold to yeast form involve induction of the heat shock response and uncoupling of oxidative phosphorylation. These are followed by a shutdown of RNA synthesis, protein synthesis, and respiratory metabolism. The cells then pass through a metabolically inactive state, emerging with enhanced enzymatic capacities involving sulfhydryl compounds (cysteine, cystine, etc) which are exclusive to the yeast stage. In the yeast stage there is recovery of mitochondrial activity and synthetic capacity but a new constellation of oxidases, polymerases, proteins, cell wall glucans, and other compounds are present.

Dimorphism in fungi is reversible, a feature that distinguishes it from developmental processes such as embryogenesis seen in higher eukaryotes. The importance of the conversion to virulence of *Histoplasma* is shown by animal studies using strains biochemically blocked from converting to the yeast phase. They neither produce disease nor persist in the host. To the extent known, these features are similar in the other dimorphic fungi.

## Histoplasmosis

### Epidemiology

Humid environmental sources, bird droppings

High prevalence in central United States

Point source outbreaks from bird roosts and bat caves

*Histoplasma capsulatum* grows in soil under humid climatic conditions, particularly soil containing bird or bat droppings. The organism has a worldwide distribution, but is particularly prevalent in certain temperate, subtropical, and tropical zones. In the United States the greatest concentration by far is in the areas drained by the Ohio and Mississippi Rivers. More than 50% of residents of states in this area show skin test evidence of previous infection. Disturbances of bird roosts, bat caves, and soil have been associated with point source outbreaks. The infection is not transmitted from person to person.

### Pathogenesis and Immunity

Reticuloendothelial system infection

Intracellular growth in macrophages

Primary lesion similar to tuberculosis

The hallmark of histoplasmosis is infection of the reticuloendothelial system with intracellular growth in phagocytic macrophages. The initial infection is pulmonary, through inhalation of infectious conidia, which convert to the yeast form in the host. They are readily phagocytosed by macrophages where they multiply in the cytoplasm, surviving the combined effects of the oxidative burst and phagolysosomal fusion.

With continued growth there is lymphatic spread and development of a primary lesion similar to that seen in tuberculosis (see Chapter 27). The extent of spread to the reticuloendothelial system within macrophages during primary infection is unknown, but such spread is presumed to occur and account for the distribution of lesions in disseminated disease; however, the vast majority of cases never advance beyond the primary stage, leaving only a calcified node as evidence of infection. Old lesions may reactivate in a small proportion of cases.

Pathologically, granulomatous inflammation with necrosis is prominent in pulmonary lesions, but *H. capsulatum* may be difficult to find even with special fungal stains. Extrapulmonary spread involves the reticuloendothelial system, with enlargement of the liver and spleen. Numerous organisms within macrophages may be found in these organs, in lymph nodes, or in bone marrow (see Fig 48–2).

Granulomatous response in liver, spleen, bone marrow

Infection with *H. capsulatum* is associated with the development of cell-mediated immunity as demonstrated by a positive delayed hypersensitivity skin test to a mycelial antigen called **histoplasmin.** Infection is believed to confer long-lasting immunity, the most important component of which is T lymphocyte mediated. In experimental infections, macrophages activated by T lymphocyte-derived cytokines are able to inhibit intracellular growth of *H. capsulatum* and thus control the disease. Immunocompromised persons, particularly those with T lymphocyte-related defects, are unable to stop growth of the organism and tend to develop progressive, disseminated disease.

Histoplasmin skin test demonstrates delayed hypersensitivity

Long-lasting Immunity derived from T cell activation of macrophages

## Histoplasmosis: Clinical Aspects

### Clinical Manifestations

Most cases of *H. capsulatum* infection are asymptomatic or show only fever and cough for a few days or weeks. Mediastinal lymphadenopathy and slight pulmonary infiltrates may be seen on x-rays. The histoplasmin skin test becomes positive after about 3 weeks. More severe cases may have chills, malaise, chest pain, and more extensive infiltrates, which usually resolve nonetheless. A residual nodule may continue to enlarge over a period of years, causing a differential diagnostic problem with pulmonary neoplasms. Progressive pulmonary disease occurs in a form similar to that of pulmonary tuberculosis, including the development of cavities, with sputum production, night sweats, and weight loss. The course is chronic and relapsing, lasting many months to years.

Primary infection lasts days to weeks

Progressive pulmonary disease similar to tuberculosis

Disseminated histoplasmosis generally appears as a febrile illness with enlargement of reticuloendothelial organs. The central nervous system, skin, gastrointestinal tract, and adrenal glands may also be involved. Painless ulcers on mucous membranes are a common finding. The course is typically chronic, with manifestations that depend on the organs involved. For example, chronic bilateral adrenal failure (Addison's disease) may develop when the adrenal glands are involved.

Disseminated histoplasmosis involves multiple organs

Mucous membrane ulcers common

### Diagnosis

In most forms of pulmonary histoplasmosis, the diagnostic yield of direct examinations or culture of sputum is low. In disseminated disease, blood culture or biopsy samples of a reticuloendothelial organ are the most likely to contain *Histoplasma*. Bone marrow culture has the highest yield. Because of their small size, the yeast cells are difficult to see in KOH preparations, and their morphology is not sufficiently distinctive to be diagnostic. Selective fungal stains such as methenamine silver demonstrate the organism, but may not differentiate it from other yeasts. Hematoxylin and eosin-stained tissue or Wright-stained bone marrow often demonstrates the organisms in their intracellular location in macrophages (see Fig 48–2). Specimens must be examined carefully under high magnification (100×, oil immersion). Identification of culture isolates requires demonstration of the typical conidia and dimorphism. Demonstration of specific mycelial antigens by immunodiffusion (exoantigen test) may be used in place of dimorphism demonstration. Nucleic acid probes have been developed for culture identification but are not yet in wide use.

Direct examination of sputum rarely helpful

Histological examination of bone marrow or affected organs requires special stains

Exoantigen test useful

Serologic tests have been developed using histoplasmin or yeast cell antigens. Antibodies can be detected by immunodiffusion or complement fixation. In histoplasmosis, complement fixation titers typically rise to 1:32 or greater, but false-negative results are common in all clinical forms of the disease. False-positive findings also occur, particularly in patients with blastomycosis. The histoplasmin skin test is useful only for epidemiologic studies. Cultural isolation or clear histologic demonstration is necessary for a firm diagnosis. A circulating polysaccharide antigen has been demonstrated by radioimmunoassay in more than 90% of patients with disseminated disease, but the test is not yet commercially available.

Culture required for firm diagnosis

### Treatment

Amphotericin B followed by azole

Amphotericin B has long been the treatment of choice for histoplasmosis. Its toxicity, however, limits its use to cases of extensive disease, such as progressive pulmonary disease and disseminated histoplasmosis. Ketoconazole, fluconazole, and itraconazole are active in vitro and produce clinical improvement but often not cure. Amphotericin B remains the most effective treatment but may be followed with a course of one of the azoles. The latter is required as ongoing suppressive treatment for AIDS patients with histoplasmosis. Primary infections and localized lung lesions usually require no treatment.

# BLASTOMYCES

## Blastomyces dermatitidis

Dimorphic fungus

Large yeast cells have broad-based buds

*Blastomyces dermatitidis* is a dimorphic fungus with some characteristics similar to those of *Histoplasma*. Growth develops in the yeast phase in tissues and in cultures incubated at 37°C. The yeast cells are typically larger (8–15 μm) than those of *H. capsulatum*, with broad-based buds and a thick wall (Fig 48–3). A smaller variant with morphologic characteristics like those of *Histoplasma* is occasionally seen. The mold phase appears in culture at 25°C. Hyphae are septate and produce round to oval conidia sufficiently similar to those produced by *H. capsulatum* to cause confusion between the two in young cultures. Although older cultures may produce chlamydoconidia, *B. dermatitidis* produces no structure as distinctive as the tuberculate macroconidium of *Histoplasma*.

## Blastomycosis

### Epidemiology

Geography similar to *Histoplasma*

Cases of blastomycosis follow a geographic distribution similar to that of histoplasmosis. Most infections occur in the middle and eastern portions of North America, but cases have been reported in South America and Africa. Again, the lack of a specific skin test limits study of the endemic area.

### Pathogenesis and Immunity

Little direct study

Much less is known about blastomycosis than the more common systemic mycoses, such as histoplasmosis and coccidioidomycosis. The lower frequency of disseminated infections and the nonspecificity of skin and serologic tests are partly responsible for this lack of information. Much of what is believed to be true of blastomycosis is based on analogy with histoplasmosis.

The primary infection is pulmonary after inhalation of conidia, which develop in soil. A mixed inflammatory response results, which ranges from neutrophil infiltration to well-organized granulomas with giant cells. The organisms appear as large yeast cells, most of

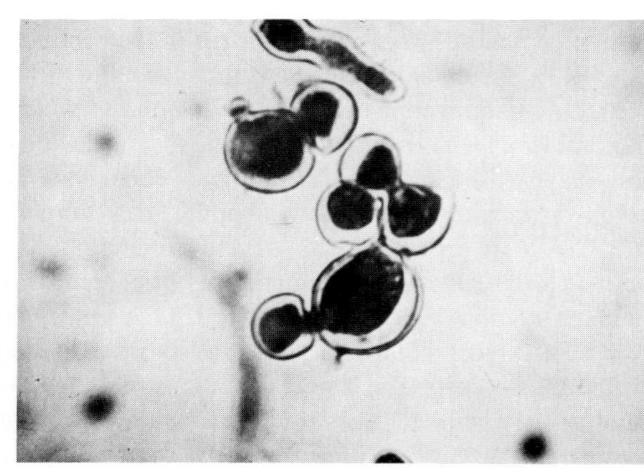

**Figure 48–3.** *Blastomyces dermatitidis.* Large thick-walled yeast are shown. Blastoconidia retain a broad attachment to the mother cell before separating. (*Reprinted with permission from Dr. E. S. Beneke and the Upjohn Company: Scope Publications, Human Mycoses.*)

which still have blastospores attached. They appear to have a double wall in hematoxylin- and eosin-stained sections because of shrinkage of the cytoplasm and dense staining of its periphery. A significant difference from *Histoplasma* is that the yeast cells are primarily extracellular rather than within macrophages. This may be due to their relatively large size, but there is little to suggest that *B. dermatitidis* shares the propensity for intracellular parasitism that is characteristic of *H. capsulatum*. The organism can spread to the skin and less often to bone and viscera. Considerable necrosis and fibrosis can lead to large, expanding lesions at infected sites.

Yeast cells primarily outside cells

Antigenic cross-reactivity with other fungi has greatly hampered the study of immunity to this organism. A number of clinical and experimental observations indicate that as with other fungi, T lymphocyte-mediated responses are the most important determinant of immunity. Macrophages activated with cytokines have enhanced capacity to kill *B. dermatitidis*.

## Blastomycosis: Clinical Aspects

### Clinical Manifestations

As mild cases are difficult to diagnose, most infections are recognized at advanced or disseminated stages of the disease. This problem was also posed by the other systemic mycoses before the development of sensitive and specific diagnostic procedures.

Pulmonary infection is evidenced by cough, sputum production, chest pain, and fever. Hilar lymphadenopathy may be present, as may nodular pulmonary infiltrates with alveolar consolidation. The total picture may mimic a pulmonary tumor, tuberculosis, or some other mycosis. Skin lesions are common and were once considered a primary form of the disease. In contrast to those in histoplasmosis, lesions develop on exposed skin; mucous membrane infection is uncommon. Extensive necrosis and fibrosis may produce considerable disfigurement. Bone infection has features similar to those of other causes of chronic osteomyelitis. The urinary and genital tracts are the most commonly affected visceral sites; the prostate is especially prone to infection.

Pulmonary blastomycosis like other mycoses

Skin lesions on exposed surfaces

### Diagnosis

Direct demonstration of typical large yeasts with broad-based buds (blastoconidia) in KOH preparations is the most rapid means of diagnosis. Biopsy specimens also have a high yield, and the organisms are visible with either hematoxylin and eosin or special fungal stains. *Blastomyces dermatitidis* grows on routine mycologic media, but culture may take as long as 4 weeks. Conidia are not particularly distinctive, and demonstration of dimorphism and typical yeast morphology is essential to avoid confusion with other fungi. The exoantigen test from mycelial-phase cultures is particularly useful in differentiation from *Histoplasma*.

Direct KOH and biopsy often diagnostic

Culture on routine media but slow

Exoantigen test particularly useful

Antigens for immunodiffusion and complement fixation serologic tests are available but lack sensitivity. They may be negative in up to 50% of cases. Skin tests have no value.

### Treatment

Although amphotericin B is the preferred therapy, it is used only for progressive or disseminated disease. As with other systemic mycoses, response to treatment is slow, and relapse is common. Ketoconazole has been effective in nonmeningeal cases, and fluconazole and itraconazole also show promise.

Amphotericin B preferred if disseminated

# COCCIDIOIDES

## Coccidioides immitis

*Coccidioides immitis* is also a dimorphic fungus, but instead of a yeast phase, a large (12- to 100-μm), distinctive, round-walled spherule (Fig 48–4) is produced in the invasive tissue form. This structure is unique among the pathogenic fungi. Its formation requires simultaneous invagination of the fungal membrane (plasmalemma) and production of new

Dimorphism involves unique spherule

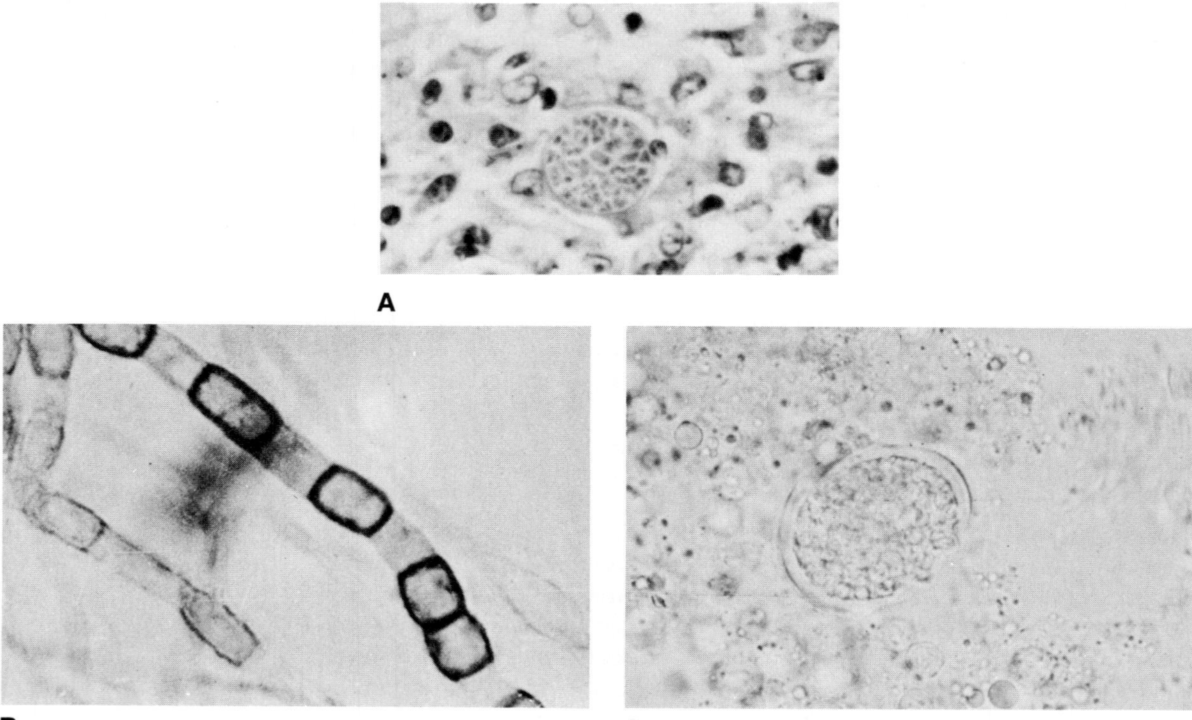


**Figure 48–4.** *Coccidioides immitis.* **A.** Tissue with thick-walled spherule containing multiple endospores. **B.** Mold phase with septate hyphae and arthroconidia. **C.** KOH preparation of sputum showing thick-walled spherule, which has just burst. (*Reprinted with permission from Dr. E. S. Beneke and the Upjohn Company: Scope Publications, Human Mycoses.*)

Spherules differentiate to form and release endospores

Mold arthroconidia form are highly infectious

cell wall to form the large multicompartmental structure. The compartments differentiate into uninucleate structures called **endospores,** each with a thin wall layer. Multiple endospores develop within each spherule and are released when the spherule ruptures. They serve as the reproductive unit in vivo. On routine culture, *C. immitis* grows only as a mold at room temperature and 37°C. Growth becomes visible in 2 to 5 days. The hyphae are septate and produce thick-walled, barrel-shaped arthroconidia (see Fig 48–4), which are the infectious unit in nature and highly infectious when they develop in the laboratory. Spherules have been produced from arthroconidia in vitro under specialized conditions.

## Coccidioidomycosis

### Epidemiology

Geography restricted to Sonoran desert

Coccidioidomycosis is the most geographically restricted of the systemic mycoses, because *C. immitis* grows only in the semiarid climates known as the Lower Sonoran life zone. These areas are characterized by hot, dry summers, mild winters with few freezes, and annual rainfall of about 10 in. during brief rainy seasons. Areas with these conditions are found scattered throughout the Americas, some as ecologic "islands." The primary endemic zones in the United States are in Arizona, Nevada, New Mexico, western Texas, and the arid parts of central and southern California. Persons living in the endemic areas are at high risk of infection, although disease is much less common. Positive skin test rates of 50 to 90% occur in longtime residents of highly endemic areas. Coccidioidomycosis is not transmissible from person to person.

Dust-borne Spread to distant areas by dust storms

Infection cannot be acquired without at least visiting an endemic area, although some interesting examples of the endemic zone itself paying a visit have been recorded. One such anecdote involves a gas station attendant with coccidioidomycosis whose only contact with an endemic area was changing a flat tire on a truck from California. In 1978, a storm originating in Bakersfield (endemic zone) carried a thick coat of dust and cases of coccidioidomycosis all the way to San Francisco. In 1992, a tenfold increase in disease in California followed an unusually wet winter with just the right drought–rain–drought pattern for growth of the mold. When the Sonoran desert blooms the arthroconidium crop is not far behind.

Climate can influence exposure

## Pathogenesis

Inhaled arthroconidia resist phagocytosis

Growing spherules produce endospores

Endospores stimulate acute inflammatory responses

Inhaled arthroconidia are small enough (2 to 6 μm) to bypass the defenses of the upper tracheobronchial tree and lodge in the alveoli. Human monocytes can ingest and kill some arthroconida on initial exposure, although the outer portion of the wall of the arthroconidium has antiphagocytic properties, which persist in the early stages of spherule development. Surviving arthroconidia convert to the spherule stage, which begins its slow growth, stimulating a macrophage and neutrophilic cellular response. As the spherule grows, its size makes effective phagocytosis difficult, although neutrophils are able to digest the wall. Later, as the spherules enlarge and multiply, the overall inflammatory response is granulomatous with some giant cells. Rupture of spherules with release of hundreds of endospores (Fig 48–5) stimulates an acute inflammatory response, which has an uncertain effect. The young endospores are released in packets with a surrounding matrix derived from the spherule, which may further protect them from destruction by the host. They then develop into new spherules.

Development of immunity and hypersensitivity associated with resolution

Enzymes have uncertain role

In most cases, this mixed inflammatory response is associated with early resolution of the infection and development of a positive delayed hypersensitivity skin test. In a few cases, the infection is not controlled. These infections may progress to a chronic pulmonary form of the disease or become disseminated to other organs. The mechanism for dissemination is not precisely known, although an elastase and a protease have been identified in spherule/endospore lysates that could aid in spherule rupture, with escape of endospores to distant sites. In animals, suppression of cellular immunity is associated with more progressive disease, and dissemination in humans is accompanied by skin test anergy.

## Immunity

PMN response and Cell-mediated immunity

Immunity to coccidioidomycosis is associated with strong polymorphonuclear leukocyte- and T lymphocyte-mediated responses to coccidioidal antigens. Progressive disease is associated with weak or absent cellular immunity. The central event appears to be the reaction

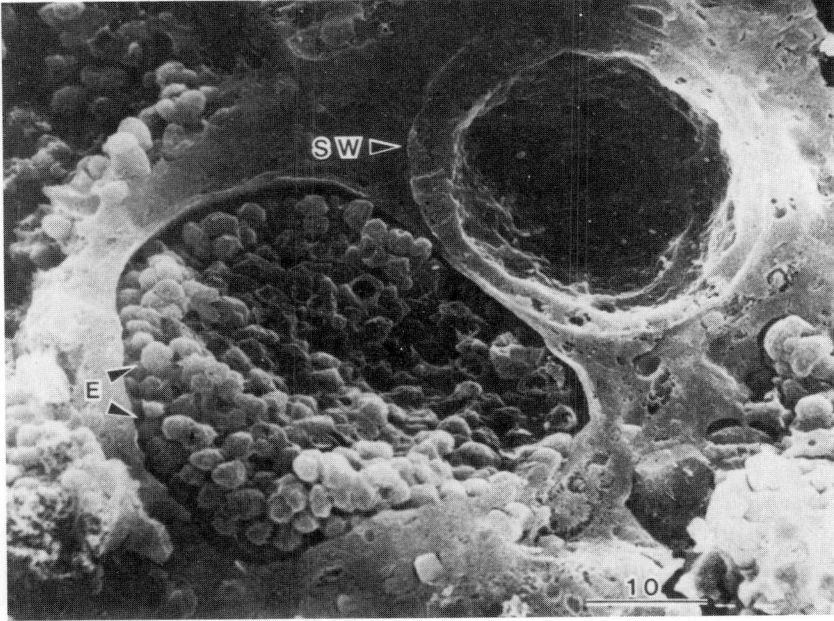


**Figure 48–5.** *Coccidioides immitis.* This electron micrograph of infected mouse lung shows a spherule filled with endospores (E) and one that has discharged its endospores into the surrounding tissue. Note the thickness of the spherule wall (SW). (*Reprinted with permission from Drutz DJ, Huppert M.* J Infect Dis. *1983;147:379, Figure 7. Copyright University of Chicago Publisher.*)

Endospores destroyed by cytokine activated macrophages

to arthroconidia or to endospores released from ruptured spherules. Arthroconidia can be phagocytosed and killed by polymorphonuclear leukocytes even before an immune response is mounted. The handling of endospores requires the additional participation of macrophages which do not become maximally effective until activated by T lymphocyte-derived cytokines. Prior to this, *C. immitis* endospores may be able to impair phagosome–lysosome fusion in the phagocyte.

Progressive disease with AIDS defects in cell-mediated immunity

In most infected persons the infection is controlled after mild or inapparent illness. The disease progresses if cell-mediated immunity and consequent macrophage activation do not develop. Such immune deficits may be a result of disease (AIDS) or immunosuppressive therapy, but may occur in patients with no other known cellular immune compromise.

Antibody production inversely related to disease progress

Antibody is not known to play any role in immunity. In fact, the presence and level of complement-fixing antibody are inversely related to the progress of disease. Persons with strong T lymphocyte responses to *C. immitis* have little if any detectable antibody to the organisms. Those with disseminated disease and absent cellular immunity have high titers of antibody.

## Coccidioidomycosis: Clinical Aspects

### Clinical Manifestations

Primary infection (valley fever) is usually asymptomatic and self-limiting

Erythema nodosum common in women

More than one half of those infected with *C. immitis* suffer no symptoms, or the disease is so mild that it cannot be recalled when skin test conversion is discovered. Others develop malaise, cough, chest pain, fever, and arthralgia 1 to 3 weeks after infection. This disease, which lasts 2 to 6 weeks, is known as **valley fever** by the local populations in the United States. Objective findings are few. The chest x-ray is usually clear or shows only hilar adenopathy. Erythema nodosum may develop midway through the course, particularly in women. In most cases, resolution is spontaneous, but only after considerable discomfort and loss of productivity. In more than 90% of cases, there are no pulmonary residua. A small number of cases progress to a chronic pulmonary form characterized by cavity formation and a slow relapsing course that extends over years. Less than 1% of all primary infections disseminate to foci outside the lung.

Chronic and disseminated disease less than 1%

Dissemination has racial, immune status risk factors

Disseminated disease is more common in men; in dark-skinned races, particularly Filipinos; and in AIDS patients and other immunosuppressed persons. Evidence of extrapulmonary infection almost always appears in the first year after infection. The most common sites are bones, joints, skin, and meninges. Coccidioidal meningitis develops slowly with gradually increasing headache, fever, neck stiffness, and other signs of meningeal irritation. The cerebrospinal fluid findings are similar to those in tuberculosis and other fungal causes of meningitis, such as *C. neoformans*. Mononuclear cells predominate in the cell count, but substantial numbers of neutrophils are often present. If untreated, the disease is slowly progressive and fatal.

Meningitis is chronic

### Diagnosis

Direct examination for spherules diagnostic

With enough persistence, direct examinations are usually rewarding. The thick-walled spherules are so large and characteristic (see Figs 48–4A and C) that they are difficult to miss in a KOH preparation. Skin and visceral lesions are most likely to be positive, cerebrospinal fluid least likely. Spherules released into expectorated sputum are often small (10–15 μm) and immature without well-developed endospores. Spherules stain well in histologic sections with either hematoxylin and eosin or the special fungal stains.

Culture usually positive except from CSF

Substantial risk of laboratory infection with arthrospores

Exoantigen for final identification

Culture of *C. immitis* from sputum, visceral lesions, or skin lesions is not difficult, but must be undertaken only by those with experience and proper biohazard protection. Cultures from cerebrospinal fluid are rarely positive. Laboratories must be warned of the possibility of coccidioidomycosis to ensure diagnosis and avoid inadvertent laboratory infection. The latter is particularly significant outside the endemic areas, where routine precautions may not be in place. Identification requires observation of typical arthroconidia and demonstration of mycelial antigens using the exoantigen test.

Skin and serologic tests very useful

Skin and serologic tests are very useful in diagnosis and management of coccidioidomycosis. The coccidioidin skin test usually becomes positive 1 to 4 weeks after the onset of symptoms of primary infection and remains so for life. Disseminated disease is frequently associated with anergy, particularly when it is severe. One half to three quarters of patients with primary infection develop serum IgM precipitating antibody in the first 3 weeks of illness. These conditions persist for 2 to 4 months. IgG antibodies detected by complement fixation tests appear somewhat later in symptomatic infections. The amount and duration depend on the extent of disease. Antibodies disappear with resolution and persist with continuing infection. The height of the complement fixation titer is a measure of the magnitude of antigenic stimulation and, thus, of the extent of disease. The presence of complement-fixing antibody in the cerebrospinal fluid is also important in the diagnosis of coccidioidal meningitis, because cultures are usually negative. Precipitating and complement-fixing antibodies may be detected by classic methods or by more recently developed immunodiffusion procedures.

IgM persists a few months

IgG antibodies a measure of antigenic stimulation

### Treatment

Primary coccidioidomycosis is self-limiting, and no antifungal therapy is indicated. Progressive pulmonary disease and disseminated disease require the use of antifungal agents, usually amphotericin B. Ketoconazole has proved effective but relapses are common. Fluconazole and itraconazole are active against *C. immitis* but need further study. With the exception of fluconazole, none of these agents have significant penetration into the central nervous system. Amphotericin B is commonly given directly into the cerebrospinal fluid for the treatment of *C. immitis* meningitis.

Amphotericin B in progressive disease

## PARACOCCIDIOIDES BRASILIENSIS

*Paracoccidioides brasiliensis* is the cause of paracoccidioidomycosis (South American blastomycosis), a disease limited to tropical and subtropical areas of Central and South America. The organism is a dimorphic fungus, the most noteworthy feature of which is the production of multiple blastoconidia from the same cell. Characteristic 5- to 40-μm cells covered with budding blastoconidia may be seen in tissue or in yeast-phase growth at 37°C. The disease manifests primarily as chronic mucocutaneous or cutaneous ulcers. The ulcers spread slowly and develop a granulomatous mulberry-like base. Regional lymph nodes, reticuloendothelial organs, and the lungs may also be involved. Little is known of the pathogenesis of the disease, although the route of infection is believed to be inhalation. Progression in experimental animals is associated with depressed T lymphocyte-mediated immune responses. The disease has a striking predilection for men despite skin test evidence that subclinical cases occur at the same rate in both sexes. This may be related to the experimental observation that estrogens but not androgens inhibit conversion of mold-phase conidia to the yeast phase. Treatment is with sulfonamides, amphotericin B, and, more recently, the azole compounds.

Produces multiple blastoconidia

Strong predilection for men

## ADDITIONAL READING

Ampel NM, Wieden MA, Galgiani JN. Coccidioidomycosis: Clinical update. *Rev Infect Dis*. 1989;11:897–911. This review remains current on all clinical, diagnostic, and treatment aspects with the exception of experience with post-ketoconazole azoles.

Levitz SM. The ecology of *Cryptococcus neoformans* and epidemiology of cryptococcosis. *Rev Infect Dis*. 1990;13:1163–1169. This brief review provides a nice discussion of the links between the soil habitat and human infection.

Maresca B, Kobayashi GS. Dimorphism in *Histoplasma capsulatum*: A model for the study of cell differentiation in pathogenic fungi. *Microbiol Rev*. 1989;53:186–209. A scholarly account of the biology of one of the best studied fungal pathogens.

Smith CE, Saito MT, Simons SA. Pattern of 39,500 serologic tests in coccidioidomycosis. *JAMA*. 1956; 160:546–552. This study is the basis for the unique application of serologic tests to the diagnosis and prognosis of coccidioidomycosis.

# Subcutaneous Fungal Pathogens

*Kenneth J. Ryan*

Assignment of fungal organisms to the category of subcutaneous fungi is somewhat arbitrary, because fungal pathogens can produce many subcutaneous manifestations as part of their disease spectrum. Those considered here are introduced traumatically through the skin and involve mainly subcutaneous tissues, lymphatic vessels, and contiguous tissues. They rarely spread to distant organs. The diseases they cause include sporotrichosis, chromoblastomycosis, and mycetoma. Only sporotrichosis has a single specific etiologic agent, *Sporothrix schenckii*. Chromoblastomycosis and mycetoma are clinical syndromes with multiple fungal etiologies (Table 49–1).

## SPOROTHRIX

### Sporothrix schenckii

*Sporothrix schenckii* is a dimorphic fungus that grows as a cigar-shaped, 3- to 5-μm yeast (Fig 49–1) in tissues and in culture at 37°C. The mold, which grows in culture at 25°C, is presumably the infectious form in nature. The hyphae are thin and septate, producing clusters of conidia at the end of delicate conidiophores (see Figure 49–1B).

Dimorphic, cigar-shaped yeast at 37°C

### Sporotrichosis

#### Epidemiology

*Sporothrix schenckii* is a ubiquitous saprophyte found in soil, in decaying organic matter, and on the surfaces of various plants. Infection is acquired by traumatic inoculation through the skin of material containing the organism. Exposure is largely occupational or related to hobbies. The skin of gardeners, farmers, and rural laborers is frequently traumatized by thorns or other material that may be contaminated with conidia of *S. schenckii*. An unusual outbreak of sporotrichosis involving nearly 3000 miners was traced to *S. schenckii* in the timbers used to support mine shafts. A 1988 outbreak covered 15 states and was traced to sphagnum moss. Infection is occasionally acquired by direct contact with infected pus or through the respiratory tract; these modes of infection, however, are much less common than the cutaneous route.

Soil saprophyte introduced by trauma

Occupational disease of gardeners, farmers, etc.

Outbreaks from raw products

#### Pathology

Local multiplication of the organism stimulates both acute pyogenic and granulomatous inflammatory reactions. The infection spreads along lymphatic drainage routes and

Pyogenic and granulomatous lesions

**TABLE 49–1. AGENTS OF SUBCUTANEOUS MYCOSES**

| Organism | Disease | Growth | | |
|---|---|---|---|---|
| | | **Tissue** | **Culture at 25°C** | **Culture at 37°C** |
| *Sporothrix schenkii* | Sporotrichosis | Yeast (rare) | Mold | Yeast |
| *Phialophora* | Chromoblastomycosis, mycetoma | Mycelia[a] | Mold | Mold |
| *Cladosporium* | Chromoblastomycosis | Mycelia[a] | Mold | Mold |
| *Petriellidium* | Mycetoma | Mycelia | Mold | Mold |

[a] Pigmented, often blunted to form round to oval bodies.

reproduces the original inflammatory lesions at intervals. The organisms are scanty in human lesions.

## Sporotrichosis: Clinical Aspects

### Clinical Manifestations

Skin papule eventually ulcerates

Lymphatic involvement yields multiple lesions

Infection rare at other sites

A skin lesion begins as a painless papule that develops a few weeks to a few months after inoculation. Its location can usually be explained by occupational exposure; the hand is most often involved. The papule enlarges slowly and eventually ulcerates, leaving an open sore. Draining lymph channels are usually thickened, and pustular or firm nodular lesions may appear around the primary site of infection or at other sites along the lymphatic drainage route. Once ulcerated, lesions usually become chronic. Multiple ulcers often develop if the disease is untreated. Symptoms are those directly related to the local areas of infection. Constitutional signs and symptoms are unusual.

Occasionally, spread occurs by other routes. The bones, eyes, lungs, and central nervous system are susceptible to progressive infection if the organisms reach these organs; such spread, however, occurs in less than 1% of all cases. Primary pulmonary sporotrichosis occurs but is also rare.

### Diagnosis

Direct examination usually negative due to small numbers of fungi

Grows readily in culture

Direct microscopic examination for *S. schenckii* is usually unrewarding because there are too few organisms to detect readily with potassium hydroxide preparations. Even specially stained biopsy samples and serial sections are usually negative, although the presence of a histopathologic structure, the asteroid body, is considered diagnostic. This structure is composed of *S. schenckii* yeast cells surrounded by amorphous eosinophilic "rays."

Definitive diagnosis depends on culture of infected pus or tissue. The organism grows within 2 to 5 days on all media commonly used in medical mycology. Identification requires demonstration of the typical conidia and of dimorphism (see Fig 49–1).

### Treatment and Prevention

Potassium iodide for cutaneous, amphetericin B or azoles for systemic

Cutaneous sporotrichosis is effectively treated with potassium iodide administered orally. Systemic infections require the use of amphotericin B. Clinical experience with itraconazole has been excellent, and it may become the treatment of choice for all but cutaneous sporotrichosis. Eradication of the environmental reservoir of *S. schenckii* is not usually practical, although the mine outbreak mentioned previously was stopped by applying antifungal agents to the mine shaft timbers.

## CHROMOBLASTOMYCOSIS

Tropical disease with multiple fungal etiologies

Wartlike, pigmented lesions

Chromoblastomycosis is primarily a tropical disease caused by multiple species of two genera of fungi, *Phialophora* and *Cladosporium*. The disease occurs typically on the foot or leg. It appears as papules that develop into scaly, wartlike structures, usually under the feet. Fully developed lesions have been likened to the tips of a cauliflower. Extension is by satel-

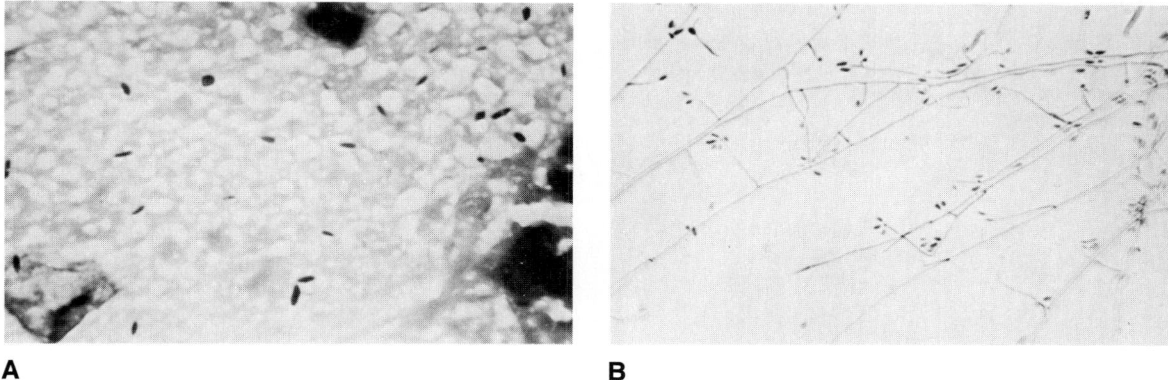


**Figure 49–1.** *Sporothrix schenckii.* **A.** The yeast form of *S. schenckii* is typically cigar-shaped but is rarely seen in human lesions. This smear is from infected mouse testis. **B.** Mold-phase cultures develop delicate hyphae and conidiophores bearing fingerlike clusters of conidia. (*Reprinted with permission from Dr. E. S. Beneke and the Upjohn Company: Scope Publications, Human Mycoses.*)

lite lesions; it is slow and painless and does not involve the lymphatic vessels. The organisms are found in the soil of endemic areas, and most infections occur in those who work barefoot.

The outstanding mycologic feature is the presence of brown-pigmented hyphae on direct examination or in culture. Branching septate hyphae, which are often blunted, can be demonstrated in KOH preparations of scrapings or in histologic sections. Cultures grow as molds, but may take weeks to appear and longer for demonstration of characteristic conidia.

Brown pigmented hyphae may be seen on KOH

Surgery and antifungal therapy have been used in chromoblastomycosis, but results in advanced disease are disappointing. Flucytosine has been the antifungal agent most frequently used.

## MYCETOMA

Multiple etiologies following traumatic inoculation

Mycetoma is another unusual infection associated with trauma to the foot and inoculation of any of several fungal species. The most common species in nontropical areas is *Petriellidium boydii*. The usual clinical appearance is of massive induration with draining sinuses. Some of the fungi that cause mycetoma are geographically widespread; most cases, however, occur in the tropics, probably because the chronically damp, macerated skin of the feet that causes predisposition toward mycetoma occurs most often in the tropical environment. This finding is illustrated by the case of a college rower in Seattle who developed mycetoma; he was the only member of his shell who insisted on rowing barefoot. Once established, the treatment of mycetoma is difficult. No antimicrobic stands out as particularly helpful.

Induration and sinuses on feet

The precise microbiologic features depend on the agent involved. Hyphae are usually present in tissue, but may be difficult to demonstrate because of a tendency to form microcolonial granules, as in actinomycosis. *Petriellidium* grows relatively rapidly, but some of the other causes may take weeks for initial growth. Identification is by morphology of the asexual conidia.

Hyphae difficult to demonstrate due to microcolonial granules

Essentially the same disease can be caused by some branching bacteria of the genus *Nocardia* (see Chapter 28).

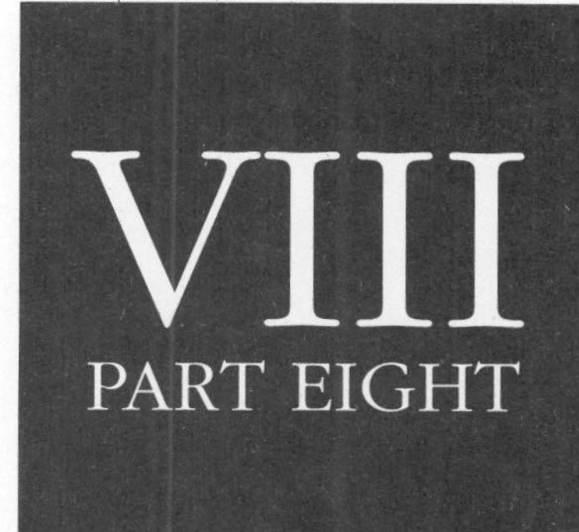


# Organisms of Uncertain Origin

# Pneumocystis carinii

James J. Plorde

Pneumocystosis is a highly lethal pneumonitis of immunocompromised patients and premature infants caused by *Pneumocystis carinii*, an organism of uncertain classification. It is now seen most frequently in patients undergoing cancer chemotherapy, organ transplant recipients receiving suppressive therapy, and patients with AIDS.

## PNEUMOCYSTIS CARINII

Originally thought protozoan

Although it was previously widely believed to be a protozoan, the taxonomic position of *P. carinii* remains unsettled. Recent studies have found similarities between the ribosomal RNA sequence of *Pneumocystis* and that of certain fungi. These sequences are highly conserved in nature, and this evidence supports its reclassification as a fungus; however, several morphologic features—the DNA content per cell, the absence of the highly conserved fungal protein elongation factor EF-3, and the organism's susceptibility to antiprotozoal, but not antifungal, chemotherapeutic agents—argue in favor of retaining its original classification. It is possible that *Pneumocystis* represents a unique evolutionary bridge between the fungi and protozoa. The organism exhibits cystic forms which are 5 to 8 μm in diameter and contain two to eight small sporozoites that are released with rupture of the cyst. These mature to pleomorphic organisms that have been termed **trophozoites.** They possess a single eccentric nucleus, a reticular cytoplasm, mitochondria, and a poorly developed cell membrane. These forms develop into the characteristic cysts. The method of replication is unknown; both sexual and asexual methods have been suggested.

Morphologic and molecular features suggest probable fungus

Cystic and noncystic forms described and named

All three forms can be demonstrated in tissue with phase or fluorescence microscopy. Methenamine silver, Gram–Weigert, and toluidine blue stains preferentially stain the cyst wall (Fig 50–1), whereas Giemsa, Wright, and Gram stains stain the sporozoite and trophozoite forms. In tissues, the cysts occur in clumps, and their walls are typically flattened at points of contact, presenting a characteristic honeycomb appearance. Organisms morphologically identical to the human parasite have been found in the lungs of several lower animals. Immunologic studies have revealed significant antigenic differences, suggesting the existence of separate strains or species.

*P. carinii* microscopic demonstration by silver and other stains

Limited in vitro cultivation, a necessary prerequisite to detailed study of any microbe, has been accomplished in a variety of cell culture lines for rodent strains of *P. carinii*. Human strains have not yet been grown.

Animal, but not human strains have been cultured

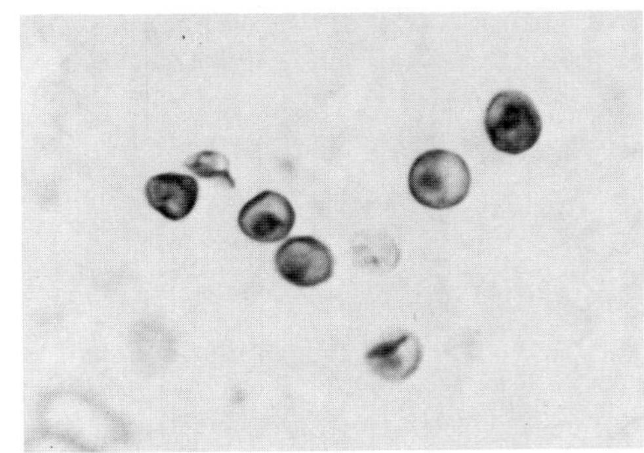

**Figure 50–1.** Cysts of *Pneumocytis carinii* in bronchial lavage fluid stained with methenamine silver.

# PNEUMOCYSTOSIS

## Epidemiology

Latent infection demonstrated in animals, possibly humans

Latent pulmonary infection occurs worldwide in a broad spectrum of animal life. Serologic and histologic evidence suggests a similar pattern in humans. Specific antibodies, detected by indirect immunofluorescence, are present in nearly all normal children by the age of 4, and autopsy studies have demonstrated organisms in the lung tissue of patients without clinical evidence of disease. Manifest illness, when it occurs, may appear in either an epidemic or a sporadic pattern.

Occasional epidemic infection in infants

Sporadic cases in immunocompromised hosts

Epidemics of pneumocystosis were first documented in Europe after World War II, when nursery outbreaks of interstitial pneumonia involving debilitated and premature infants were ultimately proved to be caused by *P. carinii*. Clinical and serologic data collected at that time suggested that the disease was contagious, possibly spreading from person to person via respiratory aerosols, a concept supported by later studies demonstrating airborne spread of the organism between animals. With economic recovery and improvement in infant nutrition, the epidemic form of disease disappeared from Europe; however, it continues to be reported occasionally from other parts of the world, most recently in orphanages in Southeast Asia. In contrast, cases in the United States have occurred sporadically among immunocompromised patients. In infants the disease is associated with congenital immunodeficiencies; in older children and adults, it has generally occurred as a complication of immunosuppressive therapy, particularly corticosteroid administration to patients with lymphoreticular malignancy, collagen vascular disease, or organ transplants.

AIDS by far the most frequent association of serious Pneumocystis infection

A leading cause of death in AIDS

In the last decade, AIDS has become the most common predisposing condition in the United States. Pneumocystosis is often the presenting manifestation of AIDS. In fact, prior to the development of effective chemoprophylactic regimens (see Treatment and Prevention), it was present in approximately half of all patients at the time of initial diagnosis. Eventually, at least 80% of AIDS patients developed one or more bouts of *P. carinii* pneumonitis, often in conjunction with another opportunistic infection, such as cytomegaloviral pneumonia. With a mortality rate of 30 to 50%, pneumocystosis was the leading cause of death in this patient population.

Unclear if latent, contagious, or both

It is generally believed that the sporadic cases in immunocompromised patients represent activation of latent infection; however, secondary cases in the families of some patients and the occasional clustering of cases in cancer wards suggest that this form of the disease may also be contagious.

## Pathogenesis and Pathology

Opportunistic pathogen

Predisposition when CD4+ T lymphocyte counts <200/mm$^3$

*Pneumocystis carinii* is evidently an organism of low virulence that seldom produces disease in a host with normal T lymphocyte function. In experimental animals, progressive infection can be initiated with starvation or corticosteroid administration, presumably by suppressing T lymphocyte function and allowing the activation of a latent infection. In AIDS patients the risk of developing pneumocystosis increases dramatically once the CD4$^+$ T lym-

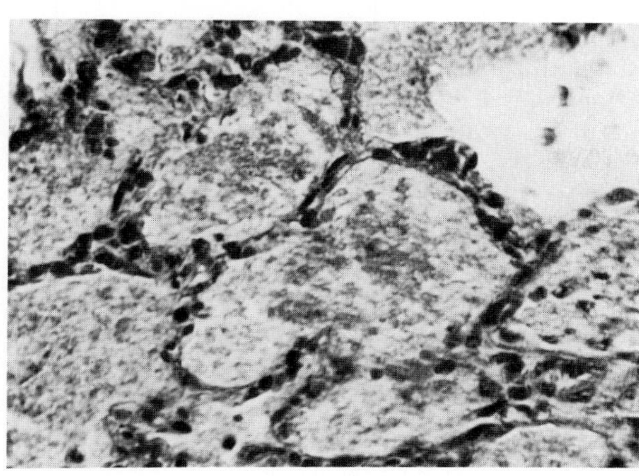

**Figure 50–2.** Lung biopsy specimen from *Pneumocystis carinii*-infected person, showing "foamy" contents of alveoli.

phocyte count has fallen to 200 cells/mm$^3$ or below. Concurrent viral, bacterial, fungal, and protozoan infections are found frequently in human cases, suggesting that *P. carinii* may require the presence of another microbial agent for its multiplication.

Histologically, latent infections are characterized by the presence of scattered, isolated cysts found in contact with one class of alveolar cells (type I pneumocytes). In clinically manifest disease, the alveoli are filled with desquamated alveolar cells, monocytes, organisms, and fluid, producing a distinctive foamy appearance (Fig 50–2); hyaline membranes may be present. Proliferation of type II pneumocytes is common and round cell infiltrates may be visible in the septa. Fibrosis, when present, is usually minimal. These changes are generally reversible with therapy, although calcification and persistent fibrosis have been documented occasionally. Lesions outside the lung were rarely seen prior to the AIDS epidemic, but are now seen with some regularity.

Pneumonia associated with foamy aveolar infiltrate

## PNEUMOCYSTOSIS: CLINICAL ASPECTS

### Clinical Manifestations

In the immunocompromised host, the disease presents as a progressive, diffuse pneumonitis. Illness may begin after discontinuation or a sudden decrease in the dose of corticosteroids or, in the case of acute lymphatic leukemia, during a period of remission. In infants and AIDS patients the onset is typically insidious, and the clinical course is 3 to 4 weeks in duration. Fever is mild or absent. In older individuals and patients who have previously been on high doses of corticosteroids, the onset is more abrupt, and the course is both febrile (38–40°C) and abbreviated. In both populations, the cardinal manifestations are progressive dyspnea and tachypnea; cyanosis and hypoxia eventually supervene. A nonproductive cough is present in one half of all patients. Clinical signs of pneumonia are usually absent, despite the presence of infiltrates on x-ray. These infiltrates are alveolar in character and spread out symmetrically from the hili, eventually affecting most of the lung. Occasionally, unilateral infiltrates, coin lesions, lobar infiltrates, cavitary lesions, or spontaneous pneumothoraces are observed. Pleural effusions are uncommon. Clinical and radiographic abnormalities are generally accompanied by a decrease in arterial oxygen saturation, diffusion capacity of the lung, and vital capacity. Death occurs by progressive asphyxia.

Progressive, diffuse pneumonitis

Progressive difficulty in breathing and hypoxia

### Diagnosis

Definite diagnosis depends on finding organisms of typical morphology in appropriate specimens. Although the organism has been found in sputum, tracheal aspirates, and gastric contents, the yield from such specimens is generally low. In AIDS patients, presumably because of the larger number of organisms present, sputum induced with hypertonic saline has been

Sputum rarely positive except in AIDS cases

Bronchial lavage and endobronchial biopsy have highest yield

reported to be positive in roughly half of all patients subsequently shown to have pneumocystosis. Bronchoalveolar lavage and transbronchial biopsies have been found more helpful, being positive in 90% of AIDS patients and 50% of those with other predisposing conditions. Percutaneous needle aspiration of the lung, needle biopsy, and open lung biopsy, although somewhat more sensitive techniques, are accompanied by more complications, including pneumothorax and hemothorax.

Immunofluorescence test recently available

Typical organisms can be visualized with any of the stains described earlier in the description of the organism. Recently, a commercial direct immunofluorescent stain using a monoclonal antibody to *P. carinii* has been shown to be equally useful. Although organism DNA can be detected in sputum and bronchoalveolar lavage specimens by polymerase chain reaction, the test is not currently available to clinical laboratories.

## Treatment and Prevention

Trimethoprim-sulfamethoxazole primary treatment

Patients with AIDS excepted, appropriate management of this disease can reduce mortality from 100 to 30%. Oxygen therapy must be administered to maintain adequate oxygenation. In some patients, mechanical ventilatory assistance may be required. Corticosteroid therapy appears to be helpful in patients with moderate to severe pneumonia. The organism is inhibited by trimethoprim–sulfamethoxazole, which should be given orally or intravenously for 14 days.

AIDS patients require longer treatment or pentamidine

Patients with AIDS respond more slowly to treatment, continue to excrete organisms after standard doses of trimethoprim–sulfamethoxazole, and suffer relapse more often. This necessitates administration for a minimum of 21 days. Unfortunately, those patients also have a high incidence of adverse effects to trimethoprim–sulfamethoxazole, frequently requiring its discontinuation and the completion of therapy with the equally effective but more toxic pentamidine. A number of secondary therapeutic regimens are available for patients who fail therapy with trimethoprim–sulfamethoxazole, pentamidine, or both.

It has recently been shown that long-term, low-dose administration of trimethoprim–sulfamethoxazole, dapsone, or atovaquone significantly decreases the incidence of *P. carinii* pneumonia in high-risk patients and prevents relapse in AIDS patients.

## ADDITIONAL READING

Bernard EM, Sepkowitz KA, Telzak EE, Armstrong D. Pneumocystosis. *Med Clin North Am.* 1992;76:107–119. A recent review on the medical management of AIDS patients with pneumocystosis.

Burke BA, Good RA. *Pneumocystis carinii* infection. *Medicine* (Baltimore). 1973;52:23–51. A classic review.

Mills J. *Pneumocystis carinii* and *Toxoplasma gondii* infections in patients with AIDS. *Rev Infect Dis.* 1986;8:1001–1011. A comprehensive review.

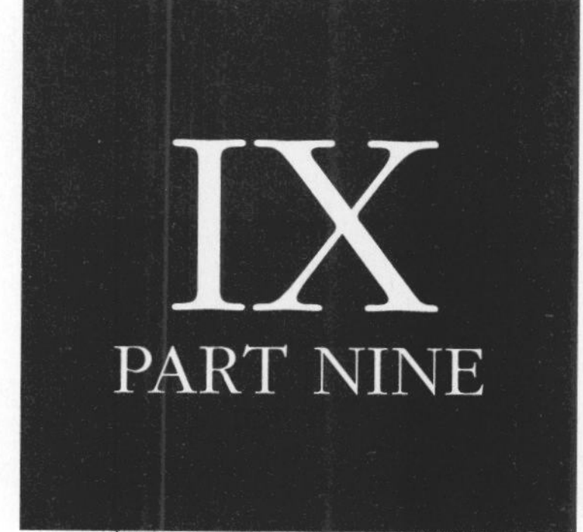


# Parasites

# Introduction to Pathogenic Parasites

## Pathogenesis and Chemotherapy of Parasitic Diseases

*James J. Plorde*

This chapter provides an overview of parasitic diseases and of antiparasitic therapy. The student may find it valuable to reread it after studying the subsequent chapters in this section.

## DEFINITION

Within the context of this section of the book, the term **parasite** refers to organisms belonging to one or two major taxonomic groups: protozoa and helminths. Protozoa are microscopic, single-celled eukaryotes superficially resembling yeasts in both size and simplicity. Helminths, in contrast, are macroscopic, multicellular worms possessing differentiated tissues and complex organ systems; they vary in length from a meter to less than a millimeter. The majority of both protozoa and helminths are free-living, play a significant role in the ecology of the planet, and seldom inconvenience the human race. The less common disease-producing species are typically obligate parasites, dependent on vertebrate hosts, arthropod hosts, or both for their survival. When their level of adaptation to a host is high, their presence typically produces little or no injury. Less complete adaptation leads to a more serious disturbance of the host and, occasionally, to death of both host and parasite.

Eukaryotic single-celled protozoa and multicellular macroscopic helminths

Most are free living

Disease-producing species usually obligate parasites

## SIGNIFICANCE OF HUMAN PARASITIC INFECTIONS

The relative infrequency of parasitic infections in the temperate, highly sanitated societies of the industrialized world has sometimes led to the parochial view that knowledge of parasitology has little relevance for physicians practicing in these areas. The continuing presence of parasitic disease among the impoverished, immunocompromised, sexually active, and peripatetic segments of industrialized populations, however, means that most physicians will regularly encounter those pathogens.

Parasitic diseases remain among the major causes of human misery and death in the

**TABLE 51–1. PREVALENCE OF PARASITIC INFECTIONS IN 1984**

| Disease | Estimated Population Involved |
|---|---|
| Amebiasis | 10% of world population |
| Malaria | |
| Population at risk | 2 billion |
| Population infected | 270 million |
| Annual deaths | 1–2 million |
| African trypanosomiasis | |
| Population at risk | 50 million |
| New cases per year | 20,000 |
| American trypanosomiasis | |
| Population at risk | 65 million |
| New cases per year | 10,000 |
| Schistosomiasis | >200 million |
| Opisthorchiasis | 28 million |
| Paragonimiasis | 5 million |
| Fasciolopsiasis | 10 million |
| Filiariasis | 90 million |
| Onchocerciasis | 17 million |
| Dracunculiasis | 5 million |
| Ascariasis | 1.5 billion |
| Hookworm | 1.0 billion |
| Trichuriasis | 800 million |
| Strongyloidiasis | 90 million |
| Cestodiasis | 65 million |

Major causes of disease and death worldwide

world today and, as such, are important obstacles to the development of the economically less favored nations (Table 51–1). Moreover, a number of recent medical, socioeconomic, and political phenomena have combined to produce a dramatic recrudescence of several parasitic diseases with important consequences to both the United States and the developing world.

Resistance of malarial parasites to chemotherapeutics

Resistance of insect vectors to insecticides

Recent increases in imported malaria

Currently, 2 billion people live in malarious areas, and of these, approximately 270 million are infected at any given time. At least a million children die of malaria each year. *Plasmodium falciparum,* the most deadly of the malarial organisms, has developed resistance to a major category of antimalarial agents, and resistant strains are now found throughout Southeast Asia, parts of the Indian subcontinent, large areas of tropical America, and, most recently, several areas of Africa. Growing resistance of the mosquito vector of malaria to the less toxic and less expensive insecticides has resulted in a cutback of many malaria control programs. In countries such as India, Pakistan, and Sri Lanka, where eradication efforts had previously interrupted parasite transmission, the disease incidence has increased 100-fold in recent years. In tropical Africa, the intensity of transmission defies current control measures. Of direct interest to American physicians is the spillover of this phenomenon to the United States. Presently, approximately 1000 cases of imported malaria are reported annually.

Amebic dysentery in 10% of world population

*Entamoeba histolytica,* an intestinal protozoan, infects 10% of the world's population, including 2 to 3% in the United States. Invasive strains produce amebiasis, a disease characterized by intestinal ulcers and liver abscesses. It is more commonly seen in the poorly sanitated areas of the world, but occurs in the United States as well, particularly in institutions for the mentally retarded and among migrant workers and male homosexuals.

Trypanosomiasis produces disease and limits food supplies

In Latin America, *Trypanosoma cruzi* infects an estimated 10 million individuals annually, leaving many with the characteristic heart and gastrointestinal lesions of Chagas' disease. In Africa, from the Sahara Desert in the north to the Kalahari in the south, a related organism, *Trypanosoma brucei,* causes one of the most lethal of human infections, sleeping sickness. Animal strains of this same organism limit food supplies by making the raising of cattle economically infeasible.

Leishmaniasis, a disease produced by another intracellular protozoan, is found in parts of Europe, Asia, Africa, and Latin America. Clinical manifestations range from a self-limiting skin ulcer, known as oriental sore, through the mutilating mucocutaneous infection of espundia, to a highly lethal infection of the reticuloendothelial system (kala azar).

In 1947 Stall, in an article entitled "This Wormy World," estimated that between the tropics of Cancer and Capricorn there were many more intestinal worm infections than people. The prevalence was judged to be far lower in temperate climates. Warren, however, recently estimated that 27% of the American population harbored worms. The most serious of the helminthic diseases, schistosomiasis, affects an estimated 200 million individuals in Africa, Asia, and the Americas. Individuals with heavy worm levels develop bladder, intestinal, and liver disease, which may ultimately result in death. Unfortunately, the disease is frequently spread as a consequence of rural development schemes. Irrigation projects in Egypt, the Sudan, Ghana, and Nigeria have significantly increased the incidence of the disease in these areas, often mitigating the economic gains of the development program itself.

Parasitic worm infections prevalent, may be spread by irrigation projects

Two closely related filarial worms, *Wuchereria bancrofti* and *Brugia malayi,* which are endemic in Asia and Africa, interfere with the flow of lymph and can produce grotesque swellings of the legs, arms, and genitals. Another filaria produces onchocerciasis (river blindness) in millions of Africans and Americans, leaving thousands blind.

Filariasis produces swellings

Toxoplasmosis, giardiasis, trichomoniasis, and pinworm infections are four cosmopolitan parasitic infections well known to American physicians. The first, a protozoan infection of cats, infects possibly one third of the world's human population. Although it is usually asymptomatic, infection acquired in utero may result in abortion, stillbirth, prematurity, or severe neurologic defects in the newborn. Asymptomatic infection acquired either before or after birth may subsequently produce visual impairment. Immunosuppressive therapy may reactivate latent infections, producing severe encephalitis.

Multiple parasitic diseases common in the United States

## BIOLOGY, MORPHOLOGY, AND CLASSIFICATION

### Protozoa

#### Morphology

Protozoa range in size from 2 to more than 100 μm. Their protoplasm consists of a true membrane-bound nucleus and cytoplasm. The former contains clumped or dispersed chromatin and a central nucleolus or **karyosome.** The shape, size, and distribution of these structures are useful in distinguishing protozoan species from one another.

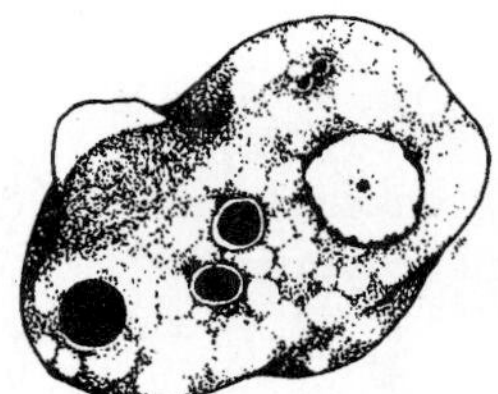

Prototypic rhizopod

The cytoplasm is frequently divided into an inner endoplasm and a thin outer ectoplasm. The granular **endoplasm** is concerned with nutrition and often contains food reserves, contractile vacuoles, and undigested particulate matter. The **ectoplasm** is organized into specialized organelles of locomotion. In some species, these organelles appear as blunt, dynamic extrusions known as pseudopods. In others, highly structured threadlike cilia or flagella arise from intracytoplasmic basal granules. Flagella are longer and less numerous than cilia and possess a structure and a mode of action distinct from those seen in prokaryotic organisms.

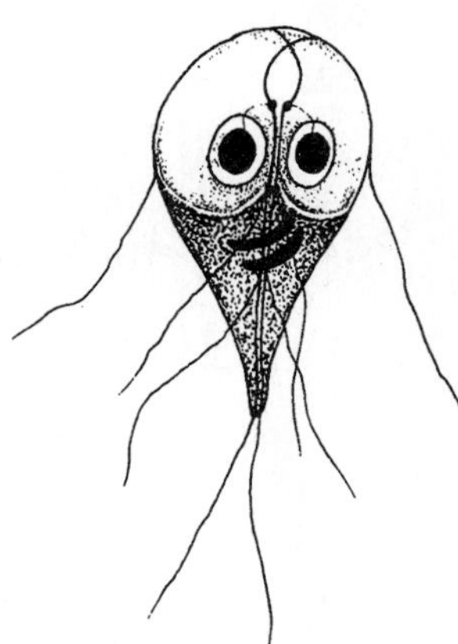

Prototypic flagellate (*Giardia*)

10 μm

#### Classification

Mode of reproduction and type of locomotive organelle are used to divide the protozoa into four major classes (Table 51–2). Although most **rhizopods** (amebas) are free-living, several are found as commensal inhabitants of the intestinal tract in humans. One of these or-

**TABLE 51–2. CLASSES OF PROTOZOA**

| Class | Organelles of Locomotion | Method of Reproduction |
|---|---|---|
| Rhizopods (amebas) | Pseudopods | Binary fission |
| Ciliates | Cilia | Binary fission |
| Flagellates | Flagella | Binary fission |
| Sporozoa | None | Schizogony/sporogony |

ganisms, *Entamoeba histolytica,* may invade tissue and produce disease. Occasionally, free-living amebas may gain access to the body and initiate illness. The majority of **ciliates** are free-living and seldom parasitize humans. **Flagellates** of the genera *Trypanosoma* and *Leishmania* are capable of invading the blood and tissues of humans, where they produce severe chronic illness. Others, such as *Trichomonas vaginalis* and *Giardia lamblia,* inhabit the urogenital and gastrointestinal tracts and initiate disease characterized by mild to moderate morbidity but no mortality. **Sporozoan** organisms, in contrast, produce two of the most potentially lethal diseases of humankind, malaria and toxoplasmosis.

### Physiology

Protozoa are facultative anaerobes

Most parasitic protozoa are facultative anaerobes. They are heterotrophic and must assimilate organic nutrients. This assimilation is accomplished by engulfing soluble or particulate matter in digestive vacuoles, processes termed **pinocytosis** and **phagocytosis,** respectively. In some species, food is ingested at a definite site, the peristome or cytostome. Food may be retained in special intracellular reserves, or vacuoles. Undigested particles and wastes are extruded at the cell surface by mechanisms that are the reverse of those used in ingestion.

Nutrients engulfed by phagocytosis or pinocytosis

Many protozoa form resistant cysts as survival form

Survival is ensured by highly developed protective and reproductive techniques. Many protozoa, when exposed to an unfavorable milieu, become less active metabolically and secrete a cyst wall capable of protecting the organism from physical and chemical conditions that would otherwise be lethal. In this form, the parasite is better equipped to survive passage from host to host in the external environment. Immunoevasive mechanisms described later under Immunity contribute to survival within the host. Reproduction is accomplished primarily by simple binary fission. In one class of protozoa, the Sporozoa, a cycle of multiple fission (schizogony) alternates with a period of sexual reproduction (sporogony).

Reproduction usually by binary fission

## Helminths

### Morphology and Classification

Great variation in size

Worms are elongated, bilaterally symmetric animals that vary in length from less than a millimeter to a meter or more. The body wall is covered with a tough acellular **cuticle,** which may be smooth or possess ridges, spines, and tubercles. At the anterior end there are often suckers, hooks, teeth, or plates used for the purpose of attachment. All helminths have differentiated organs. Primitive nervous and excretory systems and a highly developed reproductive system are characteristic of the entire group. Some have alimentary tracts; none possess a circulatory system.

Differentiated organs: no circulatory system

The common helminthic parasites of humans can be placed in one of three classes on the basis of body and alimentary tract, configuration, nature of the reproductive system, and need for more than a single host species for the completion of the life cycle (Table 51–3).

**Roundworms,** or nematodes, have a cylindrical fusiform body and a tubular alimentary tract that extends from the mouth at the anterior end to the anus at the posterior end. The sexes are separate, and the male worm is typically smaller than the female. These worms

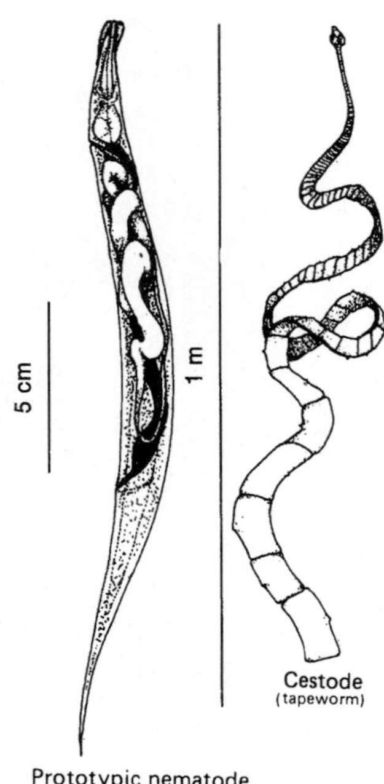


TABLE 51–3. CLASSIFICATION OF HELMINTHIC PARASITES OF HUMANS

| Characteristic | Roundworm (Nematode) | Tapeworm (Cestode) | Fluke (Trematode) |
|---|---|---|---|
| Morphology | Spindle-shaped | Head with segmented body (proglottids) | Leaf-shaped with oral and ventral suckers |
| Sex | Separate sexes | Hermaphroditic | Hermaphroditic[a] |
| Alimentary tract | Tubular | None | Blind |
| Intermediate host | Variable[b] | One[c] | Two[d] |

[a] *Schistosoma* group has separate sexes.
[b] Tissue nematodes have intermediate hosts; intestinal nematodes do not.
[c] *Diphyllobothrium* group has two.
[d] *Schistosoma* group has one.

can be divided into those that dwell within the gastrointestinal tract and those that parasitize the blood and tissues of humans. Unlike the latter, those in the gastrointestinal tract generally do not require intermediate hosts.

**Tapeworms,** or cestodes, have flattened, ribbon-shaped bodies. The anterior end, or **scolex,** is armed with suckers and frequently with **hooklets,** which are used for attachment. Immediately behind the head is a neck that generates a chain of reproductive segments, or **proglottids.** Each segment contains both male and female gonads. The worm lacks a digestive tract and presumably absorbs nutrients across its cuticle. One or sometimes two intermediate hosts are required for completion of the life cycle.

**Flukes,** or trematodes, are leaf-shaped organisms with blind, branched alimentary tracts. Particulate waste is regurgitated through the mouth. Two suckers, one surrounding the mouth and the second located more distally on the ventral aspect of the body, serve as organs of attachment and locomotion. Most are hermaphroditic and require two intermediate hosts. The blood-dwelling schistosomes, however, are unisexual and require but a single intermediate.

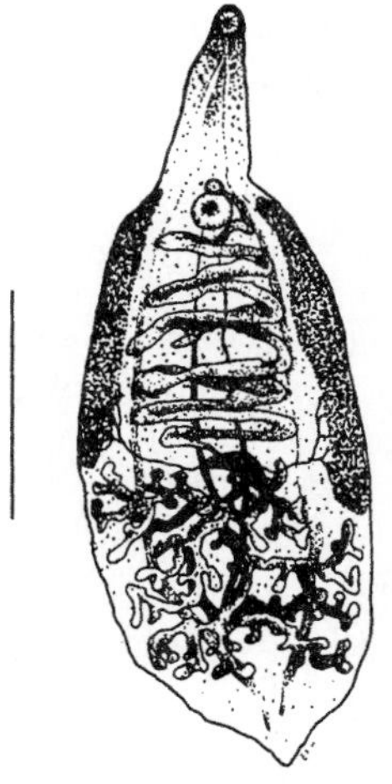


Prototypic trematode (flukes)

### Physiology

Anaerobic respiration of adult worm

Helminthic parasites are nourished by ingestion or absorption of the body fluids, lysed tissue, or intestinal contents of their hosts. Carbohydrates are rapidly metabolized, and the glycogen concentration of the worms is high. Respiration is primarily anaerobic, although larval offspring frequently require oxygen. A large part of the energy requirement is devoted to reproductive needs. The daily output of offspring can be as high as 200,000 for some worms. Typically, helminths are **oviparous** (excrete eggs), but a few species are **viviparous** (give birth to living young). The egg shells of many parasites with an aquatic intermediate host possess a lidded opening, or **operculum,** through which the embryo escapes once the egg reaches water. Whether hatched or freeborn, the resulting larva is morphologically distinct from the mature worm and undergoes a series of changes or molts before it achieves adulthood.

High fertility producing thousands of eggs

Protection from the host's digestive and body fluids is afforded by the tough cuticle and the secretion of enzymes. Some worms, such as the schistosomes, can protect themselves from immunologic attack by the incorporation of host antigens into their cuticles. The life span of the adult helminth is often measured in weeks or months, but some, such as the hookworms, filaria, and flukes, can survive within their hosts for decades.

Mechanical protection from environment and immunological attack

## LIFE CYCLES, TRANSMISSION, AND DISTRIBUTION

### Single-Host Parasites

As is evident from the previous discussion, many parasites require but a single host species for the completion of their life cycles. The method by which the parasite is transmitted from individual to individual within that species is determined in large part by its viability in the external environment and, in the case of helminths, by the conditions required for the maturation of offspring. The mode of transmission, in turn, determines the social, economic, and geographic distribution of the parasite. A few illustrative examples are summarized in Table 51–4.

**TABLE 51–4. TRANSMISSION AND DISTRIBUTION OF FOUR REPRESENTATIVE PARASITES**

| Organism | Infective Form | Mechanism of Spread | Distribution |
|---|---|---|---|
| *Trichomonas vaginalis* | Trophozoite | Direct (venereal) | Worldwide |
| *Entamoeba histolytica* | Cyst/trophozoite | Direct (venereal) | Worldwide |
| | Cyst | Indirect (fecal–oral) | Areas of poor sanitation |
| *Ascaris lumbricoides* | Egg | Indirect (fecal–oral) | Areas of poor sanitation |
| *Plasmodium falciparum* | Sporozoite | *Anopheles* mosquito | Tropical and subtropical areas |

Transmission by direct sexual contact

The protozoan *Trichomonas vaginalis* does not produce protective cyst forms. Although its active, or trophozoite, form is relatively hardy, it can survive only a few hours outside of its normal habitat, the human genital tract. Thus, for all practical purposes, transmission requires the direct genital contact of sexual intercourse. As a result, trichomoniasis is cosmopolitan, occurring wherever human hosts engage in sexual activity with multiple partners.

Fecal-oral transmission common for less fragile intestinal parasites

Another protozoan, *Entamoeba histolytica,* inhabits the human gut and produces hardy **cysts** that are passed in the stool. Transmission occurs when another individual ingests these cysts. Like *T. vaginalis,* the organism can be passed by direct physical contact, in this case by oral–anal sexual activity. This mode of transmission, in fact, accounts for the high incidence of amebic infections in male homosexuals. Unlike *T. vaginalis,* however, the cysts can survive prolonged periods in the external environment, where they may eventually contaminate food or drinking water. Thus, in environments such as mental institutions, where the level of personal hygiene is low, or in populations in which methods for the sanitary disposal of human wastes are not available, amebiasis is common.

Some require infectivity development in soil

The intestinal helminth *Ascaris lumbricoides* illustrates still another transmission pattern. In this infection, highly resistant eggs are passed in the human stool. Unlike the situation with *E. histolytica* described previously, the eggs are not immediately infective, but must incubate in soil under certain conditions of temperature and humidity before they are fully embryonated and infectious. As a result, this parasite cannot be transmitted directly from host to host. The organism spreads only when indiscriminate human defecation results in deposition of eggs on soil and subsequent exposure of that soil to the climatic conditions required for embryonation of the eggs. For this reason, *Ascaris* infections are most prevalent in poorly sanitated areas of the tropics and subtropics.

## Multiple-Host Parasites

Multiple hosts may be involved in life cycle

A few protozoa and many helminths require two or more host species in their life cycle. To avoid confusion, it is customary to refer to the species in which the parasite reproduces sexually as the **definitive host;** that in which asexual reproduction or larval development takes place is the **intermediate host.** When there is more than one intermediate, they are known simply as the first and second intermediate hosts. In some cases, such as that of *Taenia saginata,* the beef tapeworm, both host species are vertebrates; humans serve as the definitive host and cattle as the intermediate. Among parasites that inhabit the blood and tissues of humans, it is more common for a blood-feeding arthropod to serve as a second host and as the transmitting vector. An example is malaria, in which the causative plasmodium is transmitted from person to person by the bite of an infected female mosquito of the genus *Anopheles*. In this particular instance, sexual reproduction occurs in the mosquito, making it the definitive host and relegating the human host to the role of a mere intermediate.

Definitive host and one or more intermediate hosts

Distribution of nonhuman hosts influences disease occurrence

The distribution of parasites requiring a nonhuman host is limited to the ecologic niche occupied by this second host. Thus, the areas in which malaria is endemic are restricted by the distribution of *Anopheles*. The area of disease distribution is, in fact, generally smaller than that of the nonhuman host, because conditions favoring parasite transmission may also differ. For example, both the abundance of *Anopheles* and the speed with which the malarial parasite completes its development within them are directly related to the ambient temperature and humidity. Among temperate zone *Anopheles,* the number of infected mosquitoes may be insufficient to sustain parasite transmission. In tropical areas, transmission is more likely to be constant and intense. In another more obvious example, infections with *T. saginata* are found only in areas where cattle are raised for human consumption and, within those areas, only where indiscriminate human defecation and the ingestion of raw or undercooked beef are common.

## IMMUNITY

The large size, complex structure, varied metabolic activity, and synthetic prowess of most parasites provide their human host with an intense antigenic challenge. The resulting immunologic response is, generally, vigorous, but its role in modulating the parasitic invasion differs significantly from that in viral and bacterial infections. It is apparent from the chronic course and frequent recurrences typical of many parasitic diseases that acquired resistance is often absent. When present, it is generally incomplete, serving to moderate the intensity of the infection and its associated clinical manifestations rather than to destroy or expel the causative pathogen. In fact, clinical recovery and resistance to reinfection in some parasitoses require the persistence of viable organisms at low concentration within the body of the host **(premunition).** Complete sterilizing immunity with prolonged resistance to reinfection is exceptional.

Immune response to parasites vigorous but often relatively infective

This pusillanimous response does not result from any dearth of immunologic mechanisms available to the host. All those generally exercised against the more primitive microorganisms, including antibodies, cytotoxic T lymphocytes, activated macrophages, natural killer cells, antibody-dependent cell-mediated toxicity, lymphokines, and complement activation, have been shown to play a part in moderating parasitic infection. In worm infections, some of these mechanisms find unique implementation. On invasion of tissue, helminths stimulate the production of IgE, the Fc portion of which binds to mast cells and basophils. Interaction of the antibody with parasitic antigen triggers the release of histamine and other mediators from the attached cells. These may injure the worm directly or, by increasing vascular permeability and stimulating the release of chemotactic factors, may lead to the accumulation of other cells and IgG antibodies capable of initiating antibody-dependent, cell-mediated destruction of the parasite. The specific killer cell involved is often the eosinophil. These cells attach by their Fc receptor site to IgG antibody-coated parasites and degranulate, releasing a major basic protein that is directly toxic to the worm.

All elements of immune response mobilized

IgE response to worm infections attracts eosinophils

Eosinophils bind to IgG-coated parasite and release toxic protein

The techniques by which parasites have been shown to evade the consequences of the host's specific acquired immunity are numerous. Included among them are seclusion within immunologically protected areas of the body, continual alteration of surface antigens, and active suppression of the host's effector mechanisms. A number of protozoa are shielded from humoral defenses by virtue of their intracellular location. Some have even found ways to avoid or survive the normally lethal environment of the phagolysosome of the macrophage. *Trypanosoma cruzi,* for example, lyses the phagosomal membrane, providing escape into the cytoplasm, whereas *Toxoplasma gondii* inhibits fusion of the phagosome with lysosomes. *Leishmania* species, capable of neither of these feats, are resistant to the action of lysosomal enzymes and survive in the phagolysosomes.

Some intracellular protozoa avoid phagolysosome destruction

*Toxoplasma,* cestode larvae, and *Trichinella spiralis* armor themselves against immunologic attack by encysting within the tissue of the host. The gut lumen is, perhaps, the largest immunologic sanctuary within the body, because, unless the integrity of the intestinal mucosa is breached by injury or inflammation, this barrier protects lumen-dwelling parasites from most of the effective humoral and cellular immune mechanisms of the host, allowing almost unfettered growth and multiplication.

Encysted and intestinal parasites relatively inaccessible to host defenses

Most immune effector mechanisms are directed against the surface antigens of the parasite, and alteration of these antigens may blunt the immunologic attack. Many parasites undergo developmental changes within their hosts that are generally accompanied by alterations in surface antigens. Immune responses directed at an early developmental stage may be totally ineffective against a later stage of the same parasite. Such stage-specific immunity has been demonstrated in malaria, schistosomiasis, and trichinosis, accounting for the seeming paradox of parasite survival in a host resistant to reinfection with the same strain of organism. Even more intriguing is the ability of some parasites to vary the antigenic characteristics of a single developmental stage. The trypanosomes causing African sleeping sickness circulate in the bloodstream coated with a thick layer of glycoprotein. The development of humoral antibody to this coating results in the elimination of the parasite from the blood. This is followed by successive waves of parasitemia, each associated with a new glycoprotein antigen on the parasite against which the previously produced antibody is ineffective. The parasite is capable of producing more than 100 glycoprotein variants, each encoded by a different structural gene. The expression of individual genes from this large genetic repertoire is controlled by the sequential transfer of a duplicate copy of each gene to an area of the parasite responsible for gene expression.

Antigenic shifts occur with developmental changes in parasite

Trypanosomal antigenic variation outpaces immunologic response

Antigenic glycoprotein variants of trypanosomes selected from preexisting genetic repertoire

A number of protozoan and helminthic pathogens are thought to be capable of neutralizing antibody-mediated attack by shedding and, later, regenerating specific surface anti-

Antigenic shedding and masking with host antigens

gens. Adult schistosomes, in addition, may immunologically hide from the host by masking themselves with host blood group antigens and immunoglobulins.

Parasites may destroy immunologic mediators

A number of parasites can destroy or inactivate immunologic mediators. Tapeworm larvae produce anticomplementary chemicals, and *Trypanosoma cruzi* splits the Fc component of attached antibodies, rendering it incapable of activating complement. Several protozoa, most notably *Trypanosoma brucei,* the etiologic agent of African sleeping sickness, induce polyclonal B-cell activation leading to the production of nonspecific immunoglobulins and eventual exhaustion of the antibody-producing capacity of the host. This and other protozoa can produce nonspecific suppression of both cellular and humoral effector mechanisms, enhancing the host's susceptibility also to a variety of unrelated secondary infections. Patients with disseminated leishmaniasis display a specific inability to mount a cellular immune response to parasitic antigens in the absence of evidence of generalized immunosuppression.

Some parasites cause immune suppression

Finally, the thick, tough cuticle of many adult helminths renders them impervious to immune effector mechanisms designed to deal with the less robust microbes.

## PATHOGENESIS

Most adult helminths do not multiply within host

In helminthic infections, humans may serve as the definitive host to the sexually mature adult worms (eg, *Taenia saginata*) or as the intermediate host to the larval stages (eg, *Echinococcus granulosus*). Occasionally, they serve as both the definitive and the intermediate host to the same worm (eg, *Trichinella spiralis, Taenia solium*). Unlike protozoan parasites, most adult helminths are incapable of increasing their numbers within their definitive host. As a result, the severity of clinical illness is related to the total number of worms acquired by the host over time. Most small worm loads are, in fact, asymptomatic and may not require therapy. Many worms are long-lived, however, and repeated infections can result in very high worm loads with subsequent disability.

Worm load related to disease severity

The pathogenesis of both protozoan and helminthic disease is highly variable. The fish tapeworm *Diphyllobothrium latum* competes with the host for nutrients. The protozoan *Giardia lamblia* and the helminth *Strongyloides stercoralis* interfere with the absorption of food across the intestinal mucosa. Hookworm infections cause loss of iron, an essential mineral. Other helminths, such as *Clonorchis sinensis* and *Schistosoma haematobium,* compromise the function of important organs by obstruction, secondary bacterial infection, and induction of carcinomatous changes. Occasionally, as in the case of echinococcosis, disease results from pressure and displacement of normal tissue by the slow growth of the parasitic cyst. In malaria, the primary pathogenic mechanism appears to be the invasion and subsequent alteration or destruction of human erythrocytes. Similarly, many helminthic larvae are capable of tissue invasion and destruction. *Entamoeba histolytica* can destroy host cells without actual cellular invasion. Finally, immunologic mechanisms are responsible for tissue damage and clinical manifestations in many diseases. Allergic or anaphylactic reactions play a major role in the cutaneous reactions to invading hookworm, strongyloides, and schistosome larvae (ground itch, swimmer's itch) and in the fever, rash, and lymphadenopathy that accompany the therapeutic destruction of onchocercal microfilariae (Mazzotti reaction). Transient pneumonias induced by the pulmonary migration of *Ascaris* and other nematode larvae (Loeffler's syndrome), nocturnal paroxysms of asthma in some patients with filariasis (tropical pulmonary eosinophilia), and the shock, asthma, and urticaria that follow rupture of a hydatid cyst are all immunologically mediated. Hemolysis in malaria and cardiac damage in Chagas' disease are thought, at least in part, to reflect antibody-mediated cytotoxicity. Immune complex diseases are seen in schistosomiasis (Katayama syndrome) and malaria (nephrosis). The granulomatous reaction to schistosomal eggs, the muscle damage in trichinosis, and the entire clinicopathologic spectrum of the leishmanial infections appear to be caused by cell-mediated immune responses.

Wide range of direct pathogenic mechanisms

Immunopathological mechanisms contribute to parasitic diseases

## DIAGNOSIS

Although parasitic diseases are not as common in the United States as elsewhere, they do occur and may, at times, be life threatening. In addition, the continuous arrival of travelers and immigrants from endemic areas necessitates consideration of these diseases in differential diagnoses. Unfortunately, the clinical manifestations of parasitic infections are seldom sufficiently characteristic to raise this possibility in the clinician's mind. Moreover, routine laboratory tests are seldom of aid. Although eosinophilia has been recognized as an important clue to the diagnosis of parasitic disease, this phenomenon is characteristic only of helminthic infection, and even in these cases it is frequently absent. Eosinophilia, which presumably reflects an immunologic response to the complex foreign proteins possessed by worms, is most marked during tissue migration. Once migration ceases, the eosinophilia may decrease or disappear entirely. Thus, the clinician must usually rely on a detailed travel, food intake, transfusion, and socioeconomic history to raise the possibility of parasitic disease.

Need to consider indigenous and imported infections

Eosinophilia seen in helminthic infections

Once considered, diagnosis is usually straightforward. Typically, it rests on the demonstration and morphologic identification of the parasite or its progeny in the stool, urine, sputum, blood, or tissues of the human host.

Morphologic demonstration parasites primary diagnostic means

In intestinal infections, a simple wet mount or stained smear, or both, of the stool is often adequate. Some parasites, however, are passed in the feces intermittently or in fluctuating numbers, and repeated specimens are needed. Ova of worms and cysts of protozoa may be concentrated by sedimentation or flotation techniques to increase their numbers for diagnosis. Occasionally, specimens other than stool must be examined. In the case of small bowel infections such as giardiasis and strongyloidiasis, aspirates of the duodenum or a small bowel biopsy may be required to establish the diagnosis. Similarly, the recovery of large bowel parasites such as *Entamoeba histolytica* and *Schistosoma mansoni* may require proctoscopy or sigmoidoscopy, with aspiration or biopsy of suspect lesions. Eggs of pinworms (*Enterobius*) and tapeworms (*Taenia*) may be found on the perineal skin when they are absent from the stool.

Stool concentration techniques used for intestinal parasites

Parasites dwelling within the tissue and blood of the host are more difficult to identify. Direct examination of the blood is useful for the detection of malarial parasites, leishmania, trypanosomes, and filarial progeny (microfilariae). The concentration of organisms in the bloodstream often fluctuates, however, requiring the collection of multiple specimens over several days. Both wet mount and stained preparations of thin and thick blood smears (see Chapter 52) are used. Lung flukes and occasionally other helminths discharge their offspring in the sputum and may be found there with appropriate concentration techniques. In others, larvae can be recovered with skin (onchocerciasis) or muscle (trichinosis) biopsy.

Demonstration of blood and tissue parasites requires proper timing

In some infections, parasite recovery is uncommon. Immunodiagnostic and nucleic acid hybridization techniques provide diagnostic alternatives for these situations. Although tests for circulating antibodies have long been available for a number of parasitic diseases, they often lacked sensitivity and specificity. The replacement of crude, antigenically complex parasitic extracts with purified homologous antigens, together with the adaptation of highly reactive test systems, has significantly increased the sensitivity and specificity of such tests. Currently, reliable serologic procedures are available for amebiasis, cysticercosis, echinococciasis, paragonimiasis, schistosomiasis, strongyloidiasis, toxocariasis, toxoplasmosis, and trichinosis. More will undoubtedly follow in the near future.

Serologic tests available for some parasites

Techniques for the detection of parasitic antigens in blood, body fluids, tissues, and excreta also have been developed. Commercial immunofluorescent and immunosorbent kits for *Pneumocystis carinii* (pulmonary secretions), *Trichomonas vaginalis* (genitourinary fluids), and *Entamoeba histolytica, Giardia,* and *Cryptosporidium* (feces) are now commonly found in clinical laboratories. Less generally available are systems for the detection of malaria antigens in blood and *Toxoplasma gondii* in tissue.

Antigen detection becoming available

DNA probes are available for the detection of *Plasmodium falciparum, Trypanosoma cruzi, Trypanosoma brucei, Onchocerca* species, and the etiologic agents of lymphatic filariasis. The probes for *P. falciparum* and lymphatic filariae have demonstrated sensitivities that match or exceed those of traditional techniques. The major limitations of DNA probes, as diagnostic tools, relate to the technical aspects of the hybridization procedure which should soon be overcome.

## CHEMOTHERAPY

The study and management of parasitic disease were seminal to the initiation of the chemotherapeutic era. Amazonian Indians first employed quinine-containing extracts of cinchona tree bark to treat malarious patients more than 300 years ago. It was in the attempt to synthesize this same antimalarial compound that 19th-century German chemists discovered aniline dyes. The circle closed in the early years of this century when Ehrlich, while investigating the suitability of these dyes as protozoan stains, developed the concept that chemicals might be found that had the capacity to destroy microbial pathogens selectively without damage to the tissues of the human host. Although the most dramatic confirmation of that concept came with the introduction of arsenical compounds for the treatment of syphilis, his first successful chemotherapeutics were directed against protozoan agents. By 1930, chemically synthesized drugs had been marketed for the treatment of malaria, trypanosomiasis, and schistosomiasis.

Antiparasitic agents among first antimicrobics

The introduction and explosive increase in the number and variety of antimicrobic agents introduced in the second and third quarters of this century forever changed the face of medicine. Unfortunately, however, few were effective against parasites because they share the eukaryotic characteristics of their hosts. With the resources of the pharmaceutical companies directed to the development and introduction of antibacterial agents, work on antiparasitic agents lagged. Safer alternatives lacking, chemotherapeutics synthesized in the preantibiotic era remained critical elements of the parasitologist's therapeutic armamentarium until very recently. Most required prolonged or parenteral administration, the effectiveness of many was restricted to particular disease stages, and the toxicity of a few mandated that use be limited to very severe or life-threatening conditions. With time, and at a pace much slower than that seen for the antibacterial agents, newer antiparasitic agents were developed that overcame many of these problems. Their numbers are still limited, and only recently has their safety and efficacy begun to match those of their antibacterial equivalents.

Newer antiparasitics broader spectrum, less toxic

## Therapeutic Goals

The process of antiparasitic drug development and use has been shaped to a significant degree by the concentration of these diseases in the impoverished areas of the world. Community-based public health measures aimed at interrupting pathogen transmission, such as provision of sanitary facilities and clean water supplies, are still often beyond the capacity of tightly constrained budgets, and the major burden of mitigating the impact of parasitic illnesses in endemic areas often falls on medical auxiliaries or village health workers who, operating in remote and relatively primitive conditions, must examine, diagnose, and treat sick patients with whom they have only fleeting contact. Given these limitations and the large numbers of the afflicted, optimal therapy requires drugs that are effective in a single dose, easily administered, safe enough to be dispensed with limited medical supervision, and sufficiently inexpensive to be widely used. Few such agents exist. Pharmaceutical companies, faced with the enormous costs of drug development and approval, have been reluctant to expend resources they are unlikely to recover. Until the international community provides the resources needed for the development of more suitable agents, the full potential of antiparasitic chemotherapy will not be realized.

Treatment programs difficult in underdeveloped economies

Ideal agents would be cheap, of low toxicity, and effective in single doses; few exist

The practical aspects of antiparasitic therapy are illustrated in the principles governing the treatment of worm infections, which differ significantly from those applied to prokaryotic or protozoan infections. Helminths, with few exceptions, do not multiply within the human host, and severe infections thus require the repeated acquisition of infectious-stage parasites. Interestingly, the intensity of infection or worm burden does not follow a normal distribution in human populations. Most infected individuals harbor fewer than a dozen adult worms; a small minority harbor very large worm numbers. As there is a direct correlation between worm burden and clinical disease, it is only this minority that suffers significant morbidity. Concentrating treatment on those few clinically ill patients moderates the medical impact of a helminthic disease on a community at a cost dramatically lower than that required for mass treatment. Moreover, it is usually unnecessary to eradicate all worms from treated patients; a significant decrease in the worm burden is adequate to alleviate clinical symptoms. This can often be accomplished with short, subcurative doses that further reduce cost and minimize the likelihood of drug toxicity. Because this approach can dramatically decrease the total community worm burden, the number of worm progeny shed

For worms, may concentrate effort on those most heavily parasitized

into the environment is similarly reduced and the transmission of the disease slowed or, at times, eliminated.

## Structure and Action

With few exceptions, antiparasitic agents have been synthesized de novo rather than developed from naturally occurring substances. Most are relatively simple and often contain benzene or other ring structures.

Most antiparasitics are synthetic

It is believed that the majority of antiprotozoan drugs interfere with nucleic acid synthesis or, less commonly, with carbohydrate metabolism. Anthelmintics, on the other hand, apparently act by compromising the worm's glycolytic pathways or neuromuscular function. In most cases, the parasite and host cells have functionally equivalent target sites. Differential toxicity is achieved by preferential uptake, metabolic alteration of the drug by the parasite, or differences in the susceptibility of functionally equivalent sites in parasite and host.

Differential toxicity based on uptake, metabolic factors

As has been the case for antibacterial agents, the impact of many antiparasitic agents has been compromised by the development of resistance in the parasite. This seems to have resulted from mutation and selection in the face of intensive, often prophylactic, drug use. The mechanisms responsible have been studied for only a few parasites, but appear to be related to reduced uptake of drug.

Acquired mutational resistance usually involves reduced uptake of drug

## Drugs

### Heavy Metals

Arsenic and antimonial compounds have been used since ancient times. They form stable complexes with sulfur compounds and probably exert their biological effects by binding to sulfhydryl groups. They are toxic to the host as well as to the parasite and have their greatest impact on cells that are most metabolically active such as neuronal, renal tubular, intestinal epithelial, and bone marrow stem cells. Their differential toxicity and therapeutic value are due to enhanced uptake by the parasite and its intense metabolic activity. Only one trivalent arsenical, melarsoprol (Mel B), is now widely used. It is capable of penetrating the blood–brain barrier and is effective in all stages of trypanosomiasis. Because of its toxicity, it is employed only when less toxic agents have failed or the central nervous system is involved. The recently introduced less toxic trypanocides that penetrate the blood–brain barrier may soon replace this drug.

Arsenic and antimonial compounds inactivate -SH groups

Differential toxicity based on uptake

Melarsoprol is active against all stages of trypanosomiasis

Antimonial agents are now restricted to the management of leishmanial infections. Two pentavalent compounds, sodium stibogluconate (Pentostam) and meglumine antimoniate (Glucantime), are used for all forms of leishmaniasis. In disseminated disease, prolonged therapy is usually required and relapses often occur. In localized cutaneous leishmaniasis, cure is usually achieved with a relatively brief course. Toxic side effects are similar to those of the arsenicals.

Antimonials used only for leishmanial infections

### Antimalarial Quinolines

Cinchona bark was employed in Europe for the treatment of fever as early as 1640. It was only after Pelletier and Caventou isolated quinine from cinchona in 1820 that this alkaloid gained widespread acceptance as an antimalarial. Synthesis of new quinolines was stimulated by the interruption of quinine supplies during two world wars and, after 1961, by the growing impact of drug-resistant falciparum malaria in several areas of the world. Among the most effective are those that share the double-ring structure of quinine.

Quinine and quinoline analogs active against malaria

Current analogs fall into three major groups: 4-aminoquinolines, 8-aminoquinolines, and 4-quinolinemethanols. Most appear to block nucleic acid synthesis by intercalation into double-stranded DNA, but failure of the 4-quinolinemethanols to intercalate indicates that other mechanisms, perhaps interference with hemoglobin digestion by the malarial parasite, are involved. Selective destruction of intracellular parasites results from accumulation of drug by parasitized host cells. Quinine, 4-aminoquinolines, and 4-quinolinemethanols concentrate in parasitized erythrocytes and rapidly destroy the erythrocytic stage of the par-

N

Quinoline ring

Accumulate in parasitized cells, block DNA synthesis

Quinine, 4-aminoquinolines (eg, chloroquine), and 4-quinolinemethanols suppress malarial infection

8-Aminoquinolines (eg, primaquine) effect radical cure

asite that is responsible for the clinical manifestations of malaria. These agents can thus be used prophylactically to suppress clinical illness should infection occur or therapeutically to terminate an acute attack. They do not concentrate in tissue cells, and thus organisms sequestered in exoerythrocytic sites, particularly the liver, survive and may later reestablish erythrocytic infection and produce a clinical relapse. The 8-aminoquinolines accumulate in tissue cells, destroy hepatic parasites, and effect a radical cure.

Primaquine has hematologic toxicity

Chloroquine phosphate, a 4-aminoquinoline, is the most widely used of the blood schizonticidal drugs. In the doses used for long-term malarial prophylaxis, it has proven remarkably free of untoward effects. Primaquine phosphate, the 8-aminoquinoline used to eradicate persistent hepatic parasites, has toxic effects related to its oxidant activity. Methemoglobinemia and hemolytic anemia are particularly frequent in patients with glucose-6-phosphate dehydrogenase deficiency, because they are unable to generate sufficient quantities of the reduced form of nicotinamide adenine dinucleotide to respond to this oxidant stress. Typically, the anemia is severe in patients of Mediterranean and Oriental ancestry and mild in black patients.

Quinine is active against many chloroquine resistant malarial strains

Quinine is the most toxic of the quinolines and is currently used primarily to treat the strains of *Plasmodium falciparum* resistant to several blood schizonticidal agents that are spreading rapidly through Asia, Latin America, and Africa. Chloroquine resistance is the most frequent and worrisome, because suitable alternatives to this safe and highly effective agent are few. The mechanism of resistance is not clearly understood, but resistant organisms fail to accumulate chloroquine. Experimental reversal of resistance with calcium channel blockers suggests that the failure to accumulate this agent results from a rapid release mechanism. Mefloquine, a newly developed oral 4-quinolinemethanol, presently displays a high level of activity against most chloroquine-resistant parasites; however, its structural similarity to choloroquine and ready in vitro development of mefloquine resistance in *P. falciparum* raise the specter that cross-resistance to this agent may develop quickly. Such resistance has already been reported from Southeast Asia and Africa.

Phenanthrene methanols active against multidrug-resistant malaria

Phenanthrene methanols are not, in the strict sense, quinine analogs. Nevertheless, they are structurally similar to this group of agents and, together with them, were discovered to have antimalarial activity during the second World War. Halofantrine, the most effective of the group, has only recently become available. In vitro and in vivo studies demonstrated that it is an effective blood schizonticide against both sensitive and multidrug-resistant strains of *P. falciparum*. Its mechanism of action is thought to differ from that of quinine and mefloquine, but more specific information is currently lacking. Halofantrine is well tolerated and appears to be free of teratogencity. Oral absorption is both slow and erratic, reaching maximum concentrations in 5 to 7 hours; its half-life is relatively short (1 to 3 days). Clinical studies have demonstrated high failure rates when the drug is given in a single dose; cure rates with multiple-dose regimens, however, have been high. In Thailand, mefloquine-resistant strains of *P. falciparum* have demonstrated decreased sensitivity to halofantrine, raising the possibility of cross-resistance between these two agents.

## Quinones

Atovaquone stable and active against malaria, pneumocystosis, and toxoplasmosis

Atovaquone is a novel hydroxynaphthoquinone that shows promise in the treatment of malaria, pneumocystosis, and toxoplasmosis. In the search for effective antimalarial agents during World War II, a number of hydroxynaphthoquinones were found to have antimalarial activity in experimental animals; however, all were rapidly metabolized in humans and proved ineffective in the treatment of malarious patients. In the 1980s a single hydroxynaphthoquinone, atovaquone, was found to be both highly effective in vitro against *P. falciparum* and metabolically stable in humans when administered orally. Its antiparasitic activity appeared to result from the specific blockade of pyrimidine biosynthesis secondary to the inhibition of the parasite's mitochondrial electron transport chain at the ubinquinol–cytochrome c reductase region (complex III). Its long half-life (70 hours) and lack of serious adverse reactions suggested that it would be of great value in the treatment of malaria. Efficacy trials established its capacity to effect rapid clearance of parasitemia in patients with chloroquine-resistent falciparum malaria. Frequent parasitic recrudescences were eliminated when atovaquone was administered in combination with proguanil or tetracycline. Subsequently, this agent has shown to be effective for the treatment of *Pneumocystis carinii* pneumonia and toxoplasmosis in AIDS patients. Unlike other antitoxoplasmic agents, atovaquone has been found to be active against *Toxoplasma gondii* cysts as well as tachyzoites, suggesting this agent may produce radical cure. Supporting this is the infrequency with which cessation of atovaquone treatment of toxoplasmic cerebritis in AIDS patients has resulted in relapse. Relapse following atovaquone treatment of pneumocystosis in this same patient population appears similarly uncommon.

### Folate Antagonists

Folic acid serves as a critical coenzyme for the synthesis of purines and ultimately DNA. In protozoa, as in bacteria, the active form of folic acid is produced in vivo by a simple two-step process. The first, the conversion of *para*-aminobenzoic acid to dihydrofolic acid, is blocked by sulfonamides. The second, the transformation of dihydro- to tetrahydrofolic acid, is inhibited by folic acid analogs (folate antagonists), which competitively inhibit dihydrofolate reductase. Used together with sulfonamides, folate antagonists are very effective inhibitors of protozoan growth.

Sulfonamide and folate antagonists inhibit protozoa

Trimethroprim, an inhibitor of dihydrofolate reductase, is used in combination with sulfamethoxazole to treat toxoplasmosis and *Pneumocystis* infection. Another folate antagonist, pyrimethamine, has a high affinity for sporozoan dihydrofolate reductase and has been particularly effective when used with a sulfonamide in the management of malaria and toxoplasmosis. Acquired protozoal resistance is mutational and generally has been limited to species of malarial parasites.

Trimethoprim effective in Toxoplasma and Pneumocystis infections

Folate antagonists may result in folate deficiency in individuals with limited folate reserves, such as newborns, pregnant women, and the malnourished. This is of great concern when large doses are used for prolonged periods, as in the treatment of acute toxoplasmosis. When folate antagonists are used with sulfonamides, the entire range of sulfonamide toxic effects may be seen. Patients with AIDS appear to suffer an unusually high incidence of toxic side effects to trimethoprim–sulfamethoxazole.

Folate deficiency and sulfonamide toxicities occur

### Qinghaosu (Artemisinin)

This natural extract of the plant *Artemesia annua* (qing hao, sweet wormwood) is a sesquiterpenelactone peroxide that is structurally distinct from all other known antiparasitic compounds. Extracts of qing hao were recommended for the treatment of fevers in China as early as AD 341; their specific antimalarial activity was defined in 1971. Although qinghaosu has also been shown to be active against the free-living ameba *Naegleria fowleria* and several trematodes, including *Schistosoma japonicum, Schistosoma mansoni,* and *Clonorchis sinensis,* its greatest impact to date has been in the treatment of malaria. Extensive investigations showed it to be schizonticidal for both chloroquine-sensitive and chloroquine-resistant strains of *Plasmodium falciparum*. Several derivatives, among them artemether and artesunate, are significantly more active than the parent compound. All are concentrated in parasitized erythrocytes where they decompose, releasing free radicals, which are thought to be damaging to parasitic membranes. Artemisinin compounds act more rapidly than other antimalarial agents, stopping parasite development and preventing cytoadherence in falciparum malaria. Although depression of reticulocyte counts has been noted, these agents appear significantly less toxic than quinoline antimalarials. As there is some evidence that they may possess teratogenic properties, they should not be used in pregnancy. Importantly, they may be given orally, by rectal suppository and parenterally. Relapses can occur unless they are given for several days or combined with a second agent such as mefloquine or tetracycline.

Plant derivative active against malaria, amebas, and *Schistosoma*

Concentrated in parasitized erythrocytes

### Nitroimidazoles

Metronidazole, a nitroimidazole, was introduced in 1959 for the treatment of trichomoniasis. Subsequently, it was found to be effective in the management of giardiasis, amebiasis, and a variety of infections produced by obligate anaerobic bacteria. Energy metabolism in all of them depends on the presence of low-redox-potential compounds, such as ferredoxin, to serve as electron carriers. These compounds reduce the 5-nitro group of the imidazoles to produce intermediate products responsible for the death of the protozoal and bacterial cells, possibly by alkylation of DNA. Resistance, although uncommon, has been noted in strains of *Trichomonas vaginalis* lacking nitroreductase activity. Of greater concern is in vitro evidence of mutagenicity. Metronidazole is the drug of choice for trichomoniasis and

Active against protozoa at low redox potential

invasive amebiasis. It is effective in giardiasis although not yet approved by Food and Drug Administration for use in this infection. Tinidazole, a newer nitroimidazole not yet available in the United States, appears to be both a more effective and less mutagenic antiprotozoal agent.

## Benzimidazoles

Broad-spectrum anti-helminthics

As the name **benzimidazole** implies, the basic structure of these antiparasitic agents consists of linked imidazole and benzene rings. Unlike their antiprotozoal cousins discussed above, the benzimidazoles are broad-spectrum anthelmintic agents. The prototype drug, thiabendazole, acts against both adult and larval nematodes and was shown to be useful in the management of cutaneous larva migrans, trichinosis, and most intestinal nematode infections soon after its introduction in the early 1960s. The mechanism by which it exerts its anthelmintic action is uncertain. It is known to inhibit fumarate reductase, an important mitochondrial enzyme of helminths. The primary mode of action, however, may derive from the known capacity of all benzimidazoles to inhibit the polymerization of tubulin, the eukaryotic cytoskeletal protein, as described for mebendazole below. Side effects are mild, related to the gastrointestinal tract or liver, and rapidly disappear with the discontinuation of the drug. Hypersensitivity reactions, induced either by the drug or by antigens released from the damaged parasite, may occur.

Inhibit helminth fumarate reductase

Mebendazole, a carbamate benzimidazole introduced in 1972, has a spectrum similar to that of thiabendazole, but also has been found to be effective against a number of cestodes including *Taenia, Hymenolepsis,* and *Echinococcus*. It irreversibly blocks glucose uptake of both adult and larval worms, resulting in glycogen depletion, cessation of ATP formation, and paralysis or death. It does not appear to affect glucose metabolism in humans and is thought to exert its effect in worms by binding to tubulin, thus interfering with the assembly of cytoplasmic microtubules, structures essential to glucose uptake. Unlike thiabendazole, the drug is not well absorbed from the gastrointestinal tract and may owe part of its effectiveness against intestine-dwelling adult worms to its high concentrations in the gut. Toxicity is uncommon. Teratogenic effects have been observed in experimental animals; its use in infants and pregnant women is contraindicated.

Mebendazole blocks glucose uptake by adult and larval worms

Interferes with tubulin, cytoplasmic microtubules

Albendazole is a new benzimidazole carbamate, available in the United States only from the manufacturer. It has a somewhat broader spectrum than that of its close relative, mebendazole, being more active against *Strongyloides stercoralis* and several tissue nematodes. In addition to the vermicidal and larvicidal properties that it shares with other benzimidazoles, it is ovicidal, enhancing its effectiveness in tissue cestode infections such as echinococciasis and cysticercosis. Its activity against *Giardia,* one of the most common intestinal protozoa, makes it an appealing candidate for the treatment of polyparasitism. Although it shares the teratogenic potential of other benzimidazoles, it is otherwise extremely well tolerated. Single-dose therapy is effective in the management of many intestinal nematode infections.

Albendazole broader spectrum agent

## Avermectins

Avermectins are macrocyclic lactones produced as fermentation products of *Streptomyces avermitilis*. Structurally similar to the macrolide antibiotics, they are effective at extremely low concentration against a wide variety of nematodes and arthropods. The avermectins appear to induce neuromuscular paralysis by acting on a receptor of the parasites' peripheral neurotransmitter, γ-aminobutyric acid (GABA). In mammals, GABA is confined to the central nervous system, and as the avermectins do not cross the blood–brain barrier in significant concentration, they do not appear to produce significant untoward effects in the mammalian host. Ivermectin, a derivative of avermectin B1, is currently the drug of choice for the treatment of onchocerciasis. It is undergoing evaluation for the treatment of human filariasis. Its usefulness in other parasitic infections of humans remains to be established.

Antibiotics that influence nematode's neurotransmitter

Activity against filariae

## Praziquantel

Praziquantel, a heterocyclic pyrazinoisoquinoline, is an important new anthelmintic effective against a broad range of cestodes and trematodes, many of which had been poorly responsive to previously available agents. It is rapidly taken up by susceptible helminths in which it appears to induce the loss of intracellular calcium, tetanic muscular contrac-

Causes loss of intracellular calcium in cestodes and trematodes

tion, and destruction of the tegument. Its differential toxicity may be related to the inability of susceptible worms to metabolize the drug. Aside from transient, mild gastrointestinal symptoms, praziquantel appears remarkably free of side effects in humans. It is currently the drug of choice for the treatment of schistosomiasis, clonorchiasis, opisthorchiasis, and neurocysticercosis. Good activity has been demonstrated against other common trematode and cestode infections. Its effectiveness is in a single dose. Its high level of safety suggests this agent may well play a significant role in worldwide mass therapy campaigns.

Safety recommends for mass therapy campaign

### Eflornithine (Difluoromethylornithine)

Eflornithine is a specific, enzyme-activated, irreversible inhibitor of ornithine decarboxylase (ODC). In mammalian cells, decarboxylation of ornithine by ODC is a mandatory step in the synthesis of polyamines, compounds thought to play critical roles in cell division and differentiation. Originally developed as an antineoplastic agent, eflornithine proved ineffective in cancer chemotherapy trials.

Originally anticancer drug

With the discovery that polyamines of *Trypansoma* species were also synthesized from ornithine, eflornithine was successfully tested in the treatment of animal trypanosomiasis. Host survival was high and associated with decreases in parasitic polyamines and inhibition of nucleic acid synthesis. In the dosage required to treat trypanosomiasis, mammals tolerated the agent well, presumably because *Trypanosoma brucei* is 100 times more sensitive to the effects of eflornithine than are mammalian cells. Eflornithine appears to be cystostatic and requires an intact host immune system for maximum effect.

Active against trypanosomes

### Other Antiparasitic Agents

A number of antiparasitic agents used in therapy, their properties, and their clinical uses are listed in Appendix 51–1.

## Control

The control of diseases spread by the fecal–oral route depends on the improvements in personal hygiene and sanitation that accompany general economic development. In contrast, efforts at preventing the spread of multihost parasites is usually focused on the simultaneous treatment of infected humans and control or elimination of the nonhuman host.

Epidemiological control in developing countries complex

To be effective, such measures must be applied in a comprehensive and coordinated manner over large areas. Administrative problems, political imbroglios, development of resistance in parasites and intermediate hosts, technical difficulties, and funding shortages have, individually and together, limited the success of such efforts. A case in point was the failure of the worldwide malaria eradication effort launched by the World Health Organization in 1955. This has refocused attention on alternative control measures, including immunization. Until recently, the development of effective parasitic vaccines has been constrained by the complexities of their immunologic interactions with the human host. Monoclonal antibodies have helped to identify antigens responsible for the induction of immunity to a number of parasitic infections, including malaria, leishmaniasis, and schistosomiasis. The subsequent cloning of the structural genes encoding such antigens has made a large-scale production of vaccine antigen feasible. It is further possible that the entire step of antigen production and purification could be bypassed by the use of synthetic peptide or anti-idiotype vaccines. All these approaches are currently being developed. Malaria vaccines are undergoing clinical trials.

Vaccine development using cloned antigens or synthesized peptides in development

## ADDITIONAL READING

Campbell WC, Rew RS, eds. *Chemotherapy of Parasitic Diseases*. New York: Plenum; 1986. The most recent comprehensive publication on this subject.

Desowitz RS. *New Guinea Tapeworms and Jewish Grandmothers: Tales of Parasites and Peoples*. New York: Norton; 1981. A delightful look at the host–parasite relationship.

*Handbook of Antimicrobial Therapy*. New Rochelle, NY: The Medical Letter; 1988. Includes a synoptic review of antiparasitic therapy.

Horton RJ, Benzimidazole anthelmintics. *Parasitol Today*. 1990;6:105–136. The best recent review of this important group of chemotherapeutic agents.
Maddison SE. Serodiagnosis of parasitic diseases. *Clin Microbiol Rev*. 1991;4:457–469. A short but comprehensive review of current antibody and antigen detection procedures, use of monoclonal antibodies in serodiagnosis, molecular biological technology, and skin tests for parasitic diseases.
Stoll NR. This wormy world. *J Parasitol*. 1947;33:1–18.
Warren KS, ed. *Immunology and Molecular Biology of Parasitic Infections*. 3rd ed. Boston: Blackwell Scientific; 1993. This relatively comprehensive monograph discusses general immune responses to parasitic infections as well as the immunity, immunopathology, immunodiagnosis, and molecular biology of specific parasitic diseases.

## APPENDIX 51–1. MISCELLANEOUS ANTIPARASITIC AGENTS

| Compound | Drug Class | Route | Mechanism of Action | Clinical Use | Comments |
|---|---|---|---|---|---|
| Bithionol | Phenol | Oral | Uncouples phosphorylation | Paragonimiasis | Not commercially available in United States |
| Diethylcarbamazine | Piperazine | Oral | Neuromuscular paralysis | Filarial infections | Allergic reactions to filarial antigens |
| Difluoromethylornithine (DFMO) | Ornithine analog | Oral | Inhibits ornithine decarboxylase | African trypanosomiasis | Effective in central nervous system disease |
| Diloxanide furoate | Acetanilide | Oral | Unknown | Intestinal amebiasis | Used only for asymptomatic carriers |
| Iodoquinol (diiodohydroxyquin) | Halogenated quinoline | Oral | Unknown | Intestinal amebiasis; *Dientamoeba* infections | Related drug has caused optic atrophy |
| Niclosamide | Phenol | Oral | Uncouples phosphorylation | Intestinal tapeworms | Does not kill eggs |
| Nifurtimox | Nitrofuran | Oral | Alkylates DNA | Acute Chagas' disease | Toxic, therapy prolonged, effectiveness marginal |
| Pentamidine | Diamidine | IV | Binds DNA | Pneumocystosis, leishmaniasis; trypanosomiasis | Toxic |
| Pyrantel pamoate | Tetrahydropyrimidine | Oral | Neuromuscular blockade; inhibits fumarate reductase | Pinworm infection; hookworm infection; ascariasis | Single-dose therapy |
| Suramin | Sulfated naphthylamine | IV | Inhibits a glycerophosphate oxidase and dehydrogenase | African trypanosomiasis; onchocerciasis | Not effective in central nervous system disease; renal toxic |

Chapter 52

# Sporozoa

James J. Plorde

Sporozoa are a unique class of intracellular protozoa distinguished by their alternating cycles of sexual and asexual reproduction. Asexual multiplication occurs by a process of multiple fission termed schizogony. In it, the nucleus of a trophozoite divides into several parts, forming a multinucleated schizont. Cytoplasm then condenses around each nuclear portion to form new daughter cells, or merozoites, which burst from their intracellular location to invade new host cells. After the completion of one or more of these asexual cycles, some merozoites differentiate into male and female gametocytes, initiating the cycle of sexual reproduction known as sporogony. The gametocytes mature and effect fertilization, forming a zygote. Upon encysting, the zygote is known as an oocyst. Sporozoites formed within the oocyst are released, penetrate host tissue cells, and begin another asexual cycle as trophozoites.

Intracellular protozoa with alternating sexual and asexual cycles

Two sporozoan infections, malaria and toxoplasmosis, are common diseases of humans; together, they affect more than one third of the world's population and kill or deform perhaps a million neonates and children each year. A third infection, cryptosporidiosis, has only recently been found to be an important cause of diarrhea, particularly in immunocompromised hosts.

Cause malaria, toxoplasmosis, and cryptosporidiosis

## PLASMODIA

> "Of all infectious diseases there is no doubt that malaria has caused the greatest harm to the greatest number." (Laderman, 1975)

### The Malarial Parasites

#### Definition

The plasmodia are sporozoa in which the sexual and asexual cycles of reproduction are completed in different host species. The sexual phase occurs within the gut of mosquitoes. These arthropods subsequently transmit the parasite while feeding upon a vertebrate host. Within the red cells of the vertebrate, the plasmodia reproduce asexually; they eventually burst from the erythrocyte and invade other uninvolved red cells. This event produces periodic fever and anemia in the host, a disease process known as malaria. Of the many species of plasmodia, four are known to infect humans and will be considered here: *Plasmodium vivax*, *P. ovale*, *P. malariae*, and *P. falciparum*.

Sexual phase in mosquito and asexual phase in humans

Species of malarial parasites infect humans

#### Morphology

The morphology of the stained intraerythrocytic parasites is shown in Figure 52–1. In stained smears, three characteristic features aid in the identification of plasmodia: red nu-

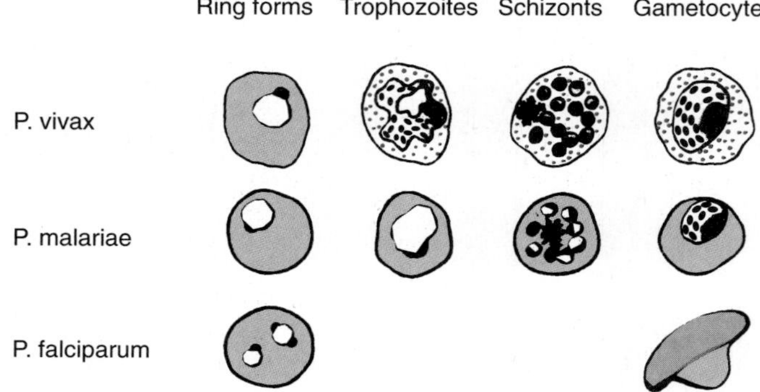


**Figure 52–1.** Examples of erythrocytic stages of malarial parasites. *Note:* Trophozoite and schizont forms of *Plasmodium falciparum* occur in visceral capillaries rather than in blood. Male and female gametocytes show distinctive morphological differences.

clear chromatin, blue cytoplasm, and brownish-black malarial pigment, or hemozoin, consisting largely of a hemoglobin degradation product, ferriprotoporphyrin IX. The change in the shape of the cytoplasm and the division of the chromatin at different stages of parasite development are obvious. Gametocytes can be differentiated from the asexual forms by their large size and lack of nuclear division. Some of the infected erythrocytes develop membrane invaginations or caveolae-vesicle complexes, which are thought to be responsible for the appearance of the pink Schüffner's dots or granules (see below).

Morphology of the parasite and the infected RBC vary by stage and species

The appearance of each of the four species of plasmodia that infect humans is sufficiently different to allow their differentiation in stained smears. The parasitized erythrocyte in *P. vivax* and *P. ovale* infections is pale, enlarged, and contains numerous Schüffner's dots. All asexual stages (trophozoite, schizont, merozoite) may be seen simultaneously. Cells infected by *P. ovale* are elongated and frequently irregular or fimbriated in appearance. In *P. malariae* infections, the red cells are not enlarged and contain no granules. The trophozoites often present as "band" forms, and the merozoites are arranged in rosettes around a clump of central pigment. In *P. falciparum* infections, the rings are very small and may contain two rather than a single chromatin dot. There is often more than a single parasite per cell, and parasites are frequently seen lying against the margin of the cell. Intracytoplasmic granules known as Maurer's dots may be present, but are often cleft shaped and fewer in number than Schüffner's dots. Schizonts and merozoites are not present in the peripheral blood. Gametocytes are large and banana shaped. These characteristics are summarized in Table 52–1.

Morphologic differences are the primary means of diagnosis

## Life Cycle of Malarial Parasites

Mosquito ingests gametocytes from blood of infected human

Sporogony, or the sexual cycle, begins when a female mosquito of the genus *Anopheles* ingests circulating male and female gametocytes while feeding upon a malarious human. In the gut of the mosquito, the gametocytes mature and effect fertilization. The resulting zy-

**TABLE 52–1. DIFFERENTIAL CHARACTERISTICS OF *PLASMODIUM* SPECIES**

| Characteristics | *P. vivax* | *P. ovale* | *P. malariae* | *P. falciparum* |
|---|---|---|---|---|
| Erythrocyte | | | | |
| Enlarged, pale | + | + | – | – |
| Oval, fimbriated | – | + | – | – |
| Schüffner's dots | + | + | – | – |
| Maurer's dots | – | – | – | + |
| Parasite | | | | |
| All asexual stages seen | + | + | + | – |
| Band forms | – | – | + | – |
| Double infections | – | – | – | + |
| Double chromatin dots | – | – | – | + |
| Banana-shaped gametocytes | – | – | – | + |

gote penetrates the mosquito's gut wall, lodges beneath the basement membrane, and vacuolates to form an oocyst. Within this structure thousands of sporozoites are formed. The enlarging cyst eventually ruptures, releasing the sporozoites into the body cavity of the mosquito. Some penetrate the salivary glands, rendering the mosquito infectious for humans. The time required for the completion of the cycle in mosquitoes varies from 1 to 3 weeks, depending upon the species of insect and parasite as well as on the ambient temperature and humidity.

Sporozoites from oocyst reach mosquito salivary glands

Schizogony, the asexual cycle, occurs in the human and begins when the infected *Anopheles* takes a blood meal from another individual. Sporozoites from the mosquito's salivary glands are injected into the human's subcutaneous capillaries and circulate in the peripheral blood. Within 1 hour they attach to and invade liver cells (hepatocytes), a process thought to be mediated by a ligand present in the sporozoites' outer protein coat (circumsporozoite protein). In *P. vivax* and *P. ovale* infections, some of the sporozoites enter a dormant state immediately after cell invasion. The remaining sporozoites initiate exoerythrocytic schizogony, each producing about 2000 to 40,000 daughter cells, or merozoites. One to two weeks later, the infected hepatocytes rupture, releasing merozoites into the general circulation.

Humans infected by mosquito bite

Rapid infection of hepatocytes starts asexual cycle in humans

The erythrocytic phase of malaria starts with the attachment of a released hepatic merozoite to a specific receptor on the red cell surface. After attachment, the merozoite invaginates the cell membrane and is slowly endocytosed. The intracellular parasite initially appears as a ring-shaped trophozoite, which enlarges and becomes more active and irregular in outline. Within a few hours, nuclear division occurs, producing the multinucleated schizont. Cytoplasm eventually condenses around each nucleus of the schizont to form an intraerythrocytic cluster of 6 to 24 merozoite daughter cells. About 48 (*P. vivax*, *P. ovale*, and *P. falciparum*) to 72 (*P. malariae*) hours after initial invasion, infected erythrocytes rupture, releasing the merozoites and producing the first clinical manifestations of disease. The newly released daughter cells invade other red cells, where most repeat the asexual cycle. Other daughter cells are transformed into sexual forms or gametocytes. These latter forms do not produce red cell lysis, and continue to circulate in the peripheral vasculature until ingested by an appropriate mosquito. The recurring asexual cycles continue, involving an ever-increasing number of erythrocytes until finally the development of host immunity brings the erythrocytic cycle to a close. The dormant hepatic sporozoites of *P. vivax* and *P. ovale* survive the host's immunologic attack, and may, after a latent period of months to years, resume intrahepatic multiplication. This leads to a second release of hepatic merozoites and the initiation of another erythrocytic cycle, a phenomenon known as relapse. The life cycle of malarial parasites is summarized in Figure 52–2.

Erythrocytic cycle begins with merozoite attachment to RBC receptor

Trophozoites multiply in RBC cytoplasm to form new merozoites

In 48–72 hours, RBCs rupture and reinfect new cells

Mosquito ingests gametocytes, which circulate without lysis of RBC

Intrahepatic dormancy causes relapses with *P. vivax* and *P. ovale*

## Physiology

Species of plasmodia differ significantly in their ability to invade subpopulations of erythrocytes; *P. vivax* and *P. ovale* attack only immature cells (reticulocytes), whereas *P. malariae* attacks only senescent cells. During infection with these species, therefore, no more than 1 to 2% of the cell population is involved. *P. falciparum,* in contrast, invades red cells regardless of age and may produce very high levels of parasitemia and particularly serious disease. In part, these differences may be related to the known differences in the red cell receptor sites available to the individual *Plasmodium* species. In the case of *P. vivax,* the site is closely related to the Duffy blood group antigens ($Fy^a$ and $Fy^b$). Duffy-negative individuals, who constitute the majority of people of West African ancestry, are therefore resistant to vivax malaria. Red cell sialoglycoprotein, particularly glycoprotein A, has been implicated as the *P. falciparum* receptor site.

Parasites vary in ability to attack subpopulations of erythrocytes

RBC Duffy antigen, glycoprotein A are RBC receptors

Certain red cell abnormalities may also effect parasitism. The altered hemoglobin (hemoglobin S) associated with the sickle-cell trait limits the intensity of the parasitemia caused by *P. falciparum* and thereby provides a selective advantage to individuals who are heterozygous for the sickle-cell gene. As a result, the sickle-cell gene, which would otherwise be disadvantageous, is found at high frequency in populations living in malarious areas. The mechanism of the increased resistance is uncertain. Parasite growth appears to be retarded in red cells heterozygous for hemoglobin S (SA) when they are exposed to conditions of reduced oxygen tension such as might be present in the visceral capillaries; the mechanism appears to involve potassium leakage from the involved erythrocytes. Sickling may also

Sickle cell trait limits intensity of *P. falciparum* infection

May retard parasite growth under reduced oxygen

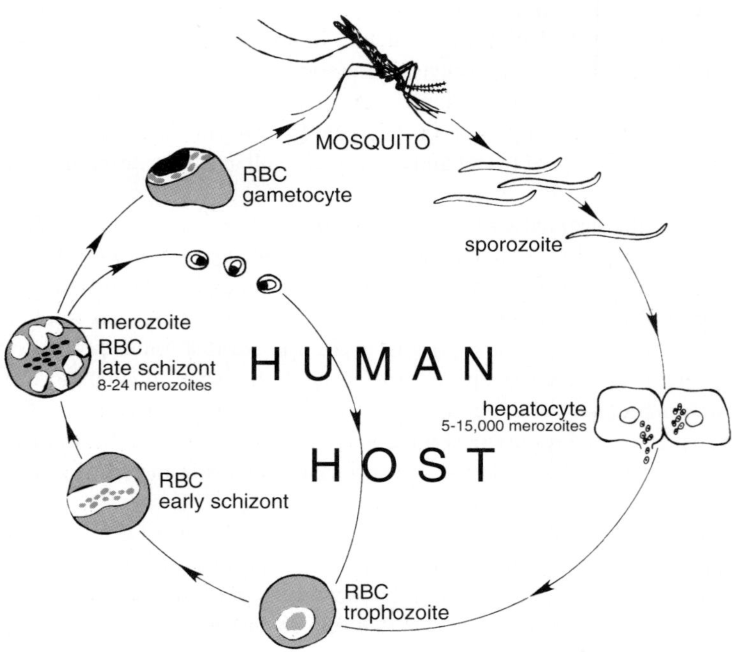


**Figure 52–2.** Life cycle of the malarial parasite.

render the erythrocyte more susceptible to phagocytosis or directly damage the parasite. A similar protective effect may be exerted by hemoglobins C, D, and E; thalassemia; and glucose-6-phosphate dehydrogenase (G6PD) or pyridoxal kinase deficiencies, as these abnormalities have also been found more frequently in malarious areas. The protection in these conditions may be related to the increased susceptibility of such red cells to oxidant stress. In thalassemia, the protection may also be related in part to the production of fetal hemoglobin, which retards maturation of *P. falciparum*, as well as an increased binding of antibodies to modified parasitic antigens (neoantigens) presenting on the erythrocytes' surface.

Other hemoglobin abnormalities in malarious areas

Once invasion has occurred, malaria parasites may induce a number of changes in the erythrocytic membrane. These include alteration of its lipid concentration, modification of its osmotic properties, and incorporation of parasitic neoantigens, rendering the red cell susceptible to immunologic attack. *P. vivax* and *P. ovale* stimulate the production of caveolae-vesicle complexes, which are visualized as Shüffner's dots in stained smears. In *P. falciparum* infections, electron-dense elevated knobs or excrescences form on the surface. These outgrowths have been shown to mediate binding to recognition glycoproteins expressed on the endothelium of capillaries and postcapillary venules. This suggests the knobs play a role in the known tendency of *P. falciparum*-infected cells to sequester in the capillaries of the deep organs, where they can produce obstruction and microinfarcts.

Changes induced in erythrocyte membrane

Binding to endothelium may cause microinfarcts

Malarial parasites generate energy by the anaerobic metabolism of glucose. They appear to satisfy their protein requirements by the degradation of hemoglobin within their acidic food vacuoles, resulting in the formation of the malarial pigment (hemozoin) mentioned previously. It has been estimated that the average plasmodium destroys between 25 and 75% of the hemoglobin of its host erythrocyte. Unlike their vertebrate hosts, malarial parasites synthesize folates de novo. As a result, antifolate antimicrobics such as pyrimethamine are effective antimalarious agents.

Malarial parasites metabolize anaerobically, synthesize their own folate

## Growth in the Laboratory

Continuous in vitro cultivation of plasmodia in human erythrocytes was first achieved in 1976. More recently, the successful in vitro completion of the entire sporogonic cycle, from ookinete to sporozoite, has been achieved. These twin developments provide new opportunities for studying the biology, immunology, and chemotherapy of human malaria. The most immediate impact of these advances has been on the introduction of methods for testing the sensitivity of *P. falciparum* to chemotherapeutic agents. Ulitmately, they will play critical roles in the development of effective antimalarial vaccines.

## Malaria

### Epidemiology

Malaria has a worldwide distribution between 45°N and 40°S latitude, generally at altitudes below 1800 m. *P. vivax* is the most widely distributed of the four species, and together with the uncommon *P. malariae*, is found primarily in temperate and subtropical areas. *P. falciparum* is the dominant organism of the tropics. *P. ovale* is rare and found principally in Africa.

Distribution in tropical areas worldwide

The intensity of malarial transmission in an endemic area depends upon the density and feeding habits of suitable mosquito vectors and the prevalence of infected humans, who serve as parasite reservoirs. In hyperendemic areas (areas where more than half of the population is parasitemic), transmission is usually constant, and disease manifestations are moderated by the development of immunity. Mortality is largely restricted to infants and to nonimmune adults who migrate into the region. When the prevalence of disease is lower, transmission is typically intermittent. In this situation, solid immunity does not develop and the population suffers repeated, often seasonal, epidemics, the impact of which is shared by people of all ages.

Intensity depends on prevalence and mosquito feeding habits

Clinical manifestations muted with hyperendemicity

At the present time, malaria infects between 200 and 300 million inhabitants of 104 countries throughout Africa, Asia, Latin America, and Oceania (Fig 52–3). One million children, primarily Africans, die of the disease each year. Although endemic malaria disappeared from the United States three decades ago, imported cases continue to be reported, and the recent worldwide resurgence of malaria combined with an increase in international travel has resulted in an increase in the US number of cases to approximately 1000 annually. Forty-five percent of patients with imported malaria have acquired the disease in Africa, 30% in Asia, and 10% in the Caribbean or Latin America. Half of recent infections have involved American travelers: nearly 60% of these acquired their infection in Africa. Clinical manifestations typically develop within 6 months of arrival of cases in the United States; however, one fourth of cases caused by *P. vivax* are delayed beyond that time. Approximately 40% of imported cases and almost all associated fatalities have been caused by the

Malaria kills a million children each year

Imported malaria may have onsets months after travel

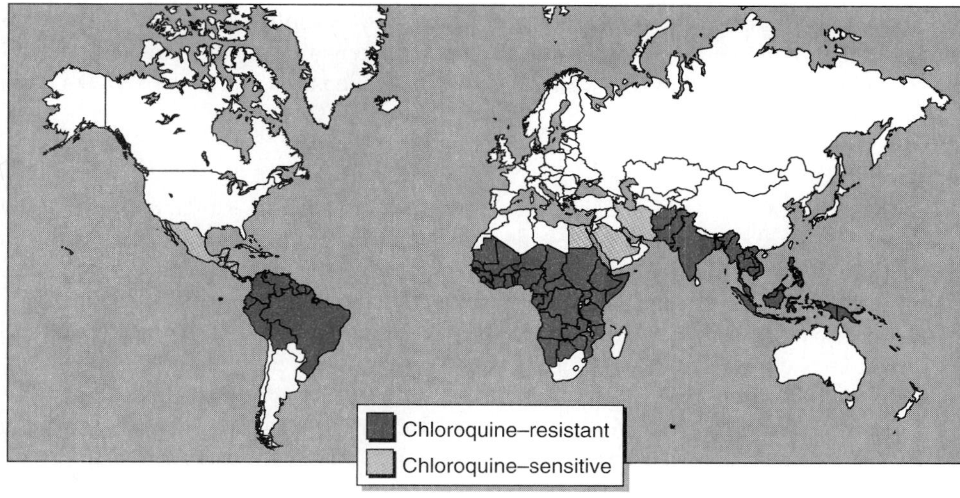


**Figure 52–3.** This map of malarious areas of the world from the Centers for Disease Control shows the few remaining regions in the world (pink) where, as of 1990, chloroquine resistance of *P. falciparum* was not a problem. In all other areas (red) where *P. falciparum* malaria is transmitted, chloroquine-resistant strains exist, and infections due to them require alternative antimalarial drugs for treatment. (*From Wyler DJ. Malaria: Overview and update.* Clin Infect Dis *1993;16(4):454, with permission.*)

Imported fatalities due to *P. falciparum*

virulent *P. falciparum*. Tragically, most of these cases could have been prevented or successfully treated. Congenital malaria in infants born in the United States of mothers from malarious areas is occasionally observed. Infections transmitted by transfusions of whole blood, leukocytes, or platelets, or by organ transplantation are, fortunately, now unusual in this country due to the improved screening procedures of blood banks.

## Pathogenesis and Pathology

The fever, anemia, circulatory changes, and immunopathologic phenomena characteristic of malaria are all the result of erythrocytic invasion by the plasmodia.

### Fever

Fever associated with red cell rupture

Fever, the hallmark of malaria, appears to be initiated by the process of red cell rupture that leads to the liberation of a new generation of merozoites (sporulation). To date all attempts to detect the factor(s) mediating the fever have been unsuccessful. It is possible that parasite-derived pyrogens are released at the time of sporulation; alternatively, the fever might result from the release of interleukin-1 (IL-1) and/or tumor necrosis factor (TNF) from macrophages involved in the ingestion of parasitic or erythrocytic debris. Early in malaria, red cells appear to be infected with malarial parasites at several different stages of development, each inducing sporulation at a different time. The resulting fever is irregular and hectic. Eventually one population dominates, sporulation is synchronized, and fever occurs in distinct paroxysms at 48-hour or, in the case of *P. malariae*, 72-hour intervals.

Synchronization of sporulation gives cyclic fever

### Anemia

Destruction of normal and parasitized erythrocytes contributes

Parasitized erythrocytes are phagocytosed by a stimulated reticuloendothelial system or are destroyed at the time of sporulation. At times, the anemia is disproportionate to the degree of parasitism. Depression of marrow function, sequestration of erythrocytes within the enlarging spleen, and accelerated clearance of nonparasitized cells all appear to contribute to the anemia. The mechanisms responsible for the latter are unclear. Intravascular hemolysis, although uncommon, may occur, particularly in falciparum malaria. When hemolysis is massive, hemoglobinuria develops, resulting in the production of dark urine. This process in conjunction with malaria is known as **blackwater fever.**

Intravascular hemolysis causes blackwater fever

### Circulatory Changes

Blood flow decreased to vital organs

The high fever results in significant vasodilatation. In falciparum malaria, vasodilatation leads to a decrease in the effective circulating blood volume and hypotension, which may be aggravated by other changes in the small vessels and capillaries. The intense parasitemias this organism is capable of producing and the adhesion of infected red cells to the endothelium of visceral capillaries can impair the microcirculation and precipitate tissue hypoxia, lactic acidosis, and hypoglycemia. Although all deep tissues are involved, the brain is the most intensely affected.

### Cytokines

Elevated levels of IL-1 and TNF are consistently found in patients with malaria. Probably released at the time of sporulation, these proteins are certainly an essential part of the host's immune response to malaria (see below). By modulating the effects of endothelial cells, macrophages, monocytes, and neutrophils, they may play an important role in the destruction of the invading parasite. However, TNF levels increase with parasite density and high concentrations appear harmful. As TNF has been shown to cause up-regulation of endothelial adhesion molecules, high concentrations might precipitate cerebral malaria by increasing the sequestration of *P. falciparum*-parasitized erythrocytes in the cerebral vascular endothelium. Alternatively, excessive TNF levels might precipitate cerebral malaria by directly inducing hypoglycemia and lactic acidosis.

Elevated cytokine levels may cause injury

### Other Pathogenic Phenomena

Thrombocytopenia and nephritis common

Thrombocytopenia is common in malaria and appears to be related to both splenic pooling and a shortened platelet lifespan. Both direct parasitic invasion and immune mechanisms may be responsible. There may be an acute transient glomerulonephritis in falciparum malaria and progressive renal disease in chronic *P. malariae* malaria. These phenomena probably result from the host immune response, with deposition of immune complexes in the glomeruli.

### Immunity

Once infected, the host quickly mounts an immunologic response that typically limits parasite multiplication and moderates the clinical manifestations of disease. There follows a prolonged recovery period marked by recurrent exacerbations in both symptoms and number of erythrocytic parasites. With time, the recrudescences become less severe and less frequent, eventually stopping altogether.

The exact mechanisms involved in this recovery are uncertain. In simian and probably in human malaria, recovery is known to require the presence of both T and B lymphocytes. It is probable that the T lymphocytes act partially through their helper effect on antibody production. Some authorities have suggested that they also play a direct role through lymphokine production by stimulating effector cells to release nonspecific factors capable of inhibiting intraerythrocytic multiplication. The B lymphocytes begin production of stage- and strain-specific antiplasmodial antibodies within the first 2 weeks of parasitemia. With the achievement of high levels of antibodies, the number of circulating parasites decreases. The infrequency with which malaria occurs in young infants has been attributed to the transplacental passage of such antibodies. It is uncertain whether they are directly lethal, act as opsonizing agents, or block merozoite invasion of red cells.

Cytokines may have direct role or through helper function

Antibody-mediated immunity clearly important

In simian malaria, the parasite can undergo antigenic variation and thereby escape the suppressive effect of the antibodies. This antigenic variation leads to cycles of recrudescent parasitemia, but ultimately to production of specific antibodies to the variants, and cure. It seems probable that similar changes occur in humans, leading to the eventual disappearance of erythrocytic parasites. With *P. falciparum* and *P. malariae*, which have no persistent hepatic forms, this results in cure. In the former, the disease typically does not exceed 1 year, but with *P. malariae* the erythrocytic infection can be extremely persistent, lasting in one case up to 53 years. How erythrocytic parasites circulating in numbers too small to be detected on routine blood films escape immunologic destruction remains a puzzle. In a closely related simian malaria, splenectomy results in rapid cure, suggesting that suppressor T lymphocytes in the spleen may play a protective role. In infection with *P. vivax* and *P. ovale*, latent hepatic infection may result in the discharge of fresh merozoites into the bloodstream after the disappearance of erythrocytic forms. This phenomenon, known as relapse, is capable of maintaining infection for 3 to 5 years.

Antigenic variation could play a role in persistence

Suppressor T lymphocytes in spleen may protect parasites

## Malaria: Clinical Aspects

### Clinical Manifestations

The incubation period between the bite of the mosquito and the onset of disease is approximately 2 weeks; that with *P. malariae* and with strains of *P. vivax* in temperate climates, however, is often more prolonged. Individuals who contract malaria while taking antimalarial suppressants may not experience illness for many months. In the United States, the interval between entry into the country and onset of disease exceeds 1 month in 25% of *P. falciparum* infections and 6 months in a similar proportion of *P. vivax* cases.

Incubation period prolonged by suppressant use

The clinical manifestations vary with the species of plasmodia, but typically include chills, fever, splenomegaly, and anemia. The hallmark of disease is the malarial paroxysm. This manifestation begins with a cold stage, which persists for 20 to 60 minutes. During this time, the patient experiences continuous rigors and feels cold. With the consequent increase in body temperature, the rigors cease and vasodilatation commences, ushering in a hot stage. The temperature continues to rise for 3 to 8 hours, reaching a maximum of 40 to 41.7°C (104 to 107°F) before it begins to fall. The wet stage consists of a decrease in fever and profuse sweating. It leaves the patient exhausted but otherwise well until the onset of the next paroxysm.

Malarial paroxysm: cold, hot, and wet stages

Typical paroxysms first appear in the second or third week of fever, when parasite sporulation becomes synchronized. In falciparum malaria, synchronization may never take place, and the fever may remain hectic and unpredictable. The first attack is often severe and may persist for weeks in the untreated patient. Eventually the paroxysms become less

Typical paroxysms after 2–3 weeks when sporulation is synchronized

regular, less frequent, and less severe. Symptoms finally cease with the disappearance of the parasites from the blood.

Cerebal malaria of *P. falciparum* may kill in 3 days

In falciparum malaria, capillary blockage can lead to several serious complications. When the central nervous system is involved (cerebral malaria), the patient may develop delirium, convulsions, paralysis, coma, and rapid death. Acute pulmonary insufficiency frequently accompanies cerebral malaria, killing about 80% of those involved. When splanchnic capillaries are involved, the patient may experience vomiting, abdominal pain, and diarrhea with or without bloody stools. Jaundice and acute renal failure are also common in severe illness. These pernicious syndromes generally appear when the intensity of parasitemia exceeds 100,000 organisms per cubic millimeter of blood. Most deaths occur within 3 days.

## Laboratory Diagnosis

Thick and thin blood smears detect parasites

Malarial parasites can be demonstrated in stained smears of the peripheral blood in virtually all symptomatic patients. Typically, capillary or venous blood is used to prepare both thin and thick smears, which are stained with Wright or Giemsa stain and examined for the presence of erythrocytic parasites. Thick smears, in which erythrocytes are lysed with water before staining, concentrate the parasites and allow detection of very mild parasitemia. Nonetheless, it may be necessary to obtain several specimens before parasites are seen. Artifacts are numerous in thick smears, and correct interpretation requires experience. The morphologic differences among the four species of plasmodia allow their speciation on the stained smear by the skilled observer.

Acridine orange may improve sensitivity of stains

A number of attempts have been made to improve on the standard thin and thick smear. One such procedure involves acridine orange staining of centrifuged parasites in quantitative buffy coat (QBC) tubes. Although it is expensive, requires a fluoroscence microscope, and permits less reliable parasite speciation, its rapidity and ease of use make it attractive to laboratories that are only occasionally called upon to identify patients with malaria. Deoxyribonucleic acid probes and antigen detection procedures have recently been described and may eventually play an important role in the diagnosis of malaria. Serologic tests for malaria are available, but are used primarily for epidemiologic purposes. They are occasionally helpful in speciation and detection of otherwise occult infections.

## Treatment

Need to destroy all forms of the parasite

The adequate treatment of malaria requires the destruction of three parasitic forms: the erythrocytic schizont, the hepatic schizont, and the erythrocytic gametocyte. The first terminates the clinical attack, the second prevents relapse, and the third renders the patient noninfectious to *Anopheles* and thus breaks the cycle of transmission. Unfortunately, no single drug accomplishes all three goals. The present strategy of chemotherapy is shown in Table 52–2.

### Termination of Acute Attack

Chloroquine inhibits hemoglobin degradation

Several agents can destroy asexual erythrocytic parasites. Chloroquine, a 4-aminoquinalone, is that most commonly used. It acts by inhibiting the degradation of hemoglobin, thereby

**TABLE 52–2. CHEMOTHERAPY OF MALARIA**

| Stage of Parasite | Clinical Goal | Drug |
|---|---|---|
| Erythrocytic schizont | Treat clinical attack | |
| | All species | Chloroquine |
| | CRFM | Quinine, antifolates, sulfonamides |
| | Suppress clinical attack | |
| | All species | Chloroquine |
| | CRFM | Antifolates, sulfonamides |
| Erythrocytic gametocyte | Prevent transmission | |
| | Relapsing malaria | Chloroquine |
| | Falciparum malaria | Primaquine |
| Hepatic schizont | Radical cure | |
| | Relapsing malaria | Primaquine |
| | Falciparum malaria | None required |

*Abbreviations:* CRFM, chloroquine-resistant falciparum malaria.

limiting the availability of amino acids necessary for growth. It has been suggested that the weak basic nature of chloroquine also acts to raise the pH of the food vacuoles of the parasite, inhibiting their acid proteases and effectiveness. When originally introduced it was rapidly effective against all four species of plasmodia and, in the dosage used, free of serious side effects.

All strains of *P. malariae*, *P. ovale*, and *P. vivax* (except a few acquired in the South Pacific) remain fully sensitive to chloroquine and should be treated with this agent. *P. vivax* infections acquired in New Guinea and Sumatra, however, should be assumed to be chloroquine-resistant and managed with mefloquine. Chloroquine-resistant strains of *P. falciparum* are now widespread; only strains acquired in Haiti, the Dominican Republic, Mexico, Central America, and the Middle East remain fully sensitive (Fig 52–3). Falciparum malaria acquired elsewhere must be treated with combinations of quinine/quinidine, antifolates, and sulfonamides. Pyrimethamine/sulfadoxine, mefloquine, halofantrine, or artemether, alone or in combination, may be more appropriate in certain circumstances.

Chloroquine resistance widespread for *P. falciparum*

Radical Cure

In *P. vivax* and *P. ovale* infections, hepatic schizonts persist and must be destroyed to prevent reseeding of circulating erythrocytes with consequent relapse. Primaquine, an 8-aminoquinalone, is used for this purpose. Some *P. vivax* infections acquired in Southeast Asia and New Guinea fail initial therapy due to relative resistance to this 8-aminoquinalone. Retreatment with a larger dose of primaquine is usually successful. Unfortunately, primiquine may induce hemolysis in patients with G6PD deficiency. Persons of Asian, African, and Mediterranean ancestry should thus be screened for this abnormality before treatment.

Primaquine used to destroy hepatic schizonts of *P. vivax* and *P. ovale*

Destruction of Circulating Gametocytes

Chloroquine destroys the gametocytes of *P. vivax, P. ovale,* and *P. malariae,* but not those of *P. falciparum.* Primaquine is, however, effective for this species.

## Prevention

Personal Protection

In endemic areas, mosquito contact can be minimized with the use of house screens, insecticide bombs within rooms, and/or insecticide-impregnated mosquito netting around beds. Those who must be outside from dusk to dawn, the period of mosquito feeding, should apply insect repellant and wear clothing with long sleeves and pants. In addition, it is possible to suppress clinical manifestations of infection, should they occur, with a weekly dose of chloroquine. In areas where chloroquine-resistant strains are common, an alternative schizonticidal agent should be used. Mefloquine or doxycycline are usually preferred. The antifolate pyrimethamine plus a sulfonamide can be taken as well. However, as use of this combination is occasionally accompanied by serious side effects, it is recommended only when mefloquine- and doxycycline-resistant strains are present in the area, and then only for individuals residing in areas of intense transmission for prolonged periods of time. On leaving an endemic area, it is necessary to eradicate residual hepatic parasites with primaquine before discontinuing suppressive therapy.

Mosquito protection with screens, repellants

Chemoprophylaxis must consider resistance in area

General

Malaria control measures are directed toward reducing the infected human and mosquito populations to below the critical level necessary for sustained transmission of disease. The techniques employed include those mentioned previously, treatment of febrile patients with effective antimalarial agents, chemical or physical disruption of mosquito breeding areas, and use of residual insecticide sprays. An active international cooperative program aimed at the eradication of malaria resulted in a dramatic decline in the incidence of the disease between 1956 and 1968. Eradication was not achieved, however, as mosquitoes became resistant to some of the chemical agents used, and today malaria still infects 200 to 300 million inhabitants of Africa, Latin America, and Asia. Tropical Africa alone accounts for 100 million of the afflicted and for most of the 1 million deaths that occur annually as a result of this disease. The long-term hope for progress in these areas now depends upon the development of new technologies.

Reduce human reservoir and eradicate mosquitos

Attempts at eradication have failed

VACCINES

Three advances in the last decade have brought the production of an effective malaria vaccine within reach of medical science for the first time. The establishment of a continuous in vitro culture system provided the large quantities of parasite needed for antigenic analysis. Development of the hybridoma technique allowed the preparation of monoclonal antibodies with which antigens responsible for the induction of protective immunity could be identified. Finally, recombinant DNA procedures enabled scientists to clone and sequence the genes encoding such antigens, permitting the amino acid structure to be determined and peptide sequences suitable for vaccine development to be identified.

Growth and molecular manipulation of malarial parasites in culture shows promise

As immunity to malaria is stage specific, the relative advantages and disadvantages of vaccines prepared against each of the plasmodial stages found in the human host (sporozoite, merozoite, and gametocyte) need to be considered. An effective sporozoite vaccine, by blocking the invasion of hepatocytes by mosquito-introduced sporozoites, would prevent the establishment of the infection within the host and, if widely administered, would interrupt parasite transmission within a community. However, to be effective, a sporozoite vaccine would have to prevent the invasion of all injected sporozoites. Theoretically, if even a single parasite reached and penetrated a liver cell, it would multiply intracellularly and later enter the bloodstream to invade erythrocytes. The patient could develop clinical disease and serve as a reservoir for subsequent transmission to others. A vaccine directed at the erythrocytic or merozoite stage, although preventing neither hepatic nor bloodstream infection, would limit the severity of the parasitemia and thus moderate or abort clinical manifestations of disease. Gametogenesis, and thus parasite transmission, would probably proceed unimpaired. Antibodies formed in response to a gametocyte vaccine might block the union of male and female gametes within the mosquito gut, interrupting parasite transmission. It would, however, neither prevent nor moderate malaria in the immunized patient. The limitations of each vaccine type has led some investigators to advocate the combination of all three in a single polyvalent preparation.

Sporozoite vaccine could help prevent initiation of infection

Erythrocytic stage vaccine could moderate disease

Gametocyte vaccine could prevent transmission

Work on a sporozoite vaccine to *P. falciparum* has been most intense. Natural immunity to this stage is induced by the circumsporozoite (CS) protein, a substance that covers the parasite surface. A major portion of the CS protein is conserved in all strains, and monoclonal antibodies prepared against it neutralize all sporozoite infectivity. Unfortunately, vaccines containing small peptide sequences within this conserved region have been poorly immunogenic. This suggests that an effective vaccine will require combinations of defined immunogens directed against several parts of the life cycle.

## TOXOPLASMA

Asexual and sexual cycles in felines

Like the plasmodia, *Toxoplasma gondii*, the cause of toxoplasmosis, is an obligate intracellular sporozoan. It differs from *Plasmodium* in that both sexual and asexual reproductive cycles occur within the gastrointestinal tract of felines, the definitive host. The disease is transmitted to other host species by the ingestion of oocysts passed in the feces of infected felines.

*Toxoplasma* can infect most warm-blooded animals, both domestic and wild; it is thus the most cosmopolitan of parasites. Approximately one half of the human population of the United States has been infected. In the overwhelming majority the infection is chronic, asymptomatic, and self-limiting. Clinical disease presents in three major forms: (1) self-limiting febrile lymphadenopathy, (2) highly lethal infection of immunocompromised patients, and (3) congenital infection of infants.

### ■ Toxoplasma gondii

#### Morphology

*T. gondii* was first demonstrated in 1908 in the gondi, an African rodent, by Nicolle and Marceaux. Its name, derived from the Greek toxo (arc), is based on the characteristic shape of the organism. All strains of this parasite appear to be closely related antigenically. The major morphologic forms of the parasite are the oocyst, trophozoite, and tissue cyst.

### OOCYST

The oocyst is ovoid, measures 10 to 12 μm in diameter, and possesses a thick wall that makes it resistant to most environmental challenges. It may be destroyed by heat in excess of 66°C and chemicals such as iodine and formalin. In its immature form, the center of the cyst lacks internal structure. With maturation two sporocysts appear, and later four sporozoites may be discerned within each sporocyst. Sporulation does not occur at temperatures below 4°C or above 37°C. This form is responsible for the spread of the parasites from felines to other warm-blooded animals via the fecal–oral route.

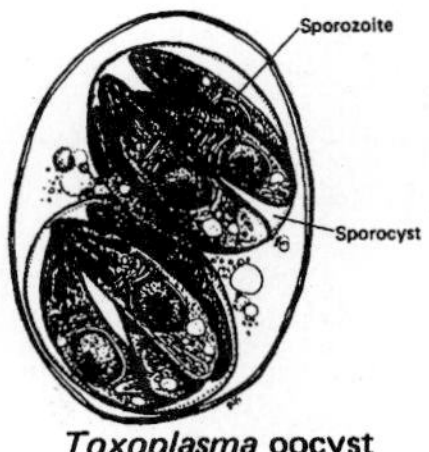


*Toxoplasma* oocyst

10 μm

### TACHYZOITE (TROPHOZOITE)

The term "trophozoite" is used in its broadest sense to refer to the asexual proliferative forms responsible for cell invasion. In different stages of the asexual cycle it is referred to by several other terms, including merozoites and tachyzoite. It is crescent or arc shaped, measures 3 by 7 μm, and can invade all nucleated cell types. Although tachyzoites are obligate intracellular organisms, they may survive extracellularly in a variety of body fluids for periods of hours to days. They cannot, however, survive the digestive activity of the stomach and therefore are not infective on ingestion.

Conoid
Rhoptry
Golgi apparatus
Nucleus
Mitochondrium

*Toxoplasma* tachyzoite (trophozoite)

3 μm

### TISSUE CYSTS

Cysts measure 10 to 200 μm in diameter. The contained organisms are similar to, but smaller than, trophozoites. Tissue cysts are resistant to digestive enzymes, and like oocysts, are infectious to the animal that ingests them. They survive normal refrigerator temperatures, but are killed by freezing and thawing and by normal cooking temperatures.

## Life Cycle

### DEFINITIVE HOST

Infection in cat ileal cells

Sexual reproduction of *T. gondii* occurs only in the intestinal tract of felines, most importantly in the domestic cat. Ingested parasites enter the epithelial cells of the ileum by mechanisms that remain poorly defined. Intracellularly, the trophozoites reside within a membrane-bound vacuole and undergo schizogony. With cell rupture, merozoites are released. The merozoites infect adjacent epithelial cells; they then repeat another asexual cycle or eventually differentiate into gametocytes, initiating sexual reproduction. Fusion of the mature male and female gametes leads to the formation of an oval, thick-walled oocyst that is then shed in the feces. In the typical infection, millions of these structures are released daily for 1 to 3 weeks. The oocysts are immature at the time of shedding and must complete sporulation in the external environment. In this process, two sporocysts, each containing four sporozoites, develop within each oocyst. The time required for sporulation varies from 1 day to 3 weeks, depending upon the ambient temperature and moisture. Once mature, the resistant oocyts may remain viable and infectious for as long as a year.

Fusion of gametes leads to oocyst formation; shed in feces

Sporulate in external environment

### INTERMEDIATE HOSTS

Mature oocysts infect hosts orally

Released sporozoites invade macrophages

After ingestion by a susceptible warm-blooded animal, sporozoites are released from the disrupted oocyst and enter macrophages. Within these cells they are transported through the lymphohematogenous system to all organ systems. Continued intracellular schizogony results in macrophage rupture and release of new parasites, which may invade any adjacent nucleated host cell and continue the asexual cycle. With the development of host immunity, many of the parasites are destroyed. Within the cells of certain organs, particularly the brain, heart, and skeletal muscle, the trophozoites produce a membrane that surrounds and protects them: within this tissue cyst, multiplication continues at a more leisurely pace. Eventually, cysts that measure up to 200 μm in diameter and contain more than a thousand organisms are produced. These cysts persist intact for the life of the host or rupture, producing parasitologic relapse. If they are ingested by a carnivore, they survive the digestive enzymes and initiate infection in the new host.

Cysts develop and persist for life

Infection from ingestion of cysts in meat

# Toxoplasmosis

## Epidemiology

PREVALENCE AND DISTRIBUTION

Worldwide distribution among mammals, birds

Toxoplasmosis is a cosmopolitan disease that occurs in almost all mammals and many birds. Human infections are found in every region of the globe; in general the incidence is higher in the tropics and lower in cold, arid regions. In the United States, the prevalence of positive serologic evidence for the disease increases with age. By adulthood, approximately 50% of Americans can be shown to have circulating antibodies against *T. gondii.*

TRANSMISSION

Although it is known that humans may acquire toxoplasmosis in a variety of ways, data on their relative frequency are both meager and conflicting. It is likely that the route of transmission varies from population to population, and perhaps from age to age, within any given area. The most important transmission mechanisms are discussed below.

Feline infections transmitted via feces

Increased hazard to children by close contact

**Ingestion of Oocysts.** Felinophobes are inclined to the view that the deposition of oocysts in the feces of cats and their subsequent ingestion by the unsuspecting owner is the most frequent way in which humans acquire this important infection. Disease epidemics associated with exposure to infected cats have been reported. Unfortunately, data from studies relating the frequency of feline exposure to the prevalence of positive serologic tests are conflicting. Acutely infected cats shed oocysts for only a few weeks. It has been shown, however, that chronically infected felines can occasionally reshed oocysts, and prevalence studies have demonstrated that 1% of domestic cats excrete oocysts at any given time. The large number of these structures passed during active shedding and their prolonged survival in the external environment greatly enhance their chance of transmission. Particularly at risk are individuals such as children at play, who may come in close contact with areas likely to be contaminated with cat feces, and adults responsible for changing a cat's litter box. It is also possible that insects can mechanically transfer oocysts to human food.

Cysts present in meat

Cysts killed by normal cooking

**Ingestion of Tissue Cysts.** Tissue cysts have been frequently demonstrated in meat produced for human consumption. They are most common in pork (25%) and mutton (10%), and less so in beef and chicken (less than 1%). Although such cysts are killed at normal (well-done) cooking temperatures, an impressive array of epidemiologic information links the handling and/or ingestion of raw or undercooked meat with serologic and, occasionally, clinical evidence of disease. Confounding these data is an Indian study that demonstrated no difference between meat eaters and vegetarians in the incidence of positive serologic tests.

Transplacental transmssion highest in 3rd trimester

**Congenital.** Approximately 1 of every 500 pregnant women acquires acute toxoplasmosis, and approximately 10 to 20% of the involved women become symptomatic. Regardless of the clinical status of the infected mother, the parasite involves the fetus in one third to one half of all acute maternal infections. The risk of transplacental transmission is independent of the clinical severity of the disease in the mother, but does correlate with the stage of gestation at which she is exposed. Fetal involvement occurs in 17% of first-trimester and 65% of third-trimester infections. Conversely, the earlier a fetal infection is acquired, the more severe it is likely to be. Overall, 20% of fetuses experienced severe consequences; a similar proportion develop mild disease. The remainder are asymptomatic.

Transmitted by blood and organ transplantation

**Miscellaneous.** In addition to causing congenital infection, trophozoites have been responsible for disease transmission in a number of other situations, including laboratory accidents, transfusions of whole blood and leukocytes, and organ transplantation. As trophozoites may survive for several hours in body fluids or exudates of acutely infected humans, it is possible for infection to occur after contact with such materials.

## Pathogenesis and Immunity

In the primary infection, the proliferation of trophozoites results in the death of involved host cells and the stimulation of a mononuclear inflammatory reaction. In immunodeficient hosts, rapid organism proliferation continues, producing numerous widespread foci of tissue necrosis. The consequences are most serious in organs such as the brain, where the potential for cell regeneration is limited.

Dissemination in immunosuppressed subjects

In normal hosts, however, acute infection is rapidly controlled with the development of humoral and cellular immunity. Extracellular parasites are destroyed, intracellular multiplication is hindered, and tissue cysts are formed. With the exception of lysis of extracellular parasites by antibody and complement, cell-mediated immunity appears to play the principal roll in this process, mediated in part by interleukin-2, interferon-γ, and cytotoxic T cells. Immunity appears to be lifelong, possibly because of survival of the parasite in the tissue cysts. The cysts, which are found most frequently in the brain, heart, and skeletal muscle, normally produce little or no tissue reaction. The suppression of cell-mediated immunity that accompanies serious illness, or the administration of immunosuppressive agents, may lead to the rupture of a cyst and the release of trophozoites. Their subsequent proliferation and the intense antibody reaction to their presence results in an acute exacerbation of the disease.

Immunity primarily cell-mediated

## Toxoplasmosis: Clinical Aspects

### Clinical Manifestations

In the vast majority of patients, infection with *T. gondii* is completely asymptomatic. Clinical manifestations, when they do appear, vary with the type of host involved. In general, they may be grouped into one of the three syndromes listed below.

#### Congenital Toxoplasmosis

Immune mechanisms are poorly developed in utero. As a result, a large proportion of fetal infections result in clinical illness. If the infection spreads to the central nervous system, the outcome is often catastrophic. Abortion and stillbirth are the most serious consequences. Liveborn children may demonstrate microcephaly, hydrocephaly, cerebral calcifications, convulsions, and psychomotor retardation. Disease of this severity is usually accompanied by evidence of visceral involvement, including fever, hepatitis, pneumonia, and skin rash. Infants infected later in prenatal development demonstrate milder disease. Many appear healthy at birth, but develop epilepsy, retardation, or strabismus months or years later. Probably the most common delayed manifestation of congenital toxoplasmosis is chorioretinitis. This condition, which is thought to result from the reactivation of latent tissue cysts, typically presents during the second or third decade of life as recurrent bouts of eye pain and loss of visual acuity. The lesions are usually bilateral but focal. If the retinal macula is not involved, vision improves as the inflammation subsides. This manifestation accounts for one quarter of all cases of granulomatous uveitis seen in the United States.

Infection in utero produces malformations, chorioretinitis, and stillbirth

#### Normal Host

The most common clinical manifestation of toxoplasmosis acquired after birth is asymptomatic localized lymphadenopathy. The cervical nodes are most frequently involved, but nontender enlargement of other regional groups, including the retroperitoneal nodes, also occurs. At times, the adenopathy is accompanied by fever, sore throat, rash, hepatosplenomegaly, and atypical lymphocytosis, thus mimicking the clinical and laboratory manifestations of infectious mononucleosis. Occasionally the normal host will develop severe visceral involvement, which may be manifested as meningoencephalitis, pneumonitis, myocarditis, or hepatitis. Chorioretinitis following postnatally acquired infection, although documented, is uncommon. Unlike congenitally acquired ocular disease, it occurs during midlife and is generally unilateral.

Fever and lymphadenopathy can mimic infectious mononucleosis

#### Immunocompromised Host

In the immunocompromised host, toxoplasmosis is a serious, often fatal disease. If primary infection is acquired while a patient is undergoing immunosuppressive therapy for malignancy or organ transplantation, widespread dissemination of the infection with necrotizing pneumonitis, myocarditis, and encephalitis may occur. More commonly, acute disease in this population results from the activation of chronic, latent infection by immunosuppres-

Primary infection or reactivation of latent infections produces severe widespread disease

sive therapy, or the acquisition of a concurrent immunosuppressive infection, particularly AIDS. Encephalitis occurs in 50% of such cases and in more than 90% of fatal cases. Toxoplasmic encephalitis is particularly common in AIDS patients, being seen in approximately 10% of those with circulating toxoplasma antibodies. As such, it is a major cause of morbidity and mortality in this patient population. Clinically, encephalitis may present as a meningoencephalitis, diffuse encephalopathy, or mass lesion.

AIDS patients develop encephalitis

## Laboratory Diagnosis

The diagnosis may be established by a variety of methods. In acute toxoplasmic lymphadenitis, the histologic appearance of the involved nodes is often pathognomonic. The trophozoite may be demonstrated in tissue with Wright or Giemsa stain. Electron microscopy and indirect fluorescent antibody techniques have also been used successfully on heart transplant or brain tissue obtained by biopsy. Although tissue cysts are selectively stained by periodic acid–Schiff, their presence is not indicative of acute disease. Isolation of the organism can be accomplished by inoculating blood or other body fluids into mice or tissue cultures. Inoculation of other tissues is not usually helpful, as a positive result may only reflect the presence of latent tissue cysts.

Demonstration of parasite in histopathologic specimens using special stains

Serologic procedures are the primary method of diagnosis. To establish the presence of acute infection, it is usual to demonstrate a fourfold rise in the IgG antibody titer between acute and convalescent serum specimens. As peak titers are often reached within 4 to 8 weeks, the acute serum must be collected early in the course of illness. Of the many tests developed for the detection of IgG antibodies, the indirect hemagglutination test and the indirect fluorescent antibody test are those most frequently used; they both are sensitive and highly specific. With these tests, titers of 1:1000 or more are usually detected after an acute infection. These levels gradually fall, but may remain high for many years.

Serodiagnosis is the primary approach

The detection of IgM antibodies provides a more rapid confirmation of acute infection. As detected by an indirect fluorescent antibody technique, these antibodies arise within the first week of infection, peak in 2 to 4 weeks, and quickly revert to negative. It also appears that IgM antibodies are produced after reactivation of latent disease. A single high titer (1:80 or more) therefore establishes the presence of acute infection or reactivation. Unfortunately, this test has been difficult to standardize, lacks sensitivity in neonates and immunocompromised (particularly AIDS) hosts, and is not widely available. Recently introduced enzyme immunoassays (EIA) for IgM antibody circumvents many of these difficulties, but still produce some false-positive results, and are not sufficiently sensitive in AIDS patients. A modification of the EIA procedure, the antibody-capture enzyme immunoassay, significantly improves both the sensitivity and specificity of the original procedure. Examination of urine and other body fluids for the presence of toxoplasma antigen, or DNA by the polymerase chain reaction (PCR), have been shown to be useful adjunctive tests in immunocompromised individuals; currently these procedures are not generally available to clinical laboratories.

Rising titers of IgG or demonstration of IgM indicate acute infection or reactivation

Antigen detection, PCR, still in development

## Treatment and Prevention

Usually patients do not require therapy unless symptoms are particularly severe and persistent or unless vital organs, such as the eye, are involved. Immunocompromised and pregnant women, however, should be treated if acute infection (or reactivation) is documented (Table 52–3). Routine serial serologic testing of such individuals would allow early detec-

Most do not require treatment

TABLE 52–3. INDICATIONS FOR TREATMENT OF TOXOPLASMOSIS[a]

| Serologic Criteria | Clinical Criteria |
|---|---|
| Elevated IgM titers | Potential laboratory acquired infection |
| Fourfold rise in IgG titers | Pregnant woman |
| Very high IgG titers (greater than 1:1000) | Neonate |
| | Immunocompromised patient (including AIDS) |
| | Severe constitutional symptoms |
| | Vital organ involvement (including active chorioretinitis) |

*Abbreviation:* Ig, immunoglobulin.
[a] Must satisfy one serologic plus one clinical criterion.

tion of infected patients and enhance the prospects of a successful outcome. It is now clear that early treatment of the acutely infected pregnant woman significantly reduces the incidence of severe congenital infections, and reduces the ratio of benign to subclinical forms in the infant. At present, the most commonly used therapeutic regimen in the United States is the combination of pyrimethamine and sulfonamides. Unfortunately, the former drug is teratogenic and should not be used in the first trimester of pregnancy; spiramycin, a cytostatic macrolide, is often substituted in this setting.

Combined sulfonamide and pyrimethamine therapy

Although the pyrimethamine/sulfonamide combination is very effective against tachyzoites, it is inactive against the cyst forms. As both parasitic forms are present in patients with toxoplasmic encephalitis, recrudescence of illness generally follows completion of standard therapy in AIDS patients. This may be prevented by initiating chronic, low-dose suppressive therapy following the completion of the standard regimen. Atovaquone, a recently introduced hydroxynaphthoquinone, posseses activity against both tachyzoite and cysts. Its use, therefore, may result in radical cure of toxoplasma encephalitis, eliminating the need chronic suppression.

AIDS patients require treatment for cyst form

Prevention should be directed primarily at pregnant women and the immunologically compromised host. Hands should be carefully washed after handling uncooked meat. Cysts in meat can be destroyed by proper cooking (56°C for 15 min) or by freezing to –20°C. Cat feces should be avoided, particularly the changing of litter boxes.

## CRYPTOSPORIDIA

Cryptosporidia are small parasites that can infect the intestinal tract of a wide range of mammals including humans. Like other sporozoan parasites, they are obligate intracellular organisms exhibiting alternating cycles of sexual and asexual reproduction. As is true for *Toxoplasma,* both cycles are completed within the gastrointestinal tract of a single host. Long recognized as an important cause of diarrhea in animals, cryptosporidia were not identified as causes of human enteritis until 1976.

### ■ Cryptosporidia ("Hidden-spore") Parasites

#### Morphology

Regardless of animal host, all strains of this tiny (2 to 6 μm) parasite appear morphologically identical. Although all strains can reasonably be regarded as a single species, that which infects humans and cattle is often referred to as *C. parvum.* They appear as small spherical structures arranged in rows along the microvilli of the epithelial cells. They are readily stained with Giemsa and hematoxylin–eosin. Although they remain external to the cytoplasm of the intestinal epithelial cell, they are covered by a double membrane derived from the reflection, fusion, and attenuation of the microvilli, and are thus, by definition, intracellular organisms. Oocysts shed into the intestinal lumen mature to contain four sporozoites; their cell wall provides the unusual property of acid fastness, allowing them to be visualized with stains generally employed for mycobacteria.

Small spherical parasites beneath surface of microvilli

Oocysts are acid-fast

#### Life Cycle

Infective oocysts are excreted in the stool of the parasitized animal. Unlike those of *Toxoplasma,* cryptosporidia oocysts are fully mature and immediately infective upon passage in the feces. Following ingestion by another animal, sporozoites are released from the oocyst and attach to the microvilli of the small bowel epithelial cells, where they are transformed into trophozoites. These divide asexually by multiple fission (schizogony) to form schizonts containing eight daughter cells known as type 1 merozoites. Upon release from the schizont, each daughter cell attaches itself to another epithelial cell, where it repeats the schizogony cycle, producing another generation of type 1 merozoites.

Mature immediately infective oocysts excreted in stool

Sporozoites, trophozoites, and merozoites all attach to epithelial cells

Eventually, schizonts containing four type 2 merozoites are seen. Incapable of continued asexual reproduction, these develop into male (microgamete) and female (macrogamete) sexual forms. Following fertilization, the resulting zygote develops into an oocyst that is shed into the lumen of the bowel. The majority possess a thick protective cell wall that ensures their intact passage in the feces and survival in the external environment.

Sexual reproduction produces oocysts which are passed in stool

Some thin walled oocysts can autoinfect

Approximately 20% fail to develop the thick protective wall. The cell membrane ruptures, releasing infective sporozoites directly into the intestinal lumen and initiating a new "autoinfective" cycle within the original host. In the normal host, the presence of innate or acquired immunity dampens both the cyclic production of type 1 merozoites and the formation of thin-walled oocysts, halting further parasite multiplication and terminating the acute infection. In the immunocompromised, both presumably continue, explaining why such individuals develop severe, persistent infections in the absence of external reinfection.

## Cryptosporidiosis

### Epidemiology

Infection rates highest in young

Animal reservoirs and person-person transmission both important

Cryptosporidiosis appears to involve most vertebrate groups. In all species, infection rates are highest among the young and immature. Experimental and epidemiologic data suggest that domestic animals constitute an important reservoir of disease in humans. However, outbreaks of human disease in day-care centers, hospitals, and urban family groups indicate that most human infections result from person-to-person transmission. In Western countries, between 1 and 4% of small children presenting to medical centers with gastroenteritis have been shown to harbor cryptosporidia oocysts; in third-world countries the rates have varied from 4 to 11%. In some outbreaks of diarrhea in day-care centers, the majority of attendees were found to have oocysts in their stool.

Asymptomatic carriage uncommon

Infection rates in adults suffering from gastroenteritis is approximately one third of that reported in children; it has been highest in family members of infected children, medical personnel caring for patients with cryptosporidiosis, male homosexuals, and travelers to foreign countries. In the United States, the parasite has been identified in 15% of patients with AIDS and diarrhea; in Haiti and Africa, 50% of such individuals may be involved. Asymptomatic carriage is uncommon. Other enteric pathogens, particularly *Giardia lamblia,* are recovered from a significant minority of infected patients.

Fecal-oral principal route of infection

Because oocysts are found almost exclusively in stool, the principal transmission route is undoubtedly by direct fecal–oral spread. Transmission via contaminated water has been documented, and the hardy nature of the oocysts makes it likely that there is also indirect transmission via contaminated food and fomites.

### Pathogenesis and Immunity

Minimal intestinal pathology

Diarrhea mechanism unknown

Although the jejunum is most heavily involved, cryptosporidia have been found throughout the gastrointestinal tract, particularly in immunocompromised subjects. Cryptosporidial cholecystitis is seen with some frequency in AIDS patients with enteritis. By light microscopy, bowel changes appear minimal, consisting of mild to moderate villous atrophy, crypt enlargement, and a mononuclear infiltrate of the lamina propria. The pathophysiology of the diarrhea is unknown, but its nature and intensity suggest that a cholera-like enterotoxin may be involved.

Prolonged disease in young, immunosuppressed

The vital role played by the host's immune status in the pathogenesis of the disease is indicated by both the enhanced susceptibility of the young to infection and the prolonged severe clinical disease seen in immunocompromised patients. Indirect evidence suggests antibodies in the intestinal lumen exert a protective effect against initial *C. parvum* infection. Experimental animal studies indicate that $CD4^+$ T lymphocytes and interferon-$\gamma$ play independent roles in the immunologic clearance of the parasite.

## Cryptosporidiosis: Clinical Aspects

### Clinical Manifestations

Explosive, self-limiting diarrhea in immunocompetent individuals

Immunocompetent patients usually note the onset of explosive, profuse, watery diarrhea 1 to 2 weeks after exposure. Typically, the illness persists for 5 to 11 days and then rapidly abates. Occasionally, purging, accompanied by a mild malabsorption and weight loss, continues for up to 1 month. A few patients complain of nausea, anorexia, vomiting, and low-grade fever. Except for its shorter duration, more prominent abdominal pain, and relative lack of flatulence, the clinical manifestations of cryptosporidiosis closely resemble those produced by *G. lamblia*. Radiographic and endoscopic examinations of the gut are either normal or demonstrate mild, nonspecific abnormalities. Recovery is complete, and neither relapse nor reinfection has been reported.

Cryptosporidiosis has been described in patients with a broad range of immunodeficiencies including childhood malnutrition in third-world countries, AIDS, and congenital hypogammaglobulinemia, and in those resulting from cancer chemotherapy and immunosuppressive management of organ transplants. In such patients, cryptosporidiosis is usually indolent in onset and manifestations are similar to those seen in normal hosts, but the diarrhea is more severe. Fluid losses of up to 25 L/day have been described. Patients with biliary cryptosporidiosis present with typical manifestations of cholecystitis and cholangitis. Unless the immunologic defect is reversed, the disease usually persists for the duration of the patient's life. Weight loss is often prominent. The prognosis depends upon the nature of the underlying immunologic abnormality; half of patients with AIDS die within 6 months. Although other intercurrent infections are usually the direct cause of death, malnutrition and complications of parenteral nutrition contribute.

Severe, prolonged diarrhea in immunosuppressed including AIDS patients

### Laboratory Diagnosis

The diagnosis of cryptosporidiosis is established by the recovery and identification of *Cryptosporidium* oocysts in a recently passed or preserved diarrheal stool. Oocyst excretion is most intense during the first week of illness, tapers during the second week, and generally stops with the cessation of diarrhea. As cryptosporidia oocysts are one of the few acid-fast particles found in feces, a definitive identification can be established with any one of the acid-fast staining procedures developed for mycobacteria. A direct immunofluorescence antibody stain using a monoclonal antibody to oocyst wall has been recently introduced that appears to be superior to acid-fast stains. When direct examinations are negative, concentration procedures are used and the concentrate restained. Immunofluorescence (IFA) and enzyme immunoassays for the detection of anticryptosporidial antibodies are now available.

Detection of oocysts by acid-fast stains and immunofluorescence

### Treatment and Prevention

In the immunocompetent patient, the disease is self-limited and attempts at specific antiparasitic therapy are not warranted; rehydration may be required in small children. In the immunocompromised host, the severity and chronicity of the diarrhea warrants therapeutic intervention. Unfortunately, there is no uniformly effective anticryptosporidial agent available at this time. Paromomycin, a luminal antimicrobic, has been shown to reduce the intensity of diarrhea in some patients, and parenteral octreotide acetate, a somatostatin analog, has been useful in decreasing stool volumes. The only uniformly successful approach has been the reversal of underlying immunologic abnormalities. When appropriate, withdrawal of cancer chemotherapy agents or immunosuppressive drugs may result in a cure.

No specific therapeutic yet in use

The stools of patients with cryptosporidiosis are infectious. Stool precautions should be instituted at the time the diagnosis is first suspected; for the immunosuppressed patient, this should be whenever diarrhea, regardless of presumed etiology, is first noted. This is particularly important in cancer chemotherapy and transplantation units where spread of the disease from a symptomatic patient to other immunosuppressed patients can have life-threatening consequences.

Precautions required to protect against infection from stools of hospital patients

## ADDITIONAL READING

Bruce-Chwatt LJ. Man against malaria: Conquest or defeat? *R Soc Trop Med Hyg* 1979;73:605–617. A leading malariologist reviews the successes and failures of the WHO-sponsored Malaria Eradication Program.

Frenkel JK, Ruiz A. Endemicity of toxoplasmosis in Costa Rica. Transmission between cats, soil, intermediate hosts and humans. *Am J Epidemiol* 1981;113:254–269. This article is the most comprehensive study on the role of cats in the transmission of toxoplasmosis. It suggests that humans are infected primarily from soil contaminated with cat feces, rather than direct contact.

Gellin BG, Soave R. Coccidian Infections in AIDS: Toxoplasmosis, cryptosporidiosis, and isoporiasis. *Med Clin North Am* 1992;76:205–234.

Heyworth MF. Immunology of *Giardia* and *Cryptosporidium* infections. *J Infect Dis* 1992;166:465–472. A current review of the immunology of these two important protozoa.

Hoffman SD. Diagnosis, treatment and prevention of malaria. *Med Clin North Am* 1992;76:1327–1355. Complete, timely summary of information needed by the physician dealing with a traveler to malarious areas of the world.

Jones TR, Hoffman SL. Immunology and pathogenic mechanisms of malaria. *Curr Opin Infect Dis* 1992;5: 310–318. A concise review of recent developments in vaccine development and other miscellaneous pathogenic mechanisms in malaria. A "quick read."

Katlama C. New perspectives on the treatment and prophylaxis of *Toxoplasma gondii* infection. *Curr Opin Infect Dis* 1992;5:833–848.

Laderman C. Malaria and progress: Some historical and ecological considerations. *Soc Sci Med* 1975; 9:587–592.

Lebech M, Petersen E. Congenital toxoplasmosis: Introduction. *Scand J Infect Dis* 1992;24(suppl 84):11–17. The introductory article in a journal supplement devoted entirely to the topic of congenital toxoplasmosis.

Luft BJ, Remington JS. Toxoplasmic encephalitis in AIDS. *Clin Infect Dis* 1992;15:211–222. A comprehensive review of an increasing common presentation of toxoplasmosis.

Soave R, Armstrong D. *Cryptosporidium* and cryptosporidiosis. *Rev Infect Dis* 1992;8:1012–1023. A recent, readable review of the topic.

Wyler DJ. Malaria: Overview and update. *Clin Infect Dis* 1993;16:449–458. A concise update on pathogenesis, epidemiology and therapy.

Zu SX, Fang GD, Fayer R, Guerrant R. Cryptosporidiosis: Pathogenesis and immunology. *Parasitol Today* 1992;18:24–27. A concise review.

Chapter 53

# Rhizopods

*James J. Plorde*

Rhizopods, or amebas, are the most primitive of the protozoa. They multiply by simple binary fission and move by means of cytoplasmic organelles called pseudopodia. These projections of the relatively solid ectoplasm are formed by streaming of the inner, more liquid endoplasm. They move the ameba forward and, incidentally, engulf and internalize food sources found in its path. Most amebas, when faced with a hostile environment, can produce a chitinous, external wall that surrounds and protects them. These forms are referred to as cysts and may survive for prolonged periods under conditions that would rapidly destroy the motile trophozoite.

The majority of amebas belong to free-living genera. They are widely distributed in nature, being found in literally all bodies of standing fresh water. Few free-living amebas produce human disease, although two genera, *Naegleria* and *Acanthamoeba,* have been implicated occasionally as causes of meningoencephalitis and keratitis.

Several genera of amebas, including *Entamoeba, Endolimax,* and *Iodamoeba,* are obligate parasites of the human alimentary tract and are passed as cysts from host to host by the fecal–oral route. Several are devoid of mitochondria, presumably because of the anaerobic conditions under which they exist in the colon. Only one, *Entamoeba histolytica,* regularly produces disease.

## ENTAMOEBA

### E. histolytica

#### Morphology and Physiology

*E. histolytica* possesses both trophozoite and cyst forms. The trophozoites are microaerophilic, dwell in the lumen or wall of the colon, feed on bacteria and tissue cells, and multiply rapidly in the anaerobic environment of the gut. When diarrhea occurs, the trophozoites are passed unchanged in the liquid stool. Here they can be recognized by their size (12 to 20 μm in diameter); directional motility; granular, vacuolated endoplasm; and sharply demarcated, clear ectoplasm with fingerlike pseudopods. Invasive strains tend to be larger and may contain ingested erythrocytes within their cytoplasm (Figure 53–1). Appropriate stains reveal a 3- to 5-μm nucleus with a small central karyosome or nucleolus and fine regular granules evenly distributed around the nuclear membrane (peripheral chromatin). Electron microscopic studies demonstrate microfilaments, an external glycocalyx, and cytoplasmic projections thought to be important for attachment.

Trophozoites passed in diarrheal stools; may contain ingested erythrocytes

With normal stool transit time, trophozoites usually encyst before leaving the gut. Initially, a cyst contains a single nucleus, a glycogen vacuole, and one or more large, cigar-shaped ribosomal clusters known as chromatoid bodies. With maturation, the cyst becomes

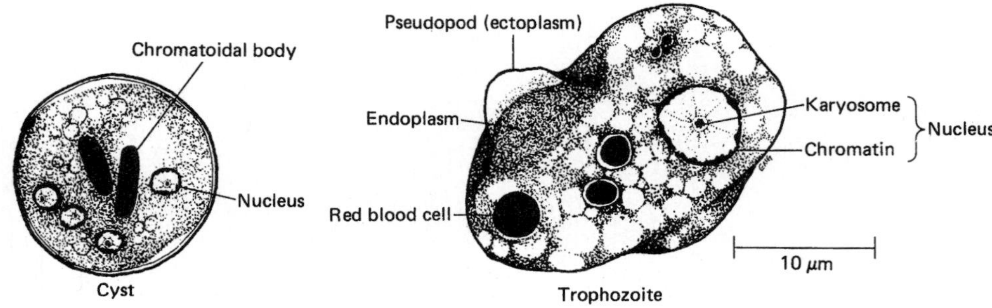


**Figure 53–1.** *Entamoeba histolytica.*

Mature quadrinucleate cysts survive in environment

quadrinucleate, and the cytoplasmic inclusions are absorbed. In contrast to the fragile trophozoite, mature cysts can survive environmental temperatures up to 55°C, chlorine concentrations normally found in municipal water supplies, and normal levels of gastric acid. *E. histolytica* can be differentiated from the other amebas of the gut by its size, nuclear detail, and cytoplasmic inclusions (Table 53–1).

## Life Cycle

Human-to-human infection by ingested cysts

Cyst releases trophozoites in small intestine

Trophozoites colonize cecum and rectosigmoid

Humans are the principal hosts and reservoirs of *E. histolytica*. Transmission from person to person occurs when a parasite passed in the stool of one host is ingested by another. Because the trophozoites die rapidly in the external environment, successful passage is achieved only by the cyst. Human hosts may pass up to 45 million cysts daily. Although the average infective dose exceeds 1000 organisms, ingestion of a single cyst has been known to produce infection. After passage through the stomach, the cyst eventually reaches the distal small bowel. Here the cyst wall disintegrates, releasing the quadrinucleate parasite, which divides to form eight small trophozoites that are carried to the colon. Colonization is most intense in areas of fecal stasis such as the cecum and rectosigmoid, but may be found throughout the large bowel.

## Laboratory Growth

Grown by feeding bacteria

Axenic cultures used for purified preparations

Trophozoites are facultative anaerobes that require complex media for growth. Most require the addition of live bacteria for successful isolation. Sterile culture techniques (axenic) have been developed, however, and are essential for the preparation of the purified antigens required for serologic testing, zymodeme typing, and characterization of virulence factors.

**TABLE 53–1. SOME DIFFERENTIAL CHARACTERISTICS OF ENTAMOEBA SPECIES**

| Characteristics | E. histolytica | E. hartmanni | E. coli |
|---|---|---|---|
| **Trophozoites** | | | |
| Cytoplasm | Differentiated[a] | Differentiated | Undifferentiated |
| Nucleus | | | |
| Peripheral chromatin | Fine | Fine | Coarse, irregular |
| Karyosome | Small, central | Small, central | Large, eccentric |
| Ingested particles | | | |
| Bacteria | No | — | Yes |
| Red blood cells | Yes | No | No |
| Size | >12 μm | <12 μm | >12 μm |
| **Cysts** | | | |
| Nuclei[b] | 1–4 | 1–4 | 1–8 |
| Chromatoid bodies | Rods | Rods | Splinters |
| Size | >10 μg | <10 μm | >10 μm |

[a] Sharp differentiation between ectoplasm and endoplasm.
[b] Fine structure similar to that of trophozoites.

## Amebiasis

### Epidemiology

*E. histolytica* is thought to infect 10% of the world's population, and to produce more deaths than any other parasite, save those caused by malaria and schistosomiasis. Although it has a worldwide distribution, infection rates are highest in warm climates and exceed 50% in areas where the level of sanitation is low. Stool surveys in the United States indicate that 1 to 5% of the population harbors this parasite; the vast majority of the involved individuals are colonized with nonpathogenic strains. Invasive disease is both less common and less widely distributed. Reports of amebic liver abscess, for instance, emanate primarily from Mexico, western South America, South Asia, and West and South Africa. For reasons apparently unrelated to exposure, symptomatic illness is much less common in women and children than in men.

Worldwide infection; highest rates in warmer climates

Invasive disease rare in United States

In the United States, the incidence of invasive amebiasis decreased sharply over several decades, reaching a nadir of 3500 cases in 1974. Since then, the numbers have steadily increased. Most cases are acquired outside the country. Invasive amebiasis is still seen in institutions for the mentally retarded, Indian reservations, migrant labor camps, and among male homosexuals and victims of AIDS.

Symptomatic amebiasis is usually sporadic, the result of direct person-to-person fecal–oral spread under conditions of poor personal hygiene. Venereal transmission appears to be particularly common among male homosexuals, presumably the result of oral–anal sexual contact. Food- and water-borne spread occur, occasionally in epidemic form. Such outbreaks, however, are seldom as explosive as those produced by pathogenic intestinal bacteria. One outbreak of intestinal amebiasis was due to colonic irrigation at a chiropractic clinic.

Fecal–oral spread linked to poor hygiene

Food, water are other modes of transmission

### Pathogenesis

In over 90% of the infected population, *E. histolytica* exists in the gut as a harmless commensal. Occasionally it invades, producing tissue damage; if the damage is sufficiently extensive, clinical disease results. This variable course appears to be mediated by both parasite and host factors. There is now a substantial body of data suggesting the existence of separate nonpathogenic and pathogenic strains or species of *E. histolytica,* distinguishable by isoenzyme patterns (zymodemes), surface antigens, DNA markers to antigens, and rRNA. Individuals harboring nonpathogenic strains seldom mount antibody responses to the organism or demonstrate physical evidence of sustained invasion.

Virulence is strain related; associated with certain zymodeme patterns

In contrast, amebic antibodies are regularly found in individuals harboring pathogenic amebas, suggesting that colonization by these strains is followed by tissue invasion. A number of virulence factors have been identified in pathogenic strains of *E. histolytica.* In an experimental setting, invasiveness correlates well with endocytic capacity, the production of extracellular proteinases capable of activating complement and degrading collagen, the presence of a galactose-specific lectin apparently capable of mediating attachment of the organism to colonic mucosa, and perhaps most importantly, the capacity to lyse host cells on contact. The latter phenomenon is initiated by the galactose-specific lectin mediated adherence of the trophozoite to a target cell. Following adherence, the ameba releases a pore-forming protein that polymerizes in the target cell membrane, forming large tubular lesions. Cytolysis rapidly follows.

Virulence determinants include lytic capacity initiated by lectin-mediated adherence

In most cases of pathogenic-strain infections, however, tissue damage is minimal, and the host remains symptom free, suggesting that host factors may modulate the invasiveness of virulent strains. These factors are still poorly understood, but changes in host resistance, the colonic milieu, or the parasite itself may amplify tissue damage and clinical manifestations. Protein malnutrition, high-carbohydrate diets, corticosteroid administration, childhood, and pregnancy all appear to render the host more susceptible to invasion. Certain colonic bacteria appear to enhance invasiveness, possibly by providing a more favorable redox potential for survival and multiplication or by facilitating the adherence of the parasite to colonic mucosa. Finally, it is known that the pathogenic strains in the tropics are more invasive than those isolated in temperate areas, possibly because poor sanitation results in more frequent passage through humans.

Most infected individuals symptom free

Colonic microflora may influence invasiveness

Virulence increased with passage through humans

### Pathology

Mucosal ulceration with little inflammatory response

Flasklike ulcers extend to submucosa

Amebomas and metastatic amebic abscesses in a few cases

Amebas contact and lyse colonic epithelial cells, producing small mucosal ulcerations. There is little inflammatory response other than edema and hyperemia, and the mucosa between ulcers appears normal. Trophozoites are present in large numbers at the junction between necrotic and viable tissue. Once the lesion penetrates below the superficial epithelium, it meets the resistance of the colonic musculature and spreads laterally in the submucosa, producing a flask-like lesion with a narrow mucosal neck and a large submucosal body. It eventually compromises the blood supply of the overlying mucosa, resulting in sloughing and a large necrotic ulcer. Extensive ulceration leads to secondary bacterial infection, formation of granulation tissue, and fibrotic thickening of the colon. In approximately 1% of patients, the granulation tissue is organized into large, tumorlike masses known as amebomas. The major sites of involvement, in order of frequency, are the cecum, ascending colon, rectum, sigmoid, appendix, and terminal ileum. Amebas may also enter the portal circulation and be carried to the liver or, more rarely, to the lung, brain, or spleen. In these organs, liquefaction necrosis leads to the formation of abscess cavities.

### Immunity

Although pathogenic strains of *E. histolytica* elicit both humoral and cellular immune responses in humans, it is still not clear which, and to what degree, these responses are capable of modulating initial infection or thwarting reinfection. In endemic areas, the prevalence of gastrointestinal colonization increases with age, suggesting that the host is incapable of clearing *E. histolytica* from the gut. However, the relative infrequency with which populations living in these areas suffer repeated bouts of severe amebic colitis or liver abscess indicates that those who experience such infections have protection against recurrent disease.

Immunity incomplete; does not correlate with antibody response

Trophozoites shed antibody and resist complement lysis

Cell-mediated immunity develops but slowly

Patients with invasive disease are known to produce high levels of circulating antibodies. Nevertheless, there is no correlation between the presence or concentration of such antibodies and protective immunity, possibly because pathogenic *E. histolytica* trophozoites have the capacity to aggregate and shed attached antibodies and are resistant to the lytic action of complement. The susceptibility to invasive amebiasis of malnourished populations, pregnant women, steroid-treated individuals, and AIDS patients indicates that cell-mediated immune mechanisms may be directly involved in the control of tissue invasion; although as measured by the onset of delayed-type hypersensitivity and T lymphocyte proliferative responses to amebic antigens, they develop slowly, often peaking weeks after recovery from invasive disease. Effector mechanisms appear to include cytotoxic T lymphocytes and lymphokine-activated macrophages, both of which have been shown capable of killing pathogenic amebas in vitro.

The role of immune mechanisms in the pathogenesis of the disease remains speculative. It is possible the presence of immune complexes and neutrophils in amebic abscess cavities contribute to tissue necrosis.

Pathogenic *E. histolytica* strains produce a lectin-like substance that is mitogenic for lymphocytes. It has been suggested that this substance could stimulate viral replication of HIV-infected lymphocytes as does another mitogen, phytohemagglutinin A. As significant numbers of homosexual males carry *E. histolytica,* it is conceivable that this parasite might accelerate the development of AIDS in HIV-infected individuals.

## ■ Amebiasis: Clinical Aspects

### Clinical Manifestations

Relationship usually commensal

Individuals who harbor *E. histolytica* are usually clinically well. In most cases, particularly in the temperate zones, the organism is avirulent, living in the bowel as a normal commensal inhabitant. Spontaneous disappearance of amebas, over a period of weeks to months, among such patients is common, and perhaps universal. Serologic data, however, suggest that some asymptomatic carriers possess virulent strains and incur minimal tissue invasion. In this population, the infection may eventually progress to produce overt disease.

Diarrhea, flatulence, and abdominal pain most common

Diarrhea, flatulence, and cramping abdominal pain are the most frequent complaints of symptomatic patients. The diarrhea is intermittent, alternating with episodes of normality or constipation over a period of months to years. Typically, the stools consist of one to four loose to watery, foul-smelling passages that contain mucus and blood. Physical findings are limited to abdominal tenderness localized to the hepatic, ascending colonic, and cecal areas. Sigmoidoscopy reveals the typical ulcerations with normal intertwining mucosa.

Fulminating amebic dysentery is less common. It may occur spontaneously in debilitated or pregnant individuals or be precipitated by corticosteroid therapy. Its onset is often abrupt, with high fever, severe abdominal cramps, and profuse, bloody diarrhea and tenesmus. Severe abdominal tenderness and a tender, enlarged liver are common. Sigmoidoscopy reveals extensive rectosigmoid ulceration. Trophozoites are numerous in stools and ulcer aspirates. A number of complications may accompany fulminant disease, including massive hemorrhage and bowel perforation with resulting peritonitis. Amebomas may project into the lumen of the bowel, where they may be mistaken for adenocarcinoma or extend circumferentially around the colon, producing partial obstruction. If tissue destruction is extensive, the colon may be left scarred and irritable despite eradication of the organism, resulting in so-called postdysenteric colitis.

Ulceration with mucus and blood in stool occur in fulminant disease

Postdysenteric colitis may be residual

Liver abscess presents either acutely or insidiously with fever and tender hepatic enlargement. Most commonly, abscesses occur singly and are localized to the upper outer quadrant of the right lobe of the liver. This localization results in the development of point tenderness overlying the cavity and elevation of the right diaphragm. Liver function is usually well preserved. Isotopic or ultrasound scanning confirms the presence of the lesion. Needle aspiration results in the withdrawal of reddish-brown, odorless fluid free of bacteria and polymorphonuclear leukocytes; trophozoites may be demonstrated in the terminal portion of the aspirate.

Hepatic abscess has insidious onset

Approximately 5% of all patients with symptomatic amebiasis present with a liver abscess. Ironically, fewer than one half can recall significant diarrheal illness. Although *E. histolytica* can be demonstrated in the stools of 72% of patients with amebic liver abscess when a combination of serial microscopic examinations and culture is employed, routine microscopic examination of the stool will detect less than half of these. Complications relate to the extension of the abscess into surrounding tissue, producing pneumonia, empyema, or peritonitis. Extension of an abscess from the left lobe of the liver to the pericardium is the single most dangerous complication. It may produce rapid cardiac compression (tamponade) and death or, more commonly, a chronic pericardial disease that may be confused with congestive cardiomyopathy or tuberculous pericarditis.

Hepatic abscess may extend to other tissues

## Laboratory Diagnosis

The diagnosis of intestinal amebiasis depends upon the identification of the organism in stool or sigmoidoscopic aspirates. As trophozoites appear predominantly in liquid stools or aspirates, a portion of such specimens should be fixed immediately to ensure preservation of these fragile organisms for stained preparations. The specimen may then be examined in wet mount for typical motility, concentrated to detect cysts, and stained for definitive identification of *E. histolytica*. Three or more specimens may be required for diagnosis. If trophozoites or cysts are seen, they must be carefully differentiated from those of the commensal parasites, particularly *E. hartmanni* and *E. coli* (Table 53–1).

Stools examined for trophozoites and cysts in stained or wet preparations

Recently, enzyme immunoassays capable of detecting *E. histolytica* antigens in stool, with a sensitivity comparable or superior to that of standard microscopic examination, have been commercially introduced; their potential value in the clinical diagnosis of amebiasis when compared to microscopic examination, remains to be established. Although the cultural detection of amebic parasites is more sensitive than either immunoassay or microscopic examination, this procedure is not currently available in most clinical laboratories. Similarly, methods for rapidly differentiating pathogenic from nonpathogenic strains of *E. histolytica* have not yet been adapted for clinical use.

EIA can detect antigen in stool

No way to distinguish pathogenic strains

The diagnosis of extraintestinal amebiasis is more difficult, as the parasite usually cannot be recovered from stool or tissue. Serologic tests are therefore of paramount importance. Typically, results are negative in asymptomatic patients, suggesting that tissue invasion is required for antibody production. Most patients with symptomatic intestinal disease and more than 90% with hepatic abscess have high levels of antiamebic antibodies. Unfortunately, these titers may persist for months to years after an acute infection, making the interpretation of a positive test difficult in endemic areas. At present, the indirect hemag-

Extraintestinal amebiasis usually demonstrates high antibody levels

glutination test and the enzyme immunoassays using antigens derived from axenically grown organisms appear to be the most sensitive. Several rapid tests, including latex agglutination, agar diffusion, and counterimmunoelectrophoresis, are available to smaller laboratories.

### Treatment

Metronidazole alone or combined with other agents

Treatment is directed toward relief of symptoms, blood and fluid replacement, and eradication of the organism. The need to eliminate the parasite in asymptomatic carriers remains uncertain. The drug of choice for eradication is metronidazole. It is effective against all forms of amebiasis, but should be combined with a second agent, such as diloxanide, to improve cure rates in intestinal disease and diminish the chance of recrudescent disease in hepatic amebiasis. Tetracycline, which apparently acts indirectly by altering the bacterial milieu of the gut, may be used as an alternative to diloxanide. Specific contraindications to the use of metronidazole are given in Chapter 54 in the section on Trichomoniasis.

### Prevention

As the disease is transmitted by the fecal–oral route, efforts should be directed toward sanitary disposal of human feces and improvement in personal hygienic practices. In the United States, this applies particularly to institutionalized patients and to camps for migrant farm workers. Male homosexuals should be made aware that certain sexual practices substantially increase their risk of this and other infections.

# NAEGLERIA AND ACANTHAMOEBA INFECTIONS

## Amebic Meningoencephalitis

Meningoecephalitis due to free-living amebas

Warm weather, brackish water favor amebas

Primary amebic meningoencephalitis is caused by free-living amebas belonging predominately to the *Naegleria* and *Acanthamoeba* genera. The disease produced by the former has been better defined; it affects children and young adults, appears to be acquired by swimming in fresh water, and is almost always fatal. *Acanthamoeba* meningoencephalitis is a subacute or chronic illness that also is usually fatal. *Naegleria* species are found in large numbers in shallow fresh water, particularly during warm weather. *Acanthamoeba* species are found in soil and in fresh and brackish water, and they have been recovered from the oropharynx of asymptomatic humans.

Naegleria infections associated with freshwater swimming

Approximately 140 cases of *Naegleria* meningoencephalitis have been reported, primarily in Great Britain, Belgium, Czechoslovakia, Australia, New Zealand, India, Nigeria, and the United States. Serologic studies suggest that inapparent infections are much more common. Most cases in the United States have occurred in the southeastern states. Characteristically, the patients have fallen ill during the summer after swimming or water-skiing in small, shallow, freshwater lakes. The Czechoslovakian cases followed swimming in a chlorinated indoor pool, and several have occurred after bathing in hot mineral water. A recent report from Africa suggests the disease may have been acquired by inhaling airborne cysts during the dry, windy season in the sub-Sahara.

Passage to central nervous system across cribriform plate

Histologic evidence suggests that *Naegleria* traverses the nasal mucosa and the cribriform plate to the central nervous system. Here the organism produces a severe purulent, hemorrhagic inflammatory reaction that extends perivascularly from the olfactory bulbs to other regions of the brain. The infection is characterized by the rapid onset of severe bifrontal headache, seizures, and at times, abnormalities in taste or smell. The disease runs an inexorably downhill course to coma, ending fatally within a few days.

Purulent bloody cerebrospinal fluid containing *Naegleria* trophozoites

A careful examination of the cerebrospinal fluid often provides a presumptive diagnosis of *Naegleria* infection. The fluid is usually bloody and demonstrates an intense neutrophilic response. The protein level is elevated and the glucose level decreased. No bacteria can be demonstrated on stain or culture. Early examination of a wet mount preparation of unspun spinal fluid will reveal typical trophozoites. Staining with specific fluorescent antibody confirms the identification. The organism can usually be isolated on agar plates seeded with a Gram-negative bacillus (to feed the amebas) or grown axenically in tissue culture. To date, only two patients have survived a *Naegleria* infection. Both were diagnosed early;

one was treated with amphotericin B, and the other with amphotericin B, miconazole, and rifampin.

Acanthamoeba affects older immunocompromised subjects

The epidemiology of *Acanthamoeba* encephalitis has not been clearly defined. Infections usually involve older, immunocompromised persons, and a history of freshwater swimming is generally absent. The ameba probably reaches the brain by hematogenous dissemination from an unknown primary site, possibly the respiratory tract, skin, or eye. Metastatic lesions have been reported. Histologically, *Acanthamoeba* infections produce a diffuse, necrotizing, granulomatous encephalitis, with frequent involvement of the midbrain. Both cysts and trophozoites can be found in the lesions.

Granulomatous encephalitis with cysts and trophozoites

More chronic disease with occasional spontaneous recovery

The clinical course of *Acanthamoeba* disease is more prolonged than that of *Naegleria* infection and occasionally ends in spontaneous recovery; the disease in immunocompromised hosts is invariably fatal. The spinal fluid usually demonstrates a mononuclear response. Amebas can seldom be visualized in or cultured from the CSF. Definitive diagnosis is made histologically after death. *Acanthamoeba* species are sensitive to a variety of agents, including sulfonamides, clotrimazole, 5-fluorocytosine, and polymyxin. Studies of clinical efficacy have not been done.

## Other Acanthamoeba Infections

Corneal ulcerations associated with contact lens use

Skin lesions, uveitis, and corneal ulcerations have also been reported. The latter are serious, producing a chronic progressive ulcerative lesion that may result in blindness. Infection commonly follows mild corneal trauma; most recently reported cases have been in users of soft contact lenses. Clinically, severe ocular pain, a paracentral ring infiltrate of the cornea, and recurrent epithelial breakdown are helpful in distinguishing this entity from the more common herpes simplex keratitis. The diagnosis can be confirmed by demonstrating typical wrinkled, double-walled cysts in corneal biopsies or scrapings using wet mounts, stained smears, and/or fluorescent antibody techniques. Culture of corneal tissue and contact lenses is frequently successful when the laboratory is given time to prepare satisfactory media. Chemotherapy has generally been ineffective unless given very early in the course of infection. Although a combination of corneal transplantation and chemotherapy may be successful later in the course of the disease, enucleation of the eye may be necessary to cure advanced infections. The drugs of choice are propamidine and neomycin eyedrops administered alternately for a period of several months. Successful use of clotrimazole has been recently reported.

Treatment usually surgical

## ADDITIONAL READING

Chesley AJ, Craig CF, Fishbein M, et al. Amebiasis outbreak in Chicago. Report of a special committee. *JAMA* 1934;102:369–372. A description of the best-known outbreak of amebiasis in the United States. Fourteen hundred clinical infections and 100 deaths resulted from an inadvertent connection between the water supply and sewage in two Chicago hotels.

Duma RJ, Helwig WB, Martinez AJ. Meningoencephalitis and brain abscess due to a free-living amoeba. *Ann Intern Med* 1978;88:468–473. A useful case report and discussion regarding the taxonomic criteria used to identify free-living amebas producing human disease.

The global problem of amebiasis: Current status, research needs and opportunities for progress. *Rev Infect Dis* 1986;8:218–272. This is a series of five papers covering the status, epidemiology, pathogenesis, immunology, and diagnosis of amebiasis. It is the most comprehensive review of *E. histolytica* infections.

Moore MB, McCulley JP, Luckenbach M. *Acanthamoeba* keratitis associated with soft contact lenses. *Am J Ophthalmol* 1985;100:396–403. A report of three patients who developed *Acanthamoeba* keratitis. It discusses the relationship between use of contact lenses and this disease, reviews the literature, and discusses diagnostic and therapeutic approaches.

Reed SL. Amebiasis: An update. *Clin Infect Dis* 1992;14:385–391. A brief, state-of-the-art summary of current concepts in amebiasis that nicely complements the 1986 review listed above.

Spice WM, Acker JP. The amoeba enigma. *Parasitol Today* 1992;8:402–406. This brief paper clearly and concisely reviews the evidence for and against the presence of distinct pathogenic and nonpathogenic forms of *E. histolytica*.

Chapter 54

# Flagellates

*James J. Plorde*

Like their amebic cousins, flagellate protozoa are widespread in nature, multiply by binary fission, and move about by means of cytoplasmic organelles of locomotion. Motility, however, is distinctly more vigorous among this group of organisms because of the efficiency of their locomotive apparatus, the flagellum. This organelle arises from an intracellular focus known as a **blepharoplast,** extends to the cell wall as a filamentous **axoneme,** and continues extracellularly as the free **flagellum.** In some species, the blepharoplast is paired with a second cytoplasmic structure known as a **parabasal body.** This structure is believed to be composed of modified mitochondria responsible for the control of flagellar movement. Both structures stain with nucleic acid stains, and they are known collectively as the **kinetoplast.**

In many flagellates the axoneme, before exiting from the cell, lifts a segment of external wall into a longitudinal fold. This undulating membrane is thrown into movement as the organism progresses, often imparting to it a characteristic rotary motion.

The long, whiplike free flagella may be single or multiple. The number is distinctive for individual species. When more than one is present, each has its own associated blepharoplast and axoneme.

Although a number of flagellate genera parasitize humans, only four, *Giardia, Trichomonas, Leishmania,* and *Trypanosoma,* commonly induce disease. The first two comprise noninvasive organisms that inhabit the lumina of the genitourinary or gastrointestinal tract and are spread without benefit of an intermediate host. Disease is of low morbidity and cosmopolitan distribution. *Leishmania* and *Trypanosoma,* on the other hand, are invasive blood and tissue parasites that produce highly morbid, frequently lethal diseases. These hemoflagellates require an intermediate insect host for their transmission. As a result, their associated disease states are limited to the semitropical and tropical niches of these intermediate hosts.

## NONINVASIVE LUMINAL FLAGELLATES

Luminal flagellates can be found in the mouth, vagina, or intestine of almost all vertebrates, and it is common for an animal host to harbor more than one species. Humans may serve as host and reservoir to eight (Table 54–1), but only two cause disease. Of these, *Giardia lamblia* inhabits the intestinal tract and *Trichomonas vaginalis* inhabits the vagina and genital tract.

Found in flora of vertebrates

These organisms are elongated or oval in shape and typically measure 10 to 20 μm in length. They often possess a rudimentary **cytostome** (mouth aperture) and organelles such as sucking discs or axostyles, which assist them to maintain their intraluminal position. They are readily recognized in body fluid or excreta by their rapid motility, and some can be specifically identified in unstained preparations. All can be cultivated on artificial media.

Morphology and rapid motility are distinctive

TABLE 54–1. LUMINAL FLAGELLATES INFECTING HUMANS

| Flagellate | Pathogenicity to Humans | Site |
|---|---|---|
| *Giardia lamblia* | + | Intestine |
| *Dientamoeba fragilis* | ? | Intestine |
| *Chilomastix mesnili* | – | Intestine |
| *Enteromonas hominis* | – | Intestine |
| *Retortamonas intestinalis* | – | Intestine |
| *Trichomonas hominis* | – | Intestine |
| *Trichomonas tenax* | – | Mouth |
| *Trichomonas vaginalis* | + | Vagina |

May or may not have cyst stage

Some luminal flagellates, most notably *T. vaginalis,* possess only a trophozoite stage and are passed from host to host by direct physical contact. Most, including *G. lamblia,* possess both trophozoite and cyst forms. The latter, which is the infective form, is transmitted via the fecal–oral route. Human-to-human infection is thus found in populations where inadequate sanitation or poor personal hygiene favors spread.

## Trichomonas

### Trichomonas vaginalis

Three *Trichomonas* species have similar morphology

Three members of the genus *Trichomonas* parasitize humans (Table 54–1), but only *T. vaginalis* is an established pathogen. The three species closely resemble one another morphologically, but confusion in identification is rare because of the specificity of their habitats.

The *T. vaginalis* trophozoite (Fig 54–1) is oval and typically measures 7 by 15 μm. Organisms up to twice this size are occasionally recovered from asymptomatic patients and from cultures. In stained preparations, a single, elongated nucleus and a small cytostome are observed anteriorly. Five flagella arise nearby. Four immediately exit the cell. The fifth bends back and runs posteriorly along the outer edge of an abbreviated undulating mem-

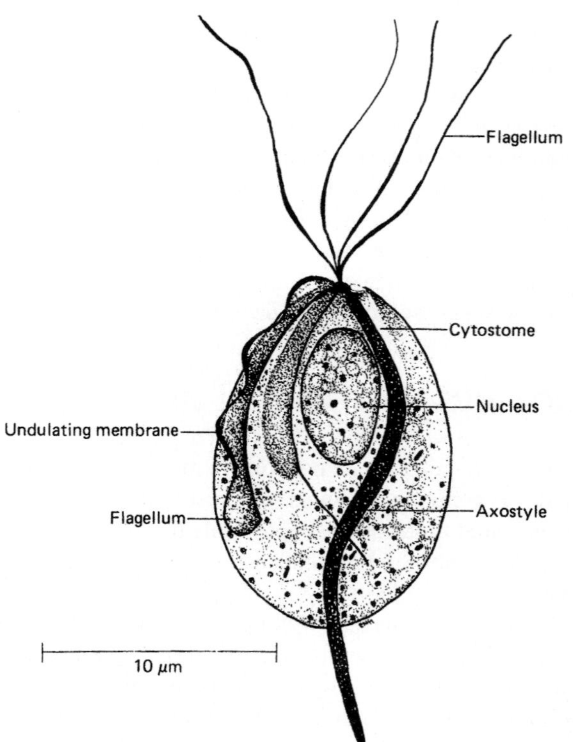


**Figure 54–1.** *Trichomonas vaginalis.*

brane. Lying along the base of this membrane is a cross-striated structure known as the costa. A conspicuous microtubule containing a supporting rod or axostyle bisects the trophozoite longitudinally and protrudes through its posterior end. It is thought that the pointed tip of this structure is useful for attachment, and it may be responsible for the tissue damage produced by the parasite. In unstained wet mounts, *T. vaginalis* is identified by its axostyle and jerky, nondirectional movements.

Protruding axostyle may mediate attachment

The organism can be grown on artificial media under anaerobic conditions at pH 5.5 to 6.0. Soluble nutrients are absorbed across the cell membrane. Particulate material, including bacteria, leukocytes, and occasional erythrocytes, may be ingested through any area of the cell surface. A variety of carbohydrates are fermented by pathways similar to those of anaerobic bacteria. Although it lacks a cyst form, the trophozoite can survive outside of the human host for 1 to 2 hours on moist surfaces. In urine, semen, and water, it is viable for up to 24 hours, making it one of the most resistant of protozoan trophozoites. Attempts to infect laboratory animals have met with limited success.

Cultivable in vitro

Lacks cyst form but survives a few hours outside host

## Trichomoniasis

### Epidemiology

Trichomoniasis is a cosmopolitan disease usually transmitted by sexual intercourse. It is estimated that 5 to 7 million women in the United States and 180 million worldwide acquire this disease annually, and 25% of sexually active women become infected at some time during their life; 30 to 70% of their male sexual partners are also parasitized, at least transiently. As would be expected, the likelihood of acquiring the disease correlates directly with the number of sexual contacts. Infection is rare in adult virgins, whereas rates as high as 70% are seen among prostitutes, sexual partners of infected patients, and individuals with other venereal diseases. In women, the peak incidence is between 16 and 35 years of age, but there is a relatively high prevalence in the 30 to 50 age group.

Transmission usually sexual

Prevalence linked to sexual activity

Nonvenereal transmission is uncommon. Transfer of organisms on shared washcloths may explain, in part, the high frequency of infection seen among institutionalized women. Female neonates are occasionally noted to harbor *T. vaginalis,* presumably acquiring it during passage through the birth canal. High levels of maternal estrogen produce a transient decrease in the vaginal pH of the child, rendering it more susceptible to colonization. Within a few weeks, estrogen levels drop, the vagina assumes its premenarchal state, and the parasite is eliminated.

Nonvenereal transmission uncommon

### Pathogenesis and Immunity

Direct contact of *T. vaginalis* with the squamous epithelium of the genitourinary tract results in destruction of the involved epithelial cells and the development of a neutrophilic inflammatory reaction and petechial hemorrhages. The precise pathogenesis of these changes are unknown. The organism is not invasive and extracellular toxins have never been demonstrated. The expression of a 200-kd parasitic glycoprotein, however, has been found to correlate with clinical manifestations. Changes in the microbial, hormonal, and pH environment of the vagina as well as factors inherent to the infecting parasite are thought to modulate the severity of the pathologic changes. Although humoral, secretory, and cellular immune reactions can be demonstrated in most infected women, they are of little diagnostic help and do not appear to produce clinically significant immunity.

Parasite damages epithelial cells on contact

## Trichomoniasis: Clinical Aspects

### Clinical Manifestations

In women, *T. vaginalis* produces a persistent vaginitis. Although up to half are asymptomatic at the time of diagnosis, most develop clinical manifestations within 6 months. Approximately 75% develop a discharge, which is typically accompanied by vulvar itching or burning (50%), dyspareunia (50%), dysuria (50%), and a disagreeable odor (10%). Although fluctuating in intensity, symptoms usually persist for weeks or months. Commonly, manifestations worsen during menses and pregnancy. Eventually, the discharge subsides, even though the patient may continue to harbor the parasite. In symptomatic patients, physical examination reveals reddened vaginal and endocervical mucosa. In severe cases, pe-

Chronic vaginitis lasting weeks to months

techial hemorrhages and extensive erosions are present. A red, granular, friable endocervix (strawberry cervix) is a characteristic, but uncommon, finding. An abundant discharge is generally seen pooled in the posterior vaginal fornix. Although classically described as thin, yellow, and frothy in character, the discharge more frequently lacks these characteristics. Recent studies have demonstrated that trichomoniasis both increases the risk of preterm birth and enhances susceptibility to HIV infections.

The urethra and prostate are the usual sites of infection in men; the seminal vesicles and epididymis may be involved on occasion. Infections are usually asymptomatic, possibly because of the efficiency with which the organisms are removed from the urogenital tract by voided urine. Symptomatic men complain of recurrent dysuria and scant, nonpurulent discharge. Acute purulent urethritis has been reported rarely. Trichomoniasis should be suspected in men presenting with nongonococcal urethritis, a history of either prior trichomonal infection or recent exposure to trichomoniasis.

Urethral and prostatic infection in men usually asymptomatic

#### DIAGNOSIS

The diagnosis of trichomoniasis rests on the detection and morphologic identification of the organism in the genital tract. Identification is accomplished most easily by examining a wet mount preparation for the presence of motile organisms. In women, a drop of vaginal discharge is the most appropriate specimen; in men, urethral exudate or urine sediment after prostate massage may be used. Although highly specific when positive, wet mounts are often negative in asymptomatic or mildly symptomatic patients and in women who have douched in the previous 24 hours. Giemsa- and Papanicolaou-stained smears provide little additional help. Cultures of urogenital specimens may increase the number of detected cases. Unfortunately, this procedure is not generally available in clinical laboratories and requires several days to complete. The recent introduction of a commercial system that allows direct, rapid microscopic examination without the need for daily sampling may ameliorate this situation. Direct detection of parasitic antigen in genital secretions may prove to be an acceptable alternative.

Wet mount examination for motile trophozoites sufficient in most symptomatic cases

Patients with trichomoniasis should be examined carefully for other venereal disease.

Positive cases should be tested for other sexually transmitted diseases

#### TREATMENT

Oral metronidazole (Flagyl) is extremely effective in recommended dosage, curing more than 95% of all infections. Simultaneous treatment of sexual partners may minimize recurrent infections, particularly when single-dose therapy is employed for the index case. Because of metronidazole's disulfiram-like activity, alcohol consumption should be suspended during treatment. Because of its potential teratogenic activity, the drug should never be used during the first trimester of pregnancy. Use in the last two trimesters is unlikely to be hazardous, but should be reserved for patients whose symptoms cannot be adequately controlled with local therapies. High-dose, long-term metronidazole treatment has been shown to be carcinogenic in rodents. No association with human malignancy has been described to date, and in the absence of a suitable alternative drug, metronidazole continues to be used.

Metronidazole cures 95% of cases

## Giardia

### ■ Giardia lamblia

*G. lamblia* was first described by Anton von Leeuwenhoek 300 years ago when he examined his own diarrheal stool with one of the first primitive microscopes. It was not until the past three decades, however, that the cosmopolitan flagellate became widely regarded in the United States as a pathogen. Of the six other flagellated protozoans known to parasitize the alimentary tract of humans, only one, *Dientamoeba fragilis,* has been credibly associated with disease. Definitive confirmation or refutation of its pathogenicity will, it is hoped, not require the passage of another three centuries.

Unlike *T. vaginalis, Giardia* possesses both a trophozoite and a cyst form (Fig 54–2). It is a sting-ray-shaped trophozoite 9 to 21 μm in length, 5 to 15 μm in width, and 2 to 4 μm in thickness. When viewed from the top, the organism's two nuclei and central parabasal bodies give it the appearance of a face with two bespectacled eyes and a crooked mouth. Four pairs of flagella—anterior, lateral, ventral, and posterior—reinforce this image by sug-

Trophozoite and cyst stages

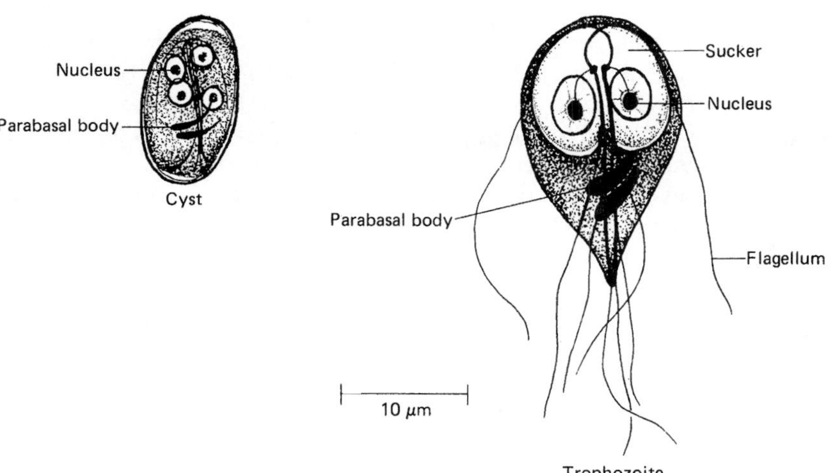


**Figure 54–2.** *Giardia lamblia.*

gesting the presence of hair and chin whiskers. These distinctive parasites reside in the duodenum and jejunum, where they thrive in the alkaline environment and absorb nutrients from the intestinal tract. They move about the unstirred mucous layer at the base of the microvilli with a peculiar tumbling or "falling leaf" motility or, with the aid of a large ventral sucker, attach themselves to the brush border of the intestinal epithelium. Unattached organisms may be carried by the fecal stream to the large intestine.

Move about duodenum and jejunum with tumbling motility

In the descending colon, if transit time allows, the flagella are retracted into cytoplasmic sheaths and a smooth, clear cyst wall is secreted. These forms are oval and somewhat smaller than the trophozoites. With maturation, the internal structures divide, producing a quadrinucleate organism harboring two sucking discs, four parabasal bodies, and eight axonemes (Fig 54–2). When fixed and stained, the cytoplasm pulls away from the cyst wall in a characteristic fashion. The mature cysts, which are the infective form of the parasite, may survive in cold water for more than 2 months and are resistant to concentrations of chlorine generally used in municipal water systems. They are transmitted from host to host by the fecal–oral route. In the duodenum of a new host, the cytoplasm divides to produce two binucleate trophozoites.

Cystic forms develop in colon

Resistant cysts transmitted from host to host

Organisms of the genus *Giardia* are among the most widely distributed of intestinal protozoa; they are found in fish, amphibians, reptiles, birds, and mammals. At first, it was assumed that *Giardia* strains found in different animals were host specific; on this basis, some 40 different species were described. As it is now recognized that some strains can infect multiple animal hosts, the practice of assigning species status by the host from which the parasite was recovered is considered invalid. Unfortunately, there is still no general agreement on an alternate method of speciation. Three morphologically distinct groups of *Giardia* have been described on the basis of their central parabasal body morphology.

Wide distribution in animal kingdom

## Giardiasis

### Epidemiology

Giardiasis has a cosmopolitan distribution; its prevalence is highest in areas with poor sanitation and among populations unable to maintain adequate personal hygiene. In developing countries, infection rates may reach 25 to 30%; in the United States, *G. lamblia* is found in 4% of stools submitted for parasitologic examination, making it this country's most frequently identified intestinal parasite. All ages and economic groups are represented, but young children and young adults are preferentially involved. Children with immunoglobulin deficiencies are more likely to acquire the flagellate, possibly because of a deficiency in intestinal immunoglobulin A. Giardiasis is also common among attendees of day-care centers. Attack rates of over 90% have been seen in the ambulatory non-toilet-trained population (age, 1 to 2 years) of these institutions, suggesting direct person-to-person transmission of the parasite. The frequency with which secondary cases are seen among family contacts

Transmission facilitated by poor hygiene, IgA deficiency

High attack rates in day-care centers

Giardiasis frequent among male homosexuals

reinforces this probability. Undoubtedly, direct fecal spread is also responsible for the high infection rate among male homosexuals. In several recent studies, the prevalence of giardiasis and/or amebiasis in that population has ranged from 11 to 40% and is correlated closely with the number of oral–anal sexual contacts

Water- or food-borne traveler's diarrhea lasts for weeks

Water-borne and, less frequently, food-borne transmission of this organism has also been documented, and probably accounts for the frequency with which American travelers to third-world nations acquire infection. Unlike the typical bacterial diarrhea syndrome seen in travelers, the diarrhea begins late in the course of travel and may persist for several weeks. More than 20 water-borne outbreaks of giardiasis have also been reported in the United States. The sources have included untreated pond or stream water, sewage-contaminated municipal water supplies, and chlorinated but inadequately filtered water. In a few of these outbreaks, epidemiologic data have suggested that wild mammals, particularly beavers, served as the reservoir hosts. Domestic cats and dogs, which have recently been shown to have a high prevalence of *G. lamblia,* may also act as reservoirs for human infections.

Beavers and other mammals possible sources

PATHOLOGY, PATHOGENESIS, AND IMMUNITY

Disease manifestations appear related to intestinal malabsorption, particularly of fat and carbohydrates. Disaccharidase deficiency with lactose intolerance, altered levels of intestinal peptidases, and decreased vitamin $B_{12}$ absorption have been demonstrated. The precise pathogenetic mechanisms responsible for these changes remain poorly understood. Mechanical blockade of the intestinal mucosa by large numbers of *Giardia,* damage to the fuzzy coat of the microvilli by the parasite's sucking disc, organism-induced deconjugation of bile salts, altered intestinal motility, accelerated turnover of mucosal epithelium with functional immaturity of transport systems, and mucosal invasion have all been suggested; none correlates well with clinical manifestations. Patients with severe malabsorption have jejunal colonization with enteric bacteria or yeasts, suggesting that these organisms may act synergistically with *Giardia*. Eradication of the associated microorganism, however, has not resulted uniformly in clinical improvement. Jejunal biopsies sometimes reveal a flattening of the microvilli and an inflammatory infiltrate, the severity of which correlates roughly with that of the of clinical disease. Generally, both malabsorption and the jejunal lesions have been reversed with specific treatment. The demonstration of occasional trophozoites in the submucosa raises the possibility that these changes reflect T lymphocyte-mediated damage. Immunologic reconstitution of experimentally infected nude (T lymphocyte-deficient) mice with lymphoid cells from previously infected animals results in similar mucosal changes.

Basis for malabsorption and jejunal pathology remains uncertain

Susceptibility to giardiasis has been related to several factors, including strain virulence, inoculum size, achlorhydria or hypochlorhydria, and immunologic abnormalities. In one experimental study, humans were challenged with varying doses from as few as 10 cysts. They were uniformly parasitized when 100 or more were ingested. Several workers have noted the frequency with which giardiasis occurs in achlorhydric and hypochlorhydric individuals. Although reinfection is common, the frequent occurrence of giardiasis in patients with immunologic diseases, plus the rarity with which it is seen in older adults, suggests that protective immunity, albeit incomplete, does develop in humans. Animal studies have demonstrated that giardia-specific, secretory IgA (sIgA) antibodies inhibit attachment of trophozoites to intestinal epithelium, perhaps by blocking parasite surface lectins. Moreover, antitrophozoite IgM or IgG antibodies, plus complement, are known to be capable of killing *Giardia* trophozoites.

Predisposing factors include hypochlorhydria, immocompromise

## ■ Giardiasis: Clinical Aspects

CLINICAL MANIFESTATIONS

In endemic situations, over two thirds of infected patients are asymptomatic. In acute outbreaks, this ratio of asymptomatic to symptomatic patients is usually reversed. When they do occur, symptoms begin 1 to 3 weeks after exposure; they typically include diarrhea, which is sudden in onset and explosive in character. The stool is foul smelling, greasy in appearance, and floats on water. It is devoid of blood or mucus. Upper abdominal cramping is common. Large quantities of intestinal gas produce abdominal distention, sulfuric eructations, and abundant flatus. Nausea, vomiting, and low-grade fever may be present.

Subclinical infections common

Diarrhea, cramping, flatus, and greasy stools

The acute illness generally resolves in 1 to 4 weeks; in children, however, it may persist for months, leading to significant malabsorption, weight loss, and malnutrition.

In many adults, the acute phase is often followed by a subacute or chronic phase characterized by intermittent bouts of mushy stools, flatulence, and "heartburn" and weight loss that persist for weeks or months. At times, patients presenting in this fashion deny having experienced the acute syndrome described previously. In the majority, symptoms and organisms eventually disappear spontaneously. It is not uncommon for lactose intolerance to persist after eradication of the organisms. This condition may be confused with an ongoing infection, and the patient may be subjected to unnecessary treatment.

Subacute and chronic infections with weight loss in adults

Lactose intolerance may persist

### Laboratory Diagnosis

The diagnosis is made by finding the cyst in formed stool or the trophozoite in diarrheal stools, duodenal secretions, or jejunal biopsy specimens. In acutely symptomatic patients, the parasite can usually be demonstrated by examining one to three stool specimens, providing appropriate concentration and staining procedures are used. In chronic cases, excretion of the organism is often intermittent, making parasitologic confirmation more difficult. Many of these patients can be diagnosed by examining specimens taken at weekly intervals over 4 to 5 weeks. Alternatively, duodenal secretions can be collected and examined for trophozoites in trichrome or Giemsa-stained preparations. There are now a number of reliable, commercially available, enzyme immunoassays for the direct detection of parasite antigen in stool. The value of serologic tests (anti-*Giardia* specific IgM) are under investigation. The organism can be grown in culture, but the methods are not currently adaptable to routine diagnostic work.

Demonstration of trophozoites and cysts in stool or duodenal aspirates diagnostic

EIA methods detect *Giardia* antigen in stool

### Treatment and Prevention

Three drugs are currently available for the treatment of giardiasis in the United States: quinacrine hydrochloride, metronidazole, and furazolidone. The latter drug is used by pediatricians because of its availability as a liquid suspension, but it has the lowest cure rate. Quinacrine and metronidazole are somewhat more effective (70 to 95%) and are preferred for patients capable of ingesting tablets. All three agents require 5 to 7 days of therapy. Tinadazole, an oral agent not yet available in the United States, is safe and effective in single-dose treatment. Albendazole may be useful in the infections refractory to the above agents. Because of the potential of giardiasis for person-to-person spread, it is important to examine and, if necessary, treat close physical contacts of the infected patient, including playmates at nursery school, household members, and sexual contacts. If possible, treatment should be withheld from pregnant women because of the potential teratogenicity of available drugs.

Several drugs available

Close contacts should be examined

Hikers should avoid ingestion of untreated surface water, even in remote areas, because of the possibility of contamination by feces of infected animals. Adequate disinfection can be accomplished with halogen tablets yielding concentrations higher than that generally achieved in municipal water systems. The safety of the latter results from additional flocculation and filtration procedures.

Avoid drinking untreated surface water

## BLOOD AND TISSUE FLAGELLATES

Of the many genera of hemoflagellates, two are pathogenic to humans: *Leishmania* and *Trypanosoma*. They reside and reproduce within the gut of specific insect hosts. When these vectors feed on a susceptible mammal, the parasite penetrates the feeding site, invades the blood and/or tissue of the new host, and multiplies to produce disease. The life cycle is completed when a second insect ingests the infected mammalian blood or tissue fluid. During the course of their passage through insect and vertebrate hosts, flagellates undergo developmental change. Within the gut of the insect (and in culture media) the organism assumes the **promastigote** (*Leishmania*) or **epimastigote** (*Trypanosoma*) form (Fig 54–3). These protozoa are motile, fusiform, and have a blunt posterior end and a pointed anterior from which a single flagellum projects. They measure 15 to 30 μm in length and 1.5 to 4.0 μm in width. In the promastigote, the kinetoplast is located in the anterior extremity and the flagellum exits from the cell immediately. The kinetoplast of the epimastigote, in contrast, is

Life cycle includes insect host stage

Promastigote and epimastigote forms in insects

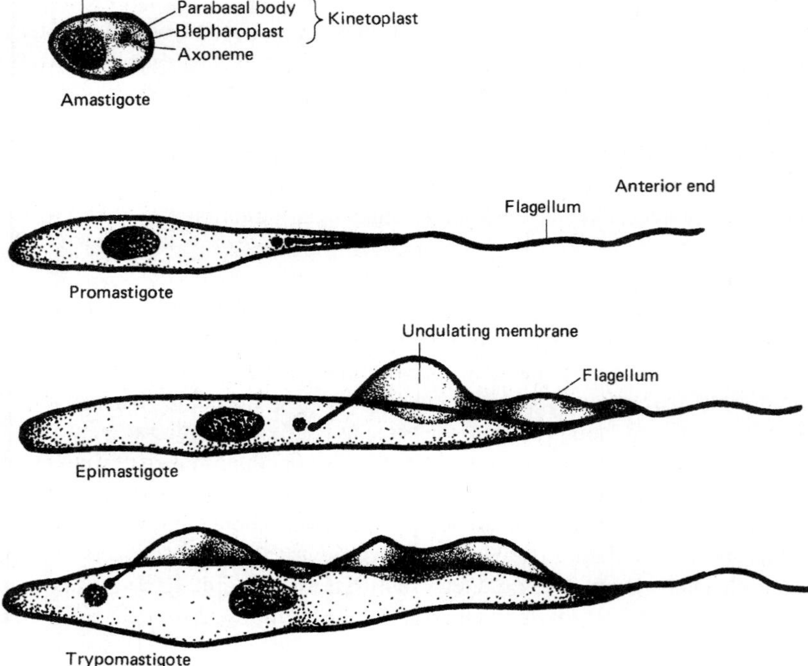


**Figure 54–3.** Stages in the life cycle of the hemoflagellates (Trypanosomidae).

located centrally, just in front of the vesicular nucleus. The flagellum runs anteriorly in the free edge of an undulating membrane before passing out of the cell. In the mammalian host, hemoflagellates appear as **trypomastigotes** (*Trypanosoma*) or **amastigotes** (*Leishmania, T. cruzi*). The former circulate in the bloodstream and closely resemble the epimastigote form, except that the kinetoplast is in the posterior end of the parasite. The amastigote stage is found intracellularly. It is round or oval, measures 1.5 to 5.0 μm in diameter, and contains a clear nucleus with a central karyosome. Although it has a kinetoplast and an axoneme, there is no free flagellum.

Trypomastigote and amastigote forms in humans

The flagellated forms move in a spiral fashion, and all reproduce by longitudinal binary fission. The flagellum itself does not divide; rather, a second one is generated by one of the two daughter cells. The organisms use carbohydrate obtained from the body fluids of the host in aerobic respiration.

## Leishmania

### Leishmania Species

*Leishmania* species are obligate intracellular parasites of mammals. Several strains can infect humans; they are all morphologically similar, resulting in some confusion over their proper speciation. Definitive identification of these strains requires isoenzyme analysis, monoclonal antibodies, kinetoplast DNA buoyant densities, DNA hybridization, and DNA restriction endonuclease fragment analysis or chromosomal karyotyping using pulse-field electrophoresis. The many strains can be more simply placed in four major groups based on their serologic, biochemical, cultural, nosologic, and behavioral characteristics. For the sake of clarity, these groups will be discussed as individual species in this chapter. Each, however, contains a variety of strains that have been accorded separate species or subspecies status by some authorities.

Species morphologically similar; differ in molecular features

The organisms can be propagated in hamsters and in a variety of commercially available liquid media.

## Disease Transmission

It is estimated that over 20 million people worldwide suffer from leishmaniasis and over 400,000 additional individuals acquire the infection annually. *Leishmania tropica* in the Old World and *L. mexicana* in the New World produce a localized cutaneous lesion or ulcer, known popularly as oriental sore and chiclero ulcer. *L. braziliensis* is the cause of American mucocutaneous leishmaniasis (espundia), and *L. donovani* is the etiologic agent of kala azar, a disseminated visceral disease.

Cutaneous ulcer or visceral infection (kala azar) the primary diseases

All four are transmitted by phlebotomine sandflies. These small, delicate, short-lived insects are found in animal burrows and crevices throughout the tropics and subtropics. At night, they feed on a wide range of mammalian hosts. Amastigotes ingested in the course of a meal assume the flagellated promastigote form, multiply within the gut, and eventually migrate to the buccal cavity. When the fly next feeds on a human or animal host, the buccal promastigotes are injected into the skin of the new host together with salivary peptides capable of inactivating host macrophages. Here, they activate complement by the classic (*L. donovani*) or alternative pathway, and are opsonized with C3 which mediates attachment to the CR1 and CR3 complement receptors of macrophages. Following phagocytosis, the promastigotes lose their flagella and multiply as the rounded amastigote form within the phagolysosome. In stained smears, the parasites take on a distinctive appearance and have been termed Leishman–Donovan bodies. Intracellular survival is mediated by a surface lipophosphoglycan (LPG) and an abundance of membrane-bound acid phosphatase, which inhibit the macrophage's oxidative burst and/or inactivate lysosomal enzymes. Continued multiplication leads to the rupture of the phagocyte and release of the daughter cells. Some may be taken up by a feeding sandfly; most invade neighboring mononuclear cells (Fig 54–4).

All four species transmitted by nocturnally feeding sandflies

Complement activation mediates attachment to macrophages

Intracellular survival by inhibiting macrophage killing mechanisms

Amastigotes released from macrophages can infect feeding sandfly

Continuation of this cycle results in extensive histiocytic proliferation. The course of the disease at this point is determined by the species of parasite and the host's immune response. In the localized cutaneous forms of leishmaniasis, a vigorous cellular immune response results in the development of a positive delayed skin (leishmanin) reaction, lymphocytic infiltration, reduction in the number of parasites, and, eventually, spontaneous disappearance of the primary skin lesion. In infections with *L. braziliensis,* this sequence may be followed weeks to months later by mucocutaneous metastases. These secondary lesions are highly destructive, presumably as a result of the host's hypersensitivity to parasitic antigens.

In localized cutaneous disease, cellular immune responses produce spontaneous cure

Mucocutaneous metastases in *L. braziliensis* infections

Some strains of *L. tropica* and *L. mexicana* fail to elicit an effective immune response in certain hosts. Such patients appear to have a selective suppressor T lymphocyte-mediated anergy to leishmanial antigens. Consequently, there is no infiltration of lymphocytes or decrease in the number of parasites. The skin test remains negative, and the skin lesions disseminate and become chronic (diffuse cutaneous leishmaniasis). In infections with *L. donovani,* there is a similar failure of cellular immunity; in this case the organisms are able to disseminate through the bloodstream to the visceral organs, possibly because of a relative resistance of *L. donovani* to the natural microbicidal properties of normal serum, and/or their ability to better survive at 37°C than strains of *Leishmania* causing cutaneous lesions. Although dissemination is associated with the development of circulating antibodies, they

Lack of cellular immune response in disseminated and chronic infections

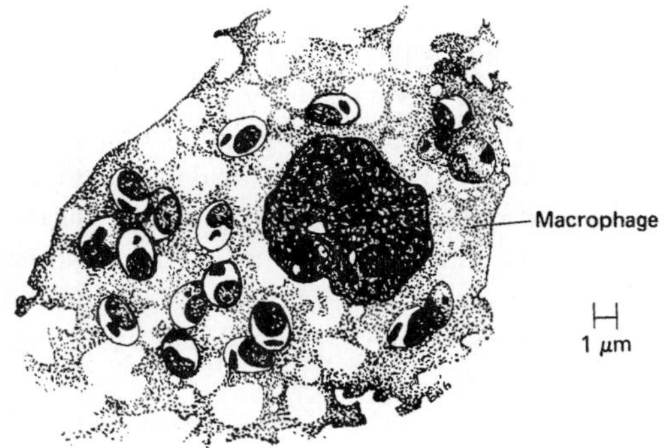


**Figure 54–4.** *Leishmania* within a mononuclear cell.

**TABLE 54–2. IMMUNE RESPONSE TO LEISHMANIASIS**

| Human Disease | Parasite | Leishmanin Skin Test | Number of Lymphocytes | Number of Parasites | Prognosis | Humoral Antibody Titer |
|---|---|---|---|---|---|---|
| Localized skin ulcer (oriental sore, chiclero ulcer, uta) | *L. tropica*<br>*L. mexicana* | Positive | Many | Few | Good | Low |
| Mucocutaneous lesions (espundia) | *L. braziliensis* | Positive | Many | Few | Poor | Low |
| Disseminated cutaneous | | | | | | |
| Ethiopian<br>American | *L. tropica*[a]<br>*L. mexicana*[a] | Negative | Few | Many | Poor | High |
| Disseminated visceral (kala azar) | *L. donovani* | Negative | Few | Many | Poor | High |

[a] Different subspecies from those causing localized skin ulcers.

do not appear to serve a protective function and may, via the production of immune complexes, be responsible for the development of glomerulonephritis. The immune responses in different forms of leishmaniasis are summarized in Table 54–2.

## Localized Cutaneous Leishmaniasis

### Epidemiology

Geographic distribution related to human and rodent reservoirs

The disease is a zoonotic infection of tropical and subtropical rodents. It is particularly common in areas of China, India, Asia Minor, Africa, the Mediterranean littoral, and Central America. In the latter area, *L. mexicana* infects several species of arboreal rodents. Humans become involved when they enter forested areas to harvest chicle for chewing gum and are bitten by infected sandflies. In the eastern hemisphere, the desert gerbil and other burrowing rodents serve as the reservoir hosts of *L. tropica*. Human infection occurs when rural inhabitants come in close contact with the burrows of these animals. In the Mediterranean area, southern Russia, and India, human disease involves urban dwellers, primarily children. In this setting, the domestic dog serves as the reservoir, although sandflies may also transmit *L. tropica* directly from human to human.

Canine reservoir in urban disease

### Clinical Manifestations

Chronic, self-limiting skin uleration

Lesions usually appear on the extremities or face (the ear in cases of chiclero ulcer) weeks to months after the bite of the sandfly. They first appear as pruritic papules, often accompanied by regional lymphadenopathy. In a few months the papules ulcerate, producing painless craters with raised erythematous edges, sharp walls, and a granulating base. Satellite lesions may form around the edge of the primary sore and fuse with it. Multiple primary lesions are seen in some patients. Spontaneous healing occurs in 3 to 12 months, leaving a pitted, depigmented scar. Occasionally the lesions fail to heal, particularly on the ears, leading to progressive destruction of the pinna. A permanent strain-specific immunity follows healing.

Strain-specific immunity

### Management

Demonstration of Leishma–Donovan bodies or culture from lesion biopsies

In endemic areas, the diagnosis is made on clinical grounds and confirmed by the demonstration of the organism in the advancing edge of the ulcer. Material collected by biopsy, curettage, or aspiration is smeared and/or sectioned, stained, and examined microscopically for the pathognomonic Leishman–Donovan bodies. Material should also be cultured in liquid media. The leishmanin skin test becomes positive early in the course of the disease and remains so for life. Recently, it has been demonstrated that small numbers of *Leishmania* may be detected in tissue by the polymerase chain reaction (PCR), and strains distinguished with probes to kinetoplast DNA. These techniques may soon permit direct, rapid, and specific diagnosis of all leishmanial infections.

Pentavalent antimonial agents, amphotericin B, and cycloguanil pamoate have all proved effective chemotherapeutic agents, but are generally reserved for extensive or multiple ulcerations. Recently, ketoconazole and allopurinol, either alone or in combination with the previously mentioned agents, have been found to be effective in some forms of cutaneous leishmaniasis. Secondary bacterial infections are treated with appropriate antibiotics.

Prophylactic measures include the control of the sandfly vector by use of insect repellents and fine mesh screening on dwellings.

## Mucocutaneous Leishmaniasis

### Epidemiology

*L. braziliensis* causes a natural infection in the large forest rodents of tropical Latin America. Sandflies transmit the infection to humans engaged in opening jungle areas for new settlements.

Rodent reservoir of *L. braziliensis*

### Clinical Manifestations

A primary skin lesion similar to oriental sore develops 1 to 4 weeks after sandfly exposure. Occasionally it undergoes spontaneous healing. More commonly, it progressively enlarges, often producing large vegetating lesions. After a period of weeks to years, painful, destructive, metastatic lesions of the mouth, nose, and occasionally the perineum, appear in 2 to 50% of patients. Sometimes, decades pass and the primary lesion totally resolves before the metastases manifest themselves. Destruction of the nasal septum produces the characteristic tapir nose. Erosion of the hard palate and larynx may render the patient aphonic. In blacks, the lesions are often large, hypertrophic, polypoid masses that deform the lips and cheeks. Fever, anemia, weight loss, and secondary bacterial infections are common.

Primary progressive lesion progresses to destructive oral and nasal lesions

### Management

The diagnosis is made by finding the organisms in the lesions as described for localized cutaneous leishmaniasis. As the propensity to metastasize to mucocutaneous sites is specific to certain species and subspecies, precise identification of the responsible organism as described in the introduction is of clinical import. The leishmanin skin test yields positive results, and most patients have detectable antibodies. As described for cutaneous leishmaniasis, it may soon be possible to provide a rapid, direct, species-specific diagnosis through the use of the polymerase chain reaction and probes to kinetoplast DNA.

Detection of organisms as with cutaneous leishmaniasis

Treatment is accomplished with the agents described later in the chapter for kala azar. Advanced lesions are often refractory, and relapse is common. Cured patients are immune to reinfection. Control measures, other than insect repellents and screening of dwellings, are impractical because of the sylvatic nature of the disease.

## Diffuse Cutaneous Leishmaniasis

Diffuse cutaneous leishmaniasis is an unusual disease seen primarily in Ethiopia, Brazil, the Dominican Republic, and Venezuela, where it is caused by variants of *L. tropica* and *L. mexicana* that do not stimulate a cellular immune response in the host. Massive dissemination of skin lesions results. The clinical picture bears a striking resemblance to that of lepromatous leprosy. The lesions contain large numbers of organisms, making the diagnosis quite simple. In contrast to all other forms of cutaneous leishmaniasis, the results of the leishmanin skin test are negative. The disease is progressive and very refractory to treatment. Pentamidine and amphotericin B may produce remissions, but cure is rare. Interferon-$\gamma$ may prove to be a useful adjunctive treatment.

Skin lesions resemble lepromatous leprosy; no cellular immune response

## Disseminated Visceral Leishmaniasis (Kala Azar)

### Epidemiology

Kala azar, which is caused by *L. donovani,* occurs in the tropical and subtropical areas of every continent except Australia. Its epidemiologic and clinical patterns vary from area to area. In Africa, rodents serve as the primary reservoir. Human cases occur sporadically, and the disease is often acute and highly lethal. In Eurasia and Latin America, the domestic dog is the most common reservoir. Human disease is endemic, primarily involves children, and runs a subacute to chronic course. In India, the human is the only known reservoir, and transmission is carried out by anthropophilic species of sandflies. The disease recurs in epidemic form at 20-year intervals, when a new cadre of nonimmune children and young adults ap-

Marked geographic differences in reservoirs and disease severity

pears in the community. There appears to be a high incidence of visceral leishmaniasis in patients with HIV infection. Presumably, HIV-induced immunosuppression either facilitates acquisition of the disease and/or allows reactivation of latent infection.

Pathogenesis and Pathology

After the host is bitten by an infected sandfly, the parasites disseminate in the bloodstream and are taken up by the macrophages of the spleen, liver, bone marrow, lymph nodes, skin, and small intestine. Histiocytic proliferation in these organs produces enlargement with atrophy or replacement of the normal tissue.

Parasites invade macrophages of reticuloendothelial system

Clinical Manifestations

Symptoms appear 3 to 12 months after acquisition of the parasite. Fever, which is usually present, may be abrupt or gradual in onset. It persists for 2 to 8 weeks and then disappears, only to reappear at irregular intervals during the course of the disease. A double-quotidian pattern (two fever spikes in a single day) is a characteristic, but uncommon, finding. Diarrhea and malabsorption are frequent in Indian cases, resulting in progressive weight loss and weakness. Physical findings include enlarged lymph nodes and liver, massively enlarged spleen, and edema. In light-skinned individuals, a grayish pigmentation of the face and hands is commonly seen, which gives the disease its name (kala azar, black disease). Anemia with resulting pallor and tachycardia are typical in advanced cases. Thrombocytopenia induces petechial formation and mucosal bleeding. The peripheral leukocyte count is usually less than 4000/mm$^3$; agranulocytosis with secondary bacterial infections contributes to lethality. Serum immunoglobulin G levels are enormously elevated, but play no protective role. Circulating antigen–antibody complexes are present and are probably responsible for the glomerulonephritis seen so often in this disease.

Delayed onset; recurrent fever; chronic disease; diarrhea

Severe systemic manifestations

Immune complex glomerulonephritis

Management

The diagnosis is made by demonstrating the presence of the organism in aspirates taken from the bone marrow, liver, spleen, or lymph nodes. In the Indian form of kala azar, *L. donovani* is also found in circulating monocytes. The specimens may be smeared, stained, and examined for the typical Leishman–Donovan bodies (amastigotes in mononuclear phagocytes) or cultured in artificial media and/or experimental animals. As described for cutaneous leishmaniasis, it may soon be possible to provide a rapid, direct, species-specific diagnosis through the use of the polymerase chain reaction and probes to kinetoplast DNA. Sensitive serologic tests are now available, but may demonstrate cross reactions in patients with *T. cruzi* infections. Results of the leishmanin skin test are negative during active disease, but become positive after successful therapy.

Demonstration of Leishman–Donovan bodies or culture

The mortality in untreated cases of kala azar is 75 to 90%. Treatment with pentavalent antimonial drugs lower this rate dramatically. Initial therapy, however, fails in up to 30% of African cases, and 15% of those that do respond eventually relapse. Resistant cases are treated with the more toxic pentamidine or amphotericin B. Allopurinol and interferon-γ have proven to be useful adjunctive therapies in resistant cases.

Up to 90% mortality without treatment

Control measures are directed at the *Phlebotomus* vector, with the use of residual insecticides, and at the elimination of mammalian reservoirs by treating human cases and destroying infective dogs.

## African Trypanosoma

African trypanosomiasis is a highly lethal meningoencephalitis transmitted to humans by bloodsucking flies of the genus *Glossina*. It occurs in two distinct clinical and epidemiologic forms: West African or Gambian sleeping sickness and East African or Rhodesian sleeping sickness. Nagana, a disease of cattle caused by a closely related trypanosome, renders over 10 million square kilometers of Central Africa unsuitable for animal husbandry.

### Trypanosoma brucei

Three recognized subspecies of *T. brucei*

The trypanosomes that produce these diseases are morphologically and serologically identical. Accordingly, they are considered varieties of a single species, *T. brucei*. The three subspecies, known as *T. brucei gambiense, T. brucei rhodesiense,* and *T. brucei brucei,* can be distinguished by their biologic characteristics, zymodeme types, mitochondrial morphology, and DNA hybridization patterns. All undergo similar development changes in the course of their passage from insect to mammalian host. Upon ingestion by the tsetse fly (*Glossina* sp.) and after a period of multiplication in the midgut, they migrate to the insect's salivary glands and assume the epimastigote form. After a period of weeks they are transformed into metacyclic trypomastigotes, which renders them infectious to mammals. When the fly again takes a blood meal, the parasite is inoculated with the fly's saliva. In the mammal, they continue to multiply extracellularly and eventually invade the bloodstream. During the initial stages of parasitemia, the trypomastigotes elongate to become graceful, slender organisms 30 μm or more in length. For reasons independent of the host's immune response, multiplication eventually slows, and some forms lose their flagella and assume a short, stumpy appearance. Near the end of the episode of parasitemia, both morphologic types may be seen in a single blood specimen. Regardless of their morphology, all trypomastigotes possess a highly immunogenic glycoprotein surface coat. Individual strains of *T. brucei* can change the antigenic character of this coat in a sequential and, at times, predictable fashion. A strain is capable of producing dozens, perhaps hundreds, of these variable antigen types, each of which is encoded in its own structural gene. The genetic repertoire seems to be strain specific. Expression of individual genes appears to be controlled by the sequential duplication and subsequent transfer of each gene (expression-linked copy) to one or more areas of the genome responsible for gene expression.

Epimastigote and trypomastigote forms develop in tsetse fly

Infectious trypomastigote form injected into the bloodstream of mammalian host from fly's saliva

Antigenic variation of glycoprotein coat of trypomastigotes is due to shifting expression of preexisting genes

## African Trypanosomiasis (Sleeping Sickness)

EPIDEMIOLOGY

The tsetse fly, and consequently sleeping sickness, is confined to the central area of Africa by that continent's two great deserts, the Sahara in the north and the Kalahari in the south. Approximately 50 million people live in this area and 10,000 to 20,000 acquire sleeping sickness annually. Major outbreaks have been reported in several locations within the endemic area over the past two decades. Riverine tsetse flies found in the forest galleries that border the streams of West and Central Africa serve as the vectors of the Gambian disease. Although these flies are not exclusively anthropophilic, humans are thought to be the major reservoir of the parasite. The infection rate in humans is affected by proximity to water, but seldom exceeds 2 to 3% in nonepidemic situations. Nevertheless, the extreme chronicity of the human disease ensures its continued transmission. Although an estimated 20,000 Americans travel to endemic areas each year, only 15 cases of African trypanosomiasis have been diagnosed in Americans since 1967.

Tsetse fly confined to central Africa

Humans major reservoir of West African sleeping sickness; chronicity ensures maintenance

Rhodesian sleeping sickness, in contrast, is transmitted by flies indigenous to the great savannas of East Africa that feed on the blood of the small antelope inhabiting these areas. The antelope serves as the major parasite reservoir, although human-to-human and cattle-to-human spread has been documented. Humans typically become infected only when they enter the savanna to hunt or to graze their domestic animals.

Savanna antelopes are reservoirs of East African trypanosomiasis; humans infected incidentally

PATHOLOGY AND PATHOGENESIS

Multiplication of the trypomastigotes at the inoculation site produces a localized inflammatory lesion. After the development of this chancre, organisms spread through lymphatic channels to the bloodstream, inducing a proliferative enlargement of the lymph nodes. The subsequent parasitemia is typically low grade and recurrent. As host antibodies (predominantly IgM) are produced to the surface antigen characteristic of a particular parasitemic wave, they bind to the organism, leading to its destruction by lysis and opsonization. The trypomastigotes disappear from the blood, reappearing 3 to 8 days later as new antigenic variants arise. The recurrences gradually become less regular and frequent, but may persist for weeks to years before finally disappearing. During the course of the parasitemia, trypanosomes localize in the small blood vessels of the heart and central nervous system. This localization results in endothelial proliferation and a perivascular infiltration of plasma cells and lymphocytes. In the brain, hemorrhage and a demyelinating panencephalitis may follow.

Local chancre at site of inoculation and lymphadenitis

Intermittent parasitemia with antigenic shifts

Parasites localize in blood vessels of heart and central nervous system with local vasculitis

The mechanism by which the trypanosomes elicit vasculitis is uncertain. The infection

High levels of IgM include specific and nonspecific antibodies

Immune complexes may cause anemia and vasculitis

stimulates the production of large quantities of immunoglobulin M (typically 8 to 16 times the normal limit). Most of this reaction represents specific protective antibodies that are ultimately responsible for the control of the parasitemia. Some, however, consists of nonspecific heterophile antibodies and rheumatoid factor. Antibody-induced destruction of trypanosomes releases invariant nuclear and cytoplasmic antigens with the production of circulating immune complexes. Many authorities believe that these complexes are largely responsible for the anemia and vasculitis seen in this disease.

## ■ Trypanosomiasis: Clinical Aspects

### Clinical Manifestations

Raised red papule on exposed surface

Parasitemic manifestations 2–3 weeks later

Central nervous system involvement late

The trypanosomal chancre appears 2 to 3 days after the bite of the tsetse fly as a raised, reddened nodule on one of the exposed surfaces of the body. With the onset of parasitemia 2 to 3 weeks later, the patient develops recurrent bouts of fever, tender lymphadenopathy, skin rash, headache, and impaired mentation. In the Rhodesian form of disease, myocarditis and central nervous system involvement begin within 3 to 6 weeks. Heart failure, convulsions, coma, and death follow in 6 to 9 months. Gambian sleeping sickness progresses more slowly. Bouts of fever often persist for years before central nervous system manifestations gradually appear. Spontaneous activity progressively diminishes, attention wavers, and the patient must be prodded to eat or talk. Speech grows indistinct, tremors develop, sphincter control is lost, and seizures with transient bouts of paralysis occur. In the terminal stage, the patient develops a lethal intercurrent infection or lapses into a final coma.

### Laboratory Diagnosis

Trypomastigotes sought in lymph node aspirates, blood, and cerebrospinal fluid

Animal inoculation may be required in Rhodesian disease

The diagnosis is made by microscopically examining lymph node aspirates, blood, or cerebrospinal fluid for the presence of trypomastigotes. Often the actively motile organisms can be seen in a simple wet mount preparation; definitive identification requires examination of an appropriately stained smear. If these tests prove negative, they are repeated after concentrating the organisms by centrifugation or filtration. Inoculation of rats or mice can also prove helpful in diagnosing the Rhodesian disease. The patient may also be screened for elevated levels of IgM in the blood and spinal fluid or specific trypanosomal antibodies by a variety of techniques. A simple card agglutination test, which can be performed on fingerstick blood, can provide serologic confirmation within minutes. Subspecies-specific DNA probes may eventually prove useful for the identification of organisms in clinical specimens.

### Treatment

Selection of drugs dependent on whether central nervous system is involved

Without CNS involvement recovery complete

Lumbar puncture must always be performed before initiation of therapy. If the specimen reveals evidence of central nervous system involvement, agents that penetrate the blood–brain barrier must be included. Unfortunately, the most effective agent of this type is a highly toxic arsenical, melarsoprol (Mel B). Although this agent occasionally produces a lethal hemorrhagic encephalopathy, the invariably fatal outcome of untreated central nervous system disease warrants its use. The ornithine decarboxylase inhibitor, eflornithine ($\alpha$-difluoromethylornithine, DFMO) appears capable, when used alone, or together with suramin, of curing central nervous system disease caused by *T. brucei gambiense* without the serious side effects associated with Mel B. Unfortunately, it is very expensive and is only variably effective in *T. brucei rhodesiense* infections. If the central nervous system is not yet involved, less toxic agents such as suramin or pentamidine can be used. In such cases, the cure rate is high and recovery complete.

### Prevention

Neither vector or reservoir control have been successful

Although a variety of tsetse fly control measures, including the use of insecticides, deforestation, and the introduction of sterile males into the fly population, have been attempted, none has proved totally practicable. Similarly, eradication of disease reservoirs by the early detection and treatment of human cases and the destruction of wild game has had limited success. Attempts to develop effective vaccines are currently under way, but are complicated by the antigenic variability of most trypomastigotes. A degree of personal protection can be achieved with insect repellents and protective clothing. Although prophylactic use of pentamidine was once advocated, enthusiasm for this treatment has waned.

## American Trypanosoma

American trypanosomiasis is a disease produced by *T. cruzi* and transmitted by true bugs of the family *Reduviidae*. Clinically, the infection presents as an acute febrile illness in children and a chronic heart or gastrointestinal malady in adults.

### Trypanosoma cruzi

The trypomastigotes of *T. cruzi* closely resemble those of *T. brucei,* and like them, disseminate from the site of inoculation to circulate in the peripheral blood of their mammalian hosts. Their developmental cycle, however, differs in several respects. Most significant, *T. cruzi* does not multiply extracellularly. The circulating trypomastigotes must invade tissue cells, lose their flagella, and assume the amastigote form before binary fission can occur. Continued multiplication leads to distention and eventual rupture of the tissue cell. Released parasites revert to trypomastigotes and regain the bloodstream. This new generation of trypomastigotes may invade other host cells, thus continuing the mammalian cycle. Alternatively, they may be ingested by a feeding reduviid and develop into epimastigotes within its midgut. Upon completion of the invertebrate cycle, the parasites migrate to the hindgut and are discharged as infectious trypomastigotes when the reduviid defecates in the process of taking another blood meal. This process can recur at each feeding for as long as 2 years. Infection in the new host is initiated when the trypomastigotes contaminate either the feeding site or the mucous membranes.

Mammalian cycle with nondividing extracellular trypomastigotes and dividing intracellular amastigotes

Invertebrate cycle produces trypomastigotes in bug

Reduviid bug may remain infectious for up to 2 years

*T. cruzi* comprises a number of strains, each with its own distinct geographic distribution, tissue preference, and virulence. They may be distinguished from one another with specific antisera and by differences in their isoenzyme and DNA restriction patterns. All are morphologically identical. In blood specimens, the trypomastigotes can be distinguished from those of *T. brucei* by their characteristic C or U shape, narrow undulating membrane, and large kinetoplast.

### American Trypanosomiasis (Chagas' Disease)

EPIDEMIOLOGY

Chagas' disease affects 15 to 20 million people living in South and Central America, producing death in 50,000 annually. Within these areas, it is the leading cause of heart disease, accounting for one quarter of all deaths in the 25- to 44-year age group. There are, currently, an estimated 100,000 infected Latin American immigrants living in the United States. *T. cruzi* has been found in both vertebrate and invertebrate hosts in the southwestern United States. Although serologic evidence suggests that the acquisition of human infections is this area is not uncommon, clinically apparent autochthonous cases have been rare.

Chagas' disease in South and Central America

Transmission occurs almost exclusively in rural areas where the reduviid can find harborage in animal burrows and in the cracked walls and thatch of poorly constructed buildings. This large (3-cm), winged insect leaves its hiding place at night to feed on its sleeping hosts. Its predilection to bite near the eyes or lips have earned this pest the nicknames of "kissing bug" and "assassin bug."

"Kissing bug" feeds at night in rural areas

In addition to humans, a number of wild and domestic animals, including rats, cats, dogs, opossums, and armadillos, serve as reservoirs. The close association of many of these hosts with human dwellings tends to amplify the incidence of disease in humans and the difficulty involved in its control. Congenital and transfusion-related infections are rapidly increasing problems in endemic areas. Transmission can more rarely be effected by breast feeding, organ transplantation and laboratory accidents.

Other wild and domestic animal reservoirs amplify transmission

PATHOGENESIS AND PATHOLOGY

Multiplication of the parasite at the portal of entry stimulates the accumulation of neutrophils, lymphocytes, and tissue fluid, resulting in the formation of a local chancre or chagoma. The subsequent dissemination of the organism with invasion of tissue cells produces a febrile illness that may persist for 1 to 3 months and result in widespread organ damage. Any nucleated host cell may be involved, but those of mesenchymal origin, especially the heart, skeletal muscle, smooth muscle, and glial nerve cells, are particularly susceptible. Cell entry is facilitated by binding to host cell fibronectin; a 60-kd *T. cruzi* surface pro-

Local chancre at site of inoculation

Entry to mesenchymal cells facilitated by fibronectin binding surface protein

Pore-forming protein aids escape from phagolysosome

Pseudocysts formed from cytoplasmic multiplication in host cells

Damage to heart may have immune mechanism

Ganglionic and smooth muscle cells last in digestive tract

tein (penetrin) appears to promote adhesion. Following penetration, the trypomastogote escapes the phagolysosome via the production of a pore-forming protein, transforms to the amastigote form, and multiplies freely within the cytoplasm to produce a pseudocyst, a greatly enlarged and distorted host cell containing masses of organisms. With the rupture of the pseudocyst, many of the released parasites disintegrate, eliciting an intense imflammatory reaction with destruction of surrounding tissue. The development of an antibody-dependent, cell-mediated immune response leads to the eventual destruction of the *T. cruzi* parasites and the termination of the acute phase of illness.

Parasitic antigens released during this acute phase may bind to the surface of tissue cells, rendering them susceptible to destruction by the host's immune response. It has been suggested by some that this results in the production of antibodies that cross-react with host tissue, initiating a sustained autoimmune inflammatory reaction in the absence of systemic manifestation of illness. In the heart, this reaction leads to changes in coronary microvasculature, loss of muscle tissue, interstitial fibrosis, degenerative changes in the mycocardial conduction system, and loss of intracardiac ganglia. In the digestive tract, loss of both ganglionic nerve cells and smooth muscle results in dilatation and loss of peristaltic movement, particularly of the esophagus and colon.

## American Trypanosomiasis: Clinical Aspects

### Clinical Manifestations

Most infections asymptomatic; acute disease usually in children

Myocardial injury indicated by tachycardia, electrocadiographic changes

Serologic studies suggest that only one third of newly infected individuals develop clinical illness. Acute manifestations, when they occur, are seen primarily in children. They begin with the appearance of the nodular, erythematous chagoma 1 to 3 weeks after the bite of the reduviid. If the eye served as a portal of entry, the patient will present with Romana's sign: reddened eye, swollen lid, and enlarged preauricular lymph node. The onset of parasitemia is signaled by the development of a sustained fever; enlargement of the liver, spleen, and lymph nodes; signs of meningeal irritation; and the appearance of peripheral edema or a transient skin rash. In a small percentage of symptomatic patients, heart involvement results in tachycardia, electrocardiographic changes, and occasionally arrhythmia, enlargement, and congestive heart failure. Newborns may experience acute meningoencephalitis. Clinical manifestations persist for weeks to months. In 5 to 10% of untreated patients, severe myocardial involvement or meningoencephalitis leads to death.

Chronic cardiomyopathy in adults leads to heart block, congestive heart failure

Dilatation of esophagus and colon seen in southern latitudes

Chronic disease, the result of end-stage organ damage, is usually seen only in adulthood. Ironically, the majority of patients with late manifestations deny a history of acute illness. The most serious of the late manifestations is heart disease. Studies of asymptomatic, seropositive patients in endemic areas have shown that a significant proportion have cardiac abnormalities demonstrated by electrocardiographic, echocardiographic, or cineangiographic techniques, suggesting that Chagas' cardiomyopathy is a progressive, focal disease of the myocardium and conduction system, leading eventually to clinical disease. This may present as arrhythmia, thromboembolic events, heart block, enlargement with congestive heart failure, and cardiac arrest. In some areas of rural Latin America, as much as 10% of the adult population may show cardiac manifestations. In the United States, chagasic heart disease in immigrants is usually misdiagnosed, initially, as coronary artery disease or idiopathic dilated cardiomyopathy. Megaesophagus and megacolon, which are less devastating than the heart disease, are typically seen in more southern latitudes. This geographic variation in clinical manifestations is thought to be attributable to a difference in tissue tropism between individual strains of *T. cruzi*. Megaesophagus leads to difficulty in swallowing and regurgitation, particularly at night. Megacolon produces severe constipation with irregular passage of voluminous stools. *T. cruzi* brain abscess has been described in a small number of AIDS patients.

### Laboratory Diagnosis

Demonstration of trypomastigotes in peripheral blood

Xenodiagnosis involves allowing bugs to feed

The diagnosis of acute Chagas' disease rests on finding the trypomastigotes from the peripheral blood and their morphologic identification as *T. cruzi*. The methods are similar to those described for diagnosis of African trypanosomiasis. If the results are negative, a laboratory-raised reduviid can be fed on the patient, then dissected and examined for the presence of parasites, a procedure known as xenodiagnosis. Alternatively, the blood may be cultured in a variety of artificial media or experimental animals. In the diagnosis of chronic disease, recovery of the organisms is the exception rather than the rule, and diagnosis depends upon the clinical, epidemiologic, and immunodiagnostic findings. A variety of serologic tests are available; small numbers of false-positive results limit their usefulness, particularly when used as screening procedures in non-endemic areas. The recent production of specific recombinant proteins and synthetic peptides for use as antibody targets may improve the reliability of these procedures. Polymerase chain reaction (PCR) techniques for the amplification of trypomastigote DNA may soon allow detection of the small numbers of circulating parasites present in patients with chronic disease.

Organisms difficult to recover in chronic disease

#### TREATMENT

The role of treatment in Chagas' disease remains unsettled. Two agents, nitrofuramox and benznidazole, effectively reduce the severity of acute disease, but appear to be ineffective in chronic infections. Both drugs must be taken for prolonged periods of time, may cause serious side effects, and do not always result in parasitologic cure. Allopurinol, a hypoxanthine oxidase inhibitor devoid of serious side effects, has recently been shown to be capable of suppressing parasitemia and reversing the sero-status of patients with acute disease. Additional studies will be required to confirm these encouraging results.

Treatment may reduce acute disease

#### PREVENTION

The reduviid vector can be controlled by applying residual insecticides to rural buildings at 2- or 3-month intervals. The addition of latex to the insecticide creates a colorless paint that prolongs activity. Fumigants can be used to prevent reinfection. Patching wall cracks, cementing floors, and moving debris and woodpiles away from human dwellings will reduce the number of reduviids within the home. Transfusion-induced disease, a major problem in endemic areas, has been partially controlled by the addition of gentian violet to all blood packs before use or by screening potential donors serologically for Chagas' disease. The large number of infected immigrants now entering non-endemic countries presents an increasing risk of transfusion-mediated parasite transmission in these areas as well. Recently, three cases of acute Chagas' disease were reported in immunosuppressed U.S. patients who received blood from donors unaware of their infection status; the resulting diseases were particularly fulminant. As immunodiagnositic tests for Chagas' disease are neither readily available nor sufficiently specific for use in non-endemic areas, prevention will probably require deferral of blood donations from persons who have recently immigrated from endemic areas. Immunoprophylaxis is not available at present.

Control of reduviid bugs in rural homes most important measure

## ADDITIONAL READING


Adler S. Darwin's illness. *Nature* (London) 1959;184:1102–1103. The author describes Charles Darwin's 40-year illness and offers convincing arguments that it represented Chagas' disease acquired during Darwin's round-the-world expedition on *H.M.S. Beagle*.

Badaro R, Johnson WD Jr. The role of interferon-γ in the treatment of visceral and diffuse cutaneous leishmaniasis. *J Infect Dis* 1993;167(suppl 1):S13–17.

Barker DC. DNA diagnosis of human leishmaniasis. *Parasitol Today* 1987;3:177–184. This article describes the techniques available for the characterization of leishmanial DNA and their utility in the separation of these organisms.

Heyworth MF. Immunology of *Giardia* and *Cryptosporidium* Infections. *J Infect Dis* 1992;166:465–472. A very recent review of the mechanisms of protective immunity in these two enteric pathogens.

Marsden PD. Selective primary health care: Strategies for control of disease in the developing world. XIV. Leishmaniasis. *Rev Infect Dis* 1984;6:736–744. An excellent concise review of the agent, clinical disease, epidemiology, and control.

Marsden PD. Selective primary health care: Strategies for control of disease in the developing world. XVI. Chagas' disease. *Rev Infect Dis* 1984;6:855–865. Another excellent review of the etiology, disease, epidemiology, and disease control methods.

Moore GT, Cross WM, McGuire CD, et al. Epidemic giardiasis at a ski resort. *N Engl J Med* 1969;281:402–407. This and the report of Walzer et al. are two of the early studies to document the pathogenicity of *Giardia lamblia* and its transmission via water supplies.

Phillips SC, Mildvan D, Williams DC, et al. Sexual transmission of enteric protozoa and helminths in a venereal-disease clinic population. *N Engl J Med* 1981;305:603–606. These authors establish that homosexual men have a higher prevalence with *Entamoeba histolytica* and *Giardia lamblia* and that the association between these infections and oral–anal sex is significant.

Rein MF, Muller M. *Trichomonas vaginalis*. In: Holmes KK, Mardh PA, Sparling PH, Wiesner PJ, eds. *Sexually Transmitted Diseases*. New York, McGraw-Hill, 1984. Most recent comprehensive review of this parasite and associated disease.

Stevens DP. Selective primary health care: Strategies for control of disease in the developing world. XIX. Giardiasis. *Rev Infect Dis* 1985;7:530–535. A brief summary of the worldwide problem with giardiasis with discussion of the relative roles of chemotherapy, sanitation, and immunization in the control of this disease.

Tanowitz HB, Kirchhoff LV, Simon D, et al. Chagas' disease. *Clin Microbiol Rev* 1992. 5:400–419. A superb recent review of this disease that emphasizes the experimental studies on pathogenesis.

Walzer PD, Wolfe MS, Schultz MG. Giardiasis in travelers. *J Infect Dis* 1971;124:235–237. One of the first articles establishing the pathogenicity of *Giardia*.

Warren KS, ed. *Immunology and Molecular Biology of Parasitic Infections.* 3rd ed. Boston, Blackwell Scientific, 1993. This relatively comprehensive monograph discusses general immune responses to parasitic infections as well as the immunity, immunopathology, immunodiagnosis, and molecular biology of specific parasitic diseases.

Werbovetz KA, Jeronimo SMB, Macdonald TL, Pearson RD. Treatment of leishmaniasis and trypanosomiasis. *Cur Opin Infect Dis* 1992;5:840–848. Recent, comprehensive literature review.

Wolf MS. Giardiasis. *Clin Microbiol Rev* 1992;5:93–100. A concise, recent review of this common disease.

# Intestinal Nematodes

*James J. Plorde*

The intestinal nematodes have cylindric, fusiform bodies covered with a tough, acellular cuticle. Sandwiched between this integument and the body cavity are layers of muscle, longitudinal nerve trunks, and an excretory system. A tubular alimentary tract consisting of a mouth, esophagus, midgut, and anus runs from the anterior to the posterior extremity. Highly developed reproductive organs fill the remainder of the body cavity. The sexes are separate; the male worm is generally smaller than its mate. The female, which is extremely prolific, can produce thousands of offspring, generally in the form of eggs. Typically, the eggs must incubate or embryonate outside of the human host before they become infectious to another person; during this time, the embryo repeatedly segments, eventually developing into an adolescent form known as a larva. In some species of nematodes, offspring develop to the larval stage in the uterus of the worm. The duration and site of embryonation differ with each worm species and determine how it will be transmitted to the new host. In many cases, eggs of nematodes that dwell within the human gastrointestinal tract are carried to the environment in the feces and embryonate on the soil for a period of weeks before becoming infectious. The egg may then be ingested with contaminated food. In some species, the egg hatches outside of the host, releasing a larva capable of penetrating the skin of a person who comes in direct physical contact with it. Obviously, intestinal nematodes are principally found in areas where human feces are deposited indiscriminately or used for fertilizer.

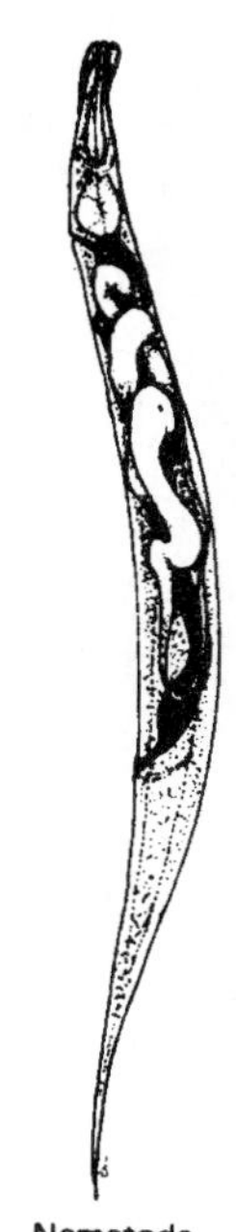

Nematode

There are six intestinal nematodes that commonly infect humans: *Enterobius vermicularis* (pinworm), *Trichuris trichuria* (whipworm), *Ascaris lumbricoides* (large roundworm), *Necator americanus* and *Ancylostoma duodenale* (hookworms), and *Strongyloides stercoralis.* Together they infect more than one quarter of the human race, producing embarrassment, discomfort, malnutrition, anemia, and occasionally death. Other closely related nematodes of animals that may occasionally infect humans are also listed in Table 55–1, but will not be discussed here.

Long survival in gut lumen

The adults of each of the six nematodes listed previously can survive for months or years within the lumen of the gut. The severity of illness produced by each depends upon the level of adaptation to the host it has achieved. Some species have a simple life cycle that can be completed without serious consequences to the host. Less well-adapted parasites, on the other hand, have more complex cycles, often requiring tissue invasion and/or production of enormous numbers of offspring to ensure their continued survival and dissemination. Within a given species, disease severity is related directly to the number of adult worms harbored by the host. The greater the worm load or worm burden, the more serious the consequences. As nematodes do not multiply within the human, small worm loads may remain asymptomatic and undetected throughout the lifespan of the parasite. Repeated infections, however, will progressively increase the worm burden and at some point induce symptomatic disease. Although humans can mount an immune response that will eventually lead to the expulsion of worms, it is slow to develop and incomplete. It is therefore the frequency

Worm load and repeated infection important to disease severity

**TABLE 55–1. INTESTINAL NEMATODES**

| Human Parasite | Animal Parasite | Human Disease |
|---|---|---|
| *Enterobius vermicularis* (pinworm) | | Enterobiasis |
| *Trichuris trichuria* (whipworm) | | Trichuriasis |
| | *Capillaria philippinensis* | Intestinal capillariasis |
| *Ascaris lumbricoides* (large roundworm) | | Ascariasis |
| | *Ascaris suum* | Ascariasis |
| | *Anisakis* sp. | Anisakiasis |
| | *Toxocara canis* *Toxocara cati* | Toxocariasis (visceral larva migrans) |
| *Necator americanus* (hookworm) | | Hookworm disease |
| *Ancylostoma duodenale* (hookworm) | *Ancylostoma braziliense* | Cutaneous larva migrans |
| *Strongyloides stercoralis* | | Strongyloidiasis |

and intensity of reinfection, more than the host's immune response, that determine the worm burden.

## LIFE CYCLES

*Enterobius vermicularis* is the best adapted intestinal nematode

The life cycles of the intestinal nematodes are summarized in Table 55–2. *Enterobius vermicularis* (pinworm), the best adapted of the intestinal nematodes, has the simplest life cycle. It feeds, grows, and copulates within the gut of its host before transiting the anus to deposit its eggs on the perineal skin. The eggs embryonate within hours and are subsequently transported to the same, or a new, host via fingers or dust. Following their inhalation or ingestion, the eggs are swallowed and hatch in the bowel lumen, completing the cycle. The only significant difference between this and the life cycle of *Trichuris trichuria* (whipworm) is that the eggs of the latter are passed in the stool and must incubate on soil before becoming infectious. This relatively minor difference has profound epidemiologic ramifications, because *Trichuris* can be passed only in populations that practice indiscriminate defecation and live in climates suitable for the maturation of eggs in the soil.

Other nematodes have increasingly complex life cycles

*Ascaris lumbricoides* is transmitted in a manner similar to *T. trichuria*. However, after hatching from the egg in the gut lumen, ascarid larvae penetrate the bowel wall and migrate through the host's liver and lung before returning, older and more sedentary, to the

**TABLE 55–2. LIFE CYCLES OF INTESTINAL NEMATODES**

| Parasite | Route of Infection | Migration in Body | Diagnostic Form | Site of Embryonation | Infective Form | Free-Living Cycle |
|---|---|---|---|---|---|---|
| *Enterobius vermicularis* | Mouth | Intestinal | Egg | Perineum | Egg | No |
| *Trichuris trichuria* | Mouth | Intestinal | Egg | Soil | Egg | No |
| *Ascaris lumbricoides* | Mouth | Pulmonary | Egg | Soil | Egg | No |
| *Necator americanus*[a] | Skin | Pulmonary | Egg | Soil | Filariform larvae | No |
| *Strongylodes stercoralis* | Skin | Pulmonary | Rhabditiform larvae | Soil; intestine[b] | Filariform larvae | Yes |

Reproduced with permission from Plorde JJ. In Isselbacher et al: *Harrison's Principles of Internal Medicine.* 9th ed. New York, McGraw-Hill, 1980, Table 206–3, p. 891.

[a] Also *Ancylostoma duodenale.*

[b] Intestine only in cases of autoinfection.

protective environment of the gut lumen. This maladaptive sojourn of juvenile worms through the host tissue is also seen in the life cycles of the hookworms and *Strongyloides stercoralis*. In contrast to *Ascaris*, however, the eggs of the latter two nematodes hatch shortly before or after they are passed in the stool of the original host, resulting in the seeding of the external environment with larval forms capable of penetrating human skin. Transmission is effected when a new host comes into physical contact with the contaminated soil. The adaptation of *S. stercoralis* is the least satisfactory of the intestinal nematodes and, in an evolutionary sense, appears to have occurred quite recently. In addition to the hookworm-like cycle described above, it has the twin capacities to complete its life cycle entirely within the body of the host or to survive in the external environment as a free-living soil organism.

*Strongyloides stercoralis* is least well adapted

## PARASITES AND DISEASES

### Enterobius

#### ■ Enterobius vermicularis (Pinworm)

The adult female is a 10-mm-long, cream-colored worm with a sharply pointed tail, characteristics that have given rise to the common name pinworm. Running longitudinally down both sides of the body are small ridges that widen anteriorly to fin-like alae. The seldom-seen male is smaller (3 mm) and possesses a ventrally curved tail and copulatory spicule. The clear, thin-shelled, ovoid eggs are flattened on one side and measure 25 by 50 µm (Fig 55–1).

Common name is pinworm

Life Cycle

The adult worms lie attached to the mucosa of the cecum. As its period of gravidity draws to a close, the female migrates down the colon, slips unobserved through the anal canal in the dark of the night, and deposits 20,000 sticky eggs on the host's perianal skin, bedclothes, and linens. The eggs are near maturity at the time of deposition and become infectious shortly thereafter. Handling of bedclothes or scratching of the perianal area to relieve the associated itching results in adhesion of the eggs to the fingers and subsequent transfer to the oral cavity during eating or other finger-mouth maneuvers. Alternatively, the eggs may be shaken into the air (for example, during making of the bed), inhaled, and swallowed. The eggs subsequently hatch in the upper intestine and the larvae migrate to the cecum, matur-

Adults inhabit cecum

Female transits anus at night to depost eggs on perineum

Eggs infectious to host and others shortly after deposition

Ingested eggs hatch and larvae mature to adults in intestine

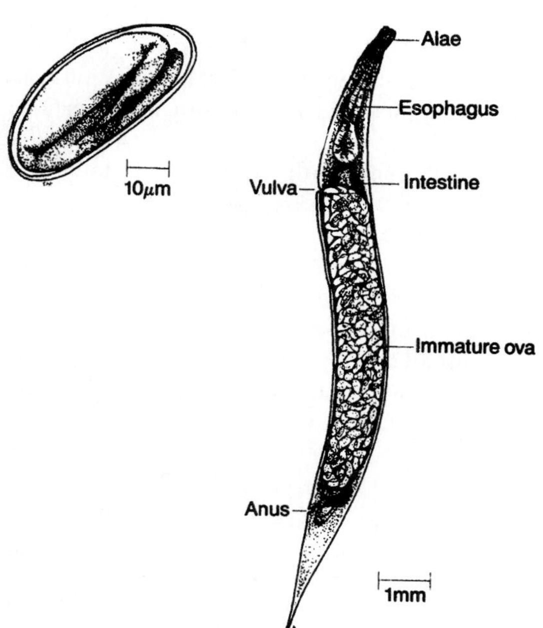


**Figure 55–1.** Female pinworm (*Enterobius vermicularis*) and embryonated egg.

ing to adults and mating in the process. The entire adult-to-adult cycle is completed in 2 weeks.

## Enterobiasis

Epidemiology

Infects 30–40 million in United States

The pinworm is the oldest and most widespread of the helminths. Eggs have been found in a 10,000-year-old coprolith, making this nematode the oldest demonstrated infectious agent of humans. It has been estimated to infect at least 200 million people worldwide, 30 to 40 million in the United States alone. Despite evidence that its prevalence is now decreasing in the United States, in both that country and in western Europe it remains the single most common cause of human helminthiasis. Infection is more common among the young and poor, but may be found in any age or economic class. The incidence in white individuals is significantly higher than that in blacks.

Resistant infective eggs

The eggs are relatively resistant to desiccation and may remain viable in linens, bedclothes, or house dust for several days. Once infection is introduced into a household, other family members are rapidly infected.

Pathogenesis and Immunity

The adult worms produce no significant intestinal pathology and do not appear to induce protective immunity.

## Enterobiasis: Clinical Aspects

Clinical Manifestations

Nocturnal pruritis ani

Occasional infection of female genitourinary tract

*E. vermicularis* seldom produces serious disease. The most frequent symptom is pruritis ani (anal itching). This symptom is most severe at night and has been attributed to the migration of the gravid female. It may lead to irritability and other minor complaints. In severe infections, the intense itching may lead to scratching, excoriation, and secondary bacterial infection. In female patients, the worm may enter the genital tract, producing vaginitis, granulomatous endometritis, or even salpingitis. It has also been suggested that migrating worms might carry enteric bacteria into the urinary bladder in young women, inducing an acute bacterial infection of the urinary tract. Although this worm is frequently found in the lumen of the resected appendix, it is doubtful that it plays a causal role in appendicitis. Perhaps the most "serious" effect of this common infection is the psychic trauma suffered by the economically advantaged when they discover that they, too, are subject to intestinal worm infection.

Laboratory Diagnosis

Anal cellophane tape test detects ova

Eosinophilia is usually absent. The diagnosis is suggested by the clinical manifestations and confirmed by the recovery of the characteristic eggs from the anal mucosa. Identification is accomplished by applying the sticky side of cellophane tape to the mucocutaneous junction, then transferring the tape to a glass slide and examining the slide under the low-power lens of a microscope. Occasionally, the adult female will be seen by a parent of an infected child or recovered with the cellophane tape procedure.

Treatment and Prevention

All family members may need treatment

Reinfection common

Several highly satisfactory agents, including pyrantel pamoate and mebendazole, are available for treatment. Many authorities believe that all members of a family or other cohabiting group should be treated simultaneously. In severe infections, retreatment after 2 weeks is recommended. Although cure rates are high, reinfection is extremely common. It need not be treated in the absence of symptoms.

# Trichuris

## Trichuris trichuria (Whipworm)

The adult whipworm is 30 to 50 mm in length. The anterior two-thirds is thin and threadlike, whereas the posterior end is bulbous, giving the worm the appearance of a tiny whip.

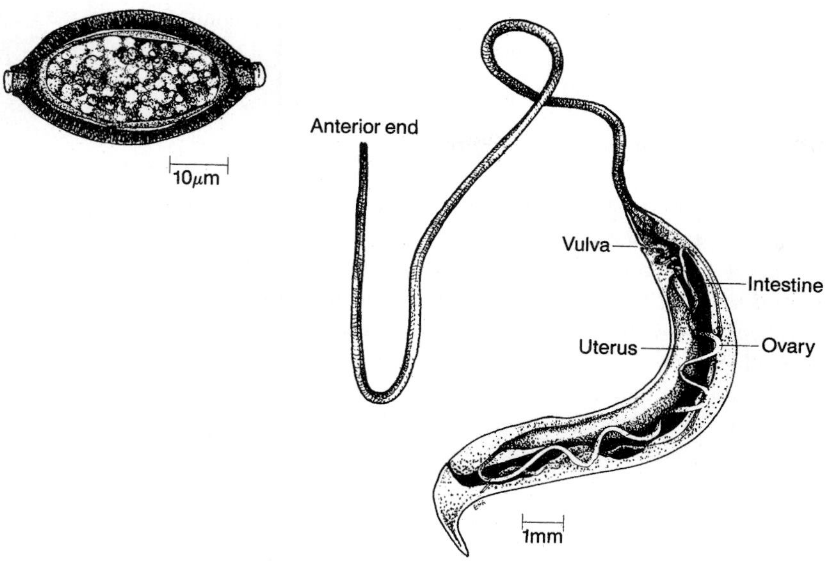


**Figure 55–2.** Female whipworm (*Trichuris trichuria*) and unembryonated egg.

The tail of the male is coiled, that of the female straight. The female produces 3000 to 10,000 oval eggs each day. They are of the same size as pinworm eggs, but have a distinctive thick brown shell with translucent knobs on both ends (Fig 55–2).

Whipworm produces up to 10,000 eggs a day

LIFE CYCLE

*Trichuris trichuria* has a life cycle that differs from that of the pinworm only in its external phase. The adults live attached to the colonic mucosa by their thin anterior end. While retaining its position in the cecum, the gravid female releases its eggs into the lumen of the gut. These pass out of the body with the feces and, in poorly sanitated areas of the world, are deposited on soil. The eggs are immature at the time of passage and must incubate for at least 10 days (longer if soil conditions, temperature, and moisture are suboptimal) before they become fully embryonated and infectious. Once mature, they are picked up on the hands of children at play or of agricultural workers and passed to the mouth. In areas where human feces are used as fertilizer, raw fruits and vegetables may be contaminated and later ingested. Following ingestion, the eggs hatch in the duodenum, and the released larvae mature for approximately 1 month in the small bowel before migrating to their adult habitat in the cecum.

Adults inhabit cecum and release eggs to lumen

Eggs must mature in soil for 10 days

## Trichuriasis

EPIDEMIOLOGY

Although it is less widespread than the pinworm, the whipworm is a cosmopolitan parasite, infecting approximately 1 billion people throughout the world. It is concentrated in areas where indiscriminate defecation and a warm, humid environment produce extensive seeding of soil with infectious eggs. In tropical climates, infection rates may be as high as 80%. Although the incidence is much lower in temperate climates, trichuriasis affects 2 million individuals throughout the rural areas of the southeastern United States. Here it occurs primarily in family and institutional clusters, presumably maintained by the poor sanitary habits of toddlers and the mentally retarded. Although the intensity of infection is generally low, adult worms may live 4 to 8 years.

Associated with defecation on soil and warm, humid climate

Adult worms live for years

PATHOGENESIS AND IMMUNITY

Attachment of adult worms to the colonic mucosa and their subsequent feeding activities produce localized ulceration and hemorrhage (0.005 mL blood per worm per day). The ulcers provide enteric bacteria with a portal of entry to the bloodstream, and occasionally a sustained bacteremia results. A decrease in the prevalence of trichuriasis in the postadolescent period and the demonstration of acquired immunity in experimental animal infections

Local colonic ulceration provides entry point to bloodstream for bacteria

suggest that immunity may develop in naturally acquired human infections. An IgE-mediated immune mucosal response is demonstrable in humans, but is insufficient to cause appreciable parasite expulsion.

## Trichuriasis: Clinical Aspects

Colonic dmage with abdominal pain, diarrhea

Colonic or rectal prolapse with heavy worm load

### Clinical Manifestations

Light infections are asymptomatic. With moderate worm loads, damage to the intestinal mucosa may induce nausea, abdominal pain, diarrhea, and stunting of growth. Occasionally, a child may harbor 800 worms or more. In these situations, the entire colonic mucosa is parasitized, with significant mucosal damage, blood loss, and anemia. The shear force of the fecal stream on the bodies of the worms may produce prolapse of the colonic or rectal mucosa through the anus, particularly when the host is straining at defecation or childbirth. The sudden appearance of a prolapsed rectum teeming with hundreds of wriggling whipworms has been known to produce nausea and lightheadedness in uninitiated obstetricians.

Stools examined for characteristic eggs

### Laboratory Diagnosis

In light infections, stool concentration methods may be required to recover the eggs. Such procedures are almost never necessary in symptomatic infections, as they inevitably produce more than 10,000 eggs per gram of feces, a density readily detected by examining 1 to 2 mg of emulsified stool with the low-power lens of a microscope. A moderate eosinophilia is common in such infections.

### Treatment

Infections should not be treated unless they are symptomatic. Mebendazole is the drug of choice. Although the cure rate is only 60 to 70%, more than 90% of the adult worms are usually expelled, rendering the patient asymptomatic. Prevention requires the improvement of sanitary facilities.

# Ascaris

## Ascaris lumbricoides

Earthworm-sized roundworm produces elipitical eggs

Eggs viable up to 6 years

*A. lumbricoides,* a short-lived worm (6 to 18 months), is the largest and most common of the intestinal helminths. Measuring 150 to 350 mm in length, it dwarfs its fellow gut roundworms and brings an unexpected richness to our mental image of a parasite. Its firm, creamy cuticle and more pointed extremities differentiate it from the common earthworm, which it otherwise resembles in both size and external morphology. The male is slightly smaller than the female and possesses a curved tail with copulatory spicules. The female passes 200,000 eggs daily, whether she is fertilized or not. Eggs are elliptic in shape; measure 35 by 55 µm; and have a rough, mamillated, albuminous coat over their chitinous shells. They are highly resistant to environmental conditions and may remain viable for up to 6 years in mild climates (Fig 55–3).

Adults inhabit small intestine

Eggs must mature for 3 weeks in soil

Larvae from ingested eggs enter bloodstream, pass through alveoli and via respiratory tract and esophagus to intestines

### Life Cycle

The adult ascarids live high in the small intestine, where they actively maintain themselves by dint of muscular activity. The eggs are deposited into the intestinal lumen and passed in the feces. Like those of *Trichuris,* the eggs must embryonate in soil, usually for a minimum of 3 weeks, before becoming infectious. The similarity to *Trichuris* ends, however, with the ingestion of the eggs by the host. After hatching, the larvae penetrate the intestinal mucosa and invade the portal venules. They are carried to the liver, where they are still small enough to squeeze through that organ's capillaries and exit in the hepatic vein. They are then carried to the right side of the heart and subsequently pumped out to the lung. In the course of this migration, the larvae increase in size. By the time they reach the pulmonary capillaries, they are too large to pass through to the left side of the heart. Finding their route blocked, they rupture into the alveolar spaces, are coughed up, and subsequently swallowed. After regaining access to the upper intestine, they complete their maturation and mate.

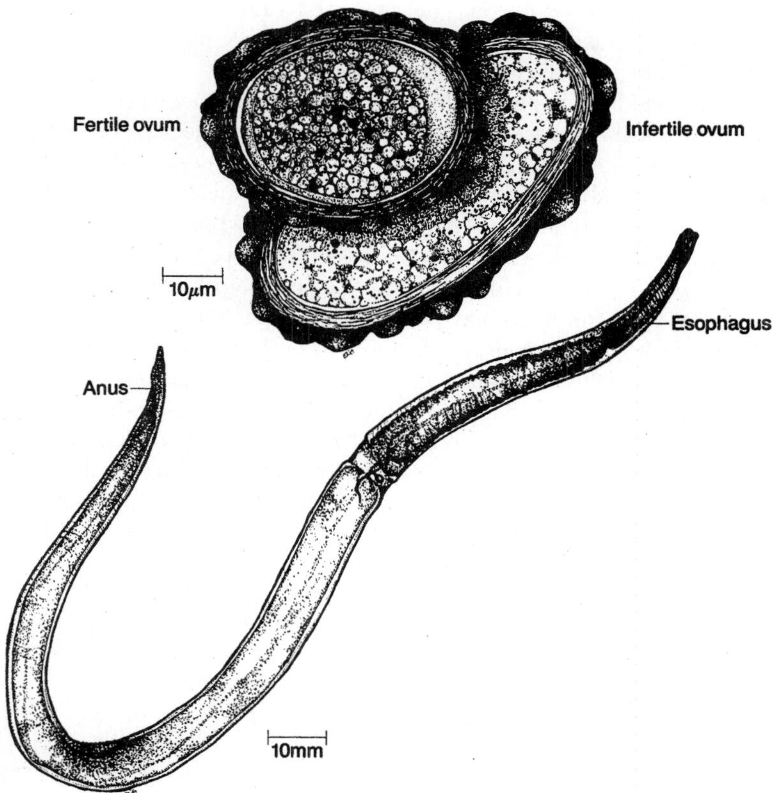


**Figure 55–3.** Female *Ascaris lumbricoides* worm and fertile and infertile egg.

## ■ Ascariasis

EPIDEMIOLOGY

More than 1 billion of the world's population, including 4 million Americans, are infected. Together they have been estimated to pass more than 25,000 tons of *Ascaris* eggs into the environment annually. Like trichuriasis, with which it is coextensive, ascariasis is a disease of warm climates and poor sanitation. It is maintained by small children who defecate indiscriminately in the immediate vicinity of the home and pick up infectious eggs on their hands during play. Geophagia is common and may result in massive worm loads. The parasite may also be acquired through ingestion of egg-contaminated food by the host; in dry, windy climates, eggs may become airborne and be inhaled and swallowed. In tropical areas, the entire population may be involved; most worms, however, appear to be aggregated in a minority of the population, suggesting that some individuals are predisposed to heavy infections. Isolated infected family clusters are more common in temperature climes.

Epidemiology similar to that of *Trichuris*

PATHOGENESIS AND IMMUNITY

There is convincing evidence that ascariasis induces a protective immune response in the host. Moreover, the severity of pulmonary damage induced by the migration of larvae through the lung appears to be related in part to an immediate hypersensitivity reaction to larval antigens.

Hypersensitive pulmonary reactions to larval migration

## ■ Ascariasis: Clinical Aspects

CLINICAL MANIFESTATIONS

Clinical manifestations may result from either the migration of the larvae through the lung or the presence of the adults in the intestinal lumen. Pulmonary involvement is usually seen in communities where transmission is seasonal; the severity of symptoms is related to the degree of hypersensitivity induced by previous infections and the intensity of the current exposure. Fever, cough, wheezing, and shortness of breath are common. Laboratory studies reveal eosinophilia, oxygen denaturation, and migratory pulmonary infiltrates. Death from respiratory failure has been noted occasionally.

Infections asymptomatic with small worm loads

If the worm load is small, infections with adult worms may be completely asymptomatic. They come to clinical attention when the parasite is vomited up or passed in the stool. This situation is most likely during episodes of fever, which appear to stimulate the worms to increase motility. Most physicians who have worked in underdeveloped countries have had the disconcerting experience of observing an ascarid crawl out of a patient's mouth, nose, or ear during an otherwise uneventful evaluation of fever. Occasionally an adult worm will migrate to the appendix, bile duct, or pancreatic duct, causing obstruction and inflammation of the organ. Heavier worm loads may produce abdominal pain and malabsorption of fat, protein, carbohydrate, and vitamins. In marginally nourished children, growth may be retarded. Occasionally a bolus of worms may form and produce intestinal obstruction, particularly in children. Worm loads of 50 are not uncommon, and as many as 2000 worms have been recovered from a single child. In the United States, where worm loads tend to be modest, obstruction occurs in 2 per 1000 infected children per year. The mortality in these cases is 3%. Estimates of annual, worldwide deaths from ascariasis range from 8000 to 100,000.

Malabsorption and occasional obstruction produced with heavy worm loads

#### Laboratory Diagnosis

Stool examination readily reveals characteristic eggs

The diagnosis is generally made by finding the characteristic eggs in the feces. The extreme productivity of the female ascarid generally makes this task an easy one, except when the atypical-appearing unfertilized eggs predominate. The pulmonary phase of ascariasis is diagnosed by the finding of larvae and eosinophils in the sputum.

#### Treatment and Prevention

Pyrantel pamoate and mebendazole are both highly effective; the latter is preferred if *T. trichuria* is also present. Communitywide control of ascariasis can be achieved with mass therapy administered at 6-month intervals. Ultimately, control requires adequate sanitation facilities.

## Hookworms

### Ancylostoma and Necator

*N. americanus* and *A. duodenale* infect humans

Two species, *N. americanus* and *A. duodenale,* infect humans. Adults of both species are pinkish-white and measure about 10 mm in length (Fig 55–4). The head is often curved in

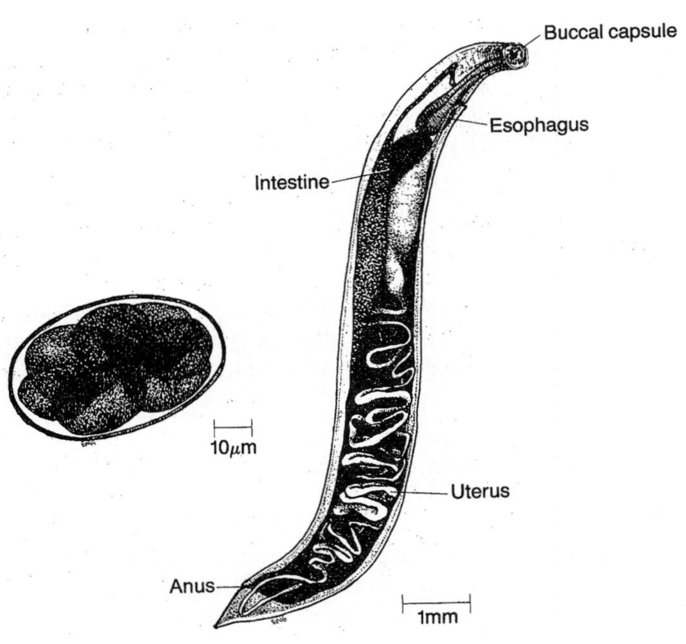


**Figure 55–4.** Female hookworm (*Necator americanus*) and egg.

a direction opposite that of the body, giving these worms the hooked appearance from which their common name is derived. The males have a unique fan-shaped copulatory bursa, rather than the curved, pointed tail common to the other intestinal nematodes. The two species can be readily differentiated by the morphology of their oral cavity. *A. duodenale,* the Old World hookworm, possesses four sharp toothlike structures, whereas *N. americanus,* the New World hookworm, has dorsal and ventral cutting plates. With the aid of these structures, the hookworms attach to the mucosa of the small bowel and suck blood. The fertilized female releases 10,000 to 20,000 eggs daily. They measure 40 by 60 μm, possess a thin shell, and are usually in the two- to four-cell stage when passed in the feces (Fig 55–4).

Species differentiated by morphology of oral cavity

#### Life Cycle

For all practical purposes, the life cycles of the two hookworms, *N. americanus* and *A. duodenale,* are identical. The eggs are passed in the feces at the 4- to 8-cell stage of development and, on reaching soil, hatch within 48 hours, releasing rhabditiform larvae. These move actively through the surface layers of soil, feeding upon bacteria and debris. After doubling in size, they molt to become infective filariform larvae, which may survive in moist conditions without feeding, for up to 6 weeks. On contact with human skin, they penetrate the epidermis, reach the lymphohematogenous system, and are passively transported to the right side of the heart and onward to the lungs. Here they rupture into alveolar spaces and, like juvenile ascarids, are coughed up, swallowed, and pass into the small intestine, where they mature to adulthood.

In soil eggs mature and release rhabditiform larvae which molt to produce infective rhabditiform larvae

Rhabditiform larvae penetrate skin; then follow same path as *Ascaris* larvae to gut

## Hookworm Disease

#### Epidemiology

Hookworm infection is found worldwide between the latitudes of 45° N and 30° S. Transmission requires deposition of egg-containing feces on shady, well-drained soil, development of larvae under conditions of abundant rainfall and high temperatures (23 to 33°C), and direct contact of unprotected human skin with resulting filariform larvae. Infections become particularly intense in closed, densely populated communities, such as tea and coffee plantations. *N. americanus* is found in the tropical areas of Asia, Africa, and America, as well as the southern United States, where it was introduced with the African slave trade. *A. duodenale* is seen in the Mediterranean basin, the Middle East, northern India, China, and Japan. It has been estimated that together these two worms extract over 7 million L of blood each day from 700 million individuals scattered around the globe, including 700,000 in the United States, effecting 50,000 to 60,000 deaths annually.

Larvae require hot moist conditions

Limited to tropical areas

#### Pathogenesis and Immunity

Each adult *A. duodenale* extracts 0.2 mL of blood daily and *N. americanus* 0.03 mL of blood. Additional blood loss may be related to the tendency of the worms to migrate within the intestine, leaving bleeding points at old sites of attachment. As the adults may survive 2 to 14 years, the accumulated blood loss may be enormous. The infection elicits both a humoral antibody response and immediate hypersensitivity reaction in the host, but evidence that these moderate the infection is lacking. The peripheral and gut eosinophilia characteristic of this disease may play a role in the destruction of worms and/or modulation of the immediate hypersensitivity reaction.

Adult worms live in gut for years

Blood loss significant

Produce peripheral and gut eosinophilia

## Hookworm Disease: Clinical Aspects

#### Clinical Manifestations

In the overwhelming majority of infected patients, the worm burden is small and the infection asymptomatic. Clinical manifestations, when they do occur, may be related to the original penetration of the skin by the filariform larva, the migration of the larva through the lung, and/or the presence of the adult worm in the gut. Skin penetration may produce a pruritic erythematous rash and swelling, popularly known as ground itch. This manifestation is more common in infection with *N. americanus,* generally occurs between the toes, and may persist for several days. It is probably the result of prior sensitization to larval antigens.

Most infections asymptomatic depending on worm load

Pruritis at site of skin penetration

Pulmonary manifestations may mimic those seen in ascariasis, but are generally less frequent and less severe. In the gut, the adult worm may produce epigastric pain and abnormal peristalsis. The major manifestations, however—anemia and hypoalbuminemia—are the result of chronic blood loss. The severity of the anemia depends upon the worm burden and intake of dietary iron. If iron intake exceeds iron loss resulting from hookworm infection, a normal hematocrit will be maintained. Commonly, however, dietary iron is ingested in a form that is poorly absorbed. As a result, severe anemia may develop over a period of months or years. In children, this condition may often precipitate heart failure or kwashiorkor. Mental, sexual, and physical development may be retarded.

Iron deficiency anemia caused by blood loss from intestinal worms

#### Laboratory Diagnosis

Eggs of both species look the same

The diagnosis is made by examining direct or concentrated stool for the distinctive eggs. As they are nearly identical in the two species, precise identification of the causative worm is generally not attempted. Quantitative egg counts can permit accurate estimation of worm load. If the stool is allowed to stand too long before it is examined, the eggs may hatch, releasing rhabditiform larvae. These larvae closely resemble those of *S. stercoralis* and must be differentiated from them.

#### Treatment and Prevention

The anemia must be corrected. When it is mild or moderate, iron replacement is adequate. More severe anemia may require blood transfusions. The two most widely used antihelminthic agents, pyrantel pamoate and mebendazole, are both highly effective. Prevention requires improved sanitation.

## Strongyloides

### Strongyloides stercoralis

Larvae differ slightly from hookworm

*S. stercoralis* may measure only 2 mm in length, making it the smallest of the intestinal nematodes. The male, which is seldom seen, is probably eliminated from the gut soon after copulation; some authorities believe that the female can conceive parthenogenetically. Be that as it may, the gravid female penetrates the mucosa of the duodenum, where she deposits her eggs. In severe infections, the biliary and pancreatic ducts, the entire small bowel, and the colon may be involved. The eggs hatch quickly, releasing rhabditiform larvae that reenter the bowel lumen and are subsequently passed into the stool. These larvae, which measure about 16 by 200 μm, can be distinguished from the similar larval stage of the hookworms by their short buccal cavity and large genital primordium (Figs 55–5 and 55–6).

#### Life Cycle

Primary cycle resembles hookworm except rhabditiform larvae develop in gut

Filariform larval development produces autoinfection

Adults can develop in soil, producing infective larvae

Three different life cycles have been described for this nematode. The first, or direct cycle, is similar to that observed with the hookworms. After rhabditiform larvae are passed in the stool, they molt on soil to become filariform larvae. Filariform larvae can penetrate human skin. After transport to the lung in the vascular system they are coughed up and swallowed and mature to adults in the small bowel. In the second, or autoinfective cycle, the rhabditiform larva's passage through the colon to the outside world is delayed by constipation or other factors, allowing it to transform into an infective filariform larva while still within the body of its host. This larva may then invade the internal mucosa (internal autoinfection) or perianal skin (external autoinfection) without an intervening soil phase. Thus, *S. stercoralis,* unlike any of the other intestinal nematodes, has the capacity to multiply within the body of the host. The worm burden may increase dramatically, and the infection persist indefinitely, without the need for reinfection from the environment, often with dire consequence to the host. In the third, or free-living cycle, the rhabditiform larvae, after passage in the stool and deposition on the soil, develop into free-living adult males and females. These adults may propagate through several generations of free-living worms before infective filariform larvae are again produced. This cycle creates a soil reservoir that may persist even without continued deposition of feces.

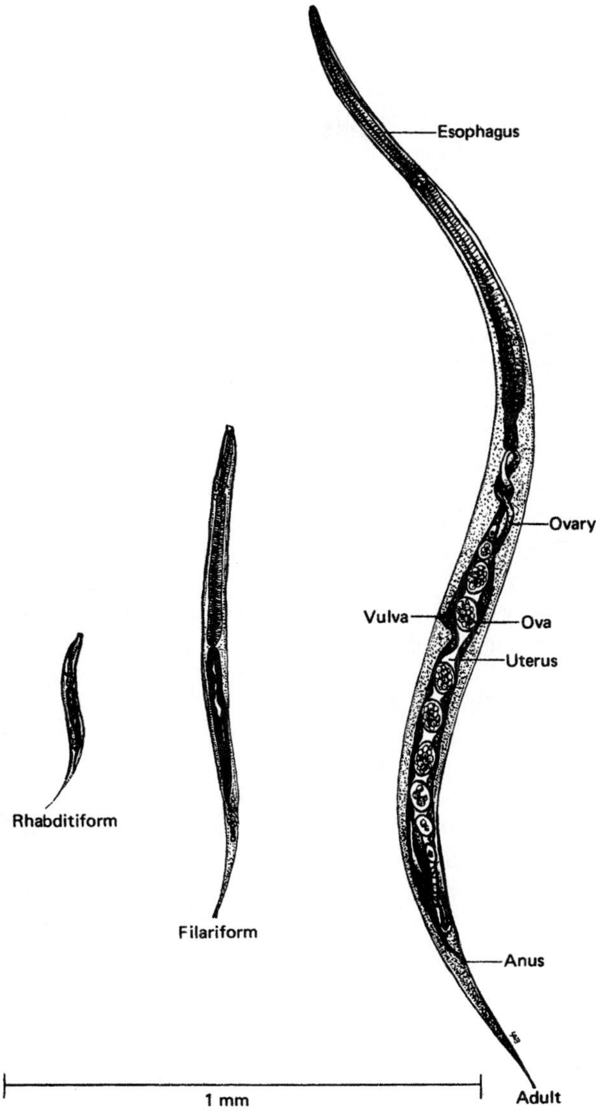


**Figure 55–5.** *Strongyloides stercoralis* worm and rhabditiform and filariform larvae.

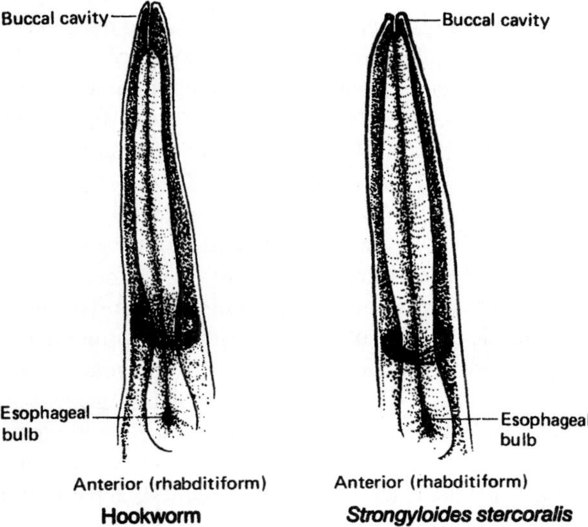


**Figure 55–6.** Anterior ends of hookworm and *Strongyloides stercoralis* rhabditiform larvae.

## Strongyloidiasis

Distribution similar to hookworm but less common

Autoinfection and infection by ingestion of filariform larvae also occur

EPIDEMIOLOGY

The distribution of *S. stercoralis* parallels that of the hookworms, although it is less prevalent in all but tropical areas. It infects 90 million individuals worldwide, including 400,000 throughout the rural areas of Puerto Rico and the southeastern sections of the continental United States. Although, like hookworm infection, it is generally acquired by direct contact of skin with soil-dwelling larvae, infection may also follow ingestion of filariform-contaminated food. Transformation of the rhabditiform larvae to the filariform stage within the gut can result in seeding of the perianal area with infectious organisms. These larvae may be passed to another person through direct physical contact or autoinfect the original host. In debilitated and immunosuppressed patients, transformation to the filariform stage occurs within the gut itself, producing marked autoinfection or hyperinfection.

Damage to intestinal mucosa may cause malabsorptive syndrome

Immunosuppression enhances risk of autoinfection by accelerating larval development

PATHOGENESIS AND IMMUNITY

Invasion of the intestinal epithelium may accelerate epithelial cell turnover, alter intestinal motility, and induce acute and chronic inflammatory lesions, ulcerations, and abscess formation, all of which may play a role in the malabsorptive syndrome that frequently characterizes clinical disease. Steroid- or malnutrition-related immunosuppression appears to accelerate the metamorphosis of rhabditiform to filariform larvae within the bowel lumen, enhancing the frequency and intensity of autoinfection. There is little evidence that protective immunity develops in the infected host.

## Strongyloidiasis: Clinical Aspects

Pulmonary and intestinal manifestations similar to hookworm

CLINICAL MANIFESTATIONS

Patients with strongyloidiasis do not generally give a history of "ground itch." They do, however, manifest the pulmonary disease seen in both ascariasis and, less often, in hookworm infection. The intestinal infection itself is usually asymptomatic. With heavy worm loads, however, the patient may complain of epigastric pain and tenderness, often aggravated by intake of food. In fact, peptic-ulcer-like pain associated with peripheral eosinophilia strongly suggests the diagnosis of strongyloidiasis. With widespread involvement of the intestinal mucosa, vomiting, diarrhea, paralytic ileus, and malabsorption may be seen.

External autoinfection gives lesions of buttocks and back

External autoinfection produces transient, raised, red, serpiginous lesions over the buttocks and lower back that reflect larval invasion of the perianal area. If the patient is not treated, these lesions may recur at irregular intervals over a period of decades; they are particularly common after recovery from a febrile illness. Over 25% of British and American servicemen imprisoned in Southeast Asia during World War II continued to demonstrate such lesions prior to diagnosis and treatment some 40 years after exposure.

Massive hyperinfection occurs in immunosuppressed but uncommon in AIDS

Massive hyperinfection may occur in immunosuppressed patients, producing severe enterocolitis and widespread dissemination of the larvae to extraintestinal organs, including the heart, lungs, and central nervous system. Inexplicably, this phenomenon has been unusual in AIDS patients, even in areas where strongyloidiasis is highly endemic. The larvae may carry enteric bacteria with them, producing Gram-negative bacteremia and occasionally Gram-negative meningitis. Unrecognized and untreated, it usually results in death.

Rhabditiform larvae detected in stool or duodenal aspirates

LABORATORY DIAGNOSIS

The diagnosis is usually made by finding the rhabditiform larvae in the stool. Preferably, only fresh specimens should be examined to avoid the confusion induced by the hatching of hookworm eggs with the release of their look-alike larvae. The number of larvae passed in the stool varies from day to day, often requiring the examination of several specimens before the diagnosis of strongyloidiasis can be made. When absent from the stool, larvae may sometimes be found in duodenal aspirates or jejunal biopsy specimens. If the pulmonary system is involved, the sputum should be examined for the presence of larvae. Agar plate culture methods may recover organisms that go undetected by microscopic examination. Serologic tests of adequate sensitivity and specificity have been recently developed, but are not generally available.

Treatment and Prevention

All infected patients should be treated to prevent the buildup of the worm burden by autoinfection and the serious consequences of hyperinfection. The drug of choice is thiabendazole. In hyperinfection syndromes, therapy must be extended for a week. The cure rate is significantly less than 100%, and stools should be checked after therapy to see if retreatment is indicated. Two recently introduced agents, albendazole and ivermectin, appear somewhat more effective than thiabendazole and may eventually replace it. Patients who have resided in an endemic area at some time in their lives should be examined for the presence of this parasite both before and during steroid treatment or immunosuppressive therapy. Medical personnel caring for patients with hyperinfection syndromes should wear gowns and gloves, as stool, saliva, vomitus, and body fluids may contain infectious filariform larvae.

Treatment essential to prevent autoinfection cycle

Medical personnel can be infected with filariform larvae

## ADDITIONAL READING

Blumenthal DS. Intestinal nematodes in the United States. *N Engl J Med* 1977;297:1437–1439.

Davis A. Intestinal helminths. In: Robinson D, ed. *Epidemiology and the Community Control of Disease in Warm Climate Countries.* 2nd ed. Edinburgh, Churchill Livingstone, 1985.

Genta RM. Dysregulation of *Strongyloidiasis:* A new hypothesis. *Clin Microbiol Rev* 1992;5:345–355. A thorough, provocative, and iconoclastic review of the factors responsible for disseminated strongyloidiasis.

Irga-Siegman Y, Kapila R, Sen P, et al. Syndrome of hyperinfection with *Strongyloides stercoralis. Rev Infect Dis* 1981;3:397–407.

Pelletier LL Jr. Chronic strongyloidiasis in World War II Far East ex-prisoners of war. *Am J Trop Med Hyg* 1984;33:55–61.

Russell LJ. The pinworm, *Enterobius vermicularis. Prim Care* 1991;18:13–24. A recent comprehensive review of this common infection.

Stevens DP. Quantitative techniques. *Clin Gastroenterol* 1978;7:231–238. The relationship of worm burden to severity of disease and need for therapy is discussed.

Chapter 56

# Tissue Nematodes

*James J. Plorde*

The nematodes discussed in this chapter induce disease through their presence in the tissues and lymphohematogenous system of the human body. They are a heterogeneous group. Three of them, *Toxocara canis, Trichinella spiralis,* and *Ancylostoma braziliense,* are natural parasites of domestic and wild carnivores. Although capable of infecting humans, they cannot complete their life cycle in this host. Humans therefore serve only as injured bystanders, rather than major participants, in the life cycle of these parasites (Table 56–1).

The remaining four major nematodes, *Wuchereria bancrofti, Brugia malayi, Loa loa,* and *Onchocerca volvulus,* are members of a single superfamily (*Filarioidea*), and all use humans as their natural definitive host (Table 56–1). The thin, threadlike adults live for years in the subcutaneous tissues and lymphatic vessels, where they discharge their live-born offspring or microfilariae. These progeny circulate in the blood or migrate in the subcutaneous tissues until they are ingested by a specific bloodsucking insect. Within this vector, they transform into filariform larvae capable of infecting another human when the invertebrate host again takes a blood meal.

The nematodes considered, diseases caused, and usual routes of infection in humans are listed in Table 56–1.

## TOXOCARA

### Toxocara canis

*T. canis* is a large, intestinal ascarid of canines, including dogs, foxes, and wolves. Each female worm discharges approximately 200,000 thick-shelled eggs daily into the fecal stream. After reaching the soil, these eggs embryonate for a minimum of 2 to 3 weeks. Thereafter, the eggs are infectious to both canines and humans and, in moist soil, may remain so for months to years. When ingested by a young dog, the larvae exit from the eggshell, penetrate the intestinal mucosa, and migrate through the liver and the right side of the heart to the lung. Here, like the offspring of *Ascaris lumbricoides*, they burst into the alveolar airspaces and are coughed up and swallowed; thereafter, they mature in the small bowel. In fully grown dogs, most of the migrating larvae pass through the pulmonary capillaries and reach the systemic circulation. These larvae eventually filter out and encyst in the tissues. Hormonal changes and/or diminished immunity in the pregnant bitch stimulate the larvae to migrate; some penetrate the placenta to infect the unborn pups. Approximately 4 weeks after parturition, both the puppies and the lactating mother begin to pass large numbers of eggs in their stools.

Cycle in canines resembles ascariasis in humans

Eggs embryonate 2–3 weeks in soil

Transplacentally infected puppies and infected lactating bitches excrete numerous ova

When humans ingest infectious eggs, the liberated larvae are small enough to pass through the pulmonary capillaries and reach the systemic circulation. Rarely does the or-

TABLE 56–1. GENERAL CHARACTERISTICS OF TISSUE NEMATODES

| Parasite | Disease | Usual Source of Human Infection |
|---|---|---|
| *Toxocara canis* | Toxocariasis (visceral larva migrans) | Ingestion of ova from canine stools |
| *Trichinella spiralis* | Trichinosis | Ingestion of improperly cooked pork |
| *Ancylostoma braziliense* | Cutaneous larva migrans | Soil contaminated with dog or cat feces |
| Major filarial worms | | |
| *Wuchereria bancrofti, Brugia malayi* | Lymphatic filariasis (elephantiasis) | Mosquito |
| *Onchocerca volvulus* | Onchocerciasis (river blindness) | *Simulium* flies |
| *Loa loa* (eye worm) | Loiasis (Calabar swellings) | Deer flies |

Transmission to humans by ingestion of ova; larvae invade tissues

ganism break into the alveoli and reach the intestine to complete its maturation to adulthood. Larvae in the systemic circulation continue to grow. When their size exceeds the diameter of the vessel through which they are passing, they penetrate its wall and enter the tissue.

## Toxocariasis

### Epidemiology

Soil extensively contaminated with ova deposited by domestic animals

Children are most often infected

Infection much more common than disease, but disease underreported

*T. canis* is a cosmopolitan parasite. The infection rate in the 50 million dogs inhabiting the United States is very high; over 80% of puppies and 20% of older animals are involved. As "man's best friend" deposits more than 3500 tons of feces daily in the streets, yards, and parks of America, there is a real health risk to our sons and daughters. In areas where studies have been done, between 10 and 30% of soil samples taken from public parks have contained viable *Toxocara* eggs. Moreover, serologic surveys of humans indicate that approximately 4 to 20% of the population has ingested these eggs at some time. The incidence of infection appears to be higher in the southeastern sections of the country; presumably the warm, humid climate prolongs survival of the eggs, thereby increasing exposure. Indeed, seroprevalence rates of more than 50% have been noted in some developing nations. The presence of puppies in the home increases the risk of infection. Clinical manifestations occur predominantly among children 1 to 6 years of age; many have a history of geophagia, suggesting that disease transmission results from direct ingestion of eggs in the soil. Most infections are subclinical, but the incidence of overt disease, although difficult to assess, is certainly underreported. Serious ocular infection by larvae is frequently seen by ophthalmologists.

## Toxocariasis: Clinical Aspects

### Clinical Manifestations

Any tissue invaded by larvae

Disease results from organ invasion and hypersensitivity

Larvae that reach the systemic circulation may invade any tissue of the body, where they can induce necrosis, bleeding, and the formation of eosinophilic granulomas. The liver, lungs, heart, skeletal muscle, brain, and eye are involved most frequently. The severity of clinical manifestations is related to the number and location of these lesions and the degree to which the host has become sensitized to larval antigens. In a subsequently criticized study in the early 1950s, investigators fed 200 embryonated eggs to each of two severely retarded young children. During the subsequent 14 months of observation, the children remained well, but demonstrated a persistent eosinophilic leukocytosis. Children with more intense infection may have fever and an enlarged, tender liver. Those who are seriously ill may develop a skin rash, an enlarged spleen, asthma, recurrent pulmonary infiltrates and abdominal pain, sleep and behavioral changes, focal neurologic defects, and convulsions. Illness often persists for weeks to months, a condition frequently referred to as visceral larva migrans (VLM). Death may result from respiratory failure, cardiac arrhythmia, or brain damage. In older children and adults, systemic manifestations are uncommon. Eye invasion by larvae (ocular larva migrans) is more common. Typically, unilateral strabismus (squint) or decreased visual acuity causes the patient to consult an ophthalmologist. Examination reveals granulomatous endophthalmitis, which is usually a reaction to a larva that is already dead; it is sometimes mistaken for malignant retinoblastoma, and an unnecessary enucleation is performed.

Ocular invasion produces granulomatous endophthalmitis

### Laboratory Diagnosis

Stool examination is not helpful, as the parasite seldom reaches adulthood in humans. Definitive diagnosis requires demonstration of the larva in a liver biopsy specimen or at autopsy. A presumptive diagnosis may be made based on the clinical picture, on eosinophilic leukocytosis, and on elevated antibody titers to blood group antigens, particularly the group A antigen. Recently, an enzyme immunoassay (EIA) using larval antigens was developed, providing clinicians for the first time with a reasonably sensitive and specific serologic test. Unfortunately, many patients with related ocular infections remain seronegative.

Tissue biopsy required for detection

Serodiagnosis using EIA reliable

### Treatment and Prevention

Corticosteroid treatment may be lifesaving if the patient has serious pulmonary, myocardial, or central nervous system involvement. Antihelminthic therapy is generally administered, although its efficacy remains uncertain. Prevention requires control of indiscriminate defecation by dogs and repeated worming of household pets. Worming must begin when the animal is 3 weeks of age and be repeated every 3 months during the first year of life and twice a year thereafter.

Corticosteroids helpful in serious disease

Worming of household pets important

## TRICHINELLA

## Trichinella spiralis

The adult *T. spiralis* lives in the duodenal and jejunal mucosa of flesh-eating animals, throughout the world, particularly swine, rodents, bears, canines, felines, and marine mammals. Although thought to be members of a single species, arctic, temperate, and tropical strains of *Trichinella* demonstrate significant biologic differences. In all cases the tiny (1.5-mm) male copulates with his outsized (3.5-mm) mate and, apparently spent by the effort, dies. Within a week, the inseminated female begins to discharge offspring. Unlike those of most nematodes, these progeny undergo intrauterine embryonation and are released as second-stage larvae. The birthing continues for the next 4 to 16 weeks, resulting in the generation of some 1500 larvae, each measuring 6 by 100 μm.

Intestinal parasite of many flesh-eating mammals

From their submucosal position, the larvae find their way into the vascular system and pass from the right side of the heart through the pulmonary capillary bed to the systemic circulation, where they are distributed throughout the body. Larvae penetrating tissue other than skeletal muscle disintegrate and die. Those finding their way to striated muscle continue to grow, molt, and gradually encapsulate over a period of several weeks. Calcification of the cyst wall begins 6 to 18 months later, but the contained larvae may remain viable for 5 to 10 years. The muscles invaded most frequently include the extraocular muscles of the eye, the tongue, the deltoid, pectoral, and intercostal muscles, the diaphragm, and the gastrocnemius. If a second animal feeds on the infected flesh of the original host, the encysted larvae are freed by gastric digestion, penetrate the columnar epithelium of the intestine, and mature just above the lamina propria.

Larvae reach striated muscle and encapsulate but are still viable

Eating infected flesh spreads the disease

## Trichinosis

### Epidemiology

Trichinosis is widespread in carnivores. Among domestic animals, swine are most frequently involved. They acquire the infection by eating rats or garbage containing cyst-laden scraps of uncooked meat. Human infection, in turn, results largely from the consumption

Swine infected by eating rats, or meat in garbage

Human infection most often from undercooked port

Wild animals (bear, walrus) also a risk

of improperly prepared pork products. In the United States, most outbreaks have been traced to ready-to-eat pork sausage prepared in the home or in small, unlicensed butcheries. Disease incidence is highest in Americans of Polish, German, and Italian descent, presumably because of their custom of producing and eating such sausage during holidays. Recent outbreaks have been reported among Indochinese refugees, apparently related to undercooking of fresh pork. Clusters have also followed feasts of wild pig in California and Hawaii. At present, approximately 10% of human cases, particularly those in Alaska and other western states, have been attributed to consumption of bear meat. Outbreaks among Alaskan and Canadian Inuit populations have followed the ingestion of raw, *Trichinella*-infected walrus. Several recent outbreaks in Europe have involved horsemeat. Each year, a few cases are acquired from ground beef intentionally but illegally adulterated with pork.

Prevalence declining due to cooking, freezing of pork

Human infections are found worldwide except in Asia and Australia. In the United States, the prevalence of cysts found in the diaphragms of patients at autopsy has declined from 16.1 to 4.2% over a period of 30 years. This decline has been attributed to decreased consumption of pork and pork products; federal guidelines for the commercial preparation of such foodstuffs; the widespread practice of freezing pork, which kills all but arctic strains of *Trichinella*; and legislation requiring the thorough cooking of any meat scraps to be used as hog feed. Nevertheless, it is estimated that more than 1.5 million Americans carry live *Trichinella* in their musculature and that 150,000 to 300,000 acquire new infection annually. Fortunately, the overwhelming majority are asymptomatic, and only about 100 clinically recognized cases are reported annually to federal officials. In other areas of the world, infection is more commonly acquired from sylvatic sources, including wild boar, bush pigs, and warthogs.

Human infections, usually are subclinical

### Pathogenesis, Pathology, and Immunity

Larvae in striated muscle, heart, and central nervous system

Acute inflammatory reaction with eosinophil-mediated destruction of larvae

The pathologic lesions of trichinosis are related almost exclusively to the presence of larvae in the striated muscle, heart, and central nervous system. Invaded muscle cells enlarge, lose their cross-striations, and undergo a basophilic degeneration. Surrounding the involved area is an intense inflammatory reaction consisting of neutrophils, lymphocytes, and eosinophils. With the development of specific IgG and IgM antibodies, eosinophil-mediated destruction of circulating larvae begins, production of new larvae is slowed, and the expulsion of adult worms is hastened. A vasculitis demonstrated in some patients has been attributed to deposition of circulating immune complexes in the walls of the vessels.

## Trichinosis: Clinical Aspects

### Clinical Manifestations

Initial abdominal pain, diarrhea as adults penetrate

Symptoms depend on number and extent of larval muscle invasion

Severe complications include hemoptysis, heart failure

One or two days after the host has ingested tainted meat, the newly matured adults penetrate the intestinal mucosa, producing nausea, abdominal pain, and diarrhea. In mild infections, these symptoms may be overlooked, except in a careful retrospective analysis; in more serious infections, they may persist for several days and render the patient prostrate. Diarrhea persisting for a period of weeks has been characteristic of outbreaks involving the Inuit population of northern Canada, a disease produced by the arctic strain of *Trichinella* present in infected walrus meat. Larval invasion of striated muscle begins approximately 1 week later and initiates the longer (6 weeks) and more characteristic phase of the disease. Patients in whom 10 or fewer larvae are deposited per gram of tissue are usually asymptomatic; those with 100 or more generally develop significant disease; and those with 1000 to 5000 have a very stormy course that occasionally ends in death. Fever, muscle pain, muscle tenderness, and weakness are the most prominent manifestations. Patients may also display eyelid swelling, a maculopapular skin rash, and small hemorrhages beneath the conjunctiva of the eye and the nails of the digits. Hemoptysis and pulmonary consolidation are common in severe infections. If there is myocardial involvement, electrocardiographic abnormalities, tachycardia, or congestive heart failure may be seen. Central nervous system invasion is marked by encephalitis, meningitis, and polyneuritis. Delirium, psychosis, paresis, and coma can follow.

### Laboratory Diagnosis

The most consistent abnormality is an eosinophilic leukocytosis that appears during the second week of illness and persists for the remainder of the clinical course. Eosinophils typically range from 15 to 50% of the white cell count and in some patients may induce extensive damage to the cardiac endothelium. In severe or terminal cases, the eosinophilia may disappear altogether.

Eosinophilia up to 50% from second week on

There are a number of valuable serologic tests, including complement fixation, indirect fluorescent antibody, and bentonite flocculation. Significant antibody titers are generally absent before the third week of illness, but may then persist for years. Recently, an EIA was developed capable of detecting specific antibody formation during the first week of illness.

Recent EIA detects antibody early

Biopsy of the deltoid or gastrocnemius muscle during the third week will usually reveal encysted larvae.

Muscle biopsy reveals larvae

### Treatment

Patients with severe edema, pulmonary manifestations, myocardial involvement, or central nervous system disease are treated with corticosteroids. The value of specific antihelminthic therapy remains controversial. The mortality of symptomatic patients is 1%, rising to 10% if the central nervous system is involved. Mebendozole and albendazole halt the production of new larvae, but in severe infection, the destruction of tissue larvae may provoke a hazardous hypersensitivity response in the host. This may be moderated with corticosteroids.

Corticosterids used in severe cases

### Prevention

Pork should be cooked to an internal temperature of at least 76.6°C, frozen at −15°C for 3 weeks, or thoroughly smoked before it is ingested. *Trichinella* in the flesh of arctic animals may survive freezing for a year or more. All strains may survive apparently adequate cooking in microwave ovens due to the variability in the internal temperatures achieved.

Thorough cooking primary prevention

## CUTANEOUS LARVA MIGRANS

Cutaneous larva migrans, or creeping eruption, is an infection of the skin caused by the larvae of a number of animal and human parasites, most commonly the dog and cat hookworm *Ancylostoma braziliense.* Eggs discharged in the feces of infected animals and deposited on warm, moist, sandy soil develop filariform larvae capable of penetrating mammalian skin on contact. In the United States, parasite transmission is particularly common in the beach areas of the southern Atlantic and Gulf states.

Caused usually by larvae of dog and cat hookworms

Although larvae do not develop further within humans, they may migrate within the skin for a period of weeks to months. Clinically, the patient notes a pruritic, raised, red, irregularly linear lesion 10 to 20 cm long. Skin excoriation from scratching enhances the likelihood of secondary bacterial infection. Half of infected patients develop Löffler's syndrome of transient, migratory pulmonary infiltrations associated with peripheral eosinophilia. The syndrome most probably reflects pulmonary migration of larvae. Larvae are rarely found in either sputum or skin biopsies, and the diagnosis must be established on clinical grounds.

Filariform larvae penetrate and migrate in human skin

Adult forms do not develop in humans

The disease responds well to oral or topical thiabendazole. Antihistamines and antibiotics may be helpful in controlling pruritus and secondary bacterial infection, respectively.

## LYMPHATIC FILARIA

Lymphatic filariasis encompasses a group of diseases produced by certain members of the superfamily *Filarioidea* that inhabit the lymphatic system of humans. Their presence induces an acute inflammatory reaction, chronic lymphatic blockade, and in some cases, grotesque swellings of the extremities and genitalia known as elephantiasis.

### Wuchereria and Brugia Species

The two agents most commonly responsible for lymphatic filariasis are *W. bancrofti* and *B. malayi.* Both are threadlike worms that lie coiled in the lymphatic vessels, male and fe-

TABLE 56–2. DIFFERENTIATION OF MICROFILARIAE

| Parasite | Location | Sheath | Size (μm) | Nuclei of Tail | Periodicity |
|---|---|---|---|---|---|
| *Wuchereria bancrofti* | Blood | Yes | 360 | None | Usually nocturnal |
| *Brugia malayi* | Blood | Yes | 220 | Two | Nocturnal |
| *Loa loa* | Blood | Yes | 275 | Continuous | Diurnal |
| *Onchocerca volvulus* | Skin | No | 300 | None | None |

Adult worms live in lymphatic vessels for a decade

Microfilariae develop from ova

Microfilariae circulate in peripheral blood once each day

Mosquito is essential vector and intermediate host

male together, for the duration of their decade-long lifespan. The female *W. bancrofti* measures 100 mm in length, and the male 40 mm. *B. malayi* adults are approximately half these sizes. The gravid females produce large numbers of embryonated eggs. At oviposition, the embryos uncoil to their full length (200 to 300 μm) to become microfilariae. The shell of the egg elongates to accommodate the embryo and is retained as a thin, flexible sheath. Although the offspring of the two species resemble each other, they may be differentiated on the basis of length, staining characteristics, and internal structure (Table 56–2). The microfilariae eventually reach the blood. In most *W. bancrofti* and *B. malayi* infections, they accumulate in the pulmonary vessels during the day. At night, in response to changes in oxygen tension, they spill out into the peripheral circulation, where they are found in greatest numbers between 9 PM and 2 AM. A Polynesian strain of *W. bancrofti* displays a different periodicity, with the peak concentration of organisms occurring in the early evening. Periodicity has an important epidemiologic consequence, as it determines the species of mosquito to serve as vector and intermediate host. Within the thoracic muscles of the mosquito, microfilariae are transformed first into rhabditiform and then into filariform larvae. These larvae actively penetrate the feeding site when the mosquito takes its next meal. Within the new host, the parasite migrates to the lymphatic vessels, undergoes a series of molts, and reaches adulthood in 6 to 12 months.

## Lymphatic Filariasis

### Epidemiology

Primarily in Asia and other tropical areas

Lymphatic filariasis currently infects about 90 million individuals in Africa, Latin America, the Pacific Islands, and Asia; more than three quarters of these cases are concentrated in Asia. *W. bancrofti,* transmitted primarily by mosquitoes of the genera *Anopheles* or *Culex,* is the more cosmopolitan of the two species; it is found in patchy distribution throughout the poorly sanitated, densely crowded urban areas of all three continents. A small endemic focus once existed near Charleston, South Carolina, but died out in the 1920s. Moreover, some 15,000 *W. bancrofti* infections were acquired by American servicemen during World War II. The same infection has recently been found in approximately 7% of Haitian refugees to the United States.

Humans are the only vertebrate hosts

*B. malayi,* transmitted by mosquitoes of the genus *Mansonia,* is confined to the rural coastal areas of Asia and the South Pacific. Strains with an unusual periodicity have been found in animals. Humans are the only known vertebrate host for most strains of *B. malayi* and for *W. bancrofti.* In the eastern Indonesian archipelago, a closely related species, *B. timori,* is transmitted by night-feeding anopheline mosquitoes.

### Pathology and Pathogenesis

Lymphatic blockade with repeated infections

Pathologic changes, which are confined primarily to the lymphatic system, can be divided into acute and chronic lesions. In acute disease, the presence of molting adolescent worms and dead or dying adults stimulates dilatation of the lymphatics, hyperplastic changes in the vessel endothelium, infiltration by lymphocytes, plasma cells, and eosinophils, and thrombus formation (that is, acute lymphangitis). These developments are followed by granuloma formation, fibrosis, and permanent lymphatic obstruction. Repeated infections eventually result in massive lymphatic blockade. The skin and subcutaneous tissues become edematous, thickened, and fibrotic. Dilated vessels may rupture, spilling lymph into the tissues or body cavities. Bacterial and fungal superinfections of the skin often supervene and contribute to tissue damage.

## Lymphatic Filariasis: Clinical Aspects

### Clinical Manifestations

Individuals who enter endemic areas as adults and reside therein for months to years often present with acute lymphadenitis, urticaria, eosinophilia, and elevated serum IgE levels; they seldom go on to develop lymphatic obstruction. A significant proportion of indigenous populations present with asymptomatic microfilaremia. Some of these spontaneously clear their infection; others go on to experience "filarial fevers" and lymphadenitis 8 to 12 months after exposure. The fever is typically low grade; in more serious cases, however, temperatures as high as 40°C, chills, muscle pains, and other systemic manifestations may be seen. Classically, the lymphadenitis is first noted in the femoral area as an enlarged, red, tender lump. The inflammation spreads centrifugally down the lymphatic channels of the leg. The vessels become enlarged and tender, the overlying skin red and edematous. In Bancroftian filariasis, the lymphatic vessels of the testicle, epididymis, and spermatic cord are frequently involved, producing a painful orchitis, epididymitis, and funiculitis; inflamed retroperitoneal vessels may simulate acute abdomen. Epitrochlear, axillary, and other lymphatic vessels are involved less frequently. The acute manifestations last a few days and resolve spontaneously, only to recur periodically over a period of weeks to months. With repeated infection, permanent lymphatic obstruction develops in the involved areas. Edema, ascites, pleural effusion, hydrocele, and joint effusion result. The lymphadenopathy persists and the palpably swollen lymphatic channels may rupture, producing an abscess or draining sinus. Rupture of intraabdominal vessels may give rise to chylous ascites or urine. In patients heavily and repeatedly infected over a period of decades, elephantiasis may develop. Such patients may continue to experience acute inflammatory episodes.

Lymphadenitis, urticaria, and eosinophilia are early findings

Acute manifectations can recur

Repeated infection leads to blockade

Elephantiasis an end result

In India, Pakistan, Sri Lanka, Indonesia, and Southeast Asia an aberrant form of filariasis is seen. This form, termed tropical eosinophilia, is characterized by an intense eosinophilia, elevated levels of IgE, high titers of filarial antibodies, the absence of microfilariae from the circulating blood, and a chronic clinical course marked by massive enlargement of the lymph nodes and spleen (children) or chronic cough, nocturnal bronchospasm, and pulmonary infiltrates (adults). Microfilariae have been found in the tissues of such patients, and the clinical manifestations may be terminated with specific antifilarial treatment. It is believed that this syndrome is precipitated by the removal of circulating microfilariae by an IgG-dependent, cell-mediated immune reaction. Microfilariae are trapped in various tissue sites where they incite an eosinophilic inflammatory response, granuloma formation, and fibrosis.

For tropical eosinophilia syndrom microfilaria not found in blood

### Laboratory Diagnosis

Eosinophilia is usually present during the acute inflammatory episodes, but definitive diagnosis requires the demonstration of microfilariae in the blood or lymphatic, ascitic, or pleural fluid. They are sought in Giemsa- or Wright-stained thick and thin smears. The major distinguishing features of these and other microfilariae are listed in Table 56–2. As the appearance of the microfilariae is usually periodic, specimen collection must be properly timed. If this procedure proves difficult, the patient may be challenged with the antifilarial agent diethylcarbamazine. This drug stimulates the migration of the microfilariae from the pulmonary to the systemic circulation and enhances the possibility of their recovery. If the parasitemia is scant, the specimen may be concentrated before it is examined. Once found, the microfilariae must be differentiated from those produced by other species of filariae. A number of serologic tests have been employed for the diagnosis of microfilaremic disease, but until recently they have lacked adequate sensitivity and specificity; even the more recent tests are of little diagnostic significance in individuals indigenous to the endemic area, as many will have experienced a prior filarial infection. Circulating filarial antigens can be found in most microfilaremic patients and also in some seropositive amicrofilaremic individuals. Antigen detection may thus prove to be a specific indicator of active disease. Tropical eosinophilia is diagnosed as described previously.

Eosinophilia during acute episodes

Timing of search for finding microfilariae in the blood requires timing or drug stimulation

### Treatment

Diethylcarbamazine eliminates the microfilariae from the blood and kills or injures the adult worms, resulting in long-term suppression of the infection or parasitologic cure. Frequently the dying microfilariae stimulate an allergic reaction in the host. This response is occa-

Killing of microfilariae may stimulate allergic response

sionally severe, requiring the use of antihistamines and corticosteroids. The role of ivermectin in the treatment of lymphatic filariasis has not yet been established. Early studies have demonstrated a high level of effectiveness in clearing microfilaremia following the administration of a single dose. The tissue changes of elephantiasis are often irreversible, but the enlargement of the extremities may be ameliorated with pressure bandages or plastic surgery. Control programs combine mosquito control with mass treatment of the entire population.

## ONCHOCERCA

Onchocerciasis or river blindness, produced by the skin filaria *O. volvulus,* is characterized by subcutaneous nodules, thickened pruritic skin, and blindness.

### Onchocerca volvulus

Adults in subcutaneous tissue, skin, and eye

Transmitted by Simulium fly

The 20- to 50-mm adults lie in coiled masses within fibrous subcutaneous nodules. The female gives birth to more than 2000 microfilariae each day of her 15-year lifespan. These progeny lose their sheaths soon after leaving the uterus, exit from the fibrous capsule, and migrate for up to 2 years in the subcutaneous tissues, skin, and eye. Ultimately they die or are ingested by black flies of the genus *Simulium,* which breed along the banks of turbulent, fast-moving streams. After transformation into filariform larvae, they are transmitted to another human host. There they molt repeatedly over 6 to 12 months before reaching adulthood and becoming encapsulated.

### Onchocerciasis

#### Epidemiology

Most cases in tropical Africa

Onchocerciasis infects approximately 20 to 40 million persons, rendering 1 to 5% of them blind. Most of the afflicted live in tropical Africa, but foci of infection are also located in Yemen, Saudi Arabia, and Latin America from southern Mexico through the northern half of South America. It has been suggested that the disease was introduced into South America by West Africans enslaved and transported to the New World for the purpose of mining gold in the mountain streams of Venezuela and Colombia. The Central American foci date from Napoleon III's use of Sudanese troops to support his invasion of Mexico in 1862. The disease still persists on the high slopes of the Sierra, where coffee plantations lie along the rapidly flowing streams that serve as breeding places for *Simulium* species.

#### Clinical Manifestations

Subcutaneous nodules may be multiple with hypersensitivity reaction to microfilariae

Important cause of blindness in affected areas

The subcutaneous nodules that harbor the adult worms can be located anywhere on the body, generally over bony prominences. In Mexico and Guatemala, where the fly vector typically bites the upper part of the body, they are concentrated on the head; in South America and Africa, they are found primarily on the trunk and legs. Although nodules may number in the hundreds, most infected individuals have less than 10. They are firm, freely movable, and measure 1 to 3 cm in diameter. Unless the nodule is located over a joint, pain and tenderness are unusual. Of greater consequence to the patient are the side effects of the presence of microfilariae in the tissues. An immediate hypersensitivity reaction to antigens released by dead or dying parasites results in acute and chronic inflammatory reaction. In the skin, this reaction is manifested as a papular or erysipelas-like rash with severe itching. In time, the skin thickens and lichenifies. As subepidermal elastic tissue is lost, wrinkles and large skin folds or hanging groins are formed. In parts of Africa, fibrosing, obstructive lymphadenitis may result in elephantiasis. Invasion of the eye, however, causes the most devastating lesions. Punctate keratitis, iritis, and chorioretinitis can lead to a decrease in visual acuity and, in time, total blindness. In Central America, eye lesions may be seen in up to 30% of infected patients. In certain communities in West Africa, 85% of the population has ocular lesions and one-half of the adult male population is blind.

### Laboratory Diagnosis

The diagnosis is made by demonstrating the microfilariae in a thin skin sample taken from an involved area. When the eye is involved, the organism may sometimes be seen in the anterior chamber with the help of a slit lamp.

Microfilariae seen in skin or eye samples

### Treatment and Prevention

Traditionally, diethylcarbamazine (DEC) has been used to kill the microfilariae. Treatment was begun with very small doses to prevent rapid parasite destruction and the attendant allergic consequences. This consideration was particularly important when the eye was involved, as a treatment-induced inflammatory reaction can damage it further. Unfortunately, diethylcarbamazine does not destroy the adult worms, which must be removed by surgical excision or killed with a second, more toxic agent, suramin. Recently, the new microfilaremic agent, ivermectin, has been demonstrated to be more effective than diethylcarbamazine. More importantly, it does not appear to induce the severe allergic manifestations seen with the latter agent. As it does not kill the adult worm, retreatment over a period of several years is necessary. No satisfactory methods of control have yet been developed. Application of insecticides to the vector's breeding waters must be sustained for decades to disrupt transmission permanently, as the parasite is so long-lived within humans. With the introduction of ivermectin, mass treatment or chemoprophylaxis may now be possible.

Treatment may cause hypersensitivity reactions

## LOA LOA

Loiasis is a filarial disease of West Africa produced by the eye worm, *Loa loa*. The long-lived adults migrate continuously through the subcutaneous tissues of humans at a maximum rate of about 1 cm/hr. During migration, they produce localized areas of allergic inflammation termed Calabar swellings. These egg-sized lesions persist for 2 to 3 days and may be accompanied by fever, itching, urticaria, and pain. At times, the adult worms may cross the eye subconjunctivally, producing intense tearing, pain, and alarm.

Adults migrate through subcutaneous tissues producing localized Calabar swellings

The female produces sheathed microfilariae, which are found in the bloodstream during daytime hours. Deer flies of the genus Chrysops serve as vectors.

The diagnosis is made by recovering the adult worm from the eye or by isolating the characteristic microfilariae from the blood or Calabar swellings. Eosinophilia is constant. Diethylcarbamazine destroys both adults and microfilariae, but must be administered cautiously to avoid marked allergic reactions. Ivermectin is less effective.

Adult worm demonstrated in eye or microfilaria in blood or tissue

## ADDITIONAL READING

Barrett-Connor E, Davis CF, Hamburger RN, Kagan I. An epidemic of trichinosis after ingestion of wild pig in Hawaii. *J Infect Dis* 1976;133:473–477.

Greene BM, Dukuly ZD, Munoz B, et al. A comparison of 6, 12, and 24 monthly dosing with ivermectin for treatment of onchocerciasis. *J Infect Dis* 1991;163:376. A study that established the dosing regimen for onchocerciasis.

Klion AD, Massougbodji A, Sadeler BC, et al. Loiasis in endemic and nonendemic populations: immunologically mediated differences in clinical presentation. *J Infect Dis* 1991;163:1318–1325. Authors note the differences in clinical presentation of loiasis in visitors to endemic areas and indigenous populations, and relate that to differences in the modulation of the immune response to parasitic antigens.

MacLean JD, Viallet J, Law C, Staudt M. Trichinosis in the Canadian Arctic: Report of five outbreaks and a new clinical syndrome. *J Infect Dis* 1989;160:513–520. This study confirms and extends the findings of Magolis et al described below. Trichinosis appears to be both common and widespread in the arctic and is characterized by a distinct clinical presentation in which gastrointestional manifestations predominate.

Margolis HS, Middaugh JP, Burgess RD. Arctic trichinosis: Two Alaskan outbreaks from walrus meat. *J Infect Dis* 1979;139:102–105. A report of two unusual outbreaks of trichinosis.

Ottesen EA. Filariasis now. *Am J Trop Med Hyg* 1989;41(suppl):9. A review of recent advances in our understanding of the immunopathogenesis, diagnosis and treatment of lymphatic filariasis.

Taylor HR. Review of the immunologic aspects of onchocerciasis: An introduction. *Rev Infect Dis* 1985;7: 787–788. This article introduces an issue of this journal devoted to a review of onchocerciasis.

Worley G, Green JA, Frothingham TE, et al. *Toxocara canis* infection. Clinical and epidemiological associations with seropositivity in kindergarten children. *J Infect Dis* 1984;149:591–597.

Chapter 57

# Cestodes

*James J. Plorde*

Cestodes are long, ribbonlike helminths that have gained the common appellation of tapeworm from their superficial resemblance to sewing tape. Their appearance, number, and exaggerated reputation for inducing weight loss have made them the best known of the intestinal worms. Although improvements in sanitation have dramatically reduced their prevalence in the United States, they continue to inhabit the bowels of many of its citizens. In some parts of the world, indigenous populations take purgatives monthly to rid themselves of this, the largest and most repulsive of the intestinal parasites.

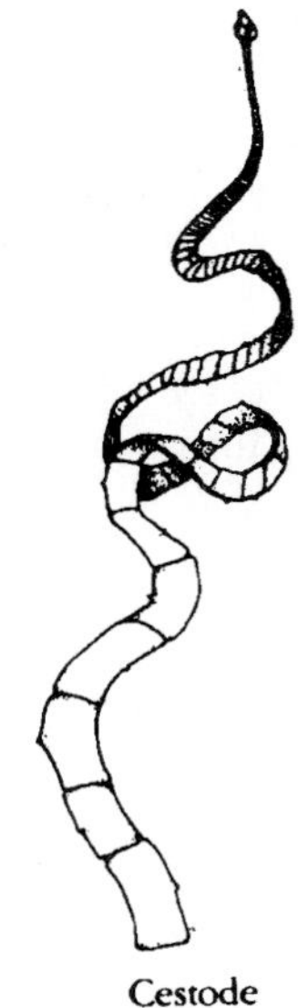

Cestode

## CESTODES

### Morphology

Like all helminths, tapeworms lack vascular and respiratory systems. In addition, they are devoid of both gut and body cavity. Food is absorbed across a complex cuticle, and the internal organs are embedded in a solid parenchyma. The adult is divided into three distinct parts: the "head" or scolex; a generative neck; and a long, segmented body, the strobila. The scolex typically measures less than 2 mm in diameter and is equipped with four muscular sucking discs used to attach the worm to the intestinal mucosa of its host. (In one genus, *Diphyllobothrium,* the discs are replaced by two grooves, or bothria.) As a further aid in attachment, the scolex of some species possesses a retractable protuberance, or rostellum, armed with a crown of chitinous hooks. Immediately posterior to the scolex is the neck from which individual segments, or proglottids, are generated one at a time to form the chainlike body. Each proglottid is a self-contained hermaphroditic reproductive unit joined to the remainder of the colony by a common cuticle, nerve trunks, and excretory canals. Its male and female gonads mature and effect fertilization as the segment is pushed farther and farther from the neck by the formation of new proglottids. When the segment reaches gravidity, it releases its eggs by rupturing, disintegrating, or passing them through its uterine pore. The eggs of the genus *Taenia* possess a solid shell and contain a fully developed, six-hooked (hexacanth) embryo. The eggs of *D. latum,* in contrast, are immature at the time of deposition and possess a covered aperture, or operculum, through which the embryo exits once fully developed.

Without gut, food absorbed from host

Divided into scolex, neck, and segmented body parts

Each proglottid a hermaphroditic unit releasing eggs via rupture or through uterine pore

### Life Cycle

With the exception of *Hymenolepis nana,* further development of all cestodes requires the passage of the larvae through one or more intermediate hosts. Eggs of the genus *Taenia* pass

TABLE 57–1. INTESTINAL AND TISSUE TAPEWORMS

| Stage | Diphyllobothrium latum | Taenia saginata | Taenia solium | Hymenolepis nana | Echinococcus granulosus | Echinococcus multilocularis |
|---|---|---|---|---|---|---|
| Adult | | | | | | |
| Definitive host | Humans, cats, dogs | Humans | Humans | Humans, rodents | Dogs, wolves | Foxes |
| Location | Gut lumen[a] | Gut lumen[a] | Gut lumen[a] | Gut lumen[a] | Gut lumen | Gut lumen |
| Length (m) | 3–10 | 4–6 | 2–4 | 0.02–0.04 | 0.005 | 0.005 |
| Attachment device | Grooves | Discs | Discs, hooklets | Discs, hooklets | Discs, hooklets | Discs, hooklets |
| Mature segment | Broad | Elongated | Elongated | Broad | Elongated | Elongated |
| Egg | | | | | | |
| Maturation status | Nonembryonated | Embryonated | Embryonated | Embryonated | Embryonated | Embryonated |
| Distinguishing characteristics | Operculate | Radial striations | Radial striations | Polar filaments | Radial striations | Radial striations |
| Larval development in humans | No | No | Yes | Yes | Yes | Yes |
| Larva | | | | | | |
| Intermediate host | Copepods, fishes | Cattle | Swine, humans | Humans, rodents | Herbivores, humans | Field mice, humans |
| Location | Tissue | Tissue | Tissue[a] | Gut mucosa[a] | Tissue[a] | Tissue[a] |
| Form | Procercoid (copepod) Plerocercoid (fish) | Cysticercus | Cysticercus | Cysticercoid | Hydatid cyst | Hydatid cyst |

[a] Site of human infection.

Eggs of Taenia must be ingested by intermediate host

Infectious cysts of Taenia form in tissues of intermediate

Definitive host ingests cysts in flesh of intermediate hosts to yield adult intestinal worms

in the stool of their definitive host, reach the soil, and are ingested by the specific intermediate. They hatch within its gut, and the released embryos penetrate the intestinal mucosa, find their way through the lymphohematogenous system to the tissues, and encyst therein. From the germinal lining of this cyst, immature scolices or protoscolices are formed. A cyst with a single such structure is known as a cysticercus (or, in the case of *H. nana,* a cysticercoid); a cyst with multiple protoscolices is known as a coenurus. In some species of tapeworm, daughter cysts, each containing many protoscolices, are formed within the mother or hydatid cyst. The cycle for all is completed when the definitive host ingests the cyst-ridden flesh of the intermediate host. After digestion of the surrounding meat in the stomach, the cyst is freed, and the protoscolex everts to become a scolex. Following attachment to the mucosa, a new strobila is generated.

*D. latum* requires two intermediates, a copepod and a freshwater fish, to complete cycle

*D. latum,* whose eggs are immature upon release, requires two intermediates to complete its larval development. The egg must reach fresh water before the operculum opens and a ciliated, free-swimming larva, or coracidium, is released. The coracidium is then ingested by the first intermediate host, a copepod, in which it is transformed into a larva (procercoid). When the copepod is, in turn, ingested by a freshwater fish, the larva penetrates the musculature of the fish to form an elongated and infectious larva, the plerocercoid. Life cycles and characteristics of important intestinal and tissue tapeworms infecting humans are summarized in Table 57–1.

## Clinical Disease

Clinical effects depend on whether humans are definitive hosts or intermediate hosts

The clinical consequences of tapeworm infection in humans depend on whether the patient serves as the primary or the intermediate host. In the former case, the adult worm is confined to the lumen of the gut, and the consequences of the infection are typically minor. Taeniasis saginata and diphyllobrothriasis are prime examples. In contrast, when the patient serves as the intermediate host (for example, for *E. granulosus*), larval development produces tissue invasion and frequently serious disease. The capacity of *H. nana* and *T. solium* to utilize humans as both primary and intermediate hosts is unique.

# BEEF TAPEWORM

## Taenia saginata

*T. saginata* inhabits the human jejunum, where it may live for up to 25 years and grow to a maximum length of 10 m. Its 1-mm scolex lacks hooklets, but possesses the four sucking discs typical of most cestodes (Fig 57.1–A). The creamy white strobila consists of 1000 to 2000 individual proglottids. The terminal segments are longer (20 mm) than they are wide (5 mm) and contain a large uterus with 15 to 20 lateral branches; these characteristics are useful in differentiating them from those of the closely related pork tapeworm, *T. solium.* When fully gravid, strings of 6 to 9 terminal proglottids, each containing approximately 100,000 eggs, break free from the remainder of the strobila. These muscular segments may crawl unassisted through the anal canal or be passed intact with the stool. Proglottids reaching the soil eventually disintegrate, releasing their distinctive eggs. These eggs are 30 to 40 µm in diameter, spherical, and possess a thick, radially striated shell (Fig 57–1B). In appropriate environments, the hexacanth embryo may survive for months. If ingested by cattle or certain other herbivores, the embryo is released, penetrates the intestinal wall, and is carried by the vascular system to the striated muscles of the tongue, diaphragm, and hindquarters. Here it is transformed into a white, ovoid (5 by 10 mm) cysticercus (*Cysticercus bovis*). When present in large numbers, cysticerci impart a spotted or "measley" appearance to the flesh. Humans are infected when they ingest inadequately cooked meat containing these larval forms.

*T. saginata* inhabits human jejunum

Gravid proglottids passed in stool

Eggs ingested by herbivore intermediates

Cysticerci in bovine striated muscle

Humans infected by eating inadequately cooked infected meat

## Beef Tapeworm Disease

### Epidemiology

In the United States, sanitary disposal of human feces and federal inspection of meat have nearly interrupted transmission of *T. saginata.* At present, less than 1% of examined carcasses are infected. Nevertheless, bovine cysticercosis is still a significant problem in the southwestern area of the country where cattle become infected in feedlots or while pastured on land irrigated with sewage or worked by infected laborers without access to sanitary facilities. Shipment of infected carcasses can result in human infection in other areas of the United States. In countries where sanitary facilities are less comprehensive and undercooked or raw beef is eaten, *T. saginata* is highly prevalent. Examples include Kenya, Ethiopia, the Middle East, Yugoslavia, and parts of the former Soviet Union and South America.

Indigenously acquired disease rare in United States

### Clinical Manifestations

Most infected patients are asymptomatic and become aware of the infection only through the spontaneous passage of proglottids. The proglottids may be observed on the surface of the stool or appear in the underclothing or bed sheets of the alarmed host. Passage may occur very irregularly and can be precipitated by excessive alcohol consumption. Some patients report epigastric discomfort, nausea, irritability (particularly after passage of segments), diarrhea, and weight loss. Occasionally the proglottids may obstruct the appendix, biliary duct, or pancreatic duct.

Clinical symptoms usually mild

### Laboratory Diagnosis

The diagnosis is made by finding eggs or proglottids in the stool. Eggs may also be distributed on the perianal area secondary to rupture of proglottids during anal passage. The adhesive cellophane tape technique described for pinworm can be used to recover them from this area. With this procedure, 85 to 95% of infections are detected, in contrast to only 50 to 75% by stool examination. As the eggs of *T. solium* and *T. saginata* are morphologically identical, it is necessary to examine a proglottid to identify the species correctly.

Adhesive cellophane tape technique and stool examination detect eggs and proglottids

### Treatment and Prevention

The drugs of choice are praziquantel or niclosamide, which act directly on the worm. Both are highly effective in single-dose oral preparations. Two other effective agents, mebendazole and the related albendazole, have not yet been approved for treatment of taeniasis.

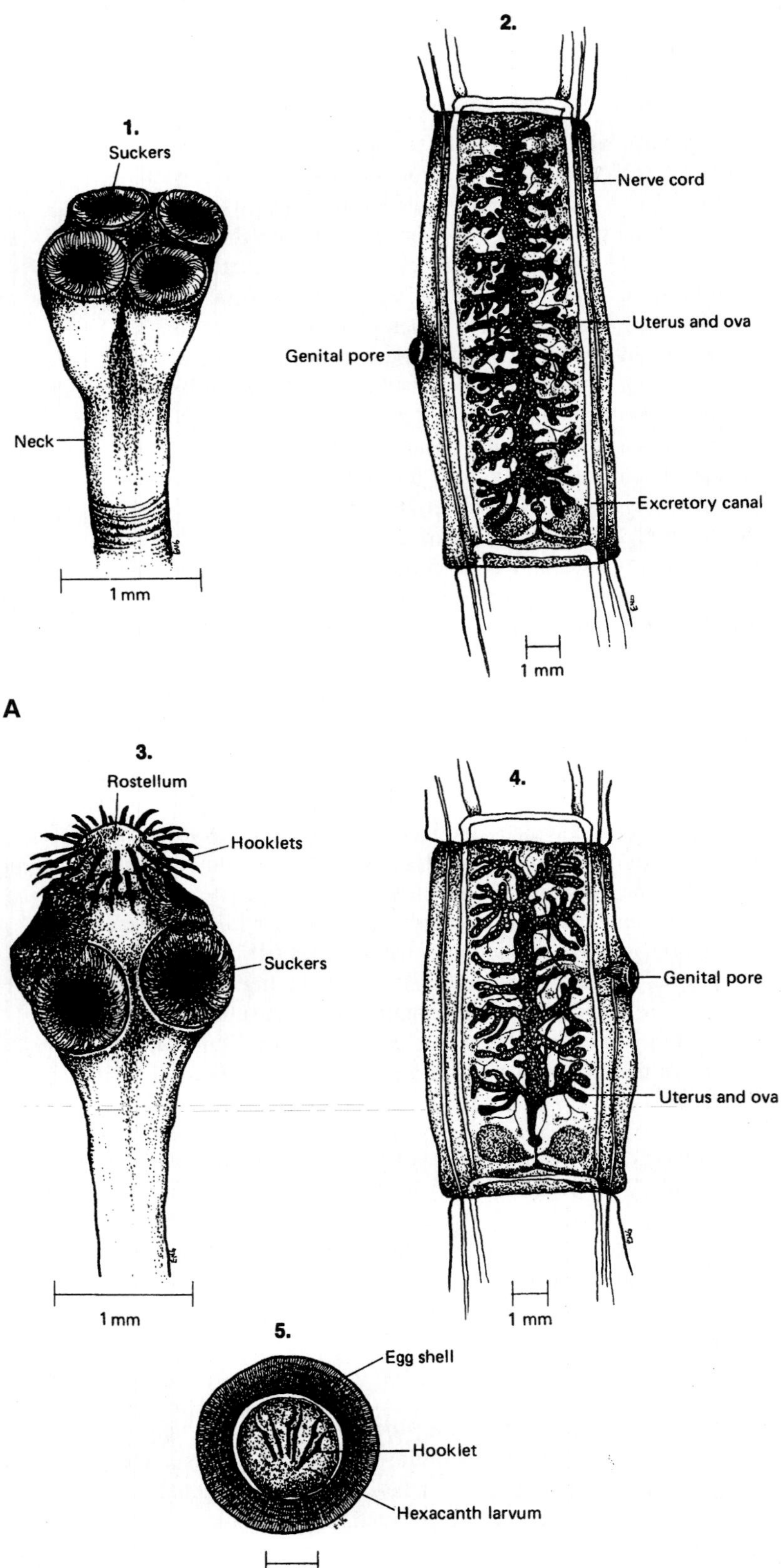


**Figure 57–1. A.** *Taenia saginata.* **B.** *Taenia solium.* (1, 3) Scolices; (2, 4) gravid proglottids; (5) ova (indistinguishable between species).

Ultimately, control is best effected through the sanitary disposal of human feces. Meat inspection is helpful, as the cysticerci are readily visible. In areas where the infection is common, thorough cooking is the most practical method of control. Internal temperatures of 56°C or more for 5 minutes or longer will destroy the cysticerci. Salting or freezing for 1 week at −15°C or less is also effective.

Sewage disposal, meat inspection, and adequate cooking

## PORK TAPEWORM

### Taenia solium

Like the beef tapeworm, which it closely resembles, *T. solium* inhabits the human jejunum, where it may survive for decades. It can be distinguished from its close relative only by careful scrutiny of the scolex and proglottids; *T. solium* possesses a rostellum armed with a double row of hooklets (Fig 57–1B3). The strobila is generally smaller than that of *T. saginata,* seldom exceeding 5 m in length or containing more than 1000 proglottids. Gravid segments measure 6 by 12 mm and thus appear less elongated than those of the bovine parasite (Fig 57–1B4). Typically, the uterus has only 8 to 12 lateral branches. Although the eggs appear morphologically identical to those of *T. saginata,* they are infective only to swine and, perhaps reflecting a genetic proximity we would prefer to overlook, humans. Both pigs and people become intermediate hosts when they ingest food contaminated with viable eggs. Some authorities have suggested that humans may be autoinfected when gravid proglottids are carried backward into the stomach during the act of vomiting, initiating the release of the contained eggs. It seems more likely that autoinfection results from the transport of the eggs from the perianal area to the mouth on contaminated fingers.

*T. solium* strobila shorter than in *T. saginata*

Eggs infective to swine and to humans

Regardless of the route, an egg reaching the stomach of an appropriate intermediate host hatches, releasing the hexacanth embryo. The embryo penetrates the intestinal wall and may be carried by the lymphohematogenous system to any of the tissues of the body. Here it develops into a 1-cm, white, opalescent cysticercus over 3 to 4 months. The cysticercus may remain viable for up to 5 years, eventually infecting humans when they ingest undercooked and "measley" flesh. The scolex everts, attaches itself to the mucosa, and develops into a new adult worm, thereby completing the cycle.

Tissue cysticerci develop in humans and swine

### Pork Tapeworm Disease

#### Epidemiology

Although infected swine are still occasionally found in the United States, most human disease are found in immigrants from endemic areas. Although this infection is widely distributed throughout the world, it is particularly common in parts of India, Indonesia, the Philippines, Asia, Africa, Mexico, Central America, and South America.

*T. solium* rarely found in United States

#### Clinical Manifestations

The signs and symptoms of infection with the adult worm are similar to those of taeniasis saginata. Clinical manifestations are totally different when humans serve as intermediate hosts. Cysticerci develop in the subcutaneous tissues, muscles, heart, lungs, liver, brain, and eye. As long as the number is small and the cysticerci remain viable, tissue reaction is moderate and the patient asymptomatic. The death of the larva, however, stimulates a marked inflammatory reaction, fever, muscle pains, and eosinophilia.

Major clinical manifestations caused by reaction to cysticerci

The most important and dramatic clinical presentation of cysticercosis results from lesions in the central nervous system. During the acute invasive stage, patients experience fever, headache, and eosinophilia. In heavy infections, a meningoencephalitic syndrome with cerebrospinal fluid (CSF) eosinophilic pleocytosis may be present. Established cysts can be found in the cerebrum, ventricles, subarachnoid space, spinal cord, or eye. Cerebral cysts are usually small, often measuring 2 cm or less in diameter; racemose lesions may be threefold larger. These parenchymal infections can induce focal neurologic abnormalities, personality changes, intellectual impairment and/or seizures; in many endemic areas, cys-

Meningoencephalitic syndrome with eosinophilia produced by CNS invasion

Multiple small cysts formed

Focal neurologic signs and epilepsy related to cysts

ticercosis is the leading cause of epilepsy. Subarachnoid lesions and cysticerci located within the fourth ventricle may obstruct the flow of cerebrospinal fluid, producing increased intracranial pressure with its associated headache, vomiting, visual disturbances, or psychiatric abnormalities. Multiple racemose lesions have a predilection for the basal cisterns, particularly in young women, from whence they rapidly spread around the base of the brain and cerebrum with catastrophic result. Spinal involvement produces cord compression or meningeal inflammation. Eye lesions incite pain and visual disturbances.

### Laboratory Diagnosis

Presence of adult worm diagnosed from proglottids

Infection with the adult worm is diagnosed as described for *T. saginata*. Cysticercosis is suspected when an individual who has been in an endemic area presents with neurologic manifestations or subcutaneous nodules. Roentgenograms of the soft tissues often reveal dead, calcified cysticerci. Viable lesions may be detected as low-density masses by computed tomograph (CT) or magnetic resonance imaging (MRI). The diagnosis is confirmed by demonstrating the larva in a biopsy sample of a subcutaneous nodule or specific antibodies in the circulating blood. Serum and CSF enzyme immunoassays and Western blot testing for specific anticysticercal antibodies have a sensitivity of 80 to 95%, but the presence of IgG antibodies alone may reflect the presence of past or inactive disease.

Biopsy required for cysticerci

### Treatment and Prevention

Infection with the adult worm is approached in the manner described for *T. saginata*. As the mortality rate in patients with symptomatic neurocysticercosis approaches 50%, aggressive management is warranted. Patients with parenchymal lesions usually respond to prolonged treatment with praziquantel or albendazole. Concomitant corticosteroid administration helps minimize the inflammatory response to dying cysticerci. Intraventricular subarachnoid and eye lesions appear relatively refractory to chemotherapy; surgery, CSF shunts, and corticosteroids may help ameliorate symptoms.

Surgery occasionally needed for cysticercosis

## FISH TAPEWORM

### Diphyllobothrium latum

The adult *D. latum* attaches to the ileal mucosa with the aid of two sucking grooves (bothria) located in an elongated fusiform scolex (Fig 57–2). In lifespan and overall length, it re-

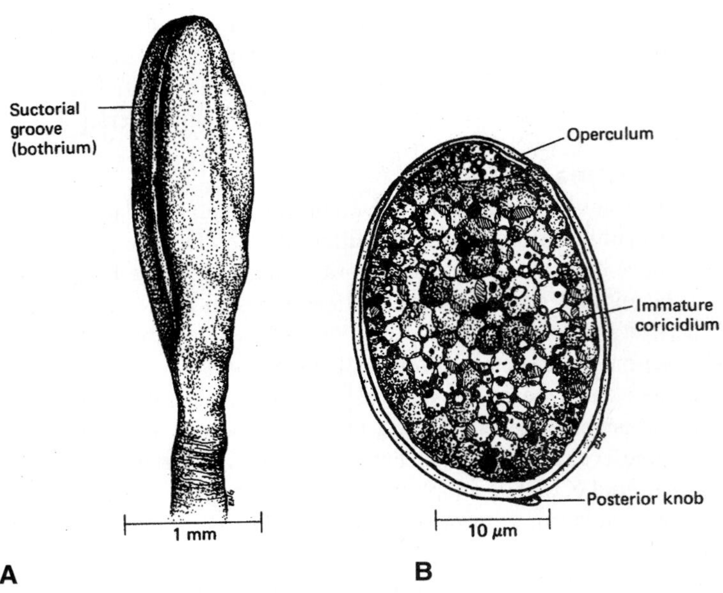


**Figure 57–2.** *Diphyllobothrium latum.* **A.** Scolex. **B.** Ovum.

sembles the *Taenia* species discussed previously. The 3000 to 4000 proglottids, however, are uniformly wider than they are long, accounting for this cestode's species designation as well as one of its common names, the broad tapeworm. The gravid segments contain a centrally positioned, rosette-shaped uterus unique among the tapeworms of humans. Unlike those of the *Taenia* species, ova are released through the uterine pore. Over 1 million oval (55 by 75 μm) operculate eggs are released daily into the stool (Fig 57–2B).

*D. latum* has broad proglottids

On reaching fresh water they hatch, releasing ciliated, free-swimming larvae or coracidia. If ingested within a few days by small freshwater crustaceans of the genera *Cyclops* or *Diaptomus,* they develop into procercoid larvae. When the crustacean is ingested by a freshwater or anadromous marine fish, the larvae migrate into the musculature of the fish and develop into infectious plerocercoid larvae. Humans are infected when they eat improperly prepared freshwater fish containing such forms.

Eggs release motile coracidia in water

Crustacean and fish intermediates; humans infected by ingesting inadequately cooked fish

## Fish Tapeworm Disease

### Epidemiology

Fish tapeworms are found wherever raw, pickled, or undercooked freshwater fish from fecally contaminated lakes and streams is eaten by humans. Human infections have been described in the Baltic and Scandinavian countries, Russia, Switzerland, Italy, Japan, and Chile. The worm, brought to North America by Scandinavian immigrants, is now found in Alaska, Canada, the midwestern states, and Florida. It was shown recently that infectious plerocercoid larvae may develop in anadromous salmon, and human cases have been traced to the ingestion of fish freshly taken from Alaskan waters. The increasing popularity of raw fish dishes such as Japanese sushi and sashimi may lead to increased prevalence of this disease in the United States. Among Ontario Indians, infection is acquired by eating fresh salted fish. Even when fish is appropriately cooked, individuals may become infected by sampling the flesh during the process of preparation.

Worldwide distribution

Worm found in Alaska, Midwest, and Florida

Eating raw fish increases risk

### Clinical Manifestations

Most infected patients are asymptomatic. On occasion, however, they have complained of epigastric pain, abdominal cramping, vomiting, and weight loss. Moreover, the presence of several adult worms within the gut has been known to precipitate intestinal or biliary obstruction. Forty percent of fish tapeworm carriers demonstrate low serum levels of vitamin $B_{12}$, apparently as a result of the competition between the host and the worm for ingested vitamin. Studies have shown that a worm located high in the jejunum may take up 80 to 100% of vitamin $B_{12}$ given by mouth. Approximately 0.1 to 2% of patients develop macrocytic anemia. They tend to be elderly, to have impaired production of intrinsic factor, and to have worms located high in the jejunum. In many, folate absorption is also diminished. Lysolecithin, a tapeworm product, may also contribute to the anemia. Neurologic manifestations of vitamin $B_{12}$ deficiency occur, sometimes in the absence of anemia. They include numbness, paresthesia, loss of vibration sense, and, rarely, optic atrophy with central scotoma.

Occasional intestinal obstruction

Vitamin $B_{12}$ deficiency related to worm consumption

### Laboratory Diagnosis

The diagnosis is established by finding the typical eggs in the stool. As *D. latum* produces large numbers of ova, identification is usually accomplished without the need for concentration techniques.

Eggs demonstrated in stool

### Treatment and Prevention

Treatment is carried out as described for *T. saginata* infections. When anemia or neurologic manifestations are present, parenteral administration of vitamin $B_{12}$ is also indicated. Personal protection can be accomplished by thorough cooking of all salmon and freshwater fish. Devotees of raw fish may choose to freeze their favorite dish at −10°C for 48 hours before serving. Ultimately, control of diphyllobothriasis is accomplished only by prohibiting the discharge of untreated sewage into lakes and streams.

Fish rendered noninfectious at −10°C for 48 hours

# ECHINOCOCCUS

Echinococciasis or hydatid disease is a tissue infection of humans caused by larvae of *Echinococcus granulosus* and *E. multilocularis*. The former, the more common infection, is that discussed herein.

## Echinococcus Species

Adult in small intestine of canines

Herbivores and humans serve as intermediates

Larvae penetrate to portal or systemic circulation

Cysts and daughter cysts develop in tissues

Cycle completed with ingestion of cysts by canine

The adult *E. granulosus* inhabits the small bowel of dogs, wolves, and other canines, where it survives for a scant 12 months. The scolex, like that of the genus *Taenia,* possesses four sucking discs and a double row of hooklets. The entire strobila, however, measures only 5 mm in length and contains but three proglottids; one immature, one mature, and one gravid. The latter segment splits either before or after passage in the stool, releasing eggs that appear identical to those of *T. saginata* and *T. solium.* A number of mammals may serve as intermediates, including sheep, goats, camels, deer, caribou, moose, and, most important, humans. When one of these hosts ingests eggs, they hatch, and the embryos penetrate the intestinal mucosa and are carried by the portal blood to the liver. Here, many are filtered out in the hepatic sinusoids. The rest traverse the liver and are carried to the lung, where most lodge. A few pass through the pulmonary capillaries, enter the systemic circulation, and are carried to the brain, heart, bones, kidneys, and other tissues. Many of the larvae are phagocytosed and destroyed. The survivors form a cyst wall composed of an external laminated cuticle and an internal germinal membrane. The cyst fills with fluid and slowly expands, reaching a diameter of 1 cm over 5 to 6 months. Secondary or daughter cysts form within the original hydatid. Within each of these daughter cysts, new protoscolices are produced from the germinal lining. Some break free, dropping to the bottom of the cyst to form hydatid sand. When hydatid-containing tissues of the intermediate host are ingested by a canine, thousands of scolices are released in the intestine to develop into adult worms.

## Hydatid Disease

### Epidemiology

Pastoral infections maintained by allowing dogs to feed on sheep viscera

Hand-to-mouth infection of humans by dog contact

Sylvatic cycle in Alaska and western Canada

There are two major epidemiologic forms of echinococciasis, pastoral and sylvatic. The more common pastoral form has its highest incidence in Australia, New Zealand, South and East Africa, the Middle East, Central Europe, and South America, where domestic herbivores such as sheep, cattle, and camels are raised in close contact with dogs. Although approximately 200 human cases are reported each year in the United States, most were acquired elsewhere. Indigenous cases do occur, however, particularly among Basque sheep farmers in California, southwestern Native Americans, and some Utah shepherds. Animal husbandry practices that permit dogs to feed on the raw viscera of slaughtered sheep allow the cycle of transmission to continue. Shepherds become infected while handling or fondling their dogs. Eggs retained in the fur of these animals are picked up on the hands and later ingested.

Sylvatic echinococciasis is found principally in Alaska and western Canada, where wolves act as the definitive host and moose or caribou as the intermediate. In two counties in California, a second cycle involving deer and coyotes has been described. When hunters kill these wild deer and feed their offal to accompanying dogs, a pastoral cycle may be established.

### Clinical Manifestations

Disease caused by mechanical effects of cysts after many years

The enlarging hydatid cysts produce tissue damage by mechanical means. The clinical presentation depends on their number, site, and rate of growth. Typically, there is a latent period of 5 to 20 years between acquisition of infection and subsequent diagnosis. Intervals as long as 75 years have been reported occasionally.

In sylvatic infections, two thirds of the cysts are found in the lung, the remainder in the liver. Most patients are asymptomatic when the lesion is discovered on routine chest x-ray or physical examination. Occasionally, the patient may present with hemoptysis, pain in the right upper quadrant of the abdomen, or a tender hepatic mass. Significant morbidity is uncommon, and death extremely rare. In the pastoral form of disease, 60% of the cysts are found in the liver, 25% in the lung. One fifth of all patients show involvement of multiple sites. The hydatid cysts, which grow more rapidly (0.25 to 1 cm/year) than the sylvatic lesions, may reach enormous size. Twenty percent eventually rupture, inducing fever, pruritus, urticaria, and, at times, anaphylactic shock and death. Release of thousands of scolices may lead to dissemination of the infection. Rupture of pulmonary lesions also induces cough, chest pain, and hemoptysis. Liver cysts may break through the diaphragm or rupture into the bile duct or peritoneal cavity. The majority, however, present as a tender, palpable hepatic mass. Intrabiliary extrusion of calcified cysts may mimic the signs of acute cholecystitis; complete obstruction results in jaundice. Bone cysts produce pathologic fractures, whereas lesions in the central nervous system are often manifest as blindness or epilepsy. Cardiac lesions have been associated with conduction disturbances, ventricular rupture, and embolic metastases. A recent study has suggested that circulating antigen–antibody complexes may be deposited in the kidney, initiating membranous glomerulonephritis.

Pulmonary cysts predominate in sylvatic disease, hepatic in pastoral

Cysts may attain large size

Rupture leads to hypersensitivity manifestations and dissemination

### Laboratory Diagnosis

On chest x-ray, pulmonary lesions present as slightly irregular, round masses of uniform density devoid of calcification. In contrast, more than one half of hepatic lesions display a smooth, calcific rim. Computed tomography, ultrasonography, and magnetic resonance imaging may reveal either a simple fluid-filled cyst or daughter cysts with hydatid sand. Endoscopic retrograde cholangiography has been valuable for determining cyst location and possible communication with the biliary tree. Because of the potential for an anaphylactoid reaction and dissemination of infection, diagnostic aspiration has been considered contraindicated. Nevertheless, in the hands of some investigators ultrasonically guided percutaneous drainage, followed by the introduction of ethanol to kill protoscoleces and germinal layer, has proven to be safe and useful, both diagnostically and therapeutically. In patients with ruptured pulmonary cysts, scolices may be demonstrated in the sputum.

Radiologic and scanning appearance characteristic

Aspiration of cysts usually contraindicated

In most cases, confirmation of the diagnosis requires serologic testing. Unfortunately, current procedures are not totally satisfactory. Indirect hemagglutination and latex agglutination tests are positive in 90% of patients with hepatic lesions and 60% of those with pulmonary hydatid cysts. When using hydatid cyst fluid or soluble scolex antigen, the presence of a precipitin line in the immunoelectrophoresis test appears to be more specific. An adaptation of this test to an enzyme-linked immunoelectrodiffusion technique appears to provide a rapid, sensitive diagnostic test. Other serologic tests are in the process of evaluation. Polymerase chain reaction assay has been shown capable of detecting picogram quantities of *Echinococcus* genomic DNA in fine-needle biopsy material from patients with suspected echinococcosis.

Serologic diagnosis important but needs improved sensitivity

### Treatment

The only definitive therapy available at this time is surgical extirpation. Patients with pulmonary hydatid cysts of the sylvatic type and small calcified hepatic lesions require surgery only if they become symptomatic or the cysts increase dramatically in size over time. All other lesions should be excised or drained and irrigated with hypertonic saline, silver nitrate, or cetrimide to kill the protoscolices and prevent metastatic infection. Medical therapy using high-dose albendazole, mebendazole, or praziquantel appears partially effective, but controlled studies are lacking. It may be considered when surgery is contraindicated.

Surgical extirpation only treatment

### Prevention

Infected dogs should be wormed, and infected carcasses and offal burned or buried. Hands should be carefully washed after contact with potentially infected dogs.

## ADDITIONAL READING

Bandres JC, White AC Jr, Samo T, et al. Extraparenchymal neurocysticercosis: Report of five cases and review of management. *Clin Infect Dis* 1992;15:799–811. A very good review of treatment of these refractory forms of neurocysticercosis.

Filice C, Di Perri G, Strosselli M, et al. Parasitologic findings in percutaneous drainage human hydatid liver cysts. *J Infect Dis* 1990;161:1290–1295. Authors demonstrate that, when appropriately done, diagnostic and therapeutic aspiration of echinococcal cysts is safe and effective.

Gottstein B. Molecular and immunological diagnosis of echinococcosis. *Clin Microbiol Rev* 1992;5:248–261. A recent reprise.

Jones TC. Cestodes. *Clin Gastroenterol* 1978;7:105–128. An extensive review.

Loo L, Braude A. Cerebral cysticercosis in San Diego. A report of 23 cases and a review of the literature. *Medicine* 1982;61:341–359.

Ruttenber AJ, Weniger BG, Sorvillo F, et al. Diphyllobothriasis associated with salmon consumption in Pacific Coast states. *Am J Trop Med Hyg* 1984;33:455–459.

Schaefer JW, Khan MY. Echinococcosis (hydatid disease): Lessons from experience with 59 patients. *Rev Infect Dis* 1991;13:243–247. Recent case presentations with thorough discussion of diagnostic and therapeutic modalities.

Schantz PM, Moore AC, Munoz JL, et al. Neurocysticercosis in an Orthodox Jewish Community in New York City. *N Engl J Med* 1992;327:692–701. An important paper that demonstrates that cysticercosis can be readily acquired from food-handlers infected with the adult tapeworm. Emigrants from countries endemic for *T. solium* infection should be screened for tapeworm infection before they are employed as housekeepers or food handlers.

Teitelbaum GP, Otto RJ, Lin M, et al. MR imaging of neurocysticercosis. *AJR* 1990;153:857. Description of an important new tool for the diagnosis of neurocysticercosis.

Wilson JF, Diddams AC, Rausch RL. Cystic hydatid disease in Alaska: A review of 101 autochthonous cases of *Echinococcus granulosus* infection. *Am Rev Respir Dis* 1968;98:1–15. The unique characteristics of sylvatic *E. granulosus* infections in Alaska are discussed.

Chapter

58

# Trematodes

*James J. Plorde*

Of the myriad relationships that have developed between helminth and human over the millennia of our mutual existence, none has proved more destructive to our health and productivity than that forged with the indomitable flukes. Typically, the adults live for decades within human tissues and vascular systems, where they resist immunologic attack and produce progressive damage to vital organs. Morphologically, trematodes are bilaterally symmetric, vary in length from a few millimeters to several centimeters and possess two deep suckers from which they derive their name ("body with holes"). One surrounds the oral cavity; the other is located on the ventral surface of the worm. These organs are used for both attachment and locomotion; movement is effected in a characteristic "inchworm" fashion. The digestive tract begins at the oral sucker and continues as a muscular pharynx and esophagus before bifurcating to form bilateral ceca that end blindly near the posterior extremity of the worm. Undigested food is vomited out through the oral cavity. The excretory system consists of a number of hollow, ciliated "flame cells" that excrete waste products into interconnecting ducts terminating in a posterior excretory pore.

Persistent flukes move through tissue and vasculature with inchworm locomotion

The reproductive systems vary and serve as a means for dividing the trematodes into two major categories: the hermaphrodites and the schistosomes. The adult hermaphrodite contains both male and female gonads and produces operculate eggs. The schistosomes have separate sexes, and the fertilized female deposits only nonoperculated offspring. The two groups have similar life cycles. The major differential features are summarized in Table 58–1. Eggs are excreted from the human host and, if they reach fresh water, hatch to release ciliated larvae called miracidia. These larvae find and penetrate a snail host specific for the

Two types of reproductive systems

Eggs hatch in fresh water to release miracidia which infects snails

TABLE 58–1. GENERAL CHARACTERISTICS OF TREMATODES

| | Trematode Type | |
|---|---|---|
| **Characteristic** | ***Blood*** | ***Tissue/Intestinal*** |
| Genus | *Schistosoma* | *Paragonimus, Clonorchis, Opisthorchis, Fasciola* |
| Morphology | | |
| Adult | Oral and ventral suckers<br>Blind gastrointestinal tract<br>Slender, wormlike | Oral and ventral suckers<br>Blind gastrointestinal tract<br>Flat, leaflike |
| Egg | Nonoperculate | Operculate |
| Biology | | |
| Sexes | Separate | Hermaphroditic |
| Intermediates | One | Two |
| Life span | Long | Long |

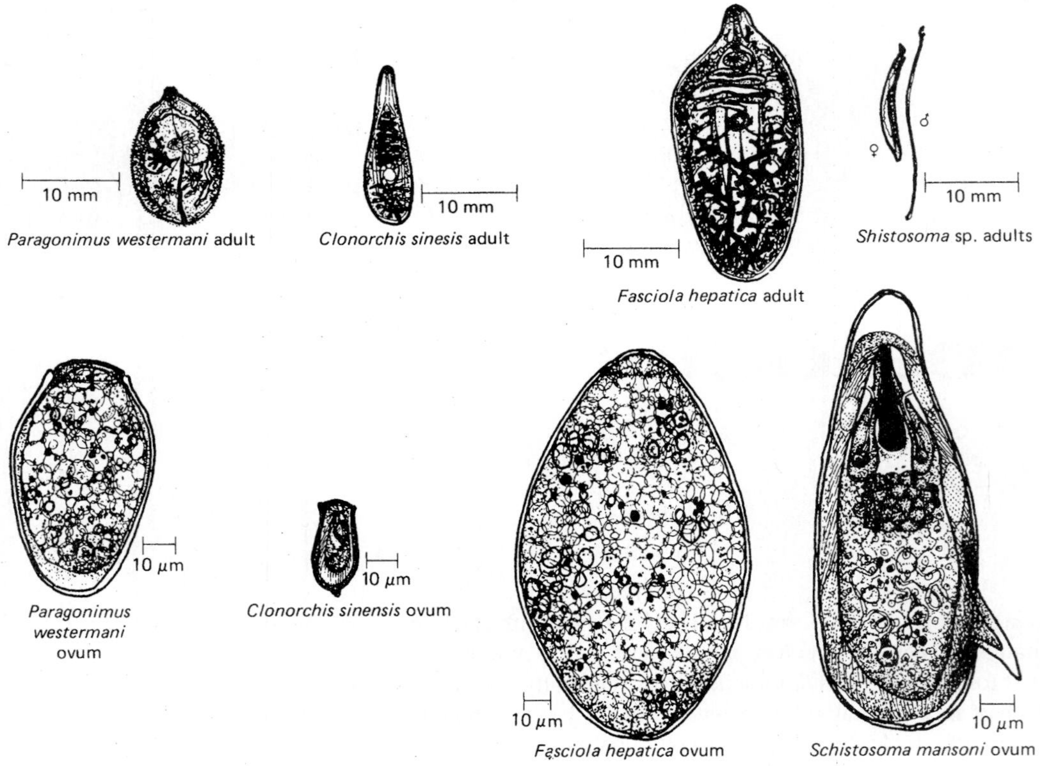


**Figure 58–1.** Adult flukes and eggs.

**TABLE 58–2. INTESTINAL AND TISSUE TREMATODES**

| | Paragonimus | Clonorchis | Opisthorchis | Fasciola | Fasiolopsis | Heterophyes/ Metagonimus |
|---|---|---|---|---|---|---|
| **Distribution** | | | | | | |
| Geographic | Asia, Africa, Central America | Japan, China, Taiwan, Vietnam | Asia, Eastern Europe | Worldwide | East and Southeast Asia | Asia, USSR, Mediterranean |
| Infected population (in millions) | 3 | 20 | 4 | — | 10 | — |
| **Adult Worms** | | | | | | |
| Reservoir hosts | Domestic and wild animals | Cats, dogs | Domestic and wild animals | Sheep and other herbivores | Pigs | Fish-eating mammals |
| Location in body | Lungs, CNS | Biliary tract | Biliary tract | Biliary tract | Small intestine | Small intestine |
| Length (mm) | 7–12 | 10–25 | 10 | 20–30 | 20–75 | 1–2 |
| Life span (years) | 4–6 | 20–30 | 20–30 | 10–15 | 0.5 | 1 |
| **Eggs** | | | | | | |
| Characteristics | Operculated | Operculated | Operculated | Operculated | Operculated | Operculated |
| Size (μm) | 80–100 | 26–30 | 26–30 | 130–150 | 130–150 | 26–30 |
| Location[a] | Sputum, stool | Bile, stool | Bile, stool | Bile, stool | Stool | Stool |
| **Larvae** | | | | | | |
| First intermediate | Snail | Snail | Snail | Snail | Snail | Snail |
| Second intermediate | Freshwater crab and crayfish | Freshwater fish | Freshwater fish | Watercress and other aquatic plants | Water chestnut and other aquatic plants | Freshwater fish |

*Abbreviation:* CNS = central nervous system.
[a] Diagnostic specimens.

trematode species. In this intermediate host, they are transformed by a process of asexual reproduction into thousands of tail-bearing larvae or cercariae, which are released from the snail over a period of weeks and swim about vigorously in search of their next host. In the case of schistosomal cercariae, this host is the human. When they come in contact with the skin surface, they attach, discard their tails, and invade, thereby completing their life cycle. The cercariae of the hermaphroditic flukes encyst in or upon an aquatic plant or animal, where they undergo a second transformation to become infective metacercariae. Their cycle is completed when the second intermediate host is ingested by a human. Of the many trematodes that infect humans, only five will be discussed: the blood flukes, all of which are members of the genus *Schistosoma* (*S. mansoni, S. haematobium,* and *S. japonicum*); and the lung (*Paragonimus* spp.) and liver (*Clonorchis sinensis*) flukes, which are hermaphroditic (Fig 58–1). Basic details of other hermaphroditic tissue and intestinal flukes are listed in Table 58–2.

Snails release motile cercariae in water

*Schistosoma cercariae* infect humans through skin

*Paragonimus* and *Clonorchis* have second intermediate host

## PARAGONIMUS

### Paragonimus westermani

Several *Paragonimus* species may infect humans. *P. westermani*, which is widely distributed in East Asia, is the species most frequently involved. The short, plump (10 by 5 mm), reddish-brown adults are characteristically found encapsulated in the pulmonary parenchyma of their definitive host. Here they deposit operculate, golden-brown eggs, which are distinguished from similar structures by their size (50 by 90 μm) and prominent periopercular shoulder. When the capsule erodes into a bronchiole, the eggs are coughed up and spat out or swallowed and passed in the stool. If they reach fresh water, they embryonate several weeks before the ciliated miracidia emerge through the open opercula. After invasion of an appropriate snail host, 3 to 5 months pass before cercariae are released. These larval forms invade the gills, musculature, and viscera of certain crayfish or freshwater crabs, in which, over 6 to 8 weeks, they transform into metacercariae. When the flesh of these second intermediate hosts is ingested by humans, the metacercariae encyst in the duodenum and burrow through the gut wall into the peritoneal cavity. The majority continue their migration through the diaphragm and reach maturity in the lungs 5 to 6 weeks later. Some organisms, however, are retained in the intestinal wall and mesentery or wander to other foci such as the liver, pancreas, kidney, skeletal muscle, or subcutaneous tissue. Young worms migrating through the neck and jugular foramen may encyst in the brain, the most common ectopic site.

Adults encapsulate in lung

Capsule erodes into bronchiole, eggs coughed up; cycle continues if eggs reach water with susceptible snail

Crayfish and freshwater crabs second intermediate hosts

In addition to humans, other carnivores, including the rat, cat, dog, and pig, may serve as definitive hosts. Immature ectopic adults in the striated muscles of the pig may infect humans after ingestion of undercooked pork.

Other carnivores are also definitive hosts

### Paragonimiasis (Lung Fluke Infection)

#### Epidemiology

Although most of the 5 million human infections are concentrated in Far Eastern nations such as Korea, Japan, China, Taiwan, the Philippines, and Indonesia, paragonimiasis has recently been described in India, Africa, and Latin America. *P. kellicotti,* a parasite of mink, is widely distributed in eastern Canada and the United States, but rarely produces human infection. Approximately 1% of recent Indochinese immigrants to this country are infected with *P. westermani*. Infection of the snail host, which is typically found in small mountain streams located away from human habitation, is probably maintained by animal hosts other than humans. Human disease occurs when food shortages or local customs expose individuals to infected crabs. When these crustaceans are prepared for cooking, juice containing metacercariae may be left behind on the working surface and contaminate other foods subsequently prepared in the same area. Fresh crab juice, which is used for the treatment of infertility in the Cameroons and of measles in Korea, may also transmit the disease. In the

Infected snails often found in mountain streams

Humans infected by ingesting infected crustaceans

Orient, crabs are frequently eaten after they have been lightly salted, pickled, or immersed briefly in wine (drunken crab), practices that are seldom lethal to the metacercariae. Children living in endemic areas may be infected while handling or ingesting crabs during the course of play.

### Clinical Manifestations

Multiple lung cysts are formed

The presence of the adult worms in the lung elicits an eosinophilic inflammatory reaction and, eventually, the formation of a 1- to 2-cm fibrous capsule that surrounds and encloses one or more parasites. The infected patient may harbor as many as 25 such lesions. With the onset of oviposition, the capsule swells and erodes into a bronchiole, resulting in expectoration of the brownish eggs, blood, and an inflammatory exudate. Secondary bacterial infection of the evacuated cysts is common, producing a clinical picture of chronic bronchitis or bronchiectasis. When cysts rupture into the pleural cavity, chest pain and effusion can result. Early in infection chest x-rays demonstrate small segmental infiltrates; these are gradually replaced by round nodules that may go on to cavitate. Eventually, cystic rings, fibrosis, and calcification occur, producing a picture closely resembling that of pulmonary tuberculosis. The confusion is compounded by the frequent coexistence of the two diseases. Adult flukes in the intestine and mesentery produce pain, bloody diarrhea, and on occasion, palpable abdominal masses. In approximately 1% of Oriental cases, more commonly in children, parasites lodge in the brain and produce a variety of neurologic manifestations, including epilepsy, paralysis, homonymous hemianopsia, optic atrophy, and papilledema.

Secondary infection of ruptured cysts produces bronchitis

Chronic pulmonary abscess may resemble tuberculosis

### Laboratory Diagnosis

Eggs difficult to find in sputum, pleural fluid, and feces

Eggs are usually absent from the sputum during the first 3 months of overt infection; however, repeated examinations will eventually demonstrate them in more than three quarters of infected patients. When a pleural effusion is present, it should be checked for eggs. Stool examination is frequently helpful, particularly in children who swallow their expectorated sputum. Approximately 50% of patients with brain lesions will demonstrate calcification on x-ray films of the skull. The cerebrospinal fluid in such cases shows elevated protein levels and eosinophilic leukocytosis. A diagnosis in these cases, however, often depends on the detection of circulating antibodies. Their presence usually correlates well with acute disease and disappears with successful therapy.

Serodiagnosis may be only means

### Treatment and Prevention

The disease responds well to bithionol or praziquantel therapy. Control requires adequate cooking of shellfish before ingestion.

## CHLONORCHIS

## ■ Chlonorchis sinensis

Adults survive decades in biliary tract

Eggs discharged in bile ducts appear in feces

Flukes of the genera *Fasciola, Opisthorchis,* and *Clonorchis* may all infect the human biliary tract and at times produce manifestations of ductal obstruction. *C. sinensis,* the Chinese liver fluke, is the most important and is discussed here (Table 58–2). The small, slender (5 by 15 mm) adult survives up to 50 years in the biliary tract of its host by feasting on the rich mucosal secretions. A cone-shaped anterior pole, a large oral sucker, and a pair of deeply lobular testes arranged one behind the other in the posterior third of the worm serve to distinguish it from other hepatic parasites. Approximately 2000 tiny (15 by 30 μm) ovoid eggs are discharged daily and find their way down the bile duct and into the fecal stream. The exquisite urn-shaped shells have a discernible shoulder at their opercular rim and a tiny knob on the broader posterior pole. On reaching fresh water, they are ingested by their intermediate snail host, transformed into cercariae, and released to penetrate the tissues of freshwater fish, in which they encyst to form metacercariae. If the latter host is ingested by a fish-eating mammal, the larvae are released in the duodenum, ascend the common bile duct, migrate to the second-order bile ducts, and mature to adulthood over 30 days.

Snails first intermediate host, fish second

Metacercariae from ingested fish migrate to biliary system

In addition to humans, rats, cats, dogs, and pigs may serve as definitive hosts.

## Clonorchiasis (Liver Fluke Infection)

### Epidemiology

Clonorchiasis is endemic in the Far East, particularly in Korea, Japan, Taiwan, the Red River Valley of Vietnam, the Southern Chinese province of Kwantung, and Hong Kong. In previous years, parasite transmission was perpetuated by the practice of fertilizing commercial fish ponds with human feces. Recent improvements in the disposal of human waste have diminished acquisition of the disease in most countries. However, the extremely long lifespan of these worms is reflected in a much slower decrease in the overall infection rate. In some villages in southern China, the entire adult population is infected. A recent survey of stool specimens from immigrants from Hong Kong to Canada showed an infection rate of more than 15% overall and 23% in adults between 30 and 50 years of age. The disease is acquired by eating raw, frozen, dried, salted, or pickled fish. Commercial shipment of such products outside of the endemic area may result in the acquisition of worms far from their original source.

Endemic in Far East

Transmission to humans related to waste disposal

Ingestion of uncooked fish infects humans

### Clinical Manifestations

Migration of the larvae from the duodenum to the bile duct may produce fever, chills, mild jaundice, eosinophilia, and liver enlargement. The adult worm induces epithelial hyperplasia, adenoma formation, and inflammation and fibrosis around the smaller bile ducts. In light infection, clinical disease seldom results. However, numerous reinfections may produce worm loads of 500 to 1000, resulting in the formation of bile stones and sometimes bile duct carcinoma in patients with severe, long-standing infections. Calculus formation is often accompanied by asymptomatic biliary carriage of *Salmonella typhi*. Dead worms may obstruct the common bile duct and induce secondary bacterial cholangitis, which may be accompanied by bacteremia, endotoxin shock, and hypoglycemia. Occasionally, adult worms are found in the pancreatic ducts, where they can produce ductal obstruction and acute pancreatitis.

Light infection usually asymptomatic

Severe hepatic and biliary manifestations from heavy worm loads

### Laboratory Diagnosis

Definitive diagnosis requires the recovery and identification of the distinctive egg from the stool or duodenal aspirates. In mild infections, repeated examinations may be required. As most patients are asymptomatic, any individual with clinical manifestations of disease in whom *Clonorchis* eggs are found must be evaluated for the presence of other causes of illness. In acute symptomatic clonorchiasis, there is usually leukocytosis, eosinophilia, elevation of alkaline phosphatase levels, and abnormal CT and ultrasonographic liver scans. Cholangiograms may reveal dilatation of the intrahepatic ducts, small filling defects compatible with the presence of adult worms, and occasionally cholangiocarcinoma.

Distinctive eggs present in feces and duodenal aspirates

Eosinophilia common in acute disease

### Treatment and Prevention

Praziquantel has proven to be an effective therapeutic agent. Prevention requires thorough cooking of freshwater fish and sanitary disposal of human feces.

# SCHISTOSOMA

## Schistosoma Species

The schistosomes are a group of closely related flukes that inhabit the portal vascular system of a number of animals. Of the five species known to infect humans, three, *S. mansoni, S. haematobium,* and *S. japonicum,* are of primary importance, infecting over 200 million individuals worldwide. The remaining two are found only in limited areas of Africa (*S. intercalatum*) and Southeast Asia (*S. mekongi*) and will not be discussed in detail.

Inhabit portal vascular system

The adults of these species can be distinguished from the hermaphroditic trematodes by the anterior location of their ventral sucker, by their cylindric bodies, and by their reproductive systems (that is, separate sexes). They are differentiated from one another only with difficulty. The 1- to 2-cm male possesses a deep ventral groove, or gynecophoral canal, in which it carries the longer, more slender female in life-long copulatory embrace. After

Different morphology and separate sexes

mating in the portal vein, the conjoined couple use their suckers to ascend the mesenteric vessels against the flow of blood. Guided by unknown stimuli, *S. japonicum* enters the superior mesenteric vein, eventually reaching the venous radicals of the small intestine and ascending colon; *S. mansoni* and *S. haematobium* are directed to the inferior mesenteric system. The destination of the former is the descending colon and rectum; the latter, however, passes through the hemorrhoidal plexus to the systemic venous system, ultimately coming to rest in the venous plexus of the bladder and other pelvic organs.

*S. mansoni* reaches colon and rectum and *S. haematobium* reaches veins of bladder and pelvic organs

On reaching the submucosal venules, the worms initiate oviposition. Each pair deposits 300 (*S. mansoni, S. haematobium*) to 3000 (*S. japonicum*) eggs daily for the remainder of its 4- to 35-year life span. Enzymes secreted by the enclosed miracidium diffuse through the shell and digest the surrounding tissue. Ova lying immediately adjacent to the mucosal surface rupture into the lumen of the bowel (*S. mansoni, S. japonicum*) or bladder (*S. haematobium*) and are passed to the outside in the excreta. Here, with appropriate techniques, they may be readily observed and differentiated. The eggs of *S. mansoni* are oval, possess a sharp lateral spine, and measure 60 by 140 μm. Those of *S. haematobium* differ primarily in the terminal location of their spine. The eggs of *S. japonicum,* in contrast, are more nearly circular, measuring 70 by 90 μm. A minute lateral spine can be visualized only with care.

Eggs deposited submucosally, rupture to lumina, and pass outside

When the eggs are deposited in fresh water, the miracidia hatch quickly. Upon finding a snail host appropriate for their species, they invade and are transformed over 1 to 2 months into thousands of forked-tailed cercariae. When released from the snail, these infectious larvae swim about vigorously for a few days. Cercariae coming in contact with human skin during this time attach, discard their tails, and penetrate. After a 1- to 3-day sojourn in the skin, the resulting schistosomula enter small venules and find their way through the right side of the heart to the lung. After a delay of several days, the parasites enter the systemic circulation and are distributed to the gut. Those surviving passage through the pulmonary and intestinal capillary beds return to the portal vein, where they mature to sexually active adults over 1 to 3 months.

In water eggs hatch to form miracidia, which invade snail

Cercariae from snail traverse human skin and vascular system

## Schistosomiasis (Blood Fluke Infection)

### Epidemiology

The widespread distribution and extensive morbidity of schistosomiasis makes it the single most important helminthic infection in the world today. Currently, more than 200 million individuals in 74 countries are infected. The continued presence of the parasite depends upon the disposal of infected human excrement into fresh water, the availability of appropriate snail hosts, and the exposure of humans to water infected with cercariae. The construction of modern sanitation and water purification facilities would break this cycle of transmission, but exceeds the economic resources of most endemic nations. Paradoxically, several massive land irrigation projects launched over the past two decades for the express purpose of speeding economic development have resulted in the dispersion of infected humans and snails to previously uninvolved areas.

Most important of helminthic infections would be stopped by modern waste disposal

Spread to areas caused by new irrigation projects

*S. mansoni,* the most widespread of the blood flukes, is the only one present in the Western Hemisphere. Originally introduced by African slaves, it is now found in Venezuela, Brazil, Surinam, Puerto Rico, the Dominican Republic, St. Lucia, and several other Caribbean islands.

As a suitable snail host is lacking, transmission does not occur within the continental United States; however, nearly half a million individuals residing there have acquired schistosomiasis elsewhere. Puerto Rican, Yemenite, and Southeast Asian populations are those predominantly involved. In the Eastern Hemisphere, the prevalence of *S. mansoni* infection is highest in the Nile Delta and the tropical section of Africa. Isolated foci are also found in East and South Africa, Yemen, Saudi Arabia, and Israel.

Geographic distribution varies with species and depends on presence of snail host

*S. haematobium* is largely confined to Africa and the Middle East, where its distribution overlaps that of *S. mansoni*. *Schistosoma japonicum* affects the agricultural populations of several Far Eastern countries, including Japan, China, the Philippines, and the Celebes. The closely related *S. mekongi* is found in the Mekong and Mun River valleys of Vietnam, Thailand, Cambodia, and Laos.

Within endemic areas, there are wide variations in both infection rates and worm loads. In general, both peak in the second decade of life and then decrease with advancing age. This finding has been explained in part by changes in the intensity of water exposure and in part by the slow development of IgE-mediated immunity. Most infected patients carry fewer than 10 pairs of worms in the vascular system and, accordingly, lack clinical manifestation of disease. Individuals who develop much heavier loads as a result of repeated infections may experience serious morbidity or mortality.

Age-related susceptibility with peak in second decade

## Pathogenesis and Clinical Manifestations

There are three major clinicopathologic stages in schistosomiasis: The first stage is initiated by the penetration and migration of the schistosomula. The second or intermediate stage begins with oviposition and is associated with a complex of clinical manifestations. The third or chronic stage is characterized by granuloma formation and scarring around retained eggs.

### Early Stage

Within a few hours of penetrating the skin, a large proportion of the schistosomula die. In *S. mansoni* and *S. haematobium* infections, immediate and delayed hypersensitivity to parasitic antigens results in an intensely pruritic papular skin rash, a manifestation that increases in severity with repeated exposures to cercariae. As the viable schistosomula begin their migration to the liver, the rash disappears and the patient experiences fever, headache, and abdominal pain for 1 to 2 weeks.

Local and systemic hypersensitivity reactions produce rash

### Intermediate Stage

One to two months after primary exposure, patients with severe *S. mansoni* or *S. japonicum* infections experience the onset of an acute febrile illness that bears a striking resemblance to serum sickness. It has been suggested that the onset of oviposition leads to a state of relative antigen excess and the formation of soluble immune complexes. Indeed, high levels of such complexes have been demonstrated in the peripheral blood and correlate well with the severity of illness. In addition to the fever and chills, patients experience cough, urticaria, arthralgia, lymphadenopathy, splenomegaly, abdominal pain, and diarrhea. Sigmoidoscopic examination reveals an inflamed colonic mucosa and petechial hemorrhages; occasionally, patients with *S. japonicum* infection will develop clinical manifestations of encephalitis. Typically, leukocytosis, marked peripheral eosinophilia, and elevated levels of IgM, IgG, and IgE immunoglobulins are present. This symptom complex is commonly termed the Katayama syndrome; it may persist for 3 months or more and occasionally results in death.

Prolonged febrile period with circulating immune complexes

Intestinal inflammation and encephalitis occur acutely

### Chronic Schistosomiasis

Approximately one half of all deposited eggs reach the lumen of the bowel or bladder and are shed from the body. Those retained induce inflammation and scarring, initiating the final and most morbid phase of schistosomiasis. Soluble antigens excreted by the eggs stimulate the formation of T lymphocyte-mediated eosinophilic granulomas. Early in the infection, the inflammatory response is vigorous, producing lesions more than 100-fold larger than the inciting egg itself. Obstruction of blood flow is common. With time, the host's inflammatory response moderates, leading to a significant decrease in granuloma size. Fibroblasts stimulated by factors released by both retained eggs and the granulomas lay down scar tissue, rendering the earlier, granuloma-induced vascular obstruction permanent. As would be expected, the severity of tissue damage is directly related to the total number of eggs retained.

Inflammatory and fibrotic reactions to retained eggs cause chronic disease

In *S. haematobium* infection, the bladder mucosa becomes thickened, papillated, and ulcerated. Hematuria and dysuria result; repeated hemorrhages produce anemia. In severe infections the muscular layers of the bladder are involved, with loss of bladder capacity and contractibility. Vesicoureteral reflux, ureteral obstruction, and hydronephrosis may follow. Progressive obstruction leads to renal failure and uremia. Calcification of the bladder wall is occasionally seen, and approximately 10% of patients harbor urinary tract calculi. Secondary bacterial infections are common. Chronic *Salmonella* bacteriuria with recurrent bouts of bacteremia have been reported from Egypt. In the same country, bladder carcinoma is frequently seen as a late complication of disease.

*S. haematobium* produces bladder lesions with hemorrhage and obstruction

Chronic urinary carriage of *Salmonella* may cause bacteremia

Severity of liver involvement linked to HLA type

Hepatitis B superinfection goes to chronic active

Salmonella focus requires eradication of parasite and bacteria

In *S. mansoni* and *S. japonicum* infections, the bowel mucosa is congested, thickened, and ulcerated. Polyposis has been reported from Egypt, but not elsewhere. Patients experience abdominal pain, diarrhea, and blood in the stool. Eggs deposited in the larger intestinal veins may be carried by the portal blood flow back to the liver, where they lodge in the presinusoidal capillaries. The resulting inflammatory reaction leads to the development of periportal fibrosis and hepatic enlargement. The frequency and severity with which the liver is involved are genetically determined and associated with the HLA type of the patient. In most cases, liver function is well preserved. Infected individuals who subsequently acquire hepatitis B virus develop chronic active hepatitis more frequently than those free of schistosomes. The presinusoidal obstruction to blood flow can result in the serious manifestations of portal obstruction. Eggs carried around the liver in the portosystemic collateral vessels may lodge in the small pulmonary arterioles, where they may produce interstitial scarring, pulmonary hypertension, and right ventricular failure. Occasionally, eggs may be deposited in the central nervous system, where they may cause epilepsy or paraplegia.

Some differences between the clinical presentation of schistosomiasis mansoni and that of schistosomiasis japonicum have been noted. Manifestations of the latter disease typically occur earlier in the course of the infection and tend to be more severe. When involvement of the central nervous system develops, it is more likely to occur in the brain than the spinal cord. On the other hand, immune complex nephropathy and recurrent *Salmonella* bacteremia are more likely to be seen in hepatosplenic *S. mansoni* infections. The latter phenomenon is apparently related to the ability of *Salmonella* to parasitize the gut and integument of the adult fluke, providing a persistent bacterial focus within the portal system of the infected patient. This focus cannot be eradicated without treatment of the schistosomal infection.

## Immunity

Major manifestations from cell-mediated immune response to eggs

Blocking anibodies and adsorption of host molecules provide antigenic disguise

Concomitant immunity prevents new infections

The major clinicopathologic manifestations of schistosomiasis result from the host's cell-mediated immune response to the presence of retained eggs. With time, the intensity of this reaction is muted; granulomas formed in the later stages of infection are smaller and less damaging than those formed early. The mechanisms responsible for this modulation are not fully understood. Present evidence suggests that both suppressor T lymphocyte activity and antibody blockade are involved. The correlation in humans between HLA types A1 and B5 and the development of hepatosplenomegaly suggests that the extent of the immunoregulation is influenced, at least in part, by the genetic background of the host.

As evidenced by their prolonged survival, the adult worms are remarkably well tolerated by their hosts. In part, this tolerance may be attributable to the formation of IgG4 blocking antibodies early in the course of infection. Tolerance may also reflect the ability of the developing parasites to disguise themselves by absorbing host molecules, including immunoglobulins, blood group glycolipids, and histocompatibility complex antigens. Antibodies formed against the immature worms before they have acquired host antigens, however, are effective in protecting the host from reinfection. Schistosomula that penetrate the skin after the primary infection are coated with specific antibody, bound to eosinophils, and destroyed. Although protection is not complete, the 60 to 80% kill rate is highly effective in controlling the intensity of parasitism. This condition, in which adult worms from a primary infection can survive in a host resistant to reinfection, has been termed concomitant immunity. Eventually, production of blocking antibodies wanes and that of protective IgE antibodies active against adult worms increases, leading to a decrease in the host's total worm population.

## Laboratory Diagnosis

*S. haemotobium* eggs found in urine

*S. mansoni* and *S. japonicum* eggs in stool; rectal biopsy

Definitive diagnosis requires the recovery of the characteristic eggs in urine, stool, or biopsy specimens. In *S. haematobium* infections, eggs are most numerous in urine samples obtained at midday. When examination of the sediment yields negative results, eggs may sometimes be recovered by filtering the urine through a membrane filter. Cystoscopy with biopsy of the bladder mucosa may be required for the diagnosis of mild infection. Eggs of *S. mansoni* and *S. japonicum* are passed in the stool. Concentration techniques such as formalin-ether or gravity sedimentation are necessary when the ova are scanty. Results of rectal biopsy may be positive when those of repeated stool examinations are negative.

Because dead eggs may persist in tissue for a long time after the death of the adult worms, active infection is confirmed only if the eggs are shown to be viable. This confirmation may be obtained by observing the eggs microscopically for movement of flame cell cilia or by hatching them in water. Quantitation of egg output is useful in estimating the severity of infection and in following response to treatment.

Determination of egg viability and output useful

Currently available serologic tests possess sensitivities exceeding 90%, but cannot reliably distinguish active from inactive disease. It is probable that this shortcoming will be alleviated by tests using defined antigens from different life stages of the schistosomes.

### Treatment

No specific therapy is available for the treatment of schistosomal dermatitis or the Katayama syndrome. Antihistamines and corticosteroids may be helpful in ameliorating their more severe manifestations. In the late stage of schistosomiasis, therapy is directed at interrupting egg deposition by killing or sterilizing the adult worms. As the severity of clinical and pathologic manifestations is related to the intensity of infection, therapy is usually reserved for patients with moderate or severe active infections.

Several anthelmintic agents may be used. Praziquantel, which is active against all three species of schistosomes, is the agent of choice for *S. japonicum*. In addition to praziquantel, metrifonate may be used for *S. haematobium* and oxamniquine for *S. mansoni*.

Multiple anthelmintic drugs are used

### Control and Prevention

It has proved both difficult and expensive to control this deadly disease. Programs aimed at interrupting transmission of the parasite by the provision of pure water supplies and the sanitary disposal of human feces are often beyond the economic reach of the nations most seriously affected. Similarly, measures to deny snails access to newly irrigated lands are expensive. Chemical molluscicides have been shown effective in limited trials, but have been less successful when used over large areas for prolonged periods. Mass therapy of the infected human population has, until recently, been severely limited by the toxicity of effective agents. It is possible that the agents developed most recently will prove more suitable for this purpose. At present, programs that have incorporated all of these control measures have been the most successful.

Sanitary disposal of feces often limited by economic state

Molluscicides effective but large scale application difficult

Currently, there is intense interest in developing a vaccine suitable for human use. A vaccine made from irradiated *S. bovis* cercariae, developed for cattle, appears to confer a significant degree of protection against infection. Similar vaccines are not available for human populations until questions concerning safety and suitability for widespread field use are satisfactorily resolved. Monoclonal antibodies have been successfully used to identify a number of schistosomula and adult antigens thought to be capable of inducing protective immunity. A number of such defined antigen vaccines are undergoing study.

Vaccines using irradiated cercariae under development

## ADDITIONAL READING

Hagen P. Reinfection, exposure and immunity in human schistosomiasis. *Parasitol Today* 1992;8:12–16. A brief, clear summary of a very complex topic.

Johnson RJ, Jong EC, Dunning SB, et al. Paragonamiasis: Diagnosis and the use of praziquantel in treatment. *Rev Infect Dis* 1985;7:200–206. Discusses the clinical presentation, diagnosis, and treatment of paragonamiasis presenting in Southeast Asian immigrants to the United States.

Nash TE, Cheever AW, Ottensen EA, Cook JA. *Schistosoma* infection in humans: Perspectives and clinical findings. *Ann Intern Med* 1982;97:740–754.

Newport GR, Colley DG. Schistosomiasis. In: Warren KS, ed. *Immunology and Molecular Biology of Parasitic Infections.* 3rd ed. Boston, Blackwell Scientific, 1993. This relatively comprehensive monograph discusses general immune responses to schistosomal infections as well as the immunity, immunopathology, immunodiagnosis, molecular biology, and vaccine development in schistosomiasis.

Rim HJ. The current pathology and chemotherapy of clonorchiasis. *Korean J Parasitol* 1986;24(suppl 3):1–141. The most comprehensive review of this disease.

Seah SK. Digenetic trematodes. *Clin Gastroenterol* 1978;7:87–104. A number of trematode infections are discussed.

Strickland GT. Schistosomiasis: Eradication or control? *Rev Infect Dis* 1982;4:951–954.

Von Lichtenberg F. Conference on contended issues of immunity to schistosomiasis. *Am J Trop Med Hyg* 1985;34:78–85. Introduction to conference dealing with the evidence for protective immunity, mechanisms of immunologic killing, and future prospects for vaccines against the schistosomes.

Warren KS. Selective primary health care: Strategies for control of disease in the developing world. I. Schistosomiasis. *Rev Infect Dis* 1982;4:715–726. This article and the Strickland article discuss lucidly the limitations of proposed control strategies and offer alternative approaches, including directed mass therapy.

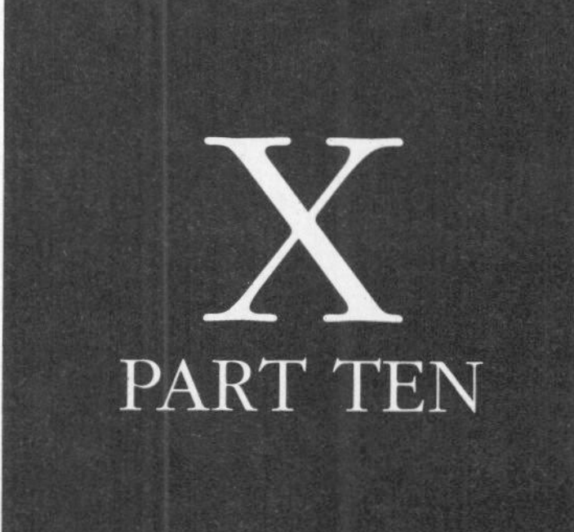


# Local and Systemic Infections

Chapter 59

# Skin and Wound Infections

*Kenneth J. Ryan*

## SKIN INFECTIONS

Infections of the skin can result from microbial invasion from an external source or from organisms reaching the skin through the bloodstream as part of a systemic disease. Blood-borne involvement is evidenced by rashes in many viral and bacterial infections, such as measles, and secondary syphilis, or may yield more chronic granulomatous skin lesions in blastomycosis, tuberculosis, and syphilis. Skin lesions remote from sites of infection can be produced by some bacterial toxins, such as the pyrogenic exotoxins of group A streptococcus and *Staphylococcus aureus.* They can also result from immunologic responses to microbial antigens that have reached the skin. Thus, there are manifold skin manifestations of infections; however, this chapter will be restricted to the discussion of direct infections that may occur in the Western Hemisphere.

The skin is an organ system with multiple functions, including protection of the tissues from external microbial invasion. Its keratinized stratified epithelium prevents direct microbial invasion under normal conditions of surface temperature and humidity, and its normal flora, pH, and chemical defenses tend to inhibit colonization by many pathogens (Chapters 9 and 10). However, the skin is subject to repeated minor traumas that are often unnoticed, but that destroy its integrity and allow organisms to gain access to its deeper layers from the external environment. The surface is also penetrated by ducts of pilosebaceous units and sweat glands, and microbial invasion can occur along these routes, particularly if the ducts are obstructed.

### Infections in Hair Follicles, Sebaceous Glands, and Sweat Glands

#### ■ Folliculitis

Staphylococci and *Pseudomonas* infect hair follicles

Folliculitis is a minor infection of the hair follicles and is usually caused by *S. aureus*. It is often associated with areas of friction and of sweat gland activity and is thus seen most frequently on the neck, face, axillae, and buttocks. Blockage of ducts with inspissated sebum, as in acne vulgaris, predisposes to the condition. Folliculitis can also be caused by *Pseudomonas aeruginosa,* and this form of the disease has become more common in recent years with the popularity of hot tubs and whirlpool baths. Unless these facilities are thoroughly cleansed and adequately chlorinated, they can grow large numbers of pseudomonads at their normal operating temperatures, causing extensive folliculitis on areas of the body that have been immersed. The lesions subside rapidly when the insult is discontinued. Occasionally folliculitis may be caused by infection with *Candida albicans*. Such cases are particularly common in immunocompromised hosts.

*Propionibacterium acnes* contributes to inflammation of acne

**Acne vulgaris** also involves inflammation of hair follicles and associated sebaceous glands. The comedo of acne results from multiplication of *Propionibacterium acnes,* the predominant anaerobe of the normal skin, behind and within inspissated sebum. Organic acids produced by the organism are believed to stimulate an inflammatory response and thus contribute to the disease process. The primary cause of the disease, however, is hormonal influences on sebum secretion that occur at puberty, and the disease usually resolves in early adult life.

### Furuncles

Staphyococcal furuncles are skin abscesses that can spread

The furuncle is a small staphylococcal abscess that develops in the region of a hair follicle. Furuncles may be solitary or multiple and may constitute a troublesome recurrent disease. Spread of infection to the dermis and subcutaneous tissues can result in a more extensive multiloculated abscess, the **carbuncle.** These lesions and their treatment are considered in Chapter 15.

#### Treatment

Folliculitis and individual furuncles are normally treated locally by measures designed to establish drainage without the use of antibiotics. Chronic furunculosis may require attempts to eliminate nasal carriage of *S. aureus,* which is sometimes the source of the infection. Antimicrobics are not usually required unless surrounding cellulitis or carbuncles develop. Severe acne can often be treated effectively with topical drying agents. Prolonged administration of low oral doses of tetracycline is often effective, although the reason for the therapeutic response is uncertain.

## Infections Through Minor or Inapparent Skin Lesions

Minor or inapparent skin lesions serve as the route of infection in many localized skin infections and in some systemic diseases, such as syphilis and leptospirosis.

### Infection of Keratinized Layers

Hypersensitivity and inflammatory response important with dermatophytes

The only organisms that can use the keratin on cells, hairs, and nails are the dermatophyte fungi. The dermatophytes are particularly well adapted to these sites, cannot grow at 37°C, and fail to invade deeper layers. The clinical manifestations of these infections result from the inflammatory and delayed hypersensitivity responses of the host, and the desquamation induced by these processes is a major factor in the ultimate control of the infection by removing infected skin. In candidiasis, control involves cell-mediated immune mechanisms, and chronic *Candida* skin and nail infections are often associated with defects in cellular immunity.

Cell-mediated immune defects in chronic candidiasis

## Infection of Other Skin Layers

### Impetigo

Pyoderma, also termed impetigo, is a common, sometimes epidemic skin lesion. This disease is caused primarily by group A streptococci. The initial lesion is often a small vesicle that develops at the site of invasion and ruptures with superficial spread characterized by skin erosion and a serous exudate, which dries to produce a honey-colored crust. The exudate and crust contain numerous infecting streptococci. *S. aureus* may occasionally produce pustular impetigo or contaminate the lesions caused by streptococci.

Epidemic impetigo is most common in childhood and under conditions of heat, humidity, poor hygiene, and overcrowding. The infection may be spread by fomites such as shared clothing and towels. It is sometimes caused by nephritogenic strains of *S. pyogenes,* particularly in the tropics, and acute glomerulonephritis may result. Rheumatic fever is not associated with streptococcal lesions of the skin. Treatment is usually with penicillin or erythromycin and topical antimicrobics or skin antiseptics to limit spread.

Bullous impetigo is a distinct disease caused by strains of *S. aureus* (usually phage type 71) that produce exfoliation. It is most common in small children, but may occur at any age. The infection is characterized by large serum-filled bullae (blisters) within the skin layers at the site of infection. Minor infections are treated topically; bullous impetigo in infants, however, is a serious disease that usually requires systemic antimicrobic treatment. Epidemic spread may occur under conditions similar to those described for streptococcal impetigo.

Staphylococcal bullous impetigo is associated with exfoliation production

### Erysipelas

Erysipelas is a rapidly spreading infection of the deeper layers of the dermis that is almost always caused by group A streptococci (*S. pyogenes*). It is associated with edema of the skin, marked erythema, pain, and systemic manifestations of infection, including fever and lymphadenopathy. As the infection is intradermal, the streptococci cannot usually be isolated from the skin surfaces. The disease can progress to septicemia or local necrosis of skin. It is serious and requires immediate treatment with penicillin or erythromycin.

*S. pyogenes* erysipelas is a spreading deep-skin infection with a high risk of bacteremia

### Cellulitis

Cellulitis is not a skin infection as such, but can develop by extension from skin or wound infections. It usually presents as an acute inflammation of subcutaneous connective tissue with swelling and pain and often with marked constitutional signs and symptoms. It can be caused by many pathogenic bacteria, but *S. aureus* and group A streptococci are most common. *Haemophilus inflenzae* type b is an important cause in infants and children. Enteric Gram-negative rods, clostridia, and other anaerobes may also cause cellulitis as a complication of wound infections, particularly in the immunocompromised host and the uncontrolled diabetic.

Cellulitis is most often caused by pyogenic cocci or *H. influenzae* in children

## Skin Ulcers and Granulomatous Lesions

Many acute and subacute skin infections are characterized by ulceration or a granulomatous response. Some are sexually transmitted and are discussed in Chapter 70. Others derive from systemic infection and are not direct infections of skin. A few examples of direct infections, which pose special diagnostic problems, are considered below.

Herpes simplex virus can invade through the skin to produce a local vesicular lesion followed by ulceration. The lesion may then recur in the infected area. Primary herpetic lesions of the finger can mimic staphylococcal paronychia very closely, as well as produce lymphangitis and local and lymph node enlargement with pain and fever. The lesions are sterile on bacterial culture.

Herpetic paronychia can mimic staphylococcal infections

Skin diphtheria, which remains common in some tropical areas, also occurred endemically among the transient population of the West Coast of the United States during the 1970s and early 1980s. The organism gains access through a wound or insect bite and causes chronic erosion and ulceration of the skin, sometimes with evidence of the systemic effects of diphtheria toxin.

Skin diphtheria seen in transients

*Mycobacterium marinum* produces a self-limiting granuloma, usually of the forearms and knees. The organism usually enters through superficial abrasions from rocks or swimming pool walls. Infections with *M. ulcerans* are more serious and produce progressive ulceration, but are limited to tropical areas and do not occur in the United States or Europe.

Swimmer's granuloma caused by *Mycobacterium marinum*

Several rare forms of necrotic spreading skin ulceration tend to develop in immunosuppressed hosts, in diabetics, and as complications of abdominal surgery. These lesions include bacterial synergistic gangrene, apparently caused by a peptostreptococcus and *S. aureus,* streptococcal gangrene associated with *S. pyogenes* infection, and infection with a variety of opportunistic fungi. Variants of these conditions produce extensive and spreading necrotic cellulitis. The major form of treatment is to excise the infected tissues widely and supplement such surgery with massive chemotherapy.

Necrotic ulcerations, bacterial synergistic gangrene may require surgery

Several primary fungal diseases are associated with cutaneous ulceration or cellulitis, including mycetoma and chromoblastomycosis, which involve the feet, and sporotrichosis,

Fungal and parastic ulcerations usually secondary to systemic infection

in which ulceration often develops from infected subcutaneous lymph nodes and vessels. Likewise, some parasites directly infect and ulcerate the skin, as in cutaneous leishmaniasis and cutaneous amebiasis. These latter two diseases are not contracted in the United States.

## WOUND INFECTIONS

Wounds subject to infection can be surgical, traumatic, or physiologic. The latter include the endometrial surface, after separation of the placenta, and the umbilical stump. Traumatic wounds comprise such diverse damage as deep cuts, compound fractures, frostbite necrosis, and thermal burns.

Sources of infection include patient, environment, and infected persons

Sources of infection include (1) the patient's own normal flora; (2) material from infected individuals or carriers that may reach the wound on fomites, hands, or through the air; and (3) pathogens from the environment that can contaminate the wound through soil, clothing, and other foreign material. Examples of such infections include contamination of a penetrating stab wound to the abdomen by colonic flora, contamination of a clean surgical wound in the operating room with *S. aureus* spread from the flora of a perineal carrier, and introduction of spores of *Clostridium tetani* into the tissues on a splinter.

### Classification of Wounds

Surgical and traumatic wounds are classified according to the extent of potential contamination and thus, the risk of infection. These criteria carry important implications regarding surgical treatment and chemoprophylaxis.

Clean, clean contaminated, and dirty wounds relate to risk of exposure

**Clean wounds** are surgical wounds made under aseptic conditions that do not traverse infected tissues or extend into sites with a normal flora. **Clean contaminated wounds** are operative wounds that extend into sites with a normal flora (except the colon) without known contamination. **Contaminated wounds** include fresh surgical and traumatic wounds with a major risk of contamination, such as incisions entering nonpurulent infected tissues. **Dirty and infected wounds** include old, infected traumatic wounds, wounds substantially contaminated with foreign material, and wounds contaminated with spillage from perforated viscera.

Infection rates in clean surgical wounds should be less than 1%, whereas untreated dirty wounds have a high probability of infection. Similar considerations apply to the chance of infection developing in a placental site or on the umbilicus. A normal delivery without retained products will rarely be followed by endometrial infection. A prolonged delivery after rupture of the membranes with retained placental fragments poses an increased risk. In some rural cultures in Africa, soil is applied to the umbilical stump, and neonatal tetanus is common, whereas it is almost unknown in the western world.

### Factors Contributing to Infection Probability

Infectious risk increases with contaminating dose of organisms

Various factors, in addition to those indicated previously, contribute to the probability of a wound becoming infected. The contaminating dose of microorganisms and their virulence can be critical and, other things being equal, the chance of infection developing increases progressively with the contaminating dose. The physical and physiologic condition of the wound also influences the probability of infection. Areas of necrosis, vascular strangulation from excessively tight sutures, hematomas, excessive edema, poor blood supply, and poor oxygenation all compromise normal defense mechanisms and substantially reduce the dose of organisms needed to initiate infection. Thus, removal of necrotic tissue and the surgeon's skill, gentleness, and attention to detail are major factors in preventing the development of infection.

Vascular integrity in wound important for defense

Nutritional and immunologic status and inflammatory response of the host

The general health, nutritional status, and ability of the patient to mount an inflammatory response are also major determinants of whether a wound infection develops. Infection rates are higher in the elderly, the obese, uncontrolled diabetics, and those on immunosuppressive or corticosteroid therapy. Nutritional deficiencies enhance the risk of infection, and new approaches to avoid protein–calorie malnutrition in patients with severe burns, for example, have led to substantial reductions in serious clinical infections.

There is strong evidence that the critical period determining whether contamination of surgical wounds proceeds to infection lies within the first 3 hours after contamination. It is for this reason that prophylactic chemotherapy of some surgical wounds and procedures can be restricted to the operative and immediate perioperative period. There is general agreement that extending such prophylaxis beyond 24 hours increases the chance of complications without reducing the risk of infection.

First 3 hours critical period for surgical wounds

### Prevention and Treatment

Epidemiologic approaches to the prevention of wound infection and the appropriate uses of chemoprophylaxis are considered in Chapter 13. There has been increasing interest in the possibilities of active or passive immunization against the types of organisms that may infect a particular patient, for example, one who has suffered a burn recently or is to undergo certain types of major surgery. Despite some encouraging experimental results, the clinical application of these findings to burns and severe trauma remains to be established.

Immunization desirable but still not possible

Severe wound infections are almost always treated with a combination of surgical and chemotherapeutic approaches. Necrotic tissue and contaminated foreign bodies, such as sutures, must be removed, pockets of pus opened, and drainage established. This approach permits access of the appropriate antibiotics to viable tissues in which they can act.

## ETIOLOGIC AGENTS

Some major causes of skin and wound infections are shown in Table 59–1. *S. aureus* remains the single most common source of infection of clean surgical wounds; however, the

*S. aureus* the most common

**TABLE 59–1. MAJOR CAUSES OF SKIN AND WOUND INFECTIONS**

| Syndrome | Bacteria | Fungi | Other |
|---|---|---|---|
| Impetigo | *Streptococcus pyogenes*<br>*Staphylococcus aureus* | | |
| Folliculitis | *Pseudomonas aeruginosa*<br>*Staphylococcus aureus* | *Candida albicans* | |
| Acne | *Propionibacterium acne* | | |
| Furuncle | *Staphylococcus aureus* | | |
| Cellulitis | group A streptococci[a]<br>*Staphylococcus aureus*<br>*Haemophilus influenzae* | | |
| Intertrigo | *Staphylococcus aureus*<br>Enterobacteriaceae | *Candida albicans* | |
| Chronic ulcers[b] | *Treponema pallidum*<br>*Haemophilus ducreyi*<br>*Corynebacterium diphtheriae*<br>*Bacillus anthracis*<br>*Nocardia*<br>*Mycobacterium* | *Sporothrix* | Herpesvirus |
| Wounds | | | |
| Trauma | *Clostridium*<br>Enterobacteriaceae<br>*Pseudomonas aeruginosa* | | |
| Surgical (clean) | *Staphylococcus aureus*<br>Enterobacteriaceae<br>group A streptococci | | |
| Surgical (dirty)[c] | *Staphylococcus aureus*<br>Enterobacteriaceae<br>Anaerobes | | |
| Burns | *Pseudomonas aeruginosa*<br>*Staphylococcus aureus*<br>Enterobacteriaceae | *Candida albicans* | |
| Animal bites | *Pasteurella multocida* | | |

[a] Including "erysipelas," an infection primarily involving the deeper layers of the dermis.
[b] Usually begin as nodules or pustules.
[c] Etiology determined by the origin of the contaminating flora (eg, abdominal vs. gynecologic surgery)

Increasing proportion of opportunistic Gram-negative infections

number of infections caused by opportunistic Gram-negative organisms is now increasing. This finding reflects the extension of surgical intervention to more patients whose defenses are compromised or who would have been unacceptable surgical risks before the introduction of new technical and therapeutic procedures. Severe invasive group A streptococcal infections have increased recently and are associated with a toxic shock-like syndrome. Many of these cases begin with skin or wound infection.

Invasive *S. pyogenes* infections have increased recently

Anaerobic Gram-negative wound infections have been reported increasingly in the last two decades or so as a result of the higher incidence of such infections in immunocompromised patients and better laboratory recognition. Most infecting organisms derive from normal floral sites and the majority are *Bacteroides* often in combination with anaerobic Gram-positive cocci and facultative aerobic bacteria. They tend to be associated with necrosis, which may spread subcutaneously, and with thrombophlebitis, which may lead to bacteremia. Most postpartum uterine infections are now caused by Gram-negative anaerobes or anaerobic Gram-positive cocci; they can range from self-limiting infections to severe infections of the uterus with pelvic thrombophlebitis. Human bite wounds are particularly subject to anaerobic infections. In contrast, infected bites of domestic animals (dogs, cats) are almost always due to *Pasteurella multocida*.

Bacteroides and anaerobic Gram-positive coccal infections derived from patients flora

Burns and areas of necrosis resulting from vascular stasis or insufficiency are subject to infection with the same organisms that predominate in postsurgical wound infections; *P. aeruginosa* causes particularly serious infections in burns, however, with loss of skin grafts and a high risk of septicemia and death. If the fluid electrolyte and nutritional deficiencies of a burned patient can be controlled, the greatest hazard to life is infection.

*P. aeruginosa* a common and virulent cause of burn infections

Tetanus remains a threat to the unimmunized or inadequately immunized individual, particularly from heavy contamination of puncture wounds or introduction of foreign bodies such as splinters, soil, or clothing into the subcutaneous tissues. *C. tetani* never spreads beyond the site of the local lesion and adequate circulating antibody from tetanus toxoid immunization will prevent the development of the disease.

Gas gangrene (clostridial myositis) can develop within a few hours of traumatic injury and lead to rapid death. *C. perfringens* is the most common cause and its alpha-toxin produces the spreading tissue damage and muscle death. Other aerobic and anaerobic bacteria are invariably present and sometimes play an important etiologic role. The disease is always associated with muscle trauma and necrosis, which provide the conditions for anaerobic multiplication. Compound fractures, gunshot wounds, and similar extensive injuries that allow entry of clostridial spores, set the stage for the disease. Prevention involves surgically debriding all necrotic or potentially necrotic tissue as soon as possible and administering high-dose penicillin.

Tetanus and gas gangrene derived from the environment

# Bone and Joint Infections

*C. George Ray*

Infections of bones and joints may exist separately or together. Both are most common in infancy and childhood. They are usually caused by blood-borne (hematogenous) spread to the infected site, but can also result from local trauma with secondary infection. Sometimes there may be local spread from a contiguous soft tissue infection, often associated with the presence of a foreign body at the site of the primary wound.

The local effect of such infections can be devastating if they are inadequately treated, because inflammation and resultant tissue necrosis may produce irreparable damage. The presence of pus under pressure can compromise normal blood flow and even cause destruction of blood vessels with avascular necrosis of tissue. When this condition develops a sequestrum can result, in which a part of the cartilage or bone becomes totally separated from its blood supply and cannot be incorporated into the healing process. In some patients, sequestrum formation can lead to a smoldering chronic infection with draining sinuses and loss of functional integrity. Normal growth of the affected site can be severely impaired in the infant or child, particularly when the epiphysis is involved. In the acute phase of infection, bacteremia may also cause sepsis and metastatic infections in sites such as the lungs and heart. The result may be fatal.

Sequestrum formation can lead to chronic infection with draining sinuses

Infection can cause growth impairment in children

Bacteremia and metastatic spread common from bone and joint infections

## OSTEOMYELITIS

The onset of acute hematogenous osteomyelitis is usually abrupt, but can sometimes be quite insidious. It is classically characterized by localized pain, fever, and tenderness to palpation over the affected site. More than one bone or joint may be involved as a result of hematogenous spread to multiple sites. With progression, the classic signs of heat, redness, and swelling may develop. Laboratory findings often include leukocytosis and elevated acute-phase reactants, such as the sedimentation rate. Osteomyelitis caused by a contiguous focus of infection is usually associated with the presence of local findings of soft tissue infection, such as skin abscesses and infected wounds.

Local pain and signs of inflammation

May come from contiguous focus

When osteomyelitis occurs in close proximity to a joint, septic arthritis may develop by direct spread through the epiphysis (usually in infants) or by lateral extension through the periosteum into the joint capsule. Such extension is particularly common in hip and elbow infections.

Extend to joints through epiphysis

### Common Etiologic Agents

The most common causes of acute osteomyelitis and those associated with special circumstances are shown in Table 60–1. It is clear that age plays a significant role in influencing

**TABLE 60–1. COMMON CAUSES OF ACUTE OSTEOMYELITIS**

| Situation | Usual Causative Organism |
|---|---|
| **Age group** | |
| Neonates (<1 mo) | *Staphylococcus aureus*; group B streptococci; Gram-negative rods (eg, *Escherichia coli, Klebsiella, Proteus, Pseudomonas*) |
| Older infants, children, adults | *Staphylococcus aureus* |
| **Special problems** | |
| Chronic hemolytic disorders (eg, sickle cell disease) | *Staphylococcus aureus; Streptococcus pneumoniae; Salmonella* species |
| Infection after trauma or surgery | *Staphylococcus aureus; Streptococcus pyogenes*; Gram-negative aerobic or anaerobic bacteria |
| Infection after puncture wound of foot | *Pseudomonas aeruginosa; Staphylococcus aureus* |

Age-related etiologies but staphylococcal osteomyelitis most common

Chronic granulomatous osteomyelitis suggests mycobacteria, fungi

the relative frequency of the various infective agents, particularly in early infancy; however, most infections are caused by *Staphylococcus aureus*.

Low-grade smoldering infections may also occur with the organisms listed in Table 60–1; however chronic granulomatous processes must also be considered, including tuberculosis, coccidioidomycosis, histoplasmosis, and blastomycosis. These latter infections usually result from systemic dissemination, and the lesions develop slowly over a period of months. Occasionally bone tumors or cysts and leukemia must also be considered in the differential diagnosis.

## General Diagnostic Approaches

The primary goals of diagnosis are to establish the existence of infection and to determine its cause. The following procedures are generally employed:

Blood cultures, direct aspirates, and bone scans

1. Blood cultures, because many infections are associated with bacteremia.
2. Radionuclide scanning or magnetic resonance imaging to demonstrate evidence of localized infection.
3. Direct staining, culture, and histology of needle aspirates or biopsies of periosteum or bone.
4. X-rays of affected sites, which often appear normal in the early stages of infection. The first changes seen are swelling of surrounding soft tissues, followed by periosteal elevation. Demineralization of bone may not become apparent for 2 weeks or more after the onset of symptoms; calcification of the periosteum and surrounding soft tissues is usually delayed even longer.

X-rays may be normal in early stages of infection

## General Principles of Management

Bactericidal antimicrobics continued for weeks

In acute infections, early intervention is important. Management includes vigorous use of bactericidal antimicrobics, which must often be continued for several weeks to ensure a bacteriologic cure and prevent progression to chronic osteomyelitis. Surgical drainage is also essential if there is significant pressure from the localized, purulent process.

Surgery and prolonged therapy required chronic osteomyelitis

In chronic osteomyelitis, sequestrum formation is frequent and sinuses may develop that drain the bone abscess to the skin surface. The infection is persistent, and treatment becomes extremely difficult. Such patients often require long-term antibiotic treatment (months to years) combined with surgical procedures to drain the abscesses and remove necrotic, infected tissues in an attempt to control infection while preserving the integrity of the affected bone.

## ■ SEPTIC ARTHRITIS

The usual clinical features of septic arthritis include onset of pain, which is often abrupt and accompanied by fever. Single or multiple joints may be involved. Tenderness and swelling of the affected joints and frequently other signs of local inflammation are present. Attempts to move the joints, either actively or passively, result in severe pain. In infants, the symptoms may be somewhat nonspecific; local swelling or excessive irritability with unwillingness to move the affected extremity (pseudoparalysis) may be the only clues to the diagnosis.

Pain on movement with swelling and fever

### Common Etiologic Agents

The major causes of septic arthritis are listed in Table 60–2. Although *S. aureus* infection can occur at any age, there are some significant age-specific relationships to other bacterial causes. There is a high frequency of group B streptococcal infections in neonates, whereas in children between 1 month and 4 years of age, pneumococci and *Haemophilus influenzae* type b are more likely to be involved, although *H. influenzae* disease is decreasing with immunization. *Neisseria gonorrhoeae* is implicated in most cases of septic arthritis in young adults.

*S. aureus* at any age

Other pyogenic cocci age, behavior related

Subacute or chronic infective arthritis should prompt consideration of tuberculosis, Lyme disease, syphilis, and fungal infections such as coccidioidomycosis or *Candida*. Arthritis attributable to *Candida* is particularly likely in immunocompromised patients.

Viruses and *Mycoplasma* can also cause acute arthritis in single or multiple joints. Such illnesses have been associated with rubella, hepatitis B, mumps, parvovirus B19, varicella, Epstein–Barr virus, Coxsackie virus, and adenovirus infections, as well as with *M. pneumoniae* and *M. hominis*. These arthritides are usually self-limiting and rarely require specific therapy. Some bacterial infections of sites other than joints may be associated with noninfectious (reactive) arthritis, possibly resulting from deposition of circulating immune complexes and complement in synovial tissues, leading to inflammation. This has occurred with intestinal infections caused by *Yersinia enterocolitica, Campylobacter jejuni,* and some *Salmonella* species and also as a delayed sequela after successful treatment of sepsis due to *N. meningitidis* or *H. influenzae*.

Tuberculous, spirochetal, and fungal arthritis have subacute or chronic course

Viral or *Mycoplasma* arthritis usually self-limiting

Immune complexes from other sites may cause reactive arthritis

Noninfectious causes of arthritis must also be considered in the differential diagnosis. They can closely mimic septic arthritis. Examples include inflammatory collagen vascular disease such as rheumatoid arthritis, gout, traumatic arthritis, and degenerative arthritis.

### General Diagnostic Approaches

In acute cases, blood cultures are often useful because bacteremia may be present. The definitive diagnosis is established by examination of synovial fluid removed from the joint by needle aspiration (arthrocentesis). As other noninfectious causes must be considered, it is important to analyze the chemical and cellular characteristics of the fluid in addition to performing a Gram stain and culture. Table 60–3 summarizes the major findings in synovial fluid in normal and various disease states. Septic bacterial arthritis is usually associated with

Blood culture particularly useful

TABLE 60–2. COMMON CAUSES OF SEPTIC ARTHRITIS

| Age Group | Usual Causative Organism |
|---|---|
| Neonate (<1 mo) | *Staphylococcus aureus*; group B streptococci; Gram-negative rods (eg, *Escherichia coli, Klebsiella, Proteus, Pseudomonas*) |
| 1 mo–4 yr | *Haemophilus influenzae* type b; *Staphylococcus aureus; Streptococcus pyogenes; Streptococcus pneumoniae; Neisseria meningitidis* |
| 4–16 yr | *Staphylococcus aureus* |
| 16–40 yr | *Neisseria gonorrhoeae; Staphylococcus aureus* |
| >40 yr | *Staphylococcus aureus* |

TABLE 60–3. FINDINGS IN SYNOVIAL FLUID IN VARIOUS FORMS OF ARTHRITIS

| Laboratory Test | Normal | Septic Bacterial Arthritis | Trauma, Degenerative Joint Disease | Rheumatoid Arthritis, Gout |
|---|---|---|---|---|
| Clarity and color | Clear | Opaque, yellow to green | Clear, yellow | Translucent, yellow; or opalescent |
| Viscosity | High | Variable | High | Low |
| White blood cells/mm³ | <200 | 25,000–100,000 | 200–2000 | 2000–20,000 |
| Polymorphonuclear cells (%) | <25 | >75 | 25–50 | ≥50 |
| Glucose level (relative to simultaneous blood glucose level) | Nearly equal | <25% | Nearly equal | 50–80% |

Needle aspiration gives characteristics of synovial fluid and material to culture

grossly purulent fluid containing more than 25,000 white blood cells per cubic millimeter, predominantly polymorphonuclear cells. The glucose level in the synovial fluid is usually less than 25% of that in the blood.

In viral, tuberculous, and fungal arthritis, as well as in partially treated bacterial arthritis, cell counts are usually lower, and mononuclear cells may constitute a greater proportion of the inflammatory cells. Occasionally, biopsy of the synovial membrane may be required to resolve the diagnosis. Histologic examination and culture of the tissue are particularly helpful in distinguishing granulomatous from rheumatoid disease.

Gonococci may be difficult to isolate from joint fluid

In most cases of acute septic arthritis, the blood culture and/or synovial fluid culture will yield the specific etiologic agent. One major exception is *N. gonorrhoeae,* which can be difficult to isolate from these sources. When this organism is suspected, it is wise to include cultures of other sites of potential infection, such as the blood, urethra, cervix, rectum, and pharynx, as well as skin lesions.

## GENERAL PRINCIPLES OF MANAGEMENT

Prompt, vigorous, systemic antimicrobial therapy is required as soon as diagnostic tests suggest a bacterial cause. This treatment usually must be continued for 3 to 6 weeks, depending upon the etiologic agent and the clinical response to therapy. Drainage of pus under pressure is also an important aspect of management. In cases of hip joint involvement, open surgical drainage is often necessary because collateral blood supply to the hip joint is relatively limited, and pus under pressure can lead to irreversible avascular necrosis of the tissues with permanent crippling. It is also difficult to evaluate the amount of pus that may be present because of the overlying muscles. Other joints can usually be managed by simple aspiration of pus whenever it reaccumulates significantly during the acute phase of infection.

Chapter 61

# Eye, Ear, and Sinus Infections

C. George Ray

## EYE INFECTIONS

Ocular infections can be divided into those that primarily involve the external structures—eyelids, conjunctiva, sclera, and cornea—and those that involve internal sites. The major defense mechanisms of the eye are the tears and the conjunctiva, as well as the mechanical cleansing that occurs with blinking of the eyelids. The tears contain secretory IgA and lysozyme, and the conjunctiva possesses numerous lymphocytes, plasma cells, neutrophils, and mast cells, which can respond quickly to infection by inflammation and production of antibody and interferon. The internal eye is protected from external invasion primarily by the physical barrier imposed by the sclera and cornea. If these are breached (for example, by a penetrating injury or ulceration), infection becomes a possibility. In addition, infection may reach the internal eye via the blood-borne route to the retinal arteries and produce chorioretinitis and/or uveitis. Such infections are a particularly common problem in immunocompromised patients.

Defenses of the eye mechanical, tears, lysozyme, sIgA

Other causes of inflammation of the external or internal eye can involve autoimmune or allergic mechanisms, which may be provoked by infectious agents or diseases such as rheumatoid arthritis.

### Common Clinical Features

**Blepharitis** is an acute or chronic inflammatory disease of the eyelid margin. It can take the form of a localized inflammation in the external margin (hordeolum or stye) or a granulomatous reaction to infection and plugging of a sebaceous gland of the eyelid (chalazion).

**Dacryocystitis** is an inflammation of the lacrimal sac. It usually results from partial or complete obstruction within the sac or nasolacrimal duct, where bacteria may be trapped and initiate either an acute or a chronic infection.

Multiple anatomic sites of infection have individual features

**Conjunctivitis** is a term used to describe inflammation of the conjunctiva; it may extend to involve the eyelids, cornea (keratitis), or sclera (episcleritis). Extensive disease involving the conjunctiva and cornea is often called keratoconjunctivitis. Progressive keratitis can lead to ulceration, scarring, and blindness. **Ophthalmia neonatorum** is an acute, sometimes severe, conjunctivitis or keratoconjunctivitis of newborn infants.

**Endophthalmitis** is rare, but often leads to blindness even when treated aggressively. The term refers to infection of the aqueous or vitreous humor, usually by bacteria or fungi.

**Uveitis** consists of inflammation of the uveal tract–iris, ciliary body, and choroid. Although most inflammations of the iris and ciliary body (iridocyclitis) are not of infectious origin, some agents have been implicated. The acute disease may be associated with severe eye pain, redness, and photophobia; other cases may progress quite silently, with decreased visual acuity as the only symptom in the late stages. The most common infective involvement of the uveal tract is chorioretinitis, in which inflammatory infiltrates are seen in the retina; this infection can lead to destruction of the choroid and inflammation of the optic nerve (optic neuritis) and may extend into the vitreous humor to cause endophthalmitis. If the disease is not treated adequately, the end result can be blindness.

## Common Etiologic Agents

Blepharitis and keratitis: staphylococcal

Acute conjunctivitis: age-related etiologies

Chronic conjuntivitis: *C. trachomatis*, herpes

Epidemic adenovirus conjunctivitis related to pools, eyedrops

Chorioretinitis usually linked to systemic disease

Endophthalmitis blood borne or contiguous spread

The major infectious causes of various inflammatory diseases of the eye are listed in Table 61–1. *Staphylococcus aureus* is the principal offender in bacterial infections of the eyelid and cornea. *Haemophilus influenzae* and *Streptococcus pneumoniae* are common causes of acute bacterial conjunctivitis. In young infants, *Neisseria gonorrhoeae* and *Chlamydia trachomatis* are significant causes of external eye disease, contracted from the mother's birth canal, that must be diagnosed and treated promptly. Chronic conjunctivitis or keratoconjunctivitis at any age must also prompt consideration of *C. trachomatis* infection. Herpes simplex is also a major cause of chronic conjunctivitis, especially in infections of the external structures, and specific therapy is available. Epidemic conjunctivitis or keratoconjunctivitis is most commonly associated with a variety of adenovirus serotypes. Outbreaks have been associated with inadequately chlorinated swimming pools, contaminated equipment or eyedrops in physicians' offices, and communal sharing of towels, which facilitates direct transmission.

Chorioretinitis is frequently a manifestation of systemic disease (for example, histoplasmosis, tuberculosis); it is particularly common in immunocompromised patients, who are liable to develop disseminated *Candida,* cytomegalovirus, or *Toxoplasma gondii* infections. Endophthalmitis may also result from blood-borne dissemination or by contiguous spread as a result of injury (for example, corneal ulcerations). In the latter situation, iatrogenic infection by agents such as *Pseudomonas* species can be induced by contaminated eye drops, and ophthalmologic examination equipment.

Infection of the soft tissues surrounding the eye (periorbital or orbital cellulitis) is po-

**TABLE 61–1. MAJOR INFECTIOUS CAUSES OF EYE DISEASE**

| Disease | Bacteria | Viruses | Fungi | Parasites |
|---|---|---|---|---|
| Blepharitis | *Staphylococcus aureus* | | | |
| Dacryocystitis | *Streptococcus pneumoniae; Staphylococcus aureus* | | | |
| Conjunctivitis; keratitis; keratoconjunctivitis | *Streptococcus pneumoniae; Haemophilus influenzae; Haemophilus aegyptius; Streptococcus pyogenes; Staphylococcus aureus; Chlamydia trachomatis; Neisseria gonorrhoeae; Neisseria meningitidis* | Adenoviruses; herpes simplex; measles; varicella–zoster | *Fusarium* species *Aspergillus* species | *Acanthamoeba* (keratitis) |
| Ophthalmia neonatorum | *Neisseria gonorrhoeae; Chlamydia trachomatis* | Herpes simplex | | |
| Endophthalmitis | *Staphylococcus aureus; Pseudomonas aeruginosa;* other Gram-negative organisms | | *Candida* species *Aspergillus* species | |
| Iridocyclitis | *Treponema pallidum* | Herpes simplex; varicella–zoster | | |
| Chorioretinitis | *Mycobacterium tuberculosis* | Cytomegalovirus; herpes simplex | *Histoplasma capsulatum; Coccidioides immitis; Candida* species | *Toxoplasma gondii; Toxocara canis* |

tentially severe and can spread to involve the functions of the eye itself. Major causes are *Staphylococcus aureus, H. influenzae,* and *Streptococcus pyogenes.*

## General Diagnostic Approaches

In external bacterial infections of the eye, etiologic diagnoses can usually be established by Gram stain and culture of surface material or, in the case of viral infections, by tissue culture. Conjunctival scrapings for *C. trachomatis* can be prepared for immunofluorescent or cytologic examination and for appropriate culture. Infections of internal sites pose a more difficult problem. Some, such as acute endophthalmitis, may require removal of infected aqueous humor for microbiologic studies. Infections involving the uveal tract may require indirect methods of diagnosis, such as serologic tests for toxoplasmosis and deep mycoses, blood cultures to demonstrate evidence of disseminated disease (for example, *Candida* sepsis), and efforts to demonstrate infection in other sites (for example, chest radiography and sputum culture to diagnose tuberculosis). Careful ophthalmologic examination using slit lamps and retinoscopy often helps to suggest specific etiologic agents based on the morphology of the lesions observed.

Gram stain for bacteria, scrapings for others

Most agents can be cultured

## General Principles of Management

Various topical antimicrobial agents have been used effectively in external eye infections of presumed or proved bacterial origin. In addition, topical antiviral treatment is available for herpes simplex infections, but has not been proved efficacious for other viral diseases of the eye.

Topical agents for superficial bacterial and herpes simplex infections

Severe infections, whether external or internal, require specialized treatment that nearly always includes ophthalmologic consultation because they may threaten vision. Systemic infection associated with eye disease (for example, fungemia, tuberculosis) must be treated vigorously with appropriate antimicrobial agents.

Ophthalmologic consultation needed with severe or deep infection

# EAR INFECTIONS

Most infections of the ear involve the external otic canal (otitis externa) or the middle ear cavity (otitis media), which contains the ossicles and is enclosed by bony structures and the tympanic membrane. Factors of importance in the pathogenesis of otitis externa include local trauma, furunculosis, foreign bodies, or excessive moisture, which can lead to maceration of the external ear epithelium (swimmer's ear). Occasionally, external otitis occurs as an extension of infection from the middle ear, with purulent drainage through a perforated tympanic membrane.

Otitis externa linked to ear canal trauma

The eustachian tube, which vents the middle ear to the nasopharynx, appears to play a major role in predisposing patients to otitis media. The tube performs three functions: ventilation, protection, and clearance via mucociliary transport. Viral upper respiratory infections or allergic conditions can cause inflammation and edema in the eustachian tube or at its orifice. These developments disturb its functions, of which ventilation may be the most important. As ventilation is lost, oxygen is absorbed from the air in the middle ear cavity, producing negative pressure. This pressure in turn allows entry of potentially pathogenic bacteria from the nasopharynx into the middle ear, and failure to clear these normally can result in colonization and infection. Other factors that can lead to compromise of eustachian tube function include anatomic abnormalities, such as tissue hypertrophy or scarring around the orifice, muscular dysfunction associated with cleft palate, and lack of stiffness of the tube wall. The latter is common in infancy and early childhood and improves with age. It may explain in part why otitis media occurs most often in infants 6 to 18 months old, then decreases in frequency as patency of the eustachian tube becomes established.

Viral infection predisposes to otitis media

Microbes enter middle ear by the eustachian tube

Failure to clear leads to otitis media

## Clinical Manifestations

P. aeruginosa causes swimming pool and malignant otitis externa

Otitis externa is characterized by inflammation of the ear canal, with purulent ear drainage. It can be quite painful, and cellulitis can extend into adjacent soft tissues. A common form is associated with swimming in water that may be contaminated with aerobic, Gram-negative organisms such as *Pseudomonas* species. "Malignant" otitis externa is a considerably more severe form of external ear canal infection that can progress to invasion of cartilage and adjacent bone, sometimes leading to cranial nerve palsy and death. It is seen most frequently in elderly patients with diabetes mellitus and in immunocompromised hosts of any age. *P. aeruginosa* is the most common causative pathogen.

Acute otitis media usually bacterial

Otitis media is arbitrarily classified as acute, chronic, or serous (secretory). Acute otitis media, nearly always caused by bacteria, is often a complication of acute viral upper respiratory illness. Fever, irritability, and acute pain are common, and otoscopic examination will reveal bulging of the tympanic membrane, poor mobility, and obscuration of normal anatomic landmarks by fluid and inflammatory cells under pressure. In some cases, the tympanic membrane will also be acutely inflamed, with blisters (bullae) on its external surface (myringitis). If treated inadequately, the infection can progress to involve adjacent structures such as the mastoid air cells (mastoiditis) or lead to perforation with spontaneous drainage through the tympanic membrane. Potential acute, suppurative sequelae include extension into the central nervous system and sepsis.

Extension to deeper structures leads to mastoiditis

Chronic otitis media follows repeated unresolved acute infections

Chronic otitis media is usually a result of acute infection that has not resolved adequately, either because of inadequate treatment in the acute phase or because of host factors that perpetuate the inflammatory process (for example, continued eustachian tube dysfunction, caused by allergic or anatomic factors, or immunodeficiency). Sequelae include progressive destruction of middle ear structures and a significant risk of permanent hearing loss.

Serous otitis media may represent either a form of chronic otitis media or allergy-related inflammation. It tends to be chronic, causing hearing deficits, and is associated with thick, usually nonpurulent secretions in the middle ear.

## Common Etiologic Agents

*H. influenzae* strains noncapsulated

The usual causes of ear infections are listed in Table 61–2. *Streptococcus pneumoniae* is the single most common cause of acute otitis media after the first 3 months of life, accounting for 35 to 40% of all cases. *H. influenzae* is also common, particularly in patients less than 5 years of age. The majority of *H. influenzae* isolates from the middle ear are non-typable; thus the current vaccine against type b strains would not be expected to markedly reduce the incidence of acute otitis media. Viruses and *Mycoplasma* are rare primary causes of

**TABLE 61–2. COMMON CAUSES OF EAR INFECTION**

| | |
|---|---|
| Otitis externa | *Pseudomonas aeruginosa* is common; occasionally *Proteus* species, *Escherichia coli*, and *Staphyloccus aureus*; bacteria found in otitis media may also be recovered if the process is secondary to middle ear infection with perforation and drainage through the tympanic membrane; fungi, such as *Aspergillus* species, are occasionally implicated |
| Acute otitis media | |
| <3 mo old | *Streptococcus pneumoniae*, group B streptococci, *Haemophilus influenzae, Staphylococcus aureus, Pseudomonas aeruginosa*, and Gram-negative enteric bacteria |
| >3 mo old | *Streptococcus pneumoniae* and *Haemophilus influenzae* are most common; others include *Streptococcus pyogenes, Moraxella catarrhalis,* and *Staphylococcus aureus* |
| Chronic otitis media | Mixed flora in 40% of cases cultured. Common organisms include *Pseudomonas aeruginosa, Haemophilus influenzae, Staphylococcus aureus, Proteus* species, *Klebsiella pneumoniae, Moraxella catarrhalis*, and Gram-positive as well as Gram-negative anaerobic bacteria |
| Serous otitis media | Same as chronic otitis media; however, many more of these effusions are sterile, with relatively few acute inflammatory cells |

acute or chronic otitis media; however, they predispose patients to superinfection by the bacterial agents.

## General Diagnostic Approaches

The diagnosis is established on the basis of clinical examination. Tympanometry can be performed in suspected cases of otitis media to detect the presence of fluid in the middle ear and to assess tympanic membrane function. The specific etiology of otitis externa can be determined by culture of the affected ear canal; one must keep in mind, however, that surface contamination and normal skin flora may lead to mixed cultures, which can be confusing. In otitis media, the most precise diagnostic method is careful aspiration with a sterile needle through the tympanic membrane after decontamination of the external canal. Gram stain and culture of such aspirates is highly reliable; however, this procedure is generally reserved for cases in which etiologic possibilities are extremely varied, as in young infants, or when clinical response to the usual antimicrobial therapy has been inadequate. Respiratory tract cultures, such as those from the nasopharynx, cannot be relied upon to provide an etiologic diagnosis.

External ear cultures often confusing

Middle ear cultures reliable but reserved for difficult cases

Respiratory tract cultures unhelpful

## General Principles of Management

Except in severe cases, otitis externa can usually be managed by gentle cleansing with topical solutions. The Gram-negative bacteria most commonly involved are often susceptible to an acidic environment, and otic solutions buffered to a low pH (3.0 or less), as with 0.25% acetic acid, will often be effective. Various preparations are available, many of which also contain antimicrobics.

Otitis externa treated with topical agents

Acute otitis media requires prompt antimicrobial therapy and careful follow-up to ensure that the disease has resolved. The choice of antimicrobic is usually empirical, designed specifically to cover the most likely bacterial pathogens because direct aspiration for diagnostic purposes is usually unnecessary. In the usual case these pathogens would be *S. pneumoniae* and *H. influenzae*.

Antimicrobic therapy for otitis media directed at common agents for age group

If there is extreme pressure with severe pain, drainage of middle ear exudates by careful incision of the tympanic membrane may be necessary.

In patients with chronic or serous otitis media, management can be more complex, and it is often advisable to seek otolaryngologic consultation to determine further diagnostic procedures as well as to plan medical and possible surgical measures.

# SINUS INFECTIONS

The paranasal sinuses (ethmoid, frontal, and maxillary) all communicate with the nasal cavity. In health, these sinuses are air-filled cavities lined with ciliated epithelium and are normally sterile. They are poorly developed in early life and, in contrast to otitis media, sinus infections are a rare problem in infancy.

The pathogenesis of sinus infection can involve several factors, most of which act by producing obstruction or edema of the sinus opening, impeding normal drainage. Consequently, bacterial infection and inflammation of the mucosal lining tissues develop. Predisposing factors may be (1) local, such as upper respiratory infections producing edema of antral tissues, mucosal polyps, deviation of the nasal septum, enlarged adenoids, or a tumor or foreign body in the nasal cavity; or (2) systemic, such as allergy, cystic fibrosis, or immunodeficiency. Occasionally, maxillary sinusitis can result from extension of a maxillary dental infection.

Factors predisposing to sinusitis involve obstruction or extension from other sites

## Clinical Manifestations

Signs and symptoms vary according to which sinuses are affected and whether the illness is acute or chronic. Fever is sometimes present; cough, nasal discharge, fetid breath, pain

**TABLE 61–3. COMMON CAUSES OF SINUS INFECTION**

| | |
|---|---|
| Acute sinusitis | *Streptococcus pneumoniae* and *Haemophilus influenzae* are most common; also *Streptococcus pyogenes, Staphylococcus aureus,* and *Moraxella catarrhalis* |
| Chronic sinusitis | Same as for acute sinusitis; also Gram-negative enteric bacteria and anaerobic Gram-negative and Gram-positive bacteria; mixed aerobic and anaerobic infections are relatively common; opportunistic fungi may be found in compromised patients (eg, those with diabetes mellitus) |

over the affected sinus, headache, and tenderness to percussion over the frontal or maxillary sinuses are all features that may appear in different combinations and suggest the diagnosis.

Complications of sinusitis can include extension of infection to nearby soft tissues, such as the orbit, and occasionally spread, either directly or via vascular pathways, into the central nervous system.

## Common Etiologic Agents

Table 61–3 summarizes the usual etiologies of sinus infections. Respiratory viruses are also occasional direct causes, but are most important as predisposing factors to bacterial superinfection of inflamed sinuses and their antral openings. Together, *S. pneumoniae* and *H. influenzae* account for more than 60% of cases of acute sinusitis. Opportunistic, saprophytic fungi, such as *Mucor, Aspergillus,* and *Rhizopus* species, are being increasingly seen in compromised hosts, such as those with severe diabetes mellitus or immune deficiency. These have a particular tendency to spread progressively to adjacent tissues and to the central nervous system and are very difficult to treat.

## General Diagnostic Approaches

Gram stain and cultures of direct sinus aspirates required

Cultures of sinus drainage unreliable

Radiographic studies of the sinuses will confirm the diagnosis. If it becomes necessary to determine the specific infectious agent, fluid should be obtained directly from the affected sinus by needle puncture of the sinus wall or by catheterization of the sinus antrum after careful decontamination of the entry site. Gram smears and cultures are then made. Cultures of drainage from the antral orifices or nasal secretions are unreliable because of contaminating aerobic and anaerobic normal flora.

## General Principles of Management

In uncomplicated acute sinusitis, prompt antimicrobial therapy is initiated. The choice of antimicrobics is usually empirical, based on the most likely bacterial causes and their usual susceptibility. For example, amoxicillin is effective against most strains of *S. pneumoniae* and *H. influenzae*.

Severe, complicated acute infections and chronic sinusitis often require otolaryngologic consultation. In such cases, it is often necessary to obtain cultures directly from the sinuses to select specific antimicrobial therapy, consider the need for surgical procedures to adequately remove the pus and inflammatory tissues, and correct any anatomic obstruction that may exist.

# Dental and Periodontal Infections

*Murray R. Robinovitch*

Dental caries, chronic marginal periodontal disease, and the sequelae of these two diseases constitute the majority of oral and dental infections. In both, the source of the causative bacteria is the microbial plaque that forms on the teeth. Thus, although dental caries and chronic marginal periodontal disease are distinctly different, the prevention and/or halting of the progression of these diseases relies upon the elimination of dental plaque from the tooth surfaces. In addition to causing caries and chronic marginal periodontal disease, the bacteria of dental plaque play a role in acute necrotizing ulcerative gingivitis (Vincent's infection), another important oral infection.

Dental plaque a deposit from bacterial colonization

**Dental plaque** is a soft, adherent dental deposit that forms as a result of bacterial colonization of the tooth surface. It is rather insoluble, as well as adherent, and thus resists removal by water spray or mouth rinsing. Only more vigorous means such as tooth brushing and flossing between the teeth will remove it. It consists almost entirely of bacterial cells ($1.7 \times 10^{11}$ cells/g wet weight).

Caries produced by plaque bacteria

**Dental caries** is the progressive destruction of the mineralized tissues of the tooth, primarily caused by the production of organic acids resulting from the glycolytic metabolic activity of plaque bacteria. The basic characteristic of the carious lesion is that it progresses inward from the tooth surface, be that the enamel-coated crown or the cementum of the exposed root surface, involving the dentin and finally the pulp of the tooth. From here, infection can extend out into the periodontal tissues at the root apex or apices.

Chronic marginal periodontal disease encompasses two separate disease entities: gingivitis and periodontitis. These diseases are believed to be related in that gingivitis, although a reversible condition, is thought to be an early stage leading ultimately to periodontitis in the susceptible subject. The term **gingivitis** is used when the inflammatory condition is limited to the marginal gingiva and bone resorption around the necks of teeth has not yet begun. **Periodontitis** is used to connote the stage of chronic marginal periodontal disease in which there is progressive loss of tooth support. Periodontitis can also lead to periodontal abscess when the chronic inflammatory state around the necks of the teeth becomes acute at a specific location.

Chronic periodontal infection causes destruction of supporting tissues

**Chronic marginal periodontitis,** or adult periodontitis as it is also called, is responsible for most tooth loss in people more than 35 to 40 years of age. The adjectives chronic and marginal indicate that the disease progresses slowly and results in the progressive destruction of the supporting tissues of the tooth (periodontal ligament and alveolar bone) from the margins of the gingiva toward the apices of the roots of the teeth. Although the accumulative effects of the disease make it appear chronic in nature, the disease may occur as a series of acute episodes separated by quiescent periods of indeterminate duration.

Acute periodontitis caused by different organisms

There is also an acute form of periodontitis that affects young children (prepubertal periodontitis), a form with an age of onset of around puberty that affects adolescents and results in more rapid loss of tooth support (juvenile periodontitis), and an adult form of the disease that progresses quite rapidly (rapidly progressive periodontitis). These diseases are thought to be caused by plaque organisms different from those responsible for chronic marginal periodontitis and/or an altered host resistance to the disease.

## DENTAL PLAQUE

Attachment of bacteria to dental pellicle begins colonization

Adhesion mechanisms are lectinlike

The formation of dental plaque is the result of a very specific colonization of tooth surfaces by oral bacteria. The mineralized tooth surface is always coated with a thin organic film called the dental cuticle or pellicle. This coating results from adsorption and binding of specific salivary macromolecules, mainly proteins and glycoproteins, to the tooth surface. As this cuticle or pellicle can form in a matter of minutes after the tooth surface is exposed to the oral fluid, bacteria never interact directly with the mineralized tooth surface. Instead, bacterial adherence to the tooth, which begins the colonization of the tooth surface, is mediated by bacterial receptors or adhesins that interact with the pellicle in some fashion, often a specific high affinity mechanism such as a lectinlike interaction. Subsequent to this initial colonization, accumulation of progeny as well as the attachment of other bacterial species occurs via a variety of coaggregation mechanisms.

Plaque comprises many species of bacteria, including anaerobes

A number of oral bacteria among the complex indigenous oral flora adhere readily to the cuticle-coated tooth above the gum line or free gingival margin. Primary among them are Gram-positive cocci, such as the sanguis group of organisms (*Streptococcus sanguis* and related species) and short Gram-positive rods, which are the initial colonizers. After 2 to 4 days, fusiform and filamentous organisms appear. Anaerobic vibrios, spirochetes, and a variety of Gram-negative, motile, anaerobic organisms appear at about 6 to 10 days. Thus, as the dental plaque increases in thickness, Gram-negative anaerobic organisms appear and multiply. In toto, there are thought to be 300 to 400 bacterial species present in mature dental plaque. The extent and complexity of involved bacteria is shown in Figure 62–1. Den-

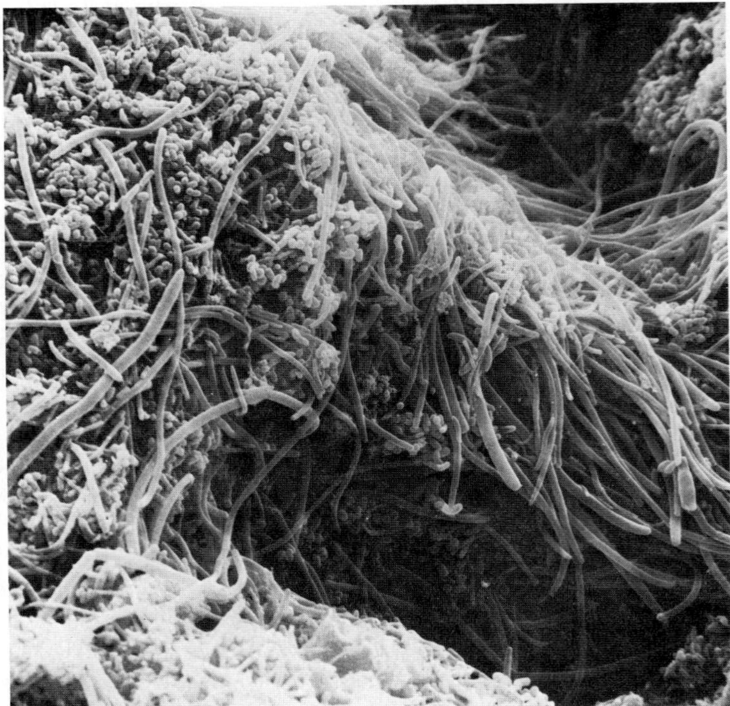

**Figure 62–1.** Scanning electronmicrograph of supragingival plaque. (*Courtesy of Dr. W. Fischlsweiger and Dr. Dale Birdsell.*)

tal plaque would coat the tooth surfaces uniformly but for its physical removal during chewing and other oral activities. Characteristically, plaque remains in the non-self-cleansing areas of the teeth such as pits and fissures, along the margins of the gingiva, and between the teeth. It is for this reason that the plaque-related diseases, caries and periodontal disease occur in their greatest frequency and severity at these locations. In addition to the supragingival plaque, the sulcus around the tooth and periodontal pockets, which are pathologic extensions of the sulcus, are colonized by subgingival bacterial plaque of somewhat different composition. This plaque has a thin adherent layer attached to the tooth surface and a nonadherent zone between that and the epithelial cells lining the sulcus, containing large numbers of Gram-negative, motile, anaerobic microorganisms. Supragingival plaque lacks such a distinct nonadherent zone.

Plaque accumulates in non-self-cleansing areas of teeth and gingiva

Supragingival and subgingival plaque differ in composition

As the causative organisms of both dental caries and chronic marginal periodontal disease are believed to be in the dental plaque, a prime method for maintaining oral health is regular home care practices for plaque removal. Dental plaque cannot be effectively removed from the teeth by chemical or enzymatic means, and the use of antibiotics for prophylactic inhibition of plaque formation cannot be clinically justified, although patients undergoing long-term antibiotic treatment for other medical reasons demonstrate a lower incidence of caries and periodontal disease. Antiseptic substances that bind to tooth surfaces and inhibit plaque formation, such as the bis-biguanides, chlorhexidine and alexidine, have been shown to be effective in reducing plaque, caries, and gingival inflammation. The U.S. Food and Drug Administration has approved a commercial preparation containing 0.12% chlorhexidine for use in controlling dental plaque and associated disease. This prescription drug along with tooth brushing and flossing constitute the available means for routine elimination of the causative organisms of caries and periodontal disease.

Removal of plaque prime element of oral hygiene

Chemicals may be used along with brushing and flossing

## DENTAL CARIES

Dental caries is the single greatest cause of tooth loss in the child and young adult. Its onset can be very soon after the eruption of the teeth. The first carious lesions usually develop in pits or fissures on the chewing surfaces of the deciduous molars and result from the metabolic activity of the dental plaque that forms in these sites. Later in childhood, the incidence of carious lesions on smooth surfaces increases; these lesions are usually found between the teeth. The factors involved in the formation of a carious lesion are (1) a susceptible host or tooth, (2) the proper microflora on the tooth, and (3) a substrate from which the plaque bacteria can produce the organic acids that result in tooth demineralization.

Greatest cause of tooth loss in child and young adult

Require microflora and suitable subtrates for organic acid production

The newly erupted tooth is most susceptible to the carious process. It gains protection against this disease during the first year or so by a process of posteruptive maturation believed to be attributable to improvement in the quality of surface mineral on the tooth.

Saliva provides protection against caries, and patients with dry mouth (xerostomia) suffer from high caries attack rates unless suitable measures are taken. In addition to the mechanical flushing and diluting action of saliva and its buffering capacity, the salivary glands also secrete several antibacterial products. Thus, saliva is known to contain lysozyme, a thiocyanate-dependent sialoperoxidase, and immunoglobulins, principally those of the secretory IgA class. The individual importance of these antibacterial factors is unknown, but they clearly play some role in determining the ecology of the oral microflora.

Saliva protects by mechanical flushing and multiple chemical actions

Proper levels of fluoride, either systemically or topically administered, result in dramatic decreases in the incidence of caries (50 to 60% reduction by water fluoridation, 35 to 40% reduction by topical application). In the case of systemic fluoridation, the protective effect is thought to result from the incorporation of fluoride ions in place of hydroxyl ions of the hydroxyapatite during tooth formation, producing a more perfect and acid-resistant mineral phase of tooth structure. Topical application of fluoride is believed to achieve the same result on the surface of the tooth by initial dissolution of some of the hydroxyapatite, followed by recrystallization of apatite that incorporates fluoride ions into its lattice structure. Another important mode of action, namely, the inhibition of demineralization, and the promotion of remineralization of incipient carious lesions by fluoride ions present in the oral fluid, has more recently been proposed as an important anticaries mechanism of fluoride. In any event, fluoridation represents the most effective means known for rendering the tooth more resistant to the carious process.

Fluoride produces more acid resistant mineral phase of tooth

Members of microflora able to produce acid can be cariogenic

The microbial basis of dental caries is well established, and Koch's postulates have been fulfilled, in general, for a number of microorganisms that cause the disease. This confirmation was achieved by using gnotobiotic (sterile) animals whose oral cavities could be colonized with a single organism. At times during the past half-century, a single microorganism was considered responsible for all caries; *Lactobacillus acidophilus* was regarded in this manner in the 1920s, and *Streptococcus mutans* enjoyed this reputation beginning in the 1960s. Currently, it is safe to say that any oral microorganism with a mechanism for colonizing the tooth surface or preexisting plaque and the ability to produce acid (acidogenic) and survive its action (aciduric) can be cariogenic. Organisms isolated from human carious lesions and shown to be cariogenic in gnotobiotic animals include some strains of *S. mutans, Streptococcus salivarius, Streptococcus sanguis, L. acidophilus, L. casei, Actinomyces viscosus,* and *A. naeslundii,* but not all strains of these species are cariogenic in humans.

Several species may be cariogenic, but *S. mutans* is most important

Studies in human subjects indicate that *S. mutans* is a major etiologic agent for smooth surface caries and possibly for pit, fissure, and root surface caries as well. When *S. mutans* strains were collected from different sources and compared, serologic and genetic heterogeneity led to designating some of these as separate species. Currently, those members of the mutans streptococci considered to be important cariogenic organisms in humans are *S. mutans* and *S. sobrinus. Lactobacillus* species may represent secondary invaders of the established caries lesion, but the mutans streptococci are thought to be the main initiator of this disease.

Demineralization is by acid production from dietary carbohydrate breakdown

Cariogenic organisms must be provided with an appropriate substrate for glycolysis in order to cause tooth demineralization, and dietary monosaccharides and disaccharides such as glucose, fructose, sucrose, lactose, and maltose are readily used by most oral bacteria. These carbohydrates permeate the dental plaque, are absorbed by the bacteria, and are metabolized so rapidly that organic acid products accumulate and cause the pH of the plaque to drop to levels sufficient to demineralize the tooth structure. Production of acid and the decreased pH are maintained until the substrate supply is exhausted. Obviously, high-sugar-content foods that adhere to the teeth and have long oral clearance times are more cariogenic than less retentive foodstuffs such as sugar-containing liquids. Once the substrate is exhausted, the plaque pH returns slowly to its resting level. Frequency of application of substrate is extremely important, as the plaque pH may never reach a normal resting level with repeated snacking between meals.

Degree and duration of acid production facilitated by sticky carbohydrates

Dietary sucrose is also used in the synthesis of extracellular polyglycans such as dextrans and levans by some microorganisms that possess glucose transferase or fructose transferase enzymes on their cell surfaces. Synthesis of polyglycans is considered an additional virulence factor for two reasons:

Extracellular polyglycans synthesized from sucrose important in adherence and carbohydrate storage

1. The polyglycan-producing microorganisms are usually aggregated in its presence, which is believed to aid in the colonization and/or accumulation of the organism on the tooth surface. *S. mutans* is a major cariogenic microorganism that acts in this way.
2. Extracellular polyglycan production may increase cariogenicity by serving as an extracellular storage form of substrate. Certain microorganisms synthesize extracellular polyglycan when sucrose is available, but then break it down into monosaccharide units to be used for glycolysis when dietary carbohydrate is exhausted. Thus, these microorganisms can prolong acidogenesis beyond the oral clearance time of the substrate.

Acidogenesis prolonged from intracellular glycogen stores

Some oral bacteria also use dietary monosaccharides and disaccharides internally to form glycogen, which is stored intracellularly and used for glycolysis after the dietary substrate has been exhausted; thus, the period of acidogenesis is again prolonged and the cariogenicity of the microorganism increased. It is therefore clear that the ability to synthesize extracellular or intracellular storage polysaccharides, to colonize tooth surfaces, and to produce and survive in acid contribute to the microorganism's cariogenicity.

Extension to pulp and periapical locations complicate infections

The most common complications of dental caries are extension of the infection into the pulp chamber of the tooth (pulpitis), necrosis of the pulp, and extension of the infection through the root canals into the periapical area of the periodontal ligament. Periapical involvement may take the form of an acute inflammation (periapical abscess), a chronic nonsuppurating inflammation (periapical granuloma), or a chronic suppurating lesion that may drain into the mouth or onto the face via a sinus tract. A cyst may form within the chronic nonsuppurating lesion as a result of inflammatory stimulation of the epithelial rests normally found in the periodontal ligament. If the infectious agent is sufficiently virulent or host resistance is low, the infection may spread into the alveolar bone (osteomyelitis) or the fascial planes of the head and neck (cellulitis) or ascend along the venous channels to cause septic thrombophlebitis. As most carious lesions represent a mixed infection by the time cavities have developed, it is not surprising that most oral infections resulting from the extension of carious lesions are mixed and frequently caused by anaerobic organisms.

More severe complications are spread to bone or local fascia

## CHRONIC MARGINAL PERIODONTAL DISEASE

Both chronic marginal gingivitis and periodontitis are now believed to be caused by certain bacteria in the dental plaque lying next to the gingival tissues. Thus, subgingival plaque found within the gingival crevice or the sulcus around the necks of the teeth is thought to house the etiologic agent(s). The characteristic histopathologic picture of gingivitis is of a marked inflammatory infiltrate of polymorphonuclear leukocytes, lymphocytes, and plasma cells in the connective tissue that lies immediately adjacent to the epithelium lining the gingival crevice and attached to the tooth. Collagen is lost from the inflamed connective tissue. There does not seem to be any direct invasion of the gingival tissues by large numbers of intact bacteria, at least in the early stages of the disease.

Subginigival plaque causes collagen loss

It has been proposed that tissue destruction is mediated by bacterial substances that pass through the epithelial barrier and cause either direct or indirect injury. Bacterial products that could cause direct injury to the tissues include toxins, such as endotoxin and leukotoxins, and enzymes, such as hyaluronidase and collagenase. Several mechanisms for indirect injury of the periodontal tissues have been proposed. These hypotheses include initiation of an unresolvable inflammatory response with excessive release of the lysosomal contents from polymorphonuclear leukocytes; activation of complement, which further magnifies the inflammatory response; and development of a host of humoral and cell-mediated immune responses, which can also magnify the inflammatory response as well as lead to tissue destruction through lymphokine release. Many oral bacteria have been found to contain potent polyclonal beta-lymphocyte activators, leading some investigators to propose that periodontal pathogens release these substances into lesions. Polyclonal beta-lymphocyte activation could promote an exaggeration of the inflammatory response and further tissue injury through enhanced antibody and lymphokine production. Regardless of the mechanisms of tissue destruction, the true source of the disease, namely, the causative bacteria, remains outside the gingival tissues in supra- and subgingival plaque, and is therefore not susceptible to the body's defense mechanisms. There is evidence that some bacteria do invade the gingival tissues, especially in the more aggressive forms of periodontitis, and this invasion may constitute a pathogenic mechanism. Nevertheless, the origin of these bacteria is the dental plaque, and so the disease continues to progress unless the dental plaque is removed and the involved tooth is kept plaque-free. If these measures are taken, chronic marginal gingivitis can resolve completely and the tissues return to normal.

Tissue destruction mediated by bacterial products

Immunological mediators play a role in tissue damage

Bacterial source of the disease is outside the affected tissues

As the disease progresses, a point may be reached at which the alveolar bone around the necks of the teeth is resorbed; the condition is then no longer termed gingivitis, but periodontitis. With resorption of the bone, the attachment of the periodontal ligament is lost and the gingival sulcus deepens into a periodontal pocket. Periodontitis is not considered to be a reversible disease in that the lost alveolar bone and periodontal ligament do not regenerate with cessation of the inflammation, even though further progression may be halted. If unchecked, bone resorption progresses to loosening of the tooth, which may ultimately fall out. Occasionally, the neck of a periodontal pocket becomes constricted, the bacteria proliferate causing an acute inflammatory response in the occluded pocket, and a periodontal abscess results. This acute exacerbation requires drainage in the same way as abscesses elsewhere for the patient to obtain relief from the symptoms.

With continued progress periodontitis and bone resorption develop

Periodontal abscess may result

Chronic marginal gingivitis will develop within 2 weeks in those who fail to practice effective tooth cleansing. It is not known whether particular species of plaque bacteria are responsible for gingival inflammation, but among those suspected of pathogenicity in the

Multiple organisms involved in chronic periodontitis

case of chronic marginal periodontitis are anaerobic Gram-negative rods (*Porphyromonas gingivalis, Prevotella intermedia, Bacteroides forsythus, Campylobacter rectus, Fusobacterium nucleatum*), *Peptostreptococcus micros, Eikenella corrodens,* and *Treponema denticola.* Many of these organisms produce periodontal disease in monoinfected animals. It has been suggested recently that the disease may be caused by the combined effects of two or more of these pathogens at a site, rather than there being only one species of microorganism responsible for the destructive lesion.

Acute juvenile periodontitis associated with *Actinobacillus*

There is some evidence that the causative agents in rapidly progressing forms of periodontitis may differ from those associated with chronic marginal disease. In the condition known as juvenile periodontitis, a small capnophylic (carbon dioxide requiring) Gram-negative rod (*Actinobacillus actinomycetemcomitans*) has been indicted based on studies of the flora of disease sites. A virulence factor found in those strains of *A. actinomycetemcometans* that are associated with this disease is the production of a leukotoxin by the bacteria. In addition, it has been found that a significant proportion of patients with this condition demonstate high serum antibody titers to *A. actinomycetemcomitans*. Also of interest is the fact that many of these patients have neutrophil chemotactic or phagocytotic defects.

## ACUTE NECROTIZING ULCERATIVE GINGIVITIS

Acute onset with painful ulcerative lesions

Fusospirochetal etiology together with other anaerobes

Acute necrotizing ulcerative gingivitis is also known as Vincent's infection or trench mouth. This disease is distinctly different from chronic marginal periodontal disease. It has an acute onset, frequently associated with periods of stress and poor oral hygiene. There is rapid ulceration of the interdental areas of the gingiva, resulting in destruction of the interdental papillae. The inflammatory condition can quickly lead to pathologic bone resorption. Unlike chronic marginal periodontal disease, acute necrotizing ulcerative gingivitis is painful. As the oral epithelium is destroyed, the causative bacteria come into direct contact with the underlying tissues and may invade them. Spirochetes and fusiform bacteria have been implicated; thus, the term fusospirochetal disease has been used to describe this infection, which can also be manifested as ulceration in other areas of the pharynx or oral cavity. *Prevotella intermedia* has also been found in high numbers, along with spirochetes, in the lesions. Morphological studies have shown that the spirochetes actually appear to invade the tissues. The disease may be treated with systemic antibiotics for immediate relief of symptoms, but resolution is dependent on thorough professional cleaning of the teeth and institution of good home care. Further discussion of fusospirochetal disease is provided in Chapter 26.

## DENTAL PLAQUE AND ORAL FLORA IN THE COMPROMISED PATIENT

Endocarditis from oral flora unless protected by prophylaxis

As it can be the source of transient bacteremia, dental plaque must be viewed as a hazard in the compromised patient. The best example is the patient with heart valve damage as a result of a congenital anomaly, rheumatic fever, or a heart prosthesis. If transient bacteremia develops, the blood-borne bacteria may form vegetative growths in the heart and cause bacterial endocarditis (Chapter 68). Such patients should always be placed on a course of prophylactic antibiotic therapy before any dental procedure is performed, including routine dental prophylaxis.

Severe opportunistic infections may develop in the immunocompromised

It has also been established that dental plaque organisms and other oral bacteria may give rise to serious systemic infections in patients whose host defense mechanisms are compromised. Patients who have undergone extensive radiation treatment of the jaw area, for example, are prone to develop osteomyelitis. Furthermore, one of the most frequent sources of fatal infections in leukemic patients is the oral cavity. Therefore, for these patients scrupulous home care and professional dental treatment are required.

## ADDITIONAL READING

Loesche WJ. Role of *Streptococcus mutans* in human dental decay. *Microbiol Rev* 1986;50: 353–380.
Newbrun E. *Cariology*. 3rd ed. Chicago, Quintessence Publishing Co, 1989.

Slots J, Taubman MA, eds. *Contemporary Oral Microbiology and Immunology.* St. Louis, Mosby Year Book, 1992.

Socransky SS, Haffajee AD. The bacterial etiology of destructive periodontal disease: Current concepts. *J Periodontol* 1992;63: 322–331.

These are authoritative reviews of caries and periodontal disease and new advances in understanding these conditions.

# Upper Respiratory Tract Infections and Stomatitis

*C. George Ray*

Upper respiratory infections usually involve the nasal cavity and pharynx, and most (more than 80%) are caused by viruses. Like middle and lower respiratory illnesses, the diseases of the upper respiratory tract are named according to the anatomic sites primarily involved. Rhinitis (or coryza) implies inflammation of the nasal mucosa, pharyngitis denotes pharyngeal infection, and tonsillitis indicates an inflammatory involvement of the tonsils. Because of the close proximity of these structures to one another, infections may simultaneously involve two or more sites (for example, rhinopharyngitis or tonsillopharyngitis). All such infections are grouped under the general term upper respiratory infections. Stomatitis is a term used to describe infections primarily localized to the mucous membranes of the oral cavity. These infections can sometimes also involve the tongue (glossitis) or the gingival and periodontal tissues (gingivostomatitis or acute necrotizing ulcerative gingivitis; see Chapter 62).

Most upper respiratory infections cuased by viruses

Other infections considered are peritonsillar abscess (quinsy), retrotonsillar abscess, and retropharyngeal abscess. These infections are the result of direct invasion from mucosal sites and localization in deeper tissues to produce inflammation and abscess formation.

## CLINICAL FEATURES

**Rhinitis** is the most common manifestation of the common cold. It is characterized by variable fever, inflammatory edema of the nasal mucosa, and an increase in mucous secretions. The net result is varying degrees of nasal obstruction; the nasal discharge may be clear and watery at the onset of illness, becoming thick and sometimes purulent as the infection progresses over several days.

The common cold

**Pharyngitis** and **tonsillitis** are associated with pharyngeal pain (sore throat) and the clinical appearance of erythema and swelling of the affected tissues. There may be exudates, consisting of inflammatory cells overlying the mucous membrane, and petechial hemorrhages; the latter may be seen in viral infections, but tend to be more prominent in bacterial infections. Viral infections, particularly herpes simplex, may also lead to the formation of vesicles in the mucosa, which quickly rupture to leave ulcers. Pharyngeal candidiasis can also erode the mucosa under the plaques of "thrush." On rare occasions, the local inflammation may be sufficiently severe to produce pseudomembranes, which consist of necrotic tissue, inflammatory cells, and bacteria. This finding is particularly common in pharyngeal diphtheria, but may be mimicked by fusospirochetal infection (Vincent's angina) and sometimes by infectious mononucleosis. In acute tonsillitis or pharyngitis of any etiology, re-

Inflammatory exudate and hemorrhages more common in bacterial infections

Vesicles and ulcerated lesions more common in viral disease

Pharyngeal pseudomembranes in diphtheria

gional spread of the infecting agents with inflammation and tender swelling of the anterior cervical lymph nodes is also common.

Herpetic and *Candida* most common causes of stomatitis

**Stomatitis** is inflammation of the oral cavity. Multiple ulcerative lesions of the oral mucosa, seen most frequently with severe primary herpes simplex infections, may extend to the tongue, lips, and face. In extreme cases, the pain may be so severe that the patient requires relief with topical anesthetics during the usual 9- to 12-day period of acute symptoms. *Candida* species can also invade oral surfaces to produce plaques identical to those of pharyngeal thrush. This infection is particularly common in young infants and immunocompromised individuals of any age.

Aphthous stomatitis (canker sores) cause unknown

**Aphthous stomatitis** is a recurrent disease of the oral mucosa characterized by single or multiple painful ulcers with irregular margins, usually 2 to 10 mm in diameter. Healing usually occurs in a few days. The term commonly used to describe this condition is **canker sore.** The cause is unknown. It can easily be confused with recurrent herpes simplex lesions and, like herpes, tends to recur in relation to stress, menses, local trauma, and other nonspecific stimuli.

Noma an extensive stomatitis of debilitated persons

A severe, gangrenous stomatitis that progresses beyond the mucous membranes to involve soft tissues, skin, and sometimes bone can complicate a variety of acute illnesses in patients who are severely debilitated and whose oral hygiene is poor. This infection, called noma or cancrum oris, is rarely seen in the United States. Typical cases occur among children with severe protein–calorie malnutrition or other immune compromise. Measles will sometimes precipitate noma. Etiologic agents thought to be involved include *Fusobacterium* and *Bacteroides* species, as well as *Pseudomonas aeruginosa*.

Milder forms of stomatitis are seen in a variety of other common viral infections. Examples include Koplik's spots in measles, buccal or palatal ulcers in chickenpox, and similar phenomena in some enteroviral infections such as hand, foot, and mouth disease.

Tonsillar asymmetry a sign of peritonsillar abscess

Peritonsillar abscesses are usually a complication of tonsillitis. They are manifested by local pain, and examination of the pharynx reveals tonsillar asymmetry with one tonsil usually displaced medially by the abscess. This infection is most common in children more than 5 years of age and in young adults. If not properly treated, the abscess may spread to adjacent structures. It can involve the jugular venous system, erode into branches of the carotid artery to cause acute hemorrhage, or rupture into the pharynx to produce severe aspiration pneumonia.

Retropharyngeal abscess causes bulging of anterior pharyngeal wall

Retropharyngeal abscesses occur most frequently in infants and children less than 5 years of age. They can result from pharyngitis or from accidental perforation of the pharyngeal wall by a foreign body. The infection is characterized by pain, inability or unwillingness to swallow, and, if the pharyngeal wall is displaced anteriorly near the palate, a change in phonation (nasal speech). The neck may be held in an extended position to relieve pain and maintain an open upper airway. Examination of the pharynx will usually reveal anterior bulging of the pharyngeal wall; if this finding is not apparent, lateral x-rays of the neck may demonstrate a widening of the space between the cervical spine and the posterior pharyngeal wall. The complications of retropharyngeal abscesses are basically the same as those described for peritonsillar abscesses; in addition, the suppurative process can extend posteriorly to the cervical spine to produce osteomyelitis or inferiorly to cause acute mediastinitis.

Oral and pharyngeal lesions accentuated in immunocompromised hosts

May be portal of entry for systemic infection

In the immunocompromised patient, all of the various forms of stomatitis and pharyngitis described previously can be accentuated. Leukemia, agranulocytosis, chronic ulcerative colitis, congenital or acquired immunodeficiency (eg, AIDS), and treatment with cytotoxic or immunosuppressive drugs are commonly associated with such lesions. The marked damage to mucosal tissues that sometimes occurs can provide a portal of entry into deeper structures and then to the systemic circulation, creating a risk of bacterial or fungal sepsis. Conversely, oral lesions may also result from dissemination of infection from other remote sites. Examples include disseminated histoplasmosis and sepsis caused by *Pseudomonas* species.

## COMMON ETIOLOGIC AGENTS

Viral infections predominate

Table 63–1 lists the more common causes of upper respiratory infections and stomatitis. Viral infections predominate. The most frequent bacterial cause to be considered are the group

**TABLE 63–1. MAJOR INFECTIOUS CAUSES OF UPPER RESPIRATORY DISEASE**

| Disease | Viruses | Bacteria and Fungi |
|---|---|---|
| Rhinitis | Rhinoviruses; adenoviruses; coronaviruses; parainfluenza viruses; influenza viruses; respiratory syncytial virus; some Coxsackie A viruses | Rare |
| Pharyngitis or tonsillitis | Adenoviruses; parainfluenza viruses; influenza viruses; rhinoviruses; Coxsackie A or B virus; herpes simplex virus; Epstein–Barr virus | *Streptococcus pyogenes; Corynebacterium diphtheriae; Neisseria gonorrhoeae* |
| Stomatitis | Herpes simplex virus; some Coxsackie A viruses | *Candida* species; *Fusobacterium* species and spirochetes |
| Peritonsillar or retropharyngeal abscess | None | *Streptococcus pyogenes* (most common); oral anaerobes such as *Fusobacterium* species; *Staphylococcus aureus* (rare); *Haemophilus influenzae* (usually in infants) |

A streptococci. *Corynebacterium diphtheriae,* although very rare in the United States, is a major pathogen that continues to cause infection in many other countries and must not be overlooked, particularly if clinical and epidemiologic findings suggest this possibility. *Neisseria gonorrhoeae,* isolated from adults with symptomatic pharyngitis in whom no other etiologic agent can be demonstrated, is now considered a pharyngeal pathogen that is usually transmitted by oral–genital contact.

*S. pyogenes* and *C. diphtheriae* bacterial pathogens

Gonococcal pharyngitis with oral–genital contact

In patients with purulent rhinitis, sinusitis should also be considered in the differential diagnosis (see Chapter 61). Unilateral and foul-smelling purulent discharge suggests the presence of a foreign body in the nose.

## GENERAL DIAGNOSTIC APPROACHES

Although viruses cause the vast majority of upper respiratory infections, they are generally not amenable to specific therapy, and laboratory tests for viral infections are usually reserved for investigating outbreaks or in cases in which the illness seems unusually severe or atypical.

The primary diagnostic approach in pharyngitis and tonsillitis is to determine whether there is a bacterial cause requiring specific treatment. The only reliable method is to collect a throat swab for culture, taking care to thoroughly swab the tonsillar fauces as well as the posterior pharynx, and to include any purulent material from inflamed areas. Cultures are usually made only to detect the presence or absence of group A streptococci. Direct antigen tests for rapidly detecting *S. pyogenes* in throat swabs have gained popularity in recent years. These are usually EIA or latex-agglutination-based methods. The most common limitation of such tests is lack of sensitivity; that is, false-negative results can occur.

Approach is to determine if there is a bacterial etiology by culture

Direct detection methods have false negatives

For the laboratory diagnosis of diphtheria or pharyngeal gonorrhea, the clinical suspicion should be indicated to the laboratory so that specific cultures for *C. diphtheriae* or *N. gonorrhoeae* may be made. *Candida* species, fusospirochetal bacteria, *Pseudomonas* species, and other Gram-negative organisms are often found in pharyngeal or oral specimens from healthy individuals as well as in certain infections. Their probable pathogenic significance in association with disease in these sites, largely based on the appearance of the lesions and the presence of the organisms in large numbers, can be supported by histologic demonstration of tissue invasion by the organisms. It is important to remember that other bacterial pathogens such as *Streptococcus pneumoniae, Staphylococcus aureus, Haemophilus influenzae,* and even *Neisseria meningitideis* may be present in the pharynx. These organisms are not primary etiologic agents in rhinitis, pharyngitis, and tonsillitis, and their presence in the throat does not implicate them as causes of the illnesses; they should instead be regarded as colonizers.

Evidence for pathogenic role of opportunists assessed by multiple means

Pathogens may be prsent in normal flora but do not cause pharyngitis

The laboratory diagnosis of causes of peritonsillar and retropharyngeal abscesses is based on Gram staining and culture of purulent material obtained directly from the lesion, including anaerobic cultures.

## GENERAL PRINCIPLES OF MANAGEMENT

Ten days of therapeutic levels of penicillin needed for *S. pyogenes* infections

Viral infections of the upper respiratory tract can only be treated symptomatically. If group A streptococci are the cause, penicillin therapy is required; if the patient is allergic to penicillin, an alternative is chosen (eg, erythromycin or a cephalosporin). Therapeutic levels of the antibiotic should be maintained for at least 10 days. Such treatment prevents suppurative or toxigenic complications (for example, pharyngeal abscess, cervical adenitis, and scarlet fever) and the development of acute rheumatic fever. The latter, a serious complication, may occur in 1 to 3% of patients in certain population groups if they are not adequately treated. In addition, treatment of acute streptococcal infections can aid in reducing spread of the organisms to other persons. When the duration of therapy is less than 10 days, the risk of relapse and failure to eradicate the organisms is significantly increased.

*C. diphtheriae* infections involve more complex management, which includes antitoxin as well as antimicrobic treatment (see Chapter 17). Infections caused by *N. gonorrhoeae* are treated with appropriate antimicrobics (Chapter 19).

The management of stomatitis includes maintenance of adequate oral hygiene. If invasive *Candida* infection is present, topical and/or systemic antifungal therapy is sometimes necessary. Vincent's angina and other fusospirochetal infections are usually treated with systemic penicillin therapy as well as with appropriate dental and periodontal care. There is no specific, widely accepted treatment for aphthous stomatitis. Peritonsillar and retropharyngeal abscesses are treated aggressively with antimicrobics and often require surgical drainage, taking care to prevent accidental aspiration of the abscess contents into the lower respiratory tract.

# Middle and Lower Respiratory Tract Infections

*C. George Ray and Kenneth J. Ryan*

## MIDDLE RESPIRATORY TRACT INFECTION

For the purpose of this discussion, the middle respiratory tract will be considered to comprise the epiglottis, surrounding aryepiglottic tissues, larynx, trachea, and bronchi. Inflammatory disease involving these sites may be localized (for example, laryngitis) or more widespread (for example, laryngotracheobronchitis). The majority of severe infections occur in infancy and childhood. Disease expression varies somewhat with age, partly because the diameters of the airways enlarge with maturation and because immunity to common infectious agents increases with age. For example, an adult with a viral infection of the larynx (laryngitis) who was exposed to the same virus in childhood will have a relatively better immune response; in addition, the larger diameter of the larynx in the adult permits greater air flow in the presence of inflammation. An infant or child with the same infection in the same site can develop a much more severe illness, known as croup, which can lead to significant obstruction of air flow.

Most severe middle tract infections occur in infancy and childhood

### Clinical Features

Epiglottitis is often characterized by the abrupt onset of throat and neck pain, fever, and inspiratory stridor (difficulty in moving adequate amounts of air through the larynx). Because of the inflammation and edema in the epiglottis and other soft tissues above the vocal cords (supraglottic area), phonation becomes difficult (muffled phonation or aphonia), and the associated pain leads to difficulty in swallowing. If this disease is not treated promptly, death may result from acute airway obstruction.

Epiglottitis carries risk of acute airway obstruction

Laryngitis or its more severe form, croup, may have an abrupt onset (spasmodic croup) or develop more slowly over hours or a few days as a result of spread of infection from the upper respiratory tract. The illness is characterized by variable fever, inspiratory stridor, hoarse phonation, and a harsh, barking cough. In contrast to epiglottitis, the inflammation is localized to the subglottic laryngeal structures, including the vocal cords. It sometimes extends to the trachea (laryngotracheitis) and bronchi (laryngotracheobronchitis), where it is associated with a deeper, more severe cough that may provoke chest pain and variable degrees of sputum production. When vocal cord inflammation is severe, transient aphonia may result.

Laryngitis and croup involve subglottic laryngeal structures

Bronchitis involves larger airways

Bronchitis or tracheobronchitis may be a primary manifestation of infection or a result of spread from upper respiratory tissues. It is characterized by cough, variable fever, and sputum production, which is often clear at the onset but may become purulent as the illness persists. Auscultation of the chest with the stethoscope often reveals coarse bubbling rhonchi, which are a result of inflammation and increased fluid production in the larger airways.

Chronic bronchitis associated with smoking, air pollution, and other diseases

Nontypable *H. influenzae* and *S. pneumoniae* found in exacerbations of chronic bronchitis

Chronic bronchitis is a result of long-standing damage to the bronchial epithelium. A common cause is cigarette smoking, but a variety of environmental pollutants, chronic infections (for example, tuberculosis), and defects that hinder normal clearance of tracheobronchial secretions and bacteria (for example, cystic fibrosis) can be responsible. Because of the lack of functional integrity of their large airways, such patients are susceptible to chronic infection with members of the oropharyngeal flora and to recurrent, acute flare-ups of symptoms when they become colonized and infected by viruses and bacteria, particularly *Streptococcus pneumoniae* and nontypable *Haemophilus influenzae*. A vicious cycle of recurrent infection may evolve, leading to further damage and increasing susceptibility to pneumonia.

## Common Etiologic Agents

Most subglottic middle airway infection are viral

With the exception of epiglottitis, acute diseases of the middle airway are usually caused by viral agents (Table 64–1). When acute airway obstruction is present, noninfectious possibilities must also be considered, such as aspirated foreign bodies and acute laryngospasm or bronchospasm caused by anaphylaxis.

## General Diagnostic Approaches

When a viral etiology is sought, the usual method of obtaining a specific diagnosis is by inoculation of cell culture with material from the nasopharynx and throat. Acute and convalescent sera can also be collected to determine antibody responses to the common respiratory viruses and *Mycoplasma pneumoniae*. In bacterial infections, the following approaches are valuable.

### Epiglottitis

*H. influenzae* type b, the most common cause of epiglottitis, produces an associated bacteremia in 85% of cases or more. Attempts to obtain cultures from the epiglottis or throat may provoke acute reflex airway obstruction in patients who have not undergone intuba-

**TABLE 64–1. MAJOR CAUSES OF ACUTE MIDDLE RESPIRATORY TRACT DISEASE**

| Syndrome | Viruses | Bacteria | Percentage Caused by Viruses |
|---|---|---|---|
| Epiglottitis | Rare | *Haemophilus influenzae* type b most common; also *Streptococcus pyogenes, Streptococcus pneumoniae, Corynebacterium diphtheriae, Neisseria meningitidis* | 10 |
| Laryngitis and croup | Parainfluenza virus, influenza virus, adenoviruses; occasionally respiratory syncytial virus, rhinoviruses, coronaviruses, echoviruses | Rare | 90 |
| Laryngotracheitis and laryngotracheobronchitis | Same as for laryngitis and croup | *Haemophilus influenzae* type b; *Staphylococcus aureus* | 90 |
| Bronchitis | Parainfluenza virus; influenza virus; respiratory syncytial virus; adenoviruses; measles | *Bordetella pertussis; Bordetella parapertussis; Haemophilus influenzae; Mycoplasma pneumoniae; Chlamydia pneumoniae* | 80 |

tion to ensure proper ventilation; furthermore, the yield is lower than that of blood culture. In addition, other bacterial agents that cause epiglottitis less frequently can often be isolated from the blood. The exception is *Corynebacterium diphtheriae* infection, in which cultures of the nasopharynx or pharynx are required.

High incidence of bacteremia in *H. influenzae* epiglottitis

### Laryngotracheitis and Laryngotracheobronchitis

Although most cases of laryngotracheitis and laryngotracheobronchitis have a viral etiology, a severe purulent process is seen occasionally. The latter is often referred to as acute bacterial tracheitis, and can be rapidly fatal if not managed aggressively. Gram staining and culture of sputum, or better yet, of purulent secretions obtained by direct laryngoscopy, help to establish the causative agent. Blood cultures are again useful in such cases when a bacterial etiology is suspected.

### Acute Bronchitis

A major bacteriologic consideration in acute bronchitis, especially in infants and preschool children, is *Bordetella pertussis*. Deep nasopharyngeal cultures plated on the appropriate media constitute the best specimens. Gram staining and examination of nasopharyngeal smears by direct fluorescent antibody methods are also useful adjuncts to establishing the diagnosis. When purulent sputum is produced, Gram staining and culture may be useful in suggesting other bacterial causes (see Table 64–1). Exceptions include *M. pneumoniae* and *Chlamydia pneumoniae* infections, which are usually diagnosed by serologic testing of acute and convalescent sera.

Nasopharyngeal specimens appropriate for diagnosis of pertussis

Serodiagnosis for *Mycoplasma* infection

## General Principles of Management

The primary initial concern is ensuring an adequate airway. It is particularly crucial in epiglottitis, but can become a major issue in laryngitis or laryngotracheobronchitis as well. Thus, some patients will require placement of a rigid tube that provides communication between the tracheobronchial tree and the outside air (a nasotracheal tube or a surgically placed tracheostomy). Other adjunctive measures, such as highly humidified air and oxygen, may also provide relief in acute diseases involving the structures in and around the larynx. In proved or suspected bacterial infections, specific antimicrobic therapy is required; other treatment, such as antitoxin administration in diphtheria, may also be necessary.

Maintenance of airway required

Antimicrobic therapy for bacterial infections

# LOWER RESPIRATORY TRACT INFECTION

Lower respiratory tract infection develops with invasion and disease of the lung, including the alveolar spaces and their supporting structure, the interstitium, and the terminal bronchioles. Infection may occur by extension of a middle respiratory tract infection, aspiration of pathogens past the upper airway defenses, or less commonly, by hematogenous spread from a distant site such as an abscess or an infected heart valve. When infection develops through the respiratory tract, there is usually some compromise of the upper airway mechanisms for filtering or clearing inhaled infectious agents. The most common are those that impair the epiglottic and cough reflexes; such as drugs, anesthesia, stroke, and alcohol abuse. Toxic inhalations and cigarette smoking may also interfere with the normal mucociliary action of the tracheobronchial tree. In healthy persons, the most common antecedent to lower respiratory infection is infection of the middle respiratory structures (usually viral), allowing an otherwise innocuous aspiration of oropharyngeal flora to reach the lower tract and progress to disease rather than undergo rapid clearance. Some small infectious particles can accomplish airborne passage through the middle airway and bypass mucociliary defenses; if they can survive or multiply in alveolar macrophages, they may produce a primary infection. Examples include arthroconidia of *Coccidioides immitis* and cells of *Mycobacterium tuberculosis.*

Infection can be by inhalation, aspiration, extension from middle tract, or bloodborne

Infection through air passages associated with compromised local defenses

## Clinical Features

### Acute Pneumonia

Sputum is purulent material generated in the alveoli

Fever, respiratory distress, and sputum production are signs of acute pneumonia

Acute pneumonia is an infection of the lung parenchyma that develops over hours to days and, if untreated, runs a natural course lasting days to weeks. The onset may be gradual, with malaise and slowly increasing fever, or sudden, as with the bed-shaking chill associated with the onset of pneumococcal pneumonia. The only early symptom referable to the lung may be cough, which is caused by bronchial irritation. In adults the cough becomes productive of **sputum,** which is purulent material generated in the alveoli and small air passages. In some cases the sputum may be blood streaked, rusty in color, or foul smelling. Labored or difficult breathing (dyspnea), rapid respiratory rate, and sometimes cyanosis are signs of increasing loss of alveolar air-exchange surface through spread of exudate. Chest pain from involvement of the pleura is common. Physical signs on auscultation reflect the filling and eventual consolidation of alveoli by fluid and inflammatory cells.

Radiologic changes confirm and refine diagnosis

The radiologic pattern of inflammatory changes in the lung is very useful in the diagnosis of pneumonia and for clinical differentiation into likely etiologic categories. The most common pattern is patchy infiltrates related to multiple foci centering on small bronchi (bronchopneumonia), which may progress to a more uniform consolidation of one or more lobes (lobar pneumonia). A more delicate, diffuse, or "interstitial" pattern, which is also common, is particularly associated with viral pneumonia.

### Chronic Pneumonia

Chronic pneumonia develops over weeks to months

Abscesses and cavities may develop

Chronic pneumonia may have noninfectious causes

Chronic pneumonia has a slow insidious onset that develops over weeks to months and may last for weeks or even years. The initial symptoms are the same as those of acute pneumonia (fever, chills, and malaise), but they develop more slowly. Cough can develop early or late in the illness. As the disease progresses, appetite and weight loss, insomnia, and night sweats are common. Cough and sputum production may be the first indication of a vague constitutional illness referable to the lung. Bloody sputum (hemoptysis), dyspnea, and chest pain appear as the disease progresses. The physical findings and radiologic features can be similar to those of acute pneumonia, except that the diffuse interstitial infiltrates of viral pneumonia are uncommon. There may be parenchymal destruction and the formation of abscesses or cavities communicating with the bronchial tree. The clinical features of chronic pneumonia may be due to a number of infectious agents or noninfectious causes such as neoplasms, vasculitis, allergic conditions, infarction, radiation or toxic injury, and diseases of unknown etiology (for example, sarcoidosis).

Pleural effusions may be infectious or noninfectious

Empyema is a purulent infection of pleural space usually by extension of bacterial infection

**Pleural effusion** is the transudation of fluid into the pleural space in response to an inflammatory process in adjacent lung parenchyma. It may result from a wide variety of causes, both infectious and noninfectious. **Empyema** is a purulent infection of the pleural space that develops when the infectious agent gains access by contiguous spread from an infected lung through a bronchopleural fistula or, less often, by extension of an abdominal infection through the diaphragm. Symptoms are usually insidious and related to the primary infection until enough exudate is formed to produce symptoms referable to the chest wall or to compromise the function of the lung. The physical and radiologic findings are characteristic, with dullness to percussion and localized opacities on x-ray that can be demonstrated by appropriate manipulation of the patient. In contrast to noninfectious effusions, empyema is frequently loculated.

### Lung Abscess

Lung abscess frequently follows aspiration pneumonia

Blood-borne infection may give multiple abscesses

Lung abscess is usually a complication of acute or chronic pneumonia caused by organisms that can cause localized destruction of lung parenchyma. It may occur as part of a chronic process or as an extension of an acute, destructive pneumonia, often after aspiration of oral or gastric contents. The symptoms of lung abscess, which are usually not specific, resemble those of chronic pneumonia or an acute pneumonia that has failed to resolve. Persistent fever, cough, and the production of foul-smelling sputum are typical. Lung abscess can be diagnosed and localized with certainty only radiologically; it appears as a localized area of inflammation with single or multiple excavations or as a cavity with an air–fluid level. Multiple abscesses may develop as a result of blood-borne infection.

## Common Etiologic Agents

The infectious agents that most frequently cause lower respiratory infection are listed in Table 64–2. The etiology of acute pneumonia is strongly dependent on age. More than 80% of pneumonias in infants and children are caused by viruses, whereas less than 10 to 20% of pneumonias in adults are viral. The reasons are probably the same as those indicated previously for middle respiratory tract infections. Influenza and other viruses, however, may provide the initial predisposition toward bacterial infection. Viruses are extremely rare as a cause of chronic as opposed to acute lower respiratory tract infections, although some symptoms of the acute infection, such as cough, may persist for weeks until the bronchial damage has healed. Influenza virus is noteworthy as a cause of acute life-threatening pneumonia, even in previously healthy young adults. Pneumonia caused by bacteria such as enteric Gram-negative rods, *Pseudomonas,* and *Legionella* is primarily limited to patients with serious debilitating underlying disease or as a complication of hospitalization and its procedures (nosocomial infection). At any age, the pneumococcus is the most common bacterial cause of acute pneumonia, and Gram-negative infections other than *Haemophilus* are rare in children unless they have cystic fibrosis. Acute and subacute pneumonia can be due to *Chlamydia*; *C. trachomatis* is almost exclusively limited to infants less than 7 months of age, while *C. pneumoniae* commonly affects school children and young adults, producing both bronchitis and pneumonia.

Most pneumonias are viral in infants and children

Viral infections predispose to acute bacterial pneumonia

Gram-negative pneumonias in debilitated hosts

Pneumococcus is most common cause of acute bacterial pneumonia

Lung abscess and empyema follow infections with the more destructive organisms or aspiration of mixed anaerobic flora from the oropharynx. Several clinical clues can suggest some of the etiologic agents, given a typical clinical syndrome. For example, *Nocardia* and mycobacteria, which are strict aerobes, tend to produce upper lobe infiltrates, whereas aspiration pneumonia caused by anaerobes tends to develop in the most dependent parts of

Lung abscess has different patterns

**TABLE 64–2. MAJOR CAUSES OF LOWER RESPIRATORY TRACT INFECTION**

| Syndrome | Viruses | Common Bacteria | Fungi | Other Agents |
|---|---|---|---|---|
| Acute pneumonia | Influenza,[a] Parainfluenza, Adenovirus, Respiratory syncytial (infants)[a] | *Streptococcus pneumoniae*, *Staphyloccus aureus*, *Haemophilus influenza*, Enterobacteriaceae *Legionella*, Mixed anaerobes (aspiration), *Pseudomonas aeruginosa*[b] | *Candida albicans*,[b] *Aspergillus* species | *Mycoplasma pneumoniae*, *Pneumocystis carinii*,[b] *Chlamydia trachomatis* (infants), *Chlamydia pneumoniae* |
| Chronic pneumonia | Rare | *Mycobacterium tuberculosis*, Other Mycobacteria; *Nocardia* | *Coccidioides immitis*,[c] *Blastomyces dermatitidis*,[c] *Histoplasma capsulatum*,[c] *Cryptococcus neoformans* | *Paragonimus westermanl*[c] |
| Lung abscess | None | Mixed anaerobes, *Actinomyces, Nocardia, Staphylococcus aureus*,[d] Enterobacteriaceae,[d] *Pseudomonas aeruginosa*[b,d] | *Aspergillus* species | *Entamoeba histolytica* |
| Empyema | None | Mixed anaerobes, *Staphyloccus aureus*,[d] *Streptococcus pneumoniae*,[d] Enterobacteriaceae, *Pseudomonas aeruginosa*[b,d] | Rare | |

[a] Occurrence limited to seasonal epidemics.
[b] Primarily infects the immunologically compromised host.
[c] Geographically limited.
[d] Infection develops during or after acute pneumonia.

the lung. Textbooks on infectious disease should be consulted for further details regarding these features.

## General Diagnostic Approaches

The degree of difficulty in establishing an etiologic diagnosis for a lower respiratory tract infection depends on the number of organisms produced in respiratory secretions, whether the causative species is normally found in the oropharyngeal flora, and how easily it is grown. In the presence of typical clinical findings, the isolation of influenza virus from the throat or of *M. tuberculosis* from sputum is sufficient for diagnosis of influenza or tuberculosis, because these organisms are not normally found in such sites. The same cannot be said for *S. pneumoniae* and most bacterial pathogens, as they may be found in the throat in a significant number of healthy persons (Chapter 9).

Sputum collection has problems of quality

The examination of expectorated sputum has been the primary means of diagnosing the causes of bacterial pneumonia, but this approach has several advantages and disadvantages. The advantages are ease of collection and absence of risk to the patient. The primary disadvantage is the confusion that results from contamination of the sputum with oropharyngeal flora in the process of expectoration and excessive contamination with saliva. Efforts have been unsuccessful to remove saliva from sputum by washing or to accomplish interpretive differentiation of infective from normal flora by quantitative culture (as with urine specimens; (see Chapter 66). The quality of a sputum sample can be enhanced by collection early in the morning (just after the patient arises), careful instruction of the patient, and occasionally by the use of saline aerosols (induced sputum) under the supervision of an inhalation therapy specialist. The worst results can be expected when the physician's only involvement is writing an order, which is then passed down the ward chain of command to an orderly, who directs the patient to put his "sputum" in a cup placed at the bedside.

Microscopic characteristics of sputum can differentiate from saliva

Salivary specimens should not be cultured

Microscopic examination before culture of direct Gram smears of specimens alleged to be sputum has proved useful. Polymorphonuclear leukocytes and large numbers of a single morphologic type of organism are typical findings in sputum from patients with bacterial pneumonia. Squamous epithelial cells from the oropharynx and a mixed bacterial population are characteristic of saliva (Fig 64–1). Unfortunately, most specimens are a mixture of both, which makes interpretation more difficult. Studies have shown that more than 10 to 25 squamous epithelial cells per low-power (×10) microscopic field are evidence of excessive salivary contamination, and such specimens should not be cultured because the results may be misleading. Thus, the direct Gram smear is crucial to the use of expectorated sputum for diagnosis of acute bacterial pneumonia. The smear may be useful in the absence

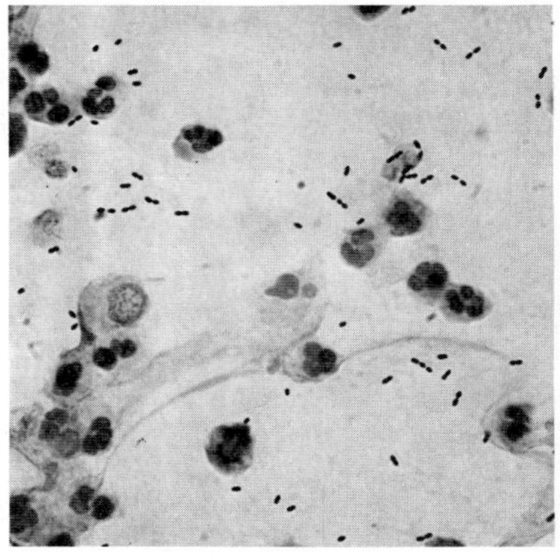

A

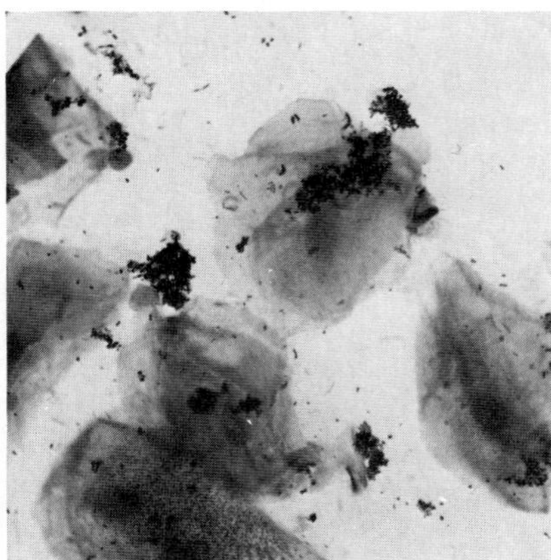

B

**Figure 64–1.** Comparison of findings in sputum and saliva. True sputum **(A)** should show an abundance of inflammatory cells and no squamous epithelial cells. In acute bacterial pneumonia, large numbers of a single organism are usually present. This Gram smear shows large numbers of polymorphonuclear leukocytes and *Streptococcus pneumonia*. Saliva **(B)** typically contains squamous epithelial cells and a mixed bacterial population.

of cultural results, but cultures are useless without a Gram smear to assess specimen quality.

Another approach is to attempt a more direct collection from the lung using methods that bypass the oropharyngeal flora. This approach may be used in patients who are not producing sputum or in cases where analysis of expectorated sputum has been inconclusive. The major techniques include transtracheal aspiration, bronchoalveolar lavage (BAL), direct aspiration, and open biopsy. In transtracheal aspiration, an incision is made in the cricothyroid membrane and a catheter advanced deep into the tracheobronchial tree to aspirate sputum directly. This method is useful in diagnosis of both pneumonia and lung abscess. BAL is a modification of bronchoscopy in which the alveoli are infused with saline which is aspirated back through the bronchoscope. Specimens obtained by BAL have been particularly useful for demonstration of organisms such as *Pneumocystis carinii* that were previously only seen in open lung biopsies. Because BAL involves initial passage of the instrument through the upper airway interpretation must take into account the possibility of some contamination with oropharyngeal secretions. Aspirates taken through tracheostomies or endotracheal tubes are of almost no value, because these sites become colonized with Gram-negative bacteria within hours of their implantation. Direct aspiration through the chest wall can be used for diagnosis of pneumonia or empyema if the involved area can be well localized and is at the lung periphery. In some cases an open lung biopsy is the only way to obtain diagnostic material.

Transtracheal aspiration, BAL, direct transpleural aspiration, and open biopsy have risks and benefits

BAL particularly useful in *P. carinii* infection

Bacteremia may occur in acute pneumonia, particularly in its early stages. A blood culture should be part of the evaluation of every acute pneumonia. If positive, it can confirm or overrule a diagnosis based on expectorated sputum culture.

Blood culture valuable in acute pneumonia

Once an appropriate specimen is obtained, diagnosis is usually readily made by culture using the methods described in Chapter 14 and in the sections on the individual etiologic agents. Only specimens collected by one of the invasive techniques should be used for anaerobic culture, because expectorated sputum is invariably contaminated with oropharyngeal anaerobes and results are meaningless. With some agents (*S. pneumoniae, H. influenzae*), detection of circulating antigen in the blood or urine by latex agglutination may establish the diagnosis. For *Mycoplasma pneumoniae* and *Chlamydia pneumoniae* infection, serodiagnosis is usually the most common procedure.

Anaerobic infections cannot be diagnosed from expectorated sputum

## Management

The general principles of management of lower respiratory tract infections are similar to those of middle tract infections. Drainage or surgical measures are needed more often as adjuncts to antimicrobial therapy in cases of chronic pneumonia, lung abscess, and empyema. When bacterial infection is considered, empirical therapy is usually given until the results of cultures and antimicrobial susceptibility tests are available. Treatment may vary from penicillin alone for a previously healthy individual in whom the most reasonable nonviral possibility is *S. pneumoniae*, to multiple drugs for a debilitated or immunocompromised patient, in whom the possibilities are much broader.

# Enteric Infections and Food Poisoning

*Kenneth J. Ryan*

Acute infections of the gastrointestinal tract are among the most frequent of all illnesses, exceeded only by respiratory tract infections such as the common cold. Diarrhea is the most common manifestation of these infections; however, because it is usually self-limiting within hours or days, most of those afflicted do not seek medical care. Nonetheless, in the United States gastrointestinal infection remains one of the three most common syndromes seen by physicians who practice general medicine. Worldwide, diarrheal disease remains one of the most important causes of morbidity and mortality among infants and children. It has been estimated that in Asia, Africa, and Latin America, depending on socioeconomic and nutritional factors, a child's chance of dying of a diarrheal illness before the age of 7 years can be as high as 50%. In developed countries mortality is very much lower, but is still significant. This chapter will summarize the known etiologies and epidemiologic circumstances of these infections, as well as diagnostic methods and some aspects of management. Chapters on the individual etiologic agents should be consulted for details.

High mortality from diarrheal diseases in developing countries

## CLINICAL FEATURES

The most prominent clinical features of gastrointestinal infections are fever, vomiting, abdominal pain, and diarrhea. Their presence varies with different diseases and different stages of infection. The occurrence of diarrhea is a central feature, and its presence and nature form the basis for classification of gastrointestinal infections into three major syndromes: watery diarrhea, dysentery, and enteric fever.

### Watery Diarrhea

The most common form of gastrointestinal infection is the rapid development of frequent intestinal evacuations of a more or less fluid character known as diarrhea (derived from the Greek "dia," for "through," and "rhein," meaning to flow like a stream). Nausea, vomiting, fever, and abdominal pain may also be present, but the dominant feature is intestinal fluid loss. Diarrhea is produced by pathogenic mechanisms that attack the proximal small intestine, the portion of the bowel in which more than 90% of physiologic net fluid absorption occurs. The purest form of watery diarrhea is that produced by enterotoxin-secreting bacteria such as *Vibrio cholerae* and enterotoxigenic *Escherichia coli,* which cause fluid loss without cellular injury. Other common pathogens that damage the epithe-

Loss of fluid from proximal small intestine

lium, such as rotaviruses, also cause fluid loss, but are more likely to cause fever and vomiting as well. Most cases of watery diarrhea run an acute but brief (1 to 3 days) self-limiting course. Exceptions are those caused by *V. cholerae,* which usually produces a more severe illness, and those caused by *Giardia lamblia,* which produces a watery diarrhea that may last for weeks.

## Dysentery

Colonic infection with inflammation and/or destruction

Pus and blood in stools

Dysentery begins with the rapid onset of frequent intestinal evacuations, but the stools are of smaller volume than in watery diarrhea and contain blood and pus. If watery diarrhea is the "runs," dysentery is the "squirts." Fever, abdominal pain, cramps, and tenesmus are frequent complaints. Vomiting occurs less often. In dysentery the focus of pathology is the colon. Organisms causing dysentery can produce inflammatory and/or destructive changes in the colonic mucosa either by direct invasion or by production of cytotoxins. This damage produces the pus and blood seen in the stools, but does not result in substantial fluid loss because the absorptive and secretory capacity of the colon is much less than that of the small bowel. Dysenteric infections generally last longer than the common watery diarrheas, but most cases still resolve spontaneously in 2 to 7 days.

## Enteric Fever

Systemic disease focus in intestine with lymphoid and reticuloendothelial invasion

Enteric fever is a systemic infection, the origin and focus of which are the gastrointestinal tract. The most prominent features are fever and abdominal pain, which develop gradually over a few days in contrast to the abrupt onset of the other syndromes. Diarrhea is usually present, but may be mild and not appear until later in the course of the illness. The pathogenesis of enteric fever is more complex than that of watery diarrhea or dysentery. It generally involves penetration by the organism of the cells of the distal small bowel with subsequent spread outside the bowel to the biliary tract, liver, mesentery, or reticuloendothelial organs. Bacteremia is common, occasionally causing metastatic infection in other organs. Typhoid fever caused by *Salmonella typhi* is the only infection for which these events have been well studied. Although it is usually self-limiting, enteric fever carries a significant risk of serious disease and significant mortality.

## ETIOLOGY

In the past three decades, great advances have been made in our understanding of gastrointestinal infections. Before the late 1960s, fewer than 20% of the infectious syndromes described previously could be linked to a specific etiologic agent by any diagnostic method. The organisms listed in Table 65–1 now account for 80 to 90% of cases, although diagnostic methods for all of them are not yet practical for clinical laboratories. The primary clinical syndrome listed for each agent in Table 65–1 should not be regarded as absolute because there are individual variations and overlap for some pathogens. For example, *Shigella* infections frequently go through a brief watery diarrhea stage before localizing in the colon, and *Campylobacter* enteritis usually begins with fever, malaise, and abdominal pain, followed by dysentery. In any single case the clinical findings may suggest a range of etiologic agents, but none are sufficiently specific to be diagnostic of any single organism.

## EPIDEMIOLOGIC SETTING

Epidemiologic setting important in preliminary diagnosis

The epidemiologic setting of the infection is of great importance in assessing the relative probability of the infectious agents. When combined with clinical findings, the differential diagnosis can often be limited to two or three organisms. The major epidemiologic settings are (1) endemic infection, (2) epidemic infection, (3) traveler's diarrhea, (4) food poisoning, and (5) hospital-associated diarrhea.

**TABLE 65–1. FEATURES OF INFECTIOUS GASTROINTESTINAL SYNDROMES**

| Organism | Common Distribution | Clinical Syndrome | Pathogenic Mechanism | Laboratory Diagnosis[a] | | | | | |
|---|---|---|---|---|---|---|---|---|---|
| | | | | | Culture | | Toxin in Stools | Serology | |
| | | | | Stool Microscopy | Stool[b] | Blood | | Antibody Detection | Antigen Detection |
| *Salmonella* serotypes | Worldwide | Dysentery | Mucosal invasion | PMNs | + | – | – | – | – |
| *Salmonella typhi* | Tropical, developing countries | Enteric fever | Penetration, spread | Monocytes | + | + | – | + | – |
| *Shigella* sp. | Worldwide | Dysentery | Mucosal invasion, cytotoxin | PMNs, RBCs | + | – | – | – | – |
| *Shigella dysenteriae* (Shiga) | Tropical, developing countries | Dysentery | Mucosal invasion, cytotoxin | PMNs, RBCs | + | + | – | – | – |
| *Campylobacter jejuni* | Worldwide | Dysentery | Unknown | PMNs, RBCs | + | – | – | – | – |
| *Escherichia coli* (EIEC) | Worldwide | Dysentery | Mucosal invasion | PMNs, RBCs | +[c] | – | – | – | – |
| *Escherichia coli* (ETEC) | Worldwide[d] | Dysentery | Enterotoxin(s) | – | +[c] | – | – | – | – |
| *Escherichia coli* (EHEC) | Worldwide | Watery diarrhea | Cytotoxin | RBCs | +[c] | – | – | – | – |
| *Escherichia coli* (EPEC) | Worldwide[d] | Watery diarrhea | Adherance | – | +[c] | – | – | – | – |
| *Vibrio cholerae* | Asia, Africa, Middle East, Central and South America, Louisiana, Texas | Watery diarrhea | Enterotoxin | – | + | – | – | – | – |
| *Vibrio parahemolyticus* | Seacoast | Watery diarrhea | Unknown | – | + | – | – | – | – |
| *Yersinia enterocolitica* | Worldwide | Enteric fever[e] | Penetration, spread | – | + | + | – | – | – |
| *Clostridium difficile* | Worldwide | Dysentery | Cytotoxin, enterotoxin | – | + | – | + | – | – |
| *Clostridium perfringens* | Worldwide | Watery diarrhea | Enterotoxin | – | + | – | – | – | – |
| *Bacillus cereus* | Worldwide | Watery diarrhea | Enterotoxin | – | + | – | – | – | – |
| Rotavirus | Worldwide | Watery diarrhea | Mucosal destruction | Electron microscopy[f] | – | – | – | – | + |
| Parvo/picornavirus | Worldwide | Watery diarrhea | Mucosal destruction | Electron microscopy[f] | – | – | – | – | – |
| *Giardia lamblia* | Worldwide | Watery diarrhea | Mucosal irritation | Flagellates, cysts | – | – | – | – | – |
| *Entamoeba histolytica* | Worldwide[d] | Dysentery | Mucosal invasion | Amebas, PMNs | – | – | – | + | – |
| *Cryptosporidium* | Worldwide | Watery diarrhea | ?toxin | Acid-fast oocysts | – | – | – | – | – |

*Abbreviations*: RBCs, red blood cells; PMNs, polymorphonuclear leukocytes; EIEC, enteroinvasive *E. coli*; ETEC, enterotoxigenic *E. coli*; EHEC, enterohemorrhagic *E. coli*; EPEC, enteropathogenic *E. coli*.

[a] Positive sign indicates procedure is useful and usually available in clinical laboratories.

[b] Which cultures are done routinely depends on the laboratory and/or physician's request.

[c] Organism may be isolated in culture, but demonstration of pathogenic potential (toxin production, etc) is limited to specialized laboratories.

[d] Organism is more common in developing countries.

[e] Infection may also manifest watery diarrhea or dysentery.

[f] Appropriate methods may be available in only a limited number of laboratories.

## Endemic Infections

Higher frequency in infants and children related to fecal–oral spread and immunity

By definition, endemic diarrheas are those that occur sporadically in the usual living circumstances of the patient (from the Greek "endemos," dwelling in a place). Some organisms are endemic worldwide, whereas others are geographically limited. There are also seasonal variations and age-related attack rates within the endemic foci. In developed countries the most common causes of endemic gastrointestinal infections are rotaviruses, parvo/picornaviruses, *Campylobacter, Salmonella,* and *Shigella.* All are more common in infants and children because they are more prone to fecal–oral spread and because development of immunity is related to age. Rotaviruses account for 40 to 60% of diarrheal infections occurring during the cooler months in infants and children less than 2 years of age, but are uncommon in older persons.

Geographic distributions are not fixed

The geographically limited agents are common only in the areas listed (Table 65–1). These distributions are not fixed, making it necessary to keep abreast of geographic changes in the distribution of established agents as well as the recognition of new ones. For example, cholera has long been limited to warm-climate river deltas in Asia, Africa, and the Middle East, but recently has spread to South and Central America and the Gulf Coast of Louisiana and Texas.

## Epidemic Infections

Typhoid, cholera, and shigellosis spread where hygiene is poor or after major disasters

Under certain epidemiologic conditions some of the organisms responsible for endemic infections can spread beyond the family unit to cause epidemics involving regional, national, and even international populations. The diarrheal diseases most frequently associated with epidemics are typhoid fever, cholera, and shigellosis. For all three, epidemics are related to the failure of basic public health sanitary measures. For example, *S. typhi* and *V. cholerae* may be spread for some distance through the community water supply, a route blocked by modern sewage and water treatment practices. When these procedures are not employed or are interrupted by equipment failure or natural disasters (floods, earthquakes), these diseases can and do recur in epidemic form. Epidemics of shigellosis may be water-borne under the same conditions, but *Shigella* dysentery is more typically a disease "of wars and armies, and of crowds and movement."* The very low infecting dose of *Shigella* can make spreading through direct contact reach epidemic proportions when crowding and poor sanitary facilities are combined. *Giardia* and *Crytosporidium* were the most frequent identified causes of waterborne epidemics in the United States in 1992.

Most current epidemic is cholera in South America

Although such epidemics are usually associated with the 19th century, it is clear that the potential remains. In the late 1970s large epidemics of both typhoid fever and shigellosis spread through Central and South America. In 1973 more than 200 cases of typhoid fever in Florida were associated with a defective chlorinator in the local water system. The current cholera epidemic has claimed thousands of lives in South America since 1991.

## Traveler's Diarrhea

Travelers from developed to less developed countries all too frequently experience a diarrheal illness in the first week that is usually brief but can be serious. The common names applied to this syndrome, such as "Delhi belly" and "Montezuma's revenge," reflect geographic associations and the cumulative frustration of those forced to spend part of their vacation next to the toilet rather than the swimming pool.

Enterotoxigenic *E. coli* predominant cause of traveler's diarrhea

The most extensive studies of traveler's diarrhea has involved travelers from the United States to Latin American countries, particularly Mexico. In nearly one-half of these cases the diarrhea is caused by enterotoxigenic strains of *E. coli* acquired during travel. *Shigella* infections account for another 10 to 20%, and the remaining cases are attributable to various pathogens or unknown causes. Ingestion of uncooked or incompletely cooked foods is

* Christie AB. *Infectious Disease, Epidemiology and Clinical Practice.* 2nd ed. New York, Churchill Livingstone, 1974; p. 137.

the most likely source of infection, but most epidemiologic studies have not shown specific food associations. An exception is the strong relationship between toxigenic *E. coli* diarrhea and the consumption of salads containing raw vegetables. "Don't drink the water" still seems like sound advice for travelers to countries where hygiene remains poor, but the adage is not well supported by studies relating infection to water or ice consumption.

Avoid salads and other uncooked foods

## Food Poisoning

Many gastrointestinal infections involve food as a vehicle of transmission. The term "food poisoning," however, is usually reserved for instances in which a single meal can be incriminated as the source. This situation typically arises when multiple cases of the same gastrointestinal syndrome develop at the same time among persons whose only common experience is a meal shared at a social event or restaurant. The probable etiologic agent can usually be assessed from knowledge of the incubation period, the food vehicle, and the clinical findings. Changes in the importation, processing, and distribution of foods have increased the complexity and potential for foodborne transmission of enteric pathogens. Outbreaks that in the past might have been limited, may now be widely distributed by fast-food chains or airline catering services.

Single-source outbreaks are becoming more complex with modern food processing

The most common causes of food poisoning are shown in Table 65–2. Some are not infections but intoxications, caused by ingestion of a toxin produced by bacteria in the food before it was eaten. Intoxications generally have shorter incubation periods than infections and may involve extraintestinal symptoms (for example, the neurologic damage in botulism). Infectious food poisoning does not differ from endemic diarrheal infections caused by the same species. The length of the incubation period and the severity of the symptoms are generally related to the number of organisms in the infecting dose.

Diseases from ingestion of preformed toxin have short incubation periods

The epidemiologic circumstances of food poisoning vary with the etiologic agent, but virtually always involve a breach in the recommended procedures for handling food. The

**TABLE 65–2. CLINICAL AND EPIDEMIOLOGIC FEATURES OF FOOD POISONING**

| Etiology | Percentage of Cases[a] | Typical Incubation Period | Primary Clinical Findings | Characteristic Foods |
|---|---|---|---|---|
| **Intoxication[b]** | | | | |
| *Bacillus cereus* (vomiting toxin) | 1–2 | 1–6 h | Vomiting, diarrhea | Rice, meat, vegetables |
| *Clostridium botulinum* | 5–15 | 12–72 h | Neuromuscular paralysis | Improperly preserved vegetables, meat, fish |
| *Staphylococcus aureus* | 5–25 | 2–4 h | Vomiting | Meats, custards, salads |
| Chemical[c] | 20–25 | 0.1–48 h | Variable | Variable |
| **Infections[b]** | | | | |
| *Clostridium perfringens* | 5–15 | 9–15 h | Watery diarrhea | Meat, poultry |
| *Salmonella* | 10–30 | 6–48 h | Dysentery | Poultry, eggs, meat |
| *Shigella* | 2–5 | 12–48 h | Dysentery | Variable |
| *Vibrio parahemolyticus* | 1–2 | 10–24 h | Watery diarrhea | Shellfish |
| *Trichinella spiralis* | 5–10 | 3–30 days | Fever, myalgia | Meat, especially pork |
| Hepatitis A | 1–3 | 10–45 days | Hepatitis | Shellfish |

[a] Based on documented outbreaks reported to the Centers for Disease Control, Atlanta (variable from year to year).
[b] Disease caused by toxin in food at time of ingestion.
[c] Includes heavy metals, monosodium glutamate, mushrooms, and various toxins of nonmicrobial origin.
[d] Disease caused by infection after ingestion.

Outbreaks associated with deficiencies in food preparation and storage

organisms may be present as contaminants in raw food before cooking or introduced by a carrier or contaminated utensil involved in preparation. Causes of bacterial food poisoning include failure to kill the organisms by adequate cooking, almost always followed by a period of warming (incubation) long enough for the organisms to multiply to infectious numbers or, in the case of toxigenic disease, to produce sufficient toxin to cause disease. In 80 to 90% of investigated outbreaks of bacterial food poisoning, the most important contributing factor is the use of improper storage temperatures for the food. This factor may obtain in home-cooked meals as well as those prepared in restaurants, in schools, or at large social events such as community picnics.

Reporting of outbreaks varies greatly

The relative frequency of each etiologic agent and the foods most frequently involved are also shown in Table 65–2. This information is based on outbreaks investigated by public health agencies, but it is generally accepted that these represent the "tip of the iceberg" due to underreporting. Large outbreaks, restaurant-associated outbreaks, and outbreaks involving serious illness with hospitalization or death are more likely to be reported to health authorities than are mild diarrheas after a dinner party or airline meal. In recent years, of the 400 to 500 outbreaks (10,000 to 15,000 cases) reported each year in the United States, fewer than 200 are "solved." Food poisoning characterized by a short incubation period (for example, *Staphylococcus aureus*) is more likely to be recognized because it can easily be associated with a specific meal and because the food itself may still be available for examination. There are also large geographic differences in reporting. For example, in 1979, New York City, in which 50% of the state population resides, reported 98% of New York state's food-borne outbreaks, and Connecticut reported more outbreaks than all of the southeastern states combined.

Determing the cause of microbial food poisoning is tailored to the circumstances

Sampling problems aside, the food poisoning syndromes listed in Table 65–2 are well recognized, with *Salmonella, Clostridium perfringens,* and *S. aureus* accounting for more than 70% of those for which a microbial etiology can be found. For bacterial infections such as *Salmonella* and *Shigella,* which are not normal members of the stool flora, establishing the diagnosis by isolating the causative organism is relatively easy. If the circumstances indicate *Clostridium perfringens* or *S. aureus* food poisoning, investigation will involve cultures of vomitus, stool from several cases, and the suspect food. In some cases, toxin detection will be required to establish the etiology and source. Such investigations are best coordinated by public health authorities, who can also address the legal and community implications of the outbreak. For example, one investigation of *Salmonella* food poisoning led to the discovery that the owner of a restaurant was keeping and slaughtering chickens at the restaurant. Although this practice may have provided very fresh chicken, it guaranteed *Salmonella* contamination of the entire kitchen.

## Hospital-associated Diarrhea

Pathogenic *E. coli, C. difficile*, and rotaviruses can cause hospital outbreaks

The hospital environment should not allow spread of the usual causes of endemic intestinal infection. When such infection occurs, it can usually be traced to an employee who continues working while ill or to contaminated food prepared outside the hospital that is "smuggled" in by the patient's friends. Two special causes of hospital-associated diarrhea are caused by *E. coli* in infants and *C. difficile* in patients treated with antimicrobial agents. Fortunately, *E. coli* outbreaks have become rare. *C. difficile* accounts for more than 90% of cases of a syndrome that ranges from mild diarrhea to fulminant pseudomembranous colitis during or after treatment with antibiotics. The responsible toxigenic *C. difficile* may be resident in the patient's intestinal flora before administration of antimicrobics or be acquired by spread from other patients in the hospital. Rotaviruses can also cause hospital outbreaks in infants.

## LABORATORY DIAGNOSIS

Laboratory diagnostic procedures (summarized in Table 65–1) include microscopic examination, culture, toxin detection, and serologic procedures. The relative value of each is different for the various etiologies. The diagnostic approach therefore requires that the physician assess the clinical and epidemiologic features of the case, decide which organisms are potential causes, and provide this assessment to the laboratory so that appropriate procedures will be used.

## Microscopic Examination

Microscopic examination is of limited value in the assessment of bacterial infections. The presence of polymorphonuclear leukocytes or blood in the stool correlates with organisms that produce disease by invasion, particularly colonic invasion. The leukocytes may be seen in unstained or methylene-blue-stained wet mount preparations; the absence of fecal leukocytes, however, does not exclude invasive diarrhea. The observation and morphologic characterization of amebas and flagellates on wet or stained preparations are the primary means by which amebic (*Entamoeba histolytica*) and flagellate (*Giardia lamblia*) infections are diagnosed. Direct electron microscopy can be used to diagnose viral diarrhea, as the rotaviruses and parvo/picornaviruses have a characteristic morphology but cannot be grown in cell culture.

Stool microsopy demonstrates WBCs, parasites

Electron microscopy detects rotaviruses and parvo/picornaviruses

## Culture

Isolation of the etiologic agent is the primary means by which bacterial enteric infection is diagnosed. In enteric fever the organism is typically present in the blood in the early stages of disease. Blood cultures are, however, usually negative in watery diarrhea and dysenteric infections, and stool culture must be relied upon for diagnosis. Fortunately, several good selective media have been developed for both direct plating and enrichment culture, which allow isolation of the infecting organism in the presence of a predominant normal flora. Selective media are then used for the various enteric pathogens (see Chapter 14). Media routinely employed may vary between clinical laboratories, but should include those appropriate for *Salmonella, Shigella,* and *Campylobacter jejuni*. Diarrhea caused by *E. coli* is a special problem, because the methods that define the enterotoxigenic, invasive, or other pathogenic mechanisms are not yet practical for clinical laboratories.

Blood cultures positive in early stages of enteric fever

Stool culture requires selective media for common agents

## Toxin Assay

The B cytotoxin of *Clostridium difficile* can be detected by its cytopathic effect in a cell culture system. In most clinical cases, enough toxin is present for direct detection in a stool specimen. This assay is currently available only in reference laboratories. A method that detects the *C. difficile* A toxin by latex agglutination has been developed, but its application to clinical illness is still controversial. A DNA probe for the toxin gene developed by recombinant DNA techniques can be applied directly to colonies to detect enterotoxigenicity.

Cytopathic effect on cell culture or antigen assays detect *C. difficile* toxin

## Antigen and Antibody Detection

At present, antibody detection is useful in the diagnosis of amebic dysentery caused by *E. histolytica* and of typhoid fever. Both are considered ancillary to the primary diagnostic tests, which involve specific detection of the organism by microscopic and cultural methods. Reagents are commercially available for the detection of rotavirus antigen in stool by latex agglutination or enzyme immunoassay. These methods have a sensitivity roughly comparable to that of electron microscopy. Serologic methods have been described for many other causes of gastrointestinal infection, but are not generally used because of lack of sensitivity, specificity, or availability of reagents.

Serology generally ancillary

Antigen detection available for a few agents

# OTHER CAUSES OF INTESTINAL INFECTION

Despite recent advances in defining the etiologies of enteric infections, there are surely more to be discovered. Organisms not listed in Table 65–1, such as *Aeromonas, Citrobacter,* and

*Plesiomonas,* have occasionally been associated with intestinal infections, but the evidence for their enteropathogenicity is not yet strong enough to interpret their isolation from individual cases. At our present state of knowledge it is not useful to attempt isolation of these organisms unless strong epidemiologic evidence, such as food-borne outbreak, supports interpretation of the results.

## TREATMENT

Maintenance of fluid and electrolyte balance always important

In most gastrointestinal infections the primary goal of treatment is relief of symptoms, with particular attention to maintaining fluid and electrolyte balance. The effect of common antidiarrheal medications such as bismuth compounds (Pepto Bismol) or antispasmodics (Lomotil) is variable depending on the etiology. In general, they may be helpful for the watery diarrhea caused by enterotoxins, but not for dysentery caused by mucosal invasion, and antispasmodics may be harmful in the latter instance. Antimicrobial agents are usually not indicated for self-limited watery diarrhea, but are required for more severe dysenteric infections. Some enteric infections, such as typhoid fever, are always treated with antimicrobics. More information on therapy is given in the individual chapters, but texts on infectious diseases should be consulted for specific recommendations.

Antimicrobic therapy not always indicated

# Urinary Tract Infections

*James J. Plorde*

> A physycyen, truely, can lyttel descerne Ony maner sekeness wythout syght of uryne.
>
> —Hawes, S. 1509. *The Pastime of Pleasure*

The examination of urine has been used to assist medical practitioners in the diagnosis and management of human illness for centuries. So great an emphasis did medieval physicians place on the color, sediment, smell, and even taste of this effluent that a urine-filled flask became the symbol of their profession. This fluid, which so faithfully reflects the maladies of the urinary tract, is produced by the kidney, collected by the renal pelvis, and transported through the ureters to the bladder for storage. Here it remains until the discomfort of bladder distention stimulates its evacuation via the urethra. Bacterial colonization of the urine within this tract **(bacteriuria)** is common and can, at times, result in microbial invasion of the tissues responsible for the manufacture, transport, and storage of urine. Infection of the upper urinary tract, consisting of the kidney and its pelvis, is known as **pyelonephritis.** Infection of the lower tract may involve the bladder **(cystitis),** urethra **(urethritis),** or prostate **(prostatitis),** the genital organ that surrounds and communicates with the first segment of the male urethra. Because all portions of the urinary tract are joined by a fluid medium, infection at any site may spread to involve other areas of the system.

Definitions of UTI depend on anatomic localization

It has been estimated that one third to one half of humans suffer a urinary tract infection (UTI) at some time during their lives. Prevalence is age and sex dependent. Approximately 1% of children, many of whom demonstrate functional or anatomic abnormalities of the urinary tract, develop infection during the neonatal period. Thereafter, infection in the male remains uncommon through the fifth decade of life; when it does occur, it is found primarily in preschool boys with intact foreskins and adult males engaged in homosexual activity. Following this period, when enlargement of the prostate begins to interfere with emptying of the bladder, infection rates rise to 20%. In contrast, the prevalence of UTI in females increases soon after infancy, stabilizing at 4 to 5% through early adolescence; a significant proportion of those affected demonstrate vesicoureteral reflux. Although most recover uneventfully, this population group is at substantially increased risk of recurrent urinary tract infection during adult life. With the onset of sexual activity, bacteriuria rates in females increase dramatically, with 20% experiencing one or more infections annually. In the elderly of both sexes, gynecologic or prostatic surgery, incontinence, instrumentation, and chronic urethral catheterization push UTI rates to 30 to 40%. These infections may be symptomatic or asymptomatic, acute or chronic, and singular or recurrent. At times they can produce permanent damage to the kidney.

Prevalence of bacteriuria varies with age, sex, and predisposing conditon

Female rates increase with sexual activity

# PATHOGENESIS

## Host Factors

Ascending infections in women of childbearing age related to bacterial of adherence and anatomic factors

Infections are seen most frequently in women of childbearing age. They are caused by gut flora, which reach the bladder via the urethra, after colonization of the vagina, external periurethral area, and distal urethra. The circumstances that lead to this colonization are not fully understood, but it is known that uropathic strains of *Escherichia coli* possess pili that allow them to adhere more readily to urinary epithelial cells. In addition, epithelial cells from the introitus of infection-prone women support bacterial adherence to a greater extent than cells from controls, suggesting a genetic predisposition of some women to UTI. This is supported by the observation that the epithelial cells of nonsecretors bind *E. coli* more avidly than do cells from secretors. Recently, colonization of the vaginal introitus has been associated with diaphragm and spermicide use, possibly due to spermicidal-induced suppression of the normal vaginal flora. Thus, both host and bacterial properties are of importance in pathogenesis. Bacteria can reach the bladder more easily in the female host than in the male because the urethra is shorter, lies in close proximity to the moist perirectal area, and is subjected to the massaging effect of sexual intercourse. Once in the bladder, organisms that cause cystitis can multiply in the contained urine.

Catheter use increases risk of infection

Bacteria can also be carried easily to the bladder in both men and women by passage of a catheter or other instrument, such as a cystoscope. This mode of transmission constitutes the most common single cause of hospital-acquired bacteriuria in either sex. A single transient catheterization of the bladder induces bacteriuria in approximately 1% of ambulatory and 10% of bed-ridden patients. An indwelling catheter, by providing a fluid-filled conduit for the migration of organisms from the external environment to the bladder, is more frequently associated with UTI. Even with meticulous attention to aseptic technique, most patients harboring a catheter for more than 2 weeks develop infection.

Concentrated urine inhibitory to some organisms

The factors that determine whether the bacteriuria persists after the removal of the initiating event include the number and type of bacteria introduced and the adequacy of the host's response to these organisms. In the overwhelming majority of cases, the number of bacteria is small and the host's defense mechanisms prove adequate. The urine itself is inhibitory to anaerobes and other fastidious organisms that are part of the normal flora of the urethral mucosa, and these bacteria seldom cause persistent infections. Even organisms known for their ability to multiply in urine may be inhibited when exposed to the very high osmolality and concentration of urea and hydrogen ions that characterize the urine of many normal individuals. It is likely that the moderation of these urinary parameters during pregnancy accounts, at least in part, for the increased incidence of bacteriuria in this population. The antibacterial properties of the bladder mucosa and the few neutrophils that reach the surface contribute to the clearance of introduced organisms.

Flushing effects of micturation an important defense

Interference with urine flow increases, risk of infection

Perhaps the most important of the host defenses, however, is the act of voiding. The constant flushing of contaminated urine from the body and its dilution with newly formed, uncontaminated urine eliminates bacteria or maintains their numbers at low levels. Any interference with this clearing mechanism results in bacterial multiplication and a greatly increased probability of developing or sustaining an infection. The interference may be by mechanical obstruction to urine flow (stone, stricture, or hypertrophied prostate), neurogenic impairment of bladder control (spinal cord injury, multiple sclerosis), or functional impairment, such as the vesicoureteral reflux seen in many children with urinary tract infections. The latter appears to result from the effect of the inflammatory reaction, which interferes with the integrity of the vesicoureteral junction and allows regurgitation of urine from the bladder into the ureters. Such reflux not only returns a pool of infected urine to the bladder after voiding is completed but also can carry bacteria to the renal pelvis and thus initiate infection in a previously uninvolved kidney.

Infections in pregnancy related to reflux

A similar functional abnormality has been described in pregnant women. The hormonal changes in pregnancy lead to a decrease in bladder tone, diminished ureteral peristalsis, and dilatation of the renal pelvis and ureters. All enhance the likelihood of reflux and explain, at least in part, the frequency with which pregnant women with bacteriuria develop upper urinary tract disease. Congenital or acquired anatomic derangements of the vesicoureteral junction produce similar results.

Occasionally, urinary tract infection occurs when bacteria seed the renal parenchyma directly from the blood. It is possible to infect the kidneys of experimental animals by intravenous injection of a variety of bacterial species other than Gram-negative bacilli. Hematogenous pyelonephritis in humans is uncommon, however, except during periods of sustained *Staphylococcus aureus* bacteremia.

Blood-borne infection an uncommon route

## Microbial Factors

Human feces contain a rich diversity of bacterial species. Surprisingly, only a few regularly produce urinary tract infection. In fact, *E. coli* accounts for more than 90% of acute infections in patients with structurally normal urinary tracts. The factors responsible for this extraordinary monopoly are incompletely understood, but the relative resistance of *E. coli* to the inhibitory effects of vaginal fluid, its possession of pili that aid its attachment to the epithelial cells of the urinary tract, and its motility appear to contribute to its effectiveness as a uropathogen. Some or all of these features, however, are found in other, less successful, enteric species. It has been shown that the relationship of *E. coli* to acute symptomatic urinary tract infection is limited to relatively few of the O/H/K serotypes of this organism found in the stool. These uropathogenic *E. coli* all possess chromosomally mediated virulence factors such as the P pilus (see Chapter 20), alpha-hemolysin, and/or siderophores such as aerobactin.

Infecting organisms usually of fecal origin

*E. coli* has features uropathogenic

Patients with urinary tract abnormalities that interfere with the free flow of urine are particularly apt to experience chronic or recurrent infection. This exposes them to multiple courses of antimicrobial therapy, which eventually leads to the replacement of antibiotic-susceptible strains of *E. coli* with more resistant pathogens. Hospitalized patients are particularly susceptible to cross-infection with nosocomial strains of *Proteus, Providencia, Pseudomonas, Klebsiella, Enterobacter, Serratia,* coagulase-negative staphylococci, and enterococci, many of which are passed directly from catheterized patient to catheterized patient on the hands of medical personnel. Once established in the urinary tract, *Proteus* strains appear to be particularly virulent. Experimental evidence suggests that *Proteus mirabilis* possesses pili that facilitate its adherence to the mucosa of the renal pelvis. In addition, urease production by all species of *Proteus* leads to hydrolysis of urea, formation of ammonium hydroxide, and alkalinization of the urine. The elevated pH in the urine is directly toxic to renal cells and stimulates the formation of magnesium and ammonium phosphate struvite urinary calculi (stones), which can contribute to the chronicity of the infection by producing ureteral obstruction and sheltering the bacteria from the patient's defensive mechanisms and the physician's antimicrobial agents. Species of *Klebsiella,* because of their more limited urease production or through production of an extracellular polysaccharide slime layer, are also associated with the presence of urinary calculi.

Chronic and recurrent infections associated with obstruction

Nosocomial infections occur with opportunists

Urease activity of *Proteus* may cause injury and stone formation

*Staphylococcus saprophyticus,* a coagulase-negative staphylococcus, is now recognized as the cause of as much as 20% of symptomatic urinary tract infections in young, sexually active women. *S. aureus* infections usually result from the bacteremic seeding of the urinary tract, as described previously.

*S. saprophyticus* infections seen in young women

Yeasts, particularly species of *Candida,* may be isolated from catheterized patients receiving antibacterial therapy and from diabetics, but they seldom produce symptomatic disease. *Chlamydia trachomatis,* in contrast, can produce the acute urethral syndrome described subsequently.

# CLINICAL FEATURES

The clinical manifestations of UTI are variable. Approximately one half of infections do not produce recognizable illness and are discovered incidentally during a general medical examination. Infections in infants produce symptoms of a nonspecific nature, including fever, vomiting, and failure to thrive. Manifestations in older children and adults, when present, often suggest the diagnosis and sometimes the localization of the infection within the urinary tract.

## Urethritis and Cystitis

Infections confined to the urethra are characterized by painful urination (dysuria) and discharge of mucoid or purulent material from the urethral orifice. They are most commonly produced by sexually transmitted agents.

Urgency, frequency, and dysuria most common symptoms

Causative bacteria multiply in urine

Suprapubic tenderness and turbid sometimes bloody urine

Acute urethral syndrome associated with lower numbers of bacteria

The symptoms of cystitis—dysuria, frequent voiding (frequency), and an imperative "call to toilet" (urgency)—are similar to those of urethritis. This symptom complex is, in fact, produced by irritation of the mucosal surface of the urethra as well as the bladder. Unlike urethritis associated with sexually transmitted agents, cystitis is produced by the multiplication of enteric organisms in the bladder urine. It is clinically distinguished from urethritis by a more acute onset, more severe symptoms, the presence of bacteriuria, and in approximately half of cases, hematuria. The urine is often cloudy and malodorous and occasionally frankly bloody; unlike patients with urethritis, those with cystitis often experience pain and tenderness in the suprapubic area. Fever and systemic manifestations of illness are usually absent unless the infection spreads to involve the kidney. Approximately one third of women presenting with dysuria and frequency lack cultural evidence of either bacteriuria or sexually transmitted disease. Use of more sensitive culturing techniques in such patients has defined an acute urethral syndrome associated with the presence in the urethra of small numbers of enteric bacteria (usually *E. coli*) or agents of sexually transmitted infections, such as *C. trachomatis*.

## Pyelonephritis

Fever, flank pain, and systemic signs indicate upper tract infection

Associated with premature delivery

The typical presentation of upper urinary infection consists of flank pain and fever that exceeds 38.3°C. These findings may be preceded or accompanied by manifestations of cystitis. Rigors, vomiting, diarrhea, and tachycardia are present in the more severely ill. Physical examination reveals tenderness over the costovertebral areas of the back and, occasionally, evidence of septic shock. In the absence of obstruction, the clinical manifestations usually abate within a few days, leaving the kidneys functionally intact. It has been estimated, however, that 20 to 50% of pregnant women with acute pyelonephritis give birth to premature infants, one of the most serious consequences of UTI. In the presence of obstruction, a neurogenic bladder, or vesicoureteral reflux, clinical manifestations are more persistent, occasionally leading to necrosis of the renal papillae and progressive impairment of kidney function with chronic bacteriuria. If a renal calculus or necrotic renal papilla impacts in the ureter, severe flank pain with radiation to the groin occurs.

## Prostatitis

Acute prostatitis causes back and perirectal pain

Chronic prostatitis associated with recurrent cystitis

Infection of the prostate is typically manifested as pain in the lower back, perirectal area, and testicles. In acute infection, the pain may be severe and accompanied by high fever, chills, and the signs and symptoms of cystitis. Inflammatory swelling can lead to obstruction of the neighboring urethra and urinary retention. On rectal palpation, the prostate is boggy and exquisitely tender. Response to antibiotic therapy is good, but occasionally abscess formation, epididymitis, and seminal vesiculitis or chronic infection develop. Typically, acute prostatitis develops in young adults; however, it can also follow placement of an indwelling catheter in an older man. Patients with chronic prostatitis seldom give a history of an acute episode. Many are totally without symptoms; others experience low-grade pain and dysuria. Periodic spread of prostatic organisms to the urine in the bladder produces recurrent bouts of cystitis. In fact, chronic prostatitis is probably the major cause of recurrent bacteriuria in men.

# GENERAL DIAGNOSTIC APPROACHES

## Specimen Collection

The diagnosis of urinary tract infection is based on examination of the normally sterile urine for evidence of bacteria or an accompanying inflammatory reaction. Critical to this examination is the use of appropriate techniques for specimen collection. Urine is most easily obtained by spontaneous micturation. Unfortunately, voided urine is invariably contaminated with urethral flora and, in the case of the female, vaginal secretions, which can confound the results of laboratory testing. Although the contaminants can never be completely eliminated, their quantity may be diminished by carefully cleansing the periurethrum before voiding and allowing the initial part of the stream to flush the urethra before collecting a specimen for examination. This **clean-voided midstream urine** collection procedure is preferred to catheterization for routine purposes because it avoids the risk of introducing organisms into the bladder. When the laboratory examination of such a specimen produces equivocal results or the patient cannot comply with the requirements of the clean-voided technique, catheterization may be needed. Alternatively, urine may be aspirated from the bladder with a needle and syringe. In this procedure, the patient refrains from voiding until the bladder is distended. The suprapubic skin is then disinfected and a small needle passed through the skin into the bladder. The procedure has proved to be safe and well tolerated.

Voided urine invarialby contaminated with perineal flora

Clean-voided urine collection safe and usually effective

Catheterization and suprapubic aspiration used when voided specimens equivocal

## Microscopic Examination

Approximately 90% of patients with acute symptomatic urinary tract infection have pyuria (that is, more than 10 white cells/mm$^3$ of urine). This finding is also common, however, in a number of noninfectious diseases. More specific is the presence of white cell casts, which occur almost exclusively, although not uniformly, in patients with acute pyelonephritis. The most sensitive and specific microscopic procedure is a Gram-stained smear of uncentrifuged urine (Fig 66–1). The presence of at least one organism per oil-immersion field is almost always indicative of bacterial infection. The absence of white cells and bacteria in several fields makes the diagnosis unlikely, but does not rule it out, especially in young women with acute, symptomatic infection who may be infected with smaller numbers of organisms.

Pyuria and white cell casts suggest UTI

Direct Gram stain detects most significant bacteriuria

## Chemical Screening Tests

A number of nonmicroscopic urinary screening tests have been commercially marketed within the past several years. The most successful detects leukocyte esterase from inflammatory cells and nitrite produced from urinary nitrates by bacterial nitrate reductase. Although technically simpler, the sensitivity and specificity of these products are similar to

Detection of leukocyte esterase and nitrite have same sensitivity as Gram stain

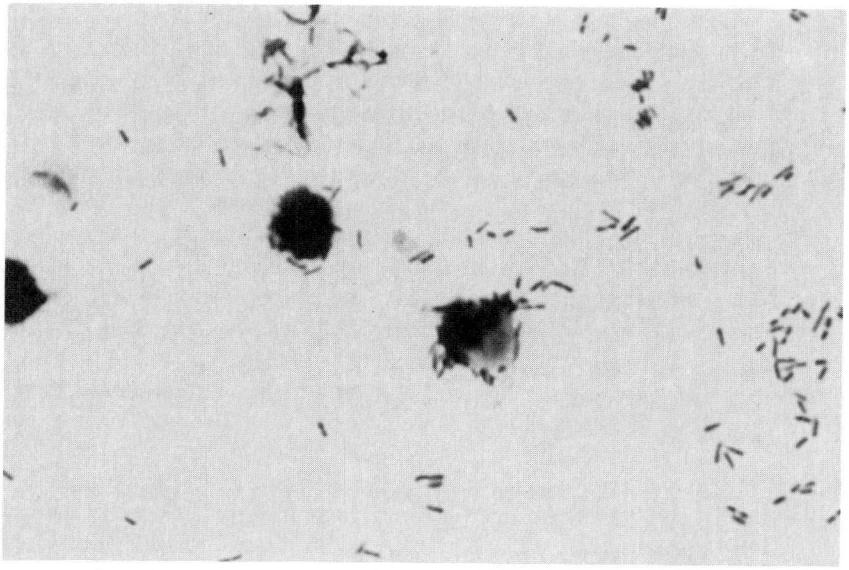

**Figure 66–1.** Gram stain of an uncentrifuged clean voided urine specimen from a patient with an acute *E. coli* urinary tract infection. Some degenerating polymorphonuclear leukocytes and numerous Gram-negative rods are present.

that of microscopic examination. Like microscopic examination, they do not reliably detect bacteriuria below the level of $10^5$ organisms/mL.

## Urine Culture

Symptomatic patients usually have >$10^5$ bacteria/mL

Urine specimens collected even by the clean-void midstream procedure contain small numbers of bacterial contaminants. This finding can be distinguished from true bacteriuria only with quantitative cultures, which allow colony counts. Contaminated specimens usually yield less than 1000 colonies of mixed bacterial flora per milliliter of urine. In urinary tract infections, in contrast, more than 100,000 colonies of a single bacterial species are generally seen. Occasionally colony counts fall between these two values. If the patient is asymptomatic, the culture should be repeated. In symptomatic patients, counts in this range are considered significant if a single bacterial species, especially a typical uropathogen, is isolated. Intermediate counts on urine specimens collected by catheterization or suprapubic aspiration are always considered significant because contamination is minimal in such specimens. Colony counts must be performed on freshly collected or refrigerated specimens to prevent bacterial growth from occurring before processing.

Intermediate counts may have to be repeated

## Miscellaneous Studies

If acute pyelonephritis or prostatitis is suspected, blood cultures should be obtained to exclude bacteremia. Infected children, men, and those who experience UTI relapse should be investigated with intravenous pyelography to allow detection and correction of any factor causing predisposition to infection.

# GENERAL PRINCIPLES OF MANAGEMENT

The principal goal in UTI treatment is eradication of the offending organism from the urine and tissues. In simple isolated instances of cystitis in a young woman, the diagnosis may be confirmed by a simple Gram smear of urine and treatment for an assumed *E. coli* infection given empirically. Many antimicrobics are successful in controlling such infections, and knowledge of the susceptibility of community-acquired *E. coli* in a particular area serves as the best guide. In many cases, 3-day therapy has been shown to be as effective as a course covering longer periods. Sulfonamides and trimethoprim alone or in combination, a fluoroquinolone, and nitrofurantoin are the agents most commonly used.

Three day treatment effective for uncomplicated cystitis

For cystitis in children, pregnant women, men, diabetics, those who have been symptomatic for more than 1 week, and in those with acute pyelonephritis, it is imperative to establish the presence of bacteriuria with one or, in asymptomatic bacteriuria, two quantitative urine cultures. Therapy must be prolonged. Except in cases of clinical emergency, it should be delayed until the diagnosis is established and susceptibility tests performed. As bacteriuria may persist despite the spontaneous abatement of symptoms, the success of treatment in patients with upper tract disease should be checked with follow-up urine cultures. The first should be obtained 48 to 72 hours after initiation of therapy. If the offending microorganism is still present at that time, the chemotherapeutic agent should be withdrawn and a substitute selected on the basis of susceptibility tests. If bacterial clearance has been achieved, the therapeutic course should be completed and repeat cultures obtained 2 weeks after termination of therapy. Sterile cultures at this time suggest eradication of the bacteriuria. A recurrence is classified as either relapse or reinfection. Relapses are infections produced by the organism responsible for the initial infection that generally occur within 2 weeks of discontinuing therapy. They usually indicate an upper UTI or, in a male case, prostatitis, and require the initiation of a urologic evaluation. If an abnormality causing predisposition to UTI is discovered, it should be corrected whenever possible. If none is found, prolonged antibiotic therapy should be administered in hopes of eradicating the residual focus of infection.

Need multiple cultures to establish microbial diagnosis in some cases

Cultural test of cure important in more complex cases

Relapses need to be separated from reinfections

Reinfections (recurrences caused by a new species or serotype) are usually indicative of a bladder infection. They respond readily to standard courses of treatment. Some patients, usually women of childbearing age, suffer repeated bladder reinfections. Those with several symptomatic episodes annually may be helped with long-term, low-dose chemoprophylaxis. In women whose recurrences are related to sexual activity, administration of the chemoprophylactic agent may be limited to immediately after intercourse.

Prophylaxis may prevent reinfection

Patients experiencing an episode of severe acute pyelonephritis should usually be hospitalized and treated, at least initially, with appropriate parenteral antibiotics. This treatment is particularly important if Gram-negative bacteremia is suspected. Milder cases can be managed with oral medications in an outpatient setting. Asymptomatic bacteriuria developing in a patient with an indwelling catheter often remits spontaneously after the removal of the catheter. It need not be treated unless the patient is at high risk of sepsis because of an underlying problem. Symptomatic infections in catheterized patients require treatment.

## ADDITIONAL READING

Gleckman RA. Treatment of urinary tract infections in adults. *Antimicrob Agents Chemother* 1987;31:1–5. This is a review of studies dealing with the appropriate treatment duration of different categories of urinary tract infections.

Johnson JR. Virulence factors in *Escherichia coli* urinary tract infections. *Clin Microbiol Rev* 1991;4:80–128. A comprehensive review of the virulence factors of recognized importance in UTI pathogenesis, including adhesions, the aerobactin system, hemolysin, K capsule, and resistance to serum killing.

Johnson JR, Stamm WE. Urinary tract infections in women: Diagnosis and treatment. *Ann Intern Med* 1989;111: 906–917.

Latham RH, Wong ES, Larson A, et al. Laboratory diagnosis of urinary tract infection in ambulatory women. *JAMA* 1985;254:3333–3336.

Lipsky BA. Urinary tract infections in men: Epidemiology, pathophysiology, diagnosis, and treatment. *Ann Intern Med* 1989;110:138–150. This article explores the several important differences in the epidemiology, pathophysiology, diagnosis, and treatment of UTI in males from that seen in the better-studied female population.

Pezzlo M. Detection of urinary tract infections by rapid methods. *Clin Microbiol Rev* 1988;1:268–280. This is a comprehensive review of recently introduced UTI screening tests.

Stamm WE, Hooten MM, Johnson JR, et al. Urinary tract infections: From pathogenesis to treatment. *J Infect Dis* 1989;159:400. A review of UTI pathogenesis.

Chapter 67

# Central Nervous System Infections

C. George Ray

The cerebrum, cerebellum, brainstem, spinal cord, and their covering membranes (meninges) constitute the central nervous system (CNS). Because of the unique anatomic and physiologic features of the CNS, infections in this site can represent unique challenges to the microbiologist and clinician. The CNS is encased in a rigid, bony vault, and it is highly vulnerable to the effects of inflammation and edema: its critical life-regulatory functions and the metabolic requirements to sustain these functions can also be easily disrupted by infection, with resultant local acidosis, hypoxia, and destruction of nerve cells. Thus, the effects of increased pressure, biochemical abnormalities, and tissue necrosis can be profound and sometimes irreversible.

One specialized defense mechanism of the CNS is the blood–brain barrier, which serves to minimize passage of infectious agents and potentially toxic metabolites into the cerebrospinal fluid (CSF) and tissues, as well as to regulate the rate of transport of plasma proteins, glucose, and electrolytes. When CNS infection develops, however, this barrier also poses difficulties in control; some antimicrobial agents and host immune factors, such as immunoglobulins and complement, do not pass as readily from the blood to the site of infection as they do to other tissues.

Blood–brain barrier affects access of microbes, immune reaction, and antimicrobics

Within the brain are the ventricles, which are cavities in which CSF is actively produced, primarily by specialized structures called the choroid plexuses. The CSF fills the lateral ventricles in each half of the brain, circulates into a central third ventricle, and then passes through the cerebral aqueduct to emerge through foramina at the brainstem. From cisterns at the base of the brain, the CSF circulates in the subarachnoid space over the entire CNS, including the spinal cord, to supply nutrients and serve as a hydraulic cushion for these tissues. It is reabsorbed primarily by the major venous system in the meninges. Obstruction of the normal flow of CSF in either the internal (ventricular) or external (subarachnoid) systems can result in increased intracranial pressure, because production of CSF by the choroid plexuses will continue within the ventricles. Such impairment of flow or normal reabsorption can occur during certain infections as a result of inflammation or subsequent fibrosis, leading to dilatation of the ventricles, compression of brain tissue, and a condition known as hydrocephalus.

## ROUTES OF INFECTION

Most CNS infections appear to result from blood-borne spread; for example, bacteremia or viremia resulting from infection of tissue at a site remote from the CNS may result in pen-

Blood-borne spread most common access to CNS

etration of the blood–brain barrier. Examples of infectious agents that commonly infect the CNS by this route are *Haemophilus influenzae, Neisseria meningitidis, Streptococcus pneumoniae, Mycobacterium tuberculosis,* and viruses such as enteroviruses and mumps. The initial source of infection leading to bloodstream invasion may be occult (for example, infection of reticuloendothelial tissues) or overt (for example, pneumonia, pharyngitis, skin abscess or cellulitis, or bacterial endocarditis). Occasionally, the route of infection is from a focus close to or contiguous with the CNS. These possible sources include middle ear infection (otitis media), mastoiditis, sinusitis, or pyogenic infections of the skin or bone. Infection may extend directly into the CNS, indirectly via venous pathways, or in the sheaths of cranial and spinal nerves.

Direct spread occurs from adjacent infected focus such as middle ear

In some cases, a contiguous or distant infectious focus may not be necessary to produce CNS infection. If an anatomic defect exists in the structures encasing the CNS, infectious agents may readily gain access to the vulnerable site and establish themselves. Such defects may be traumatically or surgically induced or result from congenital malformations. For example, fractures of the base of the skull may produce an opening between the CNS and the sinuses, nasal passages (defects in the cribriform plate), mastoid, or middle ear. All of these sites are contiguous with the upper respiratory tract, which enables a potentially pathogenic member of the respiratory flora to gain ready access to the CNS. Neurosurgical procedures also create transient communications between the external environment and the CNS that can be readily contaminated. This risk can be compounded when foreign bodies, such as shunts or external drainage tubes, must be left in place for the treatment of hydrocephalus. These foreign bodies, when colonized, can serve as chronic foci of infection. Congenital defects, such as meningomyeloceles or sinus tracts through the cranium or spine, may also be sources. The latter may be overlooked; the orifice of the sinus may be a small cleft on the skin surface, or occasionally it may open internally into the intestinal tract. Recurrent purulent meningitis or unusual pathogens in an otherwise healthy host should prompt a careful search for such defects.

Traumatic, surgical, or congential lesions may give direct access

Implanted foreign bodies such as shunts increase risk

Perhaps the least common route of CNS infection is by intraneural pathways. Agents capable of intraneural spread to the CNS include rabies virus (presumably along peripheral sensory nerves), herpes simplex virus (often, but not exclusively, via the trigeminal nerve root or sacral nerves), polioviruses, and perhaps some togaviruses.

Intraneural pathways operate with a few viruses

Abscesses of the CNS deserve special mention. Although relatively uncommon compared with other CNS infections, they represent a special microbiologic and clinical problem. Such abscesses may be within the tissues of the CNS (for example, brain abscess; Fig 67–1) or localized in the subdural or epidural spaces. They sometimes develop as a complication of pyogenic meningitis. More commonly, abscesses of the CNS result from embolization of bacteria or fungi from a distant focus, such as endocarditis or pyogenic lung abscess; extension from a contiguous focus of infection (for example, sinusitis or mastoiditis); or a complication of surgery or nonsurgical trauma.

Abscesses present diagnostic problems and may seed CSF

## CLINICAL FEATURES

Several terms commonly applied to CNS infections need to be understood. **Purulent meningitis** refers to infections of the meninges associated with a marked, acute inflammatory exudate and is usually caused by a bacterial infection. Such infections frequently involve the underlying CNS tissue to a variable degree, and it is now appreciated that often the ventricular system is also involved (ventriculitis). Most cases of purulent meningitis are acute in onset and progression and are characterized by fever, stiff neck, irritability, and varying degrees of neurologic dysfunction that, if untreated, usually progress to a fatal outcome. Large numbers of polymorphonuclear leukocytes are present in the CSF of established cases.

Acute onset and progression with stiff neck and neurologic dysfunction

Serious prognosis if untreated

**Chronic meningitis** has a more insidious onset, with progression of signs and symptoms over a period of weeks. This is usually caused by mycobacteria or fungi that produce granulomatous inflammatory changes, but occasionally protozoal agents are responsible (see Table 67–3). The cellular response in the CSF reflects the chronic inflammatory nature of the disease.

Granulomatous infections are chronic

**Aseptic meningitis** is a term used to describe a syndrome of meningeal inflammation

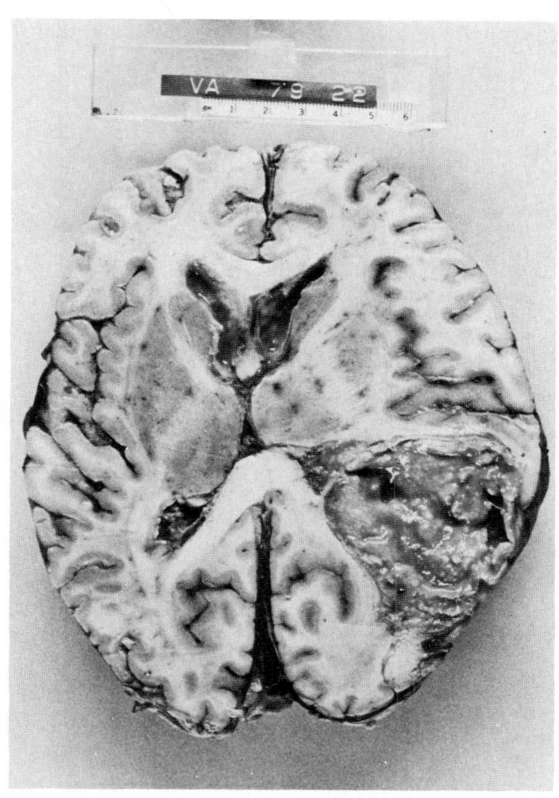


**Figure 67–1.** Coronal section of a brain demonstrating a poorly encapsulated abscess.

associated mostly with an increase (pleocytosis) of lymphocytes and other mononuclear cells in the CSF and absence of readily cultivable bacteria or fungi. It is associated most commonly with viral infections and is often self-limiting. The syndrome can also occur in syphilis and some other spirochetal diseases, as a response to the presence of drugs or radiopaque substances in the CSF, or from tumors or bleeding involving the meninges or subarachnoid space. The primary site of inflammation is in the meninges without clinical evidence of involvement of the neural tissue. Such patients may have fever, headache, a stiff neck or back, nausea, and vomiting.

Aseptic meningitis is most commonly of viral etiology

Other causes include syphilis

**Encephalitis** also implies a primary viral etiology; however, acute or chronic demyelinating diseases with or without inflammation are included. This latter group includes the postinfectious or allergic encephalomyelitis syndromes, in which the etiology and pathogenesis are not always clearly defined. Clinically, the diagnosis of encephalitis is applied to patients who may or may not show signs and CSF findings compatible with aseptic meningitis, but also show objective evidence of CNS dysfunction (for example, seizures, paralysis, and disordered mentation). Many clinicians use the term meningoencephalitis to describe patients with both meningeal and encephalitic manifestations.

Viral and post-infectious etiology most common

**Poliomyelitis** refers to the selective destruction of anterior motor horn cells in the spinal cord and/or brainstem, which leads to weakness or paralysis of muscle groups and occasionally respiratory insufficiency. It is usually associated with aseptic meningitis, sometimes with encephalitis. The polioviruses are the major causes of this syndrome, although Coxsackie viruses (primarily type A7) and other enteroviruses, such as enterovirus 71, have been implicated. The hallmark of poliomyelitis is asymmetric flaccid paralysis.

Viral destruction of anterior horn cells causes paralysis

Two other nervous system syndromes presumably associated with infection deserve brief mention. **Acute polyneuritis,** an inflammatory disease of the peripheral nervous system, is characterized by symmetric flaccid paralysis of muscles. In most cases, no specific etiology is found; some, however, have been associated with *Corynebacterium diphtheriae* toxin and infections by cytomegalovirus or Epstein–Barr virus. **Reye's syndrome** (encephalopathy with fatty infiltration of the viscera) is an acute, noninflammatory process, usually observed in childhood, in which cerebral edema, hepatic dysfunction, and hyperammonemia develop within 2 to 12 days after onset of a systemic viral infection. Although the influenza A and B and varicella–zoster viruses have been most frequently implicated in

Acute polyneuritis involves peripheral nerves

Reye's syndrome follows systemic viral infection

this syndrome, the precise pathogenesis is not yet known. Concomitant salicylate therapy is believed to be a contributory factor.

## COMMON ETIOLOGIC AGENTS

Acute purulent meningitis caused by encapsulated pathogens

The causes of CNS infections are numerous, as illustrated in Tables 67–1 through 67–3. Acute purulent meningitis is usually caused by one of three organisms: *Haemophilus influenzae* type b, *Neisseria meningitidis,* or *Streptococcus pneumoniae*. The incidence of *H. influenzae* meningitis has now fallen sharply as a result of routine immunization. In neonatal infections, *Escherichia coli* or group B streptococci are most frequently implicated. However, many other bacteria can occasionally cause the disease if they gain access to the meninges.

Acute viral disease has a variety of manifestations

Sensonality important clue

Of the viral causes of acute CNS disease, the categories most commonly encountered are the enteroviruses, mumps, herpes simplex, Epstein–Barr virus, and arthropod-borne viruses. In the United States, enteroviruses account for the greatest proportion of infections. Viral CNS infections can be manifested clinically as aseptic meningitis, encephalitis, or with poliovirus and some other enterovirus infections, poliomyelitis. The age of the patient and the season of occurrence help somewhat in predicting some of the agents that may be involved, as illustrated in Table 67–2; other epidemiologic, ecologic, and clinical factors associated with these infections are discussed in the individual chapters on specific virus groups.

Slow viral infections of the CNS, such as subacute sclerosing panencephalitis (due to measles or sometimes congenitally acquired rubella virus), AIDS encephalopathy, progressive multifocal leukoencephalopathy (due to JC polyomavirus), and Creutzfeldt–Jacob disease ("unconventional" viruses), are discussed in Chapters 33, 41, 42, and 43, respectively.

Chronic meningitis caused by slow-growing agents

Other important causes of CNS infections (Table 67–3) that must not be overlooked include *Mycobacterium tuberculosis* and the deep mycoses (especially *Cryptococcus neoformans* and *Coccidioides immitis*). These chronic infections can be insidious in onset and mimic other processes, thus delaying consideration of the proper diagnosis.

Noninfectious diseases may mimic infections

Finally, there are noninfectious causes of CNS disease to be considered in the differential diagnosis. These include (1) metabolic disturbances, such as hypoglycemia, diabetic coma, and hepatic failure; (2) toxic conditions, such as those caused by bacterial toxins (diphtheria, tetanus, botulism), insect toxins (tick paralysis), poisons (lead), and drug abuse; (3) mass lesions, such as acute trauma, hematoma, and tumor; (4) vascular lesions, such as intracranial embolus, aneurysm, and subarachnoid hemorrhage; and (5) acute psychiatric episodes.

**TABLE 67–1. COMMON CAUSES OF PURULENT CENTRAL NERVOUS SYSTEM INFECTIONS**

| Age Group | Agent |
|---|---|
| Newborns (<1 mo old) | Group B streptococci and *Escherichia coli* (most common); *Listeria monocytogenes; Klebsiella* species; other enteric Gram-negative bacteria |
| Infants and children | *Haemophilus influenzae* type b; *Neisseria meningitidis; Streptococcus pneumoniae* |
| Adults | *Streptococcus pneumoniae; Neisseria meningitidis* |
| **Special Circumstances** | |
| Meningitis or intracranial abscesses associated with trauma, neurosurgery, or intracranial foreign bodies | *Staphylococcus aureus; Staphylococcus epidermidis; Streptococcus pneumoniae;* anaerobic Gram-negative and Gram-positive bacteria; *Pseudomonas* species |
| Intracranial abscesses not associated with trauma or surgery | Microaerophilic or anaerobic streptococci, anaerobic Gram-negative bacteria (often mixed aerobic and anaerobic flora of upper respiratory tract origin) |

**TABLE 67–2. PRIMARY ACUTE VIRAL INFECTIONS OF THE CENTRAL NERVOUS SYSTEM**

| Agent | Major Age Group Affected | Seasonal Predominance |
|---|---|---|
| Enteroviruses (Coxsackie A, Coxsackie B, echoviruses, polioviruses) | Infants, children | Summer-fall |
| Mumps | Children | Winter-spring |
| Herpes simplex | | |
| Type 1 | Adults | None |
| Type 2 | Neonates, young adults | None |
| Arboviruses | | |
| Western equine encephalitis | Infants, children | Summer-fall |
| St. Louis encephalitis | Adults over 40 yr old | Summer-fall |
| California encephalitis | School-aged children | Summer-fall |
| Eastern equine encephalitis | Infants, children | Summer-fall |
| Rabies | All ages | Summer-fall |
| Measles | Infants, children | Spring |
| Varicella–zoster | Infants, children | Spring |
| Lymphocytic choriomeningitis | Adults | None |
| Epstein–Barr virus | Children, young adults | None |
| Other (myxoviruses, paramyxoviruses, cytomegaloviruses, adenoviruses, etc) | Infants, children | Variable |

## GENERAL DIAGNOSTIC APPROACHES

Except in unusual circumstances, in which severe increases in intracranial pressure make the procedure dangerous, a lumbar puncture is the first step in the workup of a patient with suspected CNS infection. The CSF pressure is determined at the time of the procedure, and CSF is removed for analysis of cells, protein, and glucose. Ideally, the glucose content of the peripheral blood is determined simultaneously for comparison with that in the CSF. Table 67–4 presents guidelines for interpretation of results of CSF analysis; these guidelines represent generalizations, however, and must not be considered as absolute findings in all cases. For example, although a patient with bacterial, mycobacterial, or fungal meningitis will usually have a glucose level in the CSF of less than 40 mg/dL, or less than half the blood glucose level (hypoglycorrhachia), this finding may not be present in the early stages of infection. Viral infections of the CNS can occasionally produce low glucose values in the CSF; in addition, the early stages of viral infection may be associated with a preponderance of polymorphonuclear leukocytes. It is clearly important to recognize that viral

Lumbar puncture gives pressure cells, protein, and glucose in CSF

CSF glucose should be compared with blood level

**TABLE 67–3. OTHER CAUSES OF CENTRAL NERVOUS SYSTEM INFECTIONS**

| Disease | Agent |
|---|---|
| Chronic granulomatous infection | *Mycobacterium tuberculosis*[a] |
| | *Coccidioides immitis* |
| | *Cryptococcus neoformans* |
| | *Histoplasma capsulatum* |
| Parasitic infection | |
| Protozoa | *Toxoplasma gondii*[b] |
| | *Trypanosoma* |
| | *Naegleria* (ameba) species |
| Nematodes | *Toxocara* species |
| | *Trichinella spiralis* |
| | *Angiostrongylus cantonensis* |
| Cestodes | *Taenia solium* (cysticercosis) |
| Other | *Leptospira* species |
| | *Treponema pallidum* |
| | *Borrelia burgdorferi* |

[a] Tuberculous meningitis can appear as acute or chronically progressive disease.
[b] Toxoplasmosis of the central nervous system is usually seen in congenital infections or immunocompromised hosts.

**TABLE 67–4. FINDINGS OF CEREBROSPINAL FLUID ANALYSIS: NORMAL VERSUS INFECTION**

| Clinical Situation | Leukocytes/mm³ | % Polymorphonuclears | Glucose (% of blood) | Protein (mg/dL) |
|---|---|---|---|---|
| **Children and Adults** | | | | |
| Normal | 0–5 | 0 | ≥60 | ≤30 |
| Viral infection | 2–2000 (80)[a] | ≤50 | ≥60 | 30–80 |
| Pyogenic bacterial infection | 5–5000 (800) | ≥60 | ≤45[b] | >60 |
| Tuberculosis and mycoses | 5–2000 (100) | ≤50 | ≤45 | >60 |
| **Neonates** | | | | |
| Normal (term) | 0–32 (8) | ≤60 | ≥60 | 20–170 (90) |
| Normal (preterm) | 0–29 (9) | ≤60 | ≥60 | 65–150 (115) |

[a] Numbers in parentheses represent mean values.
[b] Usually very low.

CNS infections can exist with a negligible CSF cell count. This sometimes also occurs in the early stages of bacterial meningitis.

Major infectious syndromes have typical CSF patterns

Realizing the limitations, it is possible to make some general interpretations that are helpful in the diagnosis. Viral CNS infections are usually associated with a preponderance of lymphocytes, a normal glucose value, and a normal or moderately elevated protein level in the CSF. In contrast, acute bacterial meningitis usually causes a CSF pleocytosis consisting primarily of polymorphonuclear cells, a low glucose value, and a high protein level. Mycobacterial and fungal infections are more commonly associated with lymphocytosis (and sometimes moderate eosinophilia) in the CSF; like the acute bacterial infections, however, they tend to lower glucose and increase protein levels markedly.

PMNs not normal in CSF

Normal values for CSF are also shown in Table 67–4. No polymorphonuclear cells should appear in normal CSF, but as many as five lymphocytes/mm$^3$ may be found in health. Neonatal CSF is considerably more difficult to interpret, as cell counts are often elevated in the absence of infection; glucose values, however, should be within the normal range.

Direct staining and culture are the definitive methods

Tests for free antigens useful in some circumstances

The other major procedures that must be performed on all CSF samples in which any infection is suspected include bacterial cultures and Gram staining. If the CSF is grossly purulent and the patient untreated, a Gram stain of the uncentrifuged CSF or of its centrifuged sediment will frequently show the infecting organism and indicate the specific diagnosis. According to the clinical indications and results of CSF cytology and chemistry, other microbiologic tests may be used, including viral cultures, special stains and cultures for fungi and mycobacteria, and immunologic methods to detect fungal or bacterial antigens (for example, latex agglutination for *Cryptococcus* or selected bacteria), and polymerase chain reactions to detect viral or bacterial nucleic acids.

Culture of blood and other sites depend on suspected etiology

Biopsy and serology useful for some agents

Tests on specimens other than CSF are selected on the basis of the clinical diagnostic possibilities. If acute bacterial meningitis is suspected, blood cultures should also be used to ensure the diagnosis. Viral cultures of the pharynx, stool, or rectal swabs may provide indirect evidence of CNS infection. Herpes simplex encephalitis poses a unique situation: to establish the diagnosis, a biopsy specimen of the brain is sometimes obtained to demonstrate viral antigen by immunofluorescence and/or growth of virus. Other studies may include acute and convalescent sera for viral serology and serologic tests to detect antibodies to certain fungi, such as *Coccidioides immitis*.

Intracranial abscesses can often be detected with radiologic techniques, such as computerized tomography or magnetic resonance imaging. A definitive etiologic diagnosis is established by careful aerobic and anaerobic culture of the contents of the abscess.

## GENERAL PRINCIPLES OF MANAGEMENT

Chemotherapy is administered immediately

In bacterial, mycobacterial, and fungal infections of the CNS, prompt and aggressive antimicrobial therapy is required. The duration of treatment varies from as little as 10 days for uncomplicated bacterial meningitis to 12 months or longer for tuberculous meningitis and several years for some cases of fungal meningitis.

In addition to antimicrobial therapy, correction of associated metabolic defects (acidosis, hypoxia, saline depletion, inappropriate antidiuretic hormone secretion) is necessary. The use of dexamethasone, a potent corticosteroid, has been advocated for initial treatment of acute purulent meningitis. Data suggest that this may reduce the risk of sequelae by minimizing early adverse inflammatory responses. Increased intracranial pressure as a result of vasogenic edema or hydrocephalus must be monitored and controlled accordingly; osmotic agents such as intravenous mannitol are often used to control acute cerebral edema, and neurosurgical shunting procedures may be needed to treat progressive hydrocephalus. Abscesses often require drainage.

Correction of metabolic defects and raised intracranial pressure important

Except for those with herpes simplex encephalitis, which may respond to early treatment with antiviral agents, patients with viral infections of the CNS receive supportive care only. This therapy includes specific attention to the metabolic and ventilatory problems that may develop in severe cases.

Chemotherapy of viral infections limited to Herpes

Chapter 68

# Intravascular Infections, Bacteremia, and Endotoxemia

*C. George Ray and Kenneth J. Ryan*

In many cases the presence of circulating microorganisms in the blood is either a part of the natural history of the infectious disease or a reflection of serious, uncontrolled infection. Depending on the class of agent involved, this process is described as viremia, bacteremia, fungemia, or parasitemia. The terms **sepsis** and **septicemia** refer to the major clinical symptom complexes generally associated with bacteremia. The clinical findings may develop acutely, as in septic shock, or slowly, as in most forms of infective endocarditis. Viremia is usually a very early, even prodromal, event accompanied by fever, malaise, and other constitutional symptoms, such as muscle aches. With the exception of a few specific infections, the detection of viremia does not play a role in the diagnosis or management of viral infections. The presence of bacteremia defines some of the most serious and life-threatening situations in medical practice, and it has a marked impact on the management and outcome of bacterial infections. This chapter will focus on the causes and implications of bacteremia and, to a lesser extent, fungemia. Diseases in which parasitemia is a feature are covered in Chapters 51 to 54.

Bacteremia or fungemia may also result from microbial growth on the inner or outer surfaces of intravenous devices. Clinical manifestations may be minor initially, but may later become severe. Because the bloodstream is sterile in health, bacteremia is considered potentially serious regardless of the symptoms present; however, transient bacteremia may occur when there is manipulation or trauma to a body site that has a normal flora. After such events, species indigenous to the site may appear briefly in the blood, but are soon cleared. Such transient bacteremias usually have no immediate clinical significance, but they are important in the pathogenesis of infective endocarditis.

## INTRAVASCULAR INFECTION

Primarily caused by bacteria

Intracardiac infections (endocarditis) and those primarily involving veins (thrombophlebitis) or arteries (endarteritis) are usually caused by bacteria although other agents including fungi and viruses have been occasionally implicated. This discussion will focus primarily on the bacterial causes, because they are the most frequent. Infections of the cardiovascular system are usually extremely serious and, if not promptly and adequately treated, can be fatal. They commonly produce a constant shedding of organisms into the bloodstream that is often characterized by continuous, low-grade bacteremia (1 to 20 organisms/mL of blood) in untreated patients.

## Infective Endocarditis

Sites of endocardial infection include prosthetic valves

The term **infective endocarditis** is preferable to the commonly used term **bacterial endocarditis,** simply because not all infections of the endocardial surface of the heart are caused by bacteria. Most infections occur on natural or prosthetic cardiac valves, but can also develop on septal defects, shunts (for example, patent ductus arteriosus), or the mural endocardium. Infections involving coarctation of the aorta are also classified as infective endocarditis because the clinical manifestations and complications are similar.

### Pathogenesis

The pathogenesis of infective endocarditis involves several factors that, if concurrent, result in infection:

Hemodynamic effects of cardiac abnormalities create sites for attachment

1. The endothelium is altered to facilitate colonization by bacteria and deposition of platelets and fibrin. Most infections involve the mitral or aortic valves, which are particularly vulnerable when abnormalities such as valvular insufficiency, stenosis, intracardiac shunts (for example, ventricular septal defect), or direct trauma (for example, catheters) exist. The turbulence of intracardiac blood flow that results from such abnormalities can lead to further irregularities of the endothelial surfaces that facilitate platelet and fibrin deposition. These factors produce a potential nidus for colonization and infection.

Transient bacteremia with normal flora is the organism source

2. Transient bacteremia is common, but usually of no clinical importance. Often seen for a few minutes after a variety of dental procedures, it has also been shown to develop after normal childbirth and manipulations such as bronchoscopy, sigmoidoscopy, cystoscopy, and some surgical procedures. Even simple activities such as tooth brushing or chewing candy can cause such bacteremia. The organisms responsible for transient bacteremia are the common surface flora of the manipulated site such as viridans streptococci (oropharynx) and are usually of low virulence. Other, more virulent strains may also be involved, however; for example, intravenous drug abuse may lead to transient bacteremia with *Staphylococcus aureus* or a variety of Gram-negative aerobic and anaerobic bacteria. Whether the organisms causing bacteremia (or fungemia) are of high virulence or not, they can colonize and multiply in the heart if local endothelial changes are suitable.

Bacteria adhere and start development of vegetation

Embolization created by dislodged parts of vegetation

3. Bacteremic organisms adhere to the damaged surface, followed by complement activation, inflammation, fibrin, and platelet deposition and further endothelial damage at the site of colonization. The resulting entrapment of organisms in the thrombotic "mesh" of platelets, fibrin, and inflammatory cells leads to a mature vegetation, which protects the organisms from host humoral and phagocytic immune defenses, and to some extent from antimicrobial agents. As a result, the infection can be exceedingly difficult to treat. The vegetation can also create greater hemodynamic alterations in terms of obstruction to flow and increased turbulence. Parts of vegetations may break off and be deposited in smaller blood vessels (embolization) with resultant obstruction and secondary sites of infection. Emboli may be transported to the brain or coronary arteries, for example, with disastrous results.

Circulating immune complexes and hyperimmune responses cause peripheral manifestations

Another phenomenon shown to contribute to the infective endocarditis syndrome is the development of circulating immune complexes of microbial antigen and antibody. These complexes can activate complement and contribute to many of the peripheral vascular manifestations of the disease, including nephritis, arthritis, and cutaneous vascular lesions.

Frequently, there is a widespread stimulus to host cellular and humoral immunity, particularly if the infection continues for more than a couple of weeks. This condition is characterized by hyperglobulinemia, splenomegaly, and the occasional appearance of macrophages in the peripheral blood. Some patients will develop circulating rheumatoid factor (IgM anti-IgG antibody), which may play a deleterious role by blocking IgG opsonic activity and causing microvascular damage. Antinuclear antibodies, which also appear occasionally, may contribute to the pathogenesis of the fever, arthralgia, and myalgia that is often seen.

In summary, infective endocarditis involves an initial complex of endothelial damage or abnormality, which facilitates colonization by organisms that may be circulating through the heart. This colonization, in turn, leads to the propagation of a vegetation, with its attendant local and systemic inflammatory, embolic, and immunologic complications.

## Clinical Features

Infective endocarditis has often been classified by the progression of the untreated disease. *Acute endocarditis* is generally fulminant with high fever and toxicity, and death may occur in a few days or weeks. *Subacute endocarditis* progresses to death over weeks to months with low-grade fever, night sweats, weight loss, and vague constitutional complaints. The clinical course is substantially related to the virulence of the infecting organism; *S. aureus,* for example, usually produces acute disease, whereas infections by the otherwise avirulent viridans streptococci are more likely to be subacute. Before the advent of antimicrobial therapy, death was considered inevitable in all cases. Physical findings often include a new or changing heart murmur, splenomegaly, various skin lesions (petechiae, splinter hemorrhages, Osler's nodes, Janeway's lesions), and retinal lesions.

Acute, subacute, and chronic infective endocarditis determined by virulence of organism

Complications include the risk of congestive heart failure as a result of hemodynamic alterations, rupture of the chordae tendinea of the valves, or perforation of a valve. Abscesses of the myocardium or valve ring can also develop. Other complications relate to the immunologic and embolic phenomena that can occur. The kidney is commonly affected, and hematuria is a typical finding. Renal failure, presumably from immune complex glomerulonephritis, is possible. Left-sided endocarditis can readily lead to coronary artery embolization and "mycotic" aneurysms; the latter will be discussed later in this chapter. In addition, more distant emboli to the central nervous system can lead to cerebral infarction and infection. Right-sided endocarditis often causes embolization and infarction or infection in the lung.

Cardiac, embolic, and immunologically mediated complications lead to death without treatment

## Etiologic Agents

Table 68–1 summarizes the most common causes of infective endocarditis. Alpha-hemolytic streptococci and enterococci are involved in just over half of the cases. In the so-called culture-negative group, infective endocarditis is diagnosed on clinical grounds, but cultures do not confirm the etiologic agent. This group of patients is difficult to treat, and the overall prognosis is considered poorer than when a specific etiology has been determined. Negative cultures may result from (1) prior antibiotic treatment; (2) fungal endocarditis with entrapment of these relatively large organisms in capillary beds; (3) fastidious, nutritionally deficient, or cell-wall-deficient organisms that are difficult to isolate; (4) infection caused by obligate intracellular parasites, such as chlamydiae (*Chlamydia psittaci*), rickettsiae (*Coxiella burnetii*), *Rochalimaea* species, or viruses; (5) immunologic factors (for example, antibody acting on circulating organisms); or (6) subacute endocarditis involving the right side of the heart, in which the organisms are filtered out in the pulmonary capillaries.

Streptococci most common cause

Many explanations for culture-negative endocarditis

Some special circumstances alter the relative etiologic possibilities, such as intravenous drug addiction, prosthetic valves, and immunocompromise. The major associations in these cases are summarized in Table 68–2.

**TABLE 68–1. COMMON ETIOLOGIC AGENTS IN INFECTIVE ENDOCARDITIS**

| Agent | Approximate Percentage of Cases |
|---|---|
| Viridans streptococci (several species) | 30–40 |
| Group D streptococci (enterococci) | 5–18 |
| Other streptococci | 15–25 |
| *Staphylococcus aureus* | 10–27 |
| *Staphylococcus epidermidis* | 1–3 |
| Enterobacteriaceae and *Pseudomonas* | 2–13 |
| Fungi (*Candida* sp., *Aspergillus* sp., etc) | 2–4 |

**TABLE 68–2. ETIOLOGIC AGENTS MORE COMMONLY OBSERVED IN SPECIAL CIRCUMSTANCES**

| Situation | Agent |
|---|---|
| Intravenous drug abuse | *Staphylococcus aureus*; group D streptococci; Enterobacteriaceae and *Pseudomonas*; fungi |
| Prosthetic valve infection | *Staphylococcus epidermidis*; *Staphylococcus aureus*; Enterobacteriaceae and *Pseudomonas*; diphtheroids; *Candida* and *Aspergillus* spp. |
| Immunocompromise, chronic illness | Any of the above organisms |

### General Diagnostic Approaches

Blood culture the most important diagnostic test

The diagnosis of infective endocarditis is usually suspected on clinical grounds; however, the most important diagnostic test for confirmation is the blood culture. In untreated cases, the organisms are generally present continuously in low numbers (1 to 20/mL) in the blood. If an adequate volume of blood is obtained, the first culture will be positive in over 95% of culturally confirmed cases. Most authorities recommend three cultures over 24 hours to ensure detection, and an additional three if the first set is negative. Multiple cultures yielding the same organism support the probability of an intravascular or intracardiac infection. In acute endocarditis, the urgency of early treatment may require collection of only two or three cultures within a few minutes so that antimicrobial therapy can begin.

Echocardiography defines vegetations

Cardiologic procedures such as transthoracic or transesophageal echocardiography can delineate the nature and size of the vegetations and progression of disease. They are also helpful in prediction of some complications such as embolization.

### General Principles of Management

Bactericidal antimicrobics required because of protective effect of the vegetation

Antimicrobic combinations often used for synergistic effect

Because of the nature of the lesions and their pathogenesis, response to therapy may be slow and cure is sometimes difficult. Therefore, specific antimicrobial therapy must be aggressive, using agents that are bactericidal (rather than bacteriostatic) and can be given in amounts that will achieve high continuous blood levels without causing toxicity to the patient. Treatment may involve a single antimicrobial if the organism is highly susceptible in vitro, or antimicrobial combinations if synergistic effects are possible (for example, a penicillin and an aminoglycoside for enterococcal endocarditis). Parenteral therapy is begun to produce adequate blood levels, and the patient may need to be monitored frequently to ensure antimicrobial activity in the serum sufficient to kill the organisms without causing unnecessary toxicity. Therapy is usually prolonged, lasting longer than 4 weeks in most cases. In some cases, surgery may be required to excise the diseased valve and replace it with a valvular prosthesis. The decision for surgery is sometimes difficult, requiring consultation with both a cardiologist and a surgeon.

Antimicrobial prophylaxis indicated for those with cardiac abnormalities

Penicillin prophylaxis used with dental work

Prophylaxis can prevent the development of endocarditis in persons with known congenital or acquired cardiac lesions that predispose to bacterial endocarditis. When they undergo procedures known to cause transient bacteremia (for example, dental manipulations or surgical procedures involving the upper respiratory, gastrointestinal, or genitourinary tracts), administration of high doses of antimicrobics is begun just before the procedure and continued for 6 to 12 hours thereafter. An example of prophylaxis is the case of a patient with rheumatic valvular disease who is planning to undergo dental work. The organism most likely to produce transient bacteremia would be a penicillin-sensitive member of the oral flora, especially viridans streptococci. Thus, an intramuscular dose of penicillin within 30 minutes before the procedure, followed by a high dose of intramuscular or oral penicillin 6 hours later, would be expected to afford protection. Several regimens similar to this approach are recommended, depending upon the patient, the nature of the procedure, and the organisms that might be expected to be involved.

## Mycotic Aneurysm

The term **mycotic aneurysm** is somewhat misleading, as it suggests infection by fungi. Originally used by William Osler to describe the mushroom-shaped arterial aneurysm that can develop in patients with infective endocarditis, the term now applies to infection with any organism that causes inflammatory damage and weakening of an arterial wall with subsequent aneurysmal dilatation. This sequence can progress to rupture, with a fatal outcome.

Arterial infection can result from direct extension of an intracardiac infection or from septic microemboli from a cardiac focus, with seeding of vasa vasorum within the arterial wall. In addition to infective endocarditis other predisposing factors include damaged arterial intima by atherosclerotic plaques, vascular thrombi, congenital malformations, trauma, or spread from a contiguous focus of infection directly into the artery. The clinical features vary according to the site of involvement. Common findings may include pain at the site of primary arterial supply (for example, back or abdominal pain in abdominal aortic infections) and fever. In many cases the initial presentation is the result of a catastrophic hemorrhage, particularly intracerebral aneurysms. The etiologic agents, diagnosis, and management are similar to infective endocarditis.

Intraarterial infection occurs at sites of vascular injury

Etiologic agents similar to those of infective endocarditis

## Suppurative Thrombophlebitis

Suppurative (or septic) thrombophlebitis is an inflammation of a vein wall frequently associated with thrombosis and bacteremia. There are four basic forms: superficial, pelvic, intracranial venous sinus, and portal vein infection (pylephlebitis). With the steadily increasing use of intravenous catheters, the incidence of superficial thrombophlebitis has risen and represents a major complication in hospitalized patients.

Thrombotic site may become seeded with organisms from blood

The pathogenesis involves thrombus formation, which may result from trauma to the vein, extrinsic inflammation, hypercoagulable states, stasis of blood flow, or combinations of these factors. The thrombosed site is then seeded with organisms, and a focus of infection is established. In superficial thrombophlebitis, an intravenous cannula or catheter may cause local venous wall trauma, as well as serve as a foreign body nidus for thrombus formation. Infection will evolve if bacteria are introduced by intravenous fluid, local wound contamination, or bacteremic seeding from a remote infected site.

Intravenous catheter often associated with thrombophlebitis

Thrombophlebitis of pelvic, portal, or intracranial venous systems most often occurs as a result of direct extension of an infectious process from adjacent structures, or from venous and lymphatic pathways near sites of infection. For example, infections of intracranial venous sinuses usually result from orbital or sinus infections (causing cavernous sinus thrombophlebitis) or from infections of the mastoid and middle ear (causing lateral and sagittal sinus thrombophlebitis). Pelvic thrombophlebitis is a potential result of intrauterine infection (endometritis), particularly after pelvic surgery or 2 to 3 weeks after childbirth. Pelvic or intra-abdominal infections may also spread to the portal venous system to produce pylephlebitis.

Local infection may extend to veins

### Clinical Features

Common features often include fever and inflammation over the infected vein. Pelvic or portal vein thrombophlebitis is usually associated with high fever, chills, nausea, vomiting, and abdominal pain. Jaundice may develop in portal vein infections. Intracranial thrombophlebitis varies in its presentation. Headache, facial or orbital edema, and neurologic deficits are variably present; for example, cavernous sinus thrombophlebitis often causes palsies of the third through sixth cranial nerves. Complications include extension of suppurative infection into adjacent structures, further propagation of thrombi, bacteremia, and septic embolization. Embolization from pelvic or leg veins is to the lungs and pulmonary embolism with infarction may be the presenting manifestation of the remote infection.

Signs and symptoms depend on anatomic site involved

### Etiologic Agents

The major infectious causes of suppurative thrombophlebitis are outlined in Table 68–3. In superficial thrombophlebitis, which often follows intravenous therapy, organisms that are common nosocomial offenders predominate (*S. aureus,* Gram-negative aerobes). Deeper infections are more frequently caused by organisms that reside on adjacent mucous membranes (for example, *Bacteroides* species in intestinal and vaginal sites) or commonly infect adjacent sites (for example, *Haemophilus influenzae* and *S. pneumoniae* in acute otitis media and sinusitis).

**TABLE 68–3. COMMON ETIOLOGIC AGENTS IN SUPPURATIVE THROMBOPHLEBITIS**

| Site | Agent |
|---|---|
| Superficial veins (saphenous, femoral, antecubital, etc) | *Staphylococcus aureus*; Gram-negative aerobic bacilli |
| Pelvic veins, portal veins | *Bacteroides* sp.; microaerophilic or anaerobic streptococci; *Escherichia coli*; β-hemolytic streptococci (group A or B) |
| Intracranial venous sinuses (cavernous, sagittal, lateral) | *Haemophilus influenzae*, *Streptococcus pneumoniae*; β-hemolytic streptococcus (group A); anaerobic or microaerophilic streptococci; *Staphylococcus aureus* |

### General Diagnostic Approaches

Direct culture or blood culture usually positive

The diagnosis is often suspected on clinical grounds and from associated events known to create predisposition to such infections (for example, surgery, presence of indwelling venous cannulas). Direct cultures of the infected site or blood cultures will usually yield the infecting organism, because bacteremia is often present. Radiologic procedures, including scanning methods, may be necessary to localize the process and support the diagnosis. In some cases, surgical exploration is required, both for definitive treatment and obtaining specimens for cultures.

### General Principles of Management

Chemotherapy and removal of catheters

The choice of antimicrobial agents is based upon culture and susceptibility test results, or in the absence of microbiologic data, the most likely possibilities listed in Table 68–3. Other important aspects of management include prompt removal of possible offending sources, such as intravenous catheters, vigorous treatment of adjacent infections, and sometimes surgical excision and drainage. Severe cases may also benefit from systemic anticoagulant therapy to prevent further propagation of thrombi and embolization.

Many cases are preventable. Unnecessary, long-term intravenous cannulation should be avoided. Whenever possible, it is better to use short needles such as "scalp vein" cannulas than venous catheters or plastic cannulas. Careful asepsis is essential with all intravenous procedures to prevent contamination of intravenous fluids, tubing, and the site of venous entry.

## Intravenous Catheter Bacteremia

Significant endocarditis and metastatic infection

A variant of intravascular infection develops when a medical device such as an intravenous catheter or any of several types of monitoring devices placed in the bloodstream becomes colonized with microorganisms. The event itself does not have immediate clinical significance but, unlike transient bacteremia from manipulation of normal floral sites, the bacteremia continues. This persistence greatly increases the chances of secondary complications such as infective endocarditis and metastatic infection, depending on any underlying disease and the virulence of the organism involved.

Skin flora most commonly involved

The organisms involved are usually those found in the skin flora, such as *S. epidermidis, Corynebacterium jeikeium,* or *S. aureus.* In debilitated patients already on antimicrobial therapy, *Candida* species may be involved. Occasionally the sources of contamination are the intravenous solutions themselves rather than the skin. In these cases, members of the Enterobacteriaceae family, *Pseudomonas,* or other Gram-negative rods are more likely.

High-level bacteremia despite mild clinical manifestations

The clinical findings in catheter bacteremia are usually mild despite large numbers of organisms in the bloodstream (Fig 68–1). Signs of inflammation may or may not be present, in addition to low-grade fever. Management is by removal of the contaminated catheter. Antimicrobial therapy often will not eradicate the organisms in the presence of a foreign body (the catheter).

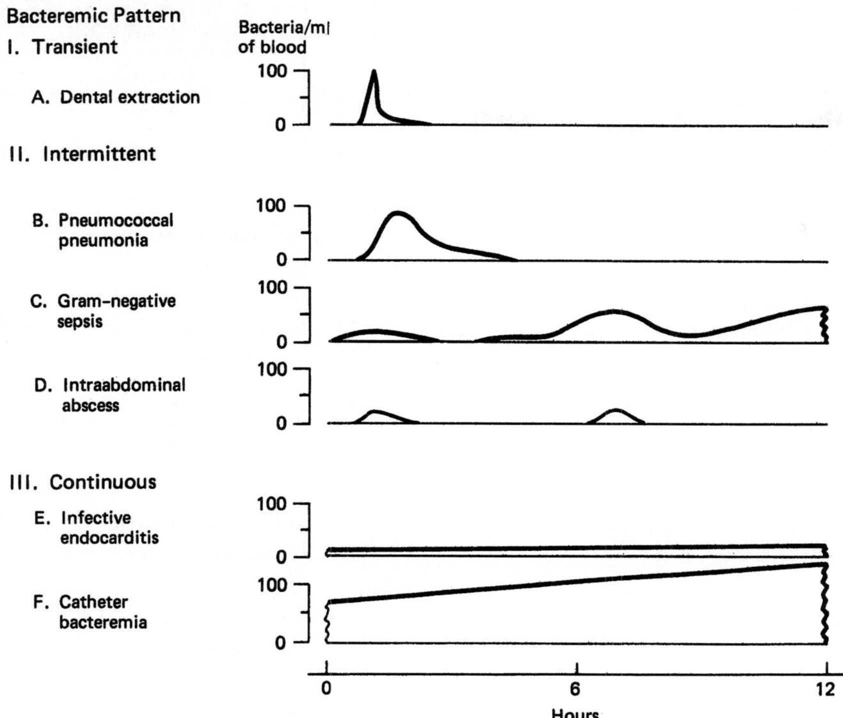


**Figure 68–1.** Patterns of bacteremia. The magnitude and timing of bacteremia for six typical patients **(A–F)** are depicted. These findings have implications for blood culture sampling plans. Cases such as **A** and **B** will only be detected by cultures taken early in their course. Cases such as **C** and particularly **D** are more variable and more likely to be detected by cultures spaced over the time period shown. Continuous bacteremia (**E** and **F**) should be detected by any sampling plan. It could be confused with transient bacteremia on single blood cultures, as both are caused by organisms of low virulence (viridans streptococci, *Staphylococcus epidermidis*); in cases such as **E** and **F**, however, bacteremia is sustained, whereas cases of transient bacteremia will yield multiple positive results only if they are collected at or near the same time.

## BACTEREMIA FROM EXTRAVASCULAR INFECTION

Although bacteremia is an integral feature of intravascular infection, most cases of clinically significant bacteremia are the result overflow from an extravascular infection. In these cases, the organisms drained by the lymphatics or otherwise escaping from the infected focus reach the capillary and venous circulation through the lymphatic vessels. Depending on the magnitude of the infection and the degree of local control, these organisms may be filtered in the reticuloendothelial system or circulate more widely, producing bacteremia or fungemia. The process is dependent on the timing and interaction of multiple events and is thus much less predictable than intravascular infection. If the infection is extensive and uncontrolled, such as an overwhelming staphylococcal pneumonia, there may be hundreds or even thousands of organisms per milliliter of blood, a poor prognostic sign. An intraabdominal abscess may only seed a few organisms intermittently until it is discovered and drained. Most infections that produce bacteremia fall between these extremes, with bloodstream invasion more common in the acute phases and intermittent at other times.

Bacteremia more variable than with intravascular infection

The causative organisms and the frequencies with which they usually produce bacteremia (or fungemia) are listed in Table 68–4. There is considerable overlap, and the probability of bacteremia is dependent on the site as well as the organism. Any organism producing meningitis is likely to produce bacteremia at the same time. Infections with *H. influenzae* type b are usually bacteremic whether the site is the meninges, epiglottis, or periorbital tissues. Meningitis caused by *S. pneumoniae* can be expected to be bacteremic, but only 20 to 30% of patients with pneumococcal pneumonia have positive blood cultures.

Frequently associated with severe infections such as meningitis

The most common sources of bacteremia are urinary tract infections, respiratory tract infections, and infections of skin or soft tissues, such as wound infections or cellulitis. The

**TABLE 68–4. FREQUENCY OF DETECTION OF BLOODSTREAM INVASION BY BACTERIA AND SOME FUNGI DURING SIGNIFICANT INFECTIONS AT EXTRAVASCULAR SITES**

| | |
|---|---|
| **Large (>90%) Proportion of Cases** | |
| *Haemophilus influenzae* type b | *Brucella*[a] |
| *Neisseria meningitidis* | *Salmonella typhi* |
| *Streptococcus pneumoniae* (meningitis) | *Listeria* |
| **Variable (10–90%) Depending on Stage and Severity of Infection** | |
| β-hemolytic streptococci | Enterobacteriaceae |
| *Streptococcus pneumoniae* | *Pseudomonas* |
| *Staphylococcus aureus* | *Bacteroides* |
| *Neisseria gonorrhoeae* | *Clostridium* (myositis and endometritis) |
| *Leptospira*[a] | Anaerobic cocci |
| *Borrelia*[a] | *Candida* |
| *Acinetobacter* | *Cryptococcus neoformans*[a] |
| *Shigella dysenteriae* | |
| **Small (<10%) Proportion of Cases** | |
| *Shigella* (except *S. dysenteriae*) | *Pasteurella multocida* |
| *Salmonella enteritidis* | *Haemophilus*, noncapsulated |
| *Campylobacter jejuni*[a] | |
| **Isolation Too Rare to Justify Attempt** | |
| *Vibrio* (intestinal infections) | *Clostridium tetani* |
| *Corynebacterium diphtheriae* | *Clostridium botulinum* |
| *Bordetella pertussis* | *Clostridium difficile* |
| *Mycobacterium*[b] | *Legionella*[c] |

[a] Isolation and/or demonstration requires special methods or prolonged incubation.
[b] *Mycobacterium avium-intracellulare* infections in AIDS patients often yield positives.
[c] Infrequent isolation may be due to inadequate cultural methods.

Bacteremia is overflow from respiratory, urinary, wound, and other primary sites of infection

frequency with which any organism causes bacteremia is related to both its propensity to invade the bloodstream (Table 68–4) and how often it produces infections. For example, cases of *Escherichia coli* bacteremia are common, attributable in part to the fact that *E. coli* is the most frequent cause of urinary tract infection.

## Sepsis and Septic Shock

Associated with bacteremic Gram-negative and Gram-positive infections

Bacteremia is the presence of viable bacteria circulating in the blood. When signs and symptoms result, further terms are used to delineate the progression of potential consequences that may occur. Both Gram-negative and Gram-positive organisms can produce the same findings, as well as fungi, protozoa, and even some viruses.

Sepsis syndrome progresses through shock to organ failure

**Sepsis** is the suspicion (or proof) of infection and evidence of a systemic response to it (eg, tachycardia, tachypnea, hyperthermia, or hypothermia). The **sepsis syndrome** includes findings of sepsis plus evidence of altered organ perfusion. These can include reduction in urine output, mental status changes, systemic acidosis, and hypoxemia. If the process remains uncontrolled, there is subsequent progression to **septic shock** (development of hypotension), **refractory septic shock** (hypotension not responsive to standard fluid and pharmacologic treatment), and **multiorgan failure** including major target organs such as the kidneys, lungs, and liver, and disseminated intravascular coagulation. Mortality is exceedingly high when patients develop refractory septic shock or multiorgan failure.

Vasodilatation followed by complex response

The initial events in the sepsis syndrome appear to be vasodilatation with resultant decreased peripheral resistance and increased cardiac output. The patient is flushed and febrile. Capillary leakage and reduced blood volume follow, leading to a whole series of events identical to those seen in shock resulting from blood loss. These manifestations include vasoconstriction, reflex capillary dilatation, and local anoxic damage. Once this stage is reached, the patient may develop hypotension and hypothermia, and acidosis, hypoglycemia, and coagulation defects ensue with failure of highly perfused organs such as the lungs, kidneys, heart, brain, and liver.

The mechanisms involved in development of septic shock have been studied extensively in experimental animals. Most of the features seen in humans can be produced with the lipopolysaccharide endotoxin of the Gram-negative cell wall, although there is some variation between animal species and with different preparations. The various events that occur are complex and still not fully understood. They include (1) release of vasoactive substances such as histamine, serotonin, noradrenaline, and plasma kinins, which may cause arterial hypotension directly and facilitate coagulation abnormalities; (2) disturbances in temperature regulation, which may be due to direct central nervous system effects or, in the case of the early febrile response, mediated by interleukin 1 and tumor necrosis factor (TNF) released from macrophages; (3) complement activation; (4) direct effects on vascular endothelial cell function and integrity; and (5) depression of cardiac muscle contractility by TNF, myocardial depressant factor, and other less-well-defined serum factors. The resultant alterations in blood flow and capillary permeability lead to progressive organ dysfunction.

Endotoxin causes release of vasoactive substances

Cytokines, complement, and other mediators cause physiological effects

Early recognition of the problem is critical, and management obviously requires considerably more than antimicrobial therapy. Other primary therapeutic measures include maintenance of adequate tissue perfusion through careful fluid and electrolyte management and the use of vasoactive amines.

## BLOOD CULTURE

The primary means for establishing a diagnosis of sepsis is by blood culture. The microbiologic principles involved are the same as with any culture. A sample of the patient's blood is obtained by aseptic venipuncture and cultured in an enriched broth or, after special processing, on plates. Growth is detected, and the organisms are isolated, identified, and tested for antimicrobial susceptibility. Because of the importance of blood cultures in the diagnosis and therapy of most bacterial and fungal infections, considerable attention must be paid to details of sampling if the prospects of obtaining a positive culture are to be maximized. The approach to blood culture must be tailored to the individual patient, as no single procedure is best for all. The important features are as follows.

Importance of blood culture demands attention to details

### Blood Culture Sampling

#### Venipuncture

Before venipuncture, the skin over the vein must be carefully disinfected to reduce the probability of contamination of the blood sample with skin bacteria. Although it is not possible to "sterilize" the skin, quantitative counts can be markedly reduced with a combination of 70% alcohol and an iodine-based antiseptic. Mechanical cleansing is as important as use of the antiseptic. Poor phlebotomy technique such as repalpating the vein after the preparation is related to introduction of contaminants. Blood is ideally drawn directly into a blood culture bottle or a sterile blood collection vacuum tube containing an anticoagulant free of antimicrobial properties. Sodium polyanethol sulfonate is currently preferred, as other anticoagulants such as citrate and ethylenediaminetetraacetic acid have antibacterial activity. Blood should not be drawn through indwelling venous or arterial catheters unless it cannot be obtained by venipuncture.

Skin decontamination removes bulk of skin flora

Some anticoagulants have antimicrobial properties

#### Volume

The number of organisms present in blood is often low (less than 1 organism/mL) and cannot be predicted in advance. Thus, small samples yield fewer positive cultures than larger ones. For example, as the volume sampled increases from 2 to 20 mL, the diagnostic yield increases by 30 to 50%. Samples of at least 10 mL should be collected from adult patients. The same principles apply with infants and young children, but the sample size must be reduced to take account of the smaller total blood volume of a child. Although it should be possible to obtain at least 1 mL, smaller volumes should still be cultured because bacteremia at levels of more than 1000 bacteria/mL is found in some infants.

Number of organisms in blood often $<1$/mL

#### Number

If the volume is adequate, it is rarely necessary to collect more than two or three blood cultures to achieve a positive result. In intravascular infections (for example, infective endo-

Two or three blood cultures usually adequate

carditis), a single blood culture will be positive in more than 95% of cases. Studies of sequential blood cultures from bacteremic patients without endocarditis have yielded 80 to 90% positive results on the first culture, more than 90 to 95% with two cultures, and 99% in at least one of a series of three cultures.

### Timing

Timing of intermittent bacteremia not predictable

Spacing cultures increases chance of detection

Antimicrobic therapy may interfere with blood culture results

The best timing schedule for a series of two or three blood cultures is dependent on the bacteremic pattern of the underlying infection and the clinical urgency of initiating antimicrobial therapy. Figure 68–1 illustrates some typical bacteremic patterns that can be related to the probability of obtaining positive blood cultures. Transient bacteremia is usually not detected, because organisms are cleared before the appearance of any clinical findings suggesting sepsis. The continuous bacteremia of infective endocarditis is usually readily detected, and timing is not critical. Intermittent bacteremia presents the greatest challenge because fever spikes generally occur after, rather than during, the bacteremia. Little is known about the periodicity of bloodstream invasion, except that the bacteremia is more likely to be present and sustained in the early acute stages of infection. Closely spaced samples are less likely to isolate the organism than those spaced an hour or more apart. In urgent situations, when antimicrobial therapy must be initiated, two or three samples should be collected at brief intervals and therapy begun as soon as possible. It is generally not useful to collect blood cultures while the patient is receiving antimicrobics unless none were collected before therapy or there is a change in the clinical course suggesting superinfection. The laboratory should be advised when such cultures are submitted, because it is sometimes possible to inactivate an antimicrobic, for example, with beta-lactamases.

## Laboratory Processing

Blood added to enriched broth

Automated and direct plating procedures now available

The basic blood culture procedure of incubating blood in an enriched broth is quite simple, but considerable effort must be expended to ensure detection of the broadest range of organisms in the least possible time. Daily examination of cultures for a week or more and a routine schedule of stains and/or subcultures of apparently negative cultures are required to detect organisms such as *H. influenzae* or *N. meningitidis,* which usually do not produce visual changes in the broth. Direct plating of blood onto blood or chocolate agar is accomplished in a system that concentrates the blood by centrifugation following lysis of the erythrocytes. This is particularly useful for bacterial quantification and rapid identification. Automated blood culture systems detect metabolic activity (primarily $CO_2$ generation) in broth culture for initial detection in place of the conventional visual and staining examinations. These systems detect growth sooner than conventional methods but still require subculture for confirmation, identification, and susceptibility testing.

Special cultural conditions required for yeasts and anaerobes

Isolation of fungi is favored by ensuring maximum aerobic conditions in direct plating systems and broth bottles. Conversely, anaerobes are recovered best when a highly reduced environment is provided for plates and broths. Some bacteria, such as *Leptospira,* will not be isolated by routine blood culture procedures. The laboratory must be notified in advance so special media can be employed.

Interpretation involves distingishing infection from normal skin floral contamination

As the blood is normally sterile, the interpretation of blood cultures growing a pathogenic organism is seldom a problem. The major decision is the differentiation of agents causing transient bacteremia and skin contamination from those opportunists associated with an intravascular or extravascular infection. Transient bacteremia is of short duration (Fig 68–1), is associated with manipulation of or trauma to a site possessing a normal flora, and involves species indigenous to that site. Despite skin disinfection, 2 to 4% of venipunctures result in contamination of the culture with small numbers of cutaneous flora such as *S. epidermidis,* corynebacteria (diphtheroids), and propionibacteria. The presence of these organisms in blood cultures can be considered a result of skin contamination unless quantitative procedures indicate large numbers (more than 5 organisms/mL) or repeated cultures are positive for the same organism. These findings should suggest diseases such as infective endocarditis or catheter bacteremia.

# Infections of the Fetus and Newborn

C. George Ray

The usual 10-month period from conception through birth and the first 4 weeks of extrauterine life is one of unusual susceptibility to infection, but also a time at which special defenses acquired from the mother are operating.

1. During normal development, the fetus is in a protected intrauterine environment, with fetal membranes serving as a physical barrier to external infection and the placenta contributing, with maternal immunity, to protection against many bloodborne infections. Transplacental transmission of specific immunoglobulins, particularly of the IgG class (IgM does not normally cross the placental barrier), continues to provide some immunologic protection to the infant for weeks to months after birth, while cytokines from the mother can provide transient cell-mediated immune support. If the infant is breast-fed, specific immunoglobulins (predominantly of the IgA class) in maternal colostrum afford some protection against pathogens that involve or invade through the infant's gastrointestinal tract.

Fetus protected in intrauterine environment

Passive immunity acquired from mother

2. On the other hand, the fetal immune system is immature, and there is relative suppression of maternal cell-mediated immunity as pregnancy progresses. These immune deficiencies serve an important biological purpose, as they protect fetus and mother from activation of specific immunologic recognition and response mechanisms to differences in their histocompatibility locus antigens. If these processes did not occur normally, the fetus could be immunologically rejected by the mother or the fetal immune mechanisms activated to respond against maternal antigens in a form of "graft versus host" disease.

Fetal immune system immature and maternal cell-mediated immunity suppressed

3. Specific and nonspecific immune responses begin to develop in early fetal life, perhaps as early as 8 weeks of gestation; however, a nearly normal immunocompetent state is usually not achieved until the infant is more than 2 years of age. Deficiencies commonly seen in the early period include poor antibody response to T-independent polysaccharide antigens, decreased phagocytic capability and variability in intracellular killing of certain infectious agents, lower levels of complement components, and decreased opsonic capacity.

Specific deficiencies of neonate include poor T-independent responses

4. Cell growth and organ differentiation are at their highest rates in the fetal–neonatal period, making the host especially susceptible to permanent damage when an infectious process intervenes.

Infection may have teratogenic effects

The actual risk of infection and the types of pathogens encountered are influenced by a variety of interacting factors, including the state of maternal health and susceptibility to specific agents, adequacy of fetal and neonatal nutrition, integrity of fetal membranes, and

Risk of infection influenced by fetal and maternal factors

degree of maturity at birth. This chapter outlines the major types of infection of concern to those caring for the fetus and neonate and the general approaches to their diagnosis. Specific biological characteristics and aspects of prevention and treatment for each of the agents have been addressed in previous chapters.

## DEFINITIONS

A number of terms are commonly used to describe the infections that can affect the fetus and newborn. **Prenatal** infections include those acquired by the mother and/or fetus at any time before birth. When fetal infection develops, it is usually either blood-borne to the placenta with subsequent spread to the fetus (transplacental), or by the ascending route from the vagina through torn or ruptured fetal membranes. **Natal** infections are those acquired during delivery. They are often caused by agents in the maternal genital tract, but occasionally by organisms introduced from exogenous sources through attendants, fetal monitors, or other instruments. **Postnatal** infections, which constitute the remainder of the group, include all infections acquired after delivery throughout the newborn (or neonatal) period, defined as the first 4 weeks of life.

Another commonly used term is **congenital** infection, which describes infection occurring at any time before or at birth (prenatal or natal). Consequently, the infection is usually still active in the newborn period and sometimes persists for months or years. **Perinatal** infection is often used to include a period extending from 20 to 28 weeks of gestation to 7 to 28 days after birth. The term will not be used in this chapter.

**Chorioamnionitis** is an inflammatory response to infectious agents involving the chorionic and amniotic fetal membranes. It usually results from entry of pathogens from the vagina through tears or ruptures in the membranes, and it places the fetus at risk of direct exposure just before or at delivery. The risk of chorioamnionitis increases rapidly when membranes have been ruptured for longer than 12 hours before birth. When infection is by the blood-borne maternal route, there may be evidence of infection of the placenta, termed **placentitis. Endometritis** may be observed occasionally if the infection is an extension from a maternal pelvic focus along venous or lymphatic pathways. **Sepsis** is a term employed to indicate a severe systemic bacterial infection associated with bacteremia.

## COMMON ETIOLOGIC AGENTS

Rarity of some childhood infections in infancy related to exposure and passive immunity

Table 69–1 lists the major pathogens affecting the fetus and newborn, according to the usual modes of acquisition. Some, such as *Mycobacterium tuberculosis* and *Plasmodium* species, are exceedingly rare, but require consideration in certain clinical and epidemiologic circumstances. It should also be noted that some pathogens that commonly affect older infants and children are quite rarely observed in newborns. This phenomenon is partially attributable to the protective effect of maternally derived immunity to organisms such as *Haemophilus influenzae* type b, *Streptococcus pneumoniae, Neisseria meningitidis,* and mumps and measles viruses, but also reflects less opportunity for exposure to some agents early in life. Some organisms, such as *Staphylococcus aureus,* very rarely cause prenatal or natal infections, but commonly colonize in the postnatal period and most often cause disease after the first week of life.

*S, aureus* infections typically postnatal

If one views the fetus as existing normally in a protected, "germ-free" intrauterine environment before emerging into a milieu of potential pathogens, it is easy to see how the newborn can be colonized with the first organisms encountered, some of which can cause disease. The external pathogenic flora initially acquired can include organisms frequently present in the maternal genital tract, such as group B streptococci and *Escherichia coli,* as well as less common *N. gonorrhoeae, Listeria monocytogenes, Chlamydia trachomatis,* and herpes simplex virus, all of which are important causes of natal infection.

First exposure is to pathogens in maternal genital flora

Postnatal infections may be late manifestations resulting from prenatal or natal colonization by pathogens such as those mentioned previously, but additional organisms may be acquired after birth. Particular risks include contamination of the nursery environment by a variety of Gram-negative bacteria, staphylococci, and some common viruses (Table

Human and environmental factors determine common neonatal infections

**TABLE 69–1. MODES OF INFECTION AND MAJOR AGENTS**

| Mode | Agents | | |
|---|---|---|---|
| | ***Bacteria*** | ***Viruses*** | ***Other*** |
| Prenatal transplacental | *Listeria monocytogenes*; *Mycobacterium tuberculosis* (rare); *Treponema pallidum* | Rubella; cytomegalovirus; enteroviruses; Epstein–Barr virus; human immunodeficiency virus; parvovirus B19 | *Toxoplasma gondii; Plasmodium* sp. |
| Ascending | Group B streptococci; *Escherichia coli; Listeria monocytogenes* | Cytomegalovirus; herpes simplex | *Chlamydia trachomatis; Mycoplasma hominis; Ureaplasma urealyticum* |
| Natal | Group B streptococci; *Escherichia coli; Listeria monocytogenes; Neisseria gonorrhoeae* | Herpes simplex; cytomegalovirus; enteroviruses; hepatitis B; varicella–zoster; human immunodeficiency virus | *Chlamydia trachomatis* |
| Postnatal | *Escherichia coli*; group B streptococci; *Listeria monocytogenes*; miscellaneous Gram-negative bacteria; *Staphylococcus aureus; Staphylococcus epidermidis; Clostridium tetani* | Cytomegalovirus; herpes simplex; enteroviruses; varicella–zoster; respiratory syncytial virus; influenza viruses | |

69–1) and attendants who are infected with or carrying such organisms. The risks are increased if the infant is born prematurely or otherwise physically compromised, and they are amplified by prolonged hospitalization and invasive procedures such as respiratory intubation, mechanical ventilation, and intravenous treatment, as well as by blood or blood product transfusions.

Prematurity, prolonged hospitalization, and invasive procedures add risk

## EFFECT OF PRENATAL INFECTION ON PREGNANCY AND INTRAUTERINE DEVELOPMENT

All of the agents indicated in Table 69–1 as causing prenatal infections have the potential of creating an adverse pregnancy outcome, either as a result of compromising the health of the mother or by directly affecting the fetus. The effect can be untimely termination of pregnancy resulting in abortion, stillbirth, or prematurity, as well as developmental defects and fetal malnutrition.

## CLINICAL FEATURES, DIAGNOSIS, AND MANAGEMENT

### Acute Bacterial Sepsis

When a physician first encounters a sick newborn, the primary concern is whether the illness represents sepsis and/or meningitis caused by bacteria. This determination is important, because treatment is both feasible and extremely urgent. Clinical disease apparent at birth or developing within the first 3 days of life (early onset) has usually been acquired prenatally. Mortality can exceed 70%, even with prompt treatment. Later onset of symptoms is commonly associated with natal or postnatal acquisition of pathogens; however, these infections can also be severe. If meningitis develops, the overall mortality, even with treatment, ranges from 10 to 25%, and permanent neurologic damage may occur in 30 to 50% of survivors. The two pathogens most commonly associated with neonatal sepsis and meningitis are group B streptococci and *E. coli*.

Early onset neonatal infections may have 70% mortality

Group B streptococci and *E. coli* sepsis and meningitis the most common

Prematurity, prolonged rupture of membranes are risk factors

Diagnostic clues subtle in newborn

The diagnosis of neonatal infections is based first on clinical suspicion. There is sometimes a history of recent maternal febrile illness immediately before or at birth. Other suggestive features include fetal distress, prolonged rupture of membranes (>12 hours), foul-smelling amniotic fluid, and premature delivery. The first signs and symptoms of illness in the infant may be subtle and extremely variable, including respiratory distress, apneic episodes, cyanosis, irritability, unexplained jaundice, tachycardia, poor feeding, abdominal distention, and fever. Initial laboratory findings often include either leukocytosis, with an increased proportion of immature neutrophils, or leukopenia. The development of seizures, hypotension, or disseminated intravascular coagulation indicates a particularly grave prognosis.

Blood and cerebrospinal fluid culture done initially

Diagnostic tests for suspected infections must be initiated as quickly as possible, followed by empirical antimicrobial therapy while waiting for culture results. The major tests include examination and culture of cerebrospinal fluid and a blood culture. The antimicrobics initially chosen are those known to be effective against the pathogens most commonly encountered. They often include ampicillin for the streptococci (also useful for *L. monocytogenes*) and an aminoglycoside such as gentamicin for *E. coli.*

## OTHER BACTERIAL AND CHLAMYDIAL INFECTIONS

*Chlamydial* and gonococci produce severe conjunctivitis

Although *N. gonorrhoeae* and *C. trachomatis* are common natally acquired infections, they are usually not associated with sepsis. Both can produce a severe conjunctivitis in the newborn that requires prompt diagnosis and treatment. Gonococcal ophthalmia is usually apparent in the first 5 days after birth, whereas the onset of chlamydial conjunctivitis is frequently delayed until after the first week of life.

Chlamydial infant pneumonia syndrome occurs up to 6 months

Another significant illness associated with natally acquired *C. trachomatis* infection is infant pneumonia syndrome. The onset of respiratory symptoms is often delayed, with most cases occurring between 2 weeks and 6 months of age. This illness is also considered in Chapter 29.

Postnatal infections by *S. aureus* may cause scalded skin syndrome

Localized infections, such as cutaneous or subcutaneous abscesses, show a particular association with postnatally acquired *S. aureus* and occasionally with various Gram-negative bacteria. If the newborn is affected by a staphylococcal strain that produces exfoliative toxin, the local lesion may be relatively trivial in contrast to the more widespread effect of circulating toxin on the skin, which is termed the staphylococcal scalded-skin syndrome. Prompt treatment with an antistaphylococcal antimicrobial agent results in resolution of the disease within 2 weeks, usually with complete healing.

### Syphilis

Congential syphilis risk reduced by serologic screening and treatment during pregnancy

Prenatal infection by *Treponema pallidum* (congenital syphilis) is unusual in the United States, but if left untreated, the organism can produce long-term damage, often without apparent signs or symptoms in the newborn period. To minimize these risks, serologic screening is recommended for all pregnant women when first seen in early gestation and at delivery. An alternative to testing the mother at delivery is to screen sera from newborn infants. In addition, serologic testing is recommended whenever clinical or epidemiologic circumstances suggest the possibility of exposure at any time during pregnancy. Prompt treatment of infected mothers during pregnancy, preferably with penicillin, will markedly reduce the risk of fetal infection. Similar treatment is also effective for the infected infant.

### TORCH Complex

Toxoplasmosis, rubella, cytomegalovirus, herpes simplex are all common congenital pathogens

When bacterial, spirochetal, and chlamydial infections have been reasonably excluded from consideration, other possibilities can best be remembered by the convenient acronym TORCH (toxoplasmosis, other, rubella, cytomegalovirus, herpes simplex). This term comprises major infections that can be particularly severe if acquired prenatally. There is often significant overlap of clinical manifestations associated with the various agents in the

TORCH complex. Common features may include low birthweight, rash, jaundice, and hepatosplenomegaly. On the other hand, many newborn infants with TORCH infections can go undiagnosed, because the clinical signs may not appear until weeks, months, or even years later. For example, congenital cytomegalovirus infection may be manifested only as mild mental retardation and/or hearing loss that may not become apparent until after the first year of life. Toxoplasmosis also presents a dilemma. It is estimated that as many as 1 in 200 pregnancies in the United States is complicated by primary infection with *Toxoplasma gondii,* which is usually subclinical. Of these cases, approximately 45% result in fetal infection, but only 8 to 11% of the infected offspring demonstrate clinical symptoms in the newborn period. The remainder are at risk, however, and can ultimately develop neurologic deterioration and/or chorioretinitis, which may not be recognized until 5 or more years later. These observations only partially illustrate the importance of TORCH complex infections and our relative impotence in controlling many of them.

Clinical manifestations may be delayed for years

Of the array of miscellaneous agents grouped in the "other" category, three viruses deserve specific mention. If the mother has active infection with hepatitis B virus during pregnancy, the risk of natal or postnatal transmission to the infant is high (range, 20 to 80%, depending on the status of virus activity). Although it is unlikely that clinical disease will be apparent in the newborn period, it is important to promptly undertake specific measures to prevent infection in the infant when the mother is infected. They include immediate administration of hepatitis B immune globulin after birth as well as immunization of the infant with hepatitis B vaccine. The chance of maternal transmission of the human immunodeficiency virus, either transplacentally or natally, is estimated to be between 12.9 and 65%. Primary varicella is infrequent in pregnancy. If the mother develops varicella less than 5 days before or 2 days after delivery, however, the risk of severe neonatal varicella is significant, with a mortality of approximately 20%. It is recommended that the infant be given varicella–zoster immune globulin (or zoster immune globulin) immediately in an attempt to prevent or modify subsequent disease. Maternal zoster infections are not associated with a significant risk to the offspring, presumably because of adequate transplacental transmission of specific antibody.

Hepatitis B infection prevented by HIB administration

HIV transmission is efficient

Neonatal varicella from infected mother severe if contracted

The approach to a suspected TORCH complex infection requires some thought in selection of appropriate tests. Appendix 69–1 summarizes the major clinical and historic features of specific agents and the diagnostic procedures that can be used. The following general comments should also be kept in mind:

1. Clinical and epidemiologic data are used as much as possible in ascertaining likely specific agents.
2. Probabilities must be weighed; for example, congenital cytomegalovirus infection is by far the most frequent TORCH complex agent encountered in the United States (more than 90% of all proved cases).
3. Potentially treatable infections must be considered first. If toxoplasmosis or herpes simplex is suggested by the historic and clinical findings, it may be controlled by prompt and aggressive therapy. Other infections, which are potentially preventable by early specific immunoglobulin therapy of the infant, include maternal varicella and hepatitis B infections. The remaining agents involved in the TORCH array are not amenable to specific therapy at present. Their importance lies more in long-term prognosis, planning of continuing care, and epidemiologic management.
4. Serologic testing, when indicated, should be done on both infant and maternal sera collected at the same time to facilitate interpretation of specific antibody titer levels in the infant. This approach is based upon the following principles: passive transplacental transmission of IgG antibodies occurs, but these maternal antibodies normally wane and disappear in the infant over 3 to 6 months. If the infant is actively infected, it usually produces its own specific antibodies to the agent, which then persist for much longer periods. Thus, a specific antibody titer in the infant's serum during the first month of life equal to or less than that of the mother may merely reflect passive transfer, and does not support a diagnosis of active infection. On the other hand, if the infant's titer is significantly higher than the mother's (fourfold or greater) or rises progressively in serial samples obtained in later months, active infection by the agent in question is suggested.

Focus on treatable conditions

Comparisons with maternal antibody titers aids diagnosis of infection in infant

Infant IgM antibodies suggest acute infection

In active congenital and neonatal infections, the infant's early responses often include IgM antibodies. As maternal IgM antibodies rarely cross the placental barrier, specific IgM antibody determinations early in life may be useful for the diagnosis of congenital toxoplasma, rubella, and cytomegalovirus infections. However, both false-positive and false-negative results have been noted. The presence of rheumatoid factor has been a major cause of false-positive results. Tests with high specificity include solid-phase IgM assays with antihuman IgM as a "capture" antibody and enzyme-linked antibody markers.

Nonspecific tests, such as quantitation of total IgM or IgA or detection of rheumatoid factor, have limited or no usefulness. Negative results do not rule out infection, and positive results must be regarded cautiously. Other tests, such as lymphocyte stimulation with specific antigens, show some promise, but are not yet available in enough centers to recommend them routinely.

5. In fetal and neonatal infections, such as those caused by human immunodeficiency virus, specific antibody testing is not usually helpful in establishing a diagnosis in the first 15 to 18 months of life. Tests for p24 antigenemia, blood culture, or polymerase chain reaction methods for viral nucleic acid detection are preferred and may need to be serially repeated if initially negative.

## CONCLUSION

Fetal and neonatal infections remain a highly significant and often frustrating challenge. They can be severe, and permanent sequelae are common. At the onset of infection, clinical signs and symptoms are often exceedingly subtle; thus, the physician must be quickly alerted to the infectious possibilities, particularly when specific treatment is available. Of all of these infections, the most preventable is rubella, and assurance of immunity before conception is a mandatory goal. Better control of the remainder may become possible in the future with newer bacterial and viral vaccines, better early diagnostic methods, and improved treatment methods.

## APPENDIX 69–1. TORCH COMPLEX: SALIENT FEATURES AND DIAGNOSTIC TESTS

### Toxoplasmosis

**Suggestive clinical findings.** Chorioretinitis (found in more than 90% of symptomatic neonatal cases); lymphadenopathy.

**Maternal history.** Usually negative; occasional cervical lymphadenopathy during pregnancy.

**Tests of choice.** Specific maternal and infant antibody titers; follow-up titers may be helpful.

### Other Infections

The list of causes includes enteroviruses, hepatitis B, human immunodeficiency virus, varicella–zoster, Epstein–Barr virus, arthropod-borne viruses, malaria, and tuberculosis. As the agents in this category most commonly encountered are the enteroviruses, the features summarized here pertain primarily to them.

**Suggestive clinical findings.** Sepsislike syndromes; meningitis; myocarditis (findings are variable).

**Maternal history.** Fever common at or near parturition.

**Tests of Choice.** Viral cultures of throat, rectum, and cerebrospinal fluid.

### Rubella

**Suggestive clinical findings.** Congenital malformations, often multiple. In severe cases, "celery stalking" of metaphyses of long bones may be seen in early radiographs (see also cytomegalovirus).

**Maternal history.** Rubellalike illness or epidemiologic history of exposure in early pregnancy is common. If available, maternal serologic and immunization history can aid in supporting or refuting this diagnostic possibility.

**Tests of choice.** Maternal and infant antibody titers, including IgM-specific antibody testing in the infant. Serial determinations over 6 months may be of additional help. Culture is not a readily available routine test in most hospitals; special arrangements must be made.

### Cytomegalovirus

**Suggestive clinical findings.** None very specific in differentiating infection from most others in the group. Statistically, cytomegalovirus is the most common congenital infection encountered. In florid cases, early radiographs of the long bones may resemble those of congenital rubella (celery stalking).

**Maternal history.** Usually none; occasionally, an account of a mononucleosislike syndrome may be elicited.

**Tests of choice.** Urine culture is the most sensitive test. If results are negative, this diagnosis is highly unlikely; if positive, the diagnosis is supported (especially if cultures are done in the first 3 weeks of life). With advancing age of the infant, however, positive cultures may require careful interpretation before an unequivocal diagnosis is made.

### Herpes Simplex

**Suggestive clinical findings.** Cutaneous vesicles and/or ocular or mucous membrane ulcerations: however, these lesions may not become apparent until other signs of illness have developed.

**Maternal history.** Up to 70% have no history of genital lesions or symptoms. Others may have a history of recent primary symptomatic infection. It is also important to ascertain whether genital lesions were known to exist in recent sexual partners.

**Tests of choice.** Culture of lesions; immunofluorescent and cytologic studies may be available for rapid diagnosis. If no lesions are present, throat culture is also a valuable source. Brain biopsy and urine and cerebrospinal cultures may also be necessary in some cases. Maternal cultures, if positive, may give indirect support regarding etiology.

Chapter 70

# Sexually Transmitted Diseases

W. Lawrence Drew

With the emergence of AIDS in the 1980s sexually transmitted diseases (STDs) received increased attention, although they have long been a major public health problem in all population groups and social strata. The most common agents are *Neisseria gonorrhoeae*, *Chlamydia trachomatis*, genital herpes simplex virus, genital papillomavirus, and now, the most worrisome, human immunodeficiency virus (HIV) and AIDS. Table 70–1 lists the major sexually transmitted pathogens and the disease syndromes associated with them. These infections are discussed in detail in chapters related to the etiologic agents.

By definition, STDs are infections transmitted by sexual activity involving contact between the genitalia of one sexual partner and the genitalia, or other mucosal surface, of the other partner. Depending on the pathogen the disease produced may be local or systemic. For the localized STDs, for example, gonorrhea and herpes, the most common manifestations are at the genital site as a focal lesion (pustule, ulcer) or inflammation (urethritis, cervicitis) which may or may not be noticed by the patient. In some cases deeper structures become involved when the infection spreads beyond the local site by direct extension (epididymitis, salpingitis). As with other infectious diseases some of these can gain access to the bloodstream and produce systemic symptoms and spread to other organs. The systemic STDs, for example, AIDS and syphilis, produce infection beyond the genital site as part of their basic pathogenesis and may or may not produce a local genital lesion. The most common clinical syndromes are discussed next.

Some STDs start as localized infection; others are primarily systemic

## GENITAL ULCERS

Single or multiple ulcerative lesions on the genitalia are one of the most common manifestations of STDs. The infection may begin as a papule or pustule and evolve into an ulcer. Table 70–2 lists the major features of genital ulcerations. The nature of the ulcer and whether it is painful are significant differential features. The ulcer (chancre) of syphilis is typically firm and indurated but painless, whereas genital herpes ulcers are more friable and quite painful. The evaluation of genital ulcers usually focuses on separation of genital herpes, the most common cause in industrialized nations, and syphilis from other causes. It should be recalled that the dark-field exam and serologic tests may be negative at the time of presentation of the syphilitic chancre and that culture for *Haemophilus ducreyi*, the cause of chancroid, requires a special selective medium.

Pain and induration are major differential features

Granuloma inguinale, a disease seen primarily in developing countries, is characterized by chronic, persistent genital papules or ulcers. It is caused by *Calymmatobacterium*

Persistent papules or ulcers

**TABLE 70–1. SEXUALLY TRANSMITTED AGENTS AND DISEASES CAUSED**

| Agent | Disease or Syndrome |
|---|---|
| Bacteria | |
| *Neisseria gonorrhoeae* | Urethritis, cervicitis, proctitis, pharyngitis, conjunctivitis, endometritis, pelvic inflammatory disease, perihepatitis, bartholinitis, disseminated gonococcal infection |
| *Chlamydia trachomatis* | Nongonococcal urethritis, epididymitis, cervicitis, salpingitis, inclusion conjunctivitis, infant pneumonia, trachoma, lymphogranuloma venereum |
| *Ureaplasma urealyticum* | Nongonococcal urethritis |
| *Treponema pallidum* | Syphilis |
| *Haemophilus ducreyi* | Chancroid |
| *Calymmatobacterium granulomatis* | Granuloma inguinale |
| Viruses | |
| HIV | AIDS, AIDS-related complex (ARC), perinatal and congenital AIDS, aseptic meningitis, subacute neurologic syndromes, persistent generalized adenopathy, asymptomatic infection |
| Herpes simplex virus | Primary and recurrent genital herpes, aseptic meningitis, neonatal herpes |
| Papillomavirus | Condylomata accuminata, laryngeal papilloma of newborn, association with cervical carcinoma |
| Cytomegalovirus | Heterophil-negative infectious mononucleosis, congenital birth defects |
| Hepatitis B virus | Hepatitis B, acute and chronic infections |
| Molluscum contagiosum virus | Genital molluscum contagiosum |
| Protozoa | |
| *Trichomonas vaginalis* | Trichomonal vaginitis |
| Fungi | |
| *Candida albicans* | Vulvovaginitis, penile candidiasis |
| Ectoparasites | |
| *Phthirus pubis* | Pubic louse infestation |
| *Sarcoptes scabiei* | Scabies |

*C. granulomatis* shows encapsulated Gram-negative bacilli on smear

*granulomatis*, an encapsulated Gram-negative bacillus which has not been grown in artificial medium. The diagnosis is usually made by examination of Wright- or Giemsa-stained impression smears from biopsy specimens of the lesion that demonstrate clusters of encapsulated coccobacilli in the cytoplasm of mononuclear cells. Tetracycline is the treatment of choice.

**TABLE 70–2. CAUSES OF GENITAL ULCERATIONS**

| Disease | Type of Lesion | Type of Inguinal Adenopathy[a] | Diagnosis |
|---|---|---|---|
| Genital herpes | Multiple grouped lesions, vesicles to coalesced ulcers, painful | Tender, discrete, nonsuppurative | Culture, enzyme immunoassay |
| Chancroid | Tender, shallow, painful, not indurated | Suppurative | Culture |
| Syphilis | Nontender, indurated | Rubbery consistency | Dark-field exam, serology |
| Lymphogranuloma venereum | Painless, small ulcer or papule, usually healed at time of presentation | Discrete progressing to suppurative, draining fistulas | Culture, serology |
| Granuloma inguinale | Chronic indolent, papular lesions | "Pseudobubo" caused by induration of subcutaneous tissue in inguinal area | Wright stain, biopsy |

[a] Involvement of inguinal lymph nodes.

## GENITAL WARTS

Genital warts may be caused by *Treponema pallidum* (condyloma latum) or human papillomavirus (condyloma accuminatum). There are over 50 genome types of human papillomavirus (HPV), of which types 6, 11, 16, 18, and 32 are the predominant causes of genital warts. In women, HPV types 16, 18, and 31 are usually associated with flat or subclinical warts and are the viral types commonly associated with cervical dysplasias, carcinoma in situ, and invasive cervical cancer. Condylomata lata are painless mucosal warty erosions that develop in warm, moist sites such as the genitals and perineum in about one third of cases of secondary syphilis. Dark-field examinations are invariably positive as are both nontreponemal and treponemal serologic tests.

Many genome types of papillomaviruses

Some types associated with carcinoma of the cervix

## URETHRITIS

Urethritis usually manifests as dysuria, urethral discharge, or both. The discharge may be prominent enough to be the chief complaint or may have to be milked from the urethra. In the absence of expressible discharge, the presence of polymorphonuclear leukocytes in a urine sediment or on a urethral swab suggests urethritis. The major causes of urethritis are *N. gonorrhoeae* and *C. trachomatis* followed by *Ureaplasma urealyticum* and herpes simplex virus. Infection with more than one organism is common, particularly dual gonococcal and chlamydial infection. Up to 20% of cases have no established etiology but are probably infectious.

*C. trachomatis* and *N. gonorrhoeae* often together

*U. urealyticum* and HSV less common

The diagnosis of gonorrhea is established primarily by culture although Gram smears may suffice in symptomatic men. Culture is the most sensitive diagnostic technique for the other agents but for technical reasons is not readily available. Direct nonculture methods have been developed for *C. trachomatis* that may meet this need in the future (see Chapter 29). The practice of simply excluding gonorrhea is responsible for the terms nongonococcal urethritis and postgonococcal urethritis, which lump together the other causes. Treatment depends on the etiologic agent and the progression of disease beyond the local site. Empiric regimens are directed at the two most common causes, *N. gonorrhoeae* and *C. trachomatis*. In cases of gonorrhea concurrent treatment for chlamydia is recommended unless the later has been specifically excluded. This might require, for example, ceftriaxone plus doxycycline. In general, the same approach is followed for epididymitis, cervicitis, and vaginitis unless another diagnosis has been established.

Gonorrhea diagnosed by culture

Nonculture methods available for *Chlamydia*

Combined treatment common

## EPIDIDYMITIS

Unilateral swelling of the epididymis is a common clinical illness seen in sexually active men. It is usually quite painful, with fever and acute unilateral swelling of the testicle that is sometimes confused with testicular torsion. In the preantibiotic era, approximately 10 to 15% of untreated gonococcal infections resulted in epididymitis. In developed countries, the two most common causes of epididymitis are *N. gonorrhoeae* and *C. trachomatis*. In men older than 35 and in homosexual men, Enterobacteriaceae and *Staphylococcus epidermidis* may also cause the disease, probably from reflux of infected urine into the epididymis. This condition is often associated with obstruction by the prostate gland. Treatment depends on demonstration of the etiologic agent in urethral specimens or epididymal aspirates.

Gonococcal and chlamydial infection in young men

Enterobacterial and *S. epidermidis* infection more common in older men

## CERVICITIS

The microbial etiology of cervical infections is varied; *N. gonorrhoeae* and *C. trachomatis* cause endocervicitis, and herpes simplex virus can infect the stratified squamous epithelium of the ectocervix. The major clinical manifestation of cervicitis is a mucopurulent vaginal discharge. The cervix is friable and inflamed, and polymorphonuclear leukocytes are present in the exudate. Viral, chlamydial, and gonococcal cultures are needed to demonstrate

Gonococcal, chlamydial, and HSV infections most common

the etiologic agent. Occasionally, other pathogens such as cytomegalovirus and *Trichomonas vaginalis* are associated with symptomatic cervicitis. Therapy depends on the etiologic agent involved.

## VAGINITIS AND VAGINAL DISCHARGE

Pelvic exam, nature of discharge define source

Symptomatic vaginal discharge may accompany salpingitis, endometritis, cervicitis, or a simple vaginitis. Evaluation includes pelvic examination, cervical cultures for *N. gonorrhoeae* and *C. trachomatis*, and microscopic examination of the discharge. Measurement of the pH of the discharge may also be helpful. Pelvic examination is valuable in determining whether uterine, adnexal, or cervical tenderness is present and whether the source of the discharge is the cervix or the vagina.

*Candida vaginitis* causes itching, thick discharge

The clinical and laboratory findings vary with the etiologic agent. *Candida albicans* generally produces a vulvovaginitis associated with pruritus and erythema of the vulvar area and a discharge with the consistency of cottage cheese. Microscopic demonstration of yeast and pseudomycelia in a potassium hydroxide preparation of the exudate confirms the diagnosis. *Candida* vaginitis can be treated with local nystatin or miconazole.

Trichomonas infection produces foamy discharge

*Trichomonas vaginalis* typically produces a foamy, purulent vaginal discharge. The pH is variable (usually greater than 5.0), and numerous polymorphonuclear cells and motile trichomonads are seen on wet mount examination. Metronidazole is effective therapy for *T. vaginalis* vaginitis. Sexual partners should also be treated.

Bacterial vaginosis a shift in flora with anaerobic overgrowth

Bacterial vaginosis (BV), previously termed *nonspecific vaginitis*, is the most common form of vaginitis in women. BV is associated with overgrowth of multiple members of the vaginal anaerobic flora, genital mycoplasmas, and a small Gram-negative rod (*Gardnerella vaginalis*) once believed to be the sole cause of the disease. BV is probably of multiple etiology and more a result of disturbance in anaerobic flora than of any specific organism. The vaginal discharge of BV is yellowish, homogenous, and adherent to the vaginal wall. The pH is greater than 5.0. Addition of KOH to the vaginal secretions produces a fishy smell as a result of volatilization of amines. The Gram stain shows a shift from the usual lactobacillary flora to one of many Gram-negative coccobacilli. Clue cells, which are vaginal epithelial cells heavily coated with *G. vaginalis*, may also be seen.

Clue cells present, lactobacilli absent

Metronidazole treatment of BV

Metronidazole is the most effective agent in treatment; clindamycin is recommended as an alternative. Relapses are common. It is uncertain whether treatment of sexual partners has any effect on the remission rate.

## PELVIC INFLAMMATORY DISEASE

Multiple etiologic agents *N. gonorrhoeae* predominant

Clinical manifestations of pelvic inflammatory disease (PID) vary, but generally include lower abdominal pain elicited by movement of the cervix or palpation of the adnexal or endometrial areas. About one half of cases are caused by *N. gonorrhoeae*. Nongonococcal PID has a complex and sometimes polymicrobial etiology, including *C. trachomatis*, *Bacteroides*, anaerobic streptococci, and *Mycoplasma hominis* alone or in various combinations. In general, nongonococcal PID is milder than that associated with *N. gonorrhoeae* infection. The incidence of PID is 5 to 10 times higher in women with intrauterine devices than in those not using this form of contraception. The diagnosis is established most reliably by culture of peritoneal aspirates from the vaginal cul-de-sac. Treatment of PID is complex because of the multiple etiologies and relative inaccessibility of the definitive diagnostic specimen. Antimicrobic combinations with predictable activity against gonococci, *C. trachomatis*, and anaerobes are usually employed. Examples include cefoxitin plus doxycycline, clindamycin plus gentamicin, and ceftriaxone plus doxycycline.

Incidence higher with use of intrauterine devices

## SYSTEMIC SYNDROMES

As indicated earlier, some STDs may manifest important pathology outside the genital tract including diseases such as cytomegalovirus which may be transmitted sexually but are not usually considered primary sexual pathogens. Syphilis and AIDS are both diseases in which the most common means of transmission is sexual, but the most devastating consequences come from infection at other sites. Both syphilis and AIDS are also highly complex, involving multiple organs and long latent periods. These organisms and diseases are best reviewed by referring back to Chapters 26 and 41.

Most serious effects of syphilis and AIDS outside of genital tract

## ADDITIONAL READING

Adimara AA, Hamilton H, Holmes KK, Sparling PF. *Sexually Transmitted Diseases*. 2nd ed. New York: McGraw-Hill; 1994. This updated pocket version of the larger treatise edited by Holmes and others is a handy synopsis of the definitive textbook on the subject.

Cates W Jr, Wasserheit JN. Genital chlamydial infections: Epidemiology and reproductive sequelae. *Am J Obstet Gynecol*. 1991;164:1771–1781. Failure to control chlamydial infections reflects four factors: (1) Many cases are mild or asymptomatic, (2) diagnostic tests are expensive and technically demanding, (3) at least 7 days of multiple-dose therapy is currently required, and (4) partner notification is not routinely performed.

Chapter 71

# Infections in the Immunocompromised Patient

*W. Lawrence Drew*

Immunocompromised patients are those whose host defense mechanisms are impaired by an underlying deficit (agammaglobulinemia), disease (AIDS), or treatment (steroids). This immunocompromised state is known to predispose these patients to infection with many of the common pathogens as well as with low-virulence organisms present in the normal flora or environment. The organisms involved are those most able to take advantage of situations such as disruption of the skin or mucosal barriers and the more specific immune defects, including (1) defects in the phagocytic response, (2) defects in the complement system, (3) defects in antibody-mediated immunity, (4) defects in cell-mediated immunity, and (5) loss of reticuloendothelial function. Each of these defects tends to be associated with infections caused by specific groups of organisms (Table 71–1). For example, neutropenia and disorders of phagocytosis are associated with infections by Gram-positive cocci, Enterobacteriaceae, *Pseudomonas*, and fungi. In contrast, patients with defects in cell-mediated immunity tend to have severe viral, parasitic, and fungal infections or disease caused by bacteria that can multiply intracellularly (eg, mycobacteria). Those with defects in antibody production, such as agammaglobulinemia, are prone to infection with encapsulated organisms such as *Streptococcus pneumoniae* and *Haemophilus influenzae* type b.

Different types of immunocompromise are associated with different infecting organisms

## IMMUNE DEFICITS ASSOCIATED WITH INFECTION

### Defects in Epithelial Barriers

Defects in mucosal barriers represent an important prelude to infection by allowing organisms that normally colonize the skin, gastrointestinal tract, or upper airway access to deeper more vulnerable tissues. Burns, extensive trauma, and decubitus ulcers remove the epithelial defense of the skin; however, less obvious factors, such as inhalation of toxic materials and cytotoxic therapy, may cause damage to mucosal surfaces that predisposes to attachment and replication of potentially pathogenic organisms and can cause loss of host-clearing mechanisms (eg, ciliary function). Defects in intestinal mucosal barriers are often associated with infections caused by Gram-negative aerobic and anaerobic enteric bacteria from the gut flora. Staphylococcal, streptococcal, and pneumococcal infections of the lung are

Burns, trauma allow access of organisms from environment or mucosal surfaces

**TABLE 71–1. INFECTIONS IN THE COMPROMISED HOST**

| Type of Compromise | Example | Pathogen |
|---|---|---|
| ↓ Leukocyte number or function | Myelocytic leukemias<br>Chronic granulomatous disease<br>Granulocytopenia<br>Acidosis<br>Burns | Extracellular bacteria[a]<br>Opportunistic fungi |
| ↓ Humoral immune response | Lymphocytic leukemias<br>Multiple myeloma<br>Nephrosis<br>Antimetabolites<br>Hypogammaglobulinemia<br>Childhood AIDS | Encapsulated bacteria[b]<br>Enteroviruses<br>*Pneumocystis*<br>*Giardia*[c] |
| ↓ Complement components | Genetic deficiencies | Extracellular bacteria[a]<br>*Neisseria*[d] |
| ↓ Cellular immune response | AIDS<br>Hodgkin's disease<br>Steroids<br>Uremia<br>Antimetabolites<br>Malnutrition | *Pneumocystis*<br>Intracellular bacteria[e]<br>*Nocardia*<br>*Candida* and fungi of systemic mycoses<br>Viruses, especially herpesviruses<br>Protozoa[f]<br>*Strongyloides* |
| ↓ Reticuloendothelial system function | Splenectomy<br>Chronic hemolysis | *Pneumococcus*<br>*Salmonella*<br>*Listeria* |

[a] Bacteria that are unable to multiply in phagocytes.
[b] For example, *Streptococcus pneumoniae*, *Haemophilus influenzae* type b.
[c] Associated with IgA deficiency.
[d] Associated with C5, C6, C7, and C8 deficiencies.
[e] Bacteria capable of multiplying in unactivated macrophage.
[f] Includes *Toxoplasma* and *Cryptosporidium*.

particularly likely when the respiratory epithelium is damaged, whereas *Pseudomonas aeruginosa* infections are a common feature of severe burns.

## Defects in Number or Function of Phagocytes

When the natural barriers of the skin and mucosal surfaces are breached, the next major line of defense is the circulating phagocytes. To defend against infection, there must be an adequate number of these cells, which must be able to move to the site of infection and ingest and kill invading organisms. Numerous defects in these processes have been described.

### Neutropenia

Neutropenia <500/mm$^3$ associated with infection; <100/mm$^3$ with bloodstream spread

Although normal neutrophil granulocyte counts vary greatly according to the age, sex, and race of the patient, the usual value is 2500 to 7500 cells/mm$^3$ of blood in adults. Neutropenia may result from inherited or acquired diseases, malignancies, use of cytotoxic drugs, or adverse reactions to therapeutic agents such as chloramphenicol. If the absolute neutrophil count decreases to fewer than 500 cells/mm$^3$, the incidence of infections increases markedly and counts below 100 cells/mm$^3$ are associated with spread to the bloodstream. Severe neutropenia is accompanied most frequently by bacterial infections caused by the pyogenic Gram-positive cocci, Enterobacteriaceae, *P. aeruginosa*, and *H. influenzae*. Fungal infections with *Candida*, *Aspergillus*, or the Zygomycetes are also common.

### Defects in Chemotaxis and Leukocytic Function

Defects in phagocytic defenses can be caused by multiple mechanisms that result in inadequate leukocyte chemotaxis or function (Table 71–2). Deficiencies of complement or immunoglobulins can decrease chemoattractants at the site of an infection, and certain

**TABLE 71–2. DISORDERS OF PHAGOCYTOSIS AND INTRACELLULAR PHAGOCYTIC KILLING**

| Chemotactic Defects | Ingestion |
|---|---|
| Complement component deficiency | Actin–myosin dysfunction |
| Immunoglobulin deficiency | Drugs (colchicine, tetracycline, cyclophosphamide) |
| Intrinsic defects | Hyperosmolar states |
| "Lazy leukocytes" | Acute infections |
| Burns | **Degranulation** |
| Hyperimmunoglobulin syndrome (Job's syndrome) | Chédiak–Higashi syndrome |
| Collagen vascular disease | |
| **Opsonization** | **Killing** |
| Immunoglobulin deficiency | Lysosomal enzyme deficiency |
| Complement component deficiency | Chronic granulomatous disease |
| Interference by immune complexes (systemic lupus erythematosus) | Glucose-6-phosphate dehydrogenase deficiency |
| Sickle cell anemia | Drugs (phenylbutazone, chloramphenicol) |
| | Glutathione reductase deficiency |

metabolic diseases such as diabetes and uremia can alter the microenvironment of leukocytes to reduce their mobility and responsiveness to tactic stimuli. This phenomenon has also been shown to occur in immune complex diseases such as lupus erythematosus. In each case, removal of the leukocyte to a normal environment restores its mobility and ability to respond chemotactically.

Diabetes, uremia can impair function

Several genetic diseases produce specific defects in granulocyte bactericidal mechanisms that result in an immunocompromised host. Because they frequently diminish life span, these illnesses are usually seen in children. That most studied is chronic granulomatous disease, a group of inherited disorders of phagocytic cell superoxide production associated with frequent pyogenic infections, usually caused by *Staphylococcus aureus*. In another disease, the Chédiak–Higashi syndrome, neutrophil lysosomes fail to fuse with the phagosome and the cells fail to destroy ingested organisms. These children also suffer recurrent infections with pyogenic organisms.

Chronic granulomatous disease due to lack of superoxide

Chédiak–Higashi disease; failure lysosome–phagosome fusion

The spectrum of infections in patients with phagocytic dysfunction is wide and includes repeated bouts of cellulitis, pharyngitis, perirectal and other abscesses, pneumonia, osteomyelitis, and bacteremia. Many pyogenic organisms other than staphylococci can be involved. Antimicrobic treatment given either therapeutically or prophylactically has helped greatly in the care of these patients, but they still suffer repeated bouts of infection that may ultimately prove fatal. Leukocyte transfusions benefit some patients.

Prophylactic antimicrobics, leukocyte transfusions may be helpful

## Antibody Deficiency

Several congenital and acquired disorders can lead to inadequate synthesis of immunoglobulins as a result of deficiency or dysfunction of B lymphocytes. The most common and least serious is immunoglobulin A deficiency, which is associated with increased risk of gastrointestinal tract infection, especially with the parasite *Giardia lamblia*. Individuals with severe defects in IgG and IgM production (hypogammaglobulinemia or agammaglobulinemia) are prone to recurrent infections with encapsulated organisms such as *Streptococcus pneumoniae* or *Haemophilus influenzae*, which require opsonization for adequate phagocytosis. Sinusitis, otitis media, bacterial pneumonia, and bacteremia are the most common types of infection. Acquired deficiency in immunoglobulin production may occur in AIDS, multiple myeloma, non-Hodgkin's lymphoma, and certain types of chronic lymphocytic leukemia that involve monoclonal proliferation of one immunoglobulin-producing cell line and relative deficiencies of cells producing other antibodies. These patients are also prone to infections by systemically invasive organisms.

IgA deficiency associated with giardiasis

IgA and IgM deficiency infection with encapsulated organisms

Acquired antibody deficiency in AIDS, multiple myeloma, and leukemia

Repeated injections of immunoglobulins (immune serum globulin) may decrease the incidence and morbidity of infections in patients with hypo- or agammaglobulinemia. In those capable of some immune responses, the use of pneumococcal vaccine (Pneumovax) may provide a degree of protection against overwhelming infection with this organism.

Immune serum globulin or some vaccines useful

## Complement Deficiency

Opsonization defects with C3 deficiency

Systemic *Neisseria* infections in C5–8 deficiencies

Defects of the complement system also predispose the patient to many infections. Individuals with deficiencies in C3 are prone to infections with encapsulated organisms that require opsonization and to a range of infections similar to those seen in patients with hypogammaglobulinemia. Those with deficiencies in later components are prone to develop recurrent bacteremia caused by *Neisseria meningitidis* or *Neisseria gonorrhoeae* if they are infected with these species. Patients with defects in the early complement components, C1, C2, or C4, have less of a problem than those with later complement deficiencies, because they retain the ability to use the alternative complement pathway to activate C3 and hence C5 to C9.

## Disorders in Cell-Mediated Immunity

Congenital CMI abnormalities rare

CD4+ lymphocytes compromised in AIDS

Glucocorticoids have multiple effects on immune cell production and function

Both congenital and acquired abnormalities of the cell-mediated immune system occur. Congenital abnormalities, which are uncommon, include thymic dysplasia syndrome, ataxia telangiectasia, and severe combined immunodeficiency (both T- and B-cell deficiency). AIDS, now the most important cause of acquired cellular immunodeficiency, acts through infection of CD4+ T lymphocytes. Another common source of acquired defects is treatment with immunosuppressive or cytotoxic agents that damage both macrophage precursors and T lymphocytes. Cytotoxic chemotherapy for cancer with cyclophosphamide and other antimetabolites has these effects and also inhibits humoral immune responses. Glucocorticoids can have multiple effects, causing neutropenia, lymphopenia, and monocytopenia through suppression of cell production, inhibition of mobilization of neutrophils to the site of inflammation, and interference with cell-mediated immune responses through alteration of the responsiveness of monocytes and macrophages to lymphokines. In addition, glucocorticoids impair the function of cells lining the mucosal surfaces, thus increasing the chance of microbial invasion by this route. Combinations of glucocorticosteroids and immunosuppressive drugs are essential in the treatment of certain diseases, but are particularly likely to interfere with the ability of a patient to combat new or established infections.

A general increased susceptibility to intracellular pathogens

Mycobacterial infections becoming epidemiologic problem in hospitals

A detailed analysis of the infections associated with the different causes of cell-mediated and combined immune deficits is beyond the scope of this chapter. In general, defects in cell-mediated immunity are associated with increased susceptibility to infection with some opportunistic pathogens, particularly facultative or obligate intracellular pathogens such as cytomegalovirus (see Table 71–1). For example, infection with *Mycobacterium tuberculosis* and other mycobacteria among AIDS patients has grown to a degree that secondary transmission of the mycobacteria to health care workers has become a major concern. Because of the wide range of potential infecting organisms, the sites of infection associated with defects in cell-mediated immunity are varied. These include superficial skin infections, lung infections, pharyngitis, otitis, sinusitis, bacteremia, and abscesses. Infections with multiple organisms are common.

# CLINICAL SITUATIONS ASSOCIATED WITH INFECTION

## Acquired Immunodeficiency Syndrome

AIDS the dominant immunocompromised state

The increasing prevalence and profound immunodeficiency of AIDS patients increasingly dominate the topic of this chapter in medical practice. AIDS is now the leading cause of death in men between the ages of 22 and 44 in the United States. Most of them die as a direct result of one of the infections mentioned earlier and discussed in more detail in Chapter 41.

## Malignancies

Although some malignancies compromise the immune system directly, the chemotherapeutic agents used to treat them are the primary cause of immunosuppression. In particular, the periods of granulocytopenia between the administration of high-dose chemotherapy and recovery of granulocyte-producing function are associated with infection. The organisms most common during this vulnerable period are generally the same as among the general population, for example, *Staphylococcus aureus* and *Escherichia coli*, but other pathogens like *Pseudomonas aeruginosa* and *Candida albicans* are more prominent than in the immunocompetent individual. As discussed earlier, chemotherapy may also compromise cell-mediated immunity, in which case the intracellular bacteria and viruses are more common.

Chemotherapy of malignancy commonly compromises granulocytes

## Transplantation

Solid organ and bone marrow transplantations are among the most important advances in modern medicine. Their success is due substantially to the ability to control and manage the desired and undesired aspects of the immunosuppressive regimens used. The undesired aspects are primarily the susceptibility to infection as long as immunosuppression is used. The pattern of microorganisms varies with the type of transplant, as does the immunosuppressive therapy, but is predominantly viral. Viruses of the herpesvirus family are the most common. The bacteria associated with both granulocyte depression and cell-mediated immune system are also involved. *Legionella* and *Nocardia* infections have been particularly prominent in kidney and heart transplant recipients. Recombinant granulocyte–macrophage colony-stimulating factor can accelerate the recovery of bone marrow myeloid elements in bone marrow transplant and some cancer chemotherapy patients and thereby shorten the period of vulnerability.

Herpesvirus family infections particularly common

*Legionella* and *Norcardia* in heart and kidney transplants

# DIAGNOSIS

Clinical recognition and treatment of infections in the immunocompromised patient are often difficult, because the infection may be relatively silent due to mutation of the immune response. Laboratory diagnosis can also be difficult, because many of the organisms involved require special culture media and grow slowly; others such as *Pneumocystis carinii* cannot be grown at all. The increased involvement of low-virulence organisms commonly found in the normal flora may make it difficult to distinguish colonization from infection. Thus, isolation of *Candida albicans* from the urine or the pharynx does not prove that it is the cause of a concurrent renal abscess or pneumonitis. Diagnostic procedures such as biopsy of involved organs are often needed to identify the causative agent.

Diagnosis often requires aggressive procedures

# TREATMENT

Successful treatment of infections in the compromised host depends on recognition of the deficit, early diagnosis, and prompt intervention. This requires recognition of the organisms most likely to be involved in the infection and is urgent in the case of classes of bacteria with short generation times. The index of suspicion must be very high, because the signs and symptoms of infection that are seen in immunocompetent individuals may be lacking. For example, in neutropenia the clinical signs of infection and even of abscess formation may not be apparent when the patient is first seen because of lack of reaction to the disease. It is thus usually necessary to initiate antimicrobic treatment before results of culture and antibiotic susceptibility tests are available. Broad-spectrum antimicrobic coverage is used initially and replaced with narrower-spectrum agents, when the etiologic agent and its susceptibility are known, to reduce the risk of superinfection. In general, bactericidal antimicrobics are needed to control infections when host defenses are inadequate, and with severe infections a combination of synergistic agents may be necessary to provide increased bactericidal action.

Early diagnosis and treatment particularly important

Bactericidal antimicrobics required

Patients with neutropenia have high rates of infection, and mortality may be as high as 20 to 30% if bacteremia develops. Therefore, short-term prophylactic antibiotic treatment has been advocated for these cases and can be effective in preventing infection until

Antimicrobic prophylaxis used during periods of neutropenia

the neutrophil count improves. Selection of resistant organisms and "breakthrough" bacteremia as a result of overwhelming infection are major risks in these susceptible patients, and the physician must be alert to the possibility of superinfection with other pathogens during treatment.

Attempts to enhance cell-mediated immune responses specifically or nonspecifically with agents that have shown some activity in animals generally have had little, if any, effect in reducing the frequency and severity of opportunistic infections in humans. There is increasing attention to prevention of opportunistic infections in patients disposed to them. For example, patients undergoing bone marrow transplantation may receive prophylactic acyclovir or ganciclovir to prevent herpesvirus and cytomegalovirus infection. AIDS patients receive prophylactic trimethoprim–sulfamethoxazole to prevent *Pneumocystis carinii* pneumonia as well as toxoplasmosis.

## ADDITIONAL READING

Drew WL. Cytomegalovirus infection in patients with AIDS. *Clin Infect Dis.* 1992;14:608–615. In patients with AIDS the array of syndromes attributable to cytomegalovirus infection is vast. The clinically important entities occurring most frequently are retinitis and gastrointestinal disease. The former is diagnosed on clinical grounds and the latter by means of biopsy. Two antiviral agents, ganciclovir and foscarnet, have been approved for the treatment of cytomegaloviral retinitis.

Dunn DL. Problems related to immunosuppression. Infection and malignancy occurring after solid organ transplantation. *Crit Care Clin.* 1990;6:955–977. This overview of the spectrum of infections that may occur after organ transplantation is one of 11 articles published together on critical care of the transplant patient.

European Organization for Research on Treatment of Cancer. Empiric antifungal therapy in febrile granulocytopenic patients. *Am J Med.* 1989;86:668–672. Overall, 47 of 68 neutropenic patients receiving amphotericin B improved compared with 34 of 64 not receiving systemic antifungal agents.

Goodrich JM, Bowden RA, Fisher L, et al. Ganciclovir prophylaxis to prevent cytomegalovirus disease after allogeneic marrow transplant. *Ann Intern Med.* 1993;118:173–178. Fourteen (45%) placebo recipients developed cytomegalovirus infection in the first 100 days after marrow transplant compared with one (3%) ganciclovir recipient ($P < 0.001$). Nine (29%) placebo recipients developed cytomegalovirus disease compared with no cases in the ganciclovir group.

Recommendations of the Advisory Committee on Immunization Practices (AICP): Use of vaccines and immune globulins in persons with altered immunocompetence. *MMWR Morb Mortal Wkly Rep.* 1993;42(RR-4):1–18.

## APPENDIX 71–1. AGENTS COMMONLY INFECTING IMMUNOCOMPROMISED PATIENTS

| Agent | Decreased Phagocytosis | Complement Deficiencies | Hypo- or Agammaglobulinemia | Defects in Cell-Mediated Immunity |
|---|---|---|---|---|
| **Bacteria** | | | | |
| *Staphylococcus aureus* and β-hemolytic streptococci | +++[a] | ++ | ++ | |
| *Streptococcus pneumoniae* | +++ | + | +++ | |
| Enterobacteriaceae | +++ | + | + | |
| *Pseudomonas aeruginosa* | +++ | ++ | + | |
| *Haemophilus influenzae* | + | + | +++ | |
| *Salmonella* species | + | + | | +++ |
| *Listeria monocytogenes* | | | | +++ |
| *Mycobacterium* species | | | | +++ |
| *Legionella* | | | | +++ |
| *Nocardia asteroides* | | | | +++ |
| *Neisseria* species | | ++ | + | |
| **Fungi** | | | | |
| *Candida* species | | | | |
| Systemic | ++ | | | |
| Chronic mucocutaneous | | | | +++ |
| *Aspergillus* species | +++ | | | |
| *Phycomyces* species | +++ | | | |
| *Cryptococcus neoformans* | | | | +++ |
| *Coccidioides immitis* | | | | +++ |
| *Histoplasma capsulatum* | | | | +++ |
| **Viruses** | | | | |
| Herpes simplex | | | + | +++ |
| Varicella–zoster | | | ++ | +++ |
| Cytomegalovirus | | | | +++ |
| Epstein–Barr | | | | +++ |
| Papovaviruses | | | | ++ |
| Enteroviruses | | | +++ | |
| Hepatitis B | | | | +++ |
| Influenza | | | + | + |
| Adenoviruses | | | + | +++ |
| **Parasites** | | | | |
| *Pneumocystis carinii*[b] | | | ++ | +++ |
| *Giardia lamblia* | | | ++ | + |
| *Toxoplasma gondii* | | | | +++ |
| *Strongyloides stercoralis* | | | | +++ |
| *Cryptosporidium* | | | | +++ |

[a] Number of pluses indicates relative susceptibility to the organisms listed according to the immune deficits.
[b] *Pneumocystic carinii* may be a fungus.

Chapter 72

# Nosocomial Infections and Hospital Infection Control

*Kenneth J. Ryan*

"Nosocomial" is a medical term for "hospital-associated." Nosocomial infections are those that arise during hospitalization as a complication of another illness. The purpose of hospital infection control is prevention of nosocomial infections by application of epidemiologic concepts and methods.

## SEMMELWEIS AND EPIDEMIOLOGY

The shining example of the fundamental importance of epidemiology in detection and control of nosocomial infections is the work of Ignaz Semmelweis (1849), which preceded the microbiologic discoveries of Pasteur and Koch by a decade. Semmelweis was assistant obstetrician at the Vienna General Hospital, where more than 7000 infants were delivered each year. Childbed fever (puerperal endometritis), which we now know was caused primarily by group A streptococci, was a major problem accounting for 600 to 800 maternal deaths per year. By careful review of hospital statistics between 1846 and 1849, Semmelweis clearly showed that the death rate in one of the two divisions of the hospital was 10 times that in the other. Division I, which had the high mortality, was the teaching unit in which all deliveries were by obstetricians and students. In division II, all deliveries were by midwives. No similar epidemic existed elsewhere in the city of Vienna and mortality was very low in mothers delivering at home.

Semmelweis and control of childbed fever

Semmelweis postulated that the key difference between divisions I and II was participation of the physicians and students in autopsies. One or more cadavers were dissected daily, some from cases of childbed fever and other infections. Hand-washing was perfunctory, which Semmelweis believed to allow the transmission of "invisible cadaver particles" by direct contact between the mother and the physician's hands during examinations and delivery. In 1847, as a countermeasure, he required hand washing with a chlorine solution until the hands were slippery and the odor of the cadaver was gone. The results were dramatic. The full effect of the chlorine hand washing can be seen by comparing mortality in the two divisions for 1846 and 1848 (Table 72–1). The mortality in division I was reduced to that of division II, and both were below 2%.

Demonstrated the critical importance of hand washing in infection control

Unfortunately, because of his personality and failure to publish his work until 1860, Semmelweis' contribution was not generally appreciated in his lifetime. As his frustration

TABLE 72–1. CHILDBED FEVER AT THE VIENNA GENERAL HOSPITAL

| | Division I (Teaching Unit) | | | Division II (Midwife Unit) | | |
|---|---|---|---|---|---|---|
| Year | Births | Maternal Deaths | Percentage | Births | Maternal Deaths | Percentage |
| 1846[a] | 4010 | 459 | 11.4 | 3754 | 105 | 2.7 |
| 1848[b] | 3556 | 45 | 1.3 | 3219 | 43 | 1.3 |

[a] No hand washing.
[b] First full year of chlorine hand washing.

mounted over lack of acceptance of his ideas, he became abusive and irrational, eventually alienating even his early supporters. Some believe that he also suffered from presenile dementia (Alzheimer's disease). He died in an insane asylum in 1865, unaware that his concept of spread via direct contact would later be recognized as the most important mechanism of nosocomial infection and that hand-washing would remain the most important means of infection control in hospitals.

## NOSOCOMIAL INFECTIONS

Community infections are present at admission

Nosocomial infections acquired in hospital

Infections occurring during any hospitalization are either community acquired or nosocomial. Community infections are those present or incubating at the time of hospital admission. All others are considered nosocomial. For example, a hospital case of chickenpox could be community acquired if it erupted on the fifth hospital day (incubating), or nosocomial if hospitalization was beyond the limits of the known incubation period (20 days). Infections appearing shortly after discharge (2 weeks) are considered nosocomial although some could have been acquired at home. Infectious hazards are inherent to the hospital environment: it is there that the most seriously infected and most susceptible patients are housed and often cared for by the same staff.

### Sources

Endogenous infections are part of the hospital risk

The infectious agents responsible for nosocomial infections arise from various sources including patients' own normal flora. In addition to any immunocompromising disease or therapy the hospital may impose additional risks by treatments that breach the normal defense barriers. Surgery, urinary or intravenous catheters, and invasive diagnostic procedures all may provide normal flora with access to usually sterile sites. Infections in which the source of organisms is the hospital rather than the patient include those derived from hospital personnel, the environment, and medical equipment.

#### Hospital Personnel

Cross-infection is preventable

Infected medical attendants particularly dangerous

Infection from carriers can transmit to patients

Physicians, nurses, students, therapists, and any others who come in contact with the patient may transmit infection. Transmission from one patient to another is called **cross-infection.** The vehicle of transmission is most often the inadequately washed hands of a medical attendant. Another source is the infected medical attendant. Many hospital outbreaks have been traced to hospital personnel, particularly physicians, who continue to care for patients despite an overt infection. Transmission is usually by direct contact, although airborne transmission is also possible. A third source is the person who is not ill but is carrying a virulent strain. For *Staphylococcus aureus* and group A streptococci nasal carriage is most important, but sites such as the perineum and anus have also been involved in outbreaks. An occult carrier is less often the source of nosocomial infection than a physician covering up a boil or a nurse minimizing "the flu." The carrier is difficult to detect unless the epidemic strain has distinctive characteristics or the epidemiologic circumstances point to a single person.

## Environmental Sources

The hospital air, walls, floors, linens, and the like are not sterile and thus could serve as a source of organisms causing nosocomial infections, but the importance of this route has generally been exaggerated. With the exception of the immediate vicinity of an infected individual or a carrier, transmission through the air or on fomites is much less important than that caused by personnel or equipment. Exceptions are instances in which organisms are numerous or the patient is particularly vulnerable (heart surgery, bone marrow transplant).

Environmental contamination least important source

## Medical Devices

Much of the success of modern medicine is related to medical devices that support or monitor basic body functions. By their very nature, devices such as catheters and respirators carry a risk of nosocomial infection, because they bypass normal defense barriers, providing microorganisms access to normally sterile fluids and tissues. Most of the recognized causes are bacterial or fungal. The risk of infection is related to the degree of debilitation of the patient and various factors concerning the design and management of the device.

Any device that crosses the skin or a mucosal barrier will allow flora in the patient or environment to gain access to deeper sites around the outside surface. Possible access inside the device (for example, in the lumen) adds another and sometimes greater risk. In some devices, such as urinary catheters, contamination is avoidable; in others, such as respirators, complete sterility is either impossible or impractical to achieve.

Infection most likely with equipment that crosses epithelial barriers

The risk of contamination leading to infection is increased if organisms that gain access can multiply within the system. The availability of water, nutrients, and a suitable temperature largely determine which organism will survive and multiply. Many of the Gram-negative rods such as *Pseudomonas, Acinetobacter,* and members of the Enterobacteriaceae family can multiply in an environment containing water and little else. Gram-positives generally require more physiologic conditions.

Bacteria grow in moist environments

Even with proper growth conditions, many hours are required before contaminating organisms become numerous. Detailed studies of catheters and similar devices show the risk of infection begins to increase after 24 to 48 hours and is cumulative even if the device is changed or disinfected at intervals. It is thus important to discontinue transcutaneous procedures as soon as medically indicated.

Need to remove transcutaneous and urethral devices as soon as possible

The medical devices most frequently associated with nosocomial infections are listed below. The infectious risk of others can be estimated from the principles discussed previously. New devices are constantly being introduced into medical care, occasionally without adequate consideration of their potential to cause nosocomial infection.

### Urinary Catheters

The infectious risk of a single urinary catheterization has been estimated at 1 to 5%. Indwelling catheters carry a risk that may be as high as 10% for each day the catheter is in place. The major preventive measure is maintenance of a completely closed system through the use of valves and aspiration ports designed to prevent bacterial access to the inside of the catheter or collecting bag. The urine itself serves as an excellent culture medium once contamination occurs.

Closed urinary drainage systems required

### Vascular Catheters

Needles and plastic catheters placed in veins (or, less often, in arteries) for fluid administration, monitoring vital functions, or diagnostic procedures are a leading cause of nosocomial bacteremia. These sites should always be suspected as a source of organisms whenever blood cultures are positive with no apparent primary site for the bacteremia. Contamination at the insertion site is generally staphylococcal, with continued growth in the catheter tip. Organisms may gain access somewhere in the lines, valves, bags, or bottles of intravenous solutions proximal to the insertion site. The latter circumstance usually involves Gram-negative rods. Preventive measures include aseptic insertion technique and appropriate care of the lines, including changes at regular intervals.

Skin primary source of intravenous contamination

### Respirators

Machines that assist or control respiration by pumping air directly into the trachea have a great potential for infection if the aerosol they deliver becomes contaminated. Bacterial

Nebulizer contamination primarily Gram negative

growth is significant only in the parts of the system that contain water; in systems using nebulizers, bacteria can be suspended in water droplets small enough to reach the alveoli. The organisms involved include *Pseudomonas, Enterobacteriaceae,* and a wide variety of environmental bacteria such as *Acinetobacter, Flavobacter,* and *Alcaligenes.* The primary control measure is periodic changing and disinfection of the tubing, reservoirs, and nebulizer jets.

### HEMODIALYSIS

Hepatitis B and HIV risk related to blood manipulation

Bacterial infections of shunts and cannulas, a possible complication of chronic hemodialysis, are generally similar in origin to other infections arising from catheterization. Contamination of the dialysis fluid or artificial kidney is now an uncommon problem, but remains possible because the fluid contains bacterial nutrients and is maintained at body temperature. A far greater problem in hemodialysis units is the risk of transmission of hepatitis B or human immunodeficiency virus (HIV) infections as a result of the many procedural manipulations involving blood. Control requires meticulous attention to procedures that prevent direct contact with blood, such as the use of gloves and gowns. Identification of hepatitis B and HIV carriers so that they can be treated separately is very important. Most units have established serologic surveillance procedures to detect both carriers and evidence of transmission among patients and staff.

## ETIOLOGIC AGENTS AND INFECTION RATES

The rates and etiologic agents of the most common forms of nosocomial infection taken from CDC surveillance statistics are shown in Table 72–2. The rates in US hospitals range between 0.8 and 8.9% with most between 3 and 5%. If extrapolated to the more than 40 million persons hospitalized in the United States each year, this percentage translates to millions of cases annually.

Differences in infection rates between hospitals reflect patient types

The ranges shown in Table 72–2 reflect differences among community, community-teaching, federal, municipal, and university hospitals. In general, the rates are lowest in community hospitals and highest in municipal and university hospitals. This finding primarily reflects differences in the types of patients treated in these institutions. For example, municipal hospitals usually have a higher proportion of elderly and debilitated patients and university hospitals a higher proportion of immunosuppressed patients. Both groups are more susceptible to infection and tend to have prolonged hospital stays. Table 72–2 also

**TABLE 72–2. NOSOCOMIAL INFECTION RATES, FREQUENCIES, AND MOST COMMON PATHOGENS**

| Infection | Infections/10,000 Hospital Discharges[a,b] | Percentage of All Nosocomial Infections[b] | Most Common Pathogens |
|---|---|---|---|
| Primary bacteremia[c] | 7–30 | 3–7 | *Staphylococcus aureus; Escherichia coli; Klebsiella* |
| Surgical wound | 52–98 | 18–27 | *Staphylococcus aureus; Escherichia coli* |
| Lower respiratory tract | 35–72 | 14–18 | *Klebsiella; Staphylococcus aureus; Pseudomonas aeruginosa* |
| Urinary tract | 112–151 | 34–46 | *Escherichia coli;* group D streptococci; *Pseudomonas aeruginosa* |
| Cutaneous | 15–33 | 4–8 | *Staphylococcus aureus* |
| All others | 23–70 | 8–16 | *Staphylococcus aureus; Escherichia coli* |

[a] Data from 1979 National Nosocomial Infection Study, published by Centers for Disease Control in March 1982.
[b] Ranges reflect differences among community, community-teaching, federal, municipal, and university hospitals.
[c] No documented site of origin.

shows that urinary tract infections are the most common nosocomial infections, constituting one third to one half of all cases. Most of these infections are associated with the use of urinary catheters.

Urinary tract infections most common

The most common pathogens isolated are *Escherichia coli* and *S. aureus,* which together account for 25 to 30% of nosocomial infections. Other members of the *Enterobacteriaceae* family, group D streptococci, *Pseudomonas aeruginosa,* and *Candida* species are also common causes. In general, the organisms most resistant to antimicrobics, such as *Klebsiella, Serratia,* and *Pseudomonas,* are much more common as causes of hospital-acquired than of community-acquired infections. For example, although Table 72–2 shows *E. coli* to be the most common cause of urinary infection in the hospital, its proportion (32%) is much smaller than its share of community-acquired urinary infections, which exceeds 90%.

Antimicrobic resistant organisms more common in hospitals

Viruses tend to be underestimated in, or excluded from, surveys of nosocomial infections, because most hospitals still lack adequate viral diagnostic laboratories. Respiratory viruses such as influenza virus and respiratory syncytial virus have been shown to spread in hospitals by droplet inhalation or direct contact. Some of the highly infectious viruses, such as varicella (chickenpox, herpes zoster) and rubella (German measles), have caused outbreaks among susceptible patients and medical staff.

Viral infections generally underreported

Hepatitis B and, less often, HIV viruses can be responsible for hospital-associated infections in which transmission is from patient to medical staff, rather than the reverse. The primary mechanism for transmission of both viruses in the health care setting is by blood or blood products. This may occur by contact of patient's blood with a mucosal surface or through accidents involving breaks in the skin, such as needle sticks. Transmission following a hepatitis B needle stick is between 10 and 35%; the HIV needle stick risk is estimated at 1 in 250. Because of its prevalence in the hospital setting, hepatitis B represents a serious risk. Between 200 and 300 health-care workers die each year from hepatitis B infection.

Hepatitis B transmission from patient to healthcare worker a significant problem

## INFECTION CONTROL

Infection control is the sum of all the means used to prevent nosocomial infections. Historically such methods have been developed as an integral part of the study of infectious diseases, often serving as key elements in the proof of infectious etiology. Semmelweis' hand washing is the first example. Later in the 19th century, Joseph Lister achieved a dramatic reduction in surgical wound infections by infusion of a phenolic antiseptic into wounds. This local destruction of organisms was known as **antisepsis,** and sometimes included liberal applications of disinfectants, including sprays to the environment. As it became recognized that contamination of wounds was not inevitable, the emphasis gradually shifted to preventing contact between microorganisms and susceptible sites, a concept called **asepsis.** Asepsis, which uses the methods of sterilization and disinfection discussed in Chapter 11, is the central concept of infection control. The measures taken to achieve asepsis vary, depending on whether the circumstances and environment are most similar to the operating room, hospital ward, or outpatient clinic.

Practices have changed from emphasis on antisepsis to asepsis

### Asepsis

#### Operating Room

The surgical suite and operating room represent the most controlled and rigid application of aseptic principles. The procedure begins with the use of an antiseptic scrub of the skin over the operative site and the hands and forearms of all who will have contact with the patient. The use of sterile drapes, gowns, and instruments serves to prevent spread through direct contact, and caps and face masks reduce airborne spread from personnel to the wound. As all students learn the first time they scrub, even the manner of dressing and moving in the operating room are rigidly specified, and those involved assume a strict aseptic attitude as well as their masks and gowns. In some hospitals the air entering the operating room is filter sterilized, but this practice is expensive and its value unproved. The level of bacteria

Surgical aseptic procedures prevent contact of organisms with wound

Contamination related primarily to personnel

in the air is generally more related to the number of persons and amount of movement in the operating room than to incoming air. The net effect of these procedures is to draw a sterile curtain around the operative site, thus minimizing contact with microorganisms. Surgical asepsis is also employed in other areas where invasive special procedures such as cardiac catheterization are performed.

### Hospital Ward

Hand washing the most important preventative measure

Although theoretically desirable, strict aseptic procedures as used in the operating room are impractical in the ward setting. Asepsis is practiced by the use of sterile needles, medications, dressings, and other items that could serve as transmission vehicles if contaminated. A "no touch" technique for examining wounds and changing dressings eliminates direct contact with any nonsterile item. Invasive procedures such as catheter insertion and lumbar punctures are done under aseptic precautions similar to those used in the operating room. In all circumstances hand washing between patient contacts is the single most important aseptic precaution.

### Outpatient Clinic

The general, aseptic practices used on the hospital ward are also appropriate to the outpatient situation as preventive measures. The potential for cross-infection in the clinic or waiting room is obvious, but has been little studied regarding preventive measures. Patients who may be infected should be segregated whenever possible using techniques similar to those of hospital ward isolation. The examining room may be used in a manner analogous to the private rooms on a hospital ward. This approach is difficult because of patient turnover, but should be attempted for infections that would require strict or respiratory isolation in the hospital.

## Isolation Procedures

Isolation segregates infectious patient

Patients with infections pose special problems, because they may transmit their infections to other patients either directly or by contact with a staff member. This additional risk is managed by the techniques of isolation, which separate the infected patient from others on the ward. The appropriate isolation techniques vary with the communicability of the infectious agent and the route(s) of transmission. These criteria have been formalized into specific isolation categories and techniques for use in hospitals (Table 72–3).

Universal precautions directed at prevention of HIV transmission

Recognition of the risk posed to health care workers by the AIDS epidemic has caused a reexamination of these category-specific isolation procedures, because there have been a number of documented transmissions of HIV to hospital personnel from patients not known to carry the virus at the time they were initially seen. Thus, limiting protective measures to known AIDS or known HIV-positive persons is no longer considered safe. This problem has been addressed by the concept of universal precautions in which the use of protective measures, such as gowns, gloves, and goggles, is determined solely by the probability of contact with blood or body fluids without regard to the patient's diagnosis. These are illustrated in Table 72–4. The category-specific measures are still appropriate for other infections when they include procedures not already implemented under universal precautions. It is the physician's responsibility to recognize the presence of infection and to institute the appropriate isolation restrictions.

## Organization

Modern hospitals are required to have formal infection control programs that include an infection control committee, epidemiology service, and educational activities. The infection control committee is composed of representatives of various medical, administrative, nursing, housekeeping, and support services. The committee establishes the institution's infection control procedures and regularly reviews information on the status of nosocomial infections in the hospital. When epidemiologic circumstances warrant it, the committee is empowered to take drastic action such as closing a hospital unit or suspending a physician's privileges.

**TABLE 72–3. CATEGORY-SPECIFIC ISOLATION TECHNIQUES USED IN HOSPITALS TO PREVENT SPREAD OF INFECTION**

| Isolation Category | Route of Transmission Blockage | Isolation Techniques | Typical Situation |
|---|---|---|---|
| Strict | All, or on clothing or fomites | Private rooms,[a] gowns, gloves, masks, all articles[b] | Congenital rubella, chickenpox, plague (pneumonic), generalized staphylococcal infections |
| Respiratory | Respiratory route | Private rooms,[a] masks; contaminated articles[b] | Measles, pertussis, tuberculosis |
| Enteric | Contact spread from stools | Private room,[a] gowns,[c] gloves,[d] contaminated articles[b] | *Salmonella; Shigella,* hepatitis |
| Contact | Contact spread from lesions: infected wounds | Private room (desirable),[d] gowns,[d] gloves,[e] masks,[e] | Infected burns,[f] draining wounds[f] |
| Blood and body fluid | Contact spread from blood or body fluids | Private room,[f] gloves | Hepatitis or HIV infections |
| Protective | Staff to patient | Private room,[a] masks | Agranulocytosis, extensive burns, immunosuppression |

[a] Door must be closed.
[b] Articles contaminated with pus or potentially infected secretions must be wrapped or otherwise handled for future sterilization or disinfection.
[c] For those touching patient.
[d] Contact with infectious material.
[e] Wound or burn infections with *Staphylococcus aureus* or group A streptococci that cannot be easily contained by dressings require strict isolation.
[f] Poor hygiene or child.

The epidemiology service is the working arm of the infection control committee. Its functions are performed by one or more epidemiologists who usually have a nursing background. This work requires familiarity with clinical microbiology, epidemiology, infectious disease, and hospital procedures, and immense tact. The main activities are surveillance and outbreak investigation.

Surveillance is conducted in hospital setting

Surveillance is the collection of data documenting the frequency and nature of nosocomial infections in the hospital to detect deviations from the institutional or national norms.

**TABLE 72–4. UNIVERSAL PRECAUTIONS USED TO PROTECT MEDICAL AND LABORATORY PERSONNEL[a,b]**

| Risk Level[b] | Route of Transmission | Isolation Techniques | Typical Situation |
|---|---|---|---|
| Low | None[c] | None[c] | General patient care, contact with intact skin |
| Moderate | Contact spread from body fluids | Gloves, gowns[d] | Blood drawing, dressing changes |
| High | Contact splash and aerosol spread from body fluids | Gloves, gowns, eye/face protection | Suctioning, bronchoscopy, emergency procedures, surgery |

[a] When infection is present, appropriate category specific measures are added.
[b] The primary determinant is the potential risk for contact with the patient's body fluids, particularly, blood.
[c] Except hand washing (appropriate for all care).
[d] If clothes could become soiled.

Although routine microbiologic sampling of the hospital environment is of no value, programs to sample some of the medical devices known to be nosocomial hazards can be useful.

Outbreak investigation aimed at preventing cross-infection

On-the-spot investigation of potential outbreaks allows early implementation of preventive measures. This activity is probably the single most important function of the epidemiology service. Suspicion of an increased number of infections leads to an investigation to verify the facts, establish basic epidemiologic associations, and relate them to preventive measures. The primary concern is cross-infection, in which a virulent organism is being transmitted from patient to patient. Solution of the problem may require additional microbiologic investigations, such as bacteriophage typing of *S. aureus*.

## SUMMARY

The prevention of nosocomial infections is contingent on basic and applied knowledge drawn from all parts of this book. Applied with common sense, these principles can both prevent disease and reduce the costs of medical care.

## ADDITIONAL READING

Gerberding LJ, Henderson DK. Management of occupational exposures to bloodborne pathogens: Hepatitis B virus, hepatitis C virus, and human immunodeficiency virus. *Clin Infect Dis.* 1992;14:1179–1185. This review focuses on what to do when a health-care worker is or may be exposed to one of these viruses.

# Appendices

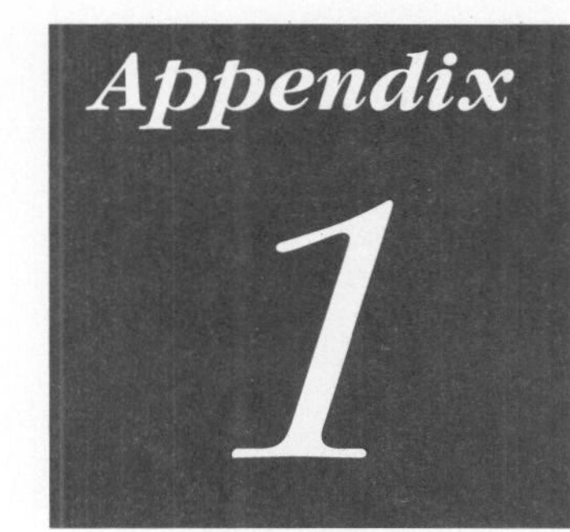

# Additional Pathogenic Organisms

SUMMARY OF SOME ADDITIONAL PATHOGENIC OR POTENTIALLY PATHOGENIC ORGANISMS NOT CONSIDERED IN THE BODY OF THE TEXT

| Organism | Disease | Comment |
|---|---|---|
| **Bacteria** | | |
| *Agrobacterium* | Various | Gram-negative bacilli that are established plant pathogens but have caused human wound, urinary, and peritoneal infections. |
| *Bartonella bacilliformis* | Verruga peruvana (skin) Oroya fever (systemic) | Small Gram-negative bacillus transmitted by Sandfly vector. Limited to Andes mountain regions. Organism invades erythrocytes producing hemolytic anemia in Oroya fever. |
| *Bordetella bronchiseptica* | Bronchitis | Animal respiratory pathogen, can cause whooping cough-like illness in humans or opportunistic infection in compromised hosts. |
| *Capnocytophagia species* | Septicemia | Gram-negative bacilli with unique gliding motility on agar plates, found in oropharyngeal flora and rare cause of disseminated infection in immunocompromised patients. |
| *Corynebacterium pseudotuberculosis* | Pneumonia, lymphadenitis | Rare cause of suppurative granulomatous pneumonia and lymphadenitis associated with handling animal products. |
| *Corynebacterium (Arcanobacterium) hemolyticum* | Pharyngitis | A hemolytic *Corynebacterium* that is a candidate cause of acute pharyngitis resembling that caused by group A streptococci |
| *Streptobacillus moniliformis* | Rat-bite fever | Highly pleomorphic Gram-negative bacillus of oropharynx of rodents. Produces high fever, rash, and septic or pneumonic complications. Most infections follow rodent bites. |
| *Spirillum minor* | Rat-bite fever | Gram-negative spiral organism with polar flagella. Habitat and epidemiology similar to *Streptobacillus moniliformis*. Disease manifests as fever, rash, and local lesion with lymphadenitis. |
| **Viruses** | | |
| Crimean–Congo hemorrhagic fever virus | Crimean–Congo hemorrhagic fever | Bunyavirus transmitted by ticks. The disease it produces is marked by lower back pain and diffuse ecchymoses. |

| Organism | Disease | Comment |
|---|---|---|
| **Viruses, (cont.)** | | |
| Junin virus | Argentine hemorrhagic fever | Arenavirus transmitted from rodent urine disseminated primarily during the spring harvest season. |
| Machupo virus | Bolivian hemorrhagic fever | Arenavirus transmitted from a rodent species found near the borders of tropical grasslands. |
| Rift Valley fever virus | Rift Valley fever | Febrile illness sometimes complicated by hemorrhage, encephalitis, and blindness. Occurs as mosquito-borne epizootics in sub-Sahara Africa and Egypt. Prduces disease in sheep, cattle, and humans. |
| **Fungi** | | |
| *Hansenula anomala* | Various | Saprophytic ascomycete recently associated with pneumonia, fungemia, and other infections in immunocompromised patients. |
| *Loboa loboi* | Lobomycosis | Chronic skin infection seen in Latin America. The lemon-shaped cells seen in lesions have not been isolated in culture. |
| *Pseudoallescheri (Petriellidum) boydii* | Pseudoallescheriasis | A free-living ascomycete that may produce infectious features similar to those of *Aspergillus* infection especially in the immunocompromised. |
| *Prototheca wickerhamii* | Chronic skin papilloma-like lesions, wound infections, and bursitis | Alga-like unicellular fungus. |
| **Protozoa** | | |
| CILIATES | | |
| *Balantidium coli* | Balantidiasis | Large colonic protozoan of swine, found primarily in tropics. Human infection may produce a diarrheal illness resembling amebiasis. |
| FLAGELLATES | | |
| *Dientamoeba fragilis* | Diamentamoebiasis | A noninvasive intestinal amebo-flagellate related to *Trichomonas.* Uncommonly, infection produces acute or recurrent diarrhea. |
| SPOROZOA | | |
| *Isospora belli* | Isosporiasis | Coccidian parasite resembling *Cryptosporidium* seen in areas of low sanitation and in patients with AIDS. Watery diarrhea is seen in acute infections, malabsorption, and weight loss in chronic disease. |
| *Sarcocystis* spp | Sarcocytosis | Coccidian parasite that produces intestinal infection in carnivores (definite hosts) and large tissue cysts in herbivores. Human infections of animal origin are seen in Latin America and Asia. They may be intestinal (producing diarrhea) or muscular (producing painful swellings). |
| *Babesia* spp | Babesiosis | Tick-transmitted intraerythrocytic parasites of animals resembling the falciparum malaria agent. In North America, human infections found primarily in off-shore islands of New England. Usually characterized by prolonged fever and mild to moderate hemolytic anemia. |
| **Helminths** | | |
| NEMATODES | | |
| *Anasakis* spp | Anasakiasis | Intestinal ascarids of sea mammals. Larval stages are found in flesh of several marine fish. Humans are infected by eating uncooked fish. Parasite may be vomited or burrow into mucosa producing abdominal pain. |

| Organism | Disease | Comment |
|---|---|---|
| *Capillaria philippinensis* | Capillariasis | Intestinal nematodes of birds related to *Trichuris.* Inhabitants of Philipines and Thailand become infected when they ingest raw fresh water crustaceans and fish, which serve as intermediate hosts. Invasion of intestinal mucosa produces severe diarrhea and malabsorption. |
| *Trichostrongylus* spp | Trichostrongyliasis | Worldwide parasite of herbivores. Humans are infected by ingesting leafy plants contaminated with larvae. Most infections are asymtomatic. Abdominal pain and diarrhea may occur. |
| *Angiostrongylus cantonesis* | Eosinophilic meningitis | Nematode parasite of mammals of the Far East and tropical areas of the Pacific. Human ingestion of raw snails or fresh water crustaceans serving as intermediate hosts results in larval invasion of the CNS and meningitis. |
| *Dracuncula mediensis* | Dracunculiasis | The "guinea worm" is the largest nematode of humans. Humans in south Asia, Middle East, and Africa are infected by drinking water containing infected fresh water fleas. Adult worm migrates to subcutaneous tissues of the legs and penetrates skin to discharge its eggs. |
| **Cestodes** | | |
| *Taenia multiceps* | Coenurosis | A dog tapeworm. Larval invasion of human subcutaneous tissues, eyes, and CNS occurs following ingestion of eggs from feces of an infected dog. |
| **Trematodes** | | |
| *Fasciolopsis buski* | Fasciolopsiasis | The largest intestinal trematode of humans inhabits duodenum and jejunum of humans and swine in the Far East and Southeast Asia. Human infection follows ingestion of fresh water plants containing infective metacercariae. Heavy infections may produce diarrhea, malabsorption and edema. |
| *Heterophyes heterophyes* | Heterophyiasis | One of several minute intestinal flukes found in the Far East, Middle East, Brazil, USSR, and Hawaii. Humans are infected by ingesting second intermediate hosts such as fresh water fish, shrimp and reptiles. Heavy infections may produce diarrhea. |
| *Fasciola hepatica* | Fascioliasis | Worldwide liver fluke of sheep and other herbivores. Human infection acquired by ingesting watercress and other water plants containing infective metacerceria. Following migration to liver, clinical manifestations resemble clonorchiasis. |
| *Opisthorchis* spp | Opisthorchiasis | Liver fluke found in eastern Europe, USSR, and Far East. Fresh water fish serve as second intermediate host. Human infection follows ingestion of raw or uncooked fish. Clinical disease resembles clonorchiasis. |

*Appendix*

2

# Historical Appendix

## Some Major Figures Contributing to Knowledge of Medical Microbiology

### Antony Van Leeuwenhoek

1670–1880

At the beginning of this period, he developed single-lensed microscopes which allowed him to see and describe microorganisms in numerous environmental and biological samples.

### Edward Jenner

In 1798 reported on the efficacy of cowpox vaccination against smallpox.

### Ignaz Semmelweiss and Oliver Wendell Holmes

1800–1860

Described the epidemiology, contagiousness, and measures for prevention of puerperal fever.

### Florence Nightingale

Showed that post-traumatic infection and epidemic diseases in hospital could be reduced by cleanliness and disinfection. Established the basis of modern hospital hygiene.

### Louis Pasteur

1860–1900

Between 1857 and 1880 demonstrated that fermentation was a microbial process, and that there was no spontaneous generation of microbes. He developed pasteurization to control contamination of wines, vinegar, and beer. He demonstrated the microbial cause of many diseases of plants, insects, and mammals, and developed attenuated vaccines for anthrax and rabies.

### Joseph Lister

Developed the techniques of antiseptic surgery for preventing surgical wound infections.

### Robert Koch

Isolated the causative agents of anthrax, tuberculosis, and cholera and conclusively demonstrated their etiologies. Developed various staining procedures and the use of solid media for pure culture techniques.

### Patrick Manson

First showed that a parasite of humans (Filaria) had a developmental phase in an insect (mosquito).

1860–1900 (continued)

**Elie Metchnikoff**
Discovered the role of phagocytic cells in immunity.

**Hans Christian Gram**
Developed the staining procedure that carries his name.

**Emil von Behring**
Discovered the neutralization of diphtheria toxin by antitoxin.

**Dmitri Ivanowksi**
Described a filterable nonbacterial agent (virus) as the cause of tobacco mosaic disease.

**Paul Ehrlich**
Postulated the side chain reaction theory of antibody production and action.

**Ronald Ross**
Conclusively demonstrated the role of the anopheline mosquito in the transmission of malaria.

**Jules Bordet**
Described the lysis of some Gram-negative bacteria by antibody and complement.

1900–1925

**August von Wasserman**
Developed the first serologic test for syphilis.

**Walter Reed**
Reported studies in 1902 that established that yellow fever virus, the first recognized human virus, could be transmitted by mosquito bites.

**Paul Ehrlich**
Defined the principles of chemotherapy and developed salvarsan as the first effective chemotherapeutic for syphilis.

**Peyton Rous**
Discovered a virally transmitted sarcoma of chickens.

**Frederick Twort and Felix d'Herelle**
Independently discovered bacterial viruses (bacteriophages).

**Alexander Fleming**
Discovered lysozyme.

1925–1945

**Fred Griffith**
Described the phenomenon of pneumococcal transformation.

**Alexander Fleming**
Reported his discovery of penicillin, and its antibacterial characteristics, in 1929.

**Max Theiler**
Developed the mouse model as a susceptible mammalian host for the isolation, propagation, and study of arboviruses.

**Ernest Goodpasture**
Showed that some viruses could be grown in the laboratory in the developing chick embryo.

**Gerhard Domagk**
Discovered the first of the sulfonamide antimicrobics.

**Max Delbrück**
Began a series of studies on bacteriophages that ultimately helped elucidate the fundamental relationships of DNA, RNA, and protein in living systems.

**Ernst Chain, Howard Florey and their Colleagues**
Produced and purified penicillin to the point of clinical trials in the early 1940s.

**Oswald Avery, Colin MacLeod, and Maclyn McCarty**
Showed that pneumococcal transformation was determined by DNA from the donor strain.

**Salvador Luria and Max Delbrück**
Showed that bacterial mutations occurred spontaneously and were not directed by the environment.

1945–1965

**Joshua Lederberg and Edward Tatum**
Demonstrated genetic exchange in bacteria by conjugation.

**John Enders, Frederick Robbins, and Thomas Weller**
Grew the poliomyelitis virus in cell culture opening the way to vaccine production.

**Norton Zinder and Joshua Lederberg**
Discovered genetic exchange mediated by bacteriophage in *Salmonella* (transduction).

**James Watson, Francis Crick, and Maurice Wilkins**
Described the double helical structure of DNA in 1953.

**Jonas Salk**
Developed the inactivated poliomyelitis vaccine in 1955.

**Albert Sabin**
Developed the live attenuated poliomyelitis vaccine.

**Alick Isaacs**
Discovered interferon.

**Jacques Monod and Francis Jacob**
Reported their studies on enzyme regulation leading to recognition of promoters, regulatory proteins, and the role of mRNA.

**Tomoichiro Akiba, Kunitaro Ochiai, Susumu Mitsuhashi, Tsutomu Wantanabe, and Others**
Discovered that multiple drug resistance was encoded on transmissible plasmids (R factors).

**Carlton Gajdusek**
Described the epidemiology of the first recognized slow virus disease (Kuru), and the unique characteristics of the etiologic agent.

1965–1994

**Baruch Blumberg**
Reported the discovery of "Australia antigen" in 1967, and later confirmed its association with hepatitis B virus.

1965–1994 (continued)

**Howard Temin and David Baltimore**
Independently described reverse transcriptase in RNA tumor viruses.

**Herbert Boyer, Stanley Cohen and Others**
Developed techniques for in vitro splicing of DNA.

**Cesar Milstein and George Köhler**
Developed the procedures for production of monoclonal antibodies.

**Luc Montagnier and Robert Gallo**
Isolated the human immunodeficiency virus (HIV) and developed the methods that define its role in AIDS.

**Kary Mullis**
Developed the polymerase chain reaction.

Appendix 3

# Glossary

The glossary is intended as an adjunct to the index for rapid reference. It includes words and phrases that have not been defined in the text or that have been defined but are used frequently in later chapters. Where a word has multiple uses, the one relevant to this text is emphasized.

The prefixes and suffixes in each alphabetical section include word elements used in combined form. The meaning of many words can be derived from the prefixes and suffixes and therefore have not been included in the glossary.

---

**A-, An-** Without.

**Acanthosis** Hyperplasia and thickening of prickle cell layer of skin.

**Accessory sinuses** Blind-ended cavities in bone draining into nasal cavity.

**Achlorhydria** Absence of hydrochloric acid in stomach.

**Acid fast** Describes an organism that resists acid decolorization after straining.

**Acidosis** Increased acidity of body fluid.

**Aciduric** Resistant to effects of acid.

**Actin** Major structural protein of the eukaryotic cell cytoskeleton.

**Addison's disease** Result of primary deficiency of production of adrenal hormones.

**Adenocarcinoma** Malignant tumor derived from glandular epithelium.

**Adhesin** Surface component of a microbe that binds to a cell receptor.

**Adnexa (uterine)** Fallopian tubes and ovaries.

**Adrenal** Important endocrine glands situated above the kidneys.

**Aerobactin** A hydroxamate siderophore produced by many bacteria.

**Agammaglobulinemia** Absence of immunoglobulins in the blood.

**Agglutinate** Clumping.

**Agranulocytosis** Failure of white blood cell production in bone marrow.

**-algia** Pain.

**Allele** Alternate forms of a gene at the same chromosomal locus.

**Alloantigen** An antigen that exists in alternate allelic forms.

**Allosteric** Property of a protein that leads to a change in conformation and function associated with attachment of a smaller effector molecule.

**Alveoli (lung)** Microscopic air sacs in lung.

**Ameboma** A local inflammatory mass caused by an amebal infection.

**Amniotic fluid** Fluid in amniotic sac surrounding the fetus.

**Anaerobe** Microorganism that multiplies only in the absence of oxygen.

**Analog** Structurally or functionally similar substance or property.

**Anamnestic** Enhanced immunological memory response on reexposure to antigen.

**Anaphylaxis** Immediate and severe antibody-mediated hypersensitivity reaction.

**Anergic** Absence of ability to respond to antigen.

**Aneurysm** Localized abnormal dilatation of blood vessel.

**Anicteric** Absence of clinical jaundice.

**Anneal** Subject to controlled heating and cooling to achieve a particular property.

**Anorexia** Loss of appetite.

**Anoxia** Lack of adequate oxygenation of blood or tissues.

**Anterior horn cell** Motor neuron in the anterior gray matter of the spinal cord.

**Anthropo-** Relationship to humans.

**Antibiogram** Pattern of in vitro susceptibilities to different antimicrobics.

**Antibody** An immunoglobulin molecule that interacts with the antigen that elicited its production.

**Antigen** A substance that elicits a specific immunological response or reacts with antibody in vitro. (*See* Immunogen *and* Hapten).

**Antiserum** Serum containing specific antibodies.

**Antitoxin** An antibody that neutralizes an exotoxin.

**Antitussive** Substance that helps control coughing.

**Aphonia** Loss of speech.

**Aplastic anemia** Failure of red cell production in bone marrow.

**Apnea** Temporary absence of breathing.

**Aqueduct of Sylvius** Canal connecting the third and fourth ventricles of the brain.

**Arachidonic acid** Precursor of prostaglandins.

**Arachnoid** The middle of three membranes that cover the brain and spinal cord (meninges).

**Arrythmia** Irregularity of heartbeat.

**Arteriole** Smallest artery leading to capillary.

**Arthralgia** Pain in a joint.

**Arthro-** Pertaining to joints.

**Aryepiglottis** Related to the epiglottis and the arytenoid cartilage.

**Ascites** Fluid in a peritoneal cavity.

**Ascus** A sac. In mycology, a specialized structure containing spores termed ascospores.

**Asepsis** Exclusion of pathogenic organisms.

**Asphyxia** Suffocation.

**Astrocyte** Connective tissue cell of the central nervous system.

**Ataxia** Disturbance of muscular coordination.

**Ataxia telangiectasia** Hereditary disorder causing ataxia and permanent dilatation of some blood vessels.

**Atelectasis** Collapse of part of lung.

**Atherosclerosis** Hardening of the arteries.

**Atrophy** Wasting.

**Attenuated** Reduced in virulence, (eg, organisms in a live vaccine).

**Auto-** Self, or arising from within.

**Autochthonous flora** Organism with intimate and permanent association with an epithelial surface.

**Autoimmunity** An immune response against the body's own tissues.

**Autolysis** Lysis of a cell by its own enzymes.

**Autonomic** Relates to involuntary nervous system controlling cardiac, vascular, intestinal, and other functions.

**Auxo-** Pertaining to growth.

**Auxotroph** Bacterial mutant that has lost the ability to synthesize an essential nutrient or metabolite.

**Avascular** Absence of blood vessels or blood supply.

**Axenic** Refers to pure cultures of a microorganism without presence of a contaminating or symbiotic organism.

**Axon** The extension of a neuron that conducts nerve impulses.

**Bacteremia** Bacteria in the blood.

**Bacteriocins** Proteins produced by one bacterium that kill another of the same or other species.

**Bacteriophage** Bacterial virus.

**Bacteriostasis** Inhibition of bacterial growth without killing.

**Bacteruria** Bacteria in the urine.

**Bartholin's glands** Lubricating glands on either side of the vaginal opening.

**Basophil** Polymorphonuclear leucocyte with basophilic granules.

**Basophilic** Stains with a basic dye.

**Biliary** Pertaining to the bile and bile ducts.

**Bilirubin** A bile pigment.

**Bio-** Pertaining to life.

**Biotype** Subtype within a species characterized by physiologic properties.

**-blast** Precursor cell.

**Bleb** *See* Bulla.

**Blepharal** Pertaining to the eyelids.

**Blepharo-** Pertaining to the eyelid.

**Blepharoplast** Basal body of a cilium or flagellum.

**Blood–brain barrier** Functional barrier preventing passage of large molecules to the brain parenchyma.

**Bolus** Rounded mass that may obstruct (eg, fecal bolus) or a concentrated mass (eg, an antibiotic) given rapidly and intravenously.

**Bothria** Paired sucking grooves in the head of the fish tapeworm (Diphyllobothrium).

**Brady-** Slowing.

**Bradycardia** Unusually slow heartbeat.

**Bronchial tree** Bronchi and bronchioles that conduct gases to and from the lung alveoli.

**Bronchiectasis** Pathological dilatation of terminal bronchi.

**Bronchiole** Smallest subdivision of bronchial tree.

**Broncho-** Pertaining to the bronchial tree.

**Bubo** Swollen, inflamed, infected lymph node.

**Buccal** Pertaining to the cheek.

**Bulla** Blister or vesicle containing semipurulent fluid.

**Bursa** Sac filled with fluid (eg, protecting a joint or tendon).

**Calculus** Pathological stone (eg, renal or gallbladder calculus).

**Calmodulin** A protein present in eukaryotic cells that activates some essential enzymes when it has bound calcium.

**Capillary** The smallest blood vessel connecting the arterial and venous systems.

**Capsid** The outer protein coat of a virus that protects its nucleic acid.

**Capsomeres** Subunits of viral capsids.

**Carbuncle** A necrotic staphylococcal infection of skin and subcutaneous tissue that has spread from infected furuncles.

**Carcinoma** Malignant growth of epithelial cells.

**Cardio-** Pertaining to the heart.

**Cardiolipin** A phospholipid occurring naturally in mitochondrial membranes against which antibodies are formed in syphilitic infection.

**Cardiomyopathy** Disease of heart muscle.

**Caseous** Cheesy in consistency.

**Catalase** Enzyme that catalyses the reduction of toxic hydrogen peroxide to oxygen and water.

**Cell-mediated immunity** Immune reactions in which T lymphocytes play the pivotal role.

**Cellulitis** Inflammation of subcutaneous tissue.

**Cementum** Layer of modified bone on tooth root.

**Cerebrospinal fluid** Fluid that fills spaces within and surrounding the central nervous system.

**Cervical** Pertaining to the neck or uterine cervix.

**Cervix** The constricted portion of an organ. Usually refers to the lower part of the uterus.

**Chancre** Sore or ulcer that develops at the site of an infection. Most often used to describe the primary syphilitic lesion.

**Chelator** Compound that binds metallic ions.

**Chemoprophylaxis** Use of antimicrobics to prevent infection.

**Chemotaxis** Attraction of a motile cell to a chemical.

**Chitin** Polysaccharide forming exoskeletons of some insects or cell walls of some fungi.

**Cholangitis** Inflammation of the bile ducts.

**Chole-** Pertaining to bile.

**Cholecystitis** Inflammation of the gallbladder.

**Cholestasis** Interruption of the flow of bile.

**Cholinergic nerves** Nerve fibers that release acetylcholine as a mediator at their effector terminals.

**Chordae tendinae** Small tendons that connect papillary muscles of the heart to the cusps of the atrioventricular valves.

**Chorea** Rapid purposeless involuntary movements.

**Chorioallantoic membrane** The outer membrane surrounding an avian embryo within the egg shell.

**Chorionic membrane** The outer extraembryonic membrane from which the placenta originates.

**Chorioretinitis** Inflammation of choroid and retina of the eye.

**Choroid plexus** Vascular invagination into the cerebral ventricles. Produces the cerebrospinal fluid.

**Chromatin** Complex of DNA and histones making up the chromosomes of eukaryotic cells.

**Chronic Granulomatous Disease** Genetic disorder causing absence of $H_2O_2$ production and myeloperoxidase activity of phagocytes. Results in repeated infections with catalase positive bacteria.

**-cidal** Killing.

**CIE** *See* Counterimmunoelectrophoresis.

**Cilia** Surface structures of some eukaryotic cells that beat rhythmically to move mucus over surfaces or confer motility on some single-celled organisms.

**Cirrhosis** Fibrosis and nodular regeneration of the liver with loss of function.

**Cistron** The smallest functional genetic unit. A gene.

**Clone** Identical progeny of a single cell, gene, or genes.

**CMI** *See* Cell-mediated immunity.

**Co-agglutination** Agglutination involving two organisms, one of which acts as an inert particle coated with specific antibody to the other.

**Co-cultivation** Process that can be used for unmasking latent virus by growing susceptible cells with those from affected tissue.

**Coarctation** Stricture or narrowing (eg, of the aorta).

**Codon** The three nucleotides encoding an amino acid or a chain termination signal.

**Collagen** Fibrous component of connective tissue.

**Coloboma** A defect of the eye.

**Colostrum** Initial secretion of the breast after delivery (contains antibodies and lymphocytes).

**Comedo** Blocked sebaceous duct with retention of sebum (blackhead).

**Commensal** Organism of the normal flora that has a symbiotic relationship with the host.

**Complement** A system of serum proteins that act in sequence to mediate inflammatory and some immune responses.

**Condyloma acuminatum** A wart-like infectious benign growth that occurs on the genitalia and in the anal canal.

**Conidia** Asexual fungal reproductive spore-like bodies.

**Conidiophore** Fungal structure that bears conidia.

**Copepod** Minute fresh water fleas that serve as intermediate hosts for some parasites.

**Coprolith** Stony, hard stool.

**Coracidium** The ciliated free swimming embryo of certain tapeworms.

**Cornea** Clear, anterior portion of the eyeball.

**Cortex** The outer layer of an organ.

**Corticosteroid** Steroid hormone from adrenal gland; some are anti-inflammatory.

**Coryza** Catarrhal rhinitis (eg, from the common cold).

**Counterimmunoelectrophoresis** A technique for increasing the sensitivity and speed of the immunodiffusion procedure by the application of an electrophoretic field (*see* Immunodiffusion).

**Crepitation** A crackling or rattling sound.

**Cribriform plate** Area of bone above nasal cavity through which pass the olfactory nerves.

**Croup** Manifestations of laryngeal obstruction from inflammation or other causes.

**CSF** *See* Cerebrospinal fluid.

**Curare** A plant extract that produces generalized paralysis by acting at neuromuscular junctions.

**Cuticle** Skin or surface layer.

**Cyanosis** Blue color of skin caused by lack of oxygen.

**Cystic fibrosis** Congenital disease of secreting glands affecting pancreas, respiratory tract, and sweat glands. Associated with viscid respiratory mucus and chronic respiratory infections.

**Cysticercus** Larval form of tapeworm enclosed in a cyst.

**Cysto-** Pertaining to the bladder.

**Cystoscope** Instrument for examining inside the urinary bladder.

**Cyto-** Pertaining to the cell.

**Cytokine** Hormone-like intercellular messenger molecule (eg, lymphokine and interleukin).
**Cytology** The study of cells rather than of tissues and organs.
**Cytoplasm** Cellular contents excluding the nucleus.
**Cytosol** Liquid portion of cytoplasm.
**Cytosome** The body of a cell apart from its nucleus.
**Cytostome** The mouth opening of certain ciliated protozoa.

**Dalton** Atomic mass unit that gives the same number as atomic weight.
**Debridement** Removing foreign matter and dead tissue.
**Decubitus ulcer** Pressure sore (bed sore).
**Defensins** A family of microbial, cationic, cystine rich polypeptides abundant in the azurophilic granules of polymorphonuclear leukocytes.
**Demyelination** Loss of nerve sheaths.
**Dendritic** Branched.
**Dermatophyte** Fungus that causes skin infections.
**Dermis** Skin connective tissue immediately below the epidermis.
**Dermo-** Pertaining to the skin.
**Desquamation** Loss of skin epithelial cells.
**Dextran** A polymer of D-glucose.
**Dimorphism** Occurring in two morphologic forms under different conditions.
**Diploid** Possessing two sets of chromosomes.
**Diverticulum** Blind-ended extrusion from a hollow organ.
**Ductus arteriosus** Fetal blood vessel connecting the pulmonary artery to the descending aorta.
**Dys-** Difficult or painful.
**Dysentery** Pain and frequent defecation resulting from inflammation of the colon or other intestines, with blood and pus in the stool.
**Dyspareunia** Difficult or painful intercourse.
**Dysphagia** Difficulty in swallowing.
**Dysplasia** Histological evidence of possible premalignant changes in cells.
**Dyspnea** Shortness of breath.
**Dysuria** Difficult or painful urination.

**Ecchymosis** Bruise.
**Ecthyma** Eroded, scabbed lesion of the skin.
**Ecto-** Outside or outer.
**-ectomy** Surgical removal of.
**Ectopic pregnancy** Fetal development outside the uterus (usually in the Fallopian tubes).
**Ectoplasm** Clear layer of cytoplasm near the cell membrane of amebas.
**Edema** Excessive fluid in tissues.
**EIA** *See* Enzyme Immunoassay
**Elastosis** Disorder of fibroelastic proteins.
**Electrophoresis** Procedure for separating charged particles by differences in their migration in an electric field.
**ELISA** Enzyme-linked immunosorbent assay (*See* Enzyme immunoassay).
**Embolism** Sudden blockage of an artery.
**-emia** Of the blood.
**Emphysema (pulmonary)** Irreversible enlargement of alveolar sacs of lung.
**Empyema** Pus in a body cavity (eg, pleural cavity).
**Encephalitis** Inflammation of brain tissue.
**Endarteritis** Inflammation of the inner coat of an artery or arteriole.
**Endemic** A disease that is continuously present at subepidemic levels in a particular region, locality, or group.
**Endo-** Within.
**Endogenous** Originating within an organism.
**Endometrium** Interior epithelial lining of the uterus.
**Endonuclease** Enzyme of a class that hydrolyzes internal bonds of DNA or RNA. Involved in synthesis and breakdown of nucleic acids.
**Endophthalmitis** Inflammation of interior tissues of the eye.
**Endoplasm** Central portion of cytoplasm of cell.
**Endoplasmic reticulum** Ramifying membranes within the cytoplasm of eukaryotic cells.
**Endospore** Bacterial spore.
**Endotoxin lipid** A toxic moiety of bacterial cell wall lipopolysaccharide.
**Entactin** Protein component of the extrcellular matrix
**Enteric** Pertaining to the intestinal tract.
**Enteric fever** Typhoid or similar systemic *Salmonella* or *Yersinia* infection.
**Entero-** Pertaining to intestines.
**Enterobactin** A phenolate siderophore produced by *E. coli* and some other enteric species of bacteria.
**Enterochelin** Synonym for Enterobactin.
**Enucleation (ocular)** Removal of an eye intact.
**Enzootic** Disease present at low levels at all times in an animal community.
**Enzyme immunoassay** A method for detecting antigen–antibody reactions by labeling one of the reagents with detectable enzyme.
**Eosinophil** Polymorphonuclear leucocyte with eosinophilic granules.
**Epi-** Upon or additional to.
**Epicardium** Outer lining of the heart.
**Epidemic** A disease that rapidly affects many people in a circumscribed period of time.
**Epididymis** Tubular structure attached to the testes in which spermatozoa mature.
**Epigastrium** Upper central region of the abdomen overlying the stomach.
**Epiglottis** Movable structure overlying and protecting the larynx.
**Epiphysis** Growing end of bone.
**Episome** Plasmid or viral DNA that can replicate extrachromosomally or can integrate into chromosome.
**Epitope** Structural part of an antigen that determines specificity of an antigen–antibody reaction (also called antigenic determinant).

**Epitrochlear node** Lymph node above inner side of elbow.

**Erythema** Red color caused by dilatation of blood vessels.

**Erythema nodosum** Red raised skin nodules usually on the legs. Usually a manifestation of a hypersensitivity reaction.

**Erythro-** Red.

**Erythrocyte** Red blood cell.

**Eschar** Necrotic scab-like area of skin.

**Etiology** Cause of a disease.

**Eukaryote** Organism comprising one or more cells containing true nuclei.

**Eustachian tube** Tube connecting the middle ear and the nasopharynx.

**Exanthem** Disease in which skin rashes are major manifestations.

**Exocrine glands** Glands excreting their products to skin, intestinal, respiratory, or genitourinary tracts.

**Exotoxin** Toxic protein liberated from a bacterial cell.

**Facultative** When describing bacteria without a qualification means ability to grow aerobically or anaerobically.

**Fallopian tubes** Tubes extending from ovaries to uterus.

**Fascia** Sheets of specialized connective tissue.

**Fauces** Area between the mouth and the pharynx. Bounded by the tonsils, soft palate, and base of tongue.

**Febrile** Having a raised temperature.

**Felinophobe** Cat hater.

**Fibrin** Insoluble protein of blood clots.

**Fibrinogen** Precursor of fibrin.

**Fibroblast** Specialized cell producing collagen and elastic connective tissue.

**Fibronectin** A glycoprotein widely distributed in connective tissue and coating cells at mucosal surfaces

**Fibrosis** Formation of collagenous connective tissue.

**Fimbriae** Very fine fibrils on the surface of a bacterium analagous to the larger pili. Often referred to as pili.

**Fistula** An abnormal passage from a hollow organ (eg, intestine).

**Flaccid** Loose; absence of muscle tone.

**Flagellum** Organelle of motion of bacteria and some eukaryotic cells.

**Fluke** Flat parasitic worm (trematode).

**Fluorochrome** A fluorescent dye.

**Follicle** A small sac or cavity.

**Folliculitis** Usually describes localized inflammation of hair follicles without the purulence of furuncles.

**Fomites** Inanimate objects transmitting infectious agents.

**Foramina** Outlets to cavities.

**Fulminant** Rapid and severe development (eg, of an infection).

**Fungemia** Fungi in the bloodstream.

**Funiculitis** Inflammation a cord-like structure, usually the spermatic cord.

**Furuncle** Purulent infection of a hair follice; a boil.

**Fusiform** Tapering at both ends.

**Gametocyte** Male or female sexual cell of the malarial parasite found in the blood of humans and transmissible to mosquitoes.

**Ganglion** Group of nerve cells outside the spinal cord.

**Gangrene** Death of tissue.

**Gastro-** pertaining to the stomach.

**-genic** arising from, origin.

**Genital primordium** First recognizable embryonic genital structure. Assists in distinguishing hookworm from Strongyloides larvae.

**Genome** The total gene complement of an organism.

**Genotype** The genetic constitution of an organism.

**Geophagia** Eating soil.

**Giemsa stain** A combination of basic and acidic dyes used to stain blood smears and to demonstrate some protozoa.

**Gingival crevice** Area between the tooth and the gums.

**Gingivo-** pertaining to the gums.

**Glaucoma** Excessive pressure in eyeball that can lead to blindness.

**Glia** Supporting cells of the central nervous system (neuroglia).

**Glomerulus** Microscopic organ of specialized capillaries in the kidney that filters waste products from the blood.

**Glottis** The sound-producing area of the larynx.

**Glucans** Polymers of glucose.

**Gnotobiotic animals** Animals reared under aseptic conditions which may either be sterile ("germ free") or in which defined microflora are introduced.

**Gonads** Ovaries or testes.

**Granulocyte** Polymorphonuclear leucocyte of the neutrophil, basophil, or eosinophil series.

**Granuloma** Chronic inflammatory lesion infiltrated with macrophages and lymphocytes and accompanied by fibroblast activity.

**Gravid** Pregnant.

**Guillain-Barré syndrome** Febrile polyneuritis with muscle weakness; may lead to paralysis.

**Gumma** Tertiary syphilitic granulomatous lesion, usually without demonstrable spirochetes.

**Halophilic** Preferring or requiring a high salt content (eg, for growth).

**Haploid** Half the number of chromosomes of eukaryotic tissue cells (*see* Meiosis) or number of chromosomes in asexual organisms.

**Hapten** A small molecule that can react with a specific antibody but does not elicit antibody production unless attached to a larger molecule.

**Helminth** A parasitic worm.

**Hemagglutination** Agglutination of erythrocytes.

**Hematocrit** Volume of erythrocytes in blood as a percentage of the total volume of blood (adult normal = 45%).

**Hematogenous** Derived from blood. Spread by the bloodstream.

**Hematoma** Extravasation of blood into the tissues causing a swelling.

**Hematopietic system** Precursor cells that produce blood cells.
**Hematoxylin–eosin stain** Commonly used histological stain. Hematoxylin stains nuclei blue. Eosin is a red counter stain.
**Hematuria** Blood in the urine.
**Hemianopsia** Loss of vision in half the visual field.
**Hemo-, Hema-** Pertaining to blood.
**Hemoglobulinemia** Free hemoglobin in the blood.
**Hemolysin** A substance or enzyme causing lysis of erythrocytes.
**Hemolysis** Liberation of hemoglobin from red cells.
**Hemolytic–uremic syndrome** A syndrome that includes hemolytic anemia, thrombocytopenia, and evidence of renal disease.
**Hemoptysis** Coughing up of blood.
**Hemothorax** Blood in the pleural cavity of the chest.
**Hepato-** Pertaining to the liver.
**Hepatocellular** Pertaining to liver cells (hepatocytes).
**Hepatocytes** Liver cells.
**Hepatoma** Malignant tumor of liver cells.
**Hetero-** Of different origin.
**Heterologous** Derived from a different clone, strain, species or tissue.
**Heterophil antibody** Antibody reacting with an antigen other than that which elicited its production.
**Heteroploid** Eukaryotic cell with abnormal number of chromosomes.
**Heterotroph** An organism that requires organic carbon for nutrition.
**Heterozygous** Possessing different alleles at a particular genetic locus in a diploid cell.
**Hexacanth** A tapeworm embryo containing six pairs of hooklets.
**Hexamer** In virology, a capsomer comprising six subunits.
**Hilar lymph nodes** Nodes at the root of the lung.
**Histiocyte** Tissue macrophage.
**Histocompatibility** Antigens on tissue cells that are recognized by the host as self or foreign.
**HIV-1 or -2** Abbreviation for human immunodeficiency viruses, the cause of AIDS.
**Hodgkin's disease** A malignant lymphoma initially affecting groups of lymph nodes.
**Homeostasis** Tendency to stability of conditions within a complex biological system.
**Homonymous hemianopsia** Blindness affecting the same half of the visual field in each eye.
**Homozygous** Possessing the same alleles at a particular genetic locus in a diploid cell.
**Humoral** Mediated by fluids. In immunonology relates to antibody mediated immunity as opposed to cellular immunity.
**Hyaline** Clear and transparent.
**Hyaluronic acid** Acid mucopolysaccharide comprising the ground substance of connective tissue. Also found in synovial fluids.
**Hybridization** Process in which denatured, single stranded nucleic acids from different sources are annealed. Homologous sequences form double strands that can be detected and quantified.
**Hybridoma** A clone derived from fused cells of different origin (eg, from an antibody producing lymphocyte and a tumor cell).
**Hydrocele** Fluid accumulation within the scrotum.
**Hydrocephalus** Pathological accumulation of cerebrospinal fluid in the ventricles of brain.
**Hydronephrosis** Accumulation of urine in the renal pelvis due to obstruction of urinary flow. Associated with atrophy of the renal parenchyma.
**Hyper-** Greater than, above normal.
**Hyperalimentation** Intravenous administration of nutrients for treatment of actual or potential malnutrition.
**Hyperammonemia** Excessive amounts of ammonia in the blood.
**Hyperbaric oxygen** Oxygen under increased pressure relative to the atmosphere.
**Hyperemia** Increased blood flow to a tissue.
**Hypernatremia** Increased serum sodium.
**Hyperplasia** Increase in the number of cells in a tissue.
**Hypersensitivity** Exaggerated and harmful immune response to a normally innocuous antigenic stimulus.
**Hypertension** Elevated blood pressure.
**Hypertonic** Of higher osmotic pressure than fluid on the other side of a semipermeable membrane (eg, cell membrane).
**Hypertrophy** Enlargement of an organ due to increase in size of its cells. Note distinction from hyperplasia.
**Hypha** A fungal filament.
**Hypo-** Less than, below normal.
**Hypochlorhydria** Reduced hydrochloric acid in the stomach.
**Hypoglycemia** Blood sugar below normal levels.
**Hypotension** Low blood pressure.
**Hypothalamus** Portion of the brain that forms the floor and part of the lateral wall of the third ventricle.
**Hypothermia** Serious reduction in body temperature.
**Hypoxia** Decreased oxygen supply to the tissues.

**Icosahedron** A solid geometric shape having 12 vertices. Serves as the structural basis for many viruses.
**Icteric** Pertaining to jaundice.
**Idiopathic** Of unknown origin.
**Ig** Abbreviation for immunoglobulin antibodies. Classes include IgG, IgM, IgA, IgD, IgE, and sIgA.
**Ileitis** Inflammation of the lower ileum.
**Ileum** Portion of the small intestine between the jejunum and the cecum.
**Immunocompromise** Deficiency in some components of the body's immune mechanisms.
**Immunocyte** Cell of the lymphoid series that responds to an antigenic stimulus by producing antibodies or initiating cell mediated immune processes.
**Immunodiffusion** A procedure involving diffusion of antigen and antibody towards each other in a gel. A vis-

ible precipitate develops where optimal concentrations interact.

**Immunofluorescence** A serologic procedure using antibody labeled with a fluorescent dye that allows visible detection of sites of reaction with antigen.

**Immunogen** An antigen that induces an immune response.

**Immunoglobulins** Large class of glycoproteins that constitute the antibodies produced in response to antigenic stimuli.

**Impetigo** Superficial purulent skin infection; pyoderma.

**In vitro** Occurring in the test tube.

**In vivo** Occurring in the living animal.

**Inclusion body** A morphologically distinct intracellular mass of viruses or virus components.

**Infarct** Interference with the blood supply producing local death of tissue.

**Integument** Skin.

**Integrins** Family of transmembrane proteins of eukaryotic cells that interact with extracellular matrix and cytoskeleton proteins

**Inter-** Between.

**Interferon** Class of cytokine proteins. When produced by virally infected cells they inhibit viral replication in these and adjacent cells.

**Interleukin** Class of cytokine produced by macrophages or T cells that mediate immune responses.

**Interstitial** Spaces between the cells of a tissue.

**Intertriginous** Pertaining to area between folds of the skin.

**Intima** Inner lining of a blood vessel.

**Intra-** Within.

**Intrapartum** Occurring during the process of childbirth.

**Intrathecal** Within the membranes of the spinal cord.

**Introitus** An opening.

**Isoantigen** Normal substance present in one individual that may elicit an antibody response in another.

**Isotonic** Of the same osmotic pressure as a solution on the other side of a semipermeable membrane.

**-itis** inflammation.

**Janeway's lesions** Painless macular lesions of palms and soles seen in acute bacterial endocarditis.

**Jejunum** Portion of small intestine between duodenum and ileum.

**Kaposi's sarcoma** Multiple malignant vascular tumors. Occur most commonly as a complication of AIDS.

**Karotype** Size, structure, and organization of chromosomes within a cell.

**Karyosome** Area of chromatin concentration in a cell nucleus.

**Keratin** Major protein of the skin, hair, and nails.

**Keratitis** Inflammation of the cornea of the eye.

**Kilobase** Unit to describe the lengths of a nucleotide sequence. One kilobase = 1000 nucleotides.

**Kinetoplast** Structure at the base of a protozoal flagellum.

**Kupffer cells** Fixed phagocytic cells of the liver sinusoids. Part of the reticulo-endothelial system.

**Kwashiorkor** Condition caused by severe protein malnutrition in children.

**Labia** Structures of the external female genitalia.

**Lactoferrin** Iron-binding protein present in milk, other secretions, and granules of neutrophil leukocytes.

**Lamina propria** Connective tissue supporting the epithelial cells of a mucous membrane.

**Laminin** Major protein component of basal lamina

**Latex beads** Used to adsorb soluble antigens. The treated beads agglutinate with specific antibody.

**Leuco-** White; relating to a leukocyte.

**Leukemia** Malignant tumor of white blood cells.

**Leukocyte** White blood cells including granulocytes, lymphocytes, and monocytes.

**Leukocytosis** Increased blood leukocyte count.

**Leukopenia** Abnormally low leukocyte count.

**Leukotrienes** Products of arachidonic acid that mediate inflammatory and allergic reactions.

**Ligand** One component of a complex involving the binding of molecules or structures.

**Lipo-** Relating to fats or lipids.

**Lobar** Related to a lobe of the lung.

**Lophotrichous** Describing several flagella at one or both ends of a bacillus.

**Lumen** Cavity within a tubular organ.

**Lupus erythematosus (systemic)** Autoimmune inflammatory disease of skin, joints, and other tissues.

**Lymph** Tissue fluid derived from the blood stream and passing to the lymphatics.

**Lymphadenitis** Enlarged, inflamed lymph nodes.

**Lymphangitis** Inflammation of lymphatic vessels.

**Lympho-** Pertaining to the lymphatic system.

**Lymphocytosis** Increased blood lymphocyte count.

**Lymphokine** Cytokine produced by lymphocytes.

**Lymphoma** Tumor of lymphatic tissues.

**Lymphoreticular** Relating to the reticuloendothelial system.

**Lysis** Dissolution of cells.

**Lysosome** Intracellular granules of cells that contain hydrolytic digestive enzymes.

**Lysozyme** Enzyme that breaks down peptidoglycan.

**-lytic** Pertaining to lysis.

**Macro-** Large.

**Macrocytic anemia** Anemia characterized by large erythrocytes.

**Macrophage** Tissue phagocyte derived from blood mononuclear cells.

**Macule** A flat lesion of skin rash.

**Masseter** Major muscle controlling movement of the lower jaw.

**Mast cell** Connective tissue cell analogous to the blood basophil. Granules contain heparin, histamine, and other vasoactive mediators.

**Mastitis** Inflammation of the breast.

**Mastoid** Process of temporal bone behind the ear that contains air cells.

**Matrix** Extracellular substance of tissues.

**Meatus** Orifice.

**Meckel's diverticulum** Congenital diverticulum of the lower part of the ileum.

**Mediastinum** Mid-portion of the chest including heart, bronchial bifurcation, and esophagus.

**Medulla** The inner portion of an organ within the cortex.

**Medulla oblongata** Portion of central nervous system between the brain and spinal cord.

**Mega-** Large.

**Megacolon** Dilatation of the colon.

**-megaly** Usually of an organ.

**Meiosis** Cellular division process yielding haploid gametes.

**Meninges** The membranes covering the brain and the spinal cord.

**Meningomyelocele** Malformation of vertebral column with protrusion of meninges.

**Mentation** Mental activity; thinking.

**Merozoite** A stage in the life cycle of a sporozoan parasite resulting from asexual division; a daughter cell.

**Mesenchymal** Derived from the embryonic mesoderm layer.

**Mesentery** Fold of peritoneum surrounding the intestinal tract and attaching it to the posterior abdominal wall.

**Mesophile** A microbe that grows best at temperatures of approximately those of the body.

**Mesosome** A complex invagination of the bacterial cell membrane.

**Metastases** Satellite tumors or infections spread through lymphatics or the blood stream from a primary site.

**-metry** measure.

**Micro-** Small.

**Microaerophilic** Can grow only in less than the atmospheric concentration of oxygen, or anaerobically.

**Microcephaly** Small head with failure of development of the brain.

**Microphthalmia** Failure to develop normal sized eyes.

**Microtubule** Cylindrical cytoskeletal element of animal and plant cells

**Mitochondria** Complex cytoplasmic organelles of eukaryotic cells involved in oxidative phosphorylation.

**Mitogen** Substance that increases the normal frequency of mutations.

**Mitral valve** Valve between the left atrium and ventricle of the heart.

**Monoclonal** Derived from a single cell.

**Monocyte** Large mononuclear phagocyte of the blood. Precursor of the macrophage.

**Monolayer** A single layer of cultured eukaryotic cells on a glass or plastic surface.

**Monotrichous** Possessing a single flagellum.

**Mordant** Substance that enhances the effect of a stain.

**Morphology** The shape, size, and form of an organism or cell.

**Mucolytic** Substance that dissolves mucus.

**Multiple sclerosis** Chronic disorder involving disseminated focal damage to nerve cells.

**Mutagen** Substance that increases the mutation rate of cells or organisms.

**Myalgia** Pain in the muscles.

**Mycelium** A mass of fungal hyphae.

**Mycetoma** A localized granuloma or lesion caused by a fungus.

**Mycosis** A fungal infection.

**Myelin** Component of the myelin sheath around the axon of a neuron that increases the conduction velocity of the nerve impulse.

**Myelitis** Inflammation of the spinal cord.

**Myeloma** Malignant tumor derived from bone marrow cells.

**Myeloperoxidase** Intracellular enzyme of professional phagocytes

**Myo-** Pertaining to muscle.

**Myocardium** Heart muscle.

**Myringitis** Inflammation of the tympanic membrane of the ear.

**Nares** Interior of the nostrils.

**Nasal turbinates** Three scroll-like bony projections from the lateral wall of the nasal cavity (nasal conchae).

**Nasolacrimal duct** Duct draining the conjunctiva into the nasal cavity.

**Necrosis** Death of tissue.

**Neo-** New.

**Neoplasm** Tumor.

**Nephrito-** Pertaining to the kidney.

**Nephritogenic** Producing inflammation of the kidneys.

**Neuro-** Pertaining to the central nervous system or nerves.

**Neuromotor synapses** Connections between nerve endings and muscle.

**Neurone** Nerve and its nerve cell.

**Neutropenia** Reduced number of circulating neutrophil leukocytes.

**Neutrophils** Major class of polymorphonuclear phagocytic leukocytes.

**NGU** Nongonococcal urethritis.

**Nidus** Focus of infection, a cluster.

**Noma** A gangrenous condition spreading from the oral cavity to the skin; seen in undernourished children.

**Nosocomial** Acquired within a hospital.

**Nucleocapsid** The nucleic acid-protein complex found inside an enveloped virus.

**Nucleoid** The double stranded circular DNA genome of a bacterium.

**Nucleolus** Round body within a eukaryotic nucleus that is the site of synthesis of ribosomal RNA.

**Occult** Hidden, inapparent.
**Olfactory** Pertaining to the sense of smell.
**Olfactory bulb** Terminal enlarged portion of the olfactory tract from which the olfactory nerves emerge.
**Oligo-** Small, few.
**Oligodendroglia** Specialized connective tissue of the central nervous system.
**Onco-** Pertaining to tumors.
**Oncogene** Gene whose activation is associated with malignant change and progression.
**Ontogeny** Origin and course of development of an individual organism.
**Operculum** A lid or cover.
**Operon** Operator gene and the adjacent structural gene(s) that it controls.
**Ophthalmia** Severe inflammation of the eye.
**Opisthotonos** Severe spasm of back muscles leading to hyperextension of the spine.
**Opportunist** A microorganism that only causes disease when the body's defenses are compromised or bypassed.
**Opsonin** Antibody or complement component that facilitates phagocytosis when bound to a microorganism.
**Orbit** Skull cavity that contains the eyeball.
**Orchitis** Inflammation of a testis.
**Organelles** Membrane-bound cytoplasmic structures of eukaryotic cells (eg, mitochondria).
**Organogenesis** Formation of the organs of the body.
**Oro-** Pertaining to the mouth.
**-oscopy** Use of an instrument to see within a viscus or vessel.
**Osler's nodes** Skin papules, usually of hands and feet, seen in bacterial endocarditis.
**Ossicles** Small bones (eg, of hearing).
**Osteo-** Pertaining to bone.
**Osteomyelitis** Inflammation of bone marrow and adjacent bone.
**Oto-** Pertaining to the ear.
**Oviparous** Producing eggs from which the embryo is released outside the body.
**Oxidase** Oxidation-reduction enzyme that catalyses transfer of electrons to molecular oxygen with formation of water.

**Pan-** All, throughout.
**Pandemic** Worldwide severe epidemic.
**Panencephalitis** Inflammation of all tissues of the brain.
**Papilla** Small nipple-like swelling.
**Papilledema** Edema of the optic nerve and adjacent retina.
**Papilloma** Warty tumor of the epithelium.
**Papule** Small, firm, elevated nodule on the skin.
**Para-** Beside, abnormal.
**Parasite** An organism that lives on and at the expense of another organism.
**Parasitism** Describes the relationship between parasite and host.
**Parenchymal** Substance of body organs in contrast to their covering.
**Parenteral** Administration by injection rather than by mouth.
**Paresis** Paralysis.
**Paresthesias** Disorders of sensation; tingling.
**Paronychia** Infection of nail fold.
**Parotid glands** Salivary glands beneath the cheek.
**Parturition** The process of giving birth.
**Pathogenic** Cause of disease.
**Pathognomonic** Diagnostic, distinctive.
**-pathy** denoting disease.
**-penia** decreased numbers.
**Pentamer** A polymer of viral capsid having five structural units.
**Peptidoglycan** High molecular weight cross-linked polymer forming the rigid structure of the bacterial cell wall.
**Peptone** Protein hydrolysed product used as a source of aminoacids in bacterial culture media.
**Peri-** Around, covering.
**Periapical** Beside the root of a tooth.
**Pericardium** Membranous lining around the heart.
**Perineum** Area between vulva or scrotum and the anus.
**Periodontal** Area around the tooth including supporting tissues.
**Perioplasm** Area between the outer and cell membranes of a Gram-negative bacterium. Contains the peptidoglycan layer.
**Periosteum** Membrane around the bone.
**Peristalsis** Normal contractile waves of a hollow organ.
**Peristome** The mouth and surrounding areas of certain ciliated protozoa.
**Peritrichous** Presence of multiple flagella around a bacterial cell.
**Permease** A protein of the bacterial cell membrane transport system.
**Petechiae** Small hemorrhages in the skin.
**Peyer's patches** Lymphoid follicles in the ileum.
**Phage** Common abbreviation for bacteriophage.
**Phagocyte** A cell that ingests foreign material.
**Phagolysosome** The digestive vacuole formed by fusion of the cell lysosomes with the phagocytic vacuole.
**Phenotype** The properties expressed by the complete genome under particular conditions.
**Pheromone** Hormone-like substance that elicits a favorable or attraction response in an individual of the same species.
**-phobia** fear of, repulsion.
**Phonation** Speech.
**Photophobia** Intolerance of light.
**-phylia** affection for.
**Phylogeny** Pertaining to the evolution of a species.
**PID** Pelvic inflammatory disease.
**Pilo-sebaceous** Unit of hair follicle and sebaceous gland.
**Pilus** Fibrillar structure on the surface of a bacterial cell.
**Pinocytosis** Uptake of fluids into a cell by a mechanism analogous to phagocytosis.
**Plaque** A patch or flat area. An area of lysis in fixed host cells by an infecting virus.
**Plasma** Noncellular component of whole blood.

**Plasmid** Extrachromosomal circular double stranded DNA molecule.

**Plasmin** Derived from plasminogen—dissolves fibrin.

**Platelet** Small anucleate cell involved in filling small holes in blood vessels and in clotting mechanisms.

**Pleo-** More.

**Pleocytosis** Increased number of cells in a particular area.

**Pleomorphism** Variation in shape and size.

**Pleura** Membrane covering the lungs and thoracic cavity enclosing the pleural space.

**Pleurisy** Inflammation of the pleura.

**Pleuro-** Relating to the pleura.

**Pleurodynia** Pain caused by inflammation or irritation of the pleura.

**Pneumonitis** Inflammation of the lung.

**Pneumothorax** Air in the pleural cavity.

**Poly-** Many, repeated.

**Polyarthralgia** Pain in several joints.

**Polycistronic** Encoding two or more proteins (eg, polycistronic mRNA).

**Polyclonal activation** Simultaneous activation of different antibody producing clones of lymphocytes.

**Polymerase chain reaction** Continuous enzyme-mediated amplification of a nucleotide sequence that allows its detection and analysis.

**Polymorphonuclear** Two or more lobes to the nucleus.

**Polymyositis** Inflammation of many muscles.

**Polyneuritis** Inflammation of many nerves.

**Polyp** A sessile benign or malignant tumor of a mucous membrane (usually of colon).

**Polyposis** Presence of many polyps.

**Porin** Protein of outer membrane pores of Gram-negative bacteria.

**Portal venous system** Veins carrying blood from the intestinal tract to the liver.

**Premenarchal** Prepubertal years in the female (before onset of menses).

**Prepuce** Foreskin.

**Pro-** Before, a precursor.

**Proctoscopy** Use of an instrument to examine interior of rectum.

**Prodromal** Initial symptoms before the characteristic manifestations of disease develop.

**Proglottid** One of the segments of the body of a tapeworm.

**Prokaryote** Organism lacking a true nucleus. Possesses a single chromosome.

**Prophage** Complete bacterial virus genome integrated in the chromosome.

**Prophylaxis** Measures or treatments designed to prevent disease.

**Prostaglandins** Derivatives of arachidonic acid that mediate a variety of biological reactions including inflammation.

**Prostate gland** Gland surrounding the male urethra that produces part of the seminal fluid.

**Prosthesis** Artificial replacement of a missing part of the body.

**Proteinuria** Protein in the urine indicating a renal abnormality.

**Prothrombin** Precursor of thrombin; thrombin activates the terminal blood clotting mechanism.

**Protomer** Protein subunit of a viral capsomere.

**Protoplasm** The viscid colloidal solution that makes up living matter.

**Protoplast** A Gram-positive bacterium that has lost its cell wall.

**Prototroph** Bacterial strains with complete synthetic pathways from which auxotrophs may be derived.

**Protozoan** A unicellular member of the animal kingdom.

**Proventriculus** An enlargement of the alimentary tract of an invertebrate that precedes the stomach.

**Provirus** Complete viral genome integrated into a eukaryotic genome.

**Pruritis** Itching.

**Pseudo-** False.

**Pseudopod** A pseudopodium. Moving extrusion of the cytoplasm of an amoeboid cell that brings about movement or ingestion of food particles.

**Psychophile** A microorganism that grows best or exclusively at low temperatures.

**Puerperal** Following childbirth.

**Purpura** Multiple hemorrhages in the skin, mucous membrane, or other organs.

**Pustule** Pus in an infected hair follicle or sweat gland producing a visible inflammatory swelling.

**Pyelonephritis** Infection of the pelvis and tissues of the kidney.

**Pylephlebitis** Inflammation in the portal venous system.

**Pyo-** Producing pus.

**Pyogenic** Producing pus and pustular lesions.

**Pyuria** Pus in the urine.

**Radioimmunoassay** A method for detecting antigen–antibody reactions that uses a radioisotope as a readily detectable label.

**Rales** Crackling respiratory sounds heard with the stethoscope.

**Receptor** Component of the cell surface to which another substance or organism attaches specifically.

**Redox potential** Oxidation–reduction potential.

**Reduviid** A large winged "cone-nosed" insect.

**Renal** Pertaining to the kidney.

**Repressor** A regulatory protein that binds to an operator sequence and inhibits expression of the adjacent gene.

**Reservoir of infection** Natural habitat or source of an infecting organism.

**Reticuloendothelial system** System of phagocytic monocytes, particularly those in the spleen, bone marrow, and lymph nodes.

**Retinoblastoma** Malignant tumor of the retina.

**Retrovirus** RNA virus, the genome of which is transcribed into DNA by its reverse transcriptase.

**Reverse transcriptase** RNA-directed DNA polymerase.

**Rhino-** Pertaining to the nose.

**Rhinorrhea** Continuous discharge of watery mucus from the nose.

**Rhonchi** Coarse snoring or rattling respiratory sounds heard with a stethoscope.

**RIA** *See* Radioimmunoassay.

**Romana's sign** Unilateral opthalmia, edema of the eyelids, and enlarged draining lymph nodes.

**Rostellum** Portion of tapeworm head that contains hooklets or other attachment organs.

**Salpingitis** Inflammation of the fallopian tubes.

**Saprophyte** Organism living on dead organic material in the environment.

**Sarcoidosis** Disease of unknown etiology characterized by granulomatous lesions of many tissues and organs.

**Sarcolemma** Membrane surrounding muscle fibers.

**Schizogany** Asexual reproduction in sporozoa producing merozoites by multiple nuclear fusion followed by cytoplasmic segregation.

**Schizont** The multinucleated stage of a sporozoan undergoing schizogany.

**Sclera** White part of the eyeball.

**Scolex** The attachment organ or head of a tapeworm.

**-scopy** Denotes use of an instrument for visual examination of a hollow viscus (eg., bronchoscopy).

**Scotoma** A blind spot in the visual field.

**Sebaceous** Relating to sebum and sebum production.

**Sebum** Waxy secretion of sebaceous glands.

**Seminal vesicles** Sacs in which semen is stored prior to ejaculation.

**Sepsis** A term often used synonymously with septicemia, but applied particularly to infants and children with severe life-threatening infections.

**Septicemia** Evidence of systemic disease associated with presence of organisms in the blood (*see* Bacteremia).

**Sequelae** Results occurring subsequent to an infection or other disease.

**Sequestrum** Necrotic bony fragment.

**Seroconversion** Development of antibodies in response to an infection.

**Serodiagnosis** Diagnosis of an infection by serologic procedures.

**Serotonin** Vasoconstricting amine usually derived from platelets

**Serotype** Subtype of species detectable with specific antisera.

**Serpiginous** Moving irregularly from one place to another, snake-like.

**Serum** Liquid part of blood separable after clotting.

**Shunt** Deviation of blood or other body fluids (eg, from artery to vein).

**Sickle cell anemia** Hereditary anemia associated with crescent-shaped erythrocytes resulting from an abnormal hemoglobin.

**Siderophore** Compound that binds iron.

**Sigmoid colon** Lower portion of the colon between descending colon and rectum.

**Sinus** 1. A tract leading from an infected area or hollow viscus to the surface. 2. A wide venous blood channel. 3. Accessory nasal sinuses that are blind sacs draining to the nasopharynx.

**Sinusoid** A wide thin-walled venous passage. Smaller than a sinus.

**Slime layer** Term sometimes used for polysaccharide surface components of bacteria that do not constitute a morphologic capsule.

**Spasticity** Excessive tone of muscles leading to awkward movement.

**Spheroplast** A circular, osmotically unstable, Gram-negative rod that has lost its peptidoglycan layer.

**Sphincter** Circular muscle controlling a natural orifice.

**Splanchnic** Pertaining to the viscera.

**Spleno-** Relating to the spleen.

**Sporogony** Sexual reproduction process in sporozoan parasites leading to formation of oocysts and sporozoites.

**Sporozoite** Motile, elongated, infective stage of sporogony.

**Sprue** A chronic form of intestinal malabsorption.

**Squamous epithelium** Composed of layers of flattened cells.

**Stasis** Stagnation or cessation of flow of body fluids.

**Stenosis** Reduction in diameter of a blood vessel or tubular organ.

**Steroids** Derivatives of cholesterol including hormones, some of which have anti-inflammatory effects.

**Sterol** Lipid-soluble steroid with long aliphatic side chains. Present in eukaryotic cell membranes as cholesterol or ergosterol.

**Stevens Johnson syndrome** A serious allergic reaction, characterized by multiple blister-like lesions of skin and mucous membrane.

**Stomatitis** Inflammation of the mouth.

**Strabismus** Squint.

**Stratum corneum** Outer keratinized part of the skin.

**Stridor** Harsh respiratory sound due to partial respiratory obstruction.

**Strobila** Chain of segments making up the body of a tapeworm.

**Sub-** Below.

**Subarachnoid** Cerebrospinal fluid containing area between the middle (arachnoid) and inner (pia mater) layers of the meninges.

**Subdural** Between the outer (dura mater) and middle (arachnoid) layers of the meninges.

**Submandibular** Below the jaw.

**Subphrenic** Below the diaphragm.

**Sulcus** Groove.

**Suppurative** Producing pus.

**Supra-** Above.

**Surfactant** A substance that acts on a surface to reduce surface tension (eg, a detergent).

**Sylvatic** Pertaining to the woods. Commonly applied to nonurban plague whether occurring in wooded or prairie land.

**Symbiont** An organism living on or in close association with another.
**Synapse** A connection between neurons for nerve impulse transmission.
**Syncytium** A multinucleate mass of fused cells.
**Syndrome** Group of clinical manifestations characterizing a particular disease or condition.
**Synergistic** Enhanced rather than additive effect of two agents or processes acting together.
**Synovium** Lining membrane of a joint, tendon, or bursa.

**T cells** Thymus derived immunocytes: helper, suppressor, and cytotoxic T cells.
**Tachy-** Increased rate, swift.
**Tachypnea** Abnormally rapid rate of breathing.
**Talin** One of the proteins that connects integrins to the actin cytoskeleton of eukaryotic cells.
**Tamponade (cardiac)** Increased fluid or constriction around the heart leading to interference in cardiac function.
**Tenesmus** Ineffective and painful straining at stool or urination.
**Tenosynovitis** Inflammation of a tendon sheath.
**Teratogenic** Causing abnormalities of fetal development.
**Thalassemia** Hereditary hemolytic anemia resulting from abnormal hemoglobin synthesis.
**Thermo-** Pertaining to heat.
**Thermophile** Bacteria with an optimal growth temperature of over 50°C.
**Thrombo-** Pertaining to thrombosis.
**Thrombocyte** See platelet.
**Thrombophlebitis** Inflammation of a vein with thrombosis; may release infected emboli.
**Thrombus** A blood clot developing in vivo.
**Thymus** A lymphoid organ located in the anterior upper portion of the mediastinum. The site of maturation of T cells.
**Titer** Highest dilution of an active substance (eg, antibody in serum) that still causes a discernible reaction (eg, an agglutination reaction).
**Tracheo-** Pertaining to the trachea.
**Tracheostomy** Surgically produced artificial air passage to the trachea.
**Trans-** Across.
**Transcriptase** DNA-directed RNA polymerase.
**Transferrin** Serum protein that binds and transports iron.
**Transovarial** Passage of infectious agents to progeny by way of the egg. Usually occurs in ticks and mites.
**Transposon** A DNA segment carrying one of more recognizable genes that can move between plasmid and between plasmid and chromosome in both directions.
**Trimester** Usually means a three-month period of pregnancy.
**Trismus** Spasm of the masseter muscle; lockjaw.
**Trophozoite** The motile feeding stage of a protozoan parasite.
**Tropism** Having an affinity for a particular organ, or moving towards or away from a particular stimulus.
**Tubulin** Protein subunit of microtubules
**Tumorigenesis** The property of causing tumors.
**Turgor pressure** Osmotic pressure of the cellular contents.
**Tympanic membrane** Eardrum.

**Ultrasonograph** Picture of deep organs of the body derived from reflection of ultrasonic waves.
**Uremia** Toxic accumulation of nitrogenous metabolites due to renal insufficiency.
**Ureter** Tube carrying urine from the kidney to bladder.
**Urethra** Tube carrying urine from the bladder to the exterior.
**-uria** Pertaining to urine.
**Uropathic** Causing disease of the urinary tract.
**Urticaria** Local edema and itching of the skin.
**Uvea** Inner vascular coat of the eyeball, including the iris.
**Uvula** Small extension hanging from the back of the soft palate.

**Vacuolate** Forming small holes of vacules.
**Vacuole** Microscopic hole or cavity.
**Vagotomy** Surgical cutting of the vagus nerve.
**Vasa vasorum** Small blood vessels in walls of veins and arteries.
**Vasculitis** Inflammation of blood vessels.
**Vaso-** Pertaining to blood vessels.
**Vector** An aminate transmitter of disease (eg, an insect).
**Venipuncture** Insertion of a hypodermic needle into a vein—usually to draw blood.
**Ventricle** Fluid cavity (eg, chamber of the heart).
**Vesicle** Small fluid filled cavity (eg, a blister-like lesion of the skin).
**Vesicoureteral junction** Junction of ureter with the urinary bladder.
**Vestibular function** Function of the vestibular branch of the eighth cranial nerve concerned with the body's equilibrium.
**Vinculin** One of the proteins that connects integrins to the actin cytoskeleton of eukaryotic cells.
**Viremia** Presence of a virus in the blood stream.
**Virion** A complete virus particle.
**Viropexis** Viral entry into the cell by phagocytosis.
**Viruria** Viruses in the urine.
**Viscera** Interior organs of the body (eg, the intestinal tract).
**Vitreous humor** The clear viscous fluid in the posterior chamber of the eye.

**Vitronectin** Protein component of extracellular matrix.

**Viviparous** Developing young within the body as opposed to oviparous.

**Weil–Felix test** Test for agglutinating antibodies to certain strains of *Proteus* that develop in the course of some rickettsial infections.

**Western blot** Test for antibodies to specific proteins separated by gel electrophoresis.

**Whitlow** Abscess of the terminal pulp of the finger. Also paronychia.

**Wright's stain** Stain for blood cells that has similar properties to Giemsa stain.

**Xenodiagnosis** Recovery of a parasite by allowing an arthropod to feed on the patient and seeking the parasite in the arthropod.

**Xerostomia** Dry mouth from dysfunction of the salivary glands.

**Zoonosis** A disease transmissable to humans from an animal host or reservoir.

**Zygote** The cell that results from fusion of male and female gamete.

**Zymodeme** An isoenzyme typing pattern.

# Index



Page numbers followed by *t* and *f* indicate tables and figures, respectively. Page numbers in **boldface** indicate major discussions.